DeGowin's

DIAGNOSTIC EXAMINATION

DeGowin's

DIAGNOSTIC EXAMINATION

Ninth Edition

Richard F. LeBlond, MD, MACP

Professor of Internal Medicine (Clinical)
The University of Iowa College of Medicine
Iowa City, Iowa

Richard L. DeGowin, MD, FACP

Professor Emeritus of Internal Medicine
The University of Iowa College of Medicine
Iowa City, Iowa

Donald D. Brown, MD, FACP

Professor of Internal Medicine
The University of Iowa College of Medicine
Iowa City, Iowa

Illustrated by

**Elmer DeGowin, MD,
Jim Abel,
and Shawn Roach**

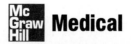

New York   Chicago   San Francisco
Lisbon   London   Madrid   Mexico City   Milan
New Delhi   San Juan   Seoul   Singapore   Sydney   Toronto

DeGowin's Diagnostic Examination, Ninth Edition

Copyright © 2009, 2004 by The McGraw-Hill Companies, Inc. All rights reserved. Printed in the United States of America. Except as permitted under the United States Copyright Act of 1976, no part of this publication may be reproduced or distributed in any form or by any means, or stored in a data base or retrieval system, without the prior written permission of the publisher.

2 3 4 5 6 7 8 9 0 DOC/DOC 12 11 10

Set ISBN 978-0-07-147898-4; MHID 0-07-147898-1
Book ISBN 978-0-07-160574-8; MHID 0-07-160574-6
Bind-in Card ISBN 978-0-07-160575-5; MHID 0-07-160575-4

The Editors were Jim Shanahan and Karen G. Edmonson.
The Production Supervisor was Phil Galea.
Project Management was provided by Samir Roy; Aptara®, Inc.
RR Donnelley was the Printer and Binder.
The Text Designer was Alan Barnett.
This book is printed on acid-free paper.

Library of Congress Cataloging-in-Publication Data

Degowin's diagnostic examination.—9th ed./[edited by] Richard F. LeBlond,
    Richard L. DeGowin, Donald D. Brown; Illustrated by Elmer DeGowin,
    Jim Abel, and Shawn Roach.
        p. ; cm.
    Includes bibliographical references and index.
    ISBN-13: 978-0-07-147898-4 (alk. paper)
    ISBN-10: 0-07-147898-1 (alk. paper)
    ISBN-13: 978-0-07-164008-4 (international ed. : alk. paper)
    ISBN-10: 0-07-164008-8 (international ed. : alk. paper)
1. Physical diagnosis.   2. Diagnosis.   3. Medical history taking.   I. LeBlond,
Richard F.   II. DeGowin, Richard L.   III. Brown, Donald D., 1940-   IV. Title:
Diagnostic examination.
    [DNLM: 1. Physical Examination.   2. Diagnosis.   3. Signs and Symptoms.
    WB 200 D3194 2008]
    RC76.D45 2008
    616.07′54—dc22   2008037098

International Edition Set ISBN 978-0-07-164008-4; MHID 0-07-164-008-8
International Edition Book ISBN 978-0-07-164023-7; MHID 0-07-164023-1
International Edition Bind-in Card ISBN 978-0-07-160575-5;
MHID 0-07-160575-4
Copyright © 2009. Exclusive rights by The McGraw-Hill Companies, Inc., for manufacture and export. This book cannot be re-exported from the country to which it is consigned by McGraw-Hill. The International Edition is not available in North America.

To our patients,
who allow us to practice our art,
encourage us with their confidence,
and humble us with their courage.
— Richard F. LeBlond

It is not easy to give exact and complete details of an operation in writing; but the reader should form an outline of it from the description.

— Hippocrates
"On Joints"

[Studies] perfect Nature, and are perfected by Experience: For Natural Abilities, are like Natural Plants, that need proyning by study: And Studies themselves, due give forth Directions too much at Large, except they be bounded in by experience. Crafty Men Contemne Studies; Simple Men Admire them; And Wise Men Use them; For they teach not their owne Use; But that is a Wisdome without them, and above them, won by Observation. Reade not to Contradict, and Confute; Nor to Beleeve and Take for granted; Nor to Finde Talke and Disourse; But to weigh and Consider.

— Francis Bacon
"Of Studies"

It is only by persistent intelligent study of disease upon a methodical plan of examination that a man gradually learns to correlate his daily lessons with the facts of his previous experience and that of his fellows, and so acquires clinical wisdom.

— Sir William Osler

Sources for Quotations:

Brecht quotation from: Bertolt Brecht. *Poems 1913–1956*. London, Methuen London Ltd., 1979.

Eliot quotation from: T.S. Eliot. *The Complete Poems and Plays, 1909–1950*. New York, Harcourt, Brace & World, Inc., 1971.

Frazer quotation from: Sir James George Frazer. *The Golden Bough, A Study in Magic and Religion*, abridged edition. New York, MacMillan Publishing Company, 1922.

Hippocrates quotation from: Jacques Jouanna (M.B. DeBevoise translator). Hippocrates. Baltimore, The Johns Hopkins University Press, 1999.

Osler quotation from: Sir William Osler. *Aequanimitas, with other Addresses to Medical Students, Nurses and Practictioners of Medicine*. Philadelphia, P. Blakistons Son and Co., 1928.

Roethke quotations from: Theodore Roethke. *On Poetry and Craft*. Port Townsend, Washington Copper Canyon Press, 2001.

CONTENTS

PART II
THE DIAGNOSTIC EXAMINATION

PART 3
PREOPERATIVE EVALUATION

PART 4
USE OF THE LABORATORY AND DIAGNOSTIC IMAGING

To The Reader:
Pray thee, take care, that tak'st my book in hand
To read it well: that is to understand.
—BEN JONSON

Far beyond being a text describing how to perform a history and physical exam, *DeGowin's Diagnostic Examination* is, uniquely, a text to assist clinicians in thinking about symptoms and physical signs to facilitate generation of reasonable, testable diagnostic hypotheses. The clinician's goal in performing a history and physical examination is to generate these diagnostic hypotheses. This was true for Hippocrates and Osler and remains true today. The practice of medicine would be simple if each symptom or sign indicated a single disease. There are enormous numbers of symptoms and signs (we cover several hundred) and they can occur in a nearly infinite number of combinations and temporal patterns. These symptoms and signs are the rough fibers from which the clinician must weave a clinical narrative, anatomically and pathophysiologically explicit, forming the diagnostic hypotheses. To master the diagnostic process, a clinician must have four essential attributes:

(1) **Knowledge:** Familiarity with the pathophysiology, symptoms, and signs of common and unusual diseases.

(2) **Skill:** The ability to take an accurate and complete history and perform an appropriate physical examination to elicit the pattern of symptoms and signs from each patient.

(3) **Experience:** Comprehensive experience with many diseases and patients, each thoroughly evaluated, allows the skilled clinician to generate a probabilistic differential diagnosis, a list of those diseases or conditions most likely to be causes of this patient's illness.

(4) **Judgment:** Knowledge of medical science and the medical literature combined with experience reflected upon hones the judgment necessary to know when and how to test these hypotheses with appropriate laboratory tests or clinical interventions [Reilly BM. Physical examination in the care of medical inpatients: an observational study. *Lancet.* 2003;362:1100–1105].

DeGowin's Diagnostic Examination has been used by students and clinicians for over 40 years precisely because of its usefulness in this diagnostic process:

(1) It describes the techniques for obtaining a complete history and performing a thorough physical examination.

(2) It links symptoms and signs with the pathophysiology of disease.

(3) It presents an approach to differential diagnosis, based upon the pathophysiology of disease, which can be efficiently tested in the laboratory.

(4) It does all of this in a format that can be used as a quick reference at the "point of care" and as a text to study the principles and practice of history taking and physical examination.

In undertaking this ninth edition of a venerable classic, my goal is once again to preserve the unique strengths of previous editions, while adding recent information and references, reducing redundancy and improving clarity. The second edition is one of the few books I have retained from medical school, 35 years ago. The reason is that *DeGowin's Diagnostic Examination* emphasizes the unchanging aspects of clinical medicine—the symptoms and signs of disease as related by the patient and discovered by physical examination.

Pathophysiology links the patient's story of their illness (the history), the physical signs of disease, and the changes in biologic structure and function revealed by imaging studies and laboratory testing. Patients describe symptoms, we need to hear pathophysiology; we observe signs, we need to see pathophysiology; the radiologist and laboratories report findings, we need to think pathophysiology. Understanding pathophysiology gives us the tools to understand disease as alterations in normal physiology and anatomy and illness as the patient's experience of these changes.

A discussion of pathophysiology (highlighted in blue) occurs after many subject headings. The discussions are brief and included when they assist understanding the symptom or sign. Readers are encouraged to consult physiology texts to have a full understanding of normal and abnormal physiology [Guyton AC, Hall JE. *Textbook of Medical Physiology.* 10th ed. Philadelphia: W.B. Saunders Company: 2000. Lingappa VR, Farey K. *Physiological Medicine: A Clinical Approach to Basic Medical Physiology.* New York, NY: McGraw-Hill; 2000]. In addition, each chapter discusses common syndromes associated with that body region, to provide you with a sense of the common and uncommon but serious disease patterns.

DeGowin's Diagnostic Examination is organized as a useful bedside guide to assist diagnosis. Part I introduces the conceptual framework for the diagnostic process in Chapter 1, the essentials of history taking and documentation in Chapter 2, and the screening physical examination in Chapter 3. Part I and Chapter 17, which introduces the principles of diagnostic testing, should be read and understood by every clinician.

Part II, Chapters 4 through 14, forms the body of the book. Two introductory chapters discuss the vital signs (Chapter 4) and major physiologic systems that do not have a primary representation in a single body region (Chapter 5). Chapters 6 to 14 are organized around the body regions sequentially examined during the physical examination and each has a common structure outlined in the Introduction and User's Guide. To avoid duplication, the text is heavily cross-referenced. I hope the reader will find this useful and not too cumbersome.

References to articles from the medical literature are included in the body of the text. We have chosen articles that provide useful diagnostic information including excellent descriptions of diseases and syndromes, thoughtful discussions of the approach to differential diagnosis and evaluation of common and unusual clinical problems, and, in some cases, photographs illustrating key findings. Most references are from the major general medical journals, the New England Journal of Medicine, the Lancet, the Annals of Internal Medicine, and the Journal of the

American Medical Association. This implies that a clinician who regularly studies these journals will keep abreast of the broad field of medical diagnosis. Some references are dated in their recommendations for laboratory testing and treatment; they are included because they give thorough descriptions of the relevant clinical syndromes, often with excellent discussions of the approach to differential diagnosis. Tests and treatments come and go, but good thinking has staying power. The reader must always check current resources before initiating a laboratory evaluation or therapeutic program.

Evidence-based articles on the utility of the physical exam are included, mostly from the Rational Clinical Examination series published over the last 15 years in the Journal of the American Medical Association. They are included with the caveat that they evaluate the physical exam as a hypothesis-testing tool, *not* as a hypothesis generating task; their emphasis on transforming the qualitative hypothesis generating task of the history and physical examination into a quantitative hypothesis testing task is misguided [Feinstein AR. *Clinical Judgement* revisited: the distraction of quantitative models. *Ann Intern Med.* 1994;120:799–805].

Each chapter was independently reviewed by faculty members of the University of Iowa Roy J. and Lucille A. Carver College of Medicine. Their feedback and assistance is gratefully acknowledged. Reviewers for this edition are Hillary Beaver MD, Associate Professor Clinical Ophthalmology (Chapter 7); Jane Engeldinger, MD, Professor, Clinical Obstetrics and Gynecology (Chapters 10 and 11); John Lee, MD, Assistant Professor, Department of Otolaryngology (Chapter 7); Christopher J. Goerdt, MD, MPH, Associate Professor, Clinical Internal Medicine, Division of General Internal Medicine (Chapters 1–3, 16, and 17); Vicki Kijewski, MD, Assistant Professor of Clinical Psychiatry and Internal Medicine (Chapter 15); Victoria Jean Allen Sharp, MD, MBA, Clinical Associate Professor, Departments of Urology and Family Medicine (Chapters 10 and 12); William B. Silverman, MD, Professor, Clinical Internal Medicine, Division of Gastroenterology and Hepatobiliary Diseases (Chapter 9); Haraldine A. Stafford, MD, PhD, Associate Professor, Clinical Internal Medicine, Division of Rheumatology (Chapter 13); Marta Vanbeek, MD, MPH, Clinical Assistant Professor, Department of Dermatology (Chapter 6); and Michael Wall, MD, Professor of Neurology and Ophthalmology (Chapters 7 and 14).

For the first time color photographs are included to supplement the drawings. Dr. Hillary Beaver supplied the eye and fundus photographs, courtesy of the University of Iowa Department of Ophthalmology. The other photos were taken by the author (RFL) in his office practice.

Once again, Mr. Shawn Roach has done an excellent job of revising many of the illustrations for this edition. I greatly appreciate his patience and cooperation. Mrs. Denise Floerchinger was instrumental in coordinating my schedule and keeping me on task. Her support in this and my many other projects and clinical activities is essential to my success and is gratefully acknowledged.

My co-authors for this edition, Donald D. Brown, MD, and Richard L. DeGowin, MD, have been instrumental in seeing that the ninth edition maintains the strengths of previous editions. Dr. Brown directed the history taking and physical examination course at the University of Iowa for over 25 years. He is annually nominated for best teacher awards by the students in recognition of his knowledge and enthusiasm for teaching these essential skills. As a practicing cardiologist, he is the primary editor for Chapters 8 and 16.

I am especially thankful for the continuing contributions and encouragement of Dr. Richard L. DeGowin during the extensive revisions for eighth edition and preparations for this ninth edition. He is a wonderful colleague and friend to whom I am ever thankful for the opportunity to edit this edition of *DeGowin's Diagnostic Examination.*

Mr. James Shanahan, our editor at McGraw-Hill, has been actively involved from the beginning in the planning and execution of the ninth edition. His encouragement and support are deeply appreciated. The McGraw-Hill editorial and publishing staff under his direction, especially Samir Roy, have been prompt and professional throughout manuscript preparation, editing, and production.

I wish to thank my colleagues who have encouraged me throughout the course of this project. I have incorporated many suggestions from my co-authors and each of the reviewers; any remaining deficiencies are mine. Ultimately, you, the reader, will determine the strengths and weaknesses of this edition. I welcome your feedback and suggestions. Email your comments to richard-leblond@uiowa.edu (please include "DeGowin's" on the subject line).

Richard F. LeBlond, MD, MACP
Iowa City, Iowa

COMMON ABREVIATIONS

CHF	congestive heart failure
COPD	chronic obstructive pulmonary disease
CLL	chronic lymphocytic leukemia
CML	chronic myelogenous leukemia
CMV	cytomegalovirus
CN	cranial nerve
CNS	central nervous system
CSF	cerebrospinal fluid
CVP	central venous pressure
DDX	differential diagnosis
DIP	distal interphalangeal joint
EBV	Epstein-Barr virus
HIT	heparin-induced thrombocytopenia
HSV	herpes simplex virus
ITP	idiopathic immune thrombocytopenia
LLQ	left lower quadrant
LUQ	left upper quadrant
LV	left ventricle
MCP	metacarpal–phalangeal joint
MI	myocardial infarction
MS	multiple sclerosis
MTP	metatarsal–phalangeal joint
NBTE	nonbacterial thrombotic endocarditis
PE	pulmonary embolism
PIP	proximal interphalangial joint
RA	rheumatoid arthritis
RLQ	right lower quadrant
RUQ	right upper quadrant
RV	right ventricle
SBE	subacute bacterial endocarditis
SLE	systemic lupus erythematosus
TTP	thrombotic thrombocytopenic purpura

INTRODUCTION AND USER'S GUIDE

Read with two objectives: first to acquaint yourself with the current knowledge on the subject and the steps by which it has been reached; and secondly, and more important, read to understand and analyze your cases.

— Sir William Osler
"The Student Life"

DeGowin's Diagnostic Examination provides the introductory knowledge base, describes the skills, and encourages the reader to acquire the experience and judgment needed to become a master clinical diagnostician. Despite recent advances in testing and imaging, the clinician's skills in taking a history and performing a physical examination are needed now more than ever. Proper use of the laboratory and imaging are based upon accurate diagnostic hypotheses generated while taking the history and performing the physical examination. The history is the patient's story of his or her illness related as the time course of their symptoms; the physical examination reveals the signs of disordered anatomy and physiology. The symptoms and signs of disease form temporal patterns, which the clinician recognizes from experience and knowledge of diseases. From the history and physical examination, the clinician generates a set of testable pathophysiologic and diagnostic hypotheses—the differential diagnosis. Acquisition of proficiency and confidence in generating this differential diagnosis is the purpose for this book. It is this differential diagnosis that is subjected to laboratory testing.

Members of the American Board of Internal Medicine have expressed concern about the atrophy of diagnostic skills among trainees and have recommended improvements in training programs [Schechter GP, Blank LL, Godwin HA Jr, LaCombe MA, Novack DH, Rosse WF. Refocusing of history-taking skills during internal medicine training. *Am J Med.* 1996;101:210–216]. They point out that overreliance on technology has contributed to loss of clinical bedside skills. *DeGowin's Diagnostic Examination* is intended to assist the student and clinician in making reasonable diagnostic hypotheses from the history and physical examination. Part I, Chapters 1 to 3, discuss the diagnostic framework in detail. Chapter 1 discusses the importance of diagnosis and the process of forming a differential diagnosis specific to each patient. Chapter 2 discusses the process of history taking and documentation of your findings in the medical record. Chapter 3 presents an outline of the screening physical examination.

The heart of *DeGowin's Diagnostic Examination* is Part II, Chapters 4 to 15. It is organized in the sequence in which the clinician traditionally performs the examination. Chapter 4 discusses the vital signs. Chapter 5 introduces some systems to keep in mind throughout the examination since they present with symptoms and signs not easily referable to a specific body region. Chapters 6 to

13 discuss the diagnostic examination by body region: the skin (Chapter 6), the head and neck (Chapter 7), the chest and breasts (Chapter 8), the abdomen (Chapter 9), the urinary system (Chapter 10), the female genitalia and reproductive system (Chapter 11), the male genitalia and reproductive system (Chapter 12), the spine and extremities (Chapter 13), the neurologic examination (Chapter 14), and the psychiatric and social evaluations (Chapter 15).

Parts III and IV provide supplemental information. Chapter 16 discusses the preoperative examination. The intent is to give the reader a framework for evaluating the medical risks of surgical procedures and an approach to communicating those risks to the patient and surgeon. Chapter 17 introduces the principles of laboratory testing and imaging. These principles are critical to an efficient use of the laboratory and radiology. Chapter 18 lists many common (not "routine") laboratory tests that provide important information about the patient's condition not accessible from the history or physical examination. More specialized tests used to evaluate specific diagnostic hypotheses are not discussed.

Chapters 6 to 14 have a uniform organization: (A) each chapter begins with a brief overview of the major organ systems to be considered; (B) next is a discussion of the superficial and deep anatomy of the body region; (C) the physical examination of the region or system is described in detail in the usual order of performance; (D) the symptoms particularly relevant to the body region and systems are presented; (E) the physical signs in the region or system exams are listed (some findings can be both symptoms and signs; discussion of a finding is in the section where it is most likely to be encountered, then cross referenced in the other section); and (F) discusses diseases and syndromes commonly in the differential diagnosis of symptoms and signs in the body region and systems under discussion. To avoid duplication, the text is heavily cross-referenced.

Brief discussions of many diseases and clinical syndromes are included so the reader can appreciate the patterns of symptoms and signs they commonly manifest. This will help the clinician determine whether that disease or syndrome should be included in the differential diagnosis of the symptoms and signs in their specific patient. Particularly useful points of differentiation are listed after the DDX symbol.

DeGowin's Diagnostic Examination is not a textbook of medicine. The reader must use this with a comprehensive textbook of medicine to fully understand the diseases and syndromes. We strongly recommend *Harrison's Principles of Internal Medicine* as a companion text [Kaspar DL, Braunwald E, Fauci AS, et al., eds. *Harrison's Principles of Internal Medicine.* 17th ed. New York, NY: McGraw-Hill; 2008].

We emphasize the characteristics of diseases because a clinician who knows the manifestations of many diseases will ask the right questions, obtain the key history, and elicit the pertinent signs that differentiate one disease from another. Instructions on how to elicit the specific signs are included in the physical examination section for each region; if the maneuver is not part of the usual exam, it is discussed with the sign itself. Following the descriptions of many symptoms and signs is a highlighted *Clinical Occurrence* section. This is a list of diseases often associated with the symptom or sign. The organization of the Clinical Occurrence section is based upon the approach to the differential diagnosis of the symptom or sign felt to be most useful clinically.

Where a broad differential exists, we have introduced an organizational scheme for the Clinical Occurrence based upon the pathophysiologic mechanisms of disease. The clinician can often narrow their differential diagnosis to one or a few basic mechanisms of disease: congenital, endocrine, idiopathic, infectious, inflammatory/immune, mechanical/traumatic, metabolic/toxic, neoplastic, neurologic, psychosocial, or vascular. This facilitates the creation of a limited yet reasonable differential diagnosis. The categories in this scheme are not mutually exclusive; a congenital syndrome may be metabolic, infections are usually accompanied by inflammation, and a neoplastic process may cause mechanical obstruction. Although not rigid, this is a useful conceptual construct for thinking about the patient's problems.

Key symptoms, signs, syndromes, and diseases are highlighted. These are important in understanding common disease processes. Critical symptoms, signs, syndromes, and diseases are noted by the ▶ marginal symbol. These are symptoms, signs, syndromes, and diseases that may indicate an emergent condition requiring immediate and complete evaluation.

By using our understanding of normal and abnormal anatomy and physiology as the basis for thinking within clinical medicine, it is possible to avoid the trap of "word space." This is the term one of us (RFL) has given to the common practice of using lists and word association as a means of thinking (or, rather not thinking) about diagnosis: associating a word (for instance, cough) with a memorized list of other words (pneumonia, bronchitis, asthma, postnasal drip, gastroesophageal reflux, etc.). The emphasis on memorization inherent in this scheme is the bane of all medical students; fortunately, it is not only unnecessary, it is counterproductive. Cough is a protective reflex arising from sensory phenomena in the upper airway, bronchi, lungs, and esophagus mediated through peripheral and central nervous system pathways and executed by coordinated contraction of the diaphragm, chest wall, and laryngeal muscles. With this physiologic context, and our understanding of the mechanisms of disease, we can hypothesize the irritants most likely to be relevant in each specific patient.

New diseases are being encountered with surprising frequency. They present not with new symptoms and signs, but with new combinations of the old symptoms and signs. It is our hope that the reader will learn to recognize the patterns of known diseases and to be alert for patterns that are unfamiliar (those not yet in their knowledge base) or previously unrecognized (the new diseases). HIV/AIDS was recognized as an unprecedented clinical syndrome with a new pattern of familiar symptoms (weight loss, fever, fatigue, dyspnea, cough) and signs (wasting, generalized lymphadenopathy, mucocutaneous lesions, Kaposi's sarcoma, opportunistic infections) in a unique population (homosexual males and IV drug users). Continuously expanding our personal knowledge of the known while welcoming the unfamiliar and unknown is the excitement of clinical practice.

The proper testing of specific diagnostic hypotheses is beyond the scope of this book. It is subject to constant change as new tests are developed and their usefulness evaluated in clinical trials. Part IV discusses the principles of laboratory testing (Chapter 17) and some common laboratory tests (Chapter 18). The reader should consult *Harrison's Principles of Internal Medicine*, 17th edition, and the current literature when selecting specific tests to evaluate their diagnostic hypotheses [Guyatt G, Rennie D, eds. *Users' Guides to the Medical Literature: A Manual for Evidence-Based Clinical Practice.* Chicago, IL: AMA Press; 2002].

User's Guide:

DeGowin's Diagnostic Examination can be read cover to cover with benefit to the student or practitioner; however, most will not, and should not, choose this strategy. As Osler said, read to understand your patients and to answer your questions.

We strongly suggest that all readers start with Chapters 1 to 3 and 17, which outline the conceptual basis for the diagnostic examination, including the approach to laboratory testing and imaging. This context is critical to an efficient use of time and resources.

If you have questions about the systems being examined in a given body region consult part A of the relevant chapter and *Harrison's Principles of Internal Medicine*, 17th edition. If your question concerns anatomy, consult part B and an anatomy textbook. If you are uncertain of the techniques of the physical examination, see Chapter 3 and part C of the body region chapters. If you are uncertain what to make of a symptom, see part D of the relevant chapter. If you are wondering how to elicit or interpret a particular sign, see part E of the relevant chapter. To find out more about the diseases mentioned in the section, consult part F of that chapter or look in the index for the page where it is discussed. Remember, the disease and syndrome discussions in this book are brief and must be complemented with reading in a textbook of medicine, e.g., *Harrison's Principles of Internal Medicine*, 17th edition.

The Table of Contents should be scanned to familiarize yourself with the structure and general content of the text. You can always consult the index to find the location of any of the material in the text.

There is no right way to use a book. The key is to use the information to inform your thinking about patients and the problems they present. No text is definitive and the reader is encouraged to consult other texts and the current and historic literature to develop a full understanding of your patients and their illnesses. The acquisition of clinical skills is a journey without end; this is an intimidating thought for the student, but is the source of lifelong stimulation for the practitioner.

After all, what we call truth is only the hypothesis which is found to work best.

— Sir James George Frazer

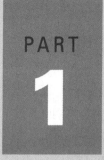
The Diagnostic Framework

To carefully observe the phenomena of life in all its phases, normal and perverted, to make perfect that most difficult of all arts, the art of observation, to call to aid the science of experimentation, to cultivate the reasoning faculty, so as to be able to know the true from the false—these are our methods.

— Sir William Osler

Don't strain for arrangement. Look and put down and let your sensibility be the sieve.

— Theodore Roethke
"Poetry and Craft"

. . . the framing of hypotheses is the most difficult part of scientific work, and the part where great ability is indispensable. So far, no method has been found which would make it possible to invent hypotheses by rule. Usually some hypothesis is a necessary preliminary to the collection of facts, since the selection of facts demands some way of determining relevance. Without something of this kind, the multiplicity of facts is baffling.

— Bertrand Russell
"A History of Western Philosophy"

Diagnosis

Why is Diagnosis Important?

The history and physical examination are the basis for diagnostic hypothesis generation; the first step in the diagnostic process. Accurate diagnosis precedes the three tasks central to the healing professions: explanation, prognostication, and therapy. These three tasks have been consistently performed by physicians throughout time and across cultures, regardless of the belief system or theory underpinning the practice: magic, faith, rationalism, or science. They provide answers to the patient's three fundamental questions: (1) What is happening to me and why? (2) What does this mean for my future? (3) What can be done about it and how will that change my future? [Cohen JJ. Remembering the real questions. *Ann Intern Med.* 1998;128:563–566; Kravitz RL, Callahan EJ. Patients' perceptions of omitted examinations and tests: A qualitative analysis. *J Gen Intern Med.* 2000;15:38–45].

Failure to pursue a diagnosis may permit a disease to progress from curable to incurable. On the other hand, for many complaints, in otherwise healthy people with no alarm symptoms or signs, a good prognosis can be ascertained without knowing the exact cause of the complaint, as, for instance, an upper respiratory infection. The experienced clinician can reassure the patient that further testing is unnecessary and will not change the prognosis or treatment. It takes experience, knowledge of the medical literature, good judgment, and an understanding of the fundamentals of clinical epidemiology and decision making to determine when pursuit of specific symptoms and signs is warranted. For an excellent review of the principles of epidemiology in a highly readable format, see Fletcher et al. [Fletcher RH, Fletcher SW, Wagner EH. *Clinical Epidemiology, the Essentials.* 3rd ed. Baltimore, MD: Williams & Wilkins; 1996].

Diseases and Syndromes: Communication and Entry to the Medical Literature

For thousands of years, physicians have recorded recurring patterns of disordered bodily structure, function, and mentation that suggest a common cause. Each pattern receives a specific name. When a common etiology and pathophysiology are confirmed, we designate the condition a *disease*. Other clusters of attributes, known by a combination of features not clearly related to a single cause, are called *syndromes*. Diseases and syndromes are intellectual constructs allowing the physicians to study groups of patients with relatively homogeneous physiologic disorders; they do not exist independently of the patients who manifest them. The diagnosis of a disease or syndrome provides an entry to the medical literature to obtain information about etiology, diagnostic findings, treatment, and prognosis.

An accurate diagnosis is indispensable to offering your patients evidence-based therapy, that is, therapy validated in clinical trials based upon accurate diagnosis of participating subjects who are similar to your patient.

The Diagnostic Examination

To reach accurate and comprehensive diagnoses the clinician must catalog each abnormality of the patient's anatomic structure, physiologic function, and mentation. Every disease has a temporal sequence of clinical and laboratory features that differentiate it from similar conditions. During the diagnostic examination, the clinician is performing two parallel tasks: (1) developing a problem list of the symptoms and signs requiring explanation; and (2) generating physiologic, anatomic, and etiologic hypotheses regarding the diagnoses.

Use a recursive process to work your way toward the diagnosis. First, from the history and physical examination, generate a problem list. Then make a list of possible diagnoses based upon the most probable anatomic sites and pathophysiologic process explaining the problems. Next, *using the specific characteristics of this patient, differentiate the probabilities of each disease on your list for this patient*: this is the differential diagnosis, each with a pretest probability. Now, choosing tests with appropriate likelihood ratios, these hypotheses are tested using laboratory and imaging tests (*this is why they call them "tests," they test the hypothesis*). The results of the testing changes the probability of each hypothesis to the posttest probability: some are now much more probable, while others are much less probable. The clinician returns to the patient, reviews the history, and repeats specific parts of the examination to reach a new, refined differential diagnosis to be tested more specifically. This process repeats, *each time returning to the patient for their ongoing history and to search for new or changing physical findings*, until one or more specific diagnoses are established that *fully explain* the patient's illness.

Stories: Listen, Examine, Interpret, Explain

The patient tells us a story of their illness. Our job is to create a story of their disease process that is congruent with their illness narrative. The key elements of a good medical story are the same as a good newspaper story: who, what, when, where, how, and why. The first three items you get directly from the patient:

WHO?: We need a history of "who this person is?" including their personal history (religion, beliefs, priorities), social history (education, sexual preferences, habits, demographics, employment, leisure activities), family history and past medical and surgical history. Without this information, we do not know this person.

WHAT?: Let them tell us what has happened to them. This is the narrative of their illness, starting with the chief complaint but going back to the beginning of the illness. Include any thoughts they have about what might be wrong and why, and any attempts at remedies they have tried. No symptom is irrelevant; often patients will dismiss symptoms or occurrences that they have thought irrelevant but which may be the key to the diagnosis. Encourage them to speak freely by not interrupting or demanding clarity prematurely.

WHEN?: Timing is everything. The sequence of events and the pattern and duration of symptoms are critical to differentiating the etiology of symptoms common to many diseases. Make sure you understand the time line for each problem.

The second set of story elements *you* have to construct from the history and your physical examination:

WHERE?: All disease processes take place somewhere. Your job is to precisely envision the anatomy of the problem. Where is the seat of illness: which organ(s), tissues, cells. Is it localized or diffuse? If diffuse, what is the pattern of tissues or fluids; which is most consistent with the story of illness?

HOW?: This is the pathophysiologic question. How, by what physiologic mechanism(s), did this illness come about? There are only a limited number of ways people become ill. A useful way of parsing pathophysiology is used in this text. Ask which of the following mechanisms is most likely: congenital, idiopathic, endocrine, inflammatory/immune, infection, metabolic/toxic, mechanical, neoplastic, psychosocial, or vascular. If we understand how the patient became ill, we can better hypothesize why.

WHY?: This is the etiologic hypothesis. We strive to have an exact diagnosis that explains the illness history and all the findings of the examination and laboratory. In addition, we want to explain why it happened to this patient at this time and make an accurate prognostic statement.

Our brains are designed to be facile with stories and images; you should use this to advantage in everyday medical practice. We are much more adept at capturing and recalling visual images than recalling words verbatim. When the patient is telling you their story, picture it and them over time experiencing the illness they describe. During the examination, create visual images of what you see, feel and hear; see the patient in imaginary 3D X-ray vision. Do not try to translate your findings into words, especially into medical jargon, until you have captured the images. You may then struggle finding the correct words, but you will be less likely to distort the image to conform to the words. Disease is a four-dimensional story, which follows the biologic imperatives of its particular pathophysiology in specific anatomic sites as influenced by the unique characteristics of this patient. Your task is not verbal, but cinematic; construct a pathophysiologic and anatomic movie of the onset and progression of the illness: the words are generated from the images, not the images from the words. After all, a picture is worth a thousand words.

Finding Clues to the Diagnosis

The diagnostic examination has four components: (1) history taking, where clues are *symptoms* (abnormalities patient perceives), (2) physical examination, where the clues are physical signs (abnormalities detected by the examiner), (3) laboratory examinations, and (4) special anatomic and physiologic examinations, such as imaging studies, electrocardiograms, electromyograms, nerve conduction studies, or polysomnography. Our focus is on the history and physical examination and the process of hypothesis generation [Boland BJ, Wollan PC, Silverstein MD. Review of systems, physical examination, and routine tests for case-finding in ambulatory patients. *Am J Med Sci*. 1995;309:194–200; Boland BJ, Wollan PC, Silverstein MD. Yield of laboratory tests for case-finding in the ambulatory general medical examination. *Am J Med*. 1996;101:142–152]. Most diagnoses result from the history, and to a lesser extent, the physical examination and laboratory testing.

The diagnostic examination begins with the first patient contact. The patient's age and sex are surrogates for diseases more or less common in that group. The duration of illness is important; for example, a disease lasting more than 3 years is unlikely to be cancer. Ethnicity is important for diagnosing some diseases; for example, sickle cell anemia rarely occurs in northern European whites. Sex-linked diseases such as hemophilia are rarely encountered in females. Males do not get pregnant. Although obvious, it is important to make each of these categorical probability decisions explicit. Sometimes, it is a disease that was excluded by using one of these criteria (usually without consciously recognizing it) that turns out to be the diagnosis, such as appendicitis in the 80-year-old with abdominal pain.

Each clue is examined closely. If it is a symptom, assess the reliability of the observer: Are the observer's perceptions accurate and consistent or are they colored by secondary considerations? Is the observer's memory accurate? What importance does the patient attach to the symptom? Does the patient regard it fearfully or with relative unconcern? Obtain history from collateral observers, family, and friends, whenever possible. Do they corroborate the patient's history?

If the clue is a *sign*, is it within the range of normal, has it changed from previous examinations or is it clearly abnormal? Is it constantly present or does it vary with position or motion? With laboratory findings, one must constantly suspect the mixing of specimens and laboratory error. Do the reports accord with what you expected? Was there opportunity for the adulteration of specimens? If the clue was found on imaging, was it present in previous studies? Was the patient properly identified when obtaining the images? Were the images interpreted by competent persons?

The Problem List: A List of Problems Needing Explanation

This is one of the most important and most frequently omitted steps in the diagnostic algorithm: list all of the problems you have identified in the history, physical examination, and initial laboratory studies. Only lump them together when you are certain they are congruent (common examples are nausea and vomiting, fever and chills), but be cautious of lumping too soon.

Select Hypotheses: Generate a Differential Diagnosis
Anatomic, Physiologic, and Diagnostic Hypotheses

Your task is to make an anatomic and physiologic story that matches in time and tempo the patient's narrative of their symptoms. Do not forget to look at the past medical and family histories for clues; the past is a good predictor of the future.

Working from your anatomic and physiologic hypotheses, select diseases that are known to cause these specific symptoms, signs, and pathophysiology. A list of all possible diagnoses is rarely of much benefit, and does not provide a guide for efficient evaluation. Rather, from this list, *we use the specific findings from the history and examination of this patient to differentiate the relative probabilities of the potential conditions* to create a short list of the most likely conditions, *the differential diagnosis.*

Because the clues that allow us to differentiate between disease of high and low probability *for this patient* are unique to this patient, a differential diagnosis is only possible for an individual patient, not a problem. For an isolated symptom or sign, we can generate a list of potential diagnoses, but have no means to differentiate their probabilities other than their population prevalence. In this book, under many symptoms and signs, we have placed a list of such *clinical occurrences.* It is up to the clinician, perhaps using this list as an organizational tool, to generate a meaningful differential diagnosis for her patient. When specific clues will help in generating the differential diagnosis, we have listed them after the DDX: symbol in the text.

The differential diagnosis is a list of the disease hypotheses to be tested. Each disease or condition is more or less probable based upon how well it explains the full range of the patient's problems. Studies show that the clinicians carry 4 or 5 diseases on their differential list a any one time, but often 13 to 15 diseases will have appeared on the list at some time during the examination.

Many patients have an acute problem occurring on the background of two or more chronic disorders. In this situation, grouping problems into clusters with a common pathophysiology is a useful technique in forming your differential diagnosis. The challenge is to account for the current problems, especially any new symptoms and signs, either by one of the known existing disorders (an exacerbation of the underlying disease process) or by a new superimposed disorder.

Hypothesis Generation

The process by which skilled clinicians arrive at hypotheses has attracted the attention of physicians, mathematicians, and psychologists. As the Bertrand Russell quote at the beginning of this section indicates, this is still a mysterious cognitive process, even to the clinician performing the task.

Pattern recognition. The whole of the patient's illness is greater than the sum of its parts and a simple mathematical summing of the sensitivity and specificity of each finding is probably far less accurate than the pattern formed in the mind of the skilled examiner by the totality of the observations. For example, it is unlikely that we could accurately identify a person by seeing separately each ear and eye, the hair, the forehead, the cheeks, the nose, the lips, or the chin. Each examination would lack the sensitivity and specificity we desire for identification. But, with just a glance at the pattern of the whole, we can identify with great accuracy literally hundreds of distinct faces. We even recognize our friends after injuries or when much of the face is covered (i.e., many of the parts are different or distorted) because of the persisting unity of the whole. We use this powerful cognitive ability in everyday life and in medical practice. It is not an exercise in reductionism: the whole is greater than the sum of the parts. This ability to recognize patterns is one of the most powerful properties of the human brain, which no computer or algorithm can match.

Most clinicians believe that composite pictures of disease, although comprising many signs, strike them at a glance. The Germans recognize this concept when they refer to Augenblick diagnoses (literally, "a blink of the eye"). Pattern recognition is the current English term describing this concept.

Among the many clinical reasoning strategies, branching, matching and probability estimates are the most commonly used conscious processes when pattern recognition has not already occurred.

Branching hypotheses.　Clinicians sequentially form anatomic and physiologic hypotheses which are tested at the bedside or in the laboratory. As specific characteristics of the disease process are confirmed, etiologic hypotheses are generated and tested. The differential diagnosis is thus revised and reviewed and each new clue may hint at other diseases for consideration. The process is iterated until all the problems have been explained and the whole story of the illness is clear.

Decisions based on probability.　The clinician must be familiar with the incidence and prevalence of all the diseases they may encounter in the general population. This is a start for determining the probability of each disease for this patient, but never the actual probability; if the examiner rigidly applied the incidence and prevalence numbers, a rare disease would never be considered. Using each individual patient's unique characteristics, you must adjust the general population probabilities to those for a population made up exclusively of patients similar to yours (age, gender, ethnicity, past history, concurrent conditions, etc.), an estimate at best. This is the list of pretest probabilities for each diagnostic hypothesis. Post-test probabilities are determined after applying tests with appropriate positive and negative likelihood ratios (see Chapter 17).

A very useful book that summarizes what is currently known about the sensitivity, specificity, and positive and negative likelihood ratios for specific physical findings is *Evidence-Based Physical Diagnosis* [McGee S. *Evidence-Based Physical Diagnosis.* Second Edition. Philadelphia, PA: WB Saunders; 2007].

Matching hypotheses.　The patient's symptoms and signs are matched with those of the hypothesized diseases. For example, suppose the examination yields findings a, d, e, k, and n. The differential begins with a list of diseases having some or all of the same attributes, adekn. The more problems that are common to the patient and the hypothesized diagnosis, the more likely that particular diagnosis. This method can be a useful adjunct to the branching pathway described above. However, with this process, it is easy to overlook the importance of temporal sequences and it easily degenerates into matching words. This strategy is based upon the abstractions of language ("word space") rather than the physiologic processes observed in the patient and is to be discouraged.

Soft Focus and Hard Focus

Pattern recognition results from a soft focus, taking in the observations without undue emphasis on any one; the observer lets the pattern emerge as their systematic observations are filtered through the lens of their knowledge and experience. Performance of the screening physical examination in a structured and relatively stereotypic sequence allows the examiner to observe each patient in a similar manner so that the repetitive patterns between patients become more evident. When the examination process becomes a routine, little or no thought is required to perform or sequence the physical acts of the examination, so the mind is free to observe. When the focus of attention is sharp, as is often the case with beginners, one thing may be seen, while much is missed.

One of the most important observations made by the experienced clinician using pattern recognition with a soft focus is the overall assessment of severity of illness: How sick is the patient? Although one could list many attributes of severe illness, for example, abnormal vital signs, pallor, diaphoresis, anxious or frightened expression, the global assessment of severity made by the experienced clinician also includes many intangibles, often based upon prior knowledge and experience with the patient. Severity of illness scores, such as Acute Physiology and Chronic Health Evaluation II scores, are attempts to systematize this global assessment. Your experience-based emotional cues are an important part of this assessment.

Use of Computers for Diagnosis

There are several areas in which computers have proven valuable in the diagnostic examination. One of these, is in the rapid communication of laboratory results and radiologic images and interpretations to clinicians. Another is in the comprehensive search of the medical literature to evaluate findings and hypotheses generated during an examination. Computer literature searches should be available on the clinical floors of every hospital and in the offices and homes of physicians.

A computer output listing the rank order of disease probability based upon a simple list of symptoms and signs may reassure physicians who fear they will forget a disease for inclusion in the differential diagnosis. Such a list might be valuable in solving complex problems of differential diagnosis, or identifying rare diseases, but its utility for an experienced clinician is probably too low to encourage its use for most problems. Moreover, you still must have the experience and judgment to evaluate the list and determine which items to pursue and how. If you have those skills, you probably do not need the computer-generated list.

Undoubtedly, technologic progress will provide physicians with new opportunities for computer assistance in the diagnostic examination. Satisfactory answers to a few basic questions should precede the adoption of a computer-assisted diagnostic system: Who developed the program and with which data? How frequently will the program be updated and by whom? Will it save time? Is it portable? How will access to confidential information be controlled? How expensive is it?

Cognitive Tests of the Diagnostic Hypotheses

In ranking your list or possible diagnoses, matching of the patient's attributes with those of the hypothetical disease is usually inconclusive. Several additional criteria should be applied to help Identify the most likely diagnosis.

Parsimony

A diagnosis has a higher probability of being correct if it can account for all of the symptoms and signs. This is Occam's razor: the simplest solution is likely to be correct. When one diagnosis does not explain all the findings, those that are able to account for the greatest proportion of the patient's signs and symptoms are more likely to be correct. Parsimony is most applicable to the previously well patient with an acute or subactue disease, the most common clinical challenge faced by Sir William Osler who introduced Occam's razor to medicine. As we care for more patients with one or more chronic disease on multiple medications, bear in mind that more than one pathologic process may be occurring in your patient;

finding one disease or condition should not stop a vigilant search for additional problems [Hilliar AA, Weinberger SE, et al. Occam's razor versus Saint's triad. *N Engl J Med.* 2004;350:599–603; Graber ML, Franklin N, Gordon R. Diagnostic error in internal medicine. *Arch Intern Med.* 2005;165:1493–1499].

Chronology

It is possible to have a perfect match of attributes between patient and disease, but if the epidemiology, onset, tempo and course of illness are not appropriate to the disease, the hypothesis is probably wrong.

Severity of Illness

Not infrequently, an inexperienced clinician will diagnose the patient's condition as, for instance, an upper respiratory infection, whereas a more experienced clinician will look at the patient and suggest the diagnosis of pneumonia, explaining that the patient looks "too sick" for the first condition. The severity of illness is valid and diagnostically useful, but it is difficult to explain or describe.

Prognosis

Often, the diagnosis is uncertain and the testing process to reach the correct diagnosis is anticipated to be prolonged. Since your initial hypothesis may be wrong, err on the side of safety: don't make the wrong mistake. The clinician should proceed first to lower the probability of life and function-threatening conditions to below a reasonable probability, then proceed in a more leisurely evaluation to the correct diagnosis. *It is more important not to miss a serious condition than to make the right diagnosis at the initial visit: the wrong mistake is one from which recovery is unlikely.* For instance, acute severe pelvic pain in fertile women is an ectopic pregnancy until proven otherwise; all other diagnoses can wait a little bit. The right mistake is erring on the side of preserving life and function.

Therapeutic Trials

If there is uncertainty between an untreatable morbid disease and one with potentially successful therapy, a therapeutic trial should be considered. Although experience shows that such trials are often inconclusive or difficult to interpret, they may save a life; for example, when appendicitis cannot be excluded, perform an appendectomy accepting that some normal appendices will be removed. Therapeutic trials, particularly medication trials, should explicitly state the drug and dose to be used, the duration of the trial, the objective and subjective end points for interpretation of the trial at the end of the stated time and the planned response to both a negative evaluation and a positive evaluation of the therapeutic trial. Failure to be explicit in stating and adhering to these parameters is a not infrequent cause of prolonged exposure of patients to hazardous treatments of little or no benefit under the poor excuse of "doing something."

Selection of Diagnostic Tests

Experienced clinicians select diagnostic tests indicated to test hypotheses generated from the history and the physical examination. They have learned that routine testing or an uncritical search for unlikely diagnostic possibilities frequently yield results that appear to require more testing, all without answering the primary diagnostic question. This "cascade effect" heightens the patient's anxiety, is hazardous, expensive and delays treatment. See Chapter 17 for a discussion of the appropriate selection of diagnostic tests. Testing should be done to answer specific diagnostic, prognostic, or therapeutic questions, and should not be a response to idle curiosity.

Rare Diseases

Some physicians, especially the inexpert, have a tendency to diagnose rare diseases with uncommon frequency. It is well to recall that rare diseases occur rarely. The old saying is, "when you hear hoofbeats think of horses, not zebras." Just remember, this works in America, not Africa, (or the zoo, perhaps an analogy for teaching hospitals which collect a disproportionate number of rare diseases). You need to know the epidemiology and demographics of your patient and the population this patient represents before you really know what is common and what is rare.

Certainty and Diagnosis

How certain should the examiner be that a diagnosis is correct before it is accepted? Unfortunately, there is no accepted scale for degrees of certainty whereby the examiner can express the extent to which the diagnosis has been established. On the one hand, the diagnosis may be defined by the image, the laboratory test, the culture, or the biopsy result. For instance, a fracture of the tibia is diagnosed when the fracture can be seen on the X-ray film with absolute assurance. Many types of neoplasia and inflammatory diseases are diagnosed by biopsy. Culture, serology or polymerase chain reaction identification of specific organisms establishes the diagnosis of specific infectious diseases. Laboratory tests are specific for endocrine and metabolic diseases. On the other hand, we speak of a diagnosis of rheumatoid arthritis, where there is much less certainty, and no definitive diagnostic tests. The diagnosis is supported by the clinical picture, and by such nonspecific tests as X-ray examinations and tests for rheumatoid factor and citrullinated proteins.

In each clinical situation, the clinician must consciously establish a "*stopping rule*." That is, the clinician must decide how much certainty is required, and stop further investigation when that point is reached. This decision is based upon the severity of the illness, an estimate of the prognosis (based upon the severity of illness and the patient's comorbidities), and whether a specific diagnosis is needed to guide a decision between mutually exclusive interventions which would harm the patient if applied to the wrong disease; for example, antibiotics or corticosteroids.

Prognostic Uncertainty

If two hypotheses with widely differing prognoses seem equally probable and neither can be proved or disproved immediately, the patient should be informed of the diagnostic and prognostic possibilities and encouraged to discuss this with his family. In these situations, we have found it best to help the patient prepare for the worst and hope for the best. Regular follow-up and frequent reevaluation are required. Often, referral to a specialist will help both the patient and the physician deal with the uncertainty.

Deferred Diagnoses

When a satisfactory diagnosis cannot be made, the clinician still must act. The following five supplementary steps should be considered.

Repeat the History and the Physical Examination

The patient or a family member may recall additional information stimulated by the first inquiry. Talk to more relatives and attendants to confirm or deny the original story and to add details. Obtain copies of patient records from all previous caregivers. Carefully repeat the physical examination to confirm your previous evaluation and to search for signs that were originally overlooked.

Repeat Laboratory Tests

Specimens may have been mixed on the initial occasion, or an error in the first test may be uncovered. As always, each test should provide the answer to a specific question; do not blindly search in the laboratory for diagnostic ideas.

Make a Provisional Diagnosis

It may be appropriate to make a provisional diagnosis, but it is difficult to avoid diagnosis creep: provisional diagnosis often become assumed diagnosis over time. Even though the meticulous physician may have qualified the diagnosis by the word "probable" or a question mark, these modifiers often get dropped when the patient has passed through several consultations. Always go back to the original information to be sure that diagnoses carried by the patient have been appropriately confirmed. Some statements of uncertainty are preliminary diagnosis, diagnostic impression, tentative diagnosis, working diagnosis, provisional diagnosis, and probable diagnosis.

Defer Diagnosis

Carefully explain the situation to secure the patient's confidence so that a return examination may be made when new symptoms or signs have appeared or time has given more perspective to the case. Retain the problem list, but mark the record "Diagnosis Deferred"; do not let medical record rules or the insurance company force a premature diagnosis.

Seek Wise Consultation

Often presenting the case to colleagues as an unknown and asking for their input, or seeking consultation with an excellent generalist or appropriate subspecialist will assist in making the diagnosis, and, even if not, may reassure the patient and physician. It is better to offer this option to the patient than to wait for the patient to insist out of frustration. However, avoid excessive consultation or visits to multiple physicians. Like excessive laboratory testing, this is more likely to add confusion than clarity.

A Summary of the Diagnostic Process

Step 1: Take a History

Elicit symptoms and the pattern of the illness to begin a problem list.

Step 2: Develop Hypotheses

Generate a mental list of anatomic sites of disease, pathophysiologic processes and diseases that might produce the symptoms.

Step 3: Perform a Physical Examination

Look for signs of the physiologic processes and diseases suggested by the history, and identify new findings for the problem list.

Step 4: Make a Problem List

List ALL the problems found during the history and physical that require an explanation.

Step 5: Generate a Differential Diagnoses

List the most probable diagnostic hypotheses with an estimate of their pretest probabilities.

Step 6: Test the Hypotheses

Select laboratory tests, imaging studies, and other procedures with appropriate likelihood ratios to evaluate your hypotheses.

Step 7: Modify Your Differential Diagnosis

Use the results of all of the tests to evaluate your hypotheses, perhaps eliminating some and adding others and adjusting the probabilities.

Step 8: Repeat Steps 1 to 7

Reiterate your process until you have reached a diagnosis or decided that a definite diagnosis is neither likely nor necessary.

Step 9: Make the Diagnosis or Diagnoses

When the tests of your hypotheses are of sufficient certainty that they meet your stopping rule, you have reached a diagnosis. If uncertain, consider a provisional diagnosis or watchful waiting. Decide whether more investigation (return to step 1), consultation, treatment, or watchful observation is the best course based upon the severity of illness, the prognosis, and comorbidities. If the diagnosis remains obscure, retain a problem list of the unexplained symptoms and signs, as well as laboratory and imaging findings, assess the urgency for further evaluation and schedule regular follow-up visits.

Caveat

The complex process we have discussed is primarily suited to the problems of chronic and relatively obscure diseases commonly encountered in the fields of internal medicine and pediatrics. A majority of patients seen by most physicians do not require such a comprehensive process. Although the principles of diagnosis hold for all patients, variations from the described process may be appropriate for a given patient's condition and the medical or surgical specialty involved. Many conditions need few or no symptoms to make a diagnosis; the situation is obvious by noting the anatomic derangement or by taking X-ray films. The dermatologist can make many diagnoses without hearing about any symptoms. On the other hand, the psychiatrist relies exclusively on the history given by the patient, friends, relatives, and attendants. It follows that the scope and length of the history vary greatly among medical specialties and with the patient's presenting complaints.

An Example of the Diagnostic Process

The objective of the diagnostic examination is to discover the physiologic cause of the patient's complaint, identify the specific disease, and determine the severity and prognosis of the disease. You need these data to counsel your patient regarding the indications for treatment.

A 21-year-old woman consults you about a painless lump in her neck (symptom). You consider her age and select hypotheses that include lymphoma, infection, and collagen vascular disease, which lead to questions about fever, itching, weight loss, exposure to pets, tuberculosis, arthralgias, and Raynaud phenomenon. Your examination reveals a single, firm, 3-cm nontender lymph node in the right cervical chain (sign), but the spleen is not palpable and there are no other signs of disease. The patient's blood counts are normal (laboratory), and a biopsy of the enlarged node (supplemental test) discloses Hodgkin disease. Bone marrow biopsy and imaging studies of the chest and abdomen fail to reveal more disease (prognosis and staging tests).

You make a diagnosis of stage I Hodgkin disease and discuss the diagnosis with your patient, informing her of the prognosis without treatment. The possibility for radiotherapy and/or chemotherapy is discussed and consultation with an oncologist is requested so the patient can have a fully informed choice of therapy taking into account the risks and benefits of each treatment program.

Other Examinations

The Autopsy

The gold standard since the mid-nineteenth century for diagnostic accuracy has been the autopsy, and it remains so today. Unfortunately, autopsy rates have declined in recent decades, and with them valuable learning experiences for physicians. The autopsy is necessary to validate or correct our diagnostic impressions. With the decline in autopsy rates, many physicians have not learned the value of an autopsy and many families have not received a full explanation of the diseases of their loved ones. Despite the abundance of laboratory tests and imaging technologies, there is considerable evidence that clinical diagnoses in difficult cases are frequently wrong, that significant disease is missed, and that the addition of technology has not substantially altered these facts [Kirch W, Schafi C. Misdiagnosis at a university hospital in 4 medical eras. *Medicine (Baltimore)*. 1996;75:29–40; Sonderegger-Iseli K, Burger S, et al. Diagnostic errors in three medical eras: A necropsy study. *Lancet*. 2000;355:2027–2031].

Physicians should work closely with patients' families to encourage autopsies in most in-hospital deaths. This is a critical part of our professional development and the continuous struggle to improve our clinical skills [McPhee SJ. The autopsy. An antidote to misdiagnosis. *Medicine (Baltimore)*. 1996;75:41–43; Combes A, Mokhtari M, et al. Clinical and autopsy diagnoses in the intensive care unit.

Arch Intern Med. 2004;164:389–392]. The issue is not one of assigning blame or responsibility; it is one of improving our diagnostic abilities through learning from our experience and that of our colleagues.

Other Varieties of Medical Examinations

There are at least seven additional forms of medical examinations that differ from one another in their purposes, their stereotyped procedures, and their diagnostic tests.

The first six examinations involve special, stereotyped routines for persons having no symptoms and who are presumed to be well. Recommendations based on yield and cost are periodically revised by various professional groups. The absence of symptoms makes the performance and interpretation of these examinations different from that of a diagnostic examination.

1. Examination of young schoolchildren: The examination usually emphasizes tests of vision and hearing, physical and social development, coordination, and language skills.
2. Examination of athletes: The examiner stresses tests of cardiopulmonary function, muscle performance, flexibility, and injury prevention.
3. Examination for military service: This resembles the examination for athletes but adds testing of the special senses and emotional stability.
4. Examination for life insurance: The routine is generally established by the insurance company; it usually consists of a history form, an abbreviated physical examination, and a few laboratory tests to exclude the presence of chronic diseases that affect longevity, substance abuse, and HIV infection.
5. Periodic health examination: For infants, follow the recommendations of the American Academy of Pediatrics for well-child examinations and immunizations. The clinician especially searches for birth defects and measures growth and social development. Annual examinations of sexually active adults with new sexual partners should be performed with Pap testing of women and screening for sexually transmitted diseases in women, and possibly men. In persons older than age 45 years, annual examinations seek to detect the early onset of cardiovascular disease, diabetes mellitus, hypercholesterolemia, hypertension, and cancer. In addition, the clinician provides counseling about age-related life changes, diet and exercise, and appropriate immunizations. The visits may foster optimal patient-physician relationships.
6. Industrial examinations: Specialized procedures detect the hazards of particular industries.
7. Preoperative screening: See Part III, Chapter 16.

History Taking and the Medical Record

... [T]here is no more difficult art to acquire than the art of observation, and for some men it is quite as difficult to record an observation in brief and plain language.

— Sir William Osler

Proper care of a patient for more than a single episode of care requires a medical record documenting the data specific to the patient and their care. Ideally, this record should be available to all providers at any site of care at any time, an ideal within grasp with electronic medical records. The record should contain, preferably in standardized formats, basic patient data, such as their demographics, list of active and past medical problems, surgical history, injury history, medication history, allergies, and drug intolerances, sexual history, family history (FH), social history (SH), personal habits, prostheses used, preventive care services, and specific counseling provided. Using standardized forms for data acquisition and filing enables the information to be recorded in a uniform way for each patient, allowing rapid review of the pertinent information at each visit. It is important to enter information in such a way that it is always current; for example, in the FH list the first names of children and siblings with their year of birth (rather than age).

Outline of the Medical Record

The parts of the medical history follow a standardized sequence, differing only in small details from one institution to another. The following sequence is suggested for adult patients. A different order giving prominence to the birth history is often preferred by pediatricians.

I. Identification
II. Informant
III. Chief complaints (CC)
IV. History of present illness (HPI)
V. Past medical and surgical history
   A. General health
   B. Chronic and episodic illnesses

Procedure for Taking a History

Definition of the Medical History

The medical history is an account of the events in the patient's life that have relevance to the patient's mental and physical health. The elements of the medical history are: (1) sensations that can never be observed by the examiner, (2) abnormalities noted by the patient at some past time so they cannot be confirmed by the PE, (3) events in the past, not readily verifiable, such as former diagnoses or treatments, and (4) the patient's FH and description of their social situation.

Much more than the patient's unprompted narrative, it is a specialized literary form in which the physician writes an account of the perceptions and events *as related by the patient* or other informants. The history may be offered spontaneously or secured by skillful probing. Often, the history is best elaborated by repeat questioning after a time, as the patient is encouraged to reflect on their experience. In taking the history, the clinician should record key statements in the patient's words. *The history is the patient's story of their illness, not the physician's interpretation of the patient's history.* The clinician should take particular care to establish the sequence of events. The clinician's task at this time is to try to understand the patient's experience and their interpretation of the illness.

Scope of the History

When patients consult their physicians for dermatitis, the necessary diagnostic history is very brief, possibly only a few sentences. For a person brought into the hospital with a fractured tibia, a long diagnostic history is unnecessary and even inhumane. In contrast, a chronic, obscure disease may require a long, careful history, perhaps repeated and expanded, with supplements from time to time as the results of further studies open new diagnostic possibilities. Writings on history taking always discuss the extended history, which is complicated and demands maximal skill. However, it would be folly to insist on an extended history for every patient; in many situations, it is unnecessary, and unnecessarily time consuming. The experienced clinician adjusts their technique to the patient's problem.

Methods in History Taking

The most accurate history is obtained by an empathetic clinician who knows the manifestations of disease and understands how patients describe the symptoms of various diseases. History taking skill improves as you learn more of people, life, and disease. The face-to-face interaction while taking a good history permits you to see the emphasis your patient puts on her symptoms, allows you to learn about your patient's personality, and provides an opportunity to develop a supportive physician-patient relationship. Use of medical intake questionnaires is encouraged to assist in obtaining a complete medical history, FH, and SH within the time constraints of practice [Ramsey PG, Curtis JR, Paauw DS, et al. History-taking and preventive medicine skills among primary care physicians: An assessment using standardized patients. *Am J Med.* 1998;104:152–158].

We believe that extensive written instructions about patient interrogation are unrewarding; you can only become proficient at history taking by actually interviewing patients. A few guidelines are useful: (1) listen actively, (2) do not interrupt, (3) ask open-ended questions, and (4) be patient, give the patient time to think and speak. Most important is to be a real person yourself; have a conversation.

Clinical experience and reflection upon your experience are necessary to link, without conscious thought, your knowledge of diseases with the history being obtained from the patient. When a disease or syndrome comes to mind, it should recall a cluster of symptoms and signs and chronologic data about which to ask the patient. When you have acquired this knowledge and experience, you can face the patient confidently and readily improvise methods of interrogation.

Taking a diagnostic history has four objectives: (1) discovering symptoms, (2) obtaining accurate quantitative descriptions, (3) securing a precise chronology of events, and (4) determining how the illness has changed the patient's life.

Conducting the Interview

Arrangement

The following describes taking an extended history in the physician's clinic, with the following caveats: the patient is not in acute distress, time limitations are not critical, and the disease is relatively obscure. Circumstances often vary greatly from these stipulations.

Address patients formally, do not use their first name unless they request it. The conversation should not be overhead by others, although the presence of the patient's spouse or a relative is often helpful in confirming the narrative and supplementing the patient's observations. Limit the interview to the patient and one other informant; more informants waste time in their disagreements on details that outweigh the slight extra yield of information.

Physician's Manner

To obtain the patient's confidence and rapport, present yourself as unhurried, interested, and sympathetic. Sit at eye level without a desk between you. In no way should you express a moral judgment on the patient's actions or beliefs. Permit patients to begin their story in their own way; listen for several minutes before gradually injecting questions to guide the interview. Gently, but firmly, keep the discussion centered on the patient's problems. By all means, avoid discussing your own health, even when a patient invites you to do so.

Note Taking

Write sparingly, while the patient talks. After you have recorded some routine data, sit back and *listen* to the narrative for a while, interjecting only a few questions.

Avoid writing the patient's narrative verbatim; it is usually too lengthy and poorly organized. Use of standardized forms for recording the past medical history, FH, and SH (which can be filled out by the patient before the interview) will greatly decrease the need for making notes. Remember that the patient is telling you a story; you should try to understand their story jotting down key words and phrases to assist recall.

Language

From the beginning, gauge the patient's meaning of the words they use; words may have different meanings for different people. Put your questions in simple, nontechnical terms. Even lay words may be misunderstood. The English vocabulary is vast and formidable, even to the scholar. Excluding your scientific and medical vocabulary, you may be able to use 100 000 words, while the adult with average education gets along with 30 000 to 60 000. So, the patient may not know half the words you use in English. Patients may leave the interview with the fear that they have presented their symptoms poorly because they have answered questions they did not understand.

Belief Systems

Physicians are trained in the scientific method and in science-based rules of evidence. For many patients, if not most, this is not the structure of their belief system. Other belief systems include magic, faith, and rationalism. It is essential to understand how the patient views cause and effect, to what sources they attribute disease and illness. The clinician's task is to understand the patient; it is not, primarily, the patient's task to understand the clinician. Education to reach a mutual understanding becomes an important part of providing proper care for many chronic diseases.

Patient's Motivation

The usefulness of the history for diagnosis depends on the assumption, frequently forgotten, that the patient's sole motive is to assist the physician in diagnosis and treatment, and, therefore, the descriptions of the patient's symptoms are complete and truthful. This is a necessary and important assumption to make, but, if the patient's history conflicts with supportive documentation or the findings of your evaluation, you must consider other motives that might prompt misrepresentation. Some patients, entirely truthful, present symptoms that are baffling until the physician learns of their resemblance to those of a friend or relative who has died of cancer, and the patient fears the same fate. The physician must ascertain whether the patient is contemplating a lawsuit for damages, claiming worker's compensation, or applying for veteran's benefits. Substance abusers may present symptoms calculated to obtain drugs. Lacking discernible motives, a few patients fabricate medical histories that may lead to extensive diagnostic examinations.

Procedure

After introducing yourself and confirming the patient's identifying data, start the patient's narrative by saying, "Tell me about your problem," or "Give me your story." Do not ask, "What is the matter with you?" or "What is troubling you?" because the patient is likely to respond, "That's what I came here to find out." Listen to the story without interruption for several minutes; use open-ended questions to encourage the patient to speak. After the general outline becomes apparent, you may need to ask specific directed questions to explore the symptoms, medications, chronology, and the extent of disability. Ask about symptoms not mentioned but that are relevant to the systems and sites likely involved with the illness. You may pause periodically to write notes, including key words and phrases.

Next, record any remaining information to complete the past medical history, surgical history, injury history, review of medications and allergies, FH, SH, sexual, obstetrical, and gynecologic history, ROS and preventive care history including procedures (e.g., mammography, colonoscopy), tests (e.g., Pap smears, tuberculin skin tests) and immunizations.

Completion of the Medical Record

It is the clinician's responsibility to see that the medical record is complete and accurate. Your signature attests to the accuracy of the information and that you have verified it to your satisfaction. *Once entered and signed, the information in the medical record cannot be altered*, although addendums and corrections can be added.

Identification

These data are frequently provided for the clinician, but should be checked for accuracy.

Patient's Name

Record the complete name, including the family and given names, being careful to obtain correct spelling and birth date. Fatal errors have occurred when patients with the same name have received treatment intended for the other. Personal identification numbers and birth date should be verified before a treatment is given. Barcoding of both patients and drugs is helping to reduce these errors.

When a married woman who has taken her husband's name, place her husband's given names in parentheses, as Brown, Mary Elizabeth (Mrs. Edward Charles), since she may sign her name as Mrs. Edward C. Brown in correspondence. Determine whether she wishes to be addressed as Ms. or Mrs.

Sex and Gender

Sex is determined by genetics, gender is the sexual identity assumed by the patient. Usually, this is obvious, but specific questions sensitively put may be required.

Residence

The address should be confirmed and recorded; occasionally, addresses are used to distinguish patients with the same name.

Birth Date and Age

Record the patient's birth date and stated age. The birth date may help distinguish between patients with the same name.

Source of Referral

When the patient was referred by another physician, confirm the name, address, telephone and FAX numbers of the referring clinician, and the reason for referral.

The Informant

Sources of the History

The history is best obtained from the patient with supportive information from others. Record your judgment of the historian's accuracy and credibility. Do not assume a normal mental status from a casual conversation. Despite conversing normally, on direct questioning the patient may be unable to tell the day, date, or even name the city.

Interpreters

Try to avoid interpreters who are not medically trained. The following is a frequent experience with a lay interpreter: You ask, "Do you have pain?" The interpreter engages the patient in animated conversation incomprehensible to you, and after 3 or 4 minutes, the interpreter turns back to you and says, "No, she doesn't have any pain." It is reasonable to assume that the interpreter has interpreted the patient's story using their own concepts of illness, as well as his words. You cannot evaluate the patient's story or specific answers unless you know what questions were asked. Your only recourse is to ask short concrete questions and insist that the resulting conversation be no longer than you judge necessary.

Chief Complaints (CC)

When recording the patient's history, begin with the CC. This is a list of the one or more symptoms of most concern to the patient and that motivated them to seek attention. The complaints should be listed as single words or short phrases with the approximate length of time they have been present: for example, nausea for 2 months; vomiting for 1 week. Always use the patient's own words free of interpretation. Do not accept a previous diagnosis as a chief complaint; patient probing may be needed before the patient relates their symptoms rather than their diagnoses or those of previous providers and family members.

CC are the starting place from which to begin making a differential diagnosis; the details of these symptoms should always be fully delineated. Furthermore, these are the symptoms that made the patient seek treatment; they require therapy or an explanation of why therapy is not given. The patient's chief complaint should be the first problem on your problem list. This would seem obvious, but occasionally the physician finds an interesting disease, unrelated to the CC; the medically attractive condition receives all the attention, and the CC are ignored.

Do not press the patient for a chief complaint too early in the interview. After they have told some of their story, they may be better able to articulate their complaints and concerns. Occasionally, when asked for their symptoms, the patient produces a long detailed list of notes. The French label this la maladie de petit papier, which may signal an inappropriate level of concern or obsession with their symptoms. However, it is appropriate for many patients to keep track of symptoms, signs, temperature, blood pressure, weight, or blood sugars to get a more accurate picture of their illness.

History of Present Illness (HPI)

The history of present illness is the patient's story of their illness experience; *it is the most important part of the diagnostic examination.* It should be written in complete sentences as a lucid, succinct, chronologic narrative. Ideally, the HPI should be brief, so that it is easily read and digested. This is only possible if the history is relatively straightforward. When story is more complex and the diagnostic possibilities broad, include more details, you cannot be certain what is pertinent and what superfluous. Because of this uncertainty, you must avoid premature interpretation of the history such as replacing their words with medical terminology or failing to record seemingly irrelevant symptoms or events.

Searching for Diagnostic Clues

The chief purpose of the history is to help you form hypotheses regarding the process unfolding in the patient. As the narrative unfolds, you should be simultaneously performing three operations: (1) accumulating data (obtaining the history), (2) evaluating the data (assessing the credibility of symptoms, seeking more details of time and quantity), and (3) preparing three sets of hypotheses. The hypotheses are anatomic (where is the problem?), physiologic (what is the pathophysiology?) and diagnostic (what diseases could account for this pathophysiology in that place?). Having formed a list of hypotheses, question the patient about other symptoms specific for processes and diseases on your lists, either to support or undermine a hypothesis. For example, when the patient complains of chest pain, ask if it is related to respiratory movements. A positive answer prompts questions about inflamed muscles, fractured ribs, and pleurisy. If the answer is negative, ask for an association with exertion or radiation suggestive of angina pectoris. Thus, each step leads to another, resulting in refinement of your hypotheses.

Symptoms

A symptom is an abnormal sensation perceived by the patient, in contrast to a physical sign that can be seen, felt, or heard by the examiner. Evaluation of a symptom can be straightforward, as when the patient says, "I've found a lump in my neck" (symptom), and the examiner can palpate a mass (physical sign). However, when the patient complains of a nonspecific symptom, such as chest pain, and no physical signs are detected, more information is required for the symptom to be diagnostically useful. Identify the attributes of each symptom, asking specifically about *P*rovocative or *P*alliative maneuvers, symptom *Q*uality, the *R*egion involved, the *S*everity and *T*emporal pattern of the symptom. The acronym PQRST is useful mnemonic for these questions (see the discussion of pain, Chapter 4, page 85).

Insist that the patients describe their symptoms, do not accept diagnoses or medical jargon as a substitute. Record the symptoms using the patient's words. When the symptoms suggest several conditions, note the absence of concomitant symptoms, ascertained by direct questioning, whose presence would favor one or another of the possibilities (pertinent negatives). For example, if the patient has had attacks of right upper abdominal quadrant pain, you should ask about jaundice, dark colored urine, pruritus, and pain radiating to the right scapula, all suggestive of hepatobiliary disease.

Nature of the Symptoms

The patient's symptoms must be clearly described and quantified; you should be forming mental images of their illness experience.

Clarification. Question the patient until sufficient details are obtained to categorize the symptom. Do not accept vague complaints such as "I don't feel well." If the patient complains of weakness, ascertain if she is weak in one or more muscle groups or if she experiences lassitude, malaise, or myalgia. When a patient says she is dizzy, have her describe the experience without using the word "dizzy." Determine whether dyspnea occurs at rest or with exertion.

Quantification. Quantification is important to the evaluation of symptoms; always record symptoms with a statement of quantity. For instance, pain cannot be measured, but the severity can be estimated by how it affects the patient. A patient may have a "terrible pain," but if the pain has never interfered with work, sleep, or other activities, "terrible" acquires a clearer meaning. Exertional dyspnea can be assessed by the amount of exertion required to produce it; for example, ask, "Can you climb a flight of stairs? Can you walk two blocks without stopping?" Neither you nor your reader can interpret what "heavy smoker" means. Heavy is a value judgment whose meaning varies from one person to another, but a record of smoking 20 cigarettes a day is a measure everyone understands. The patient who had hemoptysis should be instructed to estimate the amount of blood lost in household measures, such as teaspoonfuls or cupfuls. The amount of sputum raised should be recorded; the volume serves as an important consideration in differential diagnosis.

Chronology. The duration of a symptom and the time of its appearance in the course of illness are significant for diagnosis. When the disease is chronic and the course complicated, the patient may be unable to place events in chronologic sequence. A time-line can assist the patient in clarifying the details: draw a vertical line demarcated in appropriate units of time, days, weeks, months, or years. Indicate on the time-line the certain dates supplied by the patient, as well as anchoring dates such as birthdays, New Year's and holidays. Seeing the chart, the patient frequently recalls further details and can place the onset of symptoms more accurately. The sequence and doses of medication can also be recorded.

Current activity. Include this in the HPI. Determine how the illness has diminished the patient's quality of life and whether therapy has improved it. Obtain a detailed picture of the patient's average work and weekend day to evaluate the patient's reaction to illness, severity of the disease, and response to therapy.

Summarization. Review your understanding of the history and ask the patient for corrections and confirmation. Test the completeness of your history by asking whether your summary conveys a clear picture of the patient's experience of their illness, that is, how the illness has affected them and their family, how it has interfered with their work, and how the symptoms have progressed.

Past Medical and Surgical History

The past history helps you to understand the person you are evaluating and the preconditions that may substantially alter current and future risks for specific health conditions. When relevant, specific facts may be included in the HPI, but they must be recorded again in this section. The significance of past illnesses may be only appreciated after future developments in the patient's condition or as newly recognized disease associations are reported.

General Health

The patient's lifetime health, before the present illness, is sometimes revealing. Factors to consider include body weight (present, maximum, and minimum, with dates of each), previous physical exams (dates and findings), and any periods of medical disability.

Chronic and Episodic Illnesses

Chronic medical illness. List all illnesses, diseases or conditions for which the patient receives, or has received, chronic medical treatment.

Infectious diseases. Infectious diseases have had an important history in medicine. Knowledge of past infections is important to understand current and future infection risk. List dates and complications of measles, German measles, mumps, whooping cough, chickenpox, smallpox, diphtheria, typhoid fever, malaria, hepatitis, scarlet fever, rheumatic fever, pneumonia, tuberculosis, sexually transmitted diseases, and HIV. Give dates of chemotherapy and antibiotic treatment. Include reactions to antibiotics under the heading, "Allergies and Medication Intolerances."

Operations and Injuries

Give dates and nature of injuries, operations, operative diagnoses, and infection, hemorrhage or other complications.

Previous Hospitalizations

Record each hospitalization, including the dates and names of hospitals and their locations. If the hospital records are available, summarize the dates and diagnoses for each admission.

Family History (FH)

A FH is essential for all patients receiving more than the most cursory of care. This should include four generations, when available: grandparents, parents, aunts and uncles, siblings, and children. For parents and grandparents, record the birth year and current health or age at death and causes. For aunts, uncles, siblings, and children, record the birth year, first name, and current health or cause of death and age at death. Make note of any family history of hypertension, heart disease, diabetes, kidney disease, autoimmune diseases, gout, atopy, asthma, obesity, endocrine disorders, osteoporosis, cancer (particularly breast, colon, ovarian and endocrine cancers), hemophilia or other bleeding diseases, venous thromboembolism, stroke, migraine, neurologic or muscular disorders, mental or emotional disturbances, substance abuse, and epilepsy.

Social History (SH)

Place of birth. This information may be useful in assessing social or national incidence of disease. The examiner may gain some insight into the probability of the patient's understanding the nuances of the English language in giving a history.

Nationality and ethnicity.   The correct classification may require considerable knowledge of geography, history, and anthropology. The patient may not be able to give a precise answer. It may be helpful to learn the nationality and ethnicity of the parents. Ethnic and genetic backgrounds are of some importance in diagnosis, for example, of diseases such as hemoglobinopathies and familial Mediterranean fever.

Marital status.   Note whether the patient is single, married, divorced, or widowed, and the duration of each marriage or long term relationship and an explanation of its termination.

Occupations.   Precise knowledge of the patient's work history sheds light on education, social status, physical exertion, psychologic trauma, exposure to noxious agents, and a variety of conditions that may cause disease. Some diseases produce symptoms years after exposure, so tabulate past occupations as well as current work. Do not accept the patient's categorization of an occupation without detailed questioning about what is actually done at work. The manual laborer may actually engage in little heavy physical work on the job but may be exposed to heavy-metal poisons or silica dust. Ask the patient if coworkers recognize some disease connected with their surroundings. Some women may give their occupation as "housewife," neglecting to mention additional part-time or full-time employment. When a woman says she is a housewife, ascertain the number of rooms in the house, how many persons she cares for, and if she has assistance with her work. If the woman lives on a farm, how much fieldwork does she perform? For farmers of both sexes, learn about contacts with agricultural chemicals. With factory workers, ascertain, if other workers in the same plant or department have symptoms similar to those of the patient. Determine how much anxiety and tension accompany the job, the attitudes of superiors, and the degree of fatigue from work.

Military history.   Note admissions to the armed services, branch of service, geographic locations of service, discharge (honorable or dishonorable), and eligibility for veteran's benefits.

Gender preference.   Labels such as heterosexual, homosexual, and bisexual are often more confusing than helpful. Ask each patient if they have had sex with anyone of the same sex. For example, ask men, "Have you ever had sex with men?" If the patient answers "yes," you should ask further questions about sex with women and the patient's past and current practices and preference. Nonjudgmental inquiry about exchange of sex for drugs, money, or services can disclose high-risk behaviors.

Social and economic status.   Record the patient's years of formal education, vocational training, current housing type, living arrangements, and any special financial problems.

Habits.   Determine the patient's former and current use of tobacco, coffee, alcohol, sedatives, illicit drugs (especially any injection drug use), placement of tattoos, and body piercing.

Violence and safety.   Record the patient's use of vehicle restraints, helmets with bicycling or motorcycling, and the presence of smoke and carbon monoxide alarms in the home.

Domestic, child, and elder abuse are common problems that go unidentified unless they are asked about explicitly and discreetly. In complete privacy, inquire whether the patient has ever been in a relationship in which she felt unsafe. If the answer is "yes," ask if she feels safe in her current situation. If she answers "no," ask if she wishes you to help her find a safe environment. At no time, try to explicitly identify the individual whom the patient finds threatening, unless this information is volunteered by the patient [Felhaus KM, Koziol-McLain J, Amsbury HL, et al. Accuracy of 3 brief screening questions for detecting partner violence in the emergency department. *JAMA*. 1997;277:1357–1361].

Prostheses and in-home assistance. Record the patient's use of eyeglasses, dentures and dental appliances, hearing aides, ambulation assistance devices (cane, walker, scooter, wheelchair), braces, prosthetic footwear, and any aide or assistance received in the home (visiting nurse, physical therapy, homemaker services).

Review of Systems (ROS)

The following outline can help you make a careful review of the history by inquiring for salient symptoms associated with each system or anatomic region. Symptoms related to the patient's current problem, discovered during your ROS inquiry, should be recorded under "present illness." Become familiar with these symptoms and learn their diagnostic significance. In practice, the patient's answers are not written down except when they are positive, or when a negative response is particularly pertinent to the differential diagnosis. We suggest that you ask the questions while examining the part of the body to which the questions pertain. In taking the HPI, when one of the symptoms emerges, inquire about the associated symptoms in this outline. Use of a standardized patient questionnaire will greatly facilitate identification of positive items on a thorough system review and saves the clinician's valuable time.

Skin, Hair and Nails

Skin: Color, pigmentation, temperature, moisture, eruptions, pruritus, scaling, bruising, bleeding. *Hair:* Color, texture, abnormal loss or growth, distribution. *Nails:* Color changes, brittleness, ridging, pitting, curvature.

Lymph Nodes

Enlargement, pain, tenderness, suppuration, draining sinuses, location.

Bones, Joints, and Muscles

Fractures, dislocations, sprains, arthritis, myositis, pain, swelling, stiffness, migratory distribution, degree of disability, muscular weakness, wasting, or atrophy, night cramps.

Hemopoietic System

Anemia (type, therapy, and response), lymphadenopathy, bleeding or clotting (spontaneous, traumatic, familial).

Endocrine System

History of growth, body configuration, and weight; size of hands, feet, and head, especially changes during adulthood; hair distribution; skin pigmentation; goiter, exophthalmos, dryness of skin and hair, intolerance to heat or cold, tremor; polyphagia, polydipsia, polyuria, glycosuria; libido, secondary sex characteristics, impotence, sterility.

Allergic and Immunologic History

Dermatitis, urticaria, angioedema, eczema, hay fever, vasomotor rhinitis, asthma, migraine conjunctivitis; known sensitivity to pollens, foods, danders, X-ray contrast agents, bee stings; previous skin tests and their results; results of tuberculin tests and others; desensitization, serum injections, vaccinations, and immunizations.

Head

Headaches, migraine, trauma, vertigo, syncope, convulsive seizures.

Eyes

Loss of vision or color blindness, diplopia, hemianopsia, trauma, inflammation, glasses (date of refraction), discharge, excessive tearing.

Ears

Deafness, tinnitus, vertigo, discharge from the ears, pain, mastoiditis, operations.

Nose

Coryza, rhinitis, sinusitis, discharge, obstruction, epistaxis.

Mouth

Soreness of mouth or tongue, symptoms referable to teeth.

Throat

Hoarseness, sore throats, tonsillitis, voice changes, dysphagia, odynophagia.

Neck

Swelling, suppurative lesions, enlargement of lymph nodes, goiter, stiffness, and limitation of motion.

Breasts

Development, lactation, trauma, lumps, pains, discharge from nipples, gynecomastia, changes in nipples, skin changes, warmth.

Respiratory System

Pain, shortness of breath, wheezing, dyspnea, nocturnal dyspnea, orthopnea, cough, sputum, hemoptysis, night sweats, fevers, pleurisy, bronchitis, tuberculosis (history of contacts), pneumonia, asthma, other respiratory infections.

Cardiovascular System

Palpitation, tachycardia, irregularities or rhythm, pain in the chest, exertional dyspnea, paroxysmal nocturnal dyspnea, orthopnea, cough, cyanosis, ascites, edema;

intermittent claudication, cold extremities, thromboses, postural or permanent changes in skin color; hypertension, rheumatic fever, chorea, syphilis, diphtheria; drugs such as digitalis, quinidine, nitroglycerin, diuretics, anticoagulants, antiplatelet agents, and other medications.

Gastrointestinal System

Appetite, changes in weight, dysphagia, nausea, eructation, flatulence, abdominal pain or colic, vomiting, hematemesis, jaundice (pain, fever, intensity, duration, color of urine and stools), stools (color, frequency, incontinence, consistency, odor, gas, cathartics, pain or difficulty with passage, urge to stool), hemorrhoids, change in bowel habits.

Genitourinary System

Color of urine, polyuria, oliguria, nocturia, dysuria, hematuria, pyuria, urinary retention, urinary frequency, incontinence, pain or colic, passage of stones or gravel. *Gynecologic History:* Age of onset, frequency of periods, regularity, duration, amount of flow, leukorrhea, dysmenorrhea, date of last normal and preceding periods, date and character of menopause, postmenopausal bleeding; pregnancies (number, abortions, miscarriages, stillbirths, chronologic sequence), complications of pregnancy; birth control practices (oral contraceptive medications, barrier methods, etc.). *Male History:* Erectile dysfunction, premature ejaculation, blood in the semen, contraceptive methods and condom use. *Venereal Disease History:* Sexual activity (sex of partners and practices), chancre, bubo, urethral discharge, treatment of venereal diseases.

Nervous System

Cranial Nerves (CNs): Disturbances of smell (CN I), visual disturbances (CN II, III, IV, VI), orofacial paresthesias and difficulty in chewing (CN V), facial weakness and taste disturbances (CN VII), disturbances in hearing and equilibrium (CN VIII), difficulties in speech, swallowing, and taste (CN IX, X, XII), limitation in motion of neck (CN XII). *Motor System:* Paralyses, muscle wasting, involuntary movements, convulsions, gait, incoordination. *Sensory System:* Pain, lightning pain, girdle pain, paresthesia, hypesthesia, anesthesia, allodynia. *Autonomic System:* Control of urination and defecation, sweating, erythema, cyanosis, pallor, reaction to heat and cold, postural faintness.

Psychiatric History

Describe difficulties with interpersonal relationships (with parents, siblings, spouse, children, friends and associates), sexual adjustments, school and employment success and difficulties, impulse control, sleep disorders, mood swings, difficulty with concentration, thought or the presence of hallucinations.

Medications

In a separate section, list all medications being taken: their names, doses, effects, reason for taking, and duration. Ask the patient to bring the pharmacist's containers with the specific data on the labels. If the labels are absent, identify tablets, pills, capsules, and suppositories by asking the pharmacist who issued the drug. Be sure to list all nonprescription drugs, herbal remedies, supplements, and vitamins.

Allergies and Medication Intolerances

A notation of past medications and untoward drug reactions should be as explicit as possible. Ask for the type of reaction or intolerance experienced with each medication. Many patients list as allergies common side effects they experienced, not allergic reactions: for example, stomach upset with codeine or erythromycin. Identify all known or suspected causes of anaphylaxis, including drugs, stings, and foods (e.g., peanuts). This summary of allergies and medication intolerances must be consulted when any drugs are prescribed in the future.

Preventive Care Services

Record the patient's history of preventive care services. List the dates and results of screening tests (e.g., mammograms, Pap smears, colorectal cancer screening, tuberculin tests), insurance examinations, and immunizations using age- and sex-specific national guidelines as your standard.

Advance Directives

Each adult should be asked if they have a living will and/or durable power of attorney for health care and, if so, who is their surrogate decision maker. Each adult should be given information about advance directives and be given an opportunity to record their wishes concerning resuscitation, mechanical ventilation, and prolonged life support. Although these discussions are more likely to be particularly relevant to the frail older adults, you should initiate this discussion with all adults more than 50 years of age, before the anticipated time of need.

Physical Examination (PE)

Here you should record the finding from your PE in a systematic fashion. The sequence of presentation below is suggested as a common and practical method:

Vital signs

General appearance

Head, eyes, ears, nose, and throat

Neck and spine

Chest: breasts

Chest: chest wall and lungs

Chest: heart, major arteries, and neck veins

Abdomen

Genitourinary examination, including inguinal hernias

Rectal examination

Extremities

Lymph nodes

Neurologic examination, including the mental status examination

Skin

Laboratory

Record the results of the initial laboratory finding which you have used to assist in the development of your differential diagnosis.

Assessment

Case Summary

After recording the history and PE, analyze the chronology, symptoms, signs, and laboratory findings of the illness. It is advisable to write a brief summary of your findings as an abstract of the significant observations.

The Problem List and Assessment

Write down your list of all the diagnostic and management problems the patient presents (variously labeled as problem list, initial assessment, impression, or diagnosis). A diagnostic problem may be a symptom, a sign, a laboratory finding, or a complex of several items that experience has taught are associated with disease. A previously diagnosed disease, or one under consideration for diagnosis, may be listed as a problem. When the diagnosis is obscure, beware of lumping problems together prematurely; this may serve to obscure rather than to clarify the diagnosis.

Generate a *differential diagnosis* for each medical problem. As discussed in Chapter 1, the differential diagnosis can be pathophysiologic, diagnostic, or both. It is a good practice to keep the patient's chief complaint the first problem on your problem list. Beyond that, we do not feel that attempts to number the problem list in a prioritized or numerically consistent fashion is useful, because priorities change as the evaluation and treatment proceed and problems disappear or consolidate as more information is acquired.

A working problem list should be maintained as a separate page in the hospital or clinic chart to record the problems with notes and dates indicating the status of each. It is important to maintain, update, and revise this problem list. By constantly reviewing the problem list, you can see that every problem is being evaluated and managed. Often, the key to the diagnostic puzzle is finding how the odd problem fits the pattern. Diagnostic problem solving is much like putting together a jigsaw puzzle without the picture and with only a few pieces provided at a time. To get the pieces together correctly, you have to have all the pieces on the table at the same time and keep looking at them, as new pieces appear to see the pattern emerge. The problem list is your table full of pieces; your hypotheses are attempts to explain the pattern. It is often the odd piece that does not seem to fit anywhere that is the key to the puzzle.

The Plan

For each problem, and the patient as a whole, you need to develop a plan. The plan for each problem has three parts: (1) plans for testing your hypothesis or differential diagnosis, (2) therapy to be considered or given, and (3) education for the patient and family.

A plan is only as good as the diagnostic hypotheses that generated it. Our emphasis in this text is to help you think about the information acquired in the performance of the history and physical exam so that you can generate sound, testable hypotheses. Once you have generated a concise and thoughtful differential diagnosis, you can consult textbooks of medicine, for example, *Harrison's Principles of Internal Medicine* [Kasper DL, Braunwald E, Fauci AS, et al. eds. *Harrison's Principles of Internal Medicine.* 17th ed. New York, NY: McGraw-Hill, 2008], or directly search the medical literature to assist in the most economical and efficient methods for testing your hypotheses.

The Oral Presentation

The optimal oral presentation holds your listener's attention for 5 to 7 minutes while you identify your patient and briefly summarize the case. Start with a statement of the patient's problems or diagnoses so your listeners can analyze your subsequent narrative for the evidence used to support the diagnosis and therapeutic plan you propose. Then summarize the history and presentation, review the vital signs, and pertinent physical findings and laboratory test results, state the diagnostic impressions or problems, and then recommend a diagnostic and therapeutic plan. Excellent presentations require that you edit and organize the information you have collected, to tell the story of the illness as it appears to you. If you regurgitate all of the extensive information that you place in the medical record, you will quickly lose your audience.

The oral presentation of the diagnostic examination is not simply an academic exercise. Brief, accurate presentations will benefit your patients by clearly communicating their problems to others who will participate in their care: your teachers, fellow house officers, sign-out partners in practice, and consultants [Lehmann LS, Brancati FL, Chen M-C, et al. The effect of bedside case presentations on patient's perceptions of their medical care. *N Engl J Med.* 1997;336:1150–1155; Bergus GR, Chapman GB, Levy BT, et al. Clinical diagnosis and the order of information. *Med Decis Making.* 1998;18:412–417].

Other Clinical Notes

Inpatient Progress Notes

Progress notes are made daily and whenever necessary. Each note should be dated and the time of day recorded. Each note has four subheads. Use the mnemonic SOAP to remember them: Subjective data (symptoms and changes in symptoms, their appearance and disappearance, and their response to therapy); Objective data (changes in or new physical signs and laboratory findings and response to therapy); Assessments (updates to your problem list and hypotheses); and Plans (diagnostic tests, therapeutic interventions and instructions to the patient and nursing staff). When a problem is resolved by inclusion in another diagnosis, or by cure or disappearance, it should be so noted in the progress note and in the working problem list.

The full and legible name of the writer should be appended to each progress note. The name should be followed by a slash mark and an abbreviation indicating hospital role, that is, MD (resident), RN (student nurse or graduate), S (staff), etc.

Off-Service Note

Write a note in the chart when you leave a service and turn over the care of the patient to your successor. Customarily, a brief résumé of the case is recorded, stating the diagnosis or problems, the treatment, and response, suggestions for continuing treatment are included. Do not include statements like, "Good luck!"

Discharge Summary

When the patient leaves the hospital, the physician should enter a final note containing an abstract of the case, with the diagnosis or problem list and the treatment given in the hospital, future plans, and each medication, dose and schedule. Note the patient's condition and functional status at discharge and any information or instructions given to the patient and attendants for home and follow-up care.

Clinic Notes

Clinic notes follow the same SOAP format described for progress notes in the hospital. If the chart contains standardized forms as part of the medical record, the note may refer the reader to those forms for current information so that it need not be repeated in the written note. All clinic notes should state the expected response to interventions, when that response is anticipated and when the patient is to be seen in follow up.

The Patient's Medical Record

The patient's medical record is a document containing: (1) the medical history, (2) the findings from the physical exam, (3) the reports of laboratory tests, (4) the findings and conclusions from special examinations, (5) the findings and diagnoses of consultants, (6) the diagnoses of the responsible physician, (7) notes on treatment, including medication, surgical operations, radiation, physical therapy, and (8) progress notes by physicians, nurses, and others.

Purposes

The purposes of the patient's medical record may be classified as follows:

Medical Purposes

1. To assist the physician in making diagnoses.
2. To assist physicians, nurses, and others in the care and treatment of the patient.
3. To serve as a record for teaching medicine and for clinical research.

Legal Purposes

1. To document insurance claims for the patient.
2. To serve as legal proof in cases of malpractice claims for injury or compensation, cases of poisoning, and cases of homicide.

Reimbursement

The federal government has developed documentation guidelines for evaluation and management services that define the standards that Medicare carriers employ in reviewing documentation physicians must use to bill for history taking, PEs, and medical decision making.

Usually, the physician composes the patient's record with attention focused on the medical purposes of making diagnoses, caring for the patient, teaching medicine, and furthering research. After the illness, sometimes years later, the medical record may be consulted to fulfill the legal purposes in support of claims and the demonstration of facts in litigation. In these contingencies, the physician may belatedly discover omissions and inaccuracies. To prevent late recriminations, always completely document each patient encounter at the time of service. Addendums may be added at a later date, but the original note must never be altered.

Attempts at grading diagnoses are encountered in some hospitals and in some insurance forms that call for a primary diagnosis and a secondary diagnosis. At face value, this request seems rational but an absurdity appears, when the same records are graded by different specialists. The primary diagnosis is often different from the view of the internist, the surgeon, the orthopedist, or the otolaryngologist. Each selects the disease pertaining to his or her own specialty. The confusion is diminished when the form states that the primary diagnosis is the reason for the clinic visit or hospitalization.

The primary purposes of enabling a physician to document his or her care in the medical record are to serve the memory of the caregiver and communicate these data to other physicians caring for the patient. Uses of the record for legal and billing purposes are secondary and should not distract or interfere with good patient care. Lawyers and insurers insist on written documentation as evidence of performance, but guidelines that encourage treating charts instead of patients are bad medicine.

Physician's Signature

Each sheet, brief entry, and doctor's order composed by the physician for the medical record should be accompanied by the physician's signature and the date and time of signing as proof of authorship. In the hospital record, the physician's initials are inadequate; the complete written signature should be legible. All dates should include the month, day of the month, year and time of day. In teaching hospitals, where many persons contribute to the record, the entries of medical students and nurses should be dated and accompanied by their signatures, affixed with suitable abbreviations indicating their status in the medical organization.

Custody of the Record

The record may rest in the physician's locked office files, or it may be in the custody of the hospital where the patient received medical care. The contents of the medical record must be guarded against access by unauthorized persons. The recorded facts are privileged communications under the law; they cannot be revealed to another person without the written consent of the patient.

The medical record should be composed with the constant realization that at some future time the patient may read it or that it may become a legal document; the date and authorship of each entry may be important. The record should not contain flippant or derogatory remarks.

Electronic Medical Records

Over the past 30 years, enthusiasts of medical informatics have continued to develop the electronic medical record. Technologic advances allow recording of all patient information, including clinical documentation, laboratory tests and imaging studies directly into the electronic record. Access to the record is password protected and encrypted information is readily transmitted electronically within an institution and around the world. Multiple providers can have simultaneous access to the record from any computer terminal, allowing improved patient care simultaneously by multiple clinicians. Systems are being installed that allow referring physicians to access the records of patients they have referred to another institution, allowing them to stay involved with the daily flow of information. In addition, decision support modules allow the clinician ready access to guidelines and literature searches pertinent to the patients under their care. The use of computer-generated reminders also facilitates preventive care. Physician order entry programs avoid common transcription errors and automatically search for drug interactions and suggest dosing changes for impaired renal function. The hope is for standardization of information domains and ultimately the sharing of patient information in a nationwide medical information network so that complete patient records are accessible at the point of care, wherever that may be, any time day or night. Issues of security, standardization of computer languages and information acquisition formats and the large and uncompensated expense for hardware and software are still major obstacles to achieving the vision.

An increasing problem encountered with the electronic record is the "cut and paste" phenomena: documentation from one day is cut and pasted to the next rather than constructed anew, and a deluge of laboratory and radiologic information is pasted into daily progress notes and discharge summaries. These are both abuses of the electronic format that are to be condemned. Neither requires that the cutter-paster has actually read the material, given it any thought, or reflected upon the whole of the information to form a new and evolving clinical assessment and management plan.

Each daily note should be constructed in its entirety each day, with appropriate references to existing records. The physical findings must be ascertained and recorded daily as they change and evolve. Test results should be succinct summaries of key radiographic findings and the few key chemistry and microbiologic reports used today to make diagnoses or change the management plan. All the detailed radiologic and laboratory information is readily available to everyone reading the note in another part of the record and it need not be duplicated.

Electronic records are a boon to patient care when generated and used correctly. Unfortunately, they also facilitate sloppy, expediant but unprofessional and potentially dangerous documentation practices that discourage thought and reflection and perpetuate misstatements, erroneous conclusions and frank errors.

CHAPTER 3

The Screening Physical Examination

In our era of high technology, the continued need for the performance of a proper physical examination may surprise the uninformed [Sackett DL. The science of the art of the clinical examination. *JAMA*. 1992;267:2650–2652; Adolph RJ, Reilly BM. Physical examination in the care of medical inpatients: An observational study. *Lancet*. 2003;362:1100–1105].

The importance of a systematic history and physical examination is best understood by considering the following points. (1) Attention to the story of the patient's illness and thoughtful performance of the physical examination (the "laying on of hands") establishes a personal relationship of trust and respect between the patient and clinician which is necessary for a good medical care. (2) Performing laboratory tests and imaging studies without diagnostic hypotheses generated from the history and physical examination is expensive and often produces false-positive results, delaying proper diagnosis. (3) Conclusions drawn from the results of blood tests, imaging procedures, and even biopsy material are based upon the pretest probability of the various diagnoses under consideration. The pretest probability is derived from the history, physical examination, and knowledge of disease prevalence. (4) Additionally, many studies have shown that the history and physical examination are more sensitive and specific than imaging tests in most difficult diagnostic situations [Kirch W, Schafi C. Misdiagnosis at a university hospital in 4 medical eras. *Medicine (Baltimore)*. 1996;75:29–40].

Each physical examination is an opportunity to train the four senses: sight, touch, hearing, and smell. With reflective practice and knowledge of anatomy, physiology, and pathology, you will perceive abnormalities in structure and function overlooked by an untrained examiner. The physiologic and disease hypotheses generated during the history and physical examination are tested in the various laboratories leading to precise diagnosis with an economical use of resources.

We use each of our four senses to elicit signs of disease: inspection (sight and smell), palpation (touch), percussion (touch and hearing), and auscultation (hearing). Only minimal manual dexterity is required for percussion and palpation. Remember to be gentle on initiation of the examination; forceful palpation and percussion are rarely necessary and will cause the patient to become tense and resist your examination.

With experience, you will be able to assess the severity of illness and the urgency for treatment. To become a skillful diagnostician, you must constantly reflect on the findings from your examination, the correlations between your examination and the laboratory and imaging studies, and the accuracy of your findings and hypotheses based upon the final confirmed diagnoses. In short, you must practice and study. No one started as an expert history taker, physical examiner, or diagnostician. The experts are those who have learned from their experience and refined their senses and skills through repetition, reflection and correlation of their physical findings with the results of imaging and laboratory tests.

Methods for Physical Examination

Inspection

Inspection is the search for physical signs by observing the patient with your eyes and sense of smell. Among the examination methods, inspection is the least mechanical and the hardest to learn, but it yields many important physical signs. Because we tend to see things that have meaning for us, inspection depends entirely on the knowledge and expectations of the observer. This is epitomized in maxims such as "We see what's behind the eyes" (Wintrobe), "The examination does not wait the removal of the shirt" (Waring), and "Was Man Weiss, Man sieht" (Goethe: "What one knows, one sees"). The layperson looks at a person and concludes that there is something "peculiar" about that person; the physician sees acromegaly. The expert observer can dissect the "peculiarity" and recognize the diagnostic components, such as the enlarged supraorbital ridges, the widely spaced teeth, the macroglossia, the buffalo hump, the wide hands and feet. Practice is required to learn inspection: remember that *sight is a faculty, whereas seeing is an art*.

Smells are impossible to describe, only experience with similar sensations will give you a context for interpretation. The body odors of poor hygiene, the fetor of advanced liver disease, the putrid smell of anaerobic infections, the smell of alcohol or acetone on the breath, and many others are useful diagnostic clues apparent to the trained observer.

General Visual Inspection

The initial step in physical examination is inspection of the person as a whole. It begins at your first encounter with the patient. If possible, watch how the patient walks when moving to the examination room. Note how he is dressed and groomed; whether eye contact is established; the tone and pattern of speech; how the patient moves and changes position; facial expression; skin type; overall body form and proportions; deformities or asymmetry of face, limbs, or trunk; nutrition; specific behaviors; signs of pain or tremor. You should also bear in mind that the patient will be inspecting you at the same time.

Close Visual Inspection

Close or focused inspection concentrates on a single anatomic region; the closer you look, the more you see. The art is in seeing all that is there and distinguishing what is important from what is not.

Visual inspection usually refers to observation with the unaided eyes. Obviously, the dermatologist relies heavily on the appearance of skin lesions to make a diagnosis. Actually, however, visual signs are the principal findings in the use of the ophthalmoscope, slit lamp, otoscope, laryngoscope, bronchoscope, gastroscope, thoracoscope, laparoscope, cystoscope, anoscope, colonoscope, and sigmoidoscope. The pathologist uses the microscope; the radiologist inspects images generated in any number of ways. All are using visual inspection to elicit information.

Proper visual inspection of the body surface requires a uniform white light source to avoid color distortion. A hand-held lens or an otoscope or ophthalmoscope can be used for magnification. Oblique lighting is often very useful to detect subtle changes in surface contours and to detect motion that may be invisible with direct lighting, for example, looking for the apical impulse on the chest. As with all parts of the physical examination it is important not just to see an abnormality, you must learn to accurately describe what you see without using language that draws a conclusion or presumes a diagnosis.

Olfactory Inspection—Smell

Although some physicians seem to regard the use of the nose for diagnosis as indelicate, odors may provide valuable and immediate clues.

Breath.   Odors on the breath from acetone, alcohol, and some poisons may lead quickly to a diagnosis.

Sputum.   Foul-smelling sputum suggests bronchiectasis or lung abscess.

Vomitus.   The gastric contents may emit the odors of alcohol, phenol, or other poisons, or the sour smell of fermenting food retained overlong. A fecal odor from the vomitus may indicate intestinal obstruction.

Feces.   Particularly foul-smelling stools are common in pancreatic insufficiency.

Urine.   An ammoniacal odor in the urine may result from fermentation within the bladder.

Pus.   A nauseatingly sweet odor, like the smell of rotting apples, is evidence that pus is coming from a region of gas gangrene. A fecal odor is imparted by anaerobic bacteria. Some anaerobic bacteria in abscesses produce an odor like that of overripe Camembert cheese.

Palpation

The usual definition of palpation is the act of feeling using the sense of touch, but this is too limited. When you lay your hands on the patient, you perceive physical signs by tactile sense, temperature sense, and the kinesthetic senses of position and vibration. As with the other forms of observation, all normal persons possess these senses, but training and practice will enable you to identify findings that escape the layperson. If you doubt the influence of practice on palpation, observe a blind person reading a book printed in braille, then close your eyes and attempt to distinguish between two braille letters by touching them.

Sensitive Parts of the Hand

Tactile sense.   The tips of the fingers are most sensitive for fine tactile discrimination.

Temperature sense.   Use the dorsa of the hands or fingers; the skin is much thinner than elsewhere on the hand.

Vibratory sense.   Palpate with the palmar aspects of the metacarpophalangeal joints or the ulnar side of the hand (fifth metacarpal and fifth phalanges) rather than with the fingertips to perceive vibrations such as thrills. Prove the superiority for yourself by touching first the fingertip and then the palmar base of your finger with a vibrating tuning fork.

Sense of position and consistency. Use the grasping fingers so you perceive with sensations from your joints and muscles.

Structures Examined by Palpation

Palpation is employed on every part of the body accessible to the examining fingers: all external structures, all structures accessible through the body orifices, the bones, joints, muscles, tendon sheaths, ligaments, superficial arteries, thrombosed or thickened veins, superficial nerves, salivary ducts, spermatic cord, solid abdominal viscera, solid contents of hollow viscera, and accumulations of body fluids, pus, or blood.

Specific Qualities Elicited by Palpation

Texture. The surface characteristics of the skin and hair are noted. Are they brittle, coarse, thick, thin, roughened or smooth?

Moisture. Assess the moisture content of the skin, hair, and mucous membranes. Are they moist and supple or dry and cracked?

Skin temperature. Palpate the head, face, trunk, arms, hands, legs, and feet to assess the local skin temperature and the distribution of heat.

Characteristics of masses. When a mass or enlarged organ is discovered, record its size, shape, consistency, mobility, surface regularity and the presence or absence of expansile or transmitted pulsation.

Precordial cardiac thrust. Palpate the precordium for signs of heart action.

Crepitus. During examination of the bones, joints, tendon sheaths, pleura, and subcutaneous tissue note crepitation.

Tenderness. Elicitation of discomfort or pain on palpation of accessible tissues and over major organs should be noted. How much pressure is required to induce the uncomfortable sensation?

Thrills. Palpate the precordium for thrills. If bruits are heard in the major arteries, palpate them for thrills.

Vocal fremitus. Palpation of vocal vibrations through the chest wall provides important information about the underlying pleura and lung.

Methods of Palpation

Light palpation. Always begin palpation with a light touch. Your sense of touch is most acute when lightly applied and the patient will be put at ease. Gently sliding your fingertips over the skin surface will often detect subtle or mobile masses that are undetected by forceful palpation. You will also locate areas of particular tenderness, which should be examined last.

Deep palpation. Firm pressure is applied to displace the superficial tissues allowing palpation for deeper lesions. This is especially useful in the abdomen, but is also useful in the neck, breasts, and large muscle masses. Avoid firm palpation over nerves or other tender structures whenever possible.

Bimanual palpation. In this technique, the tissue is examined between the fingers of the two hands. It is useful for soft tissue such as the breasts, intraoral, abdominal and pelvic examinations, and examination of the muscles and joints.

Percussion

Percussion is the act of striking the surface of the body to elicit a sound. When the body surface is struck, the underlying tissues vibrate to produce percussion notes having mixed frequencies that vary with the density of the organ, the composition overlying tissue and the force of the blow [McGee SR. Percussion and physical diagnosis: Separating myth from science. *Dis Mon (United States)*. 1995;41: 641–92.

Bimanual, Mediate, or Indirect Method of Percussion

Striking the percussion blow on an inanimate object or your finger is *indirect or mediate percussion.* This is the form of percussion most commonly used. The palmar surface of the non-dominant long finger is firmly pressed onto the body surface, as a pleximeter, only the distal phalanx should touch the wall. As a plexor, the tip of the dominant long finger strikes a sharp blow on the distal interphalangeal joint of the pleximeter finger (Fig. 3–1). The examiner holds the plexor finger partly flexed and rigid and delivers the blow by bending only the wrist, so the weight of the hand lends momentum ensuring repetitive blows of equal force. The wrist must be relaxed and neither the elbow nor the shoulder should be moved. After the stroke, the plexor should rebound quickly from the pleximeter to avoid damping the vibrations. Usually, two or three staccato blows are struck in one place, and then the pleximeter is moved elsewhere for a second series of blows to compare the sounds. Most physicians employ this bimanual method for percussion of both the thorax and abdomen.

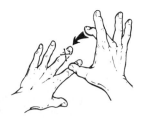

Fig. 3–1 *Method of Indirect (Bimanual) Percussion. The terminal digit of the left long finger is firmly applied to an interspace, or other body surface, as a pleximeter. The distal interphalangeal joint of that finger is struck a sharp blow with the tip of the flexed right long finger. To furnish blows of equal intensity, the fingers of the right hand are held partly flexed and the wrist is loose so that the striking hand pivots exclusively at the relaxed wrist. To avoid dampening the vibrations after striking the blow, withdraw the plexor hand rapidly from the pleximeter.*

Direct Percussion

When you elicit sound by striking the body surface directly with your fingers, hand, or reflex hammer, the procedure is called *direct or immediate percussion*. This method is not commonly used, but can be very rewarding. Since your finger is not receiving the blow, be careful to not strike the patient too firmly.

Sonorous Percussion

Sonorous percussion is used to detect alterations in the density of an organ. For example, striking an air-filled lung produces one sound; a lung filled with fluid produces quite another. The change in sounds is determined by the change in tissue densities. The different sounds are given specific names. Percussing the gastric air bubble yields a sound called *tympany*—the word is derived from the Greek for "drum"—and the sound vaguely resembles a drumbeat. The percussion note from the air-filled lung is of quite different pitch and timbre, termed *resonance*. Absent in the normal body, *hyperresonance* is emitted by the emphysematous lung; it is intermediate between resonance from the lung, filled with small air sacs and septa, and tympany from the large undivided bubble in the stomach. *Dullness* is a distinctive noise elicited by percussion over the heart when it is not covered by inflated lung. Percussion of the thigh muscles yields *flatness*.

In a nontechnical sense, the percussion sounds may be regarded as the notes of a scale, which progresses from tissues of high density to tissues of low density in the following sequence: flat, dull, resonant, hyperresonant, and tympanitic. The duration of emitted sound correlates inversely with the density producing it: flatness is a very short sound and, as the density lessens, each succeeding note in the scale is longer than its predecessor.

The pitch and timbre of the sounds must be learned by listening. Language is inadequate for description of sounds, and attempts to describe these notes are futile and confusing. Proper recognition of these distinctions must be gained by listening. Some clinicians have trained themselves to feel changes in resonance, using vibration sense, as well as to perceive them as sound.

Sonorous percussion is employed to ascertain the density of the lungs, the pleural space, the pleural layers, and the hollow viscera of the abdomen. It requires a strong blow, estimated to vibrate tissue for a radius of 6 cm in the chest, 3 cm in the thoracic wall, and 3 cm in the lung parenchyma.

Definitive Percussion

When the density of an organ is invariable and contrasts with that of the surrounding tissue, the borders of the organ can be identified as the transition site of one sound quality to the other; this is *definitive percussion*. For example, percussion of the heart is employed only to locate its boundaries with the lung; the density of neither tissue is in question. A lighter blow should be struck for definitive percussion than for sonorous percussion. Mapping of the area of greater density gives an idea of the size of the structure or the extent of its border.

Definitive percussion is commonly used to determine the location of the lung bases, the height of fluid in the pleural cavity, the width of the mediastinum, the size of the heart, the outline of dense masses in the lungs, the size and shape of the liver and spleen, the size of a distended gallbladder and urinary bladder, and the level of ascitic fluid. Caution is advised in the interpretation of definitive percussion. At best, definitive percussion provides a hypothesis to the experienced observer and at worst, it can badly mislead the inexperienced.

Auscultation

Although auscultation literally means using hearing to obtain physical signs, it has come to mean hearing through the stethoscope. There is no technical term for hearing the patient speak, cough, groan, or shriek, although all these sounds furnish diagnostic clues; this just emphasizes the importance of listening to the patient, not just the patient's words.

The uses of auscultation have expanded as the correlation of auscultatory findings to physiologic and pathophysiologic processes has been revealed by ultrasonography, echocardiography, and other diagnostic studies. As every musician knows, the ear can be trained to recognize sounds quite accurately. Each person learns to recognize the voices of many associates by patterns of pitch and overtones.

Use of the Stethoscope

The stethoscope contains a vibrating air column connecting the body wall to the ears. Because stethoscopes invariably modify sound to some extent, you should use a single instrument whenever possible. The usual stethoscope does not amplify sound; it merely assists in excluding extraneous noises. Electronic stethoscopes, which amplify and/or project the sound through a speaker, are particularly useful for teaching purposes.

Binaural instruments consist of a chest piece, plastic tubes, and two earpieces connected by a spring. Two chest pieces are needed to better detect the full range of frequencies. The bell is a hollow cone with a rim of hard rubber or plastic. The bell transmits all sounds from the chest; the low-pitched sounds come through particularly well. The low-pitched murmur of mitral stenosis and the fetal heart sounds may be audible only with the bell. A wide bell can transmit sounds of lower pitch than a narrow diameter bell. The diaphragm is a flat cup covered with a semirigid diaphragm that serves as a filter to limit low-pitched sounds, so the isolated high-pitched sounds seem louder. The diaphragm is best suited for high-pitched sounds from the heart (e.g., regurgitant aortic murmurs) and breath sounds. Cracks in the diaphragm impair its properties. The chest piece shown in Fig. 3–2 is a representative and convenient configuration of the bell and diaphragm with a valve to direct the air column from one to the other. The tubing should be thick-walled; the inside diameter should not be smaller than the

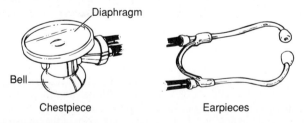

Fig. 3–2 *The Sprague Stethoscope.* *The chest piece combines the bell and diaphragm, with a valve to direct the air through either. The earpieces are connected by a spring that holds them in place.*

caliber of the connecting tubes. For optimal acoustics, the length of the rubber tubing should not exceed 30 cm, although many physicians accept a longer, more convenient length.

The stethoscope should fit the user's ears. The plastic or rubber earpiece should impinge on the external auditory meatus without discomfort or pain, yet fit tightly without air leakage. The spring, size, and design of the earpiece determine the tightness of the fit.

More art than meets the eye is required to use the stethoscope. The diaphragm should be pressed tightly against the chest wall; in contrast, the rim of the bell should touch the chest wall lightly, but seal completely. Heavy pressure with the bell stretches the underlying skin over the bell's circumference so the skin becomes a diaphragm excluding low-pitched sounds. The entire rim of the bell must touch the skin; a roaring sound from extraneous noise warns the examiner of a leak. The listener may be distracted by extraneous noises coming through the walls of the tubing before learning to ignore these completely; this subconscious editing of what is heard can lead to missing important findings if listening is not an active searching of the full spectrum of audible frequencies. The breath of the examiner on the tubing produces noise; try this, so the sound may be recognized and eliminated. Skin or hair rubbing on the chest piece produces sounds like crackles, which can be eliminated by wetting the hair or by placing a soft rubber rim on the bell. Movements of muscles, joints, or tendons sound like friction rubs; be certain that you can recognize them. If you do not hear the expected sounds with your first attempt, do not discredit your instrument or your ears; they are probably normal, but you need practice. Use the bell for narrow spaces such as the supraclavicular fossae. Thin-walled chests present difficulties in fitting the chest piece into the interspaces without leakage. Examine the instrument occasionally to ensure that it has no leaks or plugs of cerumen or other debris.

Auscultation is used to examine the heart and lungs. From the lungs, the stethoscope conveys breath sounds, whispers, and voice sounds, as well as crackles and friction rubs. The heart generates the normal heart sounds, gallops, murmurs, rhythm disturbances, and pericardial rubs and knocks. The vessels of the neck are examined for murmurs in the thyroid, carotid, and subclavian arteries and for venous hums. Auscultation of the abdomen reveals bowel sounds and murmurs from aneurysms and stenotic arteries. The skull can be auscultated for the bruit of an arteriovenous fistula. Crepitus can be heard in joints, tendon sheaths, muscles, and fractured bones, as well as in subcutaneous emphysema.

Procedure for the Screening Physical Examination

Within practical limits, there is no such thing as a routine physical examination. Like history taking, the physical examination is a structured method for eliciting observations of the patient using multiple techniques. The emphasis of each examination varies as prompted by the symptoms, physical signs, and laboratory findings of each patient; for example, the heart and circulation will be examined more carefully and thoroughly in a patient with exertional dyspnea than in a patient who has just sustained a fractured ankle.

Either unconsciously or, preferably, after careful consideration, every physician adopts a sequence of examination. The physician develops a routine or basic screening examination that is periodically performed with most patients. If significant abnormalities are encountered that focus attention on an anatomic site or some physiologic problem, a more detailed examination of that area or system should be performed. The screening examination should vary very little from patient to patient of the same gender and age. The diagnostic examination following up on problems identified in the history or abnormalities elicited on the screening examination is unique to each patient and problem. The clinician must master a structured, efficient screening examination, which, when combined with the history, is likely to identify most serious abnormalities.

For convenience, and for the patient's comfort, we examine the body by regions. In contrast, we recognize illness and disease by the physiologic systems involved. Consequently, **examine by regions, but think by systems.** This requires practice, reflection, and experience. The beginner sees all the regions and may identify many or most of the findings, but has trouble integrating those findings into a complete picture of the anatomy and physiology he has observed. This integration of findings is critical for generating unifying diagnostic hypotheses (see Problem Lists, page 5, and Hypothesis Generation, page 5ff).

A single routine that everyone should follow exactly is impractical. There are many possible sequences of examination, each with its advantages and disadvantages; none is perfect. We have based our recommendation on several observations:

1. Many physical signs are recognized and evaluated during history taking.
2. A well-organized examination room with easily accessible instruments familiar to the examiner enhances efficiency.
3. Examining each patient from head to foot in the same sequence avoids missing signs and develops an appreciation of normal variation.
4. Excessive changes of position by the examiner or patient take time and are uncomfortable for both.
5. This screening examination can be performed in 15 minutes or less.

Always keep the following points in mind:

1. Respecting your patient's modesty and retaining a professional approach encourages the patient's cooperation and diminishes the chances for misinterpretation of your intent to examine emotionally sensitive anatomy.
2. A screening examination not only discovers diagnostic signs but also reassures the patient.
3. Examining the problem area first responds to the patient's anxiety but should not distract from completing a complete examination.
4. Detailed evaluation of specific signs requires additional time.
5. In some circumstances, a full screening examination is inappropriate; a regional or special examination may be all that is indicated. This is particularly true for the patient returning for follow up after a short interval or an otherwise healthy patient with an acute limited problem.

Preparing for the Screening Examination

This example of a multisystem screening examination is designed to be performed with the patient in only four or five positions (Fig. 3–3). It should take no more than 15 minutes to complete. The following sections describe the examination sequence. The methods for each regional examination are detailed in their respective chapters.

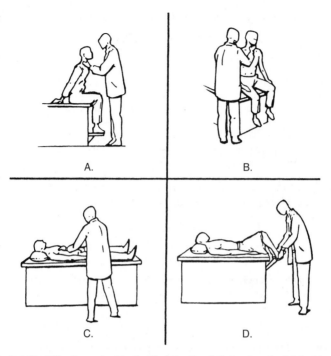

Fig. 3–3 *The Office Screening Physical Examination. **A.** Patient draped and sitting (physician facing). **B.** Patient draped and sitting (physician to right and back). **C.** Patient draped and supine (physician to right). Place the patient in the left lateral decubitus position to listen at the cardiac apex. **D.** Female pelvic examination: patient draped and supine, knees and hips flexed (physician at foot).*

Preparation: Required Equipment

A minimum list of equipment for the screening examination includes a stethoscope, sphygmomanometer, otoscope, ophthalmoscope, penlight, tongue blades, reflex hammer, tuning fork and calibrated monofilament for sensory testing, tape measure, latex or plastic gloves, lubricant for rectal and vaginal examinations, reagent for occult blood test, sterile swabs, and materials for specimen collection during the female pelvic examination. The instruments must be within easy reach. Wear gloves when examining the anus, recutum, genitalia, infected skin or when you may come in contact with body fluids.

Preparation: The Patient

The patient undresses in private, puts on an examination gown, and sits on the end of the examination table with a sheet draped over the lap and legs.

Preparation: The Clinician

The clinician of either gender should be modestly and neatly dressed; coats and ties for men and conservative attire for women are recommended. Always address patients as Mr., Mrs., Miss or Ms. and by his or her last name, unless otherwise directed by the patient. Even then, you must be comfortable with the form of address you use; excessive informality may lead to problems. Always leave the room while the patient prepares for the examination; this assures privacy and avoids potential problems. If the patient requires assistance, ask your nurse or a family member to assist. Keep the patient informed as to the plan and sequence of the examination, as you proceed, so that they can anticipate your actions. Always have a chaparone present for female genital and breast examinations; alert your staff to the need for their presence to avoid excessive delays. Preserve and protect the patient's modesty keeping genitalia and female breasts covered when not directly examining them. Always observe first without comment and control your facial and body language during the examination. Remember, the patient will be observing you as closely as you are observing them. Be sure your communications, both verbal and nonverbal, convey professionalism and inspire confidence [Gwande A. Naked. *N Engl J Med.* 2005;353:645–648].

Performance of the Screening Examination

Phase A: Vital Signs, General Inspection, Close Inspection, and Palpation of the Head, Ears, Eyes, Nose, and Throat

Patient and Examiner Positions: patient draped and sitting facing the examiner.
   To start the examination, the physician washes her hands.

Vital signs.   Obtain the vital signs or, if previously obtained by a nurse, review them and confirm any abnormal findings by rechecking them yourself.

General inspection.   Note the general appearance of the patient. Inspect the head and face, sclera and conjunctivae, external ears, scalp, skin of the head and neck, the hands and fingernails, and the skin of the arms.

Close inspection.   Examine the ears with the otoscope, check hearing, visual fields by confrontation, extraocular movements and pupillary size and reactions, examine the fundi, and inspect the oral cavity and oropharynx using the tongue blade.

Palpation.   Palpate any areas of head, face, or neck deformity, and use bimanual palpation of intraoral pathology. Palpate any areas of deformity of the hand, wrist, and elbow joints for synovitis or effusion. Palpate all skin rashes.

Phase B: Inspection of the Back of the Head, Neck, Back, and Shoulders; Palpation of the Neck, Shoulders, and Back; Percussion of the Spine and Lungs; Auscultation of the Lungs

Patient and Examiner Positions: patient draped and sitting; examiner on the patient's right side behind the patient.
   You may either stand to the patient's right side or sit on the examination table behind the patient, for part of the examination.

Inspection.   Expose the patient's back and inspect for skin lesions, scars, rashes, and the like. Observe the neck from the side and check range of neck motion.

Palpation.   Palpate the anterior neck noting the carotid pulsations, the thyroid, and the position of the trachea. Search each lymph node bed for adenopathy. Visually and by palpation, determine the position of the thoracic and lumbar vertebral spines; note any scoliosis or excessive kyphosis or lordosis. Palpate any deformities or swelling of the neck, back, shoulders, or scapulae.

Percussion. Use fist percussion to check for spinal or costovertebral angle tenderness. Percuss the chest anteriorly and posteriorly, comparing right to left and apices to bases.

Auscultation. Auscultate the chest posteriorly, laterally, and anteriorly (under the gown), comparing right to left and apices to bases.

Phase C (Female Patients Only): The Sitting Breast Examination

Patient and Examiner Positions: patient draped and sitting facing the examiner.

After proper explanation, expose the breasts while the patient sits with the arms relaxed.

Inspection. Inspect the breasts for symmetry, skin dimpling, and nipple retraction. Have the patient press her hands to her waist, and then raise her hands over her head, each time repeating the inspection.

Palpation. Pendulous breasts may be most easily examined in this position by using a bimanual technique.

Phase D: Examination of the Anterior Neck and Chest, Breasts, Axillae, Abdomen, Legs and Feet

Patient and Examiner Positions: patient draped and supine; examiner standing at the patient's right side.

Start at the neck and work toward the feet exposing one area for examination at a time: the neck, the anterior chest and each breast separately, the abdomen, the groin, and the legs. Most left-handed clinicians are able to examine a patient from the right side.

Neck. *Inspection.* Observe the neck veins for fullness and pulsations.

Chest and precordium. *Inspection.* Observe the precordium for any deformities of the sternum or ribs, and then identify the apical impulse. *Palpation.* Palpate the apical impulse and any lifts or heaves or other palpable cardiac signs. *Percussion.* Percuss the lung fields anteriorly and identify the borders of cardiac dullness. *Auscultation.* Start auscultating over the apical impulse to identify the first heart sound. Listen at the apex, the lower left and upper left sternal borders and the right second intercostal space. Auscultate the carotid arteries. Auscultate lung sounds in the anterior chest and supraclavicular fossae.

Breasts. Expose each breast separately. *Inspection.* Inspect the breasts for symmetry, skin dimpling, or nipple retraction. *Palpation.* Palpate the breasts and nipples.

Axillae. *Inspection.* Lift the arms to expose the axilla for inspection. *Palpation.* Palpate the axilla and infraclavicular lymph node beds.

Abdomen. Reposition the drape over the chest and expose the abdomen from below the breasts to the symphysis pubis. Ask the patient to flex the hips and knees to relax the abdominal musculature. *Inspection.* Observe the symmetry and shape of the abdomen. Note any scars or skin abnormalities. Have the patient tense the abdominal muscles to reveal an abdominal wall hernia (Plate 27).

Percussion. Percuss the abdomen noting any areas of tympany or tenderness with percussion. Use definitive percussion to identify the liver and look for splenomegaly. *Auscultation.* Auscultate over the epigastrium, both flanks, and both femoral triangles. *Palpation.* Perform superficial and deep palpation of the abdomen. Palpate deeply to identify the aorta and palpate both femoral pulses and the inguinal lymph nodes.

Legs and feet.   Cover the abdomen and expose the legs and feet. *Inspection.* Inspect skin, muscles, and joints, and look for edema. Flex each hip to 90 degrees and perform internal and external rotation. *Palpation.* Palpate dorsalis pedis and posterior tibial pulses. Palpate any areas of asymmetry, deformity, or joint enlargement.

Phase E: Supplementary Neurological Examination, Sitting (When Indicated)

Patient and Examiner Positions: patient draped and sitting; examiner facing the patient.

Return the patient to the sitting position. Now is a good time to do any remaining parts of the neurologic examination if they are indicated by the patient's history and examination to this point. From this position, it is easy to do precise testing of the cranial nerves, followed by testing of muscle tone and strength in the upper extremities, reflexes, and sensation (position, vibration, touch, and 10-g monofilament), followed by stance, gait, and lower extremity strength in Phase F.

Phase F: Supplemental Neurologic Examination, Standing (When Indicated)

Patient and Examiner Positions: patient standing facing examiner; supplementary neurologic and spine examinations, when indicated.

This portion of the examination is indicated, if the history or examination suggests neurologic disease or back problems.

Inspection.   Have the gowned patient stand in front of you and observe the stance. Perform the Romberg maneuver. Check the range of spinal motion. Have the patient walk away from you and then toward you first on his toes, then on his heels. Have the patient hop on the balls of both feet, and then hop on one foot at a time.

Phase G: The Urogenital Examinations

Patient and Examiner Positions: female patients in the lithotomy position, male patients standing; examiner at the foot of the table.

Female patients.   With the help of an assistant, position female patients in the lithotomy position for the female pelvic and rectal examinations (see Chapter 11, page 544 for a description of the examination).

Male patients.   Begin the examination with the patient standing facing the examiner. *Inspection.* Inspect the penis, scrotum, and inguinal areas. *Palpation.* Palpate the testes and evaluate for inguinal hernias. Next, have the patient turn and bend over the examination table, or lie on the table in the left lateral position. *Inspection.* Examine the perineum and anus and perform the rectal and prostate examinations. Test the stool for blood if indicated.

Provide tissues for the patient to clean themselves at the conclusion of the urogenital and rectal examinations.

Phase H: Concluding the Visit

Have the patient get dressed while you are out of the examination room.

When you return and the patient is comfortable, share your synopsis of the patient's history, a summary of your physical findings, your impression of the patient's problems, and your recommendations for further diagnostic tests, treatment and follow-up. Conclude, by asking if there are any questions. Be sure to set a follow-up appointment appropriate for the patient and problems.

The preceding routine is a sequence that has served us well for many years. Remember that the purpose of the screening examination is to detect significant abnormalities in any of the body regions and systems, to establish a baseline against which future findings can be compared, and to continually hone your examination skills by experiencing the range of normal findings. Truncating the examination in the interest of excessive efficiency may lead to overlooking important findings and the loss of valuable clinical experience.

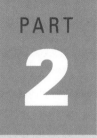

PART

2

The Diagnostic Examination

In order to observe one must learn to compare. In order to compare one must have observed. By means of observation knowledge is generated; on the other hand knowledge is needed for observation. And he observes badly who does not know how to use what he has observed. The fruit grower inspects the apple tree with a keener eye than the walker but no one can see man exactly unless he knows it is man who is the measure of man.

The art of observation applied to man is but a branch of the art of dealing with men.

— Bertolt Brecht
"Speech to Danish Working Class Actors on the Art of Observation"

Early learn to appreciate the differences between the descriptions of disease and the manifestations of that disease in an individual—the difference between the composite portrait and one of the component pictures.

— Sir William Osler

Not only to perceive the thing sharply, but to perceive the relationships between many things sharply perceived.

— Theodore Roethke
"Poetry and Craft"

This section presents the classic approach to diagnosis, evolved over 2000 years, in which the diagnostic clues to diseases and syndromes are sought as symptoms (abnormalities perceived by the patient's own senses and conveyed to the physician during the history) and physical signs (abnormalities perceived by the physician's senses and found during the physical examination).

Each chapter is organized in the following sequence:

- A brief review of the *Major Systems* to be examined, including the physiology and anatomic landmarks to keep in mind during the examination.
- The *Physical Examination* of the body region.
- The *Symptoms* commonly elicited from patients, which refer the clinician to this body region.
- The *Signs* the clinician may encounter during the examination of this region.
- The *Diseases and Syndromes* commonly encountered in this region.

The symptoms and signs are set in boldface type as paragraph heads, with or without preceding modifiers. To emphasize relative importance, certain symptoms and signs are distinguished as key symptoms, key signs, and key syndromes or diseases. These are the authors' choices for clues that are often most important in understanding the pathophysiology of the illness and in formulating diagnostic hypotheses. Most of the key symptoms commonly occur as chief complaints. The diseases and syndromes so marked are those that the generalist physician should be able to recognize.

Symptoms, signs, and syndromes marked with the icon ➤ are those of potentially extreme seriousness for the patient. The clinician needs to always be alert for these symptoms, signs, and conditions to avoid delayed diagnosis of life-threatening conditions.

Most of the physical signs are placed in order as they are encountered by the physician who conducts the head-to-foot physical examination of the patient.

When particular symptoms and signs are useful to help the clinician in differentiating between the various etiologies of a particular symptom or sign, they are discussed after the **DDX:** notation. This will help formulation of an accurate differential diagnosis.

The distinction between symptoms and signs is frequently unclear. For instance, jaundice may be a symptom that brings the patient to the physician, but it is also a sign visible to the clinician. In instances where the finding can be either a sign or a symptom, it is generally discussed where it is most likely to be found during the examination. Vomiting, although it can be witnessed, is more often a symptom, while tenderness, although it may be noted by the patient, is a sign that can be elicited by the examiner.

Diseases and syndromes in which the symptoms and signs occur are listed under *CLINICAL OCCURRENCE.*

Vital Signs, Anthropometric Data, and Pain

The vital signs, temperature, pulse, respirations, and blood pressure (BP), are discussed in the first part of this chapter. We discuss measures of body size (height, weight, and body mass index) in the second and pain assessment in the final part of the chapter. The former have direct bearing on health risk assessment, and the latter is essential in the initial evaluation and ongoing management of patients with acute or chronic illness or injury.

Vital Signs

Why are temperature, pulse, respirations, and BP called *vital* signs? These are the signs of life (L. *vitalis*, from *vita*: life); their presence confirms life and their absence confirms death. More usefully, the amount of deviation from normal is correlated, for each parameter and especially in combination, with the magnitude of threat to life. Since ancient times, practitioners have used the skin temperature, the pulse, and the respirations as prognostic signs. More recently, the BP has been found to have similar predictive strength.

These signs have played a major role in the history of medicine. In the nineteenth century, entire texts were written on the interpretation of pulse, fever, and respiratory patterns. With the advent of modern diagnostic methods, it is now apparent that most of these signs are of insufficient specificity to be of much utility in establishing a specific diagnosis. On the other hand, they are sensitive indicators of the presence of disease and are useful in generation of pathophysiologic hypotheses and differential diagnosis. They remain strongly correlated with severity of illness and outcome.

Body Temperature

Internal body temperature is tightly regulated to maintain normal cellular function of vital organs, particularly the brain. Deviation of temperature by more than 4°C above or below normal can produce life-threatening cellular dysfunction. Regulation of internal temperature is controlled by the hypothalamus, which maintains a set point for temperature. The autonomic nervous system plays a key role in maintaining body temperature by regulating blood flow conducting heat from the internal organs to the skin and innervating sweat glands. Increasing flow and dilating cutaneous capillaries radiates heat away by conductive loss while production of sweat increases evaporative heat loss. Behavioral adaptations are also important; in hot conditions, people become less active and seek shade or a cooler environment when they are able. Decreased body temperature is opposed by increased heat generation in muscles by shivering and by behavioral adaptations such as putting on clothes and seeking warmer environs. Deviations of body temperature indicate changes in the set point, increased heat production, decreased heat dissipation, failure of regulatory systems, or any combination of those.

Record the patient's temperature at each visit. Doing so, establishes an individualized baseline for future reference and detects deviations from this baseline, either fever or hypothermia. Scales on clinical thermometers are either Fahrenheit or Celsius. Conveniently remembered clinical equivalents are $35°C = 95°F$, $37°C = 98.6°F$, and $40°C = 104°F$.

Normal Temperatures

Diurnal variation of body temperature.   Daytime workers who sleep at night, register their minimum temperature at 3 to 4 AM, whence it rises slowly to a maximum between 8 and 10 PM. This pattern is reversed in nightshift workers. The transition from one pattern to the other requires several days.

Simultaneous temperatures in various regions.   Heat is produced by the chemical reactions of cellular metabolism, so a temperature gradient extends from a maximum in the liver to a minimum on the skin surface. Customarily, the body temperature is measured in the rectum, the mouth, the ear, the axilla, or the groin. Among these sites, the rectal temperature is approximately $0.3°C$ $(0.6°F)$ higher than that of the oral or groin reading, the axillary temperature is approximately $0.5°C$ $(1.0°F)$ less than the oral value.

Normal body temperature.   Internal body temperature is maintained within a narrow range, $±0.6°C$ $(1.0°F)$, in each individual. However, the population range of this set point varies from 36.0 to $37.5°C$ $(96.5–99.5°F)$ making it impossible to know an individual's normal temperature without a prior established baseline. A clinical shortcut for a patient whose normal baseline temperature is unknown is to regard as probably in the febrile range a maximum oral temperature above $37.5°C$ $(99.5°F)$ and a rectal temperature exceeding $38.0°C$ $(100.5°F)$. The minimum normal temperature is more difficult to define; the oral temperature often dips to $35.0°C$ $(95.0°F)$ during sleep.

Elevated Temperature

Increased body temperature results from excessive production of heat or interference with heat dissipation. Each of these mechanisms may be physiologic (i.e., occurring as a normal response to a physiologic challenge), or pathologic (i.e., temperature elevation as a result of damage to the normal thermoregulatory pathways). Physiologic elevation of temperature results from an elevation of the hypothalamic physiologic set point for body temperature, a fever. Pathologic elevations of body temperature, hyperthermia, result from unregulated heat generation and/or impairment of the normal mechanisms of heat exchange with the environment.

> **KEY SIGN**   **Physiologic Elevated Temperature—Fever**

Release of endogenous pyrogens, particularly interleukin (IL-1), triggered by tissue necrosis, infection, inflammation, and some tumors, elevates the hypothalamic set point leading to an increased body temperature. Onset of fever may be marked by a chill with shivering and cutaneous vasoconstriction as the body begins generating increased heat and decreasing heat loss; particularly severe chills are called *rigors*. When the new set point is reached, the skin is usually warm, moist, and flushed; but absence of these signs does not exclude fever. Occasionally, the skin temperature may be subnormal or normal while the core temperature is markedly elevated. Tachycardia usually accompanies fever, the increase in the pulse rate being proportionate to the temperature elevation. During the fever, the patient usually feels more comfortable in a warm environment. The new set point and the pattern of the fever curve depend upon the dynamics of the particular pathophysiologic process. Return of the set point to normal, either temporarily or permanently, is marked by sweat and flushing as the body dissipates the accumulated heat. Night sweats occur in many chronic infectious and inflammatory diseases, and some malignancies, particularly lymphomas. They represent an exaggeration of the normal diurnal variation in temperature, the sweat marking the decline of the temperature at night.

Some patients are unable to mount a febrile response to infection, for example, older adults patients and those with renal failure or on high doses of corticosteroids.

Fever occurring in several specific patient groups require special consideration. These include fever in immunocompromised hosts, HIV-infected patients and nosocomial fever. Discussion of these topics is beyond the scope of this text.

Patterns of Fever. The pattern of temperature fluctuations may be a useful diagnostic clue. Many patterns have been defined.

- **Continuous Fever.** A fever with a normal diurnal variation of 0.5 to 1.0°C (1.0 to 1.5°F).
- **Remittent Fever.** A fever with a diurnal variation of more than 1.1°C (2.0°F) but with no normal readings.
- **Intermittent Fever.** Episodes of fever separated by days of normal temperature. Examples include tertian fever from *Plasmodium vivax* in which paroxysms of malaria are separated by an intervening normal day; quartan fever in which paroxysms from *Plasmodium malariae* occur with two intervening normal days.
- **Relapsing Fever.** Bouts of fever occurring every 5 to 7 days from infection with spirochetes of the group Borrelia and Colorado tick fever.
- **Episodic Fever.** Fever lasts for days or longer followed by prolonged periods (at least 2 weeks) without fever and with remission of clinical illness. This pattern is typical of the familial periodic fevers [Drenth PPH, van der Meer JWM. Hereditary periodic fever. *N Engl J Med.* 2001;345:1748–1757].
- **Pel-Epstein Fever.** Occurring in Hodgkin disease, bouts of several days of continuous or remittent fever followed by afebrile remissions lasting an irregular number of days.

✔ **FEVER—CLINICAL OCCURRENCE:** *Congenital* familial Mediterranean fever, other familial periodic fevers, porphyrias; *Endocrine* hyperthyroidism, pheochromocytoma; *Infectious* bacterial, viral, rickettsial, fungal, and parasitic infections either localized or systemic (occult abscess is common); *Inflammatory* systemic lupus erythematosus (SLE), acute rheumatic fever, Still disease, vasculitis, serum sickness, any severe local or systemic inflammatory process (e.g., sarcoidosis, bullous dermatosis); *Mechanical/Traumatic* tissue necrosis (e.g., myocardial infarction, pulmonary infarction, stroke), exercise; *Metabolic/Toxic* drug reactions, gout; *Neoplastic* leukemia, lymphomas and solid tumors; *Neurologic* seizures; *Psychosocial* factitious; *Vascular* thrombophlebitis, tissue ischemia and infarction, vasculitis, subarachnoid hemorrhage.

> **KEY SYNDROME** Fever of Unknown Origin (FUO)

To qualify as an FUO, three conditions must be met: (1) the illness must be at least 3 weeks in duration, (2) the temperature must be repeatedly more than 38.3°C (100.9°F), and (3) no diagnosis should have been reached after at least three outpatient visits or at least 3 days in the hospital. The most common identified causes of FUO in immunocompetent patients in the modern era are noninfectious inflammatory diseases, infections, and malignancies, especially hematologic malignancies. Fever remains unexplained in almost 50% of patients, especially those with episodic fevers [Mourad O, Palda V, Detsky AS. A comprehensive evidence-based approach to fever of unknown origin. *Arch Intern Med.* 2003:163:545–551; Vanderschueren S, Knockaert D, Adriaenssens T, et al. From prolonged febrile illness to fever of unknown origin: The challenge continues. *Arch Intern Med* 2003;163:1033–1041; Jha AK, Collard HR, Tierney LM. Diagnosis still in question. *N Engl J Med.* 2002;346:1813–1816]. **CLINICAL OCCURRENCE:** *Noninfectious Inflammatory Diseases* Still disease, SLE, sarcoidosis, Crohn disease, polymyalgia rheumatica, vasculitis (giant cell arteritis, Wegener disease, polyarteritis nodosa); *Infections:* endocarditis, tuberculosis, urinary tract infection, cytomegalovirus, Epstein-Barr virus, HIV, subphrenic abcess, cholangitis and cholecystitis; *Neoplasms:* non-Hodgkin lymphoma, Hodgkin disease, leukemia, adenocarcinoma; *Miscellaneous:* habitual hyperthermia, subacute thyroiditis, Addison disease, drug fever.

> **KEY DISEASE** Rheumatic Fever

See page 669.

Pathologic Overproduction and Impaired Dissipation of Heat

➤ **KEY SIGN** Hyperthermia

Unregulated overproduction of heat or damage to the systems responsible for dissipation of heat leads to rapid and severe elevations of temperature without hypothalamic control or compensation. It is unusual for this to result from severe fever from the causes noted above, without primary failure of the normal control mechanisms. More commonly, environmental factors, behavioral events (bad judgment, impaired intellect), or toxin exposure results in loss of normal temperature control. **CLINICAL OCCURRENCE:** *Impaired Heat Loss:* high environmental temperature and humidity (often combined with exercise), moderately hot weather for a person with congenital absence of sweat glands, congestive heart failure, heat stroke from failure of the heat-dissipating apparatus, anticholinergic drugs and toxins. Poverty, homelessness and psychosis all inhibit the ability to adapt to environmental challenges. *Increased Heat Generation:* malignant hyperthermia, neuroleptic malignant syndrome, heavy exertion in hot and humid environment.

KEY SYNDROME   Neuroleptic Malignant Syndrome

Antagonism to the central actions of dopamine is thought to play a role. One to two days after exposure to a neuroleptic (antipsychotic) drug, the patient develops hyperthermia, rigidity, altered mental status, labile BP, tachycardia, tachypnea, and progressive metabolic acidosis. Myoglobinuria and acute renal failure can occur. It can be confused with worsening of the psychotic state leading to delayed diagnosis and administration of more neuroleptics.

KEY DISEASE   Malignant Hyperthermia

This results from an inherited disorder of muscle sarcoplasmic reticulum calcium release. Exposure to inhalational anesthetics or succinylcholine precipitates sustained muscle contraction. The patient develops rigidity, hyperthermia, rhabdomyolysis, metabolic acidosis, and hemodynamic instability. Prompt recognition and treatment is lifesaving.

KEY SYNDROME   Heat Exhaustion (Heat Prostration)

Exertion in a hot, usually humid environment leads to loss of fluid and electrolytes and decreased ability to dissipate body heat. This is classically seen in younger individuals participating in athletic events or working in hot, humid environments. Symptoms are palpitations, faintness, lassitude, headache, nausea, vomiting, and cramps. Patients have tachycardia, diminished BP, diaphoresis, ashen, cool, moist skin and dilated pupils. The core body temperature is elevated, but <40°C (104°F). Untreated it can lead to heat stroke.

KEY SYNDROME   Heat Stroke

There is failure of the thermoregulatory system producing decreased sweating and rapid increases in core body temperature. Cardiovascular disease increases the risk for heat stroke by limiting the increase in cardiac output necessary to perfuse the skin. Diuretics and anticholinergic drugs also increase the risk. The typical victim is a chronically ill patient confined in a hot, humid environment during heat waves. The patient is often delirious or comatose; the diagnostic clue is the hot dry skin [Bouchama A, Knochel JP. Heat stroke. *N Engl J Med.* 2002;346:1978–1988].

Factitious fever.   This is usually encountered in hospitalized patients attempting to malinger, although the motives are often obscure. The situation is suspected when a series of high temperatures are recorded forming an unusual pattern of fluctuation or when a recorded high temperature is unaccompanied by other signs of fever.

Some Infections Presenting as Fever

KEY DISEASE   Tuberculosis

Infection with *Mycobacterium tuberculosis* may be limited to the lung or spread via the lymph nodes or bloodstream to affect any organ.   ***Primary infection***   is in the lung and often goes unrecognized, leaving a calcified nodule in the middle or lower lung and hilar lymph nodes (Ghon complex).   ***Progressive primary*** *tuberculosis*   This is seen more commonly in HIV-infected patients and presents as progressive pulmonary infection (usually in the lower lung zones) pleural effusion, and lymphadenopathy. In immunosuppressed hosts or dark-skinned races, there is an increased risk for early hematogenous dissemination to multiple organs.   **Miliary tuberculosis**   These patients present with fever, anorexia, and weight loss, and may have hepatomegaly, splenomegaly, or lymphadenopathy.   **Reactivation tuberculosis**   Reactivation may be miliary or localized to one organ system, most commonly the apices of the lungs. Patients present with fever, malaise, night sweats, cough with sputum production, and findings of consolidation and/or cavity formation on pulmonary examination. Reactivation is not infrequently seen in the bones, especially the spine (Pott disease), the peritoneum, meninges, kidneys and urinary tract, lymph nodes, intestine, and pericardium [Tanoue LT, Mark EJ. Case records of the Massachusetts General Hospital. Case 1-2003. *N Engl J Med.* 2003;348:151–161].

> **KEY SYNDROME**   Endemic North American Fever Syndromes

Several infectious diseases are found exclusively or with significantly increased frequency in specific regions of the United States. Knowledge of these syndromes combined with a travel history from a patient presenting with an undifferentiated febrile illness will greatly assit in the timely recognition and treatment of these disorders. They all have many features in common in the first days of illness. *Clinical Occurrence:*   Rocky Mountain spotted fever (RMSF), other rickettsial infections, bebesiosis, ehrlichiosis and anaplasmosis, Lyme disease, Q fever, leptospirosis, relapsing fever, Colorado tick fever and other viral exanthems can present similarly.

> **KEY DISEASE**   Rocky Mountain Spotted Fever (RMSF)

Rickettsia rickettsii are transmitted by the bite of an infected tick (wood ticks *Dermacentor andersoni* or the wood tick *D. variabilis*). The obligate intracellular parasites infect endothelial cells producing acute systemic illness. The onset is nonspecific with headache, fever, chills, myalgias, and asthenia frequently accompanied by nausea, vomiting and abdominal pain. An erythematous macular rash spreading centrally from the wrists and ankles may be seen after the third day of illness; the palms and soles may be affected and dorsal edema of the hands and feet is characteristic. The lesions are initially blanching but progress to papules which become nonblanching purpura. Systemic involvement leads to widespread organ damage and death in 25% of untreated patients. The disease is highly endemic to the Atlantic coastal states where it may be acquired by vacationers. It can be acquired in any state and many foreign countries. **DDX:** The other rickettsial disease present in a similar fashion with severe headache, fever, myalgias, and malaise. Louse borne typhus (epidemic typhus, trench fever), endemic typhus (murine typhus), and ricketsial pox are all endemic in the United States as well as imported. The latter is seen in the Northeastern US and has a papular erythematous rash at the mite bite site that becomes a necrotic eschar with regional lymphadenopathy. Nausea and vomiting are highly characteristic of murine typhus. Confusion with babesiosis, Lyme disease and Ehrlichiosis/anaplasmosis can be reduced by careful history and examination [Cunha BA. Rocky Mountain spotted fever revisited. *Arch Intern Med.* 2004;164:221].

Babesiosis. Babesia are intracellular protozoa transmitted by infected Ixodes ticks. They parasitize red blood cells where they can be identified on blood smears. Babesiosis is a worldwide zoonotic infection in which humans are infected incidentally. It is highly endemic in the Atlantic coastal regions of New York, Connecticut, Rhode Island and Massachucetts. It has been reported from many other locals, however, and imported cases are seen. Symptoms are gradual onset of fever, headache, myalgias and fatigue. There may be hepatosplenomegaly and hemolysis. A rash does not occur. Coincident infection with other tick borne diseases (Lyme, ehrlichiosis) has been reported not infrequently.

► **Ehrlichiosis and anaplasmosis.** Ehrlichia and anaplasmas are intracellular parasites that reproduce in either mononuclear phagocytic cells in the blood and tissues (*Ehrlichia chaffeensis*) or granulocytes (*Ehrlichia ewiigi* and *Anaplasma phagocytophilia*) forming vacuolar inclusions (morula) visible on light microscopy. Human monocytotropic ehrlichiosis and erhlichiosis erwingii are transmitted by the Lone Star tick (*Amblyomma americanum*) and are most prevalent in the south-central, southeastern and mid-Atlantic states. Onset of both diseases is nonspecific with fever, headache, malaise, myalgias often accompanied by nausea, vomiting and diarrhea. Rash, cough, and confusion may be seen. *A. phagocytophilia* is transmitted by bites of the Ixodes ticks with high concentrations in the northeastern and upper midwestern states. A high index of suspicion is required to make these diagnoses promptly.

> **KEY DISEASE** Lyme Disease

Infection with *Borrelia burgdorferi* is transmitted by bites of Ixodes ticks. Initially infection is in the skin with a characteristic rash, but it disseminates within days to involve virtually all organs and tissues. The characteristic rash of erythema migrans (see page 162) may be missed or ignored so the patient presents with symptoms of systemic disease with fever, headache, myalgias, neck stiffness, arthralgias and striking fatigue and malaise. These symptoms may persist for several weeks, gradually resolving or being replaced with neurologic symptoms and signs (peripheral neuropathy, mononeuritis multiplex, cranial neuropathy, aseptic meningitis, or chorea); Bell's palsy is quite common at this stage. Cardiac conduction block with symptomatic bradycardia may be seen. The predominate late manifestation is an inflammatory oligoarthritis of the large joints, especially the knee.

Leptospirosis. Leptospirosis is a world wide zoonosis transmitted by ingestion of contaminated water or contact with urine or tissues of infected animals. The onset is abrupt with fever, headache, myalgias and malaise often accompanied by conjunctival suffusion. There may be muscle tenderness, lymphadenopathy, hepatosplenomegaly or rashes. History of contact with contaminated water in the summer or fall is a key to making the diagnosis. Men are more often exposed than women. If not recognized and treated initially, symptoms may subside or disappear for a week only to recur. Severe disease causes multiorgan failure, that is, Weil's syndrome with jaundice, renal insufficiency, and hemorrhage.

Relapsing fever: *Borrellia* spp. infect humans after louse or tick bites. The organisms can change their antigenic coating of variable major proteins causing escape from an initially effective immune response leading to relapsing illness. Tick borne relapsing fever is a zoonotic infection with *Borrelia* spp. transmitted by infected argasid ticks feeding on humans. The patient presents with fever, myalgias, chills, nausea, vomiting, and arthralgias. Abdominal pain, cough, photophobia, neck stiffness and rash are less common. Delirium can accompany the high fever and sleep may be difficult. The illness reaches a crisis within 3 to 5 days when the fever peaks with chills followed by lysis of fever, diaphoresis and hypotension. Relapse occurs with the next antigenic variant after 7 to 9 days. Each crisis is equivalent to a Jarisch-Herxheimer reaction. **DDX:** Louse borne relapsing fever is transmitted by the human body louse. The symptoms are similar. It is endemic to portions of Ethiopia, but has caused major epidemics in wartime Europe.

Q fever: This is a zoonotic infection with *Coxiella burnetii* transmitted by infected cattle, goats, and sheep, especially via products of conception during delivery, and infected milk. Both inhalation of organisms and ingestion produce infection. The illness has protean manifestations. Common symptoms are fever, severe fatigue and headache, cough, nausea, vomiting, diarrhea, and rash may be present. Several symptom complexes can develop including an influenza-like illness, pneumonia, hepatitis, meningoencephalitis or culture negative endocarditis. Chronic disease with hepatosplenomegaly implies persistent endocardial infection. Diagnosis is difficult.

Colorado tick fever: Colorado tick fever virus is transmitted by infected wood ticks (*D. andersoni*) in the northern Rocky Mountain states from late spring to fall. It causes a biphasic illness manifest as fever, myalgia, headache and occaisionally menigoencephalitis and rash. It is self-limited.

> **KEY SYNDROME** Fever in Returning Travelers

This is a common problem in our era of global travel. The patient presents with fever and a history of travel to exotic, usually tropical locations. There is the possibility of a host of unfamiliar infectious diseases as well as more common illnesses. A clinically useful approach is presented in the references [Ryan ET, Wilson ME, Kain KC. Illness after international travel. *N Engl J Med.* 2002;347:505–516; Spira AM. Assessment of travellers who return home ill. *Lancet.* 2003;361:1459–1469].

> **KEY DISEASE** Dengue

Infection with one of the four dengue viruses transmitted by mosquitos well adapted to urban environments in tropical and subtropical environments worldwide. This is the most common febrile illness in travelers returning from the Caribbean. Patients present with fever, headache, back pain and severe myalgias (break bone fever). Dengue hemorrhagic fever is potentially fatal.

> **KEY DISEASE** Malaria

Infection is with *P. vivax, Plasmodium ovale, P. malariae,* or *Plasmodium falciparum* transmitted by infected anopheline mosquitos. Infection of the liver is followed by invasion of erythrocytes. Cyclical release of mature merozoites from ruptured erythrocytes produces cyclical fever. *Plasmodium fulciparum* infection can produce severe hemolysis, hypoglycemia, and obstruction of cerebral capillaries (cerebral malaria). *P. vivax* and *P. ovale* can persist in the liver causing replapsing infections. Patients present with fever, headache, malaise, and myalgias. Nausea, vomiting, and abdominal pain may be present. Symptoms may progress to delirium and coma. Establishing a history of travel to an endemic area and prompt examination of blood smears by trained laboratory technicians are the keys to recognition. **DDX:** Dengue fever may present a similar clinical picture but blood smears are negative.

> **KEY DISEASE** **Typhoid Fever**

Disseminated infection with *Salmonella typhi* or *Salmonella paratyphi* follows ingestion of contaminated food or water. The incubation period is 3 days to as much as 60 days. Onset begins with chills and prolonged, persistent fever, prostration, cough, epistaxis, and constipation or diarrhea. There is slowly progressing lassitude, abdominal distention and tenderness, splenomegaly, and rose spots on the trunk and chest. Delirium may occur. Complications include localized infections (gallbladder, bone, liver, spleen, endocarditis, pneumonia, meningitis, and orchitis), gastrointestinal bleeding and perforation of the bowel with peritonitis.

Brucellosis: Systemic infection with aerobic gram-negative bacilli acquired from animals, a zoonosis. *Brucella abortus* (cattle), *suis* (pigs), *melitensis* (goats), or *canis* (dogs) are the causes. Exposure to nonpasteurized milk, contaminated meat or other animal tissues results in infection. Lassitude and weight loss accompany recurrent (undulant) fever and sweating. Pain in the back and joints is common. Physical findings include splenomegaly, lymphadenopathy, and tender bones or joints. The disease may be acute or chronic [Vogt T, Hasler P. A woman with panic attacks and double vision who liked cheese. *Lancet*. 1999;354:300].

Rickettsiosis: In addition to importing rickettsial diseases known in the United States (RMSF, typhus, rickesialpox), several ricketsioses endemic to other countries and regions may be imported. Fever, headache, myalgias and rash are characteristic of the spotted fever syndromes (e.g., Boutonneuse fever). An inoculation eschar with regional lymphadenopathy idicates an ulceroglandular syndrome (see Chapter 6, page 162). Scrub typhus is imported from Australia, the southern Pacific region and southern and southeast Asia. In addition to fever, headache, myalgias and malaise, cough is a prominent symptom. An inoculation eschar from the mite bite and regional lymphadenopathy may be seen.

Lowered Body Temperature

> **KEY SYNDROME** **Hypothermia**

A decreased hypothalamic set point, insufficiency of the heat-generation systems, excessive heat loss, behaviors, and environmental conditions all can lead to sustained declines in core temperature. Core temperatures are usually lower in older adults who are particularly susceptible to decreased environmental temperatures. Low body temperature impairs cellular metabolism and brain function, particularly judgment, and the combination can prevent protection from continued exposure leading to fatal hypothermia. Hypothermia also protects the tissues from ischemic injury, an observation used in prolonged surgical procedures and resuscitation from cardiac arrest, so complete recovery is possible from rapid and sustained cooling even when the patient appears clinically dead. This is especially true for cold-water immersion (drowning) where the body is cooled very rapidly. Relative or absolute hypothermia in situations where fever would be expected (e.g., severe infection) is a poor prognostic sign.

✔ *HYPOTHERMIA—CLINICAL OCCURRENCE:* **Endocrine** hypothyroidism; **Idiopathic** advanced age; **Infectious** sepsis; **Mechanical/Traumatic** exposure
and immersion, hypothalamic injury from trauma or hemorrhage, burns;
Metabolic/Toxic antipyretics, hypoglycemia, drug overdoses; **Neoplastic**
brain tumors; **Neurologic** stroke; **Psychosocial** poverty, homelessness, and
psychosis all inhibit the ability to adapt to environmental challenges; **Vascular**
stroke.

The Pulse: Rate, Volume, and Rhythm

The arterial pulse is generated by left ventricular systolic contraction ejecting
blood into the aorta. The pulse wave travels along the arteries at a rate dependent
upon the force of ejection and the elastic properties of the arterial wall. The
regularity of the pulse wave is determined by the rhythm of cardiac electrical
depolarization and muscular contraction.

The sinoatrial (SA) node lies in the right atrial wall near the entrance of the
superior vena cava (Fig. 4–1). As the normal pacemaker of the heart, it originates
regular waves of excitation that spread quickly through the wall of both atria
until they reach the atrioventricular (AV) node near the posterior margin of the
interatrial septum. Here, there is a slight delay while atrial systole is completed.
The excitation then passes down the bundle of His, dividing into right and left
branches which pass down the corresponding sides of the interventricular septum,
to excite the muscle of the right and left ventricles more or less simultaneously.
Abnormalities of atrial or ventricular excitation or AV conduction cause changes
in rate and rhythm that can be analyzed with considerable accuracy by the surface
electrocardiogram (ECG).

Examination of the Pulse

Palpation of the arterial pulse.   The pulse may be palpated in any of the accessible
arteries (Fig. 4–2). The physician at the bedside usually examines the brachial
or radial pulse. The radial artery is pressed lightly against the radius with the
examining finger. The examiner ascertains the pulse rate, and rhythm; the contour
of the pulse wave and its volume, are discussed under heart action (Chapter 8,
page 382).

Normal pulse rate and rhythm: sinus rhythm.   This is the beat of the normal
heart with a rate between 55 and 100 beats per minute (bpm). Infants and children have higher normal heart rates; consult pediatric references for the normal
ranges. Well-conditioned athletes may have resting pulses into the low forties,
while deconditioned adults may have rates approaching 100. With heart rates
<100 bpm, diastole is longer than systole; the two intervals become equal at ap-
proximately 100 bpm; above 100 bpm, systole is longer. Heart rates lower than 55
bpm are called *bradycardias* and those above 100 bpm, *tachycardias*. Exertion may
cause acceleration to almost 200 bpm in young, healthy adults; the maximum
achievable heart rate declines predictably with age. The pulse rhythm is normally
regular with slight variation caused by respirations. Vagus stimulation by breath
holding, Valsalva or carotid sinus massage slows the rate.

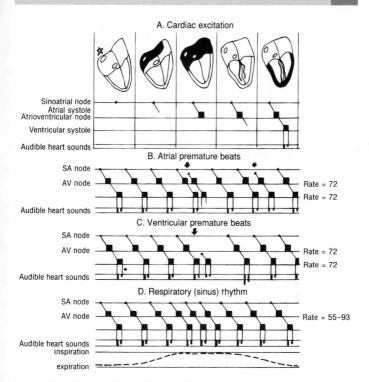

A. Cardiac excitation

Sinoatrial node
Atrial systole
Atrioventricular node
Ventricular systole
Audible heart sounds

B. Atrial premature beats

SA node
AV node
Rate = 72
Rate = 72
Audible heart sounds

C. Ventricular premature beats

SA node
AV node
Rate = 72
Rate = 72
Audible heart sounds

D. Respiratory (sinus) rhythm

SA node
AV node
Rate = 55–93
Audible heart sounds
inspiration
expiration

Fig. 4–1 *Disturbances of Cardiac Rate and Rhythm I. A. Diagram illustrating the spread of excitation over the heart.* *The stimulus starts in the SA node and spreads throughout the walls of the atria, finally reaching the AV node, where there is a short delay. The stimulus then proceeds down the His bundle by its two branches along the right and left wall of the interventricular septum to the apex, spreading from there to the muscle of the right and left ventricles. The atria contract before the impulse has left the AV node; ventricular systole occurs when the impulse has spread over the walls of the lower chambers. Note that the heart sounds that result from ventricular systole are the only perceptible physical signs of this process.* **B. Atrial premature beat is represented as originating outside the SA node, an ectopic beat.** *This is followed by a short compensatory pause that cannot ordinarily be detected.* **C. An ectopic ventricular beat with a detectable compensatory pause. D. Respiratory or sinus arrhythmia.** *There is acceleration of the heart rate near the height of inspiration; this acceleration originates in the SA node. In any dysrhythmia, the heart sounds of a beat following a shortened interval are often fainter than normal; beats following an abnormally long pause are louder than normal.* **E. Ventricular rates.**

Variations in Ventricular Rate and Rhythm

The emphasis is on ventricular phenomena since the signs of heart action are practically all ventricular (see Fig. 4–1E). The atria usually function silently, contributing no important diagnostic signs except for the atrial components of the neck vein pulsations, generation of the fourth heart sound, the variations

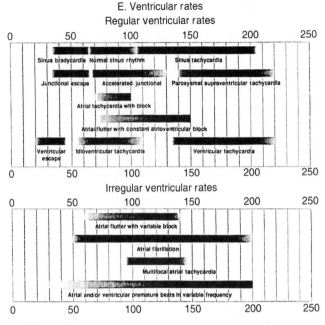

Fig. 4–1 *(Continued)*

in loudness of the first heart sound that accompany AV dissociation, and the ventricular filling sounds associated with atrial contraction sometimes heard in AV block (see Chapter 8, page 363ff).

While a rhythm abnormality may be suspected on physical examination, *none can be diagnosed with the certainty required in good clinical practice without an ECG.* Nevertheless, general groupings of disorders is possible by noting the overall heart rate (slow, normal, fast) and whether it is regular, irregular in a rather chaotic manner, or irregular but in a reproducible manner [Mangrum JM, DiMarco JP. The evaluation and management of bradycardia. *N Engl J Med.* 2000;342:705–709].

Slow regular rhythms.   Rates below approximately 55 bpm, suggest sinus bradycardia, second-degree AV block (Fig. 4–3A), and third-degree AV block with junctional or ventricular escape rhythms (Fig. 4–3B).

Regular rhythms with rates greater than 120 bpm.   Rhythms include sinus tachycardia, atrial flutter with 2:1 AV block, paroxysmal supraventricular tachycardia (Fig. 4–3C), and ventricular tachycardia. Especially with rates of more than 140, sinus tachycardia must be distinguished from atrial flutter with 2:1 block, paroxysmal supraventricular tachycardia and ventricular tachycardia. **DDX:** The response to vagus stimulation may give an indication of which rhythm is present. In flutter, the rate slows stepwise. Paroxysmal atrial tachycardia does not slow, but may convert to normal rhythm and rate. Sinus rhythm may gradually slow and ventricular tachycardia does not change.

Regular rhythms with rates of 60 to 120 bpm.   These include sinus rhythm, accelerated junctional rhythm (also known as nonparoxysmal junctional tachycardia),

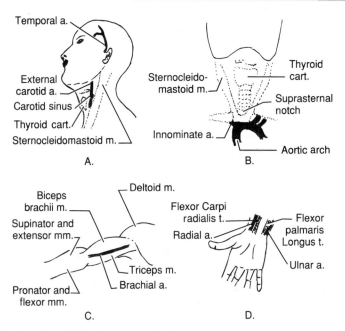

Fig. 4–2 *Sites of Palpable Arteries. A. The temporal* artery is anterior to the ear and overlies the temporal bone, one of the few normally tortuous arteries. The common carotid is deep in the neck near the anterior border of the sternocleidomastoid muscle. The bifurcation of this artery is opposite the superior border of the thyroid cartilage. The carotid sinus is at the bifurcation. ***B. Elongation or dilation of the ascending aorta and*** arch makes this vessel accessible to palpation in the suprasternal notch. With slight shifting to the right or left, the innominate or left carotid arteries may also be felt in the notch. ***C. The brachial artery*** lies deep in the biceps-triceps furrow on the medial side of the arm near the elbow. It courses toward the midline of the antecubital fossa, where it is usually just medial to the biceps tendon. ***D. The radial*** artery is just medial to the outer border of the radius and lateral to the tendon of the flexor carpi radialis, where the finger can press it against the bone. The ulnar artery is in a similar position to the ulna, but it is buried deeper, so it often cannot be felt. ***E. The abdominal aorta and parts of the iliac arteries*** can usually be felt as generalized pulsations through the abdominal wall. The femoral artery is palpable at the inguinal ligament midway between the anterior superior iliac spine and the pubic tubercle. F. The posterior tibial artery is palpable as it curves forward below and around the medial malleolus of the tibia. ***The dorsalis pedis artery*** is felt usually in the groove between the first two tendons on the medial side of the dorsum of the foot.

atrial tachycardia with block, idioventricular tachycardia (also known as accelerated ventricular rhythm and slow or benign ventricular tachycardia), and atrial flutter (Fig. 4–3D) with 3:1 or 4:1 AV block.

Rhythms that are irregular in no repetitive manner. Atrial flutter with variable AV block, atrial fibrillation, multifocal atrial tachycardia, and frequent atrial or

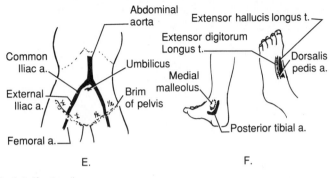

Fig. 4–2 *(Continued)*

ventricular premature beats that occur with no consistent pattern all need to be considered. The overall rates of such rhythms may vary from as slow as 50 up to 200 bpm. However, atrial flutter with variable AV block rarely exceeds 150 bpm and the range for multifocal atrial tachycardia is usually between 100 and 150 bpm.

Irregular rhythms with "reproducible irregularity". This pattern suggests either atrial or ventricular premature beats occurring at regular intervals (i.e., bigeminal, trigeminal, and quadrigeminal premature beats) or Mobitz I (Wenckebach) AV block producing grouped beats. It is necessary to obtain an ECG to reach a definitive diagnosis.

Common Dysrhythmias

Respiratory (sinus) arrhythmia. The depolarizations originate in the SA node and are conducted normally through the heart. The ventricular rate accelerates as inspiration approaches its maximum and decelerates during expiration (see Fig. 4–1D). When the overall ventricular rate is slow, the association may not be as evident as expected. This is normal and more easily demonstrable in children. **DDX:** The relation to respirations is diagnostic.

Sinus tachycardia. Exertion and increased sympathetic tone increase the rate of SA node depolarizations transmitted normally through the conducting system. The rate is between 100 and 160 bpm with a regular rhythm. Vagus stimulation produces smooth deceleration. This is normal and expected with exercise, anxiety, hyperthyroidism, anemia, fever, pregnancy, β-adrenergic medications and deconditioning from any cause. Its absence in these situations, requires explanation. **DDX:** Especially with rates higher than 140, sinus tachycardia must be distinguished from atrial flutter with 2:1 block. In flutter, vagus stimulation slows the rate in jerky fashion; paroxysmal atrial tachycardia does not slow, but may convert to normal rhythm and rate.

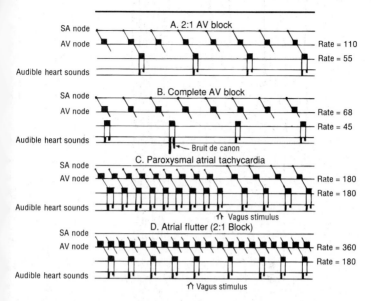

Fig. 4–3 *Disturbances of Cardiac Rate and Rhythm II.* *In all diagrams, the audible heart sounds are the only physical signs to indicate the presence and operation of the mechanisms.* ***A. Second-degree AV block*** *is depicted with a 2:1 ratio. Alternate stimuli from the atria are blocked in the AV node, so the ventricles beat only half as fast as the atria. The only physical sign is a slow regular heartbeat with first sounds of equal intensity.* ***B. Complete AV*** *block is depicted, in which the ventricles beat independently of the atria and usually assume a slow rate, below 50/min, that accelerates little with exertion. A louder-than-common first sound occurs when ventricular filling is augmented by an atrial contraction occurring by chance at the optimal time, this is called by the French—the "bruit de canon."* ***C*** *and* ***D.*** *When ventricular beats are regular with rates between 160 and 220/min, two conditions must be distinguished.* ***C. Paroxysmal atrial tachycardia.*** ***D. Atrial flutter.*** *Vagal stimulation may convert paroxysmal atrial tachycardia to normal rhythm, but there is no temporary slowing. In contrast, the only response of flutter to vagus stimulus is slowing for a few beats.*

> **KEY SIGN   Orthostatic Tachycardia**

See page 77, Orthostatic Hypotension. A pulse rise of more than 15 bpm on sitting or standing from the supine position suggests intravascular volume depletion.

Postural orthostatic tachycardia syndrome (POTS).   The cause is unknown. It usually affects women between 15 and 50 years of age, following a minor illness. Standing from a sitting or lying position is associated with an increase in the heart rate to >120 bpm or >30 bpm above the baseline rate. Tachycardia is often associated with symptoms and signs of autonomic hyperactivity (tremor, palpitations, nausea) or presyncope (light headedness, weakness, visual change).

Sinus bradycardia. The conduction is normal but the rate is slow due to vagal influence on the node or disease of the SA pacemaker cells. This is the natural rate for well conditioned athletes. Rates usually range from 40 to 55 bpm, rarely <40 bpm. The rhythm is regular. Severe hypothyroidism and sick sinus syndrome are other causes. **DDX:** The rate accelerates smoothly with exertion.

KEY SYNDROME Sinus Rhythm with Second-Degree Block

In Mobitz I (Wenckebach) AV block, there is decremental conduction in the AV node so that, after a series of conducted beats, one beat is dropped. This produces grouped beats with a P to QRS ratio of n:n-1 (e.g., 3:2, 5:4). In Mobitz II block, sinus impulses from the atria are regularly blocked in the His bundle or below and complete heart block may occur. The atrial rate is multiple of the ventricular rate, 2:1, 3:1, 4:1, or higher. For instance 3:1 block occurs when every third beat from the atrium is transmitted through the AV node. Mobitz I block is the most common type of AV block. The ventricular complexes appear in groups followed by a pause. The interval between beats shortens until a beat is dropped with a longer pause and the cycle recurs. The shortening of the R-R interval is usually only apparent on the ECG. In Mobitz II block, ventricular systoles occur at regular intervals with rates dependent upon the sinus rate and degree of block (see Fig. 4–3A). Each beat has the same intensity. The only distinctive physical sign may be faintly audible atrial contractions in the cycles not resulting in ventricular beats. In 2:1 block, two A-waves may be seen in the jugular vein for each ventricular contraction. Although 2:1 block is relatively common, 3:1 block is much less so. **DDX:** In both sinus bradycardia and second-degree heart block, the rate is accelerated with exertion, but complete heart block exhibits little response. **CLINICAL OCCURRENCE:** Acute infections (especially rheumatic fever, Lyme disease, and diphtheria), valvular heart disease, digitalis intoxication, hyperkalemia, drugs (diltiazem, verapamil, β-blockers), coronary artery disease.

► KEY SYNDROME Third-Degree (Complete) AV Block

The atria beat regularly driven by the SA node, but there is no conduction from the atria to the ventricles. Block may occur in the AV node or ventricular conduction system (His bundle or both bundle branches). Escape pacemakers in junctional tissue near the AV node or the ventricular conduction system establish an escape rhythm with rates of 25 to 60 bpm; the higher the pacemaker, the faster the escape rate. The ventricular contractions are regular; the intensity of the heart sounds is increased when an atrial systole happens to precede ventricular contraction (see Fig. 4–3B). When ventricular contraction and atrial contraction nearly coincide, there is a booming sound, *bruit de canon;* it may come infrequently, so auscultation should be prolonged for 60 seconds or more. More frequently, there are less spectacular variations in intensity of the first sounds. The causes are the same as second-degree AV block with the addition of degenerative and granulomatous diseases such as sarcoidosis. **DDX:** This is the only bradycardia in which exertion does not accelerate the ventricular rate. The variation in intensity of the first sounds is distinctive.

KEY SYNDROME   Premature Beats

A depolarization arises from an ectopic focus in the atrium or ventricle; if it arises from the atrium, it is transmitted to the ventricles, producing the premature contraction. Isolated or infrequent premature beats are usually recognized by palpation or auscultation. An atrial premature beat occurs among a series of normal beats but before its expected time (see Fig. 4–1B). The following compensatory pause is shorter than expected with ventricular premature beats, but differentiation is difficult, if not impossible, at the bedside. If the premature beat occurs shortly after a normal ventricular systole, there will be little ventricular filling, the heart sounds are less intense and the stroke volume may be insufficient to produce a palpable arterial pulse. When premature beats are very frequent, they present a diagnostic problem (Fig. 4–4A) [Wang K, Hodges M. The premature ventricular complex as a diagnostic aid. *Ann Intern Med.* 1992;117:766–770].

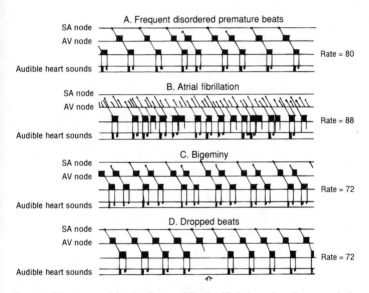

Fig. 4–4 *Disturbance of Cardiac Rate and Rhythm III.* *As in previous diagrams, only the audible heart sounds are the physical signs of these disorders.* **A.** *Normal rhythm is interspersed with two random premature beats: If such beats are very frequent, the ear may not be able to distinguish them from atrial fibrillation unless some maneuvers are employed. The rhythm becomes regular as the rate accelerates to approximately 120 beats per minute.* **B. Atrial fibrillation:** *The ventricular rhythm is grossly irregular and continues to be irregular when the rate is accelerated by exercise to more than 120/min.* **C. Bigeminy:** *A normal beat is followed by a premature beat and this pattern repeats many times. The premature beats tend to fall out when exercise accelerates the rate to more than 120/min.* **D. Dropped beats in second-degree AV block:** *Each successive impulse going through the AV node produces a longer interval until one fails to induce ventricular contraction. In contrast to premature beats, exercise tends to increase the number of dropped beats.*

KEY SIGN Coupled Rhythm: Bigeminy, Trigeminy

One or two normal beats is followed regularly by a premature beat arising from an ectopic focus in the atrium or ventricle. The ventricular beats are grouped in pairs (bigeminy) or triplets (trigeminy), the last a premature beat; the compensatory pause after the premature beat separates one group from its successor (Fig. 4–4C). Bigeminy has a regular rhythm. Since the premature beat may not be palpable, a regular rhythm at half the true ventricular rate may be suspected if only the peripheral pulse is examined; heart auscultation reveals the bigeminy. As with other premature beats, exercise may cause the rhythm to resume a normal pattern. Coupled premature ventricular contractions (PVCs) occur in normal hearts, all forms of organic heart disease and digitalis intoxication. **DDX:** A similar pulse pattern is produced by Mobitz type I second-degree AV block (Wenckebach) with 3:2 Wenckebach simulating bigeminy and 4:3 simulating trigeminy.

KEY SIGN Grouped Beats and Dropped Beats

The mechanism is sinus pauses or SA block, second-degree AV block (Mobitz type I or II), or regularly occurring premature atrial beats in a trigeminal or quadrigeminal pattern if they are blocked in the AV node. A series of two, three, four, or more beats is followed by a pause. The pattern may recur regularly. The rhythm is unchanged by acceleration of the heart rate. Electrocardiography is essential to distinguish between these rhythms.

KEY SYNDROME Atrial Fibrillation

The atria do not contract in a synchronized fashion; different muscle segments contract separately. Stimuli arrive in complete disorder at the AV node, and a variable minority are transmitted to the ventricles at irregular intervals (see Fig. 4–4B). Accordingly, the ventricular rhythm and pulse presents no pattern. The carefully evaluated pulse is "irregularly irregular." Rapid ventricular responses are irregular but difficult to distinguish by palpation. At ventricular responses of >70 bpm, the rhythm may seem regular with some premature beats. With rates <60 or >120 bpm, the irregularity of the fibrillation may be difficult to detect. Because ventricular contractions occur at all stages of chamber filling, the heart sounds and pulse volume from ventricular contractions vary in intensity. The pulse volume is longer after longer R-R intervals. The ventricular rate is accelerated by exertion. Atrial fibrillation can only be diagnosed by ECG with accurate measuring of the intervals [Falk RD. Atrial fibrillation. *N Engl J Med.* 2001;344:1067–1078]. **DDX:** In flutter with variable AV block, exercise increases the rate by large increments. ***CLINICAL OCCURRENCE:*** Organic heart disease (especially mitral and tricuspid valve disease or disorders causing congestive heart failure), hyperthyroidism, acute infections including rheumatic fever, postoperative (especially chest surgery), electrolyte imbalances, hypoxia and hypercarbia. "Lone atrial fibrillation" may occur in the absence of any structural heart disease or metabolic abnormalities.

KEY SYNDROME Atrial Flutter

Regular impulses are generated in the atria at extremely high rates by reentry circuits, causing atrial contractions from 220 to 360 times per minute (see

Fig. 4–3D). The AV node cannot respond to such rapid stimuli, so block develops, for example, 2:1, 3:1, 4:1, or higher. The ventricular contractions are usually perfectly spaced, with no differences in the intensity of heart sounds from beat to beat. In some patients, there is considerable variability in the blockade of the atrial impulses. This causes variability in the ventricular response, which may be almost as irregular as atrial fibrillation. Digitalis, verapamil, diltiazem, and β-adrenergic blocking drugs increase the degree of block in flutter, a possibility to consider in taking the history. Vagus stimulation may produce sudden drops in ventricular rate as the degree of block is increased from 2:1 to 3:1, while the atrial rate remains constant. Flutter may be seen with almost any form of organic heart disease and is especially common after heart surgery. **DDX:** In sinus tachycardia, vagus stimulation causes smooth slowing while paroxysmal atrial tachycardia will not slow but may convert to normal.

KEY SYNDROME Paroxysmal Supraventricular (Atrial) Tachycardia (PSVT, PAT, SVT)

The arrhythmia is most often a reentrant or reciprocating form of tachycardia involving the AV node. True ectopic atrial tachycardia does occur. The attack begins and ends suddenly, lasting for a few minutes to many days. The ventricular rate is usually between 150 and 225 bpm. All ventricular beats have the same intensity and are equally spaced. Vagus stimulation or intravenous adenosine does not slow the rate; either there is no response, or the attack is terminated abruptly and normal rhythm resumes within a single cycle (see Fig. 4–3C). PSVT occurs in normal hearts and with AV bypass pathways (Wolf-Parkinson-White syndrome). **DDX:** PSVT must be distinguished from sinus tachycardia, which exhibits smooth vagus slowing, and from atrial flutter, in which vagus slowing is often associated with varying AV block.

KEY SYNDROME Ventricular Tachycardia (VT)

VT is usually a reentry dysrhythmia triggered by a PVC and sustained by the dispersion of conduction and repolarization in damaged ventricular muscle. Diagnosis is urgently needed since ventricular fibrillation may supervene leading to sudden death. There is usually complete AV dissociation, with the ventricles beating faster than the atria. The onset and, when self-limited, the ending are abrupt. The ventricular rate usually is between 150 and 250 bpm; occasionally, the ventricular rate <150 bpm. The rhythm is regular, and is not influenced by vagal stimulation; it must be distinguished from atrial flutter and PSVT. The variable relationship of atrial to ventricular systole produces the most distinctive sign: variation in the intensity of the first sounds. Some sounds are especially loud cannon sounds resulting from superimposition of atrial systole with ventricular systole. The cannon sounds are absent when the atria are fibrillating. Only the first heart sound may be audible. **CLINICAL OCCURRENCE:** Acute myocardial ischemia and infarction, coronary artery disease, drugs (digitalis, quinidine, procaine amide). Trauma to the heart from surgery or catheterization. Inherited causes include right ventricular dysplasia, long QT syndrome, hypertrophic cardiomyopathies and Brugada syndrome.

➤ **KEY SYNDROME** Ventricular Fibrillation (VF)

Ventricular muscle fibers depolarize and contract in a chaotic fashion which cannot produce effective ventricular contraction. No ventricular emptying occurs, so no heart sounds are produced. The diagnosis is made by ECG. Unless the dysrhythmia is interrupted by prompt electrical defibrillation, death follows rapidly.

Abnormal Pulse Contour

Pulse Contour Changes. See Chapter 8, page 382.
Pulse Volume Changes. See Chapter 8, page 383.

Respirations: Respiratory Rate and Pattern

Respiratory Rate

Normal respirations. In the newborn, the normal respiratory rate is approximately 44 cycles per minute; it decreases gradually the rate until maturity when the rate in adults is between 14 and 18 cycles per minute. Women have slightly higher rates than men. Since people tend to breathe faster when their breathing is being observed, the respiratory rate should be counted unobtrusively, such as pretending to count the pulse.

KEY SIGN Increased Respiratory Rate—Tachypnea

Increased respiratory rate occurs with central nervous system (CNS) stimulation and as compensation for increasing $PaCO_2$, decreases in tidal volume or metabolic acidosis. Hypoxia, increased oxygen demands, and increased CO_2 generation each lead to an increase in respiratory rate and tidal volume. Minute ventilation is maintained in restrictive disease of the lung or chest wall by increasing the respiratory rate to compensate for the reduced tidal volume. Tachypnea occurs with exertion, fear, fever, cardiac insufficiency, pain, pulmonary embolism, acute respiratory distress from infections, pleurisy, anemia, and hyperthyroidism. Breathing is faster when restricted by weakness of the respiratory muscles, emphysema, pneumothorax, or obesity. An arterial blood gas is required to distinguish pathological from compensatory tachypnea: a primary respiratory alkalosis indicates a pathological state.

KEY SIGN Decreased Respiratory Rate—Bradypnea

Minute ventilation is preserved when slow rates are accompanied by an increased tidal volume (hyperpnea). Slow rates without an increase in tidal volume produce alveolar hypoventilation indicating an abnormality of the medullary respiratory center. A slower than usual respiratory rate is not abnormal if gas exchange is preserved as demonstrated by arterial blood gas determination. When alveolar hypoventilation occurs ($PaCO_2 > 45$ mm Hg), metabolic encephalopathy as a result of CNS-depressant drugs (e.g., opiates, benzodiazepines, barbiturates, alcohol) or uremia, or structural intracranial lesions (especially conditions with increased intracranial pressure) are most likely.

Respiratory Pattern

> **KEY SIGN   Deep Breathing—Hyperpnea (Kussmaul Breathing)**

An increased tidal volume produces increased alveolar ventilation, which increases excretion of CO_2. This is an appropriate compensatory response to metabolic acidosis of any cause and is a direct toxic effect of salicylates. It is also seen with hypoxia. The term Kussmaul breathing is applied to deep, regular respirations, whether the rate be normal, slow, or fast. Common examples of precipitating metabolic acidoses are diabetic ketoacidosis and uremia. Hypoxemia (e.g., pneumonia, pulmonary embolism) and decreased oxygen delivery as a result of severe anemia or hemorrhage also lead to hyperpnea.

> **KEY SIGN   Shallow Breathing—Hypopnea**

Decreased depth of breathing results from decreased medullary respiratory center drive, weakness of the respiratory muscles, or loss of alveolar volume from any cause. Depression of the medullary respiratory center occurs as in bradypnea. Muscular weakness can result from myasthenia gravis, amyotrophic lateral sclerosis, Guillain-Barré syndrome, drugs (e.g., paralyzing agents, rarely aminoglycosides) and exhaustion when the work of breathing is increased due to decreased chest wall and/or lung compliance as in severe asthma. Decreased lung volumes can result from alveolar filling disorders (congestive heart failure with pulmonary edema, acute lung injury, alveolar hemorrhage, pneumonia, etc.), severe restrictive disease of the lung or chest wall or severe airways obstruction (asthma, emphysema).

> **KEY SIGN   Periodic Breathing—Cheyne-Stokes Respiration**

The pattern results from cyclic hyperventilation followed by compensatory apnea caused by phase delay in the feedback controls trying to maintain a constant PCO_2. This is the most common periodic breathing pattern. Respirations are interrupted by periods of apnea. In each cycle, the rate and amplitude of successive breaths increase to a maximum, then progressively diminish into the next apneic period. Pallor may accompany the apnea. The patient is frequently unaware of the irregular breathing. Patients may be somnolent during the apneic periods and then arouse and become restless during the hyperpneic phase. *CLINICAL OCCURRENCE:*   It may be seen during the sleep of normal children and the aged. *Disorders of the Cerebral Circulation*   stroke, atherosclerosis;   *Heart Failure* low cardiac output of any cause;   *Increased Intracranial Pressure*   meningitis, hydrocephalus, brain tumor, subarachnoid hemorrhage, intracerebral hemorrhage; *Brain Injury*   stroke, head injury;   *Drugs*   opiates, barbiturates, alcohol;   *High Altitude*   during sleep, before acclimatization.

Irregular breathing—biot breathing.   An uncommon variant of Cheyne-Stokes respiration, periods of apnea alternate irregularly with series of breaths of equal depth that terminate abruptly. It is most often seen in meningitis.

Irregular breathing—painful respiration.   Otherwise normal respirations are interrupted by the pain of thoracic movement from pleurisy, injured or inflamed muscles, fractured ribs or cartilage, or subphrenic inflammation, such as liver or subdiaphragmatic abscess, acute cholecystitis, or peritonitis.

> **KEY SYNDROME**   Irregular Breathing—Sleep Apnea

Obstructive sleep apnea results from obstruction of the extrathoracic airway caused by relaxation of the pharyngeal muscles and tongue with ineffective inspiratory efforts often terminating with a loud snort or snore. Central apnea occurs when respiratory effort ceases because of absence of medullary respiratory drive. The periods of apnea are accompanied by hypoxia, acidosis, and cardiac dysrhythmias (bradycardia, tachycardia, especially ventricular) that sometimes cause sudden death. The classic patient is a morbidly obese male with daytime somnolence, polycythemia, alveolar hypoventilation, pulmonary hypertension producing right ventricular failure; this is the picture of advanced disease. The daytime somnolence is the result of nocturnal interruptions of sleep by many arousals resulting from intervals of apnea lasting more than 10 seconds. Symptoms of early disease include early morning headaches, depression or irritability from chronic sleep deprivation, and systemic hypertension. Physical examination findings predictive of obstructive sleep apnea are increased Mallampati grade of oropharyngeal narrowing (see Chapter 7, page 271), tonsil size and BMI. [Netzer MC, Stoohs RA, Netzer CM, et al. Using the Berlin questionnaire to identify patients at risk for the sleep apnea syndrome. *Ann Intern Med*. 1999;131:485–491].

Irregular breathing—sighing respirations.   The normal respiratory rhythm at rest is occasionally interrupted by a long, deep sigh. The patient briefly senses shortness of breath without limitations of exertion when active. This is commonly encountered in anxious individuals.

Blood Pressure and Pulse Pressure

Every patient's BP should be checked at each visit to detect hypertension and to establish a benchmark for future comparison. The BP should be taken in both arms at the first office visit and again in both arms when the patient has new cardiovascular or neurologic complaints. When elevated arm pressures are found in young persons, the pressures in both legs should be checked. Many circumstances temporarily raise BP in the absence of disease, for example, anxiety, the "white-coat syndrome," rushing to make the appointment on time, bladder distention, chronic alcoholism, amphetamines, cocaine, and recent caffeine intake or cigarette smoking. Frequent BP checks are encouraged [Bailey RH, Bauer JH. A review of common errors in the direct measurement of blood pressure: Sphygmomanometry. *Arch Intern Med*. 1993;153:2741–2748].

Measurement of Arterial BP

The intraarterial BP can be measured directly, but this is only done in intensive care units. Clinically, the indirect method is used, in which external pressure is applied to the overlying tissues and the pressure (measured in millimeters of mercury) necessary to occlude the artery is assumed equal to the intraarterial pressure. The arm cuff should be at least 10 cm wide; for the thigh, a width of 18 cm is preferable. The tension to compress the overlying tissues is usually regarded as negligible, but a thick arm will yield readings 10 to 15 mm Hg higher than the actual pressure unless a wide cuff is used [Reeves RA. The rational clinical examination. Does this patient have hypertension? How to measure blood pressure. *JAMA*. 1995;273:1211–1218].

In some situations, the BP measured by the arm cuff may be higher than the actual intraaortic pressure; this can lead to further efforts to lower an already low BP with tragic consequences. It is important for the clinician caring for critically ill patients to understand this possibility [O'Rourke MF, Seward JB. Central arterial pressure and arterial pressure pulse: new views entering the second century after Korotkov. *Mayo Clin Proc.* 2006;81:1057–1068; Moser, M, Setaro JF. Resistant or difficult-to-contol hypertension. *N Engl J Med.* 2006;355:385–392]. Finding that the radial artery remains palpable after the BP cuff is inflated above systolic pressure (the Osler maneuver) demonstrates the calcified arteries that may produce this condition [Messerli FH, Ventura, HO, Amodeo C. Osler's maneuver and pseudo-hypertension. *N Engl J Med.* 1985;312:1548–1551].

(STOP) *In hypotensive states with coincident intense peripheral vasoconstriction, the sphygmomanometric method may seriously underestimate the true intraarterial pressure. This often occurs in shock. With smaller degrees of vasoconstriction the Korotkoff sounds underestimate the systolic pressure and overestimate diastolic values.*

Measurement of the brachial artery pressure. The patient may be either sitting or lying supine; a 10-minute rest before determining the BP is advisable. Bare the arm and affix the collapsed cuff snugly and smoothly, so the distal margin of the cuff is at least 3 cm proximal to the antecubital fossa. Rest the supinated arm on the table or bed with the antecubital fossa approximately at the level of the heart. Palpate for the exact location of the brachial arterial pulse; it is usually medial, but occasionally lateral, to the insertion of the biceps tendon. Inflate the cuff to a pressure approximately 30 mm Hg above the point where the palpable pulse disappears. Open the valve slightly so the pressure drops gradually (no more than 2 mm Hg/s) while auscultating over the brachial artery.

Vibrations from the artery, called Korotkoff sounds, are used to determine the pressures. With the bell of the stethoscope pressed lightly over the brachial artery, note the pressure at which sounds first appear: this is the systolic pressure. As deflation proceeds, the sounds become louder and maintain a maximum for a considerable range before becoming muffled and finally disappearing. Note the pressures at the point of muffling and where the sounds disappear. Record the readings, for example, 130/80/75. The highest value is the systolic pressure, but disagreement exists as to whether the second or third value represents the closest approximation to the intraarterial diastolic pressure. With all three values recorded, readers can draw their own conclusions, and they are not forced to guess at the criterion employed by the examiner for the diastolic pressure. The American Heart Association now recommends the point of disappearance for the diastolic pressure in most instances. Occasionally, as in hyperthyroidism and aortic regurgitation, the sounds persist to zero pressure. In such cases, accept the second value, since a diastolic pressure of zero is impossible. Palpation is an alternate method, employed to check the results by auscultation or when Korotkoff sounds are imperceptible. Palpate the brachial or radial artery distal to the cuff, and record as the systolic pressure; the pressure at which pulse waves first appear. Alternatively, a hand-held Doppler ultrasound device can be used to identify the pulse and the systolic pressure.

In some patients the Korotkoff sounds appear then disappear before reappearing again as the cuff pressure is lowered, producing an *auscultatory gap*. This is observed more commonly in older individuals with hypertension and may indicate increased arterial stiffness. It is important to inflate the cuff to well above the putative systolic pressure in order to not miss the initial sounds, which would result in recording a falsely low systolic pressure.

The *pulse pressure* is the difference between the arterial systolic and diastolic pressures. The normal mean value is 50 mm Hg in men and women.

Wrist BP.   It is often difficult to get an accurate BP in a short fat arm in which case the BP should be checked at the wrist. The cuff is wrapped around the forearm and the stethoscope bell is placed over the radial artery.

Femoral artery BP.   When taking the arterial pressure in the femoral artery, have the patient lie prone on a table or bed. Wrap a wide cuff (18 cm or more) around the thigh so that the lower margin of the cuff is several centimeters proximal to the popliteal fossa. Inflate the cuff and auscultate the popliteal artery. It is often difficult to get even compression with the cuff on a conical thigh.

Ankle BP.   This may is more convenient than the femoral BP. With the patient supine, apply the cuff just above the malleolus. Place the chest piece of the stethoscope distal to the cuff and behind the medial malleolus on the posterior tibial artery or on the dorsal extensor retinaculum of the ankle over the dorsalis pedis artery. In patients with unobstructed arteries BP by this method is comparable to brachial artery BP.

Manometric detection of pulse wave disturbances.   During measurement of the BP, changes in the volume of individual pulse waves may be detected that are too subtle to be detected by palpation. This may be found in atrial fibrillation, pulsus paradoxus (tamponade, chronic obstructive pulmonary disease), and pulsus alternans (page 383).

> **KEY SIGN**   **Inequality of BP in Arms**

BPs normally differ by < 10 mm Hg between the arms; the right arm is usually greater than the left. Inequality is frequent and sometimes cannot be explained. Conditions to be considered are obstruction in the subclavian artery, thoracic outlet syndrome and aortic dissection. [Eguchi K, Yacoub M, Jhalani J, et al. Consistency of blood pressure differences between the left and right arms. *Arch Intern Med.* 2007;167:388–393].

Normal Arterial Pressure

The precise bounds of the normal BP are difficult to define and definitions of normal and hypertension continue to evolve (Table 4–1). The risk for cardiovascular disease begins to increase with pressures >115/75 and doubles for each 20/10 mm Hg thereafter. Statistical data show an increase in the average systolic pressure with age. Normal adults exhibit a circadian variation in the BP; it is highest at midmorning, falls progressively during the day, and reaches its lowest point at approximately 3 AM. The Seventh Report of the Joint National Committee on Prevention, Detection, Evaluation, and Treatment of High Blood Pressure has defined the ranges for the description of BP [Chobanian AV, Bakris GL, Black HR, et al. The seventh report of the joint national committee on prevention,

Table 4–1   JNC-7 BP Classification

Classification	Systolic Pressure mm Hg	Diastolic Pressure mm Hg
Normal	<120	<80
Prehypertension	120–139	80–89
Hypertension		
Stage 1	140–159	90–99
Stage 2	>159	>100

detection, evaluation, and treatment of high blood pressure. *JAMA*. 2003;289: 2560–2572].

High Blood Pressure

> **KEY SYNDROME   Hypertension**

Most hypertension is of unknown cause and is termed "essential hypertension." The primary lesion is suspected to be in the kidney. Increased diastolic pressure results from increased peripheral resistance, either by vasoconstriction or intimal thickening. Increased systolic pressure can result from increased stroke volume or decreased compliance of the aorta (in which case the pulse pressure is widened) and with increased diastolic pressure (with a normal or increased pulse pressure). The systolic pressure may be elevated with a normal diastolic pressure: isolated systolic hypertension. More commonly, both the systolic and diastolic pressures are elevated. If only the diastolic pressure is elevated, the pulse pressure is narrowed and one should suspect impaired cardiac output. The diastolic pressure represents the minimal continuous load to which the vascular tree is subjected and makes the greatest contribution to the mean arterial pressure. Both isolated systolic and systolic combined with diastolic hypertension are strongly correlated with stroke, heart failure, left ventricular hypertrophy, and chronic kidney failure. In patients older than 50 years of age, elevated systolic BP is more important than diastolic BP as a risk factor for cardiovascular disease. Discovery of sustained hypertension should lead you to search for hypertensive retinopathy, left ventricular hypertrophy and ischemia, and renal insufficiency.

✔ **HYPERTENSION—CLINICAL OCCURRENCE:** Essential hypertension is a diagnosis of exclusion, so alternative explanations need to always be considered. **Congenital** coarctation of the aorta, congenital adrenal hyperplasia (early or late onset), polycystic kidney disease; **Endocrine** pheochromocytoma, aldosteronoma, adrenal hyperplasia, hypercortisolism (Cushing disease and syndrome), hyperthyroidism, hypothyroidism, hyperparathyroidism, acromegaly; **Idiopathic** essential hypertension, toxemia of pregnancy; **Inflammatory/Immune** atherosclerosis, vasculitis; **Metabolic/Toxic** renal insufficiency, medications (NSAIDs estrogens, oral contraceptives, cyclosporine), drug abuse (cocaine, amphetamines, etc.), porphyria, lead poisoning, hypercalcemia; **Mechanical/Trauma** obstructive sleep apnea; **Neoplastic** adrenal adenoma, pheochromocytoma, pituitary adenoma, brain tumors; **Neurologic** stroke, diencephalic syndrome, increased intracranial pressure, acute spinal cord injury; **Psychosocial** substance abuse (cocaine, amphetamines, alcohol); **Vascular** renal artery stenosis (atherosclerosis, fibromuscular dysplasia).

KEY SYNDROME   Isolated Systolic Hypertension

The increased systolic pressure is the result of either increased stroke volume or increased rigidity of the aorta its branches. The systolic pressure is elevated but the diastolic pressure is normal. It is correlated with an increased risk for stroke, left ventricular hypertrophy, and heart failure. Systolic hypertension is seen with increased cardiac output (hyperthyroidism, anemia, arteriovenous fistulas, aortic regurgitation, anxiety), a rigid aorta as a result of atherosclerosis, and is particularly common in the older adults.

KEY SYNDROME   Malignant Hypertension

Severely elevated BP leads to end-organ dysfunction with positive feedback loops as a result of ischemia, which further aggravates the pressure. Patients present with headache, confusion, dyspnea, seizures, angina or rapidly progressive renal insufficiency; diastolic pressures are >120 mm Hg and systolic pressures usually >200 mm Hg. Rapid reduction of pressures is required to prevent irreversible damage to the brain, heart, eyes and kidneys.

KEY SYNDROME   Paroxysmal Hypertension: Pheochromocytoma

A benign tumor of the adrenal or sympathetic chain secretes epinephrine or norepinephrine. In one-third of the patients, the tumor secretes intermittently. The patient's BP may be normal except for episodes of hypertension associated with pallor, anxiety, sweating, palpitation, nausea, and vomiting. However, most patients have sustained hypertension. Orthostatic hypotension is common due to intravascular volume depletion. The condition must be distinguished from panic attacks and the "white-coat syndrome" in which some anxious patients register hypertensive readings only when their BP is taken by a physician or nurse [Lenders JWM, Pacak K, Walther MM. Biochemical diagnosis of pheochromocytoma: Which test is best? *JAMA*. 2002;287:1427–1434].

KEY SYNDROME   Paroxysmal Hypertension: Neuroleptic Malignant Syndrome

See page 54.

Low BP

KEY SYNDROME   Hypotension

Hypotension results from a loss of blood volume, loss of vascular tone, or decreased cardiac output. Both the systolic and diastolic pressures are diminished below the patient's normal: note that values within the normal range are hypotensive for the patient who has previously had sustained hypertension. Signs of hypoperfusion (cool skin, decreased urine output, decreased mental alertness) and compensatory cardiovascular responses (peripheral vasoconstriction, tachycardia) indicate that low BP is pathologic. *CLINICAL OCCURRENCE:*   *Loss of Blood Volume*   bleeding, capillary leak syndrome (anaphylaxis, sepsis, IL-2, idiopathic), third-spacing (ascites, burns, secretory diarrheas), polyuria (diabetes mellitus, diabetes insipidus, diuretics), inadequate fluid intake, excessive sweating (heat prostration and heat stroke), adrenal insufficiency; *Loss of Vascular Tone* sepsis, drugs (vasodilators, tricyclic antidepressants, ganglionic blockers), fever, autonomic insufficiency (multisystem atrophy), acute spinal cord injury (spinal shock), arteriovenous malformations; *Decreased Cardiac Output* acute myocardial infarction, ischemic cardiomyopathy, idiopathic dilated cardiomyopathy, aortic stenosis, pulmonary embolism, pericardial tamponade and severe mitral insufficiency.

KEY SIGN   Orthostatic (Postural) Hypotension

The patient is hypovolemic, sympathetic drive to the heart and blood vessels is diminished, or venous return to the heart is deficient. The BP is normal in the recumbent position, but when the patient stands there is a fall, within 3 minutes, of 20 mm Hg in the systolic or 10 mm Hg in the diastolic BP and/or the heart rate rises by $\geq$15 bpm. This is an early sign of intravascular volume loss [McGee S, Abernethy WB III, Simel DL. The rational clinical examination. Is this patient hypovolemic? *JAMA.* 1999;281:1022–1028]. When the drop in BP is not accompanied by a rise in pulse rate, autonomic insufficiency is suggested. Patients with chronic orthostatic hypotension frequently have postprandial hypotension and reversal of the normal circadian BP pattern (i.e., higher BP at night than during the day) [Ejaz AA, Haley WE, Wasiluk A, Meschia JF, Fitzpatrick PM. Characteristics of 100 consecutive patients presenting with orthostatic hypotension. *Mayo Clin Proc.* 2004;79:890–894]. CLINICAL OCCURRENCE: *Loss of Blood Volume* see Hypotension above; *Loss of Vascular Tone* deconditioning after long illnesses, autonomic insufficiency (multisystem atrophy), peripheral neuropathies (diabetes, tabes dorsalis, alcoholism), drugs (vasodilators, tricyclic antidepressants, ganglionic blockers); *Impaired Venous Return* ascites, pregnancy, venous insufficiency, inferior vena cava obstruction or hemangiomas of the legs.

Postprandial hypotension.   In some individuals, especially older adults on vasoactive medications, the BP drops by 20 mm Hg or more following meals. The exact mechanisms are unclear, but the result is an increased risk for falls, syncope, dizziness and fatigue. Careful questioning of patients about the relationship of their symptoms to meals will help identify this syndrome [Jansen RWMM, Lipsitz LA. Postprandial hypotension: epidemiology, pathophysiology, and clinical management. *Ann Intern Med.* 1995;122:286–295].

► KEY SYNDROME   Anaphylactic Shock

IgE-mediated mast cell degranulation leads to release of histamine and other vasoactive substances, producing vasodilatation and opening of endothelial tight junctions with loss of plasma volume. This is a fulminant and life-threatening hypersensitivity reaction occurring on exposure to a specific allergen. Sudden vascular collapse is preceded or accompanied by malaise, pruritus, pallor, stridor, cyanosis, syncope, vomiting, diarrhea, tachypnea, tachycardia, and distant heart sounds. Angioedema and urticaria may be present, but are often absent. CLINICAL OCCURRENCE: Hymenoptera stings, drugs (e.g., penicillin and other antibiotics), peanut ingestion, and many others. Anaphylaxis may occur with exercise, cold exposure, heat exposure or without evident cause (idiopathic anaphylaxis). Clinically identical reactions occur when mast cell release is stimulated by non-IgE-mediated mechanisms such as radiographic contrast agents.

➤ **KEY SYNDROME**   Septic Shock

This is a complex physiologic reaction to endotoxin release into the systemic circulation with activation of inflammatory and thrombotic pathways. Patients present with hypotension, often, but not always, accompanied by fever and prostration. Initially, the skin is warm and flushed, despite the low BP. As the condition worsens, peripheral vasoconstriction, decreased urine output, confusion, progressive hypotension and acidosis ensue. Prompt recognition, location, and appropriate treatment of the source of infection are essential.

➤ **KEY SYNDROME**   Toxic Shock Syndrome

A toxin produced by certain strains of *Staphylococcus aureus* produces hypotension with high cardiac output and generalized erythroderma. This was originally described when highly absorbent vaginal tampons became infected with the organism. Now, surgical wounds containing infected foreign bodies (sutures) and sinusitis are the most common identified sites of infection. The patient suddenly develops high fever, myalgia, nausea, vomiting, and diarrhea. A diffuse erythematous rash (like sunburn) is followed by confusion, acute respiratory distress syndrome, hypotension, and shock. Exfoliation of skin from the palms and soles may occur in convalescence.

Pulse Pressure

KEY SIGN   Widened Pulse Pressure

Pulse pressure increases when the peak systolic pressure is increased (increased stroke volume, increased rate of ventricular contraction, decreased aortic elasticity) and/or there is a decreased diastolic pressure (decreased peripheral resistance, arteriovenous shunts, aortic insufficiency). A pulse pressure of ≥ 65 mm Hg is abnormal. With a large stroke volume, the pulse is often described as bounding or, in the case of aortic regurgitation, collapsing. The head may bob with each heart beat. Thrills may be palpable and murmurs audible over AV shunts, either congenital/traumatic, or iatrogenic. With decreased peripheral resistance from vasodilation, the skin is usually warm and flushed. Widened pulse pressure is associated with increased cardiovascular morbidity and mortality [Asmar R, Vol S, Vrisac A-M, Tichet J, Topouchian J. Reference values for clinical pulse pressure in a nonselected population. *Am J Hyperens.* 2001;14:415–418]. An increased pulse pressure is an important risk factor for new onset atrial fibrillation [Mitchell GF, Vasan RS, Keyes MJ, et al. Pulse pressure and risk of new-onset atrial fibrillation. *JAMA.* 2007;297:709–715]. *CLINICAL OCCURRENCE:* *Increased Systolic Pressure* systolic hypertension, atherosclerosis, increased stroke volume (aortic regurgitation, hyperthyroidism, anxiety, bradycardia, heart block, post-PVC, after a long pause in atrial fibrillation, pregnancy, fever, systemic arteriovenous fistulas); *Increased Diastolic Runoff* aortic regurgitation, sepsis, vasodilators, patent ductus arteriosus, hyperthyroidism, arteriovenous fistulas, beriberi.

> ### KEY SIGN   Narrowed Pulse Pressure

Pulse pressure narrows with decreased stroke volume and decreased rate of ventricular ejection. Pulse pressures less than 30 mm Hg may occur with tachycardia and many other conditions associated with a low stroke volume. *CLINICAL OCCURRENCE: Decreased Stroke Volume* severe aortic stenosis, dilated cardiomyopathy, restrictive heart disease, constrictive pericarditis, pericardial tamponade, intravascular volume depletion, venous vasodilatation; *Decreased Rate of Ventricular Contraction* ischemic and dilated cardiomyopathy, aortic stenosis, myocarditis.

Anthropometric Data

Height

Linear growth occurs throughout infancy, childhood and adolescence, ending with closure of the long bone epiphyses. Mature height is determined by both genetic and environmental factors, especially nutrition. Linear growth requires the presence of growth hormone, adequate nutrition (protein, calories, vitamin D, calcium, and phosphorus) and a skeleton able to respond to these signals. After achieving mature height, height should not change throughout the years of maturity into old age. With aging, there is a hormone-independent loss of bone mineral density, particularly of trabecular bone, leading to a slow and gradual loss of height. The latter is aggravated in many cases by loss of muscle tone and strength affecting posture. Addition of pathologic states such as osteoporosis and spinal compression fractures produce sometimes dramatic loss of height.

Height should be measured and recorded regularly as part of well-child examinations throughout infancy and childhood. Growth is plotted on standardized growth charts, which give a rapid, visual indication of current stature and growth trends over time. Once stable mature height is reached, it need not be measured more than once every few years until the person reaches age 60 when annual measurement should begin.

Measurement of height.   Height is measured standing with bare feet. The patient should be erect (e.g., heels, buttocks, and scapulae touching a wall) and the head in a neutral position (normally, the occiput will not touch the wall). The height is recorded by the vertical distance between the floor and a point horizontal with the highest point of the scalp. Compress the hair, or separate especially thick hair, to eliminate overestimating height. The height is recorded in inches (to 0.25 in) or in centimeters (to 0.5 cm).

> ### KEY SIGN   Short Stature

Short stature indicates a failure of growth hormone production, decreased tissue receptivity, or impaired nutrition. Expected stature can be estimated from standard scales or by adding 6.5 cm (2.6 in) for boys and subtracting 6.5 cm (2.6 in) for girls from the mid-parental height. Consult textbooks of pediatrics for discussions of the evaluation of short stature in children [Israel EJ, Levitsky, Anupindi SA, et al. Case 3-2005: a 14-year-old boy with recent slowing of growth and delayed puberty. *N Eng J Med.* 2005;352:393–403].

✔ *SHORT STATURE—CLINICAL OCCURRENCE:* **Congenital** intrauterine growth retardation, pseudohypoparathyroidism, vitamin D-resistant rickets, familial short stature, Turner syndrome, achondroplasia, Noonan syndrome, Prader-Willi syndrome; **Endocrine** growth hormone deficiency, hypothyroidism, hyperthyroidism, diabetes mellitus, Cushing disease, hypogonadism; **Idiopathic** constitutional delay in growth; **Infectious** any chronic debilitating infection; **Inflammatory/Immune** juvenile rheumatoid arthritis, SLE, chronic glomerulonephritis; **Mechanical/Traumatic** brain injury; **Metabolic/Toxic** chronic glucocorticoid use, malnutrition; **Neoplastic** cancer treatment during childhood, including brain irradiation; **Neurologic** suprasellar masses; **Psychosocial** chronic emotional deprivation, misassigned paternity; **Vascular** pituitary infarction.

KEY SIGN Accelerated Linear Growth

This can only occur before the epiphyses are closed in late adolescence and is a result of increased growth hormone from a pituitary tumor. Linear growth normally goes through an early and a late growth acceleration. Deviations from the expected growth rate are detected by the routine use of growth charts during childhood. Significant deviations from the expected rate of linear growth should initiate a search for a growth hormone-producing pituitary adenoma.

Excessive height—gigantism. Growth hormone accelerates linear bone growth at open epiphyses. Linear growth in excess of that predicted by parental height, especially if a significant deviation from the previous record, suggests an overproduction of growth hormone from a pituitary tumor, gigantism. Note that excessive growth hormone production after epiphyseal closure results in acromegaly (enlarged hands, feet, skull, mandible, and soft-tissue thickening) without increase in height. See Chapter 13, page 663.

KEY SYNDROME Abnormal Body Proportions: Marfan Syndrome

See Chapter 13, page 664. Affected individuals are tall, of extremely slender build, and with an arm span that exceeds their height.

KEY SYNDROME Abnormal Body Proportions: Klinefelter Syndrome

See Chapter 12, page 584.

KEY SIGN Loss of Height

Decreased height after reaching skeletal maturity can only result from loss of long bone length, cartilage in lower extremity joints (especially the hip and knee), vertebral height, or intervertebral disc spaces (especially lumbar), or excessive spinal curvatures. A careful history and physical examination, combined with a minimum of radiographic investigation, can quickly identify the specific conditions affecting an individual. Unless height is measured regularly, the slow progression of height loss may go undetected until changes are severe and significant disability brings the patient to attention. *CLINICAL OCCURRENCE:* **Long Bones** trauma, surgery, osteomalacia; **Cartilage** osteoarthritis, rheumatoid arthritis (RA); **Intervertebral Discs** herniated discs, desiccated disks, disk infection; **Vertebrae** osteoporosis, osteomalacia, Paget disease, traumatic compression fracture, multiple myeloma; *Spinal Curvature* scoliosis, pregnancy, abdominal muscle weakness, myositis, polio.

Weight

Total body weight is usually thought of as a series of compartments. Gain or loss of weight should be thought of in terms of how much is added to or lost from each compartment.

One scheme is to think of the body as water and everything else: water makes up approximately 60% of the total body mass in men, slightly less in women, and it decreases with age in both sexes. The higher the proportion of body fat, the lower the proportion of water. Body water is divided into two large compartments, the intracellular water (66%) and the extracellular water (34%); it is important to note that the extracellular water is essentially saline with a sodium concentration of approximately 140 mEq/L, while the intracellular water is rich in potassium and relatively low in sodium. The extracellular compartment is further divided into the extravascular fluid (75%) and the intravascular fluid (25%) most of which is in the capacitance veins.

Another scheme is to visualize the body as a series of tissue compartments. There is a relatively stable component forming the visceral organs and skeleton, which vary little in mass, and a variable component made up largely of extracellular fluid, skeletal muscle and fat. Therefore, when faced with inappropriate or unexpected changes in weight, the clinician should try to determine which combinations of changes in body water, muscle and fat have occurred. This will help in determining the specific etiology of the change observed.

Weight should be measured at each visit to establish a baseline range and to detect any significant changes. Weight is measured on a scale, the most accurate being a calibrated balance scale. Properly calibrated electronic scales are quite accurate. Weight is recorded in pounds or kilograms, preferably without heavy clothing or shoes.

Body Mass Index

The body mass index (BMI) is a standardized measure of the relationship of body mass to height. It has allowed for the calculation of the risk for adverse events of populations with different BMIs. The BMI is calculated by dividing the weight in kilograms by the (height in meters)^2; the units are thus kg/m^2. The upper limit of normal was identified as the point at which the risk for adverse health outcomes began to rise; the lower limit was similarly determined (Table 4–2). The BMI does not distinguish increases in lean body mass from increases in fat mass.

Growth charts using the BMI have been developed and are being used increasingly in well-child care. Calculation of BMI and setting weight loss goals based on the BMI are clinically useful; it allows patients to compare themselves with other individuals and the population risks associated with their current and target BMI.

Waist-Hip Ratio

Women have more subcutaneous fat than men, and they tend to distribute increased adipose tissue more diffusely, predominately in the subcutaneous fat. Men, especially those who gain weight in mid-life, tend to develop visceral adiposity in the internal organs and omentum; this adipose tissue is metabolically different from the subcutaneous fat and appears to play a pathophysiologic role

Table 4–2   Interpretation of BMI

BMI	Description
<18.5	Underweight
18.5–25	Normal
>25–30	Overweight
>30–35	Class I: Obese
>35–40	Class II: Very obese
>40	Class III: Extremely obese

in the increased incidence of hyperlipidemia and insulin resistance in these individuals. The waist:hip ratio (the ratio of the body circumference at the hip and waist) has been used to quantify this type of fat distribution. Abnormal waist-hip ratio is >0.9 for women and >1.0 for men; abnormal waist circumference is >40 inches (90 cm) for men or >35 inches (80 cm) for women. An increased waist-hip ratio or waist circumference correlates with risks of adverse health events, and appears to be a better predictor than BMI [Yusuf S, Hawken S, Ounpuu S, et al. Obesity and the risk of myocardial infarction in 27 000 participants form 52 countries: A case-contol study. *Lancet*. 2005;366:1640–1649; Romero-Corral A, Montori VM, Somers VK, et al. Association of bodyweight with total mortality and with cardiovascular events in coronary artery disease: A systematic review of cohort studies. *Lancet*. 2006;368:666–678].

KEY SYNDROME   Growth Retardation—Cystic Fibrosis

Any of several autosomal recessive mutations of the epithelial chloride channel gene leads to production of viscous mucus by the exocrine glands. This results in chronic progressive disfunction of the pancreas and lungs. Patients are usually diagnosed in childhood, although some, with more mild mutations, escape detection until adulthood. Symptoms include bulky, foul-smelling stools, cough, and dyspnea. Pancreatic obstruction leads to maldigestion and growth retardation. Lung involvement produces cough and recurrent pulmonary infections, often leading to chronic infection with *Pseudomonas aeruginosa* and bronchiectasis. Involvement of the sweat glands makes affected individuals very susceptible to salt and water losses in warm environments. Complications include fecal impactions, intussusception, volvulus, and chronic bronchitis. With advanced pulmonary disease, cardiomegaly and clubbing of the fingers are present.

KEY SIGN   Weight Loss

Weight loss occurs when energy (calorie) utilization or loss exceeds intake. It can arise from decreased effective intake (net of ingestion, emesis and stool losses), maldigestion, malabsorption, increased metabolic utilization, or increased losses of calories. Failure to gain weight and grow appropriately in childhood and adolescence has the same significance as weight loss in the adult. The history is most useful in formulating a probable pathophysiology. Ask the patient's estimate of the weight lost over a specific time and obtain records of weight to validate the history. Ask whether the patient's clothes fit differently or if family or friends have noted a change in appearance. Review the patient's daily intake of food and drink, and determine if there has been a change in activities. Look at the patient's belt to see if there is a change in the pattern of wear. Look for striae and loose skin over the abdomen and arms. Often more than one mechanism is at work, for example, decreased intake and increased utilization [Bouras EP, Lange SM, Scolpaio JS. Rational approach to patients with unintentional weight loss. *Mayo Clin Proc.* 2001;76:923–929; Detsky AS, Smalley PS, Chang J. The rational clinical examination. Is this patient malnourished? *JAMA.* 1994;271: 54–58]. **DDX:** Weight loss without a decrease in intake suggests impaired nutrient assimilation (maldigestion, malabsorption), glucosuria (diabetes mellitus), or increased metabolic rate (hyperthyroidism, pheochromocytoma). Cancer and psychosocial problems, especially depression, are the two most prevalent explanations.

✔ *WEIGHT LOSS—CLINICAL OCCURRENCE:* **Endocrine** hyperthyroidism, adrenal insufficiency, diabetes (especially type 1); **Idiopathic** advanced age (normal adults lose weight gradually after age 60 years), any debilitating disease; **Inflammatory** any systemic inflammatory disease, for example, SLE, RA, vasculitis; **Infectious** chronic disseminated infection or advanced local infection, for example, tuberculosis, chronic active hepatitis, AIDS, intestinal parasites; **Metabolic/Toxic** organ failure (uremia, advanced liver disease, emphysema, congestive heart failure), increased physical activity, maldigestion and malabsorption, dieting, decreased intake and starvation; **Mechanical/Traumatic** bowel obstruction, dysphagia, odynophagia, dental and chewing problems, decreased mobility, paralysis, apraxia; **Neoplastic** cancers decrease appetite and increase utilization, especially when disseminated or involving the liver; **Neurologic** hypothalamic disorders; **Psychosocial** dieting, dementia, depression, anorexia nervosa, bulimia, abuse, isolation, poverty; **Vascular** vasculitis, multiinfarct dementia.

Cachexia: Cytokines released in chronic infections and in the presence of malignancies lead to wasting of muscle protein and increased metabolic demands resulting in profound weight loss and redistribution. Cachexia is physiologically distinct from starvation and cannot be reversed by refeeding. Cachexia is classically seen in chronic tuberculosis ("consumption") and slow growing visceral malignancies (e.g., advanced pancreatic and colon cancers), but any chronic disease with persistent activation of the immune system may produce the syndrome [Kotler, DP. Cachexia. *Ann Intern Med.* 2000;133;622–634]. *CLINICAL OCCURRENCE:* common associations are HIV-AIDS, CHF, advanced liver and renal disease, RA, Addison disease, chronic obstructive pulmonary disease and advance age.

> **KEY SIGN** Weight Gain

Weight increases whenever the intake of calories exceeds the metabolic demands, or when calorie-free salt and water are retained. Therefore, weight gain can occur from increased intake, decreased metabolic demands, and/or renal retention of salt and water. Weight gain is a part of normal growth and failure to gain weight appropriately during childhood and adolescence is abnormal. Once skeletal maturity is reached, weight gain continues for a variable length of time as skeletal muscle mass increases to adult size, this is especially true in men. After reaching adult mass in the early twenties, any further increase in weight indicates a pathologic condition, a decrease in physical exercise, or an increase in caloric intake. Fats and alcohol have the highest energy content, 9 and 7.5 kcal/g respectively, whereas the energy content of carbohydrates and protein is 4.5 kcal/g. A careful dietary and exercise history should be obtained. Also, inquire about changes in appetite, libido, skin, hair, and bowel habits. Note the pattern of weight gain during the physical examination and any evidence of retention of extracellular fluid as edema. **CLINICAL OCCURRENCE:** *Increased Intake* overeating, mild hyperthyroidism, insulinoma, hypothalamic injury, treatment of diabetes, anabolic steroids; *Decreased Metabolic Demands* hypothyroidism, hypogonadism, inactivity, confinement; *Salt and Water Retention* congestive heart failure, kidney failure, nephrotic syndrome, hepatic insufficiency, portal hypertension with ascites, idiopathic edema, diuretic rebound, venous insufficiency with dependent edema.

KEY SYNDROME   Obesity

Genetics and lifestyle each play important roles in the development of obesity. Caloric intake in excess of expenditures will lead to weight gain, but obesity requires the failure of a feedback loop to control intake; the cause(s) of this failure are unknown. Obesity is epidemic in the United States; fully a third or more of the adult population is obese. There is a strong correlation of obesity with insulin resistance and the development of hypertension, diabetes, heart disease, cancer, and overall mortality. Obesity is readily recognized and diagnosed, but is very difficult to treat, especially if onset is in childhood or adolescence. Obesity can result from the causes of weight gain (see above, page 83), but more commonly the exact factors leading to the marked gain in body weight, beyond dietary and exercise habits, are obscure [Haslam DW, James WPT. *Obesity* Lancet. 2005;366:1197–1209; Yanovski SZ, Yanovski JA. Obesity. *N Engl J Med.* 2002:346:591–602]. DDX The *distribution of adipose tissue* assists diagnosis. Truncal obesity with thin limbs, round facies and a prominent hump of fat over the upper back are characteristic of Cushing disease, iatrogenic steroid use and, more recently, the use of protease inhibitors in the treatment of HIV-AIDS. Localized accumulations of fat are seen at sites of repetitive insulin injection (*lipodystrophy*). *Abdominal obesity* tends to be seen in men with mid-life weight gain ("beer belly").

KEY SYNDROME   Metabolic Syndrome

The clustering of specific conditions with an increased risk for diabetes and cardiovascular disease has been labeled the metabolic syndrome. The cause is unknown, but obesity and insulin resistance play large roles. The definitions have been evolving and a new consensus definition was published in 2005. The diagnosis is based upon increased waist circumference (ethnically specific, Table 4–3), plus any two of the following: elevated triglycerides (>150 mg/dL) or treatment of hypertriglyceridemia; reduced HDL-cholesterol (men <40 mg/dL, women <50 mg/dL) or treatment for low HDL; elevated BP (systolic ≥130 mm Hg, diastolic ≥85 mm Hg) or treatment of hypertension; elevated fasting plasma glucose (≥100 mg/dL) or previously diagnosed type 2 diabetes [Alberti KG, Zimmet .P, Shaw J. The metabolic syndrome—a new worldwide definition.

Table 4–3   Waist Circumference Norms by Ethnic Group*

	Waist Circumference (cm)	
Ethnic Group	Men	Women
European descent	≥94	≥80
South Asians	≥90	≥80
Chinese	≥90	≥80
Japanese	≥85	≥90
Ethnic South and Central Americans	Use South Asian recommendations	
Sub-Saharan Africans	Use European recommendations	

*Based upon *Lancet.* 2005;366:1059–1062.

Lancet. 2005;366:1059–1062; Eckel RH, Grundy SM, Zimmet PZ. The metabolic syndrome. *Lancet.* 2005;365:1415–1428].

Pain

Pain is a complex subject beyond the scope of this text. The reader is encouraged to explore pain texts to gain a more complete understanding of pain pathways and the pathophysiology of acute and chronic pain.

Pain can be roughly classified as *acute* or *chronic.* Acute pain is an event; chronic pain is a persistent experience. The mechanism of most acute pain is related to direct tissue injury, ischemia or release of inflammatory mediators. Adequate treatment of acute pain not only makes the patient more comfortable, but decreases the likelihood of progression to chronic pain. Unremitting pain leads to remodeling of the central pain pathways and facilitates the persistence of pain as a chronic pain syndrome. Chronic pain is frequently accompanied by functional impairment and depression. A recent review [Woolf CJ. Pain: Moving from symptom control toward mechanism-specific pharmacologic management. *Ann Intern Med.* 2004;140:441–451] is recommended to the reader. An excellent series of articles in the Lancet on the pathophysiology and management of pain will greatly increase your understanding of pain physiology, experience of pain by patients and how they report symptoms, and your management of acute and chronic pain: Loeser, JD, Melzack R. Pain: An overview. *Lancet.* 1999;353:1607–1609; Besson JM. The neurobiology of pain. *Lancet.* 1999;353:1610–1615; Portenoy RK, Lesage P. Management of cancer pain. *Lancet.* 1999;353:1695–1700; Turk DC, Okifuji A. Assessment of patients' reporting of pain: An integrated perspective. *Lancet.* 1999;353:1784–1788; Ashburn MA, Staats PS. Management of chronic pain. *Lancet.* 1999;353:1865–1869; Woolf CJ, Mannion RJ. Neuropathic pain: Aetiology, symptoms, mechanism, and management. *Lancet.* 1999;353:1959–1964; Carr DB, Goudas LC. Acute Pain. *Lancet.* 1999;353:2051–2058; Cervero F, Laird JMA. Visceral pain. *Lancet.* 1999;353:2145–2148.

Diagnostic Attributes of Pain

Pain directs attention to a specific anatomic region and often, although not always, indicates tissue injury. You can obtain diagnostic precision by eliciting the pain attributes using PQRST as a mnemonic explained below. The same questioning is useful for other symptoms.

P: Provocative and Palliative Factors

The occurrence of pain with specific movement implicates the structures displaced by the motion. The location may be confirmed by pressure eliciting tenderness. Conversely, if resting a part relieves the pain; those tissues are likely the source of the pain. Therapeutic interventions can be used diagnostically: chest pain relieved by nitroglycerin suggests angina pectoris while relief by antacids suggests acid-peptic disease.

Q: Quality

The quality of pain also assists the clinician in reaching a diagnosis. Somatic pain, arising from the skin, skeletal muscles, bones, ligaments, tendons, and soft tissues, is usually described as sharp or stabbing and is well localized; the patient can point with one finger to the site of maximal pain. Visceral pain, arising from ischemia; inflammation; or other injury to the viscera in the body cavities is poorly localized, the patient can only indicate a general area or areas of the pain, often described as deep or inside. It is aching, pressing, or squeezing in quality, and often accompanied by autonomic symptoms such as nausea, vomiting, diaphoresis, and intestinal ileus. Neuropathic pain arises from damage to the nerve cells themselves, rather than to other tissues; it is usually described as a burning or hot pain in the distribution of the affected nerve or nerves. These distinctions are far from exact, but are clinically useful. Shooting pain usually results from irritation of a nerve trunk. Displacement of inflamed tissues surrounding a pulsating artery causes throbbing pain.

R: Region and Referral

Pain is usually confined to one or more anatomic regions to which the patient can point. Because each region comprises a separate group of tissues and organs, the diagnostic significance of pain is conveniently discussed in this book in the chapters dealing with the examination of each region. Pain is also referred into nearby anatomic areas following developmental and neurological organizational principles. Nerve injury will refer pain, and often paresthesias, in the distribution of the dermatome(s) subserved by the sensory components of the nerve (page 700ff). Muscular pain is referred towards muscles innervated by or derived from the same spinal segments (the myotome). Similarly, skeletal pain is radiated to structures innervated by or derived from the same spinal segments (the sclerotome).

S: Severity

Tests with a painful stimulus of measured intensity indicate that individuals have remarkably similar thresholds for pain. However, individuals vary greatly in their reactions to pain and fear may aggravate pain. Assessment of pain severity is mandated by Medicare at each visit. Pain is a subjective sensation so the patient's statement should be accepted without debate. It is useful to calibrate pain on a 0 to 10 scale: with 0 being no pain and 10 being the worst possible pain. The pain scores are used to follow pain progression and the response to its management. It is useful to communicate the caregiver's goals for pain relief: "We should be able to reduce your pain to a 3/10." Intense pain is usually accompanied by physiologic signs such a look of apprehension, bodily postures (protecting a limb, abdominal guarding), sweating, pallor, pupillary dilatation, hypertension, tachycardia, nausea and vomiting.

T: Timing

The timing and duration of pain often indicates its cause. Pain that is insidious in onset and relentlessly progressive without palliative features suggests cancer pain or increasing pressure in a closed space (e.g., intracranial pressure, toothache). Intermittent episodic pain suggests an underlying predisposition with specific episodic events (e.g., passing kidney stones, intermittent intestinal obstruction). A single episode may be short or prolonged, steady, worsening or relenting in waves. Daytime pain is common to conditions in which muscle movement causes pain; daytime relief suggests muscle or joint stiffening, which improves with motion. Nighttime pain is likely to result when muscle spasm relaxes its protection of tender tissues or the absence of competing sensory inputs allows the persistent pain of an unremitting process to become predominant; this is typical of bone pain.

Pain Syndromes

Site-specific pain is discussed in each of the chapters dealing with a specific region of the body.

> **KEY SYNDROME** **Complex Regional Pain Syndrome (CRPS)—Reflex Sympathetic Dystrophy, Causalgia**

Minor injury initiates a complex series of spinal and CNS responses that result in altered autonomic function and pain perception. CRPS occurs after surgery or injury to an extremity, especially of the hands or feet. The pain may involve an entire anatomic region and can occur days to weeks after the event. The patient usually describes the pain as constant, burning, aching, and/or throbbing and it is disproportionate to the injury. Examination may reveal hyperalgesia, hyperesthesia, edema, erythema, and changes in skin temperature. Progression leads to vascular changes, including cyanosis and mottling, atrophy of skin, muscle and subcutaneous tissue, contractures, and altered sweating. Two forms are recognized: CRPS type 1 occurs without nerve injury and CRPS type 2 (causalgia) is associated with major nerve injury. Early recognition and treatment is necessary [Kaplan PE. Complex regional pain syndrome. *Lancet.* 2001;358:1552].

> **KEY SYNDROME** **Postherpetic Neuralgia**

Reactivation of latent varicella-zoster virus in the dorsal root ganglia produces clinical herpes zoster and can result in a subacute or chronic painful neuropathy. Most patients with acute herpes zoster have intense pain which abates over a period of weeks to months. The pain is sometimes very severe, burning in quality, and associated with severe allodynia where the slightest disturbance of the skin induces lancinating pain. Older adults are at increased risk for persistent postherpetic neuralgia.

Non-Regional Systems and Diseases

Several body systems are located diffusely or within multiple regions of the body. As a result, the clinician assesses these systems continuously throughout the examination to a greater extent than the more localized systems. Although disease predominately arising in a single body system can present with constitutional symptoms, this is generally more true of the systems discussed here. It is important to keep these systems in mind throughout the examination process. Diseases and syndromes within these systems are exemplars of the need to integrate the findings from all parts of the diagnostic examination into your hypothesis generating process. This concept is reflected in the century-old saying that "he who knows syphilis, knows medicine." This is analogous to knowing human immunodeficiency virus (HIV)/acquired immunodeficiency syndrome (AIDS) today.

Constitutional Symptoms

Constitutional symptoms are those that relate to the body or person as a whole, generally excluding psychological symptoms. Many of these symptoms are very nonspecific, but may be clues to serious systemic illness. Because of their nonspecific nature, they must be combined with other physical examination findings and laboratory tests before a specific set of physiologic and diagnostic hypotheses can be generated. It may, however, be possible to posit a class or two of general physiologic processes. For instance, the middle-aged patient who presents with anorexia, weight loss, and night sweats suggests the presence of neoplastic or chronic infectious or inflammatory disease, or possibly Addison disease.

KEY SYMPTOM Fatigue

Fatigue is a nonspecific symptom that can result from serious organic disease, neuropsychiatric disease, or deconditioning. Patients describe decreased energy, decreased endurance for normal activities, and a feeling of increased effort in usual tasks. It is important to distinguish fatigue from shortness of breath and excessive sleepiness. Fatigue can complicate any chronic disease or medical condition; especially common causes are anemia, hypothyroidism, and hyperthyroidism, autoimmune and neurologic disorders [Chaudhuri A, Behan PO. Fatigue in neurological disorders. *Lancet*. 2004;363:978–988]. **DDX:** When a complete history, physical examination, and screening laboratory evaluation do not find a specific explanation consider deconditioning, depression, sleep disorders, and chronic fatigue syndrome.

✔ *FATIGUE—CLINICAL OCCURRENCE:* These are examples only. *Congenital* muscular dystrophies, mitochondrial myopathy; *Endocrine* hypothyroidism, hyperthyroidism, Addison disease, hypopituitarism, hypoparathyroidism, hypogonadism; *Idiopathic* chronic fatigue syndrome, inclusion body myositis; *Infectious* tuberculosis, infectious mononucleosis, hepatitis, following other viral illnesses, hookworm infestation, HIV infection; *Inflammatory/Immune* systemic lupus erythematosis (SLE), rheumatoid arthritis (RA), polymyositis, dermatomyositis, vasculitis; *Metabolic/Toxic* hypokalemia, hypocalcemia, hypomagnesemia, hyponatremia, anemia, uremia, hypoglycemia, congestive heart failure, drugs (e.g., β-blockers, sedatives, anticholinergics), alcohol; *Neoplastic* acute and chronic leukemia, myelodysplastic syndromes, myeloproliferative syndromes, solid tumors, lymphomas; *Neurologic* myasthenia gravis, amyotrophic lateral sclerosis, multiple sclerosis, dementia; *Psychosocial* disordered sleep, depression, deconditioning, overwork and overtraining, chronic anxiety; *Vascular* claudication, strokes.

KEY SYNDROME   Chronic Fatigue Syndrome

The cause is unknown, but frequently follows a viral infection. This usually is seen in young to middle-aged adults. The case definition requires new onset of fatigue not related to exertion and not relieved by rest, which results in substantial limitation of previous occupational, educational, social, or personal activities. Four or more of the following should have started with the fatigue and recur or persist for at least 6 months: impaired short-term memory, sore throat, tender cervical or axillary nodes, muscle pain, polyarthralgias without arthritis, headaches, unrefreshing sleep, and postexertional malaise that lasts longer than 24 hours [Fukuda K, Straus SE, Hickie I, et al. The chronic fatigue syndrome. *Ann Intern Med.* 1994;121:953–959].

KEY SYMPTOM   Disturbance of Appetite

Appetite is controlled by the hypothalamus under the influence of hormones (insulin, cortisol, leptin, grehlin, incretins-GLP-1), metabolites, neural afferents (especially from the viscera via the vagus), and cortical inputs reflecting emotional and cognitive state. Change in appetite can result from a disturbance in any of these systems.

Anorexia.   A lack of appetite for food is anorexia. Although anorexia lacks specificity, it is sensitive to the presence and severity of many diseases; few patients with significant illness have normal appetites. When the caloric expenditure is unchanged, anorexia results in weight loss.

✔ *ANOREXIA—CLINICAL OCCURRENCE:* *Endocrine* adrenal insufficiency, hypothyroidism, hypopituitary; *Inflammatory/Immune* inflammatory cytokines (interleukin-1, tumor necrosis factor) suppress appetite, so any systemic inflammatory process can depress appetite; *Infectious* hepatitis, any acute or chronic systemic infection; *Metabolic/Toxic* uremia, advanced liver disease, amphetamines, and stimulants; *Mechanical/Traumatic* gastrointestinal obstruction, dysphagia, odynophagia; *Neoplastic* malignancy, especially when metastatic to the liver or regionally advanced; *Neurologic* dementia, delirium, anosmia;   *Psychosocial*   depression, poverty, social isolation, abuse, school problems, anorexia and bulimia nervosa;   *Vascular*   vasculitis, stroke.

Polyphagia.   Increased or insatiable appetite is uncommon and causes weight gain if caloric intake exceeds losses, weight loss when losses exceed intake, or no change in weight when intake and losses remain in balance. It is important to remember that losses include caloric expenditures, ingested calories not absorbed because of vomiting, maldigestion, or malabsorption, and calories absorbed but lost to the body's economy (glucosuria, proteinuria).   *Clinical Occurrence: Endocrine*   diabetes, hyperthyroidism, insulinoma;   *Metabolic/Toxic*   malnutrition (protein, essential fatty acids) iron deficiency;   *Neoplastic*   insulinoma;   *Neurologic*   hypothalamic lesions;   *Psychosocial*   bulimia, binge eating syndrome, night eating syndrome.

> **KEY SYMPTOM**   Abnormal Eating Behaviors

Behaviors associated with the selection, acquisition, preparation, serving, and eating of food are culturally determined and socially important. Changes in food-related behaviors suggest medical, psychiatric, and social problems. See Chapter 15, pages 774 and 781.   *Clinical Occurrence: Endocrine*   pregnancy;   *Idiopathic*   anosmia;   *Infectious*   hookworm infestation;   *Metabolic/Toxic*   iron deficiency, trace metal deficiency;   *Neoplastic*   food preferences and taste are frequently disturbed with malignant disease, especially with liver involvement;   *Psychosocial*   psychosis, delusions.

Pica.   An unusual craving or appetite leading to the ingestion of unnatural foods such as clay, chips of old paint, plaster, laundry starch (with pregnancy), and ice chips (with iron deficiency). The symptoms depend upon the substance eaten: ingestion of paint may cause lead poisoning, while ingestion of laundry starch may cause obesity and hypochromic anemia.

> **KEY SYMPTOM**   Thirst

Thirst is triggered by water depletion (increased osmolarity and serum sodium concentration) or moderate to severe extracellular volume depletion; normally, both produce increased release of antidiuretic hormone (ADH) leading to increased water intake and increased water absorption by the collecting ducts. A defect in the production of ADH or the response of the renal collecting duct to ADH leads to water loss and persistent thirst. The sudden development of thirst is a reliable indication of dehydration when it appears with hemorrhage, traumatic shock, the polyuria of diabetes insipidus, and in some cases of severe electrolyte or fluid imbalance. It is important to distinguish between isolated water loss (increased osmolarity with normal extracellular volume), loss of extracellular saline alone (normal osmolarity, but decreased volume), and combined losses of saline and water (increased osmolarity and decreased volume).   *Clinical Occurrence:*   Diabetes insipidus (central or nephrogenic), diabetes mellitus, hemorrhage, hypotension of any cause, overuse of diuretics, dry mouth of any cause, psychogenic polydipsia.

Diabetes Insipidus.   Decreased production of ADH (vasopressin) or unresponsiveness of the renal collecting duct to ADH results in an excessive, constant water diuresis. Patients present with an unquenchable thirst, polydipsia, and polyuria with a low urine specific gravity.

The Immune System

To understand the disorders of the immune system and how they present, it is essential to understand the normal physiology of the immune system. The reader should consult *Harrison's Principles of Internal Medicine*, 17th edition for a complete discussion of the subject [Kasper DL, Braunwald E, Fauci AS, et al., eds. *Harrison's Principles of Internal Medicine*. 17th ed. New York, NY: McGraw-Hill; 2008]. For practical purposes, the immune system is thought of as having an innate, nonspecific component, and an adaptive component. The latter has evolved more recently. Disorders of innate immunity are often quantitative or qualitative disorders of neutrophils and macrophages. These are discussed under the hematopoietic system. Here, we are concerned with disorders of adaptive immunity.

Serious congenital disorders of the immune system present in infancy or childhood and are beyond the scope of this book. See *Harrison's Principles of Internal Medicine* for a complete discussion of these topics. Acquired immunologic deficiencies can present to the clinician at any age. Immunologic disorders are conceptually divided into defects in antibody production (humoral immunity) and defects in cell-mediated immunity. Because humoral immunity requires functioning T cells for proper regulation, defects in cell-mediated immunity are often accompanied by impaired humoral immunity.

Patients with altered immune systems present with a variety of illnesses. Most commonly, they have infections, neoplastic diseases, or autoimmune illnesses. Combinations of these disorders are not uncommon. This can be the result of a common primary problem (e.g., immunosuppressive drugs), or the cause of the immune disturbance may be the presence of a neoplastic disease (e.g., multiple myeloma), severe autoimmune disease (e.g., SLE), or a chronic infection (e.g., HIV/AIDS, tuberculosis). Treatment of many neoplastic and autoimmune disorders is highly immunosuppressive. In practice, iatrogenic immunosuppression is the most common form of immunodeficiency encountered.

Defects in humoral immunity are most commonly manifest by infections with organisms that require opsonizing antibodies for recognition and elimination. These are the encapsulated bacteria such as *Streptococcus pneumonia*, *Haemophilus influenzae*, *Neisseria meningitidis* and gonorrhea. Because the spleen is the major site of clearance of opsonized bacteria from the blood, overwhelming infections with these organisms are more likely in patients with normal immune systems following splenectomy. All patients in whom splenectomy is contemplated should be immunized for these organisms, before the procedure if possible.

Patients with defects in cellular immunity have an increased risk for neoplastic diseases and infections with intracellular pathogens (e.g., tuberculosis) and opportunistic bacterial, viral, and fungal organisms.

The major autoimmune diseases (SLE, RA, vasculitis syndromes, Addison disease, etc.) are discussed elsewhere in this text. It is important to recall that autoimmune endocrine deficiency is common and may present as an autoimmune polyglandular syndrome with multiple insufficiencies.

Two Common Syndromes

> **KEY SYNDROME   HIV and AIDS (Acquired Immunodeficiency Syndrome)**

Infection with HIV leads to progressive destruction of CD4 cells and impaired cellular and humoral immunity. AIDS is defined by <200 CD4 cells/mm^3 or the presence of an AIDS-defining illness, either opportunistic infection or AIDS-associated neoplasm. Risk factors for infection are unprotected sexual intercourse (male homosexuals and heterosexuals of both sexes) intravenous drug use with needle sharing, contact with infected blood or body fluids, and vertical transmission from mother to newborn. Opportunistic infections include parasites (*Pneumocystis pneumonia*, toxoplasmosis encephalitis, and cryptosporidium enteritis), viruses (cytomegalovirus, Epstein-Barr virus, herpes simplex, herpes zoster, and human herpes type 8, the cause of Kaposi sarcoma), fungi (candidiasis, cryptococcal meningitis, coccidioidomycosis, histoplasmosis, aspergillosis), bacteria (salmonellosis, *Streptococcus pneumoniae, H. influenzae*), mycobacteria (*Mycobacterium tuberculosis, M. avium* complex), listeriosis, *Treponema pallidum*, and nocardiosis. ***Symptoms and Signs.*** Acute HIV infection presents a nonspecific viral syndrome often with an exanthem; it may be mistaken for Ebstein-Barr virus infection. After a latent period of several years, the patient develops an immunosuppressive syndrome manifest as lymphadenopathy, weight loss, dermatitis, opportunistic infections, and malignancies (e.g., Kaposi sarcoma, central nervous system lymphoma, human papillomavirus-associated anal and cervical carcinomas).

> **KEY SYNDROME   Common Variable Immunodeficiency**

An acquired defect in the maturation of B cells leads to decreased immunoglobulin production and decreased circulating levels of immunoglobulin IgG, IgM, and/or IgA. Patients are usually adults who present with chronic and recurrent infections of the upper and lower airways, especially sinusitis and pneumonia. They have an increased risk of developing non-Hodgkin lymphomas.

The Lymphatic System

The lymph vessels and their nodes are part of a discontinuous circulation whose efferent loop is the arteries, arterioles, and capillaries of the vascular system, and whose afferent loop is the network of lymphatic vessels that drain centrally through the regional lymph nodes to the thoracic duct, which empties into the left subclavian vein. The lymphatic system plays a major role in the recognition and response to foreign antigens. Macrophages and Langerhans cells from the periphery (antigen-presenting cells) migrate from peripheral sites with processed antigen, which they present to T cells and B cells in the lymph nodes. T cells circulate from the capillary circulation to the lymphatics and nodes and back into the circulation until they are presented with an antigen specific to their T-cell receptor; recognition leads to activation and proliferation, generating an immune response. Disorders of the lymphatics produce only three physical signs: palpable lymph nodes, red streaks in the skin from superficial lymphangitis, and lymphedema. Palpable lymph nodes indicate lymphadenopathy.

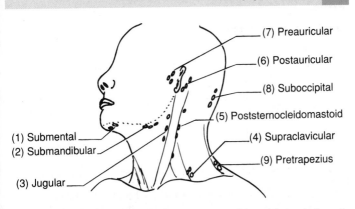

Fig. 5–1 *Superficial Lymph Nodes of the Neck.* *Palpation of the neck for lymphadenopathy is accurate when the region of each group of nodes is examined in systematic fashion. The drawing contains a numbered scheme for examining nine groups of nodes in sequence.*

Examination of the Lymph Nodes

Enlarged nodes may be visible by inspection, especially with oblique light. Examination is primarily by palpation. The following characteristics of palpable lymph nodes should be noted: number, size, consistency, mobility, tenderness, warmth, and whether they are discrete or matted together. Procedures for examining the major lymph node beds are described below, but all lymph node-bearing areas should be palpated when searching for generalized lymphadenopathy. The spleen should always be examined as part of the examination of the lymphatic system.

Palpation of the Cervical Lymph Nodes. Seat the patient in a chair, stand behind the patient to palpate the neck with your fingertips. Examine, in sequence, the various lymph node sites (Fig. 5–1): (1) submental, under the chin in the midline and on either side, (2) submandibular, under the jaw near its angle, (3) jugular (anterior triangle), along the anterior border of the sternocleidomastoid, (4) supraclavicular, behind the midportion of the clavicle, (5) poststernocleidomastoid (posterior triangle), behind the posterior border of the upper half of the sternocleidomastoid, (6) postauricular, behind the pinna on the mastoid process, (7) preauricular, slightly in front of the tragus of the pinna, (8) suboccipital, in the midline under the occiput and to either side, and (9) pretrapezius, in front of the upper border of the trapezius. When an enlarged lymph node is found, carefully examine the drainage region for a primary lesion: anterior cervical triangle—the anterior third of the scalp and face, posterior cervical triangle and occiput—the posterior two-thirds of the scalp.

Palpation of Axillary, Infraclavicular and Supraclavicular Lymph Nodes. Examine the sitting patient by palpating the left axilla with your right hand and vise versa (Fig. 5–2A). Relax the patient's left arm and axillary muscles by holding the left wrist with your left hand and elevating the upper arm toward the chest wall. Place your hand in the axilla with the fingers together and the palm toward the chest wall. Point your fingers obliquely toward the apex of the axilla. Now have the patient rest their left hand on your examining right arm, while your left hand supports the shoulder. Gently, but firmly, rake the pulps of your examining

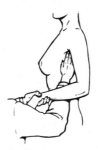
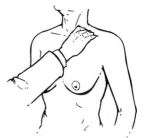

A. Search for axillary nodes B. Search for supraclavicular nodes

Fig. 5–2 *Palpation of Axillary and Supraclavicular Lymph Nodes.* **A.** *Axilla: In palpation of the left axilla, the examiner slides his right hand toward the axillary apex, with palm toward the chest wall and approximated fingers extended so the pulps feel the structures on the thoracic cage. With his left hand, he directs the patient's upper arm close to the chest to relax the axillary muscles. He asks the patient to rest her arm on his examining arm and he supports her shoulder with his left hand. The positions are reversed to examine the right side.* **B.** *Supraclavicular Fossa.*

fingers along the thoracic cage to feel for enlarged lymph nodes. Note the size, location, consistency, and mobility of the nodes. The central group of nodes occurs near the middle of the thoracic wall of the axilla (Fig. 5–3). The lateral axillary group is located near the upper part of the humerus and is best demonstrated by having the patient's arm elevated so that you can feel along the axillary vein. With the patient's arm still elevated, feel along beneath the lateral edge of the pectoralis major muscle for the pectoral group. Palpate the subscapular nodes from behind the patient with the arm raised, palpating with the left hand under the anterior edge of the latissimus dorsi muscle. Palpate under the clavicle for the infraclavicular group. Enlargement in the supraclavicular group is sought by feeling the soft tissues above and behind the clavicle (Fig. 5–2B).

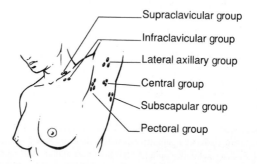

Supraclavicular group
Infraclavicular group
Lateral axillary group
Central group
Subscapular group
Pectoral group

Fig. 5–3 *Axillary Lymph Node Groups.* *Note that the lateral axillary group is on the inner aspect of the upper arm, near the axillary vein. The subscapular group lies deep to the anterior edge of the latissimus dorsi muscle. The pectoral group is behind the lateral edge of the pectoralis major muscle.*

Palpation of the Inguinal Nodes.   Palpate at and just below the inguinal ligament then distally along the course of the greater saphenous vein.

Lymph Node Signs

> **KEY SIGN**   **Lymphadenopathy**

Lymph node enlargement results from a stimulated regional or systemic immune response, direct infection of the node, which can lead to suppuration, deposition of intracellular or extracellular material, or infiltration with neoplastic cells. Physical examination of the nodes should describe their distribution, number in each location, size, mobility, consistency (fluctuant, soft, firm, hard), surface (smooth, irregular), and the presence of tenderness, warmth, and/or sinus tracts draining to the skin. A meticulous examination of the skin and soft tissues of the involved region is mandatory when looking for signs of regional inflammation, infection, or neoplasm. Pain and tenderness suggests inflammation and/or infection, while painless lymphadenopathy is more likely to be neoplastic. Fluctuant nodes suggest suppuration from bacterial, mycobacterial, or fungal infection. Fixation of the nodes to underlying tissue is most common with metastatic carcinoma, but may occur with chronic inflammation. Matting together of nodes suggests lymphoma or chronic inflammation. Lymph node enlargement may be the presenting sign in many diseases. Lymphadenopathy, which is widespread, involving several lymph node regions both above and below the diaphragm, suggests a widespread systemic disease.

Lymph Node Syndromes

> **KEY SIGN**   **Generalized Lymphadenopathy**

Lymphadenopathy occuring simultaneously in multiple lymphatic beds, especially above and below the diaphragm, suggests a systemic process, usually infectious, inflammatory or neoplastic.

CLINICAL OCCURRENCE: *Congenital*   Niemann-Pick disease, Gaucher disease; *Idiopathic*   sarcoidosis, sinus histiocytosis with massive lymphadenopathy (Rosai-Dorfman disease); *Inflammatory/Immune*   RA, Still disease, dermatomyositis, SLE, amyloidosis, serum sickness, drug allergy, graft-vs-host disease, hyper IgM syndrome; *Infectious bacterial*   scarlet fever, brucellosis, Lyme disease, secondary syphilis, tularemia, bubonic plague, cat-scratch fever, Whipple disease, melioidosis, scrub typhus; *mycobacterial*   tuberculosi, atypical mycobacteria; *viral*   rubella, rubeola, infectious mononucleosis, HIV; *protozoal*   African trypanosomiasis, Chagas disease, kala-azar, toxoplasmosis; *fungal*   sporotrichosis; *helminths*   filariasis; *ectoparasites*   scabies; *Metabolic/Toxic*   drugs (e.g., diphenylhydantoin), berylliosis, silicosis; *Neoplastic*   Hodgkin disease, non-Hodgkin lymphoma, chronic lymphocytic leukemia, systemic mastocytosis, metastatic carcinomas.

> **KEY DISEASE**   **Non-Hodgkin Lymphoma**

Clonal proliferation, usually of B-lymphocytes at a specific stage of maturation and with specific surface markers identifies these disorders. Patients may present

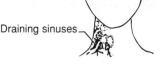

Draining sinuses

A. Cervical lymphadenopathy
of Hodgkin disease

B. Cervical lymphadenopathy
of tuberculosis

Fig. 5–4 *Cervical Lymphadenopathy.* ***A.*** *Hodgkin Disease: There is no specific pattern of involvement of the nodes. The neck is frequently affected first, often unilaterally. The nodes are large, firm, discrete, nontender, and nonsuppurative.* ***B.*** *Tuberculosis: One finds a matted mass of nontender lymph nodes. The nodes are firm, but some have suppurated and formed draining sinuses.*

with systemic symptoms of fever, weight loss, and night sweats, with abdominal pain or fullness, or with palpable lymphadenopathy. These diseases involve multiple sites and may arise in nonlymphoid tissue such as the lung, stomach, intestine, and central nervous system. Clinically, they are separated into high-grade disease that tends to be rapidly progressive, but potentially curable, and low-grade disease for which curative therapy is not generally available.

KEY DISEASE   Hodgkin Disease

This is a malignant disease of B cells of unknown etiology that spreads to contiguous lymph node beds, the spleen, liver, and bone marrow. There are two age peaks, in the third and eighth decades. Symptoms include pruritus, painless enlargement of lymph nodes, abdominal pain, and occasionally periodic or continuous fever (Pel-Epstein fever, page 53) and cachexia. Although the disease may involve any lymph nodes in the body, only a single group is affected frequently, most often in the neck (Fig. 5–4A). The lymph nodes may enlarge rapidly over 1 to 3 weeks, or slowly over a few months; the enlargement is much greater than in acute adenitis. The nodes are resilient or rubbery. Hepatomegaly and splenomegaly may accompany or precede the diagnosis. A thorough examination of all accessible nodes is required. DDX: The ingestion of alcohol may rarely produce severe pain in the nodes so severe and predictable that patients voluntarily abstain from alcohol. Lymphadenopathy in non-Hodgkin lymphoma is usually generalized and rarely confined to the neck.

KEY DISEASE   Chronic Lymphocytic Leukemia

A clonal proliferation of mature lymphocytes (90% B cell, 10% T cell) leads to infiltration of the lymph nodes and bone marrow with progressive cytopenias and impaired humoral or cellular immunity. Patients are often asymptomatic until relatively late in the disease. They present with lymphadenopathy and progress to anemia, neutropenia and thrombocytopenia with recurrent infections. Death usually results from infection or hemorrhage.

> **KEY DISEASE   HIV Infection**

See page 92.

> **KEY SYNDROME   Lymphedema**

Obstruction of lymphatic drainage by whatever cause leads to the accumulation of interstitial fluid with a high protein content. Massive enlargement of the part may occur and fibrosis develops over time. Patients present with progressive painless swelling of a body part. Common causes are surgical, irradiation or traumatic injury to lymphatics, and neoplastic obstruction. Longstanding lymphedema is associated with an increased risk for lymphangiosarcoma. DDX: The edema may pit at first, but characteristically is not pitting.

Filariasis (Wuchereriasis). Lymphatic infestation with larvae of *Wuchereria bancrofti* or *Brugia malayi* follows the bite of an infected mosquito. There is inflammation and later scarring with lymphatic obstruction, and lymphedema. Headache, photophobia, vertigo, fatigue, low-grade fever, and myalgia are common symptoms. Signs include conjunctivitis, orchitis, lymphangitis, and lymphadenopathy acutely; later, obstruction of lymphatic and venous drainage with edema, hydrocele, elephantiasis of breasts, scrotum, vulva, or legs.

Important Regional Lymph Node Syndromes

More limited, regional lymphadenopathy may be an early sign of a generalized disease, or might represent regional or local disease. Two specific signs involving regional lymphadenopathy are worthy of special consideration:

> **KEY SIGN   Inoculation Lesion with Regional Lymphadenopathy**

See also, Chapter 6, Ulceroglandular syndromes, page 162. Cutaneous inoculation of infectious agents is followed by spread through the subcutaneous lymphatics, with varying degrees of inflammation and induration, to regional lymph nodes. The cutaneous inoculation site may show minimal signs, or may be marked by local inflammation, ulceration, and/or necrosis with eschar formation. A careful history, including the time of year and occupational or avocational exposures, is essential to an accurate and timely diagnosis.

✔ *INOCULATION LESION WITH REGIONAL LYMPHADENOPATHY—CLINICAL OCCUR-RENCE: Infectious bacterial* streptococcal infections, syphilitic chancre, anthrax, erysipeloid, tularemia (ulceroglandular type), bubonic plague, rat-bite fever, cat-scratch disease, nocardia, actinomycosis, glanders; ***mycobacterial*** inoculation tuberculosis, atypical mycobacteria; ***fungal*** sporotrichosis; ***rickettsial*** scrub typhus, boutonneuse fever, South African tick fever, Kenya typhus, rickettsialpox; ***viral*** herpes simplex; ***helminths*** filariasis, trypanosomiasis, leishmaniasis; ***Neoplastic*** melanoma, squamous cell carcinoma, lymphangioleiomyomas.

Nodular lymphangitis. See Chapter 6, page 163.

> **KEY SYNDROME** Suppurative Lymphadenopathy

The following diseases commonly cause suppuration of lymph nodes: strepto-coccal infections, staphylococcal infections, tuberculosis (bovine type) actino-myces lymphogranuloma venereum, coccidioidomycosis, anthrax, cat-scratch fever, sporotrichosis, plague, and tularemia.

Syndromes of Specific Regional Lymph Nodes

Infectious, inflammatory, or neoplastic lesions within the regional drainage give rise to regional lymphadenopathy. Since each of the causes of generalized lym-phadenopathy may cause regional adenopthy, we will avoid repetition by only mentioning singular or unusual entities specific to a given region as etiology in this section:

The Head and Jaw

Suboccipital nodes. *Location:* Midway between the external occipital protu-berance and the mastoid process (see Fig. 5–1), near the great occipital nerve. *Drainage:* Afferents from back of scalp and head; efferents to deep cervi-cal nodes. *Symptoms:* Impingement of the enlarged nodes on the great oc-cipital nerve may produce headache. *Clinical Occurrence:* Ringworm of the scalp, pediculosis capitis, seborrheic dermatis, secondary syphilis and metastatic cancer.

Postauricular nodes. *Location:* On mastoid process and at insertion of stern-ocleidomastoid muscle, behind pinna (see Fig. 5–1). *Drainage:* Afferents from external acoustic meatus, back of pinna, temporal scalp, efferents to superior cer-vical nodes. *Symptoms:* Mastoid tenderness simulating mastoiditis. *Clinical Occurrence:* Bacterial or herpetic infection of the acoustic meatus, rubella (not rubeola), leishmaniasis.

Preauricular nodes. *Location:* In front of the tragus of the external ear (see Fig. 5–1). *Drainage:* Afferents from lateral portions of eyelids and their palpebral conjunctivae, skin of temporal region, external acoustic meatus, ante-rior surface of pinna. *Clinical Occurrence:* Ulcerating basal cell carcinoma, epithelioma, chancre of face, erysipelas, ophthalmic herpes zoster, rubella, trachoma. *Ocular-Glandular Syndrome:* Gonorrheal ophthalmia, tuberculo-sis, syphilis, sporotrichosis, glanders, chancroid, epidemic keratoconjunctivitis, adenoidal-pharyngeal-conjunctival virus, Leptothrix infection, lymphogranu-loma venereum, tularemia, cat-scratch fever, Chagas disease.

Mandibular nodes. *Location:* Under the mandible (see Fig. 5–1). *Drainage:* Afferents from tongue, submandibular gland, submental nodes, medial con-junctivae, mucosa of lips and mouth; efferents to superficial and deep jugular nodes.

Submental nodes. *Location:* In midline under apex of mandibular junc-tion (see Fig. 5–1). *Drainage:* Afferents from central lower lip, floor of mouth, tip of tongue, skin of cheek; efferents to mandibular nodes, deep jugular nodes.

The Neck

> ### KEY SIGN Acute Cervical Lymphadenopathy—Localized Lymphadenitis

Infections of the scalp, face, mouth, teeth, pharynx, or ear cause localized lymphadenitis of the neck in the particular group of nodes draining the involved region. Included in localized lesions is chancre of the face with its regional lymphadenitis. Cervical adenopathy is also common in erythema nodosum, although the subcutaneous lesions are almost always limited to the legs. If the patient is toxic and tenderness is severe, consider Lemierre's syndrome (page 276).

> ### KEY DISEASE Chronic Localized Cervical Lymphadenopathy: Tuberculosis (Scrofula)

Usually the disease is caused by the bovine strain of tubercle bacilli, although human strains have been implicated. The disease has a predilection for the cervical lymph nodes. The nodes are large, multiple, and nontender. Classically, they are matted together, but this is often difficult to determine by palpation (Fig. 5–4B). Frequently the nodes suppurate and form indolent sinus tracts. Extensive scarring of the neck often results.

> ### KEY DISEASE Chronic Localized Cervical Lymphadenopathy: Kikuchi Lymphadenitis

This unusual syndrome affects young women who present with cervical lymphadenopathy. It is benign, but often confused with other entities [Dorfman RF, Berry GJ. Kikuchi's histiocytic necrotizing lymphadenitis: An analysis of 108 cases with emphasis on differential diagnosis. *Semin Diagn Pathol*. 1988;5:329–345].

> ### KEY DISEASE Chronic Localized Cervical Lymphadenopathy: Actinomycosis

Infection by bacteria of the genus Actinomyces from the oral flora involve the mouth, face, and cervical lymph nodes. The infection crosses tissue planes. The nodes are prone to suppurate, forming sinuses with a bright-red hue. The pus contains sulfur granules, 1 to 2 mm in diameter.

> ### KEY SIGN Subacute Localized Cervical Lymphadenopathy: Metastatic Carcinoma

Asymptomatic cancers of the head and neck frequently present as metastases in a cervical lymph node. The nodes are usually stony hard, nontender, and nonsuppurative. Epidermoid carcinoma predominates. With anterior triangle involvement, primary malignancies are found in the upper aerodigestive tract, including the maxillary sinus, oral cavity, tongue, tonsil, hypopharynx, and larynx. In the submental region, metastases occur from primary neoplasms in the lower lip, anterior tongue, and floor of the mouth. In the posterior triangle, the nasopharynx and scalp are common sites of origin. Carefully examine suspicious areas and the remainder of the upper aerodigestive tract. Never surgically biopsy a solitary cervical lymph node suspicious for metastatic cancer. Violation of the tissue planes of the neck may preclude surgical cure. Always refer such a patient for direct examination of the aerodigestive tract by an experienced observer to search for the primary tumor.

Jugular nodes. *Location:* Along anterior border of the sternocleidomastoid, from angle of mandible to clavicle (see Fig. 5–1). *Drainage:* Afferents from tongue except apex, tonsil, pinna, parotid gland; efferents to deep jugular nodes. *Clinical Occurrence:* Infection or neoplasm of the tonsils and oral cavity; thyroid cancer.

Poststernocleidomastoid nodes. *Location:* Along the posterior border of the sternocleidomastoid muscle are the posterior cervical and inferior deep cervical nodes which are not readily separated clinically (see Fig. 5–1). *Drainage:* Afferents from the scalp and neck, upper cervical nodes, axillary nodes, skin of arms and pectoral region, surface of the thorax. *Clinical Occurrence:* Trypanosomiasis (Winterbottom sign).

Scalene nodes. *Location:* These are part of the inferior deep cervical nodes that lie deep in the supraclavicular fossa behind the sternocleidomastoid muscle. *Drainage:* Afferents from the thorax. Although not palpable, they are easily biopsied. *Clinical Occurrence:* Intrathoracic granulomatous disease and neoplasms.

The Chest, Axilla, and Arms

Supraclavicular nodes. *Location:* Part of the inferior deep cervical chain, behind the origin of the sternocleidomastoid muscle (see Fig. 5–1). *Drainage:* Afferents from head, arm, chest wall, breast. *Clinical Occurrence:* Granulomas and neoplasms of the lung and esophagus on the right and left; in addition on the left, neoplasms in the abdomen.

KEY SIGN   Sentinel Node (Virchow Node)

The node is the site of metastasis via the thoracic duct from a primary carcinoma in the upper abdomen. There is enlargement of a single lymph node, usually in the left supraclavicular group and frequently behind the clavicular head of the left sternocleidomastoid. It is often so deep that it escapes casual examination. A purposeful search requires the patient to be erect; examine behind the muscle head while facing the patient. The node may be better appreciated as the patient performs a Valsalva. When a primary carcinoma is found in the abdomen, demonstration of the sentinel node is proof of distant metastasis. Breast and lung cancers spread to the supraclavicular nodes, usually more laterally in the supraclavicular fossa.

Axillary nodes. *Location:* Five groups lie on the medial aspect of the humerus, the axillary border of the scapula, and the lateral border of the pectoralis major (see Fig. 5–3). *Drainage:* Afferents from the upper limb, the thoracic wall, and the breast. In women, enlarged axillary nodes on the thoracic wall must be distinguished from axillary tail of the breast. *Clinical Occurrence:* Small mobile axillary nodes are common in normal individuals.

Epitrochlear nodes. *Location:* Approximately 3 cm proximal to the medial humeral epicondyle, in the groove between the biceps and triceps brachii. *Drainage:* Afferents from ulnar aspect of forearm and hand, and entire little and ring fingers, the ulnar half of the long finger. *Clinical Occurrence:* Cat-scratch disease, secondary syphilis (father-in-law sign); a common inoculation site of systemic infections.

Mediastinal nodes. *Location:* These are not accessible to palpation. Chest radiographs show widening of the mediastinum, a mass in the anterior mediastinum, and masses in the hilar regions. *Clinical Occurrence:* Tuberculosis, coccidioidomycosis, histoplasmosis, anthrax, sarcoidosis, silicosis, beryllium poisoning, erythema nodosum, Hodgkin disease, non-Hodgkin lymphoma (lymphoblastic lymphoma), chronic lymphocytic leukemia, testicular cancer.

The Abdominal and Inguinal Nodes

Abdominal nodes. *Location:* Distinction between intraabdominal and retroperitoneal nodes cannot be made clinically. Occasionally, large nodes may be palpated as vague masses in the abdomen. Calcified nodes may be seen in the X-ray films. *Clinical Occurrence:* Lymphoma and testicular carcinoma.

> **KEY SIGN**   **Genital Lesion with Satellite Nodes**

Syphilis, gonorrhea, chancroid, herpes simplex, lymphogranuloma venereum, tuberculosis, and cancer of penis need to be considered.

Inguinal nodes. *Location:* A horizontal group lies along the inguinal ligament and a vertical group is beside the great saphenous vein in the proximal thigh. *Drainage:* Afferents of the horizontal group come from the skin of the lower anterior abdominal wall, retroperitoneal region, penis, scrotum, vulva, vagina, perineum, gluteal region, and lower anal canal; afferents of the vertical group come from the lower limb, along the great saphenous vein, penis, scrotum, and gluteal region. *Clinical Occurrence:* Many persons have moderately enlarged nodes from recurrent infections or trauma. Remember that tumors of the testis metastasize directly to the paraaortic nodes and do not involve the inguinal nodes; scrotal cancer spreads to inguinal nodes.

Disorders of B Cells

> **KEY DISEASE**   **Chronic Lymphocytic Leukemia**

See page 96.

> **KEY DISEASE**   **Waldenström Macroglobulinemia**

Proliferation and infiltration of the bone marrow, spleen, and liver by plasmacytoid lymphocytes producing excessive monoclonal IgM (macroglobulin) leads to hemolytic anemia, immune thrombocytopenia, and increased blood viscosity. Symptoms are insidious in onset with anorexia, malaise, and weakness, nasal and gingival bleeding, and exertional dyspnea. Signs include any combination of pallor, petechiae, ecchymoses, retinal hemorrhages, lymphadenopathy, hepatosplenomegaly, edema, and signs of heart failure. The disease runs a very prolonged course.

KEY DISEASE Multiple Myeloma

A clonal proliferation of plasma cells produces intact immunoglobulins and/or light chains that are detected in the serum and urine. Humoral activation of osteoclasts leads to bone resorption without healing, hypercalcemia, and pathologic fractures. Symptoms include bone and muscle pain, backache, weakness, weight loss, and fatigue. There are no specific signs; bone pain may indicate pathologic fractures [Case Records of the Massachusetts General Hospital: Case 6-2002. *N Engl J Med.* 2002;346603–346610].

KEY SYNDROME Amyloidosis

Deposition of the fibrillar amyloid proteins leads to organ enlargement and dysfunction. Several specific types exist, identified by the specific protein in the deposits. AL amyloidosis results from deposition of immunoglobulin light chains. AA amyloidosis occurs in chronic inflammatory diseases. The hereditary amyloidoses have specific fibrillar proteins depending upon the specific familial syndrome. Deposition of amyloid proteins, either generally or locally, can be asymptomatic or can cause organ dysfunction. Symptoms are nonspecific with constitutional complaints of weakness and fatigue. Specific complaints are referable to the organ system involved: diarrhea, dysphagia, and weight loss (GI involvement); paresthesias (peripheral nerves); dyspnea, orthopnea, and pleural effusions (restrictive cardiomyopathy). The signs depend upon the organs involved: macroglossia, eyelid plaques, hypertension, lymphadenopathy, hepatomegaly, splenomegaly, purpura, nephrotic syndrome, edema, shoulder-pad sign, joint and muscle pain, neuropathy, and fluid in serous cavities [Dember LM, Shepard J-A, Nesta F, et al. Case 15-2005: An 80-year-old man with shortness of breath, edema, and proteinuria. *N Engl J Med.* 2005;352:2111–2119].   *Clinical Occurrence:* AL Amyloidosis—multiple myeloma, monoclonal gammopathies, primary idiopathic amyloidosis; AA amyloidosis—chronic inflammatory diseases (e.g., osteomyelitis, tuberculosis, leprosy), familial Mediterranean fever, other familial periodic fevers.

The Hematopoietic System and Hemostasis

The hematopoietic system is intimately linked to the immune system through the production of B cells and T cells and the production of cells of the innate immune system (monocytes, macrophages, neutrophils, eosinophils, and basophils). In practice, disorders of the hematopoietic system are those that affect the major cellular elements of the blood (red blood cells, neutrophils and platelets). Hematopoietic disorders can be thought of as quantitative, an increase or decrease in the specific cell type, or qualitative, a disorder of function with, usually, a normal numbers of cells. It is useful to think of the presentations of the diseases by the cell type involved.

Red Blood Cell (Erythrocyte) Disorders

KEY SYNDROME   Anemia

Anemia is caused by a decreased production of erythrocytes from hypoproliferation or ineffective erythropoiesis as a result of defects in normoblast maturation, increased erythrocyte destruction (hemolysis), hemorrhage, or sequestration of erythrocytes in an enlarged spleen. Patients present with nonspecific symptoms of fatigue, dyspnea, decreased exercise tolerance, and weakness. Pallor is evident on examination when the hemoglobin is <10 gm/dL, and is especially notable in the conjunctivae and the palmar skin creases [Sheth TN, Choudhry NK, Bowes M, Detsky AS. The relation of conjuctival pallor to the presence of anemia. *J Gen Intern Med.* 1997;12:102–106]. The examiner should look for jaundice, lymphadenopathy, enlargement of the spleen or liver, and signs of hemorrhage. DDX: Patients with dyspnea on exertion due to anemia do not have orthopnea, unlike patients with congestive heart failure.

✔ ANEMIA—CLINICAL OCCURRENCE: *Hypoproliferation*   iron deficiency, anemia of chronic disease, hypothyroidism, kidney failure, marrow damage (tumor infiltration, granulomatous disease, myelofibrosis);   *Ineffective erythropoiesis* thalassemias, sickle cell disease, vitamin B_{12} and folate deficiency, myelodysplastic syndrome;   *Hemolysis*   congenital erythrocyte disorders (hereditary spherocytosis, hereditary elliptocytosis, glucose-6-phosphate dehydrogenase deficiency, pyruvate kinase deficiency), autoimmune hemolytic anemias (warm-reacting, IgG; cold-reacting, IgM), paroxysmal nocturnal hemoglobinuria, microangiopathic states (thrombotic thrombocytopenic purpura, hemolytic-uremic syndrome, malignant hypertension), infections, hemophagocytic syndromes, hypersplenism;   *Sequestration*   massive splenomegaly (chronic myelogenous leukemia, portal hypertension);   *Hemorrhage*   this is usually obvious, but occult gastrointestinal hemorrhage is common.

KEY DISEASE   Sickle Cell Disease

This is an autosomal recessive disease with affected patients homozygous for hemoglobin S. This hemoglobin is unstable in low-oxygen tensions, leading to aggregation and "sickling" deformity of erythrocytes, which then obstruct the microcirculation and produce tissue ischemia and hemolysis. Patients of African ancestry are most commonly affected. Compound heterozygotes with other hemoglobinopathies may present with more mild symptoms. The disease becomes apparent in childhood with painful crises associated with fever, malaise, headache, epistaxis, and pains in legs and abdomen associated with hemolysis. Abnormalities of growth include tower skull, short trunk, thoracic kyphosis, and small stature. Additional physical findings are abdominal and bone tenderness, pallor, yellow–green sclerae, cardiomegaly, hepatomegaly, splenomegaly, and ulcers on shins.

KEY DISEASE β-Thalassemia Major

There is a homozygous defect of hemoglobin A β-chain synthesis leading to hemolysis and ineffective erythropoiesis. There is expansion of the marrow, extramedullary hematopoiesis, and increased production of hemoglobin F. The disease is evident in childhood with mongoloid facies, prominent frontal bosses, hepatomegaly, splenomegaly, pallor, cardiac dilatation, and failure to grow normally.

KEY DISEASE β-Thalassemia Minor

There is a heterozygous defect of the β-globulin gene leading to a mild hypochromic, microcytic anemia. The patients are generally asymptomatic or may have mild fatigue. They are often misdiagnosed as having iron deficiency on the basis of the hypochromic microcytic anemia. Iron overload can occur if iron is given inappropriately.

KEY DISEASE   Paroxysmal Nocturnal Hemoglobinuria

There is increased sensitivity of erythrocytes to complement as a result of acquired loss of a membrane anchor protein. Symptoms include abdominal, retrosternal, or lumbar pain. There is chronic anemia, superficial migratory thrombophlebitis, and hemoglobinuria at night. There is an increased risk for developing acute leukemia.

KEY DISEASE   Pernicious Anemia and Vitamin B_{12} Deficiency

In pernicious anemia, autoimmune gastritis leads to decreased production of intrinsic factor and vitamin B_{12} malabsorption. Other causes of B_{12} malabsorption from the terminal ileum are more common. Patients present with fatigue, glossitis, or proprioception deficits caused by posterior column disease or dementia. A high index of suspicion is required. Up to 5% of persons older than 75 years of age are B_{12} deficient. Other causes of B_{12} deficiency include postgastrectomy, celiac disease, bacterial overgrowth of the small intestine, intestinal parasites, distal ileal resection, dietary deficiency.

KEY SYNDROME   Erythrocytosis—Polycythemia

Increased production of erythrocytes results from clonal proliferation (polycythemia vera) or is secondary to either hypoxemia, abnormal hemoglobins, renal tumors or drugs (testosterone, erythropoietin). Patients present with plethora and dyspnea. In secondary polycythemia, there may be signs of advanced chronic lung disease. Congestive heart failure with edema occurs with hematocrits >60% and hyperviscosity of the blood can produce signs of organ dysfunction, stroke, and thrombosis. DDX: In polycythemia vera, there is splenomegaly and the plasma volume is elevated, along with the increase in red blood cell volume. Usually there is also a leukocytosis and thrombocythemia.

Neutrophil Disorders

Neutropenia. Decreased production of neutrophils (granulocytes, segmented polymorphonuclear leukocytes) results from aplastic anemia, a myeloproliferative syndrome, leukemia, infection, or drug toxicity. Hypersplenism reduces the circulating PMNs. The patient is asymptomatic until the neutrophil count is <500 per mm³ when infection with their own flora, especially *Staphylococcus aureus, Streptococcus pyogenes*, and gram-negative flora from the gastrointestinal tract, is greatly increased. Patients may present with fever and signs of septicemia as the first indication of a problem. Febrile neutropenia is especially common with cancer chemotherapy and presents a diagnostic and therapeutic challenge.

Leukocytosis. Increased production of neutrophils is a normal response to infection and hemorrhage. Early release of band forms is most consistent with infection. Epinephrine and corticosteroids cause neutrophils adherent to the vessel walls (the marginated pool) to demarginate and may increase the neutrophil count by 50–100%. Increases in mature leukocyte counts are asymptomatic, even at levels greater than 200,000 per mm³. The keys to the diagnosis are the symptoms and signs of the underlying disease. Persistent neutrophilia without evident cause, especially with immature forms circulating suggests chronic myelogenous leukemia.

Myeloproliferative Disorders and Acute Leukemia

KEY DISEASE   Chronic Myelogenous Leukemia

An acquired balanced genetic translocation of the bcr gene on chromosome 9 and the abl gene on chromosome 22 leads to a fusion bcr-abl functional tyrosine kinase which causes the disease. Symptoms begin gradually with fatigue, malaise, loss of appetite, and abdominal fullness. There is usually palabable splenomegaly which may become massive. With progression, anemia and thrombocytopenia occur; the disease terminates in a "blast crisis" with transformation to a relatively refractory acute leukemia.

KEY DISEASE   Polycythemia Vera

There is a clonal proliferation of erythrocytes, neutrophils and platelets. Increases in both the red cell mass and the plasma volume lead to increased blood volume, increased hematocrit, and decreased blood flow in the capillaries as a consequence of increased viscosity of the blood. Patients present with fatigue, neurologic symptoms, aquagenic pruritus, and thromboses. Spontaneous thrombosis of the hepatic vein (Budd-Chiari syndrome) and portal or mesenteric vein thrombosis should trigger an evaluation for P.vera even in the absense of elevated hematocrit. Physical findings are plethora and splenomegaly.

KEY DISEASE   Essential Thrombocytosis

There is unregulated proliferation of platelets leading to very high platelet counts (>500,000 and often >1,000,000 per mm³). Patients are usually asymptomatic until they present with bleeding or thrombosis. They may present with headache, transient ischemic attacks, or hemorrhage.

KEY DISEASE   Myelofibrosis (Myeloid Metaplasia)

Fibrosis of the bone marrow obliterates the marrow space. There is extramedullary hematopoiesis in the spleen and liver and progressive pancytopenia. The cause is unknown. Patients complain of weakness, increased fatigability, weight loss, pallor, fullness in the left upper quadrant. Splenomegaly and hepatomegaly are usually evident, and dependent edema, bone pain, and fever may be present.

KEY DISEASE   Acute Leukemias

Several different forms occur, all presenting with clonal proliferation of very immature myeloid or lymphoid precursors leading to marrow replacement, neutropenia and thrombocytopenia. The onset and progression are acute and rapid. Symptoms may be fever, bleeding, or malaise. Prompt recognition and treatment are required. Acute promyelocytic leukemia is associated with a high risk for disseminated intravascular coagulation; recognition of this entity and treatment with all-trans retinoic acid has greatly improved survival.

Platelet Disorders

Disorders of platelet function.   See Intradermal Hemorrhage, Chapter 6, page 146ff.

KEY SYNDROME   Thrombocytopenia

Decreased platelet production, increased platelet consumption, immune-mediated platelet destruction, or hypersplenism are the common causes. Patients present with a hemostatic disorder manifest as bleeding from the gums, bruising, epistaxis, or bleeding following trauma or minor surgical procedures. Signs include purpura, from petechiae to large ecchymoses. The examiner should look for splenomegaly, hepatomegaly, and lymphadenopathy. Spontaneous intracranial hemorrhage is a significant risk with counts below 10,000 per mm^3.

THROMBOCYTOPENIA—CLINICAL OCCURRENCE: *Decreased Production*   cytotoxic chemotherapy, other drugs (e.g., heparin, thiazides, ethanol, quinine); *Increased Consumption*   massive hemorrhage, hypertransfusion syndrome, thrombotic thrombocytopenic purpura, disseminated intravascular coagulation; *Immune Destruction*   immune thrombocytopenic purpura, lymphomas, monoclonal gammopathy of unknown significance, systemic lupus erythematosus, HIV infection, heparin-induced thrombocytopenia (HIT);   *Hypersplenism*   portal hypertension, lymphoma.

Idiopathic Thrombocytopenic Purpura.   Antibodies directed against platelets lead to destruction in the spleen with very low platelet counts despite an increase in bone marrow megakaryocytes. This can present at any age, and is especially common in women with other autoimmune diseases especially SLE. Monoclonal gammopathies of unknown significance may be found in association. It is asymptomatic and the signs are those of purpura. Large platelets are seen on the peripheral smear.

Heparin-induced thrombocytopenia (HIT). Antibodies to platelet factor 4-heparin complex lead to rapid agglutination of platelets either directly (HIT-I) or secondary to immune mechanisms (HIT-II). Patients receiving heparin for several days develop acute and worsening thrombosis often of major arteries in association with thrombocytopenia. It may occur within hours on reexposure to heparin in a previously treated patient. The symptoms and signs are related to the sites of thrombosis and infarction.

KEY SYNDROME   Thrombocytosis

Increased production of platelets occurs with myeloproliferative diseases, iron deficiency, chronic inflammatory disorders, and hemorrhage. This is usually asymptomatic until the platelet counts are >750,000 per mm^3. Hemorrhage is the most common complication, although thrombosis also occurs. See Essential Thrombocytosis, page 105.

Coagulation Disorders

Disorders of blood coagulation may be congenital or acquired. Congenital abnormalities usually are deficiencies of specific factors or decreased factor function. Acquired disorders may be factor deficiencies or functional inhibition of coagulation. In either case, patients present with delayed bleeding from sites of trauma, spontaneous hemorrhage into joints and severe hemorrhage following surgical procedures.

Hypoprothrombinemia. Warfarin administration, vitamin K deficiency (dietary or absorptive), or hepatic insufficiency lead to loss of the vitamin K-dependent coagulation factors (II, VII, IX, X) and to loss of proteins S and C. Patients present with visceral bleeding including epistaxis, bleeding from gums, easy bruising, ecchymoses hematuria, melena, and/or menorrhagia. Symptoms and signs of malabsorption may be present if the cause is malabsorption of fat soluble vitamins (A, D, E, and K).

Hemophilias: factor VIII deficiency (hemophilia A and antibodies to factor VIII) and factor IX deficiency (hemophilia B). The hemophilias are X-linked disorders with decreased synthesis of physiologically active factor VIII or IX. Clinically they are indistinguishable. Symptoms and signs begin in childhood with spontaneous bleeding or excessive hemorrhage following dental extractions and surgery. Hemarthroses lead to joint deformities and contractures. Antibodies to factor VIII may be acquired in the older adults, postpartum, with drugs and in SLE.

KEY DISEASE   von Willebrand Disease

These are autosomal dominant defects in factor VIII von Willebrand factor production or function. Patients present with signs of platelet dysfunction as a result of ineffective platelet adhesion. The use of aspirin by these patients greatly augments their symptoms. The pastial thromboplastin time (PTT) is prolonged. Many affected people are never recognized.

KEY SYNDROME   Thrombophilia

Congenital or acquired disorders of coagulation and fibrinolytic pathways lead to an increased risk for thromboembolism. Patients present with venous, and less commonly arterial, thromboembolism. Often there is no identifiable risk factor (e.g., trauma, surgery, immobility) other than a family history of thromboembolic disease. Common causes are factor V Leiden, deficiencies of antithrombin III and of proteins C and S, prothrombin gene mutations, and the antiphospholipid syndrome. DDX: Arterial thromboembolism suggests antiphospholipid syndrome, nonbacterial thrombotic endocarditis, or Trousseau syndrome associated with cancer [Bessis D, Sotto A, Viard JP, et al. Trousseau's syndrome with nonbacterial thrombotic endocarditis: Pathogenic role of antiphospholipid syndrome. *Am J Med.* 1995;98:511–513].

KEY SYNDROME   Antiphospholipid Syndrome

Antibodies to phospholipids are associated with inappropriate activation of the clotting system leading to arterial and venous thrombosis. Patients present with in-situ arterial thrombosis, venous thromboembolic disease, livedo reticularis, evidence of cardiac valvular abnormalities and/or frequent miscarriage. This syndrome is frequently seen in association with SLE and greatly increases the risk of end organ damage and death. Primary antiphospholipid syndrome rarely progresses to SLE [Levine JS, Branch DW, Rauch J. The antiphospholipid syndrome. *N Engl J Med.* 2002;346:752–763].

The Endocrine System

Endocrine disorders are common and the clinician should always think of endocrine disorders when patients present with systemic symptoms, such as fatigue, weakness, anorexia, change in weight, and malaise, especially in the absence of fever or other localizing symptoms and signs.

Diabetes and Hypoglycemia

KEY DISEASE   Diabetes Mellitus Type 1

Immune destruction of β-cells in the pancreatic islets produces an absolute insulin deficit resulting in hyperglycemia, osmotic diuresis, impaired energy metabolism and reliance on oxidation of fatty acids for energy, leading to ketosis and ketoacidosis. With chronic disease, there is progressive injury to the microvasculature in the eyes, glomeruli, and nerves, and large vessel atherosclerosis. Symptoms include polydipsia, polyuria, polyphagia, weight loss and weakness. Physical findings are dryness of the skin and acetone on the breath. With chronic disease, the symptoms and signs of peripheral neuropathy, atherosclerosis, renal insufficiency, and retinopathy are seen.

KEY DISEASE   Diabetes Mellitus Type 2

Insulin resistance is the primary disorder with hyperglycemia despite elevated circulating insulin levels resulting from persistant hepatic gluconeogenesis. Patients are usually obese adults, although it is seen increasingly in children. There is a strong familial predisposition, and an increased risk in some racial groups (e.g., Hispanics, Pima Indians). The metabolic abnormalities are similar to those of type 1 diabetes, but less acute, so many patients escape detection until complications (e.g., myocardial infarction, neuropathy, retinopathy, renal insufficiency) bring them to medical attention. Polyuria and polydipsia are gradual in onset and less pronounced than in type 1.

> **KEY SYNDROME** Hypoglycemia

Low blood glucose results from increased insulin effects or a decreased ability to produce glucose from other substrates in the liver. Patients frequently give a history of "hypoglycemia" in themselves or relatives. Often the complaints are nonspecific and related to autonomic activity (sweating, shakiness, flushing, anxiety, or nausea). True symptoms of hypoglycemia are classified as neuroglycopenic (dizziness, confusion, tiredness, dysarthria, headache, and thinking difficulty). Inadvertent or surreptitious use of insulin or hypoglycemia-inducing medications is the most common cause of true hypoglycemia, usually in patients with known diabetes. Insulinoma is rare and reactive hypoglycemia (alimentary hypoglycemia) is an unproven concept.

Disorders of Thyroid Function

Thyroid Disorders Anatomic alterations of the thyroid gland are frequently associated with disturbances of function. Excesses or deficits of thyroid hormone alter the physical structure of the body to produce physical signs. Therefore, examine your patient (1) to determine the size and morbid anatomy of the thyroid gland, (2) to assess thyroid function, and (3) to judge the likelihood of cancer. The mass effect of the thyroid is assessed by history, inspection and palpation. Thyroid function is evaluated by seeking symptoms and signs of hypothyroidism and hyperthyroidism. Pay particular attention to the pulse, pulse pressure, appearance of the eyes and face, voice, skin and hair, neuromuscular function (especially the stretch reflexes), affect, and mood. Confirm the diagnosis by laboratory tests. The presence or absence of malignancy can only be evaluated by obtaining tissue. See Chapter 7, page 299ff. for discussion of goiters and thyroid nodules.

Abnormalities of thyroid function. Thyroid production of T4 is controlled by thyrotropin (thyroid stimulating hormone, TSH) which is released by the anterior pituitary under the control of the hypothalamic hormone, thyrotropin-releasing hormone (TRH). l-Thyroxine (T4) and triiodothyronine (T3) are released into the circulation from the thyroid follicles in a ratio of. 20:1. In peripheral tissues, T4 is converted to the active hormone, T3, at a rate determined within each tissue. T4 and T3 inhibit TRH release from the hypothalamus and TSH release by the pituitary. Thyroid hormones bind to nuclear thyroid hormone receptors, which affect transcription of multiple genes affecting cellular metabolism through binding to thyroid response elements.

> **KEY SYNDROME** Hypothyroidism

Underproduction of thyroid hormone slows the metabolism of all tissues producing cellular, organ, and whole-body hypofunction. The most severe form is known as myxedema, from the soft-tissue thickening consequent to interstitial mucopolysaccharide accumulation. Symptoms: Patients complain of fatigue, loss of energy, decreased concentration, coldness, constipation, and weight gain despite decreased food intake. The onset is often gradual and overlooked. Signs: The face is rounded, relaxed, and indefinably puffy without frank edema. The expression is placid and good-natured. Responses are slow. The speech is slow and the voice is frequently hoarse from vocal cord edema. There is a paucity of motion (hypokinesia), movements are slow and deliberate. There is generalized weakness, but muscle atrophy or paralysis is absent. When testing the knee and ankle reflexes, the slow muscle relaxation can be seen and felt; it is as if the reflex were "hung up." The tongue may be large and awkward. The skin is cool, dry, and thick; often there is scaling that is difficult to distinguish from ichthyosis. The palms and circumoral skin may be yellow from carotenemia. The hair is dry, coarse and easily broken. The nails are also dry and brittle. The only ocular sign is periorbital edema. Cardiovascular signs include a reduced strength of myocardial contraction manifest as a reduced apical impulse and pulse contour. Angina and heart failure may occur initially or with thyroid hormone replacement. Pericardial effusion (with low-voltage QRS complexes on the ECG), ascites, and edema of the ankles occur without heart failure. The ventricular rate is normal or slow. Dysrhythmias are rare. The blood pressure is normal or there is moderate elevation of both systolic and diastolic pressure. Constipation is very common; the resulting tympanites may suggest ileus. Menorrhagia is common. There are changes in the mental status. The patient often complains of thinking more slowly (bradyphrenia), is irritable and emotionally labile. Patients may develop depression. Myxedema coma is a rare but grave occurrence.

KEY SYNDROME   Hyperthyroidism

Overproduction of thyroid hormone, or ingestion of excessive thyroid medication, increases the metabolic rate, producing changes in all organ systems. Increased stimulation of the sympathetic nervous system produces many of the symptoms and signs. *Symptoms:* Patients initially feel energetic and are often happy to be losing weight. As the symptoms progress, they develop tremor, sweaty skin, frequent defecation, and progressive weight loss despite increased food intake. *Signs:* The face is thin, the features sharp, the expression alert and vigilant. Responses to questions are quick and the emotions are labile. The voice is normal in hyperthyroidism. Movement is increased (hyperkinesia) and faster than normal. Speech cadence is accelerated. There is often some generalized muscle weakness, with the quadriceps femoris most often affected; the patient must push with the arms to rise from a chair. The reflexes in hyperthyroidism are normal or hyperactive with unsustained clonus; in patients incidentally taking β-blockers, this may be the only sign of hyperthyroidism. There is almost always a fine tremor. The skin is thin, moist, and sweaty; the hair is fine and oily. The fingernails may separate from the matrix (onycholysis); usually only one or two pairs of nails are involved. Lid lag is frequent. Cardiovascular signs include tachycardia and an increased strength of myocardial contraction, manifest by an accentuated apex beat and sharp heart sounds. Angina and congestive failure may be precipitated in patients with coronary artery disease. The systolic blood pressure is slightly elevated, the diastolic diminished, so the pulse pressure is widened; thus, a pistol-shot sound is often present in the femoral arteries. There is a high incidence of atrial fibrillation. Defecation may be more frequent; the onset of true diarrhea is a grave prognostic sign. Extracellular fluid does not accumulate unless cardiac failure occurs. Menses are usually normal; occasionally there is oligomenorrhea. Changes in mental status commonly include irritability, emotional lability, and depression in hyperthyroidism; occasionally, manic states develop.

KEY DISEASE   Graves Disease (Diffuse Toxic Goiter)

Thyroid-stimulating antibodies react with the TSH receptor to produce TSH-independent hyperplasia and increased release of thyroid hormone. Myxomatous infiltration of the extraocular muscles produces exophthalmos and abnormalities of gaze. Graves disease is an autoimmune disease characterized by goiter, exophthalmos, pretibial myxedema, and hyperthyroidism. The thyroid is diffusely enlarged, usually less than twice normal size. Usually, the right lobe is larger than the left. Asymmetry may occur from congenital absence of a lobe or the isthmus. A bruit may be heard over the thyroid as a result of the increased blood flow through the tortuous thyroid arteries. The eye signs may be absent or occur any time in the course of the disease; they also can occur without abnormalities of thyroid hormone secretion. The entire spectrum of eye lesions may not occur in a single individual. Often the signs are initially unilateral. The signs are lid lag, lid spasm, lacrimation, chemosis, periorbital edema, periorbital infiltration with mucopolysaccharides, and exophthalmos (proptosis) (see Fig. 7–36). Often there is paresis of extraocular muscles, usually involving one or two symmetrical pairs; isolated weakness of the two superior recti is common. The skin over the shins may be have circumscribed elevated areas that are firm, nontender, and pink. Paradoxically, this is called pretibial myxedema; it usually occurs in association with the ophthalmopathy. A similar finding is thickening of the skin on the dorsa of the fingers or toes (thyroid acropachy) [Weetman AP. Grave's disease. *N Engl J Med*. 2000;343:1236–1248].

KEY SYNDROME   Hashimoto Thyroiditis

Lymphocytic inflammation of the gland leads to induration and gradual loss of function. This is the most common cause of hypothyroidism; it occurs most commonly in women after the fifth decade. The gland is firm, only slightly enlarged; nontender and nodules may be present [Pearce EN, Farwell AP, Braverman LE. Thyroiditis. *N Engl J Med*. 2003;348:2646–2655].

KEY SYNDROME   Postpartum Thyroiditis

Painless inflammation of the thyroid gland is common following normal pregnancy. Onset is usually 3–6 months postpartum and is signaled by signs of either hyperthyroidism or hypothyroidism. The latter is often confused with the fatigue and stress of caring for a newborn. The gland is diffusely enlarged and nontender. The condition usually resolves completely over a period of months.

> **KEY SYNDROME** De Quervain Thyroiditis, Viral Thyroiditis

Acute inflammation of the thyroid from viral infection or postinfectious inflammation results in release of thyroid hormone from the damaged follicles producing hyperthyroidism with depressed TSH and iodine uptake. The patient may complain of pain with swallowing. The pain is frequently referred to the ear, so the physician may be consulted for earache. The gland is unusually firm and rather small (20–30 g), but it frequently contains one or more, often tender, nodules. The patient may be euthyroid or hyperthyroid in the acute phase.

Disorders of Adrenal Function

> **KEY SYNDROME** Corticosteroid Excess: Cushing Syndrome

Hypercortisolism results from adenoma or adenocarcinoma of the adrenal cortex, excess adrenocorticotropic hormone (ACTH) from a pituitary adenoma, therapy with corticosteroids or ectopic ACTH production. Patients present with complaints of weakness, weight gain, amenorrhea, and/or back pain. Physical findings include hypertension, moon face, acne, thoracic kyphosis, supraclavicular fat pads, hypertrichosis, wide purple striae on the abdomen and thighs, and peripheral edema [Raff H, Findling JW. A physiologic approach to diagnosis of the Cushing syndrome. *Ann Intern Med.* 2003;138:980–991].

➤ > **KEY DISEASE** Primary Adrenal Insufficiency: Addison Disease

Primary adrenal failure results from autoimmune, ischemic or hemorrhagic destruciton of the adrenal. The result is cortisol and mineralocorticoid (aldosterone) deficiency and increased circulating ACTH. Increased stimulation of proopiomelanocortin synthesis and ACTH release from the pituitary causes secondary increase in melanocyte-stimulating hormone. Symptoms include weakness, fatigue, lethargy, nausea and vomiting, diarrhea, weight loss, abdominal pain, and craving for salt. Physical examination may reveal mottled skin pigmentation, pigment in buccal mucosa (in whites), lips, vagina, rectum, reduced growth of hair, hypotension (especially orthostatic), and signs of dehydration [Salvatori R. Adrenal Insufficiency. *JAMA.* 2005;294:2481–2488; Dorin RI, Qualls CR, Crapo LM. Diagnosis of adrenal insufficiency. *Ann Intern Med.* 2003;139:194–204]. *Clinical Occurrence:* tuberculosis, fungal infection, other granulomatous processes, amyloidosis, hemochromatosis, tumor, or autoimmune destruction.

> **KEY SYNDROME** Secondary Adrenocortical Insufficiency

Pituitary insufficiency with decreased production of ACTH or inadequate recovery of ACTH responsiveness following prolonged corticosteroid administration leads to inadequate cortisol levels. Symptoms and signs are less prominent than with primary adrenal failure because the mineralocorticoid axis remains intact. Symptoms are often precipitated by infections, trauma, and surgery, which lead to relative cortisol deficiency in a setting of increased cortisol demands.

Disorders of Parathyroid Function

> **KEY SYNDROME** Hyperparathyroidism

An adenoma, hyperplasia, or neoplasia of the parathyroid gland leads to excessive secretion of parathyroid hormones causing bone resorption and inhibition of the renal tubular reabsorption of phosphate. Hyperparathyroidism may be primary or secondary to hypocalcemia (renal insufficiency, hypercalciuria) leading to secondary activation of the parathyroid glands. In some cases of secondary hyperparathyroidism, the gland becomes autonomous and not suppressible with correction of the underlying disorder, tertiary hyperparathyroidism. Primary hyperparathyroidism is most common in women in the 3rd to 5th decades. The onset is insidious and is often detected by abnormal calcium on serum chemistries drawn for another reason. The clinical triad of peptic ulcer, urinary calculi, and pancreatitis suggests the diagnosis. Symptoms can include muscle weakness or stiffness, loss of appetite, nausea, constipation, polyuria, polydipsia, weight loss, deafness, paresthesias, bone pain, and renal colic. Signs include band (calcific) keratitis, hypotonia and weakness, osteopenic fractures, and skeletal deformities.

> **KEY SYNDROME** Hypoparathyroidism

This occurs spontaneously or results from removal of the parathyroid glands during thyroidectomy. Inadequate parathyroid hormone secretion leads to hypocalcemia and hyperphosphatemia. Symptoms are nervousness, weakness, paresthesias, muscle stiffness and cramps, headaches, and abdominal pain. Tetany with spontaneous carpopedal spasm may be seen. Classic signs of hypocalcemia are carpal spasm induced by inflation of a blood pressure cuff on the arm (Trousseau sign) and a facial twitch caused by light percussion over the facial nerve (Chvostek sign). Other signs are loss of hair, cataracts, and papilledema.

> **KEY SYNDROME** Vitamin D Deficiency

Vitamin D_3 is synthesized in the skin under the influence of sunlight. It is converted to the active 1,25-dihydoxycholecalciferol form sequentially in the liver (25-hydorxylation) and kidney (1-hydroxylation). Vitamin D deficiency is very common especially in older and/or chronically ill patients in the more northern latitudes. African Americans and darkly pigmented individuals of other ethnic backgrounds are especially at risk. Diets low in milk products (supplemented with vitamin D) are another risk factor. In addition to osteomalacia manifest as low bone density and leading to secondary hyperparathyroidism, these patients frequently complain of diffuse persistent musculoskeletal pain. Anyone presenting with these risk factors or complaints should be evaluated for vitamin D deficiency [Plotnikoff GA, Quigley JM. Prevalence of severe hypovitaminosis D in patients with peristent, nonspecific musculoskeletal pain. *Mayo Clin Proc.* 2003;78:1463–1470].

Disorders of Pituitary Function

> **KEY SYNDROME** Acromegaly and Gigantism

See Chapter 13, page 663.

> **KEY DISEASE** **Cushing Disease**

See Cushing Syndrome, page 112.

> **KEY SYNDROME** **Prolactinoma**

Increased secretion of prolactin by a functioning pituitary micoadenoma or macroadenoma suppresses FSH and LH secretion and produces lactation. Women present with galactorrhea and amenorrhea. Men present with decreased libido and hypogonadotrophic hypogonadism. Headache suggests a macroadenoma.

> **KEY SYNDROME** **Hypopituitarism**

The pituitary gland is destroyed by tumor, injury, infarct, or granuloma, leading to progressive pituitary insufficiency with decreased function of the thyroid, adrenal cortex and gonads. Symptoms are those of multiple endocrine failure; hypogonadal symptoms are a common early indication. Cold intolerance, weakness, nausea, vomiting, impotence, and amenorrhea are characteristic. Signs include hypothermia, bradycardia, hypotension, atrophy of skin, pallor, hypotonia, areolar depigmentation, loss of axillary and pubic hair, and atrophy of sex organs [Vance ML. Hypopituitarism. *N Engl J Med.* 1994;330:1651–1662].

Sheehan syndrome.   Hemorrhage and shock during obstetrical delivery causes hypopituitarism secondary to pituitary necrosis. Symptoms include failure of lactation, amenorrhea, lethargy, sensitivity to cold, and diminished sweating. There is fine wrinkling of the skin, hair loss, depigmentation of the skin and areola, and mammary and genital atrophy.

The Skin and Nails

Every clinician should be able to examine the skin and nails identifying the primary skin diseases and cutaneous signs of systemic disease. This chapter will help you characterize lesions sufficiently to either make a diagnosis or determine that referral to a dermatologist is indicated. The assistance of dermatologic atlases and textbooks listed in the bibliography is encouraged.

Physiology of the Skin and Nails

The skin covers the entire body surface protecting the underlying tissues from injury, infection, heat and fluid loss, and supporting the peripheral nerve endings. It is contiguous with the orifice mucous membranes at sharply demarcated borders. It is essential for temperature regulation dissipating heat via radiation, conduction, and convection (aided by the production of sweat), and providing insulation with the dermal and subcutaneous fat. Integrity of the epidermis depends upon tight intercellular adhesion to form an impermeable barrier. The dermis is rich in blood vessels, which dilate or constrict to dissipate or conserve body heat. Integrity of the dermis depends upon interlacing collagen bundles and elastic tissue.

In addition to its physical protective functions, the skin forms an immunologic barrier as well. Within the epidermis are *Langerhans cells*, antigen-presenting cells that migrate to the regional lymph nodes when activated by foreign antigens.

The skin also contains many specialized structures. Some of these are skin appendages, including the hair and glands and special sensory organs of the nervous system, often uniquely aggregated in specific locations. So, in addition to its protective functions, the skin and hairs also function as a sensory organ.

Functional Anatomy of the Skin and Nails

Morphologically, the three chief layers of the skin are the epidermis, the dermis, and the subcutaneous tissue.

Epidermis

The epidermis (cuticle) (Fig. 6–1) is the most superficial layer. It has four strata. The *keratin layer* (*stratum corneum*) is made of overlapping stratified keratinized nonliving cells that sequentially separate and drop off (*desquamation*). Underlying

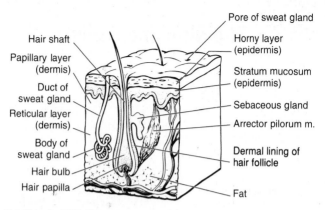

Fig. 6–1 *Principal Skin Structures.*

the horny layer are the *granular layer* (*stratum granulosum*), the *spinous layer* (*stratum spinosum*), and the *basal layer* (*stratum basale*). These layers consist mostly of keratinocytes, living cells deriving their nourishment from the dermis, since the epidermis is avascular. *Melanocytes* in the lower epidermis contain *melanin*, a brown or black pigment whose concentration is determined by heredity, exposure to sunlight, injury and repair, and hormonal control. The epidermis contains a network of furrows or rhomboid lines, visible with the unaided eye through the keratin layer; on relaxed surfaces the furrows are narrow, while over joints they are widened. The epidermis is thickest in areas of high friction, such as the palms and soles. The epidermis is separated from the dermis by the basement membrane and attached to it through hemidesmosomes.

Dermis and Subcutaneous Tissue

The superficial dermis is thrown into a series of papillae into which the epidermis is molded, the *papillary dermis*. The deeper *reticular layer* consists of dense connective tissue containing blood vessels, lymphatics, nerves, and considerable elastic tissue. In its deeper portion are collagenous bundles mixed with elastic fibers. Between the meshes of this layer are sweat glands, sebaceous glands, hair follicles, and fat cells. The reticular layer merges with the deeper and looser *subcutaneous layer*. The dermis is thickest over the back; it is extremely thin over the eyelids, scrotum, and penis. In general, the dermis is thicker over dorsal and lateral than over ventral and medial surfaces. Dermal appendages include hair apparatus as well as eccrine, apocrine, and sebaceous glands.

The Fingernails

The astute diagnostician always examines the fingernails. With the exception of the eye, there is no region of comparable size in which so many physical signs of generalized disease can be found. The nails continue to grow throughout life, providing a record of brief or prolonged disturbances of nutrition. They also serve as windows through which to view capillary changes associated with constitutional disease.

The *nail plate* is a horny, semitransparent rectangle, convex rectangle, with a smaller radius of curvature transversely (Fig. 6–2). The nail plate rests on and

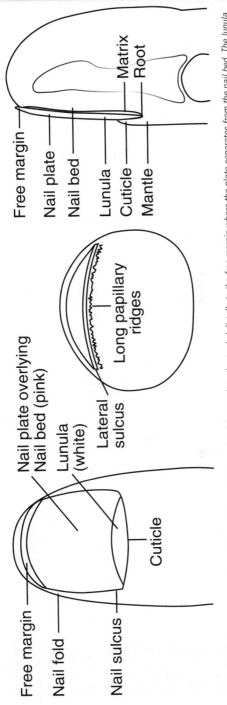
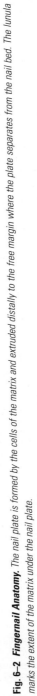

Free margin
Nail fold
Nail sulcus

Nail plate overlying
Nail bed (pink)
Lunula
(white)
Lateral
sulcus

Long papillary
ridges

Cuticle

Free margin
Nail plate
Nail bed
Lunula
Cuticle
Mantle

Matrix
Root

Fig. 6-2 Fingernail Anatomy. The nail plate is formed by the cells of the matrix and extruded distally to the free margin where the plate separates from the nail bed. The lunula marks the extent of the matrix under the nail plate.

adheres to the *nail bed*, a layer of modified skin on the dorsal aspect of the terminal phalanx. The bed is studded with small longitudinal ridges containing a rich capillary network that shows through the nail plate as a pink surface. Roughly, the proximal third of the nail bed is composed of partially cornified cells containing granules of *keratohyalin*; this specialized layer is the *matrix* where new nail is made and added to the nail plate, forcing it distally. The matrix is viewed through the nail plate as the white *lunula*. The proximal part of the nail plate, buried in a dermal pouch, is the *root*. The dermal lip of the pouch is called the *mantle*; it terminates in the *cuticle*, a sharp cornified rim. The distal nail plate not adherent to the bed is the *free edge* and the *body* is the intervening portion. The sides of the nail plate are buried in lateral *nail folds* of skin and cuticle.

The nail plate grows continuously by elongation from the root and thickening from the matrix. The average time for growing a new fingernail is approximately 6 months; growth is faster in youth than in old age. Most changes in the fingernails have accompanying counterparts in the toenails, but signs in the latter are not so evident.

The Toenails

The toenails undergo the same changes as the fingernails, but most of the signs are less pronounced. It takes 12 to 18 months for a toenail to regrow. Painful lesions are accentuated by weight bearing and by ill-fitting footwear.

Skin Coloration

In human beings, skin color is determined by four pigments: melanin (brown), carotene (yellow), oxyhemoglobin (red), and reduced hemoglobin (bluish-red). Except in albinos, melanin content is the primary determinant of normal skin color. In persons with dark skin, melanin may obscure colorations obvious in patients with light skin. Therefore, examine conjunctivae, buccal mucosa, nail beds, and palms to assess pallor, cyanosis, or erythema. Melanin pigmented lesions lying deep in the dermis appear blue due to the altered spectrum of light reflecting up through the overlying skin, a phenomenon known as the Tyndall effect.

Physiology of melanin pigmentation.   Dermal melanocytes positioned along the dermal-epidermal conjunction convert tyrosine to melanin. Each melanocyte contacts approximately 30 keratinocytes via dendrites. The melanin-containing organelles (*melanosomes*) are transported from the melanocytes to epidermal keratinocytes and hair as melanin granules. The number of melanocytes is similar from person to person regardless of whether an individual's skin is dark or light. Hereditary factors control constitutive skin color by determining the number, aggregation, and maturity of the melanosomes. Individual differences in pigmentation are determined by the baseline amount and the type of melanin produced. Eumelanin and pheomelanin are the two most common types, with eumelanin appearing brown to black and pheomelanin yellow to red. Eumelanin is superior to pheomelanin in its photoprotective abilities. Facultative changes in response to hormones, ultraviolet light, medications, and local stimuli such as inflammation lead to acquired changes in pigmentation.

Hair

The skin is covered with hairs except on the palms, soles, dorsa of the distal phalanges, glans penis, inner surface of the prepuce, and labia minora. The hair follicle is a long tubular invagination of epidermis and dermis often extending into the subcutaneous tissue [Paus R, Cotsarelis G. The biology of hair follicles. *N Engl J Med.* 1999;341:491–497]. At its blind end, the follicle cups a component of the dermis known as the *papilla.* A complex interchange of molecular signals between papilla and follicle determine whether the hair is in a stage of active growth (anagen), regression (catagen) or rest (telogen). The *hair shaft* is long and slender—in a straight hair, its cross section is round or oval; in a curled hair, it is flattened. The shaft consists of a *medulla*, which is frequently absent, and a *cortex*, whose cells contain *pigment* in colored hairs. On its surface is the *cuticle*, a single layer of flat scales. The proximal end of the shaft is the root, terminating in a hollow bulb that fits over the hair papilla; the root is softer and lighter in color than the shaft. The hair follicle penetrates the dermis obliquely forming an obtuse angle with the undersurface of the skin; in this angle is an involuntary muscle, the *arrector pili*, extending from near the hair bulb to the superficial dermis. Its contraction pulls the hair to a perpendicular position producing "goosebumps" or "gooseflesh."

Adults have two types of hair. Both sexes are covered in soft, colorless, short *vellus hairs. Terminal hairs* are longer, coarser, and darker than vellus hairs. Terminal hair is found on the scalp, in the pubic region, and in the axillae of both sexes. Males often exhibit terminal hair on the trunk, face, and extremities.

Sebaceous Glands

A group of specialized cells in the dermal lining of the hair follicle produce sebum through holocrine secretion into a duct emptying into the follicle near its distal end; one or more sebaceous glands are associated with each follicle. Sebaceous glands are most densely distributed on the face and the back.

Eccrine (Sweat) Glands

The body of the gland is a coiled tube in the deep dermis or subcutaneous tissue from which a straight duct leads to the epidermis, emerging on the skin surface in a funnel-shaped opening or pore known as the acrosyringium. Eccrine glands are present in the entire skin with the exception of the vermilion border of the lips, the nailbeds, the labia minora, the male prepuce, and glans penis. They are necessary for cooling of the body through the evaporation of the sweat they produce from the skin surface. These glands receive primarily cholinergic innervation from the autonomic nervous system.

Apocrine Glands

Apocrine glands are associated with hair follicles, are almost exclusively limited to the skin of the axillae, pubic and perianal skin, and become active during puberty. They have both cholinergic and adrenergic innervation. The exact composition of their products is unknown. The function of the apocrine gland in humans is also uncertain. The most widely held belief is that they serve(d) as scent glands. Ceruminal, ciliary, circumanal, and mammary glands are modified sweat glands.

Nerves

The skin contains a variety of nerves transmitting a multiplicity of stimuli. Meissner corpuscles are found in the dermal papillae and convey light touch. Pacinian corpuscles found in the deep dermis, and sometimes in the subcutaneous tissues, transmit pressure and vibration. Other more noxious sensations such as pain, itch, and temperature are transmitted by a variety of unmyelinated fibers. No area of the skin is insensate, unless it is the result of injury, disease or developmental anomaly. The density of the different types of nerves varies greatly by location, with the fingertips and lips being two of the more sensitive body areas, and the back one of the least sensitive.

Circulation of the Skin and Mucosa

Most lesions of the skin and mucous membranes involve the vascular system to some extent. The skin has a rich anastomotic network of vessels, so ischemia implies obstruction of the larger proximal arterioles or arteries.

Cutaneous Wound Healing and Repair

The skin has a remarkable ability to repair injury. Injury into the dermis heals with scarring, while epidermal wounds typically heal without scarring. Healing occurs in three phases: inflammation, proliferation, and maturation. In the initial inflammatory phase, platelets provide hemostasis and release pro-inflammatory cytokines. Neutrophils are the first immune cells to infiltrate the wound, while macrophages derived from circulating monocytes arrive later but contribute more significantly to wound healing. Along with neutrophils, they debride the wound and help prevent infection. In addition, by releasing growth factors and cytokines, they affect tissue remodeling. Two weeks after injury and appropriate closure wound strength is approximately 10% of that of normal skin prior to injury. Collagen produced by fibroblasts is remodeled in the scar for up to a year after injury. By 1 year, the scar is fully remodeled and its strength is around 80% of normal skin.

Multiple factors can adversely affect wound healing. Chief among these is infection, which may delay or even halt healing of the skin. Adequate perfusion of the injured tissues is also important. Well-vascularized tissue heals better and more quickly than relatively ischemic tissue as evidenced by the relatively rapid healing of scalp and facial injuries with their rich blood supplies compared to the slower healing of the less well-vascularized lower legs. Some patients are genetically prone to slow healing and/or poor scar formation. Both oral and topical corticosteroids inhibit collagen synthesis, and, as a result, dramatically impede wound healing. Finally, the wound care regimen affects the speed and quality of healing. Following gentle cleansing and debridement, petrolatum and an occlusive bandage should be applied to most wounds to reduce or prevent eschar formation and provide an environment optimal for re-epithelialization.

Examination of the Skin and Nails

The history should include complete characterization of the lesions including: symptoms such as pain, burning, and itching with attention given to the onset, intensity, and duration, as well as alleviating and aggravating factors; the initial site; a description of the lesion(s); the chronology of any changes; any exposure, injury, medication, or systemic disease; and response to therapy.

The skin is examined by inspection, including compression and magnification, supplemented by palpation to detect nodularity and induration. A systematic examination is essential noting especially the anatomic distribution of lesions, the configuration of grouped lesions, if present, and the morphology of the individual lesions [Schwarzenberger K. The essentials of the complete skin examination. *Med Clin North Am*. 1998;82:981–999].

Evaluation of skin turgor. Pinch the skin over the back of the hand with the thumb and index finger, and then release it (Fig. 6–3). Normal turgid skin rapidly resumes its customary shape. Loss of turgor is indicated by persistence of the fold for a time after pinching.

Examination of nail fold capillaries. Nail fold capillaries are examined with an ophthalmoscope. This technique may be useful in patients with clinical findings suggestive of dermatomyositis, lupus, scleroderma, or other connective tissue disease. Practice is required for proper examination. Select a finger without recent trauma. Place a small drop of immersion oil or lubricating jelly on the nail fold to decrease skin reflection. Use the 15 to 40 magnification to visualize the capillaries. Normally, the capillary arcs are fine, parallel, narrow loops extending from the base of the nail fold toward the nail and returning. Dilation, irregularity, and dropout of loops are abnormal [Houtman PM, Wouda AA, Kallenber CGM. The diagnostic role of nail fold capillary microscopy. *VASA*. 1987;(suppl 18): 21–27].

Tourniquet test for impaired initial hemostasis. Moderately increased venous pressure produces few petechial hemorrhages in normal skin. When the capillaries are fragile many more petechiae, known as the *Rumpel-Leede* or *Hess test*. Venous hypertension is produced with a blood pressure (BP) cuff, which has replaced the tourniquet. Inscribe a 2.5 cm diameter circle on the volar surface of the forearm, 4 cm distal to the antecubital fossa. Place the BP cuff on the upper arm and

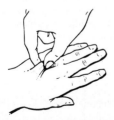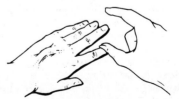

Fig. 6–3 *Testing for Skin Turgor.*

inflate to a pressure halfway between systolic and diastolic pressure for 5 minutes. Release the pressure, wait at least 2 minutes then count the petechiae within the circle. The normal number does not exceed 5 in men or 10 in women and children. A positive test is commonly seen in platelet disorders (e.g., immune thrombocytopenic purpura and platelet dysfunction) and vascular disorders, such as scurvy and actinic purpura. This test is quite uncomfortable for the patient and is of limited clinical utility.

Supplemental Aids to Dermatologic Diagnosis

Magnification. A standard magnifying glass serves as a useful aid in the characterization of skin lesions. Other tools that provide both magnification and illumination, such as dermatoscopes and dermlights, are available and commonly used by dermatologists.

Diascopy. Compress red lesions with a magnifying glass or a glass slide, to see, if they blanche indicating dilated vessels. Extravasated blood will not blanch. See Plate 1.

KOH preparation. KOH preparations allow visualization of dermatophyte hyphae, *Candida* pseudohyphae and budding yeasts and the spores and fragmented hyphae of tinea versicolor. Scrape skin scales from the lesion and place them on a glass slide. Add 2 drops of a 10% to 20% solution of KOH to dissolve keratin, allowing the fungal elements to be more easily seen microscopically. Gentle heating with a flame will catalyze this process, but care should be taken to avoid boiling the solution. First, examine the slide at scanning magnification, followed by a higher power view. Hyphae appear as thin, elongated filaments, often best seen just slightly out of the plane in which the keratinocytes are in focus. To the inexperienced eye, hyphae may be difficult to distinguish from the outline of a keratinocyte. Other confounders include hair and clothing fibers.

Tzanck smear. To identify herpes simplex or varicella-zoster viruses in vesicular lesions, firmly scrape the base of an unroofed early vesicle with a scalpel and air dry the specimen on a glass slide. Stain it with Wright or Giemsa stain and examine microscopically for characteristic cytopathic changes such as multinucleated giant cells or ballooning keratinocytes. Culture a fresh specimen for virus identification.

Wood light. Ultraviolet illumination (360 nm) demonstrates a characteristic fluorescence in scalp infections caused by some (but not all) dermatophytes such as *Microsporum canis* (yellow), *Pseudomonas* abscesses (pale blue), or intertriginous infections with *Corynebacterium minutissimum* (coral red). Keep in mind that recent bathing may decrease the presence of the fluorescent substance and lead to falsely negative results.

Skin biopsy. Skin biopsy is easily performed. Techniques include use of a skin punch, shaving with a scalpel or razor blade, and sharp excision. Some training is required for selection of the technique appropriate for each lesion and technical performance of the biopsy.

Skin and Nail Symptoms

> ### KEY SYMPTOM   Itching (Pruritus)

Itching is a common symptom and treatment may prove frustrating in the absence of a specific diagnosis. Ask what induces and relieves the itching, if it is related to a recent exposure or beginning a new medication, where it itches, whether it inhibits sleep, when it started, and whether it is constant and progressive. Excoriations and lichenification (thickening of the skin with accentuation of the skin lines, often in a rhomboid pattern) are telltale signs of scratching. *CLINICAL OCCURRENCE:*   *Local Causes:*   contact dermatitis (e.g., poison ivy), insect bites, chigger bites (red larva of Trombiculidae mites), scabies, tinea, candidiasis, trichomoniasis, atopic dermatitis, neurodermatitis, seborrheic dermatitis, lichen simplex, urticaria, pruritus ani, pruritus vulvae, stasis dermatitis, dermatitis herpetiformis, miliaria (heat rash); *Generalized Causes:*   asteatosis ("winter itch"), pruritus of pregnancy, pityriasis rosea, psoriasis, drug reactions, uremia, obstructive jaundice, biliary cirrhosis, myxedema, polycythemia vera (aquagenic pruritus), Hodgkin disease, cutaneous and other lymphomas, diffuse cutaneous mastocytosis, pediculosis (body lice), hookworm, onchocerciasis, filariasis.

Skin and Nail Signs

Diagnosis is greatly facilitated by learning to accurately and completely describe your observations using precise terminology. This facilitates use of reference materials, helps to provide adequate, accurate information when referring a patient for consultation with a dermatologist or filling out a pathology requisition for examination of a biopsy. Following the description of the signs are examples of conditions that cause the lesion.

Anatomic Distribution of Lesions

Many skin diseases have characteristic anatomic patterns. Some patterns are determined by regional skin features and others by selective exposure to noxious agents; the explanation for many patterns is unknown. A few examples follow (Fig. 6–4).

Head and neck. *Acne:*   face, neck, and shoulders; *Actinic Keratoses:*   face; *Amyloidosis:*   eyelids; *Atopic Dermatitis:*   face, neck; *Cancer:*   face, nose, ears, lips; *Contact Dermatitis:*   eyelids, face; *Discoid Lupus Erythematosus:*   nose, cheeks; *Herpes Zoster:*   trigeminal nerve distribution in face; *Psoriasis:*   scalp; *Rosacea:*   face; *Seborrhea:*   scalp, eyebrows, eyelids, nasal alae; *Secondary Syphilis:*   face; *Spider Angiomata:*   cheeks, neck; *Tinea Capitis:*   scalp; *Xanthelasma:*   eyelids; *Variola (Smallpox):*   head and face extremities trunk.

Trunk. *Candidiasis:*   under breasts, axillae, inguinal and gluteal folds; *Dermatitis Herpetiformis:*   scapulae, sacrum, buttocks; *Drug Eruption:*   front and back of thorax and abdomen; *Petechiae:*   abdomen; *Pityriasis Rosea:*   front and back of trunk; *Secondary Syphilis:*   thorax and abdomen; *Spider Angiomata:*   chest, shoulders, abdomen; *Varicella (Chickenpox):*   trunk extremities and face.

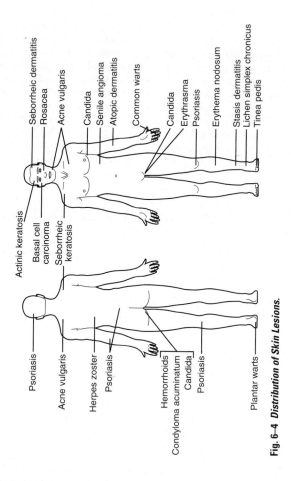

Fig. 6-4 *Distribution of Skin Lesions.*

Seborrheic dermatitis
Rosacea
Acne vulgaris
Candida
Senile angioma
Atopic dermatitis
Common warts
Candida
Erythrasma
Psoriasis
Erythema nodosum
Stasis dermatitis
Lichen simplex chronicus
Tinea pedis

Actinic keratosis
Basal cell carcinoma
Seborrheic keratosis

Psoriasis
Acne vulgaris
Herpes zoster
Psoriasis
Hemorrhoids
Condyloma acuminatum
Candida
Psoriasis
Plantar warts

Extremities. *Actinic Keratoses and Cancer:* backs of the hands; *Atopic Dermatitis:* antecubital fossae; *Contact Dermatitis:* arms, hands, legs; *Erythema Multiforme:* arms, hands, legs, feet, palms, soles; *Erythema Nodosum:* legs, shins; *Granuloma Annulare:* backs of hands and fingers; *Onychomycosis:* fingernails, toenails; *Petechiae:* forearms, hands, legs, feet; *Pityriasis Rosea:* upper arms, upper legs; *Plantar Warts:* soles; *Psoriasis:* elbows, hands, fingernails; *Secondary Syphilis:* palms, soles.

Pattern of Lesions

Single lesions may have distinctive shapes and patterns, some quite large (e.g., erythema chronicum migrans of Lyme disease). In other conditions, individual, smaller lesions are grouped into more-distinctive or less-distinctive configurations (e.g., herpes zoster). Multiple single lesions often coalesce into larger less-distinctive patterns, so a careful history of the evolution of lesions is critical. In pruritic diseases, attempts to relieve symptoms by the patient may result in the presenting pattern differing significantly from that of the primary lesions.

Annular, arciform and polycyclic pattern. The individual lesions are arranged in circles, arcs, or irregular combinations of the two. *CLINICAL OCCURRENCE:* Drug eruptions, erythema multiforme, urticaria, psoriasis, granuloma annulare, tinea.

Serpiginous pattern. The lesions occur in wavy lines or have wavy, indented margins. *CLINICAL OCCURRENCE:* Granuloma annulare, nodular lesions of late syphilis, larva migrans.

Target (Iris) pattern. A bull's-eye pattern occurs with an encircled round spot; more than one ring may be present. *CLINICAL OCCURRENCE:* Erythema multiforme, erythema migrans.

Irregular pattern. Groups of individual lesions with no distinct pattern. *CLINICAL OCCURRENCE:* Urticaria and insect bites.

Dermatomal pattern. Lesions conform to the distribution of the spinal root sensory dermatome; they do not cross the midline. *CLINICAL OCCURRENCE:* Herpes zoster, rarely in metastatic breast carcinoma.

Linear pattern. Lesions follow linearly arranged cutaneous and subcutaneous structures (e.g., nerves, lymphatics, or blood vessels), or result from contact with a linear irritant. *CLINICAL OCCURRENCE:* Lymphangitis, superficial phlebitis, contact dermatitis (e.g., poison ivy), jellyfish envenomation, trauma.

Retiform pattern. The individual lesions form a net-like pattern consistent with the cutaneous arterial or venous anatomy. The venous pattern is a lacey network; arteriolar occlusion results in infarcts with finger-like borders. *CLINICAL*

OCCURRENCE: *Venous Pattern:* erythema ab igne, livedo reticularis. *Arterial Pattern:* necrotizing vasculitis, cutaneous emboli, arteriolar thrombosis.

Extrinsic pattern. The lesions follow no anatomic pattern and often have relatively straight borders and/or a prominent geometric shape suggesting that the pattern is impressed upon patient from the outside. *CLINICAL OCCURRENCE:* Radiation injury, including sunburn and X-ray dermatitis, contact dermatitis.

Morphology of Individual Lesions

After noting the anatomic distribution and pattern, carefully examine and characterize several individual lesions. Have the patient identify individual lesions in each stage of development: new, mature, and resolving. Palpate the lesions to identify papules, nodules, plaques, and infiltration. View the skin through a compressing magnifying glass (diascopy, see above) to disclose deep lesions obscured by erythema and to determine whether red lesions blanch or persist; this helps distinguish vasodilation from extravasation of blood.

Individual Lesion Types

Macules and patches. These localized changes in the skin color or appearance are, by definition, not palpable (Fig. 6–5A). The areas may be small or large: macules <1 cm and patches are 1 cm or larger. They occur in many shapes and colors and the borders may be sharp or indistinct. There may be desquamation or scaling. *CLINICAL OCCURRENCE:* Freckles, exanthems (rubeola, rubella, secondary syphilis, rose spots of typhoid fever), drug eruptions, petechiae, first-degree burns, systemic lupus erythematosus (SLE), pityriasis rosea, café-au-lait spots, vitiligo.

Maculopapules. Parts of the otherwise macular lesion are slightly elevated. *CLINICAL OCCURRENCE:* Pityriasis rosea, erythema multiforme, fixed drug eruptions, exanthems.

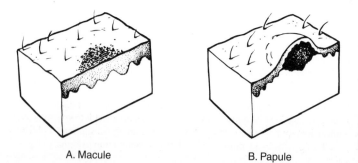

A. Macule
B. Papule

Fig. 6–5 *Macules and Papules. A.* Macules are visible but not palpable. *B.* Papules are palpable and <5 mm in diameter.

Papules. The lesions are elevated; they are defined as <1 cm in diameter (Fig. 6–5B). Their borders and tops may be distinctive. **CLINICAL OCCURRENCE:** **Acuminate or Pointed** bites, acne, physiologic gooseflesh; **Flat-topped** psoriasis, atopic eczema, lichen planus, molluscum contagiosum, condyloma latum; **Round or Irregular** angiomas, melanoma, eczematous dermatitis, papular secondary syphilis; **Filiform** condyloma acuminatum; **Pedunculate** skin tags, neurofibromas.

Plaques. Any diffusely elevated area of 1 cm in diameter or greater is called a plaque, usually formed from confluent papules. Characteristically, plaques are flat topped and much broader than high, like a plateau. **CLINICAL OCCURRENCE:** Cutaneous lymphomas (mycosis fungoides, Sézary syndrome); **Red, Scaling** psoriasis, pityriasis rosea, discoid lupus erythematosus (with atrophy); **Yellow** xanthomas; **Brown** seborrheic keratoses; **Hyperkeratotic** plantar warts; **Lichenified** atopic dermatitis.

Nodules. The lesions are solid and elevated and distinguished from papules by extensioin deeper into the dermis or subcutaneous tissue (Fig. 6–6A). They are usually >1 cm in diameter. The depth may be inferred by palpation; when below the dermis, the skin slides over them; lesions within the dermis move with the skin. **CLINICAL OCCURRENCE:** Gummas, rheumatoid nodules, lipomas, cancer, lymphoma cutis, xanthomas, gouty tophi, erythema nodosum, panniculitis, Dercum's disease.

Wheals. Cutaneous edema produces circumscribed, irregular, and relatively transient plaques (Fig. 6–6B). Their color varies from red to pale, depending on the amount of fluid in the skin. Hives (urticaria) often itch. **CLINICAL OCCURRENCE:** Urticaria, insect bites.

Vesicles. Fluid accumulates in and dissects the epidermis producing an elevation covered by translucent epithelium that is easily punctured to release the fluid (Fig. 6–7A). By definition, vesicles are <5 mm in diameter. Umbilicated

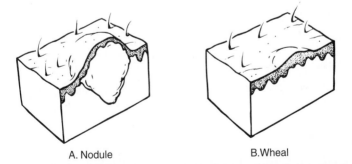

A. Nodule   B.Wheal

Fig. 6–6 *Nodules and Wheals. A. Nodules are persistent, discrete and firm lesions in the skin or subcutaneous tissue. **B.** Wheals are transient, discrete areas of edema in the epidemis and dermis.*

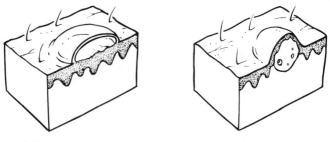

A. Vesicle, bulla, or pustule   B. Cyst

Fig. 6–7 *Fluctuant Skin Lesions.* A. *Vesicle, bullae, and pustules involve the epidermis.* **B.** *Cysts are subepidermal and may extend into the subcutaneous tissues.*

vesicles usually result from viral infections.   ***CLINICAL OCCURRENCE:***   Acute contact dermatitis, second-degree burns, varicella, herpes simplex and zoster, smallpox.

Bullae.   Accumulation and dissection of fluid within or under the epidermis >5 mm in diameter are bullae (Fig. 6–7A). If the separation is below the basal layer, the bullous will be tense; if it is superficial to the basal layer, it will be flaccid and more easily ruptured with minor trauma. Patients with flaccid bullae may present with superficial erosions and no intact bullae.   ***CLINICAL OCCURRENCE:***   Contact dermatitis, second-degree burns, bullous impetigo, pemphigus, pemphigoid, dermatitis herpetiformis, erythema multiforme (rarely), diabetic bullae.

Pustules.   Vesicles or bullae that become filled with pus and tiny abscesses in the skin are termed pustules (Fig. 6–7A). The contents appear milky, orange, yellow, or green. Pustules frequently arise from hair follicles or sweat glands.   ***CLINICAL OCCURRENCE:***   Folliculitis, acne, furuncles, variola, pustular psoriasis, bromide, and iodide eruptions.

Cysts.   Cysts are papules or nodules containing fluid or viscous material surrounded by an epithelial layer (Fig. 6–7B). Similar lesions without an epithelial lining are *pseudocysts*; the distinction is made histologically, after excision.   ***CLINICAL OCCURRENCE:***   epidermal inclusion and pilar (trichilemmal) cysts;   ***Pseudocysts***   cystic acne.

Vegetations.   Elevated irregular growths are called vegetations (Fig. 6–8A). When their covering is keratotic or dried, they are verrucous; when covered by normal epidermis, they are *papillomatous.* ***CLINICAL OCCURRENCE:***   ***Verrucous*** verruca vulgaris (common wart), seborrheic keratosis;   ***Papilloma*** condyloma acuminatum.

Scales.   Thin plates of partly separated dried cornified epithelium clinging to the epidermis (Fig. 6–8B).   ***CLINICAL OCCURRENCE:***   ***Large Scales*** psoriasis, exfoliative dermatitis;   ***Small Scales***   pityriasis rosea, seborrheic dermatitis.

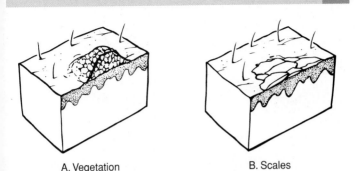

A. Vegetation   B. Scales

Fig. 6–8 *Vegetations and Scales. A. Vegetations are irregular growths above the skin surface. B. Scales are small or large flakes of cornified epithelium loosely adherent to the skin surface.*

Hyperkeratosis. Keratotic cells don't separate and slough normally, so they are piled up producing elevated thick skin. *CLINICAL OCCURRENCE:* Calluses, seborrheic keratoses and actinic keratoses are all common. Arsenic produces punctate keratoses of the palms and soles.

Lichenification. Repeated rubbing of the skin produces hyperplasia of all layers (Fig. 6–9A). This appears as a dry plaque in which the normal skin furrows or rhomboid lines are accentuated. *CLINICAL OCCURRENCE:* Atopic dermatitis, lichen simplex chronicus.

Crusts. A plate of dried serum, blood, pus, or sebum forms on the surface of an underlying vesicular or pustular lesion when it ruptures (Fig. 6–9B) or may accumulate on the surface of chronically inflamed skin. *CLINICAL OCCURRENCE:* The honey-colored crusts of impetigo are typical.

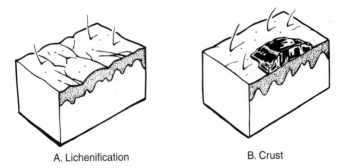

A. Lichenification   B. Crust

Fig. 6–9 *Lichenification and Crusts. A. Lichenification is a leathery thickening of all skin layers with prominent furrows. B. Crusts form from dried blood, serum, pus or other secretions from the skin.*

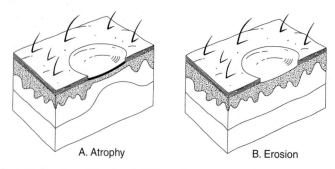

Fig. 6–10 *Atrophy and Erosion*. A. *With atrophy, all skin layers are present but thin.* **B.** *Erosions represent traumatic loss of the stratum corneum.*

Atrophy. The skin is thinned and lacks resilience, skin furrows or rhomboid lines (Fig. 6–10A). ***CLINICAL OCCURRENCE:*** Actinic atrophy, striae, discoid lupus erythematosus, prolonged application of potent topical steroids, steroid injections, and insulin lipodystrophy.

Sclerosis. Increased amounts of collagen and/or calcium salts are deposited in the cutaneous and subcutaneous tissues, often resulting from chronic inflammation. ***CLINICAL OCCURRENCE:*** Keloid, stasis dermatitis, scleroderma (systemic and localized), nephrogenic fibrosing dermopathy, calciphylaxis, scleroderma, and variants.

Erosions. Erosions are lesions with partial thickness loss of the epidermis (Fig. 6–10B). Erosions ooze and heal without scarring. ***CLINICAL OCCURRENCE:*** After rupture of vesicles or bullae or following mechanical or thermal trauma.

Fissures. A vertical cleavage of the epidermis extending into the dermis is a fissure (Fig. 6–11A). Commonly, it occurs from trauma to thickened, dry, and

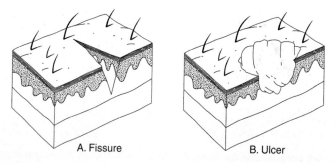

Fig. 6–11 *Fissures and Ulcers*. A. *Fissures are vertical splits extending through the epidermis into the dermis.* **B.** *Ulcers are actual loss of epidermal and dermal tissues that may extend into the subcutaneous tissue and muscle down to bone.*

inelastic skin, especially on the hands and feet. *CLINICAL OCCURRENCE:* Chapped lips, with diabetes and neuropathy.

Ulcers. A locally excavated lesion results from loss of epidermis and the papillary layer of the dermis (Fig. 6–11B). *CLINICAL OCCURRENCE:* Trauma, pressure over bony prominences (pressure ulcers), pyoderma gangrenosum, burns, stasis ulcers, necrotizing infections (bacterial, fungal).

Generalized Skin Signs

Petechiae and purpura. See pages 146ff. Blood is extravasated into the skin from disruption of the dermal vessels producing non-blanching red macules and patches.

Telangiectasia. Dilated small blood vessels that blanch with pressure. *CLINICAL OCCURRENCE:* Spider angiomata, Osler-Weber-Rendu disease, rosacea, sun and irradiation damage.

> **KEY SIGN** Gangrene

Ischemic necrosis of the skin and subcutaneous tissues creates a blackened, atrophic eschar. If the primary problem is arterial insufficiency, the lesions are atrophic and dry (dry gangrene). If the primary lesion is a local necrotizing process, the lesion may be edematous and weeping (moist gangrene). *CLINICAL OCCURRENCE:* *Dry Gangrene* arterial insufficiency. *Moist Gangrene* Aspergillosis, pyoderma gangrenosum, necrotizing fasciitis.

> **KEY SIGN** Urticaria

Inflammatory mediators produce local capillary dilation and leak leading to dermal and epidermal erythema and edema. The lesions are discrete raised erythematous papules and plaques, often intensely pruritic. Precipitating factors may be allergic, mechanical or physical. By definition, individual urticarial lesions should be present no more than 24 hours; their transient nature helps to distinguish urticaria from other conditions that may have a similar appearance, such as erythema multiforme. However, outbreaks of urticaria may last for years. True urticaria lesions lasting more than 24 hours are likley urticarial vasculitis, a condition requiring additional work up of collagen vascular disease. [Greaves MW. Chronic urticaria. *N Engl J Med.* 1995;332:1767–1772] *CLINICAL OCCURRENCE:* These are examples only, see dermatologic texts for more complete lists. *Allergic:* drug eruptions, topical sensitivity; *Physical:* cold, exercise, dermatographia; *Systemic Diseases:* mastocytosis, SLE.

> **KEY SIGN** Dermatographia

Dermatographia is a form of urticaria stimulated by stroking the skin. Normally, a light scratch produces linear macular blanching limited to the skin directly scratched. An urticarial response produces a bright-red macular line that becomes more purple with time. In more severe reactions, a red mottled flare develops laterally to the red line and a wheal may develop.

Mastocytosis. Mast cells infiltrate the skin producing brown macules that urticate when stroked (Darier sign). Mastocytosis may be limited to the skin (urticaria pigmentosa) or produce systemic disease with hepatosplenomegaly and signs of systemic histamine release (abdominal pain, diarrhea, peptic ulcer, hypotension, flushing).

KEY SIGN **Angioedema**

Localized interstitial edema in the dermis and subcutaneous tissues can be caused by immunoglobulin (Ig) E-mediated allergy, complement activation, or nonimmunologic mast cell activation, or it may be idiopathic. Single or multiple pruritic nonpitting swellings appear on the face, tongue, larynx, hands, feet, and/or genitalia that subside with or without treatment. Nausea, vomiting, and diarrhea may be seen with gastrointestinal involvement. Laryngeal angioedema can cause fatal airway obstruction. *CLINICAL OCCURRENCE:* *IgE Mediated* hymenoptera (bee) stings, drugs (e.g., penicillin and other antibiotics), food allergens (e.g., peanuts, shellfish), foreign proteins used therapeutically, many others; *Non-IgE Mediated* angiotensin-converting enzyme inhibitors, radiologic contrast agents, cold exposure; *Complement Mediated* hereditary angioedema (C1-esterase deficiency), serum sickness, vasculitis.

KEY SIGN **Dry Skin—Xerosis and Anhydrosis**

Loss of adequate sebaceous and/or sweat gland function leads to excessive drying of the skin. The skin is dry, often cracked and leathery in texture. Xerotic skin is more permeable to water because it lacks the normal protective oils. Normal aging results in progressively more xerotic skin. *CLINICAL OCCURRENCE:* Ichthyosis, anticholinergic drugs, denervation in peripheral neuropathies such as diabetes.

KEY SIGN **Decreased Skin Turgor—Extracellular Fluid Deficit**

Loss of extracellular fluid leads to increased viscosity of the interstitial space fluid. This should not be confused with a decrease in cutaneous elastic tissue (Decreased Skin Elasticity, below). In evaluating for dehydration, check the lying, sitting, and standing BP and pulse for postural changes; check for loss of skin turgor and longitudinal furrowing of the tongue. Loss of total body water does not result in loss of skin turgor. Technically, the term dehydration (loss of water) is an inaccurate description of this condition.

KEY SIGN **Decreased Skin Elasticity**

Destruction or disruption of the elastic fibers in the skin results in decreased elasticity. Decreased elasticity is evident as wrinkling and redundancy of the skin. *CLINICAL OCCURRENCE:* Sun exposure (solar elastosis), actinic cutaneous atrophy, excessive stretching of the skin (e.g., pregnancy, obesity), glucocorticoid excess (Cushing syndrome), pseudoxanthoma elasticum.

KEY SIGN Scars

Injury to the epidermis can heal without scarring, but may leave alterations in pigmentation. Injury to the elastic and collagen fibers in the dermis results in scarring. Deeper injury to the subcutaneous fat and muscle can result in visible depressions or masses. All cutaneous scars are initially raised and red; they fade through pink to a pallid hypopigmented hue over months to years as the vascularity of the fibrous tissue diminishes. Sutured wounds healing without infection or tension produce thin scars because there is a minimum of bridging fibrosis. Wounds healing by secondary intention leave wide, inelastic scars similar to burns, but following the contour of the surgical incision. The pattern of scarring indicates the mechanism (sharp trauma, burn, excessive tension, scarification, etc.) and etiology (e.g., surgery, obesity).

KEY SIGN Striae

Stretching normal skin ruptures the elastic fibers in the reticular dermis. In adrenal hypercorticism, the epidermis itself becomes fragile and easily breaks under normal tension. Striae are permanent even after removal of the precipitating condition. Multiple scars, 1 to 6 cm long, run axially under the epidermis. When recent, they are pink or blue; older striae are silvery. They occur in skin regions under chronic tension. Although striae are most common on the abdomen, deposition of adipose tissue or edema also produces them on the shoulders, thighs, and breasts. Striae should be differentiated from traumatic and therapeutic scarring, and self-inflicted injury. *CLINICAL OCCURRENCE:* Abdominal distention (pregnancy, obesity, ascites, tumors), subcutaneous edema, Cushing syndrome (usually exhibits fresh-appearing purple striae), traumatic stretching.

KEY SIGN Surgical And Traumatic Scars

Identify each scar, relating it to surgery or trauma. Without a history, the cause may only be inferred by the size, pattern, location, and contour (smooth or jagged) of the scar. The presence of suture marks indicates surgical repair of the skin, but not the depth of injury or incision. Full thickness burns cause deep, irregular, broad, inelastic scars.

KEY SIGN Hypertrophic scars and keloids

In some individuals, cutaneous injury variably produces persistent raised, red, hypertrophic scars. When scars extend beyond the boundary of the inciting wounds they are called keloids. Keloids may progressively thicken over time. Keloids are more prevalent in dark-skinned persons and after complicated wounds. They can occur anywhere on the body and after minor injury.

KEY SIGN Crepitus

When gas bubbles are present in the subcutaneous tissues or underlying muscle, pressure on the skin produces a peculiar sensation caused by the sliding of bubbles under the fingers. This may be accompanied by a crackling sound. The bubbles feel like small fluctuant nodules that move freely with palpation. They are not painful or tender. DDX: Subcutaneous crepitus is pathognomonic of subcutaneous emphysema or gas gangrene. In subcutaneous emphysema, the bubbles contain air that has entered the tissues through operative wounds or from trauma, such as a fractured rib piercing the lung. Infection with anaerobic and microaerophilic microorganisms may produce gas by fermentation; the signs of severe local infection with systemic toxicity distinguish it from subcutaneous emphysema.

Changes in Skin Color

Constitutive Diffuse Brown Skin—Normal Melanin Pigmentation: This is the inherited constitutive skin color. Persons of African descent have the greatest melanin density; lesser amounts occur, in order, from Asian Indians, Native Americans, Indonesians, Oriental Asians (Chinese and Japanese) to Western Europeans who have the least. There is also variation within anthropologic ethnic groups of related genetic background: for example, among whites, the natives of India are often very dark, while the inhabitants of the Mediterranean region are darker than the Northern Europeans. Individual variation within a family is also large. DDX: The inheritance of skin color can usually be established by questioning patients or their acquaintances about the origin and appearance of their relatives.

> **KEY SIGN** **Tattoos**

Tattoos are common and indicate an increased risk for blood-borne disease, if not placed using sterile technique. Determine, whether the tattoos were placed professionally or by amateurs and the degree of sterility and any sharing of instruments. Inquire about other high-risk behaviors such as intravenous drug use and high-risk sexual behaviors.

> **KEY SIGN** **Malignant Melanoma**

See page 175.

> **KEY SIGN** **Nevi—Moles**

See page 174.

> **KEY SIGN** **Acquired Diffuse Brown Skin—Melanism**

Multiple mechanisms can augment melanin production including increased production of adrenocorticotropic hormone and melanocyte-stimulating hormone, and increased iron deposition in the skin. Melanism is a darkening of the skin from augmented production of melanin in the facultative pigment deposits. The brown color is diffuse, with accentuation in palmar creases, recent scars, and pressure points at elbow, knee, and knuckles. Pigmentation appears in the oral mucosa (this is abnormal when found in whites). A history of a definite onset establishes that the pigmentation was acquired. Its presence should prompt a search for underlying disease.

✔ **MELANISM—CLINICAL OCCURRENCE:** *Congenital* hemochromatosis, porphyria, alkaptonuria; *Endocrine* Addison disease, Nelson syndrome, Graves disease, hypothyroidism, pregnancy (melasma—primarily on the face), contraceptive hormones; *Infectious* Whipples disease; *Inflammatory/Immunologic* scleroderma; *Metabolic/Toxic* cirrhosis, pernicious anemia, B_{12} and folic acid deficiency, drugs (busulfan, arsenicals, dibromomannitol); *Neoplastic* hormone-secreting neoplasms; *Psychosocial* tanning.

Hemochromatosis. The actual color may be bronze, blue-gray, brown, or black, accentuated in the flexor folds, the nipples, recent scars, and in parts exposed to the sun. The pigment is melanin, although hemosiderin is also increased. Skin color change may antedate hepatic cirrhosis and diabetes mellitus by several years.

> **KEY SIGN** **Blue-Grey Color**

Deposition of foreign substances discolors the skin. DDX: Increased concentrations of unsaturated or abnormal hemoglobin in the cutaneous vessels gives cyanosis (page 144), but this blanches with pressure. **CLINICAL OCCURRENCE:** Use of amiodarone or minocycline; deposition of silver (argyria), gold, or bismuth salts; hemochromatosis, cyanosis, sulfhemoglobinemia, methemoglobinemia arsenic poisoning.

Silver (Argyria): Silver salts from ingestion or intranasal absorption are deposited in the skin producing a blue-gray or slate color, accentuated in the areas exposed to sunlight. The mucosa and nail lunulae may be deposition sites. The pigmentation may appear years after exposure and is typically permanent. It is easily differentiated from cyanosis by the failure to blanch with pressure [Tomi NS, Kranke B, Aberer W. A silver man. *Lancet.* 2004;363: 532].

Arsenic: The ingestion of arsenic, therapeutically or with chronic poisoning, produces a diffuse gray background with superimposed dark macules 2 to 10 mm in diameter. This is often accompanied by punctate hyperkeratoses of the palms and soles. The skin manifestations may appear from 1 to 10 years after ingestion of the chemical.

Alkaptonuria (Ochronosis): An inherited metabolic error of homogentisic acid oxidase causes black polymers of homogentisic acid in the connective tissues and urine. The black accumulations shine through the skin, giving a faint blue-gray color to the skin, especially over the pinnae, the tip of the nose, and in the sclerae. The blackened extensor tendons of the hands may shine through the skin. Often a dark butterfly pattern will appear on the face; the axillae and genitalia will be pigmented. Exogenous ochronosis (pseudoochronosis) is a rare result of prolonged use of certain topical medications, most notably the skin bleaching preparation hydroquinone. The treated areas develop a blue-gray appearance similar to endogenous ochronosis.

Gold (Chrysoderma, Chysiasis): Occasionally, the parenteral administration of gold salts to treat rheumatoid arthritis causes a blue-gray pigmentation of the periocular skin and regions exposed to the sun.

KEY SIGN   Acquired Diffuse Yellow Skin

Yellow discoloration results from deposition of pigments in the skin. The most common causes are jaundice and carotenemia, which are easily distinguished on clinical grounds by their different distributions and presentations.

KEY SIGN   Jaundice (Icterus, Bilirubinemia)

See Jaundice, Chapter 9, page 470.

KEY SIGN   Carotenemia

Fat-soluble carotene is concentrated in the stratum corneum of the palms and soles and is excreted in the sebum. The liver fails to metabolize carotene in conditions such as myxedema (carotene is converted to vitamin A in the liver with the assistance of thyroid hormone) and diabetes. Excessive deposition of carotene appears as yellow skin, especially on the forehead, the nasolabial folds, behind the ears, and on the palms and soles. The carotene comes from chronic ingestion of large quantities of carrots, squash, oranges, peaches, apricots, and leafy vegetables. DDX: The water-soluble pigments of bilirubinemia are more uniformly distributed, including discoloration of the sclerae and thin skin.

KEY SIGN   Erythema

Erythema is a reddening of the skin caused by dilation of the cutaneous vasculature; it is often accompanied by increased skin temperature.   *CLINICAL OCCURRENCE:*   Local inflammatory lesions, local infection (e.g., cellulitis, lymphangitis), scarlet fever, scarlatiniform drug eruptions, polycythemia, porphyria, pellagra, lupus erythematosus, first-degree burns. Transient erythema occurs in blushing and in some cases of metastatic carcinoid.

KEY SIGN   Hypopigmentation and Depigmentation

Loss of normal skin pigmentation may be patchy or diffuse, usually with discrete borders. The distribution and pattern of depigmentation is important in identification of the specific etiology.   *CLINICAL OCCURRENCE: Depigmentation*   Vitiligo, albinism;   *Hypopigmentation*   tinea versicolor, scars, stria, and sites of subcutaneous steroid injection or topical steroid application on ethnically dark skin.

KEY SIGN   Hyperpigmentation

Increased melanin deposition in the skin can result from either local or systemic factors.   *CLINICAL OCCURRENCE:*   Addison disease, hemochromatosis, porphyria, arsenic poisoning, progressive systemic sclerosis (scleroderma), sun exposure, post-inflammatory hyperpigmentation, chronic local irritation from burning or scratching.

> **KEY SIGN** Acanthosis Nigricans

These asymptomatic hyperpigmented lesions with a velvety texture are most commonly seen on the neck, axillae groin, and other body folds. **CLINICAL OC-CURRENCE:** *Congenital* hereditary benign; *Endocrine* diabetes, increased androgens, acromegaly, Cushing syndrome, Addison disease, insulin resistance syndromes, hypothyroidism; *Metabolic/Toxic* obesity, drug induced, for example, nicotinic acid, glucocorticoids; *Neoplastic* paraneoplastic with adenocarcinomas or lymphoma.

Changes in the Hair

Excessive hair growth is termed *hypertrichosis* or *hirsutism*. This may occur locally over a nevus or generally. The presence of less hair than normal is *hypotrichosis*, as in some congenital ectodermal defects.

Telogen Effluvium: The hair growth cycle shifts from anagen to telogen due to physiologic stressors such as pregnancy, illness or emotional distress. The hair follicles remain in the resting phase (telogen) for up to a few months. Upon return to the growth phase (anagen), the newly growing hair causes the extrusion of the previous hair, resulting in diffuse shedding. The resultant hair thinning is temporary, although it may be quite distressing to the patient.

Anagen Effluvium: Anti-metabolites such as chemotherapeutic agents cause arrest of the hair growth phase and diffuse hair loss. Cessation of the offending agent will result in regrowth of the hair.

> **KEY SIGN** Alopecia

Alopecia is the loss of hair in either congenital or acquired conditions. The pattern and history of hair loss assist in the diagnosis. A male pattern in women suggests androgenic alopecia. Local trauma and traction on hairs or obsessive pulling or twisting on the hair (trichotilllomania) also cause alopecia [Springer K, Brown M, Stulberg DL. Common hair loss disordes. *Am Fam Physician.* 2003;68:93–102,107–108]. **CLINICAL OCCURRENCE:** Androgenic alopecia in the male (male pattern baldness), alopecia areata, telogen effluvium, anagen effluvium, hypothyroidism, thallium intoxication, drugs.

> **KEY SYNDROME** Alopecia Areata

This form of hair loss is thought to be an autoimmune phenomenon, but the exact pathophysiology is uncertain. Sudden loss of hair may be associated with emotional disturbances or infections, but can occur without associated illness. There is painless loss of hair in patches or complete denudation of body without other visible changes to the skin. Associations with other autoimmune disorders such as thyroiditis have been reported.

> **KEY SIGN** Graying of the Hair

Loss of pigmentation in the hair is a normal event; the age of occurrence is variable and to some extent familial. **CLINICAL OCCURRENCE:** Normal aging, premature aging syndromes, pernicious anemia, chloroquine therapy; localized graying occurs in vitiliginous lesions.

> **KEY SIGN**   **Hirsutism and Hypertrichosis**

True hirsutism is excess growth of terminal hairs from androgen-sensitive pilosebaceous units. It may result from excess androgen secretion or genetically determined increased androgen sensitivity. Hirsutism is especially distressing to women, as the hair tends to grow in a masculine pattern, including on the face, shoulders, back, chest, abdomen, thighs, and buttocks. The challenge is to discern normal variation from the rare conditions associated with androgen excess. Hypertrichosis is excess "nonsexual" hair growth. The hairs are of the vellus type and cover the body evenly [Rosenfield RL. Hirsutism. *N Engl J Med.* 2005;353:2578–2588]. **CLINICAL OCCURRENCE:** **Hirsutism** androgen-secreting tumors, polycystic ovary, late-onset congenital adrenal hyperplasia, glucocorticoid excess, prolactinemia, carcinoma, drugs (e.g., certain oral contraceptives, testosterone, anabolic steroids); **Hypertrichosis** congenital, anorexia nervosa, hypothyroidism, dermatomyositis, malnutrition, drugs (minoxidil, phenytoin, hydrocortisone, cyclosporine, penicillamine, and streptomycin).

Fingernail Signs

Absence of Nails: The nails may be congenitally absent, sometimes in association with ichthyosis. A traumatized nail may be shed and damage to the matrix may prevent regrowth.

Malnourished Nails: The nails grow slowly or not at all. They are dry, brittle, and contain transverse ridges; they thicken with time.

Irregular, Short Nails—Bitten Nails: The free edge of the nail plate may be absent from the nervous habit of biting the nails (Fig. 6–12A).

Square, Round Nail Plates—Acromegaly and Cretinism: Disproportionate lateral growth produces nail plates more wide than long.

Long, Narrow Nail Plates—Eunuchoidism and Hypopituitarism: The nails are longer and narrower than usual and may resemble those in Marfan syndrome.

Brittle Nail Plates—Onychorrhexis: The cut edges of the various keratin layers may be delaminated and present a step-like appearance. Borders may be frayed and torn (Fig. 6–12B). **CLINICAL OCCURRENCE:** Malnutrition, iron deficiency, thyrotoxicosis, or calcium deficit; many times the cause is unknown.

Longitudinal Ridging in Nail Plate—Reedy Nail: An exaggeration of normal, it has been attributed to many conditions, but the diagnostic significance is meager (Fig. 6–12C).

Friable Nail Plates—X-ray Irradiation: The edges may be frayed, the growth stunted. They are often softened (Fig. 6–12D).

> **KEY SIGN**   **Transverse Furrow in Nail Plate—Beau Line**

Decreased nail growth caused by an acute illness manifests as a transverse furrow whose width reflects the duration of illness. As the nail elongates, the furrow

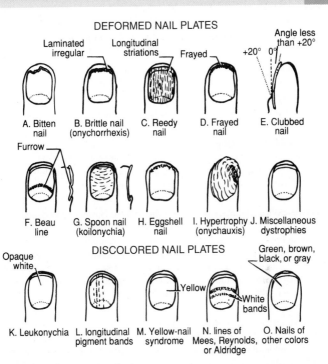

DEFORMED NAIL PLATES

Laminated irregular — Longitudinal striations — Frayed — +20° 0° Angle less than +20°

A. Bitten nail B. Brittle nail (onychorrhexis) C. Reedy nail D. Frayed nail E. Clubbed nail

Furrow

F. Beau line G. Spoon nail (koilonychia) H. Eggshell nail I. Hypertrophy (onychauxis) J. Miscellaneous dystrophies

DISCOLORED NAIL PLATES

Opaque white Green, brown, black, or gray Yellow White bands

K. Leukonychia L. longitudinal pigment bands M. Yellow-nail syndrome N. lines of Mees, Reynolds, or Aldridge O. Nails of other colors

Fig. 6–12 *Diagnosis of Fingernail Lesions I. Many nail lesions are depicted here. It is necessary to know whether the lesion is in the nail plate or in the nail bed. The distinction can usually be made, by noting, if the abnormal color is changed by pressure on the nail plate, indicating a lesion of the nail bed. See text for descriptions.*

moves into view from beneath the mantle, progresses distally, and is finally pared off (Fig. 6–12F).

Concave nail plate—spoon nails (Koilonychia). The natural convexity is replaced by concave, saucer nails (Fig. 6–12G). Often the nail plate is thin. *CLINICAL OCCURRENCE:* Most often encountered with iron deficiency; rare in rheumatic fever, lichen planus, and syphilis.

Hypertrophy of the Nail Plates—Onychauxis: The nail plate becomes greatly thickened by piling up of irregular keratin layers (Fig. 6–12I). It may be familial or the result of chronic fungal infections.

KEY SIGN Nail Pitting

Occasional pits in the nails are normal. Large numbers of pits are seen in psoriasis, especially psoriatic arthritis; other skin signs of psoriasis may be subtle or absent. Nail pitting in transverse bands is associated with alopecia areata.

Dystrophy of the Nail Plates: Under this head are grouped many ill-defined changes including opacities, furrowing, ridging, pitting, splitting, and fraying, all testaments to poor nail growth (Fig. 6–12J). ***CLINICAL OCCURRENCE:*** Chronic infections of the nails, lesions of the nerves supplying the limb, vascular deficits of the extremity, amyloidosis, and the collagen diseases.

White Nail Plates—Partial Leukonychia: Irregular white areas in the nail plates are common and most often indicate a history of minor trauma.

White Nail Plates—Total Leukonychia: The nail plates are completely chalk white (Fig. 6–12K). The condition is inherited as a dominant character with varying penetrance.

Yellow Nail Plates—Yellow-Nail Syndrome: The disorder results from impeded lymphatic circulation and often antedates lymphedema elsewhere. The nail plates become yellow or yellow-green, thicken, and grow more slowly (Fig. 6–12M) with excessive transverse curvature. Occasionally, ridging and onycholysis occur.

Transverse White Banded Nail Plates—Mees Lines: The nail plates contain transverse white bands that are laid down during a generalized illness or poisoning. The formation ceases with recovery, producing a white band that moves distally with growth of the nail plate (Fig. 6–12N, Plate 2). The bands are probably evidence of a lesser degree of injury than Beau lines. ***CLINICAL OCCURRENCE:*** Poisoning (arsenic, thallium, and fluoride), chemotherapy, infectious febrile illnesses, renal insufficiency, cardiac failure, myocardial infarction, Hodgkin disease, sickle cell disease and many others.

Longitudinal Brown Banded Nail Plates: This may be a normal variant in persons with black skin, most commonly with more than one nail affected (Fig. 6–12L). Similar longitudinal bands are seen in patients receiving some antiretroviral medications. Melanoma should be considered if the longitudinal brown banding affects a single nail, irrespective of skin pigmentation.

Discolored Nail Plates: Various drugs, infections, and stains occasionally color the nail plates (Fig. 6–12O), the color giving a clue to etiology: blue-green = infection with *Pseudomonas*; brown-yellow = ingestion of phenindione; brown or black = fungal infections, fluorosis, quinacrine; and blue-gray = argyria.

White Banded Nail Beds—Muehrcke Lines in Hypoalbuminemia: Paired, narrow, arcuate bands of pallor, parallel to the lunulae, appear in the nail beds (Fig. 6–13A). They occur during periods of hypoalbuminemia (less than 2.0 g/dL) and resolve when the deficit has been corrected. Because they are not in the nail plates, they do not move distally with nail growth.

Red Lunula—Heart Failure: Red lunulae rather than normal white (Fig. 6–13B) are associated with cardiac failure.

Azure Lunula—Hepatolenticular Degeneration (Wilson Disease): The lunulae are light blue (Fig. 6–13C). Examine the eyes for Kayser-Fleischer rings.

White Proximal Nail Beds—Terry Nails: The mechanism is unknown. The proximal 80% or more of the nail bed is white (Fig. 6–13D), leaving a distal band of normal pink. The nail findings are associated with hepatic cirrhosis.

White Proximal Nail Beds—Half-and-Half Nail (Lindsay Nails): The proximal 40% to 80% of the nail beds is white but the distal portion is red, pink, or brown (Fig. 6–13E). The colored portion is sharply demarcated, usually by a curved line parallel to the free edge. Constriction of the venous return deepens the color of the

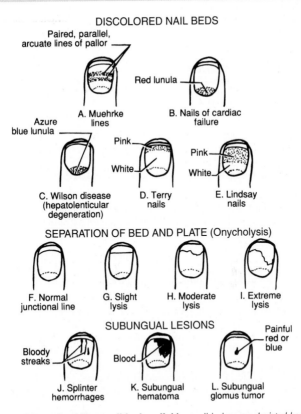

Fig. 6–13 *Diagnosis of Fingernail Lesions II. Many nail lesions are depicted here. It is necessary to know whether the lesion is in the nail plate or in the nail bed. The distinction can usually be made, by noting, if the abnormal color is changed by pressure on the nail plate, indicating a lesion of the nail bed. See text for descriptions.*

distal portion, but only a slight pink is induced in the proximal bed. Most patients have renal disease, usually advanced. This is somewhat similar in appearance to Terry nails.

Separation of the nail—onycholysis. Normally, the line of adhesion of plate to bed is a smooth curve (Fig. 6–13F); in onycholysis, the plate separates from the nail bed more proximally, collecting debris underneath, inaccessible to cleaning (Fig. 6–13G-I). *CLINICAL OCCURRENCE:* Hyperthyroidism, psoriasis, and mycotic diseases of the nails.

Subungual Hemorrhage—Splinter Hemorrhage: Bleeding from the capillaries in the nail plate is confined to the longitudinal ridges giving a longitudinal linear appearance. These lesions are asymptomatic (Fig. 6–13J). *CLINICAL OCCURRENCE:* Trauma is most common. Local skin diseases, and systemic thrombotic and embolic illness (e.g., endocarditis, antiphospholipid syndrome, vasculitis) should be considered.

> ### KEY SIGN   Subungual Hemorrhage—Subungual Hematoma (Fig. 6–13K)

This traumatic lesion is intensely painful; relief of pain is achieved either by dissection of the hemorrhage to the distal nail plate (resulting in lifting and subsequent loss of the nail) or by therapeutic drainage through the nail plate to preserve the nail.

> ### KEY SIGN   Subungual Pigmentation—Ungual Melanoma

An unusual location for malignant melanoma (2.5% of melanomas), ungual melanoma is most frequently found under the nails of the thumb or great toe. Its characteristic sign is leaching of melanin from under the nail to its border and into the paronychial area.

Painful Red or Violet Subungual Spot—Glomus Tumor: Tumors arising from sensory glomus bodies are especially common in the nail bed, where they are exquisitely painful. It is seen through the nail plate as a round red or violet spot (Fig. 6–13L). It resembles a hemangioma, but the latter is not tender.

Inflammation of the Nail Fold—Paronychia: Bacterial infection of the nail fold, most commonly with staphylococci, produces pain, redness, fluctuance and purulent drainage. Chronic infection at the base of the nail damages the matrix causing permanent nail deformity. *Candida* infection of the nail folds is common in individuals whose hands are frequently exposed to warm moist environments or who bite their cuticles. The cuticle is retracted from the nail plate and is rounded, erythematous and thickened, but not tender. Several nails may be involved.

Foot and Toenail Signs

Certain lesions of the feet and toenails need special mention.

> ### KEY SIGN   Thickening of Skin—Callus

A well circumscribed area of thickened epidermal keratin develops at locations of repeated pressure or friction. Callus is normal under the first and fifth metatarsal heads and the heel. Occurrence at other locations, usually with a decrease in the normal callosities, indicates unusual weight distribution or pressure from footwear. Calluses are infrequently painful in themselves, but pressure on underlying structures, especially periosteum, may cause pain. Hard callus transmits pressure from footwear to the underlying soft tissues impinged between the callus and the underlying bone. Calluses may be distinguished from verrucae by the preservation of skin lines (dermatoglyphics) in the former.

> ### KEY SIGN   Hard Corn

Pressure on thin skin overlying bone, especially on the toes, produces a conical callus pointing into the dermis. Pain is produced by pressure on the callus, usually from footwear. There is a central core that is seen when the top is pared away.

> **KEY SIGN Soft Corn**

This is a corn on an interdigital surface that undergoes maceration from moisture and infection. It is quite painful.

> **KEY SIGN Plantar Wart (Verruca Pedis or Plantaris)**

This wart is caused by human papilloma virus infection. The lesions are frequently multiple. Disruption of the skin lines is seen and black spots of hemorrhage may appear as dark pearls. Weight bearing may cause pain.

> **KEY SIGN Ulcer of the Sole—Perforating Neurotrophic Ulcer**

Normal pressure and pain sensation are essential to protect the foot from excessive and prolonged pressure over boney prominences. In the insensitive foot (e.g., diabetic neuropathy) pressure can lead to painless ischemic necrosis of the soft tissue, infection, and/or ulceration. A punched-out, indolent, painless ulcer occurs under a metatarsal head, at the tip of the toe, over the proximal interphalangeal joint of a hammertoe or on the heel. Test for sensation to pressure by using graded monofilament (page 703). If bone is exposed or reached by a probe osteomyelitis is likely [Sumpio BE. Foot ulcers. *N Engl J Med*. 2000;343:787–793; Caputo GM, Cavanagh PR, Ulbrecht JS, et al. Assessment and management of foot disease in patients with diabetes. *N Engl J Med*. 1994;331:854–860; Grayson ML, Gibbons GW, Balogh K, et al. Probing to bone in infected pedal ulcers: A clinical sign of underlying osteomyelitis in diabetic patients. *JAMA*. 1995;273:721–723; Edelman D, Hough DM, Glazebrook KN, Oddone EZ. Prognostic value of the clinical examination of the diabetic foot ulcer. *J Gen Intern Med*. 1997;12:537–543].

Ingrown Toenail: Excessive transverse growth of the nail plate causes the lateral edge to lacerate the nail fold. Usually the lateral nail fold of the great toe is affected. An ulcer is formed and maintained by repeated trauma and infection. Weight bearing is painless, but any pressure on the nail plate, as from shoe or sock, elicits tenderness. Exuberant granulation tissue may form in the nail fold.

Subungual Pain—Subungual Exostosis: The great toe is usually involved. An exostosis arises from the dorsal surface of the distal phalanx to penetrate the distal half of the nail bed and subsequently the nail plate itself. Early, a painless discoloration under the nail is visible; later, the nail is pushed upward and split. The protruding surface becomes covered with granulations that form painful ulcers.

Overgrowth of the Toenail—Ram's Horn Nail: The nail becomes thickened, conical, and curved like a ram's horn; it may assume grotesque shape and size. This condition may be a source of significant discomfort, particularly with closed footwear.

Vascular Signs

Some disorders of dermal vessels furnish signs of generalized disease. These are considered together with local abnormalities, from which they must be distinguished. These lesions contain enough blood that their red or blue color readily identifies them as vascular disorders.

> **KEY SIGN** **Pallor**

Pallor is the absence of the normal red color of the skin and mucous membranes imparted by blood in the superficial vessels. Inspection for generalized pallor requires observing the conjunctivae, the oral mucosa and palmar creases. In deeply pigmented persons, these may be the only reliable physical signs. Pallor can be produced by edema or myxedematous tissue surrounding the superficial blood vessels, vasoconstriction, anemia, or any combination. ***CLINICAL OCCURRENCE:*** *Localized Pallor* cold exposure, vasoconstriction (e.g., Raynaud phenomenon), arterial insufficiency (narrowed lumina, thrombosis, embolism), edema; ***Generalized Pallor generalized vasoconstriction***—exposure to cold, severe pain, hypoglycemia, volume depletion or low cardiac output syndrome; ***chronic pallor***—normal in some persons, anemia, renal failure (anemia may contribute); ***Paroxysmal Pallor*** apneic periods in periodic breathing, hypertensive periods from pheochromocytoma, vertiginous periods in Ménière disease, migraine; ***Obscuration of Skin Vessels*** edema, myxedema (anemia may contribute), scleroderma.

> **KEY SIGN** **Cyanosis**

Cyanosis is the blue color seen through the skin and mucous membranes when the reduced hemoglobin concentrations in capillary blood exceed 4.0–5.0 g/dL, 0.5 to 1.5 g of methemoglobin, or 0.5 g of sulfhemoglobin. The amount of oxyhemoglobin does not affect the color. Local cyanosis occurs when blood is deoxygenated in the vessels in venous stasis or in the tissues from extravasation. Many normal persons have localized venous stasis in some parts of the body. Generalized cyanosis is seen in the lips, nail beds, ears, and malar regions. DDX: Central cyanosis usually becomes more prominent with exertion or exposure to a warm environment, but peripheral cyanosis does not. Because the blue color is within the venules, capillaries, and arterioles of the subpapillary plexus, it fades with superficial pressure, distinguishing it from argyria. ***CLINICAL OCCURRENCE:*** *Local Cyanosis* localized venous stasis or arterial obstructions, Raynaud phenomenon, extravasations of blood in superficial tissues; ***Central Cyanosis*** hypoxemia (right-to-left shunt, impaired oxygenation as a result of lung disorders), presence of abnormal hemoglobin pigments (methemoglobin or sulfhemoglobin); ***Peripheral Cyanosis*** (implies normal arterial oxygen concentration but increased oxygen extraction because of sluggish flow in the capillaries of the cutaneous vessels) cutaneous vasoconstriction secondary to cold exposure, reflex response to decreased cardiac output.

> **KEY SIGN** **Abnormal Nail Fold Capillaries—Scleroderma**

Episodic digital vasospasm is common in scleroderma (Raynaud phenomena) or in otherwise normal persons (Raynaud disease). Finding abnormal nail fold capillaries is strongly associated with later appearance of scleroderma.

Arterial Circulation Signs

The tissue effects of arterial blood flow must be distinguished from those of venous drainage. Arterial deficits cause dermal pallor, coldness, and tissue atrophy. Small-vessel disturbances are recognizable as specific patterns in the skin. Diseases of the larger vessels cause regional hypoperfusion syndromes; diseases which affect smaller vessels, such as the vasculitides, tend to be more diffuse [McGee SR, Boyko EJ. Physical examination and chronic lower-extremity ischemia: A critical review. *Arch Intern Med*. 1998;158:1357–1364].

Warm Skin: Normal skin temperature indicates adequate arterial flow. The normal color of the nail beds is red or pink. If warm feet have blue nail beds, the warmth has been externally applied to feet with inadequate arterial flow.

Skin Pallor and Coldness—Chronic Arterial Obstruction: See Chapter 8, page 387. Pallid cool skin strongly suggests regional hypoperfusion. It is normal in a cold environment, but should rapidly resolve on exposure to warm air or water.

Dependent Rubor and Coldness—Chronic Arterial Obstruction: The skin and nail beds are blue or purple due to the inadequate arterial flow which is unable to displace venous blood containing reduced hemoglobin from venous capillaries which are dilated distal to the arterial obstruction. Raise the part above heart level to drain the blue venous blood away unmasking tissues made pallid by insufficient arterial flow (Fig. 6–14). When the elevated foot is lowered, the pink color normally returns in 20 seconds. Return of color in 45 to 60 seconds confirms an arterial deficit. See page 387.

Acute Pain with Skin Pallor and Coldness—Arterial Embolus or Thrombosis: Acute occlusion of a major peripheral artery causes cutaneous and muscular ischemia producing skin and nail bed pallor, decreased temperature, and ischemic pain. See page 427.

Malnourished Skin: The skin is thinner than normal, as demonstrated by its shiny appearance and the fine texture of the wrinkles produced when it is pinched. The

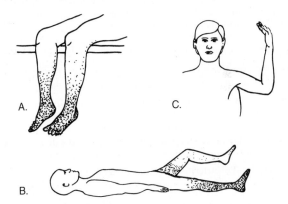

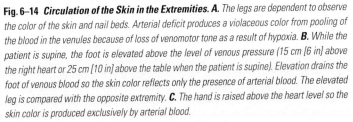

Fig. 6–14 *Circulation of the Skin in the Extremities.* **A.** *The legs are dependent to observe the color of the skin and nail beds. Arterial deficit produces a violaceous color from pooling of the blood in the venules because of loss of venomotor tone as a result of hypoxia.* **B.** *While the patient is supine, the foot is elevated above the level of venous pressure (15 cm [6 in] above the right heart or 25 cm [10 in] above the table when the patient is supine). Elevation drains the foot of venous blood so the skin color reflects only the presence of arterial blood. The elevated leg is compared with the opposite extremity.* **C.** *The hand is raised above the heart level so the skin color is produced exclusively by arterial blood.*

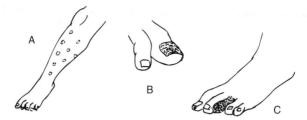

Fig. 6–15 Dermal Lesions from Arterial Deficit. A. Atrophy. *The skin over the legs contains round areas of dermal atrophy, with or without pigmentation. These result from small superficial infarctions.* **B. Dystrophic nails.** *The toenails grow more slowly than normal and the nail plates become thickened and laminated; the layers form transverse ridges.* **C. Necrosis.** *Gangrene of the distal parts may develop from arterial deficit. The sketch shows a round spot of gangrene on the tip of the great toe, and the middle toe blackened from dry gangrene.*

normal fine epidermal furrows are absent. The lanugo hair on the backs of the hands and feet and the dorsa of the fingers and toes fails to grow.

Skin Scars: The skin on the extremities contains round scars, covered with atrophied skin that may be pigmented (Fig. 6–15A). These develop without trauma as the result of obstruction of small arteries.

Malnourished Nails: The nails grow slowly or not at all. They are dry, brittle, and contain transverse ridges. Later, they become thickened (Fig. 6–15B).

Skin Ulcers: Ischemic ulcers occur over the tips of the toes, the malleoli, the heels, the metatarsal heads, and the dorsal arches. They are termed cold ulcers because they lack the warm erythematous areola characteristic of warm ulcers caused by infection. Frequently, the borders of cold ulcers appear punched out. They are also seen in diabetes mellitus with severe neuropathy and sickle cell disease.

Retiform Necrosis: Necrotic skin in a scalloped (retiform) pattern suggests obstruction of the dermal arteriole feeding the area. Vasculitis should be suspected.

Skin Gangrene: In the earliest stage, the lesions are round, less than 1 mm in diameter, with pitted centers of black skin (Fig. 6–15C). The areas may spread to involve the entire foot. When the skin is black, wrinkled, and dry, the condition is termed dry gangrene. If secondary infection occurs, the dead area becomes swollen with fluid oozing onto the surface; this is wet gangrene.

Nodular Vessels—Polyarteritis Nodosa: See page 414.

Purpura

> **KEY SIGN** **Intradermal Hemorrhage**

In general, mucocutaneous bleeding occurs with platelet abnormalities (number or function) or problems of the vessel wall (e.g., scurvy); bleeding into joints or viscera is more likely related to deficiencies or inhibitors of clotting factors. Extravasation of blood into the skin produces an area that is first red, then blue; in a few days, the degradation of hemoglobin changes the color to green or yellow and fades. Because the blood in the area is extravascular, the color does not blanch with pressure. A **petechia** (plural, petechiae) is a round, discrete hemorrhagic area less than 2 mm in diameter. Doubtful spots can be circled with ink; their disappearance in a few days rules out angioma. A larger spot is an **ecchymosis** (plural, ecchymoses). When hemorrhages of either size occur in groups, the condition is termed **purpura**. Purpuric lesions may become confluent and they usually do not elevate the skin or mucosa (macules and patches). Spontaneous purpura from platelet or vessel defects usually occurs on the lower extremities, although slight trauma to the skin may induce it elsewhere. A **hematoma** is an area in which underlying hemorrhage causes elevation of the skin or mucosa (nodule); extravasated blood frequently colors the surface and dissects along tissue planes. DDX: When the capillaries are involved by infectious disease, the resulting purpura may predominate on the thorax and abdomen. *Palpable purpura* suggests a cutaneous or systemic vasculitis; larger nodules may be palpable in polyarteritis nodosa. In subacute bacterial endocarditis, isolated petechiae from bacterial emboli may occur anywhere. In the skin, they may be distinguished from small angiomas by not blanching under pressure. Septic emboli frequently appear in the mucosa of the palate, buccal surfaces, and conjunctiva, where changes in color during resolution are not evident; in the conjunctiva, the petechiae sometimes have gray centers. **CLINICAL OCCURRENCE:** *Vascular Abnormalities* eroded or traumatized large vessels, hereditary hemorrhagic telangiectasia, vasculitis, infections (Rocky Mountain spotted fever), scurvy, Schamberg disease, Cushing syndrome; *Blood Abnormalities* *quantitative platelet defects* (e.g., autoimmune thrombocytopenic purpura, heparin-induced thrombocytopenia, hypersplenism), *qualitative platelet defects* (e.g., aspirin, von Willebrand disease, Glanzmann syndrome), thrombotic thrombocytopenic purpura (TTP), bone marrow failure (e.g., aplastic anemia, leukemia, chemotherapy), meningococcemia, cryoglobulinemia, disseminated intravascular coagulation (DIC).

> **KEY SYNDROME** Immune Thrombocytopenic Purpura (ITP)

Immunologic destruction of platelets leads to thrombocytopenia and increased size of circulating platelets; the bone marrow shows megakaryocyte hyperplasia. Easy bruising, petechiae, menorrhagia, epistaxis, or other mucocutaneous bleeding signals the onset of ITP. The spleen is not palpable. Children with acute ITP frequently recover without treatment. Adults with very low platelet counts are at risk for intracranial hemorrhage and are more likely to develop chronic thrombocytopenia. DDX: The history, physical examination, and selected tests should exclude SLE, HIV infections, cytomegalovirus, Epstein-Barr virus, drug-induced thrombocytopenia, hypersplenism, malignant lymphoma, and other hematologic disorders.

> **KEY SYNDROME** Purpura, Abdominal Pain and Arthralgia—Schönlein-Henoch Purpura (Anaphylactoid Purpura)

See Chapter 8, page 416. This vasculitis is most commonly encountered in children, often coincident with streptococcal infections. A purpuric rash occurs in association with urticaria, arthralgias, abdominal pain, gastrointestinal blood loss, nausea and vomiting, and glomerulitis. The platelet count remains normal.

The disease is self-limited in children; corticosteroids are believed helpful in severe cases.

KEY DISEASE   Scurvy

Punctate perifollicular hemorrhages occur in the skin. The lesions are most common in the lower extremities. Close inspection discloses that each petechia surrounds a hair follicle (perifollicular hemorrhage). The hair is tightly coiled (corkscrew hairs). Mucous membrane bleeding and loosening of the teeth also occur.

➤ KEY DISEASE   Rocky Mountain Spotted Fever And Typhus

See Chapter 4, page 56. On approximately the fourth day of fever, an eruption of erythematous blanching macules 2 to 6 mm in diameter appears on the wrists, ankles, palms, and soles. It spreads centripetally to the trunk, face, axillae, and buttocks. In 2 or 3 days, the lesions become maculopapular, assume a deep-red color, and finally become petechial hemorrhages that resolve with the usual color changes. DDX: In contrast, the eruption of **typhus fever**, with similar individual lesions, begins on the trunk and extends centrifugally, rarely involving the face, palms, or soles.

➤ KEY DISEASE   Meningococcemia

Three-quarters of patients with meningococcal meningitis develop meningococcemia. The eruption involves the trunk and extremities with petechial hemorrhages, together with bright-pink, tender maculopapules 2 to 10 mm in diameter. Some maculopapules develop hemorrhagic centers. Large ecchymoses and hemorrhagic vesicles may form. Gangrene of soft tissues, especially fingers and toes, may occur. Livedo reticularis may be present.

➤ KEY SYNDROME   Disseminated Intravascular Coagulation (DIC) (Consumption Coagulopathy)

Persistence of activated clotting factors and other procoagulants in the circulation leads to deposition of platelet-fibrin thrombi in multiple vessels with depletion of intravascular clotting factors. Simultaneous activation of the fibrinolytic system leads to dissolution of fibrin and a hemorrhagic diathesis. The onset may be sudden or gradual. It may be characterized by shock, the appearance of ecchymoses, purpura, or petechiae, fever, and bleeding from multiple sites. It usually occurs as a complication of preexisting multisystem disease.   *CLINICAL OCCURRENCE:* Septicemia, malignancy (especially acute promyelocytic leukemia, certain adenocarcinomas, and sarcomas), extensive surgery, trauma, complications of pregnancy (dead fetus, amniotic fluid embolism, abruptio placenta, septic abortion, preeclampsia, and eclampsia), envenomation, hepatic failure.

➤ KEY DISEASE   Thrombotic Thrombocytopenic Purpura (TTP) and Hemolytic Uremic Syndrome (HUS)

In TTP, large multimers of von Willebrand factor circulate because of a metallo-protein enzyme inhibition that appears to be immunologically mediated. Arteriolar platelet-rich thrombi produce fragmentation of circulating erythrocytes and ischemic infarcts in vital organs. The mechanism of HUS is less-well understood. Rapid diagnosis and treatment are necessary; examination of the peripheral blood smear for schistocytes is the most rapid way to establish the diagnosis. Without treatment, the mortality is >90%. Most patients with **TTP** are young adults, more often women, with a history of recent viral infection. Other known risk factors are pregnancy, bee sting, AIDS, SLE, chemotherapy with mitomycin C, or recent organ transplantation. Petechiae from thrombocytopenia may be the first sign noted by the patient. The classic pentad of the syndrome is: (1) thrombocytopenia, (2) microangiopathic hemolytic anemia, (3) renal insufficiency, (4) diffuse nonfocal neurologic deficits, and (5) fever, which is variably present. Headache, confusion, delirium, seizures, and other mental status changes develop in 90% of those who die. Relapses of TTP following successful treatment are common. The **HUS** in children produces the same arteriolar lesions and laboratory findings without signs of CNS involvement. The specific metalloprotein enzyme inhibition of TTP is not found in HUS. HUS occurs sporadically and in epidemics associated with gastroenteritis from *Escherichia coli* 0157:H7.

Schamberg Disease (Progressive Pigmentary Dermatosis): A benign chronic disorder with repeated crops of nonblanching petechiae and orange ("cayenne pepper") to fawn-colored macules on feet and legs.

> **KEY SYNDROME** Atheroembolic Disease

Embolization of cholesterol-rich contents of atherosclerotic plaques causes ischemic infarction with hemorrhage in the skin and organs distal to the site of plaque rupture. Patients frequently have had an endovascular procedure with mechanical disruption of plaques on the vessel wall. They present hours to 1 to 2 days later with pain and erythema followed by retiform ecchymoses and purpura, which may progress to frank infarction. The lesions, which may be palpable, range from 1 mm to 2 cm in size; toes and fingertips may become necrotic (Plate 3). Livedo reticularis is common [O'Keefe ST, Woods BO'B, Breslin DJ, Tsapatsaris NP. Blue toes syndrome: Causes and management. *Arch Intern Med.* 1992;152:2197–2202]. *CLINICAL OCCURRENCE:* This most commonly follows passage of intravascular catheters during diagnostic or therapeutic procedures, or follows the initiation of warfarin therapy.

Palpable Purpura—Vasculitis: Inflammation of the small arterioles or venules in the skin associated with immune complex deposition produces inflammation with punctate edema and hemorrhage, palpable purpura. The patient may be well or have symptoms and signs of a systemic disease, including visceral involvement. The pattern and size of involved arteries and/or veins is characteristic of each vasculitis syndrome (see page 413).

Non-Purpuric Vascular Lesions

Pink Papules—Rose Spots of Typhoid Fever: These are erythematous papules, 2 to 4 mm in diameter, that blanch with pressure. They appear in the second week of the fever, usually in crops, but few in number. They are commonly seen on the upper abdomen and lower thorax; each lesion persists for 2 or 3 days and then disappears, leaving a faint brown stain.

Red Macule or Papule—Cherry Angioma (Papillary Angioma): Usually less than 3 mm in diameter and often no larger than a pinhead, the cherry angioma is bright red, discrete, and irregularly round. Larger lesions may be slightly elevated; occasionally they are pedunculated. The growth is surrounded by a narrow halo of pallid skin. Pressure induces only partial or no blanching. Small lesions may be distinguished from petechiae only by their permanence when observed for several days. The angiomas occur more often on the thorax and arms than on the face and abdomen; they are less frequent on the forearms and on the lower extremities. With advancing age, some lesions become atrophic and faded. Everyone has a few; the number increases after the age of 30 years. They have no clinical significance.

Blue Papule—Venous Lakes: Thin-walled papules are filled with venous blood. Gentle pressure forces them to empty, leaving lax indentations beneath skin level. They rarely occur before the age of 35 years; their numbers increase with age. They are 10 times more common in men than in women. Lakes are more frequent on the ears and face than on the lips and neck; they are uncommon elsewhere. Sun exposure is the only condition with which they are associated.

Blue Papules—Scrotal Venous Angioma (Fordyce Lesion): (Fig. 6–16B) and Chapter 12, page 576.

KEY DISEASE **Punctate Red Macules—Hereditary Hemorrhagic Telangiectasia (Osler-Weber-Rendu Disease)**

The disease is transmitted as a mendelian dominant trait. Most lesions develop after puberty and are probably permanent. Affected children often have repeated epistaxis before diagnostic lesions appear in the skin and mucosa. The skin may be pale from anemia due to continual gastrointestinal blood loss and spotted with dull red lesions. The average lesion is punctate, approximately 1 to 2 mm in diameter. Usually, it is not elevated; some appear slightly depressed. The overlying skin may be covered with a fine silvery scale. Pressure causes fading, although blanching is sometimes incomplete. With diascopy, the spots may be seen to pulsate. Occasionally, one or two fine, superficial vessels may radiate from the punctum, but the radicles in arterial spiders are more numerous and the centers smaller. The mucosa is practically always involved; lesions are almost invariably found in the anterior portion of the nasal septum, giving rise to frequent epistaxis. The tip and dorsum of the tongue are favorite sites. Most frequently affected in the skin are the palmar surfaces of the hands and fingers, the skin under the nail plates, the lips, ears, face, arms, and toes. The trunk is least involved. Because any structure may be the site of these lesions, bleeding may cause epistaxis, hemoptysis, hematemesis, melena, or hematuria. There is a high incidence of pulmonary arteriovenous fistulas, which can lead to polycythemia and clubbing of the fingers; arteriovenous fistulae in the liver should be suspected if a RUQ abdominal bruit is heard [Guttmacher AE, Marchuk DA, White RI Jr. Hereditary hemorrhagic telangiectasia. *N Engl J Med.* 1995;333:918–924].

Blue Nodule—Rubber-Bleb Nevi of Skin and Gastrointestinal Tract: There are three types of lesions: a large disfiguring angioma, a fluctuant thin-skinned bleb containing blood that leaves a rumpled sac when compression empties it into venous channels, and an irregular blue area that gradually merges with the surrounding skin, fading only partially with pressure. Nevi of the skin may be accompanied by similar lesions in the gastrointestinal tract that are sites of serious

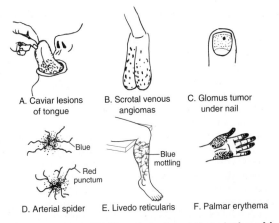

A. Caviar lesions of tongue

B. Scrotal venous angiomas

C. Glomus tumor under nail

D. Arterial spider

E. Livedo reticularis

F. Palmar erythema

Fig. 6–16 *Some Named Superficial Vascular Lesions. A. Caviar Lesions of the Tongue:* Varicose veins under the tongue form bluish masses that appear as bunches of caviar. *B. Scrotal venous angiomas:* When the scrotum is spread out, multiple papules may be demonstrated, 3 to 4 mm in diameter, dark red or blue. *C. Glomus tumor under the nail:* An elevated nodule, 2 to 10 mm in diameter, may occur any place in the skin, frequently under the nail plate. It is extremely painful. *D. Venous stars and arterial spiders:* One form of venous star is depicted; the lesions may also appear as cascades, flares, rockets, comets, or tangles. A typical form of arterial spider, with punctum and radicles, is presented. While venous stars are bluish, spiders are fiery red. Both lesions fade with pressure. Pressing the center with a pencil tip will not blanch the branches of a star; the radicles of the spiders will fade with pressure on the punctum. The star always overlies a large vein; the spider is not associated with a visible large vessel. As seen through a pressing glass slide, the venous star does not pulsate; the arterial spider fills from the center with pulsatile spurts. *E. Livedo reticularis:* Seen most often on the legs, the skin is mottled, with deeply cyanosed areas interspersed with round pale spots. In one type, the discoloration disappears with warming; in others, it does not. *F. Palmar erythema:* An intense diffuse erythema occurs, which is deepest over the hypothenar eminence and less pronounced on the thenar eminence and the distal segments of the fingers. The erythema is not mottled.

hemorrhage. The dermal lesions may be few, or they may be scattered throughout the body. The condition is not hereditary.

Painful Red or Blue Nodule—Glomus Tumor: This a benign neoplasm, thought to arise from the pericyte in the vessel walls of the glomus body. The lesions are more common in the hands and fingers, especially beneath the nail (Fig. 6–16C). The red or blue tumor is an elevated nodule, from 2 to 10 mm in diameter. It is exquisitely painful, completely disproportionate to its size. The pain may occur in paroxysms. Relief may be obtained by surgical excision.

> **KEY DISEASE**   **Irregular Spongy Tumor—Cavernous Hemangioma**

The tumor occurs in any tissue and varies in size from microscopic to huge, with an entire extremity involved. Usually present at birth, it tends to enlarge with age. The tumor may involve skin, subcutaneous tissue, muscle, and even bone. The surface presents an irregular nodular mass, frequently bluish, and fluctuant. Raising the involved extremity above heart level may result in partial emptying. The hemangioma may consume platelets and procoagulants to produce a picture of DIC (*Kasabach-Merritt syndrome*).

Stellate Figure—Venous Star: The lesion occurs as part of the aging process or as a result of venous obstruction. Branches of small superficial veins radiate from a central point (Fig. 6–16D). The patterns include stars, angular Vs, cascades, flares, rockets, and tangles. The entire figure may vary from a few millimeters to several centimeters in diameter. The vessels are bluish, whereas arterial spiders are bright red. When pressed upon, the color fades; the figure refills from the center when pressure is released, as do arterial spiders. Venous stars are more common in women. The predominant sites are the dorsum of the foot, the leg, the medial aspect of the thigh above the knee, and the back of the neck. They also occur in the skin swollen from superior vena cava obstruction. Their clinical importance is to distinguish them from arterial spiders. DDX: In contrast to arterial spiders, pressure on the central point with a pencil does not blanch the radicles. The figure always overlies a larger vein, whereas the spider is not associated with a larger vessel.

> **KEY SIGN**   **Stellate Figure—Arterial Spider (Spider Angioma, Spider Telangiectasis)**

The cause of arterial spiders is unknown. Anatomic studies demonstrate that a coiled vessel arises perpendicularly from a deep artery, its distal end forming the central body from which the legs radiate in the plane of the skin, branching, and rebranching. Typically, the fiery red vascular figure in the skin consists of a central body or punctum, varying from a pinpoint to a papule, 5 mm in diameter (Fig. 6–16D). The "body" is an arteriole from which radiates arterialized capillaries forming the "legs" (radicles) of the "spider." The vessels may dip into the tissue to reappear further on, forming short, visible segments. An area of erythema surrounds the body and extends several millimeters beyond the radicular tips. The lesion feels warmer than the surrounding skin. Rarely, the body is visibly pulsatile; occasionally the pulsation may be felt. Invariably, pressure over the body with a glass slide discloses the blood emerging from the punctum in pulses. When the body is pressed with a pencil tip, the radicles fade; they fill centrifugally when pressure is released. Spiders occur commonly on the face and neck and, in diminishing order of frequency, on the shoulders, anterior chest, back, arms, forearms, and dorsa of the hands and fingers; rarely are they found below the umbilicus. DDX: Spiders are frequently accompanied by palmar erythema in liver disease and pregnancy. *CLINICAL OCCURRENCE:*   cirrhosis, hyperestrinism, pregnancy (disappearing after delivery) and occasionally following significant cumulative sun exposure.

Reticular Pattern—Costal Fringe: Particularly in older men, the superficial veins near the anterior rib margins and the xiphoid process form networks, sometimes in the pattern of bands with rough correspondence to the attachments of the diaphragm. The lesion is usually associated with aging, but has been seen as evidence of collateral blood flow in a patient with superior vena cava obstruction.

Reticular Pattern—Facial Telangiectasis: The vessels of the nose and face may be dilated in older persons. They are common in rosacea and in patients with hepatic disease. They are associated with exposure to the wind and cold, as in farmers and sailors.

Reticular Pattern—Radiation Telangiectasis: Therapeutic X-irradiation produces skin changes months after exposure. The chief signs are pigmentation, skin atrophy, and telangiectasis; the last is the most conspicuous. Fine red or blue vessels form a disordered network. The sharp border in the shape of the radiation port establishes the diagnosis.

> **KEY SIGN   Reticular Pattern—Livedo Reticularis**

The skin of the arms and legs is mottled, with a circinate bands of cyanosis surrounding patches of normal skin (Fig. 6–16E, Plate 4). Three types are described. In *cutis marmorata* the mottling appears on exposure to cold and disappears with warming. The other types persist when warmed. They are *livedo reticularis idiopathica*, which is not associated with other disease, and *livedo reticularis symptomatica*, a frequent accompaniment of the antiphospholipid syndrome, cryoglobulinemia, and polyarteritis nodosa. Ulceration is sometimes a complication of the two types that persist with warming. Livedo reticularis is also seen with atheroembolic events (page 149).

> **KEY SIGN   Palmar Erythema**

A fixed, diffuse erythema involves the hypothenar eminence and, with less intensity, the thenar prominence (Fig. 6–16F). In severe cases, the palmar surfaces of the terminal digits and the thumb are similarly reddened. Rarely, the normal mottling of the palms becomes accentuated and fixed.   ***CLINICAL OCCURRENCE:*** Liver disease and pregnancy (disappearing after delivery).

> **KEY SIGN   Generalized Erythroderma**

Diffuse dilation of the cutaneous capillaries may result from systemic inflammation, fever, or release of bacterial toxins. The patient presents with generalized cutaneous erythema, which may be asymptomatic in benign conditions, or intensely painful and burning with systemic inflammation (Plate 5).   ***CLINICAL OCCURRENCE:***   Fever, viral exanthems, staphylococcal or streptococcal toxic shock syndrome, staphylococcal scalded-skin syndrome, scarlet fever, drug eruptions (exfoliative dermatitis), Stevens-Johnson syndrome, toxic epidermal necrolysis, psoriasis, SLE cutaneous T-cell lymphoma.

Acute Generalized Exanthematous Pustulosis: A generalized acute erythroderma is accompanied by fever, chills and leukocytosis. The erythroderma progress over hours to a widespread pustulosis. The condition is self-limited and appears to follow exposure to viruses or certain drugs (nonsteroidal anti-inflammatory drugs).

> **KEY SYNDROME   Paroxysmal Flushing, Blanching, and Cyanosis—Metastatic Carcinoid**

Usually a benign tumor of the ileum, carcinoid may metastasize to the liver, where it produces large amounts of serotonin (5-hydroxytryptamine). Circulating serotonin causes paroxysms of cutaneous erythema intermixed with areas of pallor and cyanosis. A given area of skin may exhibit all three colors in rapid succession.

The eruption is most pronounced on the face and neck, although it may extend to the chest and abdomen. The excessive serotonin also causes hypotension, abdominal cramps, diarrhea, and bronchospasm. Fibrosis in the right heart may result in tricuspid stenosis, tricuspid insufficiency and pulmonary stenosis.

> **KEY SYNDROME**   Red Burning Extremities Erythromelalgia

The patient complains of painful red skin on the extremities, especially the feet and hands, aggravated by dependency. Ambient temperatures above 31°C (87.8°F) usually initiate the attacks; they are relieved by cold exposure. During a paroxysm, the limbs are red, warm, swollen, and painful. The arterial pulses are present and normal. DDX: Similar lesions, but not true erythromelalgia, occur with atherosclerosis, hypertension, frostbite, immersion foot, trench foot, peripheral neuritis, disseminated sclerosis, hemiplegia, chronic heavy metal poisoning and gout [Kurzrock R, Cohen PR. Erythromelalgia: Review of clinical characteristics and pathophysiology. *Am J Med*. 1991;91:416–422]. *CLINICAL OCCURRENCE:* An autosomal dominant or acquired syndrome associated with drugs (e.g., nifedipine, bromocriptine) or myeloproliferative diseases (may antedate by years polycythemia vera or essential thrombocytosis).

Signs of Systemic Lipid Disorders

> **KEY SIGN**   Xanthomas

Systemic disorders of lipid metabolism lead to deposition of lipid in cutaneous and subcutaneous structures, including tendons. The asymptomatic lesions are macules, papules, plaques, or nodules, often brown to orange in color. The distribution of the lesions is highly suggestive of the underlying disorder.

Xanthelasma: There are soft, elevated beige-colored plaques on the eyelids, usually symmetrical, and often coalescent. This is an increasingly common condition after the sixth decade. It may occur in otherwise normal people, or be a sign of elevated low-density lipoprotein cholesterol.

Eruptive Xanthomas: Hypertriglyceridemia leads to rather sudden appearance of multiple closely packed red-to-brown cutaneous papules and nodules. They are common on the elbows and buttocks, but may occur anywhere.

Palmar Xanthomas: Infiltration of the volar creases of the hands produce yellowish ridges. This is pathognomonic for familial dysbetalipoproteinemia.

Tendinous Xanthomas: These relatively large nodules are palpable along tendons and ligaments particularly the Achilles tendon and tendons of the hands. They are associated with marked elevations of the serum cholesterol.

Common Skin and Nail Syndromes

Common Skin Disorders

> **KEY DISEASE**   Acne Vulgaris

The interaction of sebaceous gland obstruction, androgens, and *Propionibacterium acnes* in the pilosebaceous unit leads to inflammation. The lesions are papular, pustular, and may progress to inflammatory pseudocysts with scarring. The distribution is that of the sebaceous glands, especially the face, chest, and upper back. The earliest lesion are *comedones*, which are either open to the air (leading to oxidation of the sebum in the gland orifice, a blackhead) or closed (which produces a white papule). Comedones are not inflamed. Rupture of the obstructed pilosebaceous unit leads to inflammatory papules, pustules and nodules. [James WD. Acne. *N Engl J Med*. 2005;353:1463–1472.

> **KEY DISEASE   Rosacea**

Patients often have a history of easy flushing. After years, acneform papules and telangiectasia develop in the central face (forehead, cheeks, chin), which may progress to chronic edema and skin thickening. Women are more affected than men, although *rhinophyma*, the chronic deformity of the nose, is more common in men. [Powell FC. Rosacea. *N Engl J Med*. 2005;352:793–803.

> **KEY DISEASE   Eczema—Dermatitis**

Dermatitis literally means inflammation of the skin; in practice it is synonymous with eczema, a specific class of epidermal inflammation. Several types are distinguished by their etiology, pattern, and appearance. Consult dermatologic textbooks for more specific information.

> **KEY DISEASE   Atopic Dermatitis**

This an inherited condition often seen in association with a history of seasonal allergies or asthma in the presenting patient, or with a history of atopic dermatitis, seasonal allergies or asthma in first-degree relatives. The condition begins in infancy or childhood and may be life long. The lesions are erythematous intensely pruritic papules or plaques with a predisposition for the flexor surfaces of the elbows, neck, and wrists, as well as the face, feet, and hands. Scratching temporarily relieves the itch, only to increase the inflammation and pruritus, ultimately producing lichenification [Williams HC. Atopic dermatitis. *N Engl J Med*. 2005;352:2314–2324; Leung DY, Bieber T. Atopic dermatitis. *Lancet*. 2003;361:151–160].

> **KEY SIGN   Lichen Simplex Chronicus**

Chronic rubbing or scratching of the skin leads to hyperkeratotic plaques in disposed persons. The lesions are intensely pruritic plaques. Nodular lesions, *prurigo nodularis*, occur at spots of persistent picking. Atopic individuals are predisposed.

> **KEY SIGN   Stasis Dermatitis**

Increased venous and capillary pressures leads to inflammation, edema, subcutaneous fibrosis, and skin atrophy with hemosiderin staining. Any cause of venous insufficiency or elevated central venous pressure can produce the syndrome. There is prominent edema, erythema, and warmth, often with tenderness; it is often mistaken for cellulitis. With chronic disease, the subcutaneous tissues become fibrotic and the edema no longer pits (brawny edema or lipodermatosclerosis). The skin becomes thin and easily injured, leading to ulceration and secondary infection. DDX: When erythema and warmth are present it is often confused with cellulitis; the rapidly advancing border of erythema distinguishes cellulitis.

KEY DISEASE   Contact Dermatitis

This is either a cell-mediated response to prior sensitization or an inflammatory response to skin irritants. The lesions are erythematous, intensely pruritic plaques. The distribution of the individual lesions and the history of specific exposures are critical to making a correct diagnosis (Plate 6). DDX: Irritant disease often forms vesicles early in the course (but so does rhus dermatitis) and evolve more rapidly than allergic disease. Irritant disease will occur in anyone given sufficient exposure to an adequate concentration of the agent (e.g., chemical burns), but allergic contact dermatitis requires prior exposure with sensitization. *CLINICAL OCCURRENCE:* ***Allergic*** rhus dermatitis (poison ivy and oak), many other plant and animal sources, drugs (neomycin, sulfonamides), chromate, solvents, latex, metals especially nickel (commonly found in earrings, belt buckles, snaps of jeans/pants), cosmetics, clothing dyes, industrial oils, and many others; ***Irritants*** acids and alkali, cement, solvents, cutting oils, detergents, and the like.

KEY DISEASE   Dyshidrotic Eczema

This is an acute condition of the hands and feet, especially the intertriginous areas, palms, and soles. Deep pruritic vesicles form and coalesce. Scratching may produce lichenification. DDX: Consider contact allergens and autosensitization from dermatophyte infection on the feet (see below).

KEY DISEASE   Asteatotic Eczema

This is common on the extremities and trunk, especially in cold dry climates. It is exacerbated by excessive exposure to soap and water. The skin is dry and cracked into irregular rhomboidal plates with erythematous margins, like a drying lakebed; marginal scaling is common. The patient complains of intense pruritis.

KEY DISEASE   Papular Eczema

The lesions are pruritic erythematous papules occurring on the extremities, especially of older adults. They may be similar to guttate psoriasis, but without the scale.

KEY DISEASE   Nummular Eczema

The nummular (coin-like) lesions are 1 to 3 cm in diameter plaques with sharp borders and a raised edge. They may weep, especially with excoriation. They are most common on the legs and trunk in older men.

KEY SYNDROME   Autosensitization Dermatitis

Sensitization to antigens at the site of a primary dermatitis, often infectious or infected, leads to distant lesions. The classic example is the "id" reaction, a vesicular eruption on the hands in patients with chronic dermatophyte infection of the feet. Characteristically, the secondary lesions only heal with treatment of the primary site of infection or inflammation.

KEY DISEASE   Seborrheic Dermatitis

This very common disorder produces erythema and scaling in areas of sebaceous gland activity: the scalp (dandruff, cradle cap), eyebrows, nasolabial folds, external acoustic meatus, and chest (Plate 7). The skin may be mildly pruritic. *CLINICAL OCCURRENCE:*   It occurs frequently with Parkinson disease and sudden severe disease may be sign of HIV infection, although usually it is of no diagnostic significance.

Photodermatitis: Sensitization of the skin by either topical or systemic chemicals leads to a dermatitis triggered by exposure to sunlight. The rash appears within hours to a day or two of sunlight exposure and only in sun-exposed areas. It is erythematous and may have a burning quality. Blistering may occur. Polymorphic light eruption refers to a delayed sensitivity reaction to sunlight exposure. *CLINICAL OCCURRENCE:*   Only partial lists. Drugs: antibiotics (tetracyclines, sulfonamides), antidepressants, antihypertensives, diuretics (thiazides especially), nonsteroidal anti-inflammatory drugs, sunscreens; polymorphic light eruption; porphyria.

KEY SIGN   Intertrigo

The intertriginous areas, the skin folds between the buttocks, under the breasts, and in the skin creases, especially of morbidly obese persons, are common sites of superficial erythema and discomfort caused by persistent warmth, moisture, and occlusion. Secondary infections may occur with streptococci, *Pseudomonas aeruginosa*, *Candida albicans*, and other fungi. DDX: Psoriasis, especially inverse psoriasis, can be confused with intertrigo.

KEY DISEASE   Psoriasis

Inflammation of the dermis is associated with increased epithelial cell division leading to thickening of the skin. This is a common disorder that occurs in approximately 1% to 3% of the population and varies from mild to severe. A family history may be found. It is bilateral and symmetrical, involves the extensor surfaces (e.g., elbows, knees) more than the flexor surfaces, and frequently involves the scalp and gluteal crease. Trunk and extremities may be involved in any combination. Occasionally, the pattern is the opposite of that expected, *inverse psoriasis*. Individual lesions vary from papules to huge plaques. They have a characteristically adherent scale; the surface bleeds when the scales are removed. The nails are frequently involved with pits and dystrophy. Skin trauma may precipitate a new lesion (*Koebner phenomena*). A severe mutilating arthritis with characteristic involvement of the axial skeleton (spondyloarthropathy) and distal interphalangeal joints may accompany or occur independently of the skin and nail disease [Schön MP, Boehncke W-H. Psoriasis. *N Engl J Med*. 2005;352:1899–1912].

Guttate Psoriasis: Following an infectious disease, often streptococcal pharyngitis, 2- to 10-mm pink papules appear diffusely on the trunk and extremities; the face and scalp are relatively spared and the palms and soles rarely involved.

The lesions resolve spontaneously over weeks. Classic plaque psoriasis may occur several years after remission of guttate psoriasis. DDX: The lesions may be difficult to distinguish from papular dermatitis.

Pustular Psoriasis: Sudden onset of intense painful erythema is followed within 24 hours by deep pustular dermal lesions, which rupture to form erosions. The patient has fever and leukocytosis. Patients may be severely ill. This frequently results from withdrawal of systemic corticosteroid therapy.

Palmoplantar Pustulosis: Pustules appear sporadically on the palms and soles associated with burning pain. The lesions heal with crusting. The cause is unknown; it is considered by some localized forms of pustular psoriasis. Palmoplantar pustulosis has been described with metal allergies and as a reaction to tumor necrosis factor inhibitors.

KEY SYNDROME   Infectious Exanthems

An *exanthem* is a diffuse skin eruption associated with bacterial or viral illness (See also Erythroderma, page 153). The viral exanthems are often accompanied by mucosal involvement, an *enanthem*. The individual lesions may take many forms: diffuse erythroderma (*scarlatiniform*), maculopapules (*morbilliform*, measles-like), or vesicles that may evolve to pustules. The diffuse erythrodermas often heal with desquamation. *CLINICAL OCCURRENCE:* *Viral (most common)* rubella, rubeola, parvovirus B19, adenoviruses, cytomegalovirus, Epstein-Barr virus, herpes simplex virus 6 (exanthem subitum) and 7 (roseola infantum), enteroviruses, HIV, Colorado tick fever, and many others; *Bacterial* Group A streptococcus (scarlet fever), staphylococcus (toxic shock syndrome), leptospirosis, meningococcemia; *Rickettsial* Rocky Mountain spotted fever, rickettsial pox, typhus.

KEY DISEASE   Scarlet Fever

Pharyngitis from a group A streptococcus with toxin production causes generalized cutaneous erythema. Excruciating sore throat, often with vomiting and malaise, is accompanied by a brilliant-red edematous pharynx with gray or white exudate or membrane and cervical adenopathy. The tongue becomes denuded and beefy red (see Strawberry Tongue, page 268) and a maculopapular erythematous blanching eruption appears on the neck, axillae, and groin, and later becomes generalized. The skin may feel slightly rough, like fine sandpaper. The rash heals with desquamation beginning around the nails.

KEY SYNDROME   Ichthyosis

These are hereditary diseases of the keratinocytes leading to hyperkeratosis and excessive drying of the skin. The skin is thickened and dry and, in severe forms, cracking hexagonally like dried clay. Hyperkeratosis of the hair follicles produces pointed follicular papules, *keratosis pilaris.*

KEY DISEASE   Granuloma Annulare

Rubbery papules and plaques, often with annular or serpiginous sharply demarcated borders appear on the hands, feet, elbows, knees, and distal extremities.

The lesions are pink, purple, or skin colored, and asymptomatic and are typically self-limited. The exact cause is unknown and the localized forms have no diagnostic significance.

KEY DISEASE   Lichen Planus

Purple, flat-topped, sharply demarcated pruritic papules appear on the wrists, ankles, eyelids, and shins. Other forms exist, including hypertrophic and bullous lichen planus. Mucous membrane involvement is common, appearing as white linear lesions in the mouth or genital mucosa (Wickham's striae); erosions, papules and plaques may also be seen in the oral mucosa. Erosive lichen planus has been assoicated with hepatitis C [Case records of the Massachusetts General Hospital: Case 24-2002. *N Engl J Med.* 2002;347:430–436].

KEY DISEASE   Genital White Patches—Lichen Sclerosis

White atrophic lesions with sharp borders appear most often on the vulva and penis, although other areas may be involved. The skin is thin and erosions may occur. Pruritus and dyspareunia are not uncommon [Powell JJ, Wojnarowska F. Lichen sclerosus. *Lancet.* 1999;353:1777–1783].

KEY DISEASE   Verrucous Papules—Warts

Infection of the skin or mucous membranes with human papilloma virus leads to verrucous hyperplasia; uterine cervix infection with specific strains is the cause of cervical cancer. The common wart is a well-demarcated papule with a verrucous surface, commonly on the fingers. Genital involvement is particularly troublesome. Flat confluent lesions without the verrucous surface occur, *flat warts*. Areas of particular difficulty are the sole of the foot, *plantar warts*, and around the nails, *periungual warts*.

KEY DISEASE   Pityriasis Rosea

This common disorder affects primarily adolescents and young adults in the fall. The eruption is asymptomatic to mildly pruritic. It primarily involves the trunk and proximal extremities although an inverse form may occur in the axillae and groin. The general eruption is often preceded by a larger single lesion, the *herald patch*. The lesions are ovate, with the long axis in the skin folds classically creating a "Christmas tree" pattern on the back. They vary from 0.5 to 3 cm in diameter, and have a slightly raised border with a collar of fine superficial scales and an erythematous base. Resolution is spontaneous over weeks.

KEY SIGN   Actinic Keratoses

Mildly erythematous papules with an adherent hyperkeratotic scale occur in sun-exposed areas. They are premalignant lesions; squamous cell carcinoma may arise in chronic lesions.

KEY SIGN Seborrheic Keratoses

These are hereditary lesions that begin to appear in midlife as brown macules. They gradually enlarge to 1- to 3-cm plaques with an adherent hyperkeratotic raised surface. They give the appearance of being stuck on the skin (Plate 8). DDX: Pigmented lesions may be confused with malignant melanoma and macular lesions with moles or lentigines.

KEY SIGN Dermatofibroma

The lesions are 3 to 8 mm, variably colored papules, usually on the extremities. They are hard intradermal lesions attached to the epidermis. Pinch the lesion and it will retract rather than elevate, the dimple sign. DDX: May be confused with melanoma.

KEY SIGN Skin Tags (Acrochordons)

These dermal polyps are most prevalent on the neck, axillary folds, and perineum. They are more common with obesity. They are of no clinical significance but are often a cosmetic concern or may be irritated by clothing or jewelry. DDX: Large skin tags may be confused with neurofibromas.

KEY SIGN Vitiligo

Destruction of melanocytes through what is most likely an autoimmune process results in complete loss of pigmentation (depigmentation) in affected areas. The macular lesions are symmetrical with sharp borders. They cause significant cosmetic discomfort in dark-skinned individuals. DDX: Vitiligo may be confused with hypopigmented lesions (e.g., discoid lupus erythematosus, leprosy), depigmentation from burns or scars, or ash leaf spots of tuberous sclerosis. *CLINICAL OCCURRENCE:* More common in families with other autoimmune disorders, for example diabetes, Addison disease, Hashimoto thyroiditis.

KEY SYNDROME Body Piercing

This has a long and rich cultural history. Western societies have seen a dramatic increase in piercing in the late 20th century. Piercing is done for many reasons. Importantly for medical professionals are the recognition of the medical risks associated with piercing, the types of piercing and their significance and the personality issues that may be involved in caring for these individuals [Stirn A. Body piercing: Medical consequences and psychological motivations. *Lancet.* 2003;361:1205–1215].

Skin Infections and Infestations

Arthropod Bites and Stings

Mosquito and other arthropod bites. These common lesions present as painful or pruritic papules with erythema and variable cutaneous edema. The central punctum marking the bite is evident with close inspection of early lesions. Most are minor and self-limited; severe local reactions with expansive erythema and edema are not uncommon with hymenoptera stings. Severe systemic allergic reactions occur in sensitized hosts to hymenoptera (bees, hornets, and wasps) and to certain ant species. *Black flies* leave a 1- to 2-mm hemorrhagic mark. Extensive bites may cause systemic toxicity.

KEY SYNDROME   Spider Bites

Most are benign and no cause for concern. Bites of the *common aggressive house spider* cause moderate necrosis of the skin with scarring. The bites are usually on the face, hands, arms, or feet. The spider attacks the victim while sleeping. The *brown recluse spider* is common, but not aggressive. It will bite in defense when disturbed in old buildings, woodpiles, and similar habitats. The bite is initially painless, but may become intensely painful with progressive severe necrosis and scarring. The *black widow spider* bite is a minor lesion with minimal erythema; the adverse effects are caused by a systemic neurotoxin. [Swanson DL, Vetter RS. Bites of brown recluse spiders and suspected necrotic arachnidism. *N Engl J Med.* 2005;352:700–707].

KEY SYNDROME   Myiasis

Some diptera deposit eggs on the skin when they bite. The larva may invade wounds or the bite and grow in the subcutaneous tissue. Since they breath air, an opening in the skin is always present. The patient may complain of feeling movement under the skin [Feder HM Jr, Mitchell PR, Seeley MZ. A warble in Connecticut. *Lancet.* 2003;361:1952].

Bacterial Infections

KEY DISEASE   Impetigo

Superficial erythematous erosions with crusts caused by staphylococcus and streptococcus organisms are common on the face of children. It may occur at any area of breaks in the skin. The crust is characteristically amber. Bullae may form in severe cases, *bullous impetigo*. Localized painful ulcerations, *ecthyma*, may occur with poor hygiene. Secondary infection of other skin lesions is termed *secondary impetiginization*; impetigo commonly complicates eczematous dermatitis.

KEY SYNDROME   Folliculitis

Pustular infection of the hair follicles commonly occur in the beard area of men, but also occur on the scalp, trunk, legs, and buttocks. Organisms include *Staphylococcus aureus*, *P. aeruginosa* (hot tub folliculitis), herpes simplex, and several fungi. DDX: *Pseudofolliculitis barbae* occurs in men with tightly curled hair who shave. Papules caused by retained hairs are present; pustules indicate secondary staphylococcal infection.

KEY SYNDROME   Cellulitis

Infection of the dermis spreads radially within the skin and subcutaneous structures. The warm, raised, and tender lesions are usually caused by streptococci or staphylococci. The borders are indistinct and a break in the skin may be seen at the entry site. Cellulitis is most common on legs and arms at sites of trauma. Fever may or may not be present. [Swartz MN. Cellulitis. *N Engl J Med.* 2004;350:904–912] DDX: Less-common causes of cellulitis are nocardia, mycobacteria, *P. aeruginosa*,

Haemophilus influenzae, and vibrios (especially in patients with liver disease). *Pasteurella multocida* is common following cat and dog bites and has a propensity to cause osteomyelitis. *Erysipeloid* is caused by *Erysipelothrix rhusiopathiae.* *Erythema chronicum migrans* is caused by Lyme borreliosis (see page 57). Noninfectious inflammation is often confused with cellulitis, for example, stasis dermatitis, superficial and deep thrombophlebitis, panniculitis, erythema nodosum, nephrogenic fibrosing dermopathy, tibial stress fracture [Falagas ME, Vergidis PI. Narrative review: Diseases that masquerade as infectious cellulitis. *Ann Intern Med.* 2005;142:47–55].

> ### KEY SYNDROME   Erysipelas

Streptococcal infection of the dermal lymphatics produces intense dermal and epidermal edema and inflammation. The lesion is intensely erythematous with a sharp, raised border. The lesions are common on the face and often a break in the skin is not evident.

> ### KEY SIGN   Skin Abscess—Furuncle, Carbuncle

Skin infections with *S. aureus* produce collections of pus and necrotic debris. The pattern is determined by the skin structure in the area of infection. *Furuncles* (boils) are single collections that are relatively superficial. *Carbuncles* are deep collections extending into the subcutaneous tissues and involve interconnected collections arising from involvement of the deep hair follicles. Carbuncles arise in areas of especially thick fibrotic skin such as the posterior neck.

> ### KEY SYNDROME   Hidradenitis Suppurative

This occurs most commonly in obese women and involves the axilla and perineum, rarely the scalp. It is more common in people with cystic acne. Inflammation of the apocrine gland areas leads to chronic, painful draining lesions that heal with scarring. Infection is probably not the primary problem, but occurs secondarily.

> ### KEY DISEASE   Erythema Migrans—Lyme Disease

See Chapter 4, page 57. At the site of inoculation an asymptomatic erythema appears, which expands progressively, often with an annular configuration. Vesiculation is uncommon. The lesions may reach several centimeters in size; more than one lesion may be present. Bell palsy, heart block, and arthritis of large joints are late manifestations of the disease [Steere AC. Lyme disease. *N Engl J Med.* 2001;345:115–125].

> ### KEY SYNDROME   Ulceroglandular Syndromes

The inoculation site of the organism develops an ulcer that is often minimally symptomatic. Dissemination via the lymphatics leads to regional lymphadenopathy. Finding regional lymphadenopathy should always initiate a search for an inoculation lesion. The history of the type and location of exposure is key to establishing an accurate diagnosis. See also page 97. ***CLINICAL OCCURRENCE:***   Tularemia, plague, syphilis, rat-bite fever, ricketsial pox, cat-scratch disease, anthrax,

Mycobacterium marinum, scrub typhus, sporotrichosis, nocardia, lymphogranuloma venereum, herpes simplex, cowpox, trypanosomiasis.

Tularemia (Rabbit Fever): *Francisella tularensis* is inoculated by fly or tick bites
or skin contact with an infected rabbit. The incubation period is 1 to
10 days followed by lassitude, headache, chills, nausea and vomiting, and
myalgia accompanied by a rather benign-looking ulcer at the inoculation
site with surrounding erythema, but little pain. Regional fluctuant painful
lymphadenopathy develops, which may suppurate. Splenomegaly may be
present. Inoculation into the eye causes an *oculoglandular syndrome* with
lacrimation, photophobia, edema of the lids, and preauricular and cervical
lymphadenopathy.

Syphilis: The chancre is the primary lesion of syphilis. A painless, shallow ulcer
appears at the site of innoculation (penis, glans, vulva, lip, tongue, pharynx,
finger, etc.). The underlying induration is peculiarly discoid, giving it the feel
of a small coin. Painless, nonsuppurating swelling of regional lymph nodes
follow.

Anthrax: Infection with *Bacillus anthracis* is transmitted from infected wild or
domestic animals by contact with hides or by ingestion or inhalation of the
spores. Malaise and a painless pruritic pustule on the skin may be followed
by dyspnea and hemoptysis during dissemination. The painless "malignant
pustule" begins on an exposed surface as an erythematous papule which
then vesiculates, ulcerates, and is surrounded by characteristic nontender
brawny edema; despite the name, it is not pustular unless superinfected. A
black eschar may form. Regional lymphadenopathy is occasionally present.
Inhalational exposure leads to a rapidly progressive pneumonia with hilar
lymphadenopathy and mediastinal widening. Because anthrax has been used
as a bioterrorism agent, a high index of suspicion is required and public
health authorities should be contacted immediately [Dixon TC, Meselson
M, Guillemin J, et al. Anthrax. *N Engl J Med.* 1999;341:815–826; Swartz
MN. Recognition and management of anthrax—An update. *N Engl J Med.*
2001;345:1621–1626].

Nodular Lymphangitis: If the infecting organism is not associated with an inoculation lesion or the inoculation site is not evident nodular lymphangitis occurs
with erythema, induration and nodular thickening of the cutaneous and subcutaneous lymphatics. Regional lymphadenopathy may or may not be found
[Kostman JR, DiNubile MJ. Nodular lymphangitis: A distinctive but often unrecognized syndrome. *Ann Inten Med.* 1993;118:883–888]. This may easily be
misdiagnosed as cellulitis; failure of skin lesions to resolve with an appropriate course of antibiotics for *Staph.* and *Strep.* should raise clinical suspicion
for one of these organisms. A complete travel and exposure history is the
key to identifying the organism. ***CLINICAL OCCURRENCE:*** Sporotrichosis,
mycobacteria marinum, *Nocardia,* leishmaniasis, tularemia, coccidioidosis,
histoplasmosis, blastomycosis, crytococcosis, *Pseudomonas pseudomallei* and
anthrax.

KEY DISEASE **Cat-Scratch Disease**

Gram-negative bacilli (*Bartonella henselae*) are inoculated by the scratch, lick,
or bite of a healthy cat. The organisms travel to the regional lymph nodes and
then disseminate. Symptoms are nonspecific with malaise and headache. Signs

include fever, a papule or pustule at the inoculation site, followed by painful fluctuant regional lymphadenopathy with overlying reddened skin. Dissemination in immunocompromised hosts can lead to hepatitis (peliosis hepatitis), osteomyelitis or meningoencephalitis. Conjunctival infection produces preauricular lymphadenopathy (Parinaud oculoglandular syndrome) [Koehler JE, Duncan LM. Case 30-2005: A 56-year-old man with fever and axillary lymphadenopathy. *N Engl J Med*. 2005:353:1387–1394; Pael UD, Hollander H, Saint S. Index of suspicion. *N Engl J Med*. 2004;350:1990–1995].

> **KEY SYNDROME**   **Rickesttsial Spotted Fever Syndromes**

See Chapter 4, page 56. These syndromes present with an inoculation eschar, high fever, myalgias, and malaise. A thorough travel and residential history is the key to accurate diagnosis.

> ➤ **KEY SYNDROME**   **Necrotizing Soft-Tissue Infections**

Anaerobic or microaerophilic organisms are inoculated deeply into the tissues by a puncture wound, or may ascend into the tissues via the lymphatics from an open wound on an extremity. The infection spreads longitudinally along the adipose tissue septa and the muscle fascia and vertically into the deeper structures via the neurovascular bundles that penetrate the tissue planes. The patient complains of severe pain disproportionate to the injury or the evident cutaneous erythema, which may be minimal at onset. The soft tissues are edematous, indurated, and very tender. These infections progress rapidly, causing extensive tissue necrosis, edema, hypoperfusion, compartment syndromes, systemic hypotension, and death. Rapid diagnosis and extensive surgical debridement are essential to save life and limb. If the infection extends into the fascia and muscle, compartment syndromes may develop. The most common organisms are group A or microaerophilic streptococci. Less common are gas-forming organisms, for example, *Clostridium perfringens (gas gangrene)*.

> **KEY DISEASE**   **Erysipeloid**

The disease is probably caused by *E. rhusiopathiae* and acquired by handling infected mammals and fish. A localized dermal infection of the fingers or hands, it produces an area of swollen, slightly tender, violaceous skin defined by sharp borders, rarely extending above the wrist. The inflammation resolves in a few days, leaving pigmentation.

Mycobacterial Infections

Infection with tuberculous or nontuberculous mycobacterium may present as progressive skin infections unresponsive to antibiotics and with negative cultures on routine media. A high index of suspicion is required to make the diagnosis. Fungal infections (e.g., cryptococcus) can mimic these infections.

Digital Infection—Tuberculosis Verrucosa Cutis (Prosecutor's, Pathologist's, or Butcher's Wart): A bluish-red patch appears on the skin; later it becomes papillomatous and warty; pus may exude from the tissues. The lesion results from inoculation with *Mycobacterium tuberculosis*. The pathologist is infected at the autopsy; butchers and packinghouse workers handle infected meat. Usually, the lesions are indolent with no constitutional symptoms.

Fish-Tank Granuloma—*M. marinum*: A small nodule or nodules develop on the fingers after exposure to contaminated aquariums. The lesions may ulcerate or form small abscesses. With lymphatic spread, the lesions may appear in a sporotrichoid pattern.

Tropical Ulcer—Buruli Ulcer: This is limited to tropical countries. A pruritic nodule breaks down to form a chronic, shallow, nonhealing ulcer. *Mycobacterium ulcerans* is the cause [Wansbrough-Jones M, Phillips R. Buruli ulcer: Emerging from obscurity. *Lancet.* 2006;367:1849–1858; Millay OJ, Connell TG, Bryant PA, et al. Skin ulceration: What lies beneath. *Lancet.* 2006:367:1874].

Viral Infections

> **KEY SIGN   Human Papilloma Virus—Warts**

See page 159.

> **KEY DISEASE   Herpes Simplex**

Herpes simples virus is common. Initial infection may be marked by a severe stomatitis with gingival involvement. Recurrent lesions of grouped vesicles on an erythematous base occur at the site of initial inoculation, most commonly on the lips (herpes labialis), buttocks, or elsewhere (Plate 9). Recurrent lesions are often preceded by 1 to 3 days of pruritic discomfort at the site of subsequent outbreak. Genital ulceration is more commonly caused by type 2 (genital herpes strain) than type 1.

> **KEY DISEASE   Varicella-Zoster**

Infection with varicella zoster virus usually in childhood disseminates initially producing a symptomatic exanthem controlled by the humoral immune response. Infection of the spinal and cranial nerve senory ganglia leads to lifelong latent infection held in check by cell mediated immunity. Reactivation of productive infection as a consequence of age related immunosuppression, severe concurrent disease or immunosuppressive drug therapy produces herpes zoster (shingles) and, rarely, disseminated infection.

Chickenpox: Initial varicella infection leads to a mild systemic disease and crops of pustules. The rash and fever begin simultaneously. The initial lesion is a red papule that becomes a superficial vesicle on an erythematous base (dew drop on a rose petal). Vesicles occur in successive crops, so lesions at various stages of development and healing are present. The lesions are most common on the trunk, less so on the face and extremities. They rapidly turn to pustules that heal by crusting and leave little or no scar.

Herpes Zoster (Shingles): Initially, the patient complains of severe burning pain and dysesthesia in a dermatomal distribution. In 1 to 3 days, clustered herpetic vesicles on an intensely erythematous base appear in the cutaneous distribution of the spinal or cranial sensory nerve. The vesicles burst, crust, and slowly heal. The lesions are always unilateral and do not cross the midline unless dissemination has occurred. The pain may subside in days or persist for months as *postherpetic neuralgia*. Before the rash appears, the diagnosis remains uncertain. A Tzanck preparation or culture of varicella virus from a vesicle confirms the diagnosis. Recurrent zoster is rare [Gnann JW Jr, Whitley RJ. Herpes zoster. *N Engl J Med*. 2002;347:340–346].

➤ **KEY DISEASE**   **Variola—Smallpox**

Infection with variola virus produces a severe systemic illness and pustular skin eruption. The rash is always preceded by 2 to 3 days of fever and severe myalgias and arthralgia. Unlike varicella, the skin lesions arise synchronously, occurring predominantly on the face and extremities. They progress from vesicles to tense deep pustules that break, crust, and heal with scarring. The mortality rate is high [Breman JG, Henderson DA. Diagnosis and management of smallpox. *N Engl J Med*. 2002;346:1300–1308].

Monkeypox: This disease of African monkeys can cross mammalian species. This infection was imported to North America in the spring of 2003. It was transmitted to humans from infected prairie dogs. The illness is acute with fever and malaise, followed by a macular rash with vesicles, which may be umbilicated. The lesions may be asynchronous.

KEY DISEASE   **HIV and AIDS**

HIV/AIDS has many skin findings that may be clues to the diagnosis. Acute HIV infection can be associated with a morbilliform or papular exanthem and enanthem. Herpes zoster can occur relatively early in the course of chronic HIV infection. Severe seborrheic dermatitis is common. *Candida* skin and vulvovaginal infections occur more frequently. Dermatophyte infections may be more common and difficult to treat. An eosinophilic folliculitis is associated with HIV infection and its treatment. Commonly, AIDS patients have a pruritic dermatitis with dry skin. Human papillomavirus-associated dysplastic changes and cervical cancer are more common in HIV-infected women than in non-HIV-infected women. In advanced disease, Kaposi sarcoma (KS) lesions may be present on the skin and oral and genital mucous membranes. Hairy leukoplakia is a characteristic oral lesion. Abnormalities of subcutaneous fat distribution, lipodystrophy, is associated with use of protease inhibitors in the treatment of HIV/AIDS.

Human Herpes Virus 8—Kaposi Sarcoma (KS): See page 176.

Fungal Infections

KEY DISEASE   **Superficial Fungal Infections—Dermatophytosis, Tinea**

Dermatophytes infect the dead keratin layer of the skin, nails, and hair. The specific fungus can be cultured, but clinically the lesions are classified by their location. The clinical picture is variable, but usually involves thickening of the skin with scaling and mild erythema. In chronically moist areas, maceration and secondary bacterial infection may occur. DDX: Mycetomas (soil fungi), chromomycosis, sporotrichosis, and disseminated deep fungal infections affect the skin. Chronic non-infectious dermatitis is often confused with tinea.

Tinea Pedis—Athlete's Foot: This occurs in the intertriginous spaces, usually between the lateral toes, as a white raised patch with fissures that may ulcerate. It may be painful or asymptomatic. It may involve the entire sole of the foot, with a sharp demarcation at edge of the sole. Vesicular forms can occur, especially on the instep.

Tinea Manuum: This is infection of the palm of one or both hands, often occurring in association with tinea pedis.

Tinea Unguium: Dermatophyte infection of the nail plate. See onychomycosis.

Tinea Capitis: This involves of the scalp and hair. The hair is brittle. The circular areas may become inflamed and ulcerate, leading to permanent loss of hair.

Tinea Barbae: This involves the beard area of men; the hair shafts are infected. The lesions are inflammatory papules or pustular folliculitis.

Tinea Corporis—Ringworm: The erythematous lesions are usually circular or arcuate, slowly spreading with a raised scaling border and central clearing. Large plaques may form.

Tinea Cruris—Jock Itch: This is often a chronic infection of the groin, proximal thighs and pubis. The tan or reddish scaling lesion is well demarcated and may be asymptomatic.

> **KEY DISEASE   Tinea Versicolor (Pityriasis Versicolor)**

Infection by *Pityrosporum ovale* (*Malassezia furfur*) causes a very superficial mildly scaling rash usually on the trunk or arms. There are hypopigmented scaly macules and patches in some patients, and hyperpigmented scaly macules and patches in others. The lesions are asymptomatic but are cosmetically important.

> **KEY DISEASE   Candidiasis**

Skin infection is common in moist areas, especially the mouth (thrush), vagina and vulva, under pendulous breasts, and on the perineum and groin of incontinent patients. The lesions are raised, intensely erythematous, and coalesce into large plaques with smaller satellite lesions. *C. albicans* is the most common species identified.

> **KEY DISEASE   Sporotrichosis**

This is a slowly progressive infection with *Sporothrix schenckii*, a soil fungus implanted under the skin by trauma or abrasion. An ulcer at the inoculation site is followed by nodular cutaneous or subcutaneous lesions that suppurate, ulcerate, and drain through multiple sinuses. Regional lymph node enlargement is expected and dissemination to viscera or bone can occur.

Deep fungal infections.   Fungi most commonly associated with deep tissue infections may give rise to skin disease. The lesions may be papules, nodules, ulcers, or confluent masses. A travel and history of places of residence is critical to establishing the most likely organism. Reactivation of latent infection shortly after initiation of anti-TNF therapy for rheumatoid arthritis is not uncommon. Biopsy and culture based on clinical suspicion of fungi in nonhealing lesions is required for diagnosis.   *CLINICAL OCCURRENCE:*   Cryptococcosis, histoplasmosis, blastomycosis, aspergillosis, coccidioidomycosis.

Infestations

> **KEY DISEASE** **Scabies**

The mite, *Sarcoptes scabiei*, burrows in the epidermis, laying eggs and depositing feces, both of which incite an inflammatory reaction. The infestation is passed between persons. The lesions are erythematous papules that are intensely pruritic; linear burrows may be seen. The mite favors areas with thin skin and few hair follicles, especially the intertriginous areas of the hands, wrists, elbows, and genitalia. A KOH preparation will reveal scabies mites, eggs, or excreta.

> **KEY DISEASE** **Pediculosis—Lice**

The patient complains of pruritus and close inspection or combing the hair with a fine comb reveals the lice; the egg sacs are cemented to hair shafts forming nits. Two species are described: *Pediculosis humanus*, which inhabits the head (pediculosis capitis) or body (pediculosis corporis), and *Phthirus pubis*, which lives in the pubic hair (pediculosis pubis).

Larval migrations—cutaneous larval migrans. Roundworm eggs hatch in the soil into motile larvae that penetrate the skin and migrate in the skin and subcutaneous tissues to their final destinations. The lesions are linear red serpiginous and raised, migrating with time. *CLINICAL OCCURRENCE:* *Ancylostoma braziliense*, *A. caninum* and hookworm. There are similar findings with strongyloidiasis (larva currens), fascioliasis, dracunculiasis, and others.

> **KEY SYNDROME** **Swimmer's Eruption**

Penetration of the skin by the larval forms of many organisms for which humans are not the primary host (bird schistosome, jellyfish or sea urchin larvae, etc.) incites a cutaneous reaction. Patients present with an intensely pruritic rash hours after emerging from the water. Bathers in salt water have often showered in fresh water with their bathing suits on; freshwater exposure triggers a sting by some free-swimming larvae. The pattern of the rash may be diffuse or restricted to the area of contact with wet clothing, which held the parasites next to the skin [Freudenthal AR, Joseph PR. Seabather's eruption. *N Engl J Med*. 1993;329:542–544].

Bullous Skin Diseases

> **KEY DISEASE** **Hereditary Epidermolysis Bullosa**

This group of hereditary disorders leads to loss of epidermal cohesion resulting in blister formation with minor trauma. Large superficial blisters develop and break leaving shallow erosions. The severity depends upon the specific genetic defect and depth of the blistering.

> **KEY DISEASE** **Pemphigus Vulgaris**

An acquired disease with IgG antibodies to epidermal desmosomes leading to loss of epidermal cell adhesion [Stanley JR, Amagai M. Pemphigus, bullous impetigo, and the staphylococall scalded-dkin syndrome. *N Engl J Med*. 2006;355:

1800–1810]. The first lesions are often in the oral mucosa with cutaneous bullae appearing later. There are vesicles and flaccid bullae which rupture easily leaking serous fluid. Slight lateral pressure on the skin may cause blistering and a subsequent erosion (Nikolsky sign) [Bystryn J-C, Rudolph JL. Pemphigus. *Lancet*. 2005;366:61–73]. *Paraneoplastic pemphigus* has histologic findings of both pemphigus and pemphigoid.

> **KEY DISEASE** Bullous Pemphigoid

Antibodies form against hemidesmosomes of the basal layer of the epidermis and subsequent complement activation leads to separation of the basal layer from the dermis. The lower legs, axillae, abdomen, legs, and groin are affected. Mucous membranes are involved. Early lesions may be erythematous papules or appear urticarial. Tense bullae develop that may be serous or hemorrhagic; they may rupture or heal by drying and crusting [Nousari HC, Anhalt GJ. Pemphigus and bullous pemphigoid. *Lancet*. 1999;354:667–672].

> **KEY DISEASE** Dermatitis Herpetiformis

This is common in celiac disease (gluten sensitive enteropathy). The exact pathophysiology is uncertain. Symmetrically distributed vesicles, papules, and/or urticaria appear on the extensor surfaces of the arms and trunk. Pruritus is severe. Symptoms may precede the skin lesions by several hours. DDX: **Linear IgA dermatosis** appears similar but is not associated with celiac disease and is immunopathologically distinct.

Bullous diabetic dermopathy. The cause is not known. The lesions are sterile noninflamed bullae that occur without trauma on the lateral aspects of the fingers in patients with poorly controlled diabetes. The blisters are tense and nontender.

Skin Manifestations of Systemic Diseases

> **KEY SYNDROME** Erythema Multiforme

Target lesions appear on the palms and soles, feet, forearms, and face; mucous membranes may be involved. The lesions evolve over several days and may be painful or pruritic. They may progress to bullae (erythema multiforme bullosa). DDX: Psoriasis, secondary syphilis, urticaria. *CLINICAL OCCURRENCE:* Herpes simplex infection, drug reactions (sulfonamides, anticonvulsants, penicillin), idiopathic.

> **KEY SYNDROME** Panniculitis

Sterile inflammation of the subcutaneous fat takes two forms: *lobular*, in which the fat lobule is primarily involved and *septal*, in which the vascular and fibrous septa separating lobules is involved. Patients present with tender erythematous swellings of the skin and subcutaneous tissues, usually over areas of abundant subcutaneous fat. The epidermis is intact and the lesions are not fluctuant [Naschitz JE, Boss JH, Misselevich I, et al. The fasciitis-panniculitis syndromes. Clinical and pathologic features. *Medicine (Baltimore)*. 1996;75:6–16]. DDX: Angioedema can give a similar appearance, but the lesions are more transient and are not restricted to adipose areas. Pyomyositis looks similar, but the lesions are within the muscle, not the fat. *CLINICAL OCCURRENCE:* **Septal Panniculitis** erythema nodosum, eosinophilic fasciitis, eosinophilia myalgia syndrome, scleroderma (localized and diffuse), polyarteritis nodosa; *Lobular* trauma, cold injury, steroid induced, idiopathic lobular panniculitis, acinar pancreatic carcinoma, SLE, sarcoidosis, vasculitis.

KEY SYNDROME   Erythema Nodosum

Tender subcutaneous nodules appear on the anterior shins. They are violaceous and slightly warm. *CLINICAL OCCURRENCE:* *Infections* mycobacteria (tuberculosis, leprosy), bacteria (cat-scratch disease, leptospirosis, tularemia, salmonellosis, yersiniosis), deep fungal infections, viruses (Epstein-Barr virus, lymphogranuloma venereum, hepatitis B); *Noninfectious* pregnancy, drug reactions, inflammatory bowel disease, sarcoidosis, paraneoplastic, Sweet syndrome, Behçet syndrome.

Adiposis dolorosa (dercum disease). In this rare form of obesity, symmetrical adipose tissue masses on the trunk and limbs are painful and tender. If inflammation is present, consider one of the forms of panniculitis [Campen RB, Sang CN, Duncan LM. Case 25-2006: A 41-year-old woman with painful subcutaneous nodules. *N Engl J Med.* 2006;355:714–722].

KEY SYNDROME   Serum Sickness

Deposition of antigen-antibody complexes in the subendothelial space elicits a local inflammatory reaction. This is a hypersensitivity vasculitis caused by antibody formation against an exogenous widely disseminated antigen, most often penicillin. Headache and pruritus are accompanied by wheal formation at the site of subcutaneous or intramuscular injection. The urticaria spreads, and large areas of skin may become edematous. An erythematous rash is often present. Myalgias and arthralgias may be severe; nausea and vomiting may occur. Generalized lymphadenopathy is frequent.

KEY SYNDROME   Scleroderma

In scleroderma, the skin and underlying tissues become contracted and fibrosed. Movements of the digits are inhibited, but there is no ankylosis or joint swelling. The distribution of the lesions and the pattern of other organ involvement defines the particular syndrome. *CLINICAL OCCURRENCE:* Diffuse cutaneous scleroderma, limited cutaneous scleroderma, CREST syndrome, morphea, toxic oil syndrome, arthralgia-myalgia syndrome, graft-vs-host disease, polyvinyl chloride exposure.

Diffuse Cutaneous Scleroderma. Tight shiny skin is present on the distal extremities and face and progresses to involve the more proximal extremities and to a lesser extent the trunk. Raynaud phenomena is common. Cutaneous sclerosis leads to joint immobility, limited mouth opening, and poorly healing ulcers following minor trauma. Dysphagia, hypertension, acute renal failure, and, less commonly, pulmonary involvement occur.

Limited Cutaneous Scleroderma. The skin lesions are less extensive and favor the trunk. Severe pulmonary involvement with refractory pulmonary hypertension and respiratory failure are common, and kidney disease is less common.

Crest Syndrome. CREST stands for the first letters of its cardinal features: Calcinosis cutis, Raynaud phenomenon, Esophageal dysfunction, Sclerodactyly, and Telangiectasia.

Morphea. Localized areas of erythema and induration progress to plaques of sclerosis on the limbs, or head. They may be linear on the extremities. Women are more affected than men. Visceral sclerosis does not occur.

Nephrogenic fibrosing dermopathy.   Patients on dialysis for end-stage renal disease develop diffuse cutaneous and subcutaneous fibrosis most prominent on the lower extremities. Systemic involvement is common with fibrosis of muscles, including the myocardium, and lung. The disease course is progressive with loss of joint mobility. The face is spared. [Mendoza FA, Artlett CM, et al. Description of 12 cases of nephrogenic fibrosing dermopathy and review of the literature. *Semin Arthritis Rheum.* 2006;35:238–249].

Scleromyxedema.   The skin is thickened, indurated and tight, and thrown into prominent folds. There is decreased mobility of the mouth and joints. It is usually found in association with a monoclonal gammopathy of unknown significance (MGUS) [Schanz S, Fierlbeck G. *N Engl J Med.* 2004;351:2218].

> **KEY SYNDROME**   **Dermatomyositis**

There is atrophy, edema, or fibrosis of the skin and nonsuppurative inflammation of skin and striated muscle; the cause is unknown. Malaise, weight loss, muscle stiffness, and dysphagia are presenting symptoms; pruritus is especially characteristic. Heliotrope discoloration of the upper lids and bridge of the nose and flat-topped violaceous papules (*Gottron papules*) over the backs of the interphalangeal joints of the hands are classic signs. In addition, erythematous rashes or exfoliative dermatitis may be seen. Proximal muscle weakness and stiffness are indicative of muscle involvement. Synovial and tendon friction rubs, lymphadenopathy, and splenomegaly may be found. Dermatomyositis may occur as a paraneoplastic syndrome. The variant of amyopathic dermatomyositis presents with skin signs and symptoms without the proximal muscle weakness [Callen JP. Dermatomyositis. *Lancet.* 2000;355:53–57].

> **KEY SYNDROME**   **Lupus Erythematosus**

This is a group of inflammatory disorders thought to share similar autoimmune pathophysiologies.

Acute Cutaneous Lupus: Several lesions occur: an acute malar or generalized rash appears, precipitated by sunlight exposure; erythematous scaling papules and plaques on the extensor surface of the fingers (sparing the interphalangeal joints); urticaria with purpura; hypersensitivity vasculitis.

Subacute Cutaneous Lupus: The skin lesions are psoriasiform plaques or annular erythematous lesions on the trunk, shoulders, extensor surfaces of the arms, or other sun-exposed areas. Systemic involvement is uncommon.

Chronic Cutaneous Lupus—Discoid Lupus: Sharply marginated plaques with adherent scales gradually expand in circles or ovals with central atrophy. The lesions may occur on the face, scalp, forearms, and phalanges. The trunk is less commonly involved. Follicular plugging is seen. DDX: Psoriasis, lichen planus, confluent actinic keratoses, and polymorphic light eruptions may be confused.

Systemic Lupus Erythematosus (SLE): See page 668. This is a systemic disease with prominent, life-threatening involvement of other organs, including the brain and kidneys. The skin findings are those of acute cutaneous lupus and subacute cutaneous lupus.

KEY SYNDROME   Pyoderma Gangrenosum

Painful skin nodules progress to necrotic ulcers with undermined edges most commonly on the lower extremities, buttocks and abdomen; the face may be involved. The base of the wound does not granulate and the ulcers heal with thin scars [Callen JP. Pyoderma gangrenosum. *Lancet.* 1998;351:581–585]. DDX: Ecthyma gangrenosum, necrotic soft-tissue infections, Wegener granulomatosis, stasis ulcers [Weenig RH, Davis MDP, et al. Skin ulcers misdiagnosed as pyoderma gangrenosum. *N Engl J Med.* 2002;347:1412–1418]. ***CLINICAL OCCUR-RENCE:*** Most often idiopathic; when an association is identified, inflammatory bowel disease (ulcerative colitis Crohn disease) is most common. Other associations are with paraproteinemia (myeloma and MGUS), leukemia, and chronic active hepatitis.

KEY SIGN   Sweet Syndrome

Painful papules and nodules appear rapidly and coalesce to form large plaques infiltrated with neutrophils, most commonly on the arms and face. The lesions heal with minimal scarring. It may be chronic and recurrent. ***CLINICAL OC-CURRENCE:*** Hematologic malignancies, myelodysplasia, MGUS, administration of granulocyte-macrophage colony stimulating factor, *Yersinia* infections, idiopathic.

KEY DISEASE   Porphyrias

Inherited or acquired enzyme defects in the metabolism of aminolevulinic acid to heme results in the tissue accumulation of specific porphyrins. Photosensitivity is the hallmark of the porphyrias with cutaneous manifestations. Severe mutilating photosensitivity and hypertrichosis occurs in *hereditary erythropoietic protoporphyria. Porphyria cutanea tarda* is an acquired or inherited disorder. The acquired form is associated with liver disease (cirrhosis, hepatitis C, hemochromatosis) and chemical exposures; it presents as burning erythematous vesicles or blisters on sun-exposed areas, often the backs of the hands or wrists; the lesions heal with atrophic hypopigmented scars. *Variegate porphyria* is inherited; the skin signs are like porphyria cutanea tarda, but systemic disease similar to acute intermittent porphyria does occur. Acute intermittent porphyria does not have skin lesions.

Paraneoplastic Skin Disease: Several skin diseases are seen in association with known or occult malignant neoplasms. The clinician should consider the possibility of an underlying cancer in each of the following conditions: neutrophilic dermatosis (Sweet syndrome, pyoderma gangrenosum); reactive erythemas (erythroderma, exfoliative dermatitis); vascular dermatoses (vasculitis, erythromelagia); papulosquamous disorders (ichthyosis); and vesiculobulous diseases (pemphigus, pemphigoid) [Ahmed AR, Avram MM, Duncan LM. Case 23-2003: A 79-year-old woman with gastric lymphoma and erosive mucosal and cutaneous lesions. *N Engl J Med.* 2003;349:382–391].

KEY SYNDROME   Sarcoidosis

Granulomatous skin lesions present as purple or brown asymptomatic papules or plaques on the torso and extremities; nodules may be more common on the face and eyelids. They do not completely blanch with pressure. See page 396.

KEY DISEASE   Diabetes

Diabetes is associated with a wide variety of skin lesions. *Necrobiosis lipoidica* is most often seen in diabetics. It begins as a brownish-red papule on the shin that enlarges to a plaque, which spreads with a raised rolled border surrounding a depressed atrophic center which commonly has a yellowish coloration. Lesions may be single or multiple and merge by expansion. Diabetic hand syndrome (*diabetic cheiropathy*) is a thickening of the subcutaneous tissues in the palmar aspect of the hand, leading to inability to completely extend the fingers as demonstrated by the prayer sign. *Diabetic dermopathy* is a chronic condition with crops of erythematous papules appearing on the shins and forearms that heal with atrophic scars. *Diabetic bullous dermopathy* presents with painless bland bullae often on the sides of the fingers; it is associated with poor diabetes control. *Mucocutaneous candidiasis* is much more common in diabetics with poor blood sugar control.

KEY SYNDROME   Calciphylaxis

It is believed to be an ischemic injury resulting from calcium deposition in the small arterioles in patients with advanced renal insufficiency and secondary hyperparathyroidism with abnormal calcium-phosphate metabolism. This uncommon disorder presents with painful indurated plaques with vascular mottling or livedo which progress to infarction and ulceration. The lesions gradually enlarge circumferentially.

KEY DISEASE   Pseudoxanthoma Elasticum

This is an inherited disorder of elastic connective tissue. The skin lesions are yellowish papules which may form plaques on the skin folds of the neck, axillae, groin, and abdomen. The skin bruises easily.

KEY DISEASE   Tuberous Sclerosis

This is an autosomal dominant disorder of ectodermal and mesodermal tissues with hamartoma formation in the skin, brain, and kidneys. The skin signs are hypopigmented skin spots that may be multiple and small or larger elongated macules, *ash-leaf spots*. Pink, fleshy nodules up to 5 mm in size appear on the central face. Similar lesions are common around the nails. *Shagreen patches* are plaques on the back or buttock that represent connective tissue nevi.

KEY DISEASE   Neurofibromatosis (NF)

Two forms, NF-1 and NF-2, are inherited as autosomal dominant disorders affecting the skin, bones, nervous system, and endocrine organs. Café au lait (coffee with milk) spots occur in childhood as uniform pigmented macules from a few millimeters to several centimeters in size. The lesions are often innumerable and particularly common in the axilla. *Neurofibromas* are brown, rounded, raised, often pedunculated, lesions that can be reduced below the skin surface with finger pressure (button-hole sign). *Plexiform neuromas* are larger, soft, sagging, subcutaneous lesions that protrude from the skin surface; they may become huge.

Vascular Disorders

> **KEY SYNDROME** **Raynaud Disease and Phenomenon**

Digital artery vasospasm involves one or several fingers or toes and can involve an entire hand. It starts with pallor and progresses to suffusion with cyanosis. It is recurrent and precipitated by cold exposure. If it occurs alone, it is termed Raynaud disease; if it occurs as part of a systemic illness, it is Raynaud phenomenon. Abnormalities of the fingernail capillaries in patients with Raynaud phenomenon is associated with systemic sclerosis [Klippel JH. Raynaud's phenomenon. *Arch Intern Med.* 1991;151:2389–2393]. Raynaud disease is associated with an increased incidence of migraine and Prinzmetal angina. See page 429 for a complete discussion.

> **KEY SYNDROME** **Warfarin Skin Necrosis—Protein C Deficiency**

Protein C deficiency leads to intravascular coagulation and skin necrosis on exposure to warfarin. Painful, indurated lesions appear within 1 to 2 days after starting warfarin and progress to necrosis and sloughing. Areas with large amounts of adipose tissue (and hence poor circulation) are primarily involved, for example, the breast, abdomen, buttocks, and thighs.

Skin Neoplasms

A high index of suspicion is required to diagnose skin cancers at an early stage. They are often picked up incidentally at the time of a visit for another problem. Always survey the visible skin in all patients and perform a complete skin examination on all patients periodically.

Lipomas. Benign tumors of mature adipose tissue can arise in any area of adipose tissue. Lipomas are common and occur mostly on the trunk and proximal extremities. They can be tender when they first appear or if over boney prominences where they are traumatized. They are smooth or lobular, soft, and mobile within the subcutaneous tissue, not attached to the epidermis. Most are 1 to 3 cm in size, but they can become very large causing functional and cosmetic problems. Large size is associated with an increase risk for liposarcoma. They are multiple and appear to be hereditary. Multiple lipomas are associated with several rare diseases (Cowden's disease, Proteus syndrome, multiple endocrine neoplasis type 1, NF-1). DDX: Sebaceous and epidermal inclusion cysts are attached to the epidermis.

> **KEY SYNDROME** **Cutaneous Nevi—Moles**

Nevi are benign proliferations of melanocytes within the epidermis or at the dermal-epidermal junction; there is a hereditary influence on the number and type of moles. Moles may be congenital; more commonly they begin to appear during puberty and adolescence. Congenital *hairy nevi* are large pigmented plaques with prominent hairs. Several different types of acquired nevi are described. *Junctional nevi* are brown to black macules a few millimeters in diameter. *Dermal nevi* are skin colored to reddish domed papules or nodules less than 1 cm in size. Compound nevi have features of both junctional and dermal nevi (Plate 10). Halo nevi are surrounded by a halo of depigmented skin; they may undergo complete regression. *Blue nevi* are deep purple to almost black, firm nodules; the blue color is the result of their deeper location in the dermis. *Atypical moles* have unusual features (asymmetry, irregular border, mixed colors, >6 mm in diameter), which raise the suspicion of melanoma; if they have abnormal histologic features on biopsy, they are *dysplastic nevi* [Naeyaert JM, Brocke ZL. Dysplastic Nevi. *NEJM*. 2003;349:2233–2240]. Serial photography is the best way to follow multiple atypical moles; dermatology referral is advised.

KEY DISEASE   Malignant Melanoma

Malignant proliferation of melanocytes initially is within the epidermis then progressively invades the reticular and papillary dermis; prognosis is related to the depth of invasion measured from the basal layer of the epidermis. Melanomas are usually pigmented, but amelanotic melanoma is not rare. The lesions are macules (*lentigo maligna*) or papules that become nodules which may ulcerate in advanced disease. Melanoma may arise from preexisting nevi or appear on otherwise normal skin. Risk factors include a family history of malignant melanoma, blond or red hair, marked freckling on the upper back, three or more blistering sunburns before the age of 20 years and the presence of actinic keratoses. The American Cancer Society uses the mnemonic ABCD to help distinguish between melanoma and benign moles. Melanomas have *A*symmetry, *B*order irregularity, *C*olor variegation, and a *D*iameter greater than 6 mm. Inquire about and observe for changes in color, shape, elevation, texture, surrounding skin, sensation, and consistency that are ominous characteristics of melanoma [Abbasi NR, Shaw HM, Rigel DS, et al. Early diagnosis of cutaneous melanoma: Revisiting the ABCD criteria. *JAMA*. 2004;292:2771–2776]. Any suspicious lesion should be referred to a dermatologist. *Never use shave biopsy for lesions that might be melanoma; a full thickness punch is required for staging* [Whited JD, Grichnik JM. The rational clinical examination. Does this patient have a mole or a melanoma *JAMA*. 1998;279:696–701].

KEY DISEASE   Basal Cell Carcinoma

This is the most common type of skin cancer. It arises on sun-exposed skin, most commonly the face and upper back, without a precursor lesion. The lesions are pearly papules, often with surface telangiectasias. They slowly enlarge and may ulcerate. They may have considerable local extension and tissue destruction, but do not metastasize. *Superficial basal cell cancers* are flat, indurated, pink plaques with a rolled border. Uncommonly, basal cell cancer presents as areas of sclerosing skin atrophy, termed *morpheaform basal cell carcinomas*. When advanced, they are erosive with elevated borders [Rubin AI, Chen EH, Ratner D. Basal-cell carcinoma. *N Engl J Med*. 2005;353:2262–2269].

KEY DISEASE   Actinic Keratosis

Abnormal keratinocytes arise in areas of sun damage and are considered by many to be "pre-cancerous" lesions with the potential for transformation to squamous cell carcinoma. Clinically, actinic keratoses arise on sites of prior sun exposure as erythematous macules or even patches, each typically with some degree of overlying sharp adherent scale. They may be asymptomatic or be associated with a tingling or burning sensation.

KEY DISEASE   Squamous Cell Carcinoma

These cancers arise on areas of sun damage from preexisting actinic keratoses or in the genital region as a result of human papillomavirus infection. When limited to the epidermis (*squamous cell carcinoma in situ, Bowen disease*) they present as sharply demarcated, slightly scaling plaques that may be several centimeters in diameter. Invasive squamous cell carcinoma may present as an ulcerated area of indurated skin (common on the lip) or as an eroded exophytic growth. These cancers invade the dermis and metastasize to regional lymph nodes. In advanced stages, squamous cell carcinoma produce fungating lesions.

KEY DISEASE   Kaposi Sarcoma (KS)

Infection with human herpes virus type 8 is the cause. Endemic disease is described in Italy and Africa; this is limited to the feet and extremities, with thickened scaling skin, enlargement of the extremity, and ulceration. HIV infection greatly increases the risk for development of KS; the pattern is distinct from endemic disease. HIV-associated Kaposi frequently involves the mucous membranes (hard palate) and viscera (lungs and gut). The initial lesions are nonblanching, red-blue or bluish-brown papules, plaques, and nodules anywhere on the skin surface; some of the lesions become spongy or compressible tumors moving centripetally from the extremities. Lymphadenopathy and lymphedema are late findings.

KEY DISEASE   Keratoacanthoma

This lesion is difficult to distinguish from squamous cell cancer. It appears as a solitary lesion, which grows rapidly to become an exophytic nodule with a central keratin plug. Some keratoacanthomas spontaneously regress over weeks to months.

KEY SYNDROME   Cutaneous T-Cell Lymphoma—Mycosis Fungoides, Sézary Syndrome

This is a multifocal proliferation of malignant T cells within the dermis and epidermis. In *mycosis fungoides*, the lesions are indurated, often scaling, plaques, reaching several centimeters in size. They may be brown or pink and may appear eczematous. The papules and plaques progress to nodules or large masses, the tumor stage of disease. The disease is limited to the skin and may be confused with eczema and psoriasis. In *Sézary syndrome*, there is systemic disease with leukocytosis and lymphadenopathy; the skin infiltration produces erythematous indurated thickening of the dermis prominently in the face and brows (leonine facies).

KEY SYNDROME   Metastatic Cancer

The skin may be involved with a metastatic lesion from carcinomas or lymphomas. Breast, lung and colon cancers, B-cell lymphomas, and metastatic melanomas are particularly common in the skin. Any suspicious cutaneous nodule or plaque should be biopsied.

ADDITIONAL READING

Klaus Wolff, Richard Allen Johnson, Dick Suurmond. *Fitzpatrick's Color Atlas and Synopsis of Clinical Dermatology.* 5th ed. New York, NY: McGraw-Hill; 2005.

Thomas P. Habit, James L. Campbell Jr., M. Shane Chapman, James GH Dinulos, Kathryn A. Zug. *Skin Disease Diagnosis and Management.* Second Edition Philadelphia, PA: Elsevier Mosby, 2005.

The Head and Neck

At least nine clinical specialties have a major focus on the head and neck: neurology, neurosurgery, ophthalmology, otolaryngology, plastic surgery, radiology, radiation oncology, oral surgery, and dentistry. Each specialty has developed detailed examinations to meet their needs, often with the use of specialized instruments. We describe examinations that can be made with the resources available to the general clinician. Presentation of the entire range of potential diagnoses is beyond the scope of this book. *Traumatic disorders are not considered.*

Examination of the head, neck, and cranial nerves is an essential part of the neurologic examination. Interpretation of physical examination findings is done with an eye to both the local findings and the pattern of neurologic abnormalities. This chapter discusses the physical examination, symptoms, and signs of the head and neck; for signs of primarily neurologic significance, we refer the reader to the appropriate section of the neurologic examination in Chapter 14 to discuss the finding and its interpretation. The major syndromes specific to the head and neck organs, exclusive of the central nervous system, are discussed in this chapter, while the neurologic syndromes are discussed in Chapter 14. By necessity, these distinctions are somewhat arbitrary.

In the general head and neck examination, the examiner should: (1) identify signs of generalized disease, (2) recognize local lesions within the purview of the generalist, and (3) recognize local lesions requiring specialist care.

Major Systems of the Head and Neck

The head and neck contain a complicated grouping of major structures all within close proximity to one another. The examiner must always be aware of the anatomy and functional physiology of the superficial and deep structures being examined.

The skull, facial bones, and scalp provide *protection and insulation* to the deeper structures. The scalp and face are rich in blood vessels that vasodilate in response to cold to maintain normal body temperatures within these vital structures. The head contains the *organs of special sense*: the eyes, ears, olfactory nerve, and taste buds of the tongue. Impairment of the special senses suggests either problems with the sensory organs, their cranial nerves, or the brain. The tongue, pharynx, and larynx are the *organs of speech.* Changes in articulation suggest anatomic or functional problems with these structures. The nose, mouth, pharynx, larynx, and trachea form *the upper airways*; any compromise of these structures may impair effective respiration and effect changes in the tone or volume of voice. The mouth, teeth, mandible and maxilla, tongue, salivary glands, pharynx, and upper esophagus are the *upper alimentary tract* necessary for mastication and swallowing of food. Impairment of these structures may result in nutritional deficiency. The head and neck structures are *highly vascular*. The superficial structures have rich anastomoses from branches of the external carotid, so ischemic injury is unusual. The internal carotid and vertebral arteries supply blood to the brain. The head and neck have a rich *lymphatic network* draining to several discrete regional lymph node beds. In addition, the tonsils and adenoids are lymphatic organs surrounding the upper aerodigestive tract. The neck contains the thyroid and parathyroid glands, major structures of the *endocrine system*.

Functional Anatomy of the Head and Neck

The Scalp and Skull

The scalp has five layers: the skin, subcutaneous connective tissue, epicranius, a subfascial cleft with loose connective tissue, and the pericranium (Fig. 7–1). Functionally, the outer three are a single thick, tough, and vascular layer. The *epicranius*, covering the vertex of the skull, is formed by the *frontalis muscle* attached to the occiput by a large central aponeurosis; the *galea aponeurotica*. The skin and subcutaneous tissue are tightly bound to the galea by many fibrous bands that sharply limit the spread of blood and pus. The *pericranium* is the periosteal layer of the bones of the skull; it dips into the suture lines, limiting subperiosteal blood or pus to the surface of a single bone. Between the pericranium and the galea is a fascial cleft containing loose connective tissue. Because of this layer, the lacerated scalp can be lifted from the skull with minimal effort and blood or pus can spread widely beneath it. A useful pneumonic for remembering this structure is SCALP: Skin, Connective tissue, Aponeurosis, Loose connective tissue, Periosteum.

The scalp has three areas of *lymphatic drainage*. The forehead and the anterior portion of the parietal bone drain to the *preauricular lymph node*. The

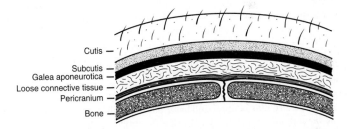

Cutis —
Subcutis —
Galea aponeurotica —
Loose connective tissue —
Pericranium —
Bone —

Fig. 7–1 *Layers of the Scalp.* *For practical purposes, the cutis, subcutis, and galea aponeurotica constitute a single, thick, tough layer with fibrous bands compartmentalizing the more superficial tissue and binding it to the galea. Between the galea and the pericranium is a potential space with a little areolar tissue. Fluid and infection spread slowly through the compartments above the galea, but spread easily through the space beneath the galea and its attached muscles (the epicranius). The pericranium is the periosteal layer that covers the bones of the skull and dips inward at the suture lines. Subperiosteal fluid is limited to the area over a single bone.*

mid-parietal region drains first to the postauricular node and then into the nodes of the *posterior cervical triangle*. The occipital area drains first into the nodes at the origin of the trapezius, and then into the *posterior cervical triangle*.

The Face and Neck

The facial contour is determined by the frontal bone, forming the forehead and the brows; the maxilla; and zygomatic arch forming the cheeks and inferior orbital rim, the bony and cartilaginous nose, external ears, and the mandible. The mandible articulates with the temporal bone anterior to the acoustic canal. The ramus drops inferiorly to the angle of the jaw from which the mandible turns anteriorly and medially with the two halves meeting in the midline to form the chin. The upper and lower teeth are important in determining vertical facial proportions. This bony superstructure is overlaid with muscles and soft tissues, including the lips, which give the face its rounded contours. Mild facial asymmetry is common. The anterior neck is dominated by the thyroid cartilage, which is more prominent in men (the Adam's apple), the cervical trachea, and the two bands of the sternocleidomastoid muscle arising on the mastoid process and inserting on the clavicle and manubrium. The posterior neck is enveloped in thick longitudinal muscles covering the cervical spine from the occiput to the upper back and the fan-shaped trapezius that forms the posterior lateral contour of the neck.

The Ears

The pinna, or auricle, and the external acoustic canal compose the *external ear*; the *middle ear* consists of the tympanic membrane (TM) and the tympanic cavity with its three ossicles. The *internal ear*, or bony labyrinth, is composed of the cochlea, the organ of hearing, and the semicircular canals, the sensory organ for maintaining balance; it is not accessible to direct examination.

The External Ear

The *pinna or auricle* is a flattened funnel with crinkled walls of yellow fibroelastic cartilage. It has a wide external brim that narrows internally to the external *acoustic meatus*. Several prominent folds are readily identified, although there is considerable individual variation (Fig. 7–2A). The *helix* originates as the *crus*, which courses anteriorly and then winds upward, backward, and downward posteriorly to form the funnel's brim. Above the midpoint of its posterior vertical portion, a fusiform swelling occasionally develops, the *Darwinian tubercle*. An inner concentric fold, the *antihelix*, partially surrounding an ovoid cavity, the *concha*, is divided into an upper and lower portion by the transverse *helical crus*. From the anterior brim of the funnel, below the crus, the tragus points backward toward the lower concha as a small eminence. From the lower portion of the antihelix, another eminence, the *antitragus*, points forward across the *intertragal notch* to the tragus. The deep lower concha forms the *external acoustic meatus*. At the junction of the inferior limbs of the helix and antihelix is a pendant lobule of adipose and areolar tissue without cartilage, the *earlobe*.

The external acoustic meatus or canal is approximately 2.5 cm long, extending from the bottom of the concha to the TM (Fig. 7–2B). The lateral one-third of the superficial canal is walled with cartilage; the medial two-thirds runs through the temporal bone. From the concha, the canal forms a gentle S, tending inward, forward, and upward. Approximqately 20 mm inside from the concha is a bony

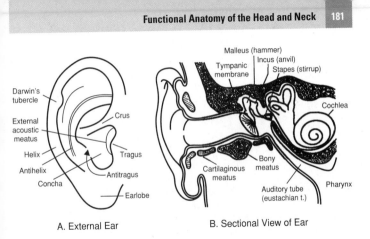

Fig. 7–2 *Pinna and Middle ear Anatomy. A. Surface of pinna.* *The main features are depicted, but there are many individual variations. Darwin tubercle is only occasionally present.* ***B. Middle ear:*** *a vertical section through the ear. Note the flexible cartilaginous and fixed bony segment of the external acoustic meatus. The plane of the TM slants outward approximately 35 degrees from vertical; the conical apex points inward and upward.*

constriction in the canal, the *isthmus*. Ear wax, produced in the cartilaginous portion of the canal, acidifies and protects the epithelium by suppressing bacterial overgrowth and capturing particles. The wax migrates to the concha with the epithelial migration of the canal skin in that direction.

The Middle Ear

Within the petrous portion of the temporal bone, the acoustic canal widens to form the tympanic cavity, surmounted by an attic providing room for movements of the ossicles. Separating the *tympanic cavity* and the external acoustic meatus is the *TM*, an ovoid biconcave disk slanting across the canal in a plane 35 degrees from the vertical, its posterior superior portion more superficial than the anterior inferior attachment (Fig. 7–2B). The *manubrium of the malleus* is firmly attached to the inner tympanic membrane; viewed from outside, the attached portion appears as a smooth ridge forming a radius of the membrane, slanting upward and slightly anterior.

The Inner Ear

The inner ear, or *labyrinth*, consists of the spiral *cochlea* (the organ of hearing), the semicircular canals, ampullae, utricle and saccule (the organs of balance), and the acoustic nerve endings carnial nerve (CN) VIII. These structures are contained in the bony labyrinth within the temporal bone adjacent to the middle ear. Two windows connect the middle and inner ear: the oval window contains the footplate of the stapes and communicates mechanical vibrations to the inner ear via the scala vestibuli; the round window covers the origin of the scala tympani.

The Eyes

The bony *orbits* are quadrilateral pyramids with bases facing anteriorly and apices pointing backward and medially. Their medial sides are parallel, while the lateral

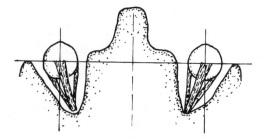

Fig. 7–3 *Relationship of the Orbits and Globes.* *A horizontal section through the orbits. The medial orbital walls are parallel. When the globes are in the primary position, the parallel optic axes are parallel with the medial orbital walls. Because the orbital apices and origins of the ocular muscles are medial to the optic axes in the primary position, the lateral rectus muscles are longer than the medial and the superior and inferior recti pull medially.*

walls form a 90-degree angle (Fig. 7–3). Seven bones comprise each orbit. The orbital roof is formed by the frontal bone and the lesser wing of the sphenoid bone. The medial wall is formed from portions of the ethmoid, maxillary, lacrimal, and sphenoid bones; the front of this wall contains the lacrimal groove for the lacrimal sac. The lateral wall is composed of the zygomatic bone and the greater wing of the sphenoid bone. The orbital floor contains the maxillary, palatine, and zygomatic bones. Several *foramen* open into the orbit. The *optic foramen* is at the posterior apex of the pyramidal orbit within the lesser wing of the sphenoid. This foramen leads into the optic canal, through which pass the optic nerve (CN II), the ophthalmic artery, and the sympathetic nerves. The *superior orbital fissure* separates the orbital roof from the lateral wall, dividing the lesser and greater wings of the sphenoid; it carries the orbital branches of the middle meningeal artery, the superior ophthalmic vein, and four cranial nerves including the oculomotor (CN III), the trochlear (CN IV), the first (ophthalmic) division of the trigeminal (CN V-1), and the abducens (CN VI) nerves.

Extraocular Movements

The optical axis of the globe passes from the midpoint of the cornea to the fovea. The globe is suspended at the orbital rim by a fascia that is continuous with the orbital septum and orbital periosteum. This method of floating suspension allows the globe to rotate about three axes intersecting perpendicularly at the center of rotation. The gaze can therefore be directed to any anterior location combining any of these planes. Rotation about the vertical axis through the equatorial plane of the globe permits *abduction* and *adduction*; rotation about the horizontal axis through the equator produces *elevation* and *depression*; rotation about the optic axis allows intorsion (toward the nose) and extorsion (away from the nose).

Six muscles rotate the globe around the three axes. The *four recti* originate in a fibrous ring around the optic foramen in the orbital apex (Fig. 7–4); these muscles insert slightly anterior to the global equator, spaced 90 degrees apart; the *superior* and *inferior recti* attach to the superior and inferior meridian, while the *lateral* (external) and *medial* (internal) recti are opposed on the horizontal meridians. The *superior oblique* muscle originates above the four recti at the optic foramen and then runs anteriorly and medially to the trochlea, a fibrous

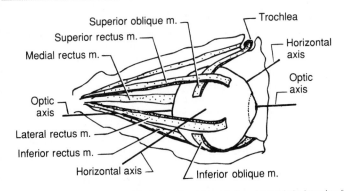

Fig. 7–4 *The Extraocular Ocular Muscles. The right orbit viewed through the lateral wall.*

pulley in the medial side of the anterior orbit, from which it runs laterally and posteriorly under the superior rectus to insert behind the equator in the upper lateral quadrant of the posterior globe. Its physiologic point of action is at the pulley. The *inferior oblique muscle* originates anteriorly near the medial lacrimal groove, passes posteriorly and laterally between the inferior rectus and the orbital floor to its insertion in the posterior lower lateral quadrant. The superior oblique is innervated by the trochlear nerve (CN IV), the lateral rectus by the abducens nerve (CN VI) and the other three recti and inferior oblique by the oculomotor nerve (CN III).

In the primary position, the globes are suspended with their optic axes horizontal in the sagittal plane. Because the rectus muscles pull toward the orbital apex, the lateral recti are longer than the medial recti. The superior and inferior recti do not pull exactly in the direction of the optic axes (Fig. 7–5A). Study Figure 7–5

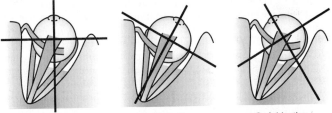

A. Primary Position   B. Abduction   C. Adduction

Fig. 7–5 *Positions of the Right Globe in Relation to the Ocular Muscles. In all positions, the lateral rectus produces abduction and the medial rectus causes adduction. With the optic axis in the* **A. primary position***, the superior rectus elevates and intorts, the inferior oblique elevates and extorts, the inferior rectus depresses and extorts, and the superior oblique depresses and intorts.* **B. With the globe abducted***, so the optic axis coincides with the pull of the superior and inferior recti, these muscles produce elevation or depression without extorsion or intorsion.* **C. When adduction causes the optic axis to coincide with the pull of the oblique muscles along the equator***, these muscles produce elevation and depression without intorsion or extorsion.*

to visualize the movements of the globe imparted by the six muscles starting from the primary position. Contraction of the medial rectus, with relaxation of the opposed lateral rectus, produces adduction; contraction of the lateral rectus and relaxation of the medial rectus results in abduction. Contraction of the superior rectus elevates and *intorts* the globe because the angular pull produces some rotation about the optic axis. Similarly, the inferior rectus causes depression and *extorsion*. The superior oblique depresses and intorts, assisting the depression while countering the extorsion of the inferior rectus. The inferior oblique assists the superior rectus in elevation, while its extorsion counters the intorting action of the superior rectus. Deviation from the primary position changes the relative effects of various muscles. When the eye is abducted (Fig. 7–5B) to a position where the direction of pull of the superior and inferior recti coincides with the optic axis, the recti produce pure elevation and depression, respectively. Similarly, adduction can attain a position where the oblique muscles pull along the equator to produce pure intorsion or extorsion (Fig. 7–5C). Convergence is accomplished by contraction of the two medial recti.

The Eyelids

The area between the opened upper and lower eyelids is the *palpebral fissure* (Fig. 7–6); the two angles of the fissure are the *lateral* (temporal) and the *medial* (nasal) *canthi*. In the medial canthus is a small protuberance of modified skin, the caruncle; posterior to the *caruncle* is a tissue fold, the *plica semilunaris*. Each lid has a *punctum* along the nasal aspect of the lid margin. These puncta open into the superior and inferior canaliculi, which meet as the common canaliculus and drain into the lacrimal sac. The *upper lid* extends superiorly from the superior lid margin to the superior rim of the bony orbit, where the lid tissue merges with the periosteum. The skin overlying the eyelids is the thinnest skin of the body; it is readily moved and picked up. During elevation, the upper eyelid invaginates between the globe and the upper border of the orbit. The lower lid extends inferiorly from the inferior lid margin to merge with the periosteum of the inferior orbital rim; the lower lid is shorter and does not infold. Extension of edema fluid into and from the orbit is limited by these firm attachments to the orbital rim. Within the lids are the circular fibers of the *orbicularis oculi muscle*, supplied by the facial nerve (CN VII). The upper lid also contains the vertical tendons of the *levator palpebrae superioris* muscle, which originates in the optic foramen and inserts into the tarsal plate; the levator palpebrae is innervated by the oculomotor

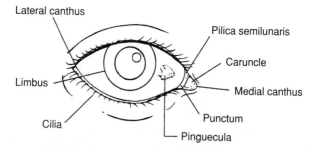

Fig. 7–6 *External Landmarks of the Normal Right Eye.*

nerve (CN III). The upper lid also contains Müller's muscle, which lies posterior to the levator and is innervated from the cervical sympathetic chain. The lids are stiffened by *tarsal plates*, transverse dense plaques of elastic and connective tissue; the upper tarsus is much taller than the lower. Both tarsi are adherent posteriorly to the palpebral conjunctiva and contain many *meibomian glands*, modified sebaceous glands that run perpendicularly to the palpebral margins and empty through pinpoint openings in the lid margins. At the skin border of the lid margins is a double row of cilia or *eyelashes* with their hair follicles. The hairs are deeply pigmented and curve outward. Deep to the temporal side of the upper lid, beneath the frontal bone, lies the *lacrimal gland* that produces tears that flush the conjunctival surfaces; the many accessory lacrimal glands that provide baseline tear production are within the conjunctiva. The epicanthal fold is a semicircular fold of skin oriented vertically over the nasal aspect of the lids and partially covering the medial canthus. It is present in approximately 20% of newborn white children, but it disappears by the age of 10 years in all but 3%. The epicanthus must be distinguished from the fold of skin that originates in the upper lid and partially or completely overhangs the superior tarsus to a variable degree in Asian patients; this is horizontal, while the epicanthal fold is vertical. Epicanthus should also not be confused with esotropia, in which there is excessive deviation of the visual axes toward each other.

The Conjunctiva and Sclera

The *palpebral conjunctiva* joins the skin at the anterior edge of the lid margins. It follows the inner surface of the lids into the *superior* and *inferior* fornices. Although firmly attached to the tarsal plates, it is quite loose in the fornices permitting movement of the globe. At the fornices, the membrane is reflected anteriorly to cover the sclera as the *bulbar conjunctiva*. The larger *episcleral vessels* are, normally, visible peripherally through the transparent bulbar conjunctiva; they may be moved by sliding the conjunctiva over the sclera. The conjunctiva is firmly attached to the sclera at the corneal limbus. The epithelial surface of the cornea is produced from limbal stem cells and is different from the epithelium of the conjunctiva. The superficial vessels of the bulbar conjunctiva run radially in tortuous courses (see Fig. 7–39). The deeper vessels are not individually visible; they radiate near the limbus. A raised yellow plaque, the *pinguecula*, resulting from sun damage to the conjunctival elastic tissue, occurs commonly and is located on either side of the limbus within the interpalpebral fissure along the horizontal plane.

The Cornea

The cornea and anterior ocular structures are best examined by binocular magnified examination with a slit lamp using a mobile, variably sized light source, allowing examination of individual cellular layers. The cornea is a clear, convex structure composed of five transparent, avascular layers, through which may be seen the anterior chamber, iris, pupil, and lens. The junction of the cornea with the sclera is called the *limbus*. The diameter of the adult cornea is approximately 12 mm. The anterior chamber is the space between the endothelial surface of the cornea and the anterior surface of the iris; the anterior chamber is filled with aqueous fluid produced by the ciliary body and drained, peripherally, through the anterior chamber angle at the circumferential junction of the iris and the cornea.

The Sclera

Beneath the bulbar conjunctiva, the ocular globe is covered by a tough, dense, avascular fibrous coat, the *sclera*. It is china white except for spots of brown melanin, varying in number with the individual's complexion and race. The sclera is pierced by the *scleral foramen*, for the optic nerve, the *long ciliary arteries* and *nerves*, the *short ciliary nerves*, and the venae vorticosae. The tendons of the ocular muscles insert into the sclera.

The Iris and the Pupil

The iris is a muscular diaphragm composed of a radial dilating muscle, the dilator pupillae, and a central, circumferential muscle, the *sphincter pupillae*. These muscles work in concert to control the aperture of the iris, the *pupil*, in order to regulate the amount of light that passes through the lens to the retina.

The Lens

The lens is a flexible; transparent structure which focuses light on the retina. The anterior and posterior lens surfaces are convex; the junction of the two curved surfaces is the equator. The lens is located behind the iris, suspended at its equator by the *zonula ciliaris*, which insert into the *ciliary body* (Fig. 7–7). When the eye is at rest for distant vision, the *ciliary muscle* relaxes increasing tension on zonula peripherally which flattens the flexible crystalline lens centrally and decreases the refractive power of the lens. During near focus the ciliary muscle contracts decreasing the tension on the zonules allowing the elastic lens to become more spherical and thicken centrally which increases the power of the lens; this process is called accommodation.

The Vitreous Body

The clear, gelatinous tissue behind the crystalline lens is the vitreous. Anteriorly, the vitreous is attached in a circumferential fashion to the peripheral pars plana and retina (vitreous base), and posteriorly it is attached to the optic nerve head, vessels, and macula. The collagenous vitreous partially liquefies with age. Traction at the vitreous base can tear the retina, allowing liquid vitreous to access the subretinal space and causing a retinal detachment. The collagenous vitreous also provides a scaffold for fibrous tissue and proliferating blood vessels in ischemic retinal disease, which can contract and tear the retina.

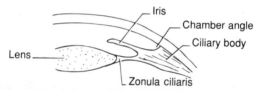

Fig. 7–7 *Cross-Section of the Lens and Ciliary Body.*

The Retina, Choroid, and Optic Nerve

To understand the anatomy of the posterior ocular segment, consider the structures from the inside out. The retina loosely lines the inside of the globe, attaching anteriorly to the peripheral ciliary body at the pars plana. The nerve fiber layer of the retina coalesces to form the optic nerve, which runs through a lattice-like opening in the posterior sclera, the lamina cribrosa, to exit the globe. The central retinal artery and vein run within the optic nerve, branching out on the retina to form a superior and inferior temporal arc around the macula. The center of the macula, the fovea, allows the eye to have detailed vision. The nasal vascular arcades supply the nasal retina, which provides indistinct temporal peripheral vision. The deepest retinal structure, the retinal pigment epithelium, shuttles nourishment and waste between the overlying retinal ganglion cells and the net-like, underlying choroidal blood vessels. Deep (external) to the choroid is the fibrous sclera.

The Nose

The external nose is a triangular pyramid with one side adjoining the face (Fig. 7–8). The upper angle of the facial side is the *root*, connected with the forehead. The two lateral sides join in the midline to form the *dorsum nasi*; its superior portion is the *bridge* of the nose. The free angle or apex forms the tip of the nose. The triangular base is pierced on either side by an elliptic orifice, the *naris* (plural *nares*), separated in the midline by the *columella*, which is continuous internally with the *nasal septum*. Lining the margins of the nares, still hairs, the *vibrissae*, inhibit inhalation of foreign bodies. The lateral nasal surface ends below in a rounded eminence, the *ala nasi* (plural, *alae nasi*).

The upper third of the lateral nasal wall is supported medially by the nasal bone and laterally by the nasal process of the maxilla. The lower two-thirds is supported by a framework of lateral cartilage, *the greater alar cartilage*, and several lesser alar cartilages. The nasal passages are separated anteriorly by the cartilaginous *nasal septum* and posteriorly by bone, the *vomer*.

The nasal septum divides the *nasal cavity* into symmetrical air passages. Each passage begins anteriorly at the naris (Fig. 7–9) and widens into a *vestibule* before passing into a high, narrow passage that communicates posteriorly with the *nasopharynx* by an oval orifice, the *choana*. The septum is a vertical plane, while the lateral nasal surface has three horizontal, parallel, downward curving bony plates,

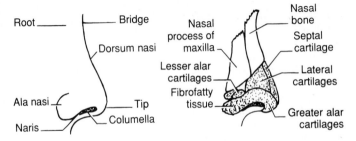

Fig. 7–8 *The External Nose.* These diagrams show the topographic features and the skeleton. Note that the proximal half of the nose is bone and the distal half (stippled) is cartilage.

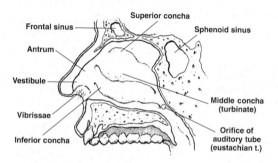

Fig. 7–9 *Lateral Nasal Wall.* This parasagittal section shows the superior, middle, and inferior conchae; under each is its corresponding meatus. Posterior to the inferior meatus is the orifice of the auditory (Eustachian) tube.

the *superior, middle,* and *inferior turbinates* or *conchae*. The mucous membranes of the inferior turbinate are highly vascular and semi-tumescent: vasoconstrictor drugs reduce blood flow thereby decreasing tumescence. Under each turbinate is a groove, the superior, middle, and *inferior meatus*. Superior and posterior to the superior turbinate is the opening of the *sphenoid sinus*. The superior meatus contains the orifices of the *posterior ethmoid cells*. The middle meatus receives drainage from the *maxillary sinus*, the *frontal sinus*, and *the anterior ethmoid cells*. The inferior meatus contains the orifice of the *nasolacrimal duct*. The *auditory* (*Eustachian*) tube opens into the nasopharynx just behind and lateral to the choana at the level of the middle meatus. In the posterior nasopharynx is an aggregation of lymphoid tissue, the *pharyngeal tonsil*, or *adenoids*.

The endings of the *olfactory nerve* (CN I) are located high in the nasal chamber, above the superior turbinate. A vascular network on the anterior nasal septum called *Kiesselbach plexus* is noteworthy because it is the site of most nosebleeds.

The Mouth and Oral Cavity

The mouth is surrounded by two fleshy *lips*; the *vermillion border* marks the transition from cornified epithelium of the skin to the noncornified squamous epithelium of the mouth. The *philtrum* is a vertical groove from columnella downward to vermilion border of the upper lip. Contraction of the *orbicularis oris*, a circular band of muscle surrounding the mouth and innervated by the facial nerve (CN VII) closes and protrudes the lips. Each lip is anchored to its adjacent gum by a fold of mucosa, the *labial frenulum*. The *oral cavity* is a short tunnel with an arched roof formed by the *hard and soft palate*, walls of the cheeks and lateral teeth, and with a floor formed by the tongue. The lips and teeth are separated by a shallow *vestibule*. The tunnel's exit is the isthmus *faucium* between the *faucial pillars*; it opens into a vertical passage, the *oropharynx*, continuous above with the *nasopharynx*.

The anterior two-thirds of the roof is formed by the hard palate, comprised of maxilla and palatine bone covered by mucosa with a *median raphe*. A fold of mucosa and muscle, the *soft palate*, continues the roof posteriorly. It hangs free forming a curtain in the *isthmus faucium*. From the midline of its free border is suspended the conical or bulbous uvula. The lateral border of the soft palate splits

Table 7–1 Age at Tooth Eruption

	Deciduous (mo)	Permanent (y)
First molars	15–21	6
Central incisors	6–9	7
Lateral incisors	15–21	8
First premolars		9
Second premolars		10
Canines	16–20	12
Second molars	20–24	12–13
Third molars		17–25

into two vertical folds, the tonsillar pillars. Between the anterior and posterior pillars lies the *palatine tonsil*, a mass of lymphoid tissue containing deep crypts or clefts. Similar lymphoid tissue lies in the base of the tongue, the *lingual tonsil.*

The Teeth

Upper and lower semicircles of *teeth* are set in the maxilla and mandible. The bony *dental ridges* and necks of the teeth are covered by tough fibrous tissue and mucosa; the *gums.* The gum borders are called the *gingival m*argins.

A child develops 20 *deciduous teeth*: from the midline on each side, uppers and lowers, they are two *incisors*, one *canine*, and a first and second *molar.* Gradually, these teeth are lost that are to be replaced by *permanent teeth* with the addition of a first and second *premolar* or bicuspid and a third molar, making a total of 32 (Table 7–1). Dentists use a universal numbering system starting with the right upper third molar as 1 and counting left to the opposite upper third molar as 16, then continuing down to the left lower third molar as 17 and counting right to 32 at the mandibular third molar. The eruption times of various teeth are shown in Table 7–1.

The Tongue

The *tongue* lies within the horseshoe curve of the mandible; its dorsal surface forms the floor of the oral cavity. The *tip* or apex is thin and narrow, resting against the lingual surface of the lower incisors. Posteriorly and inferiorly is the *root,* composed of muscle masses and their bony attachments. The tip and dorsal surface of the tongue is the visible portion of a much larger muscular mass. The *extrinsic muscles* extend between the *symphysis mentis* of the mandible, the *hyoid bone,* and the *styloid process* of the temporal bone; they cause protrusion and retraction of the tip, convex and concave curving of the dorsum, and move the root upward and downward. The *intrinsic muscles* alter the length, width, and curvature of the dorsal surface. The lingual muscles are innervated by the hypoglossal nerve (CN XII).

The tongue is free at its tip, dorsum, sides, and anteroinferior surface (Fig. 7–10). A midline fold of mucosa, the *lingual frenulum,* attaches the tongue to the floor of the mouth and the lingual surface of the lower gum. Near its base, the frenulum swells to form twin eminences, the *carunculae sublingualis,* each

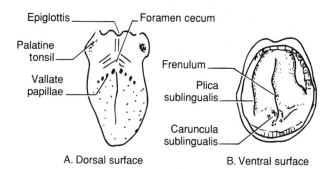

A. Dorsal surface   B. Ventral surface

Fig. 7–10 *Tongue Surfaces.* The dorsal surface from the tip of the epiglottis is depicted, showing the position of the palatine tonsils. The ventral surface is viewed from the outside of the mouth. The caruncula sublingualis is at the base of the frenulum; it contains the orifices of the submaxillary salivary ducts. In the plica, sublingualis are some sublingual salivary gland orifices.

surmounted by the orifice of a *submandibular duct* (Wharton duct). Running from the carunculae laterally and posteriorly around the base of the tongue is a ridge of mucosa, the *plica sublingualis*, punctured at intervals by the duct orifices from the sublingual gland, lying deep to the ridges.

The *dorsum* of the tongue extends from its tip to the epiglottis. The *median sulcus* bisects the dorsum from tip to the posterior third, where it ends in a depression, the *foramen cecum*, at the closure site of the embryonal *thyroglossal duct*. A *sulcus terminalis* extends forward and laterally from either side of the foramen cecum to form a V whose apex is posterior. Slightly anterior and parallel is another V formed by a row of 8 to 12 *vallate papillae*. The vallate papillae are round, discrete eminences with concentric fossae. The anterior two-thirds of the dorsum is textured like velvet by microscopic *filiform papillae*. These papillae catch desquamated cells, bacteria, and particles of food to form the coating of the normal tongue. Scattered among the filiform papillae, at the tip and sides of the tongue, are the less numerous *fungiform papillae*. They are readily identified with the unaided eye as large, raised, rounded, and deeper red. Microscopic taste buds are numerous in the vallate and fungiform papillae, on the sides and back of the tongue, in the soft palate, and on the posterior surface of the epiglottis. The sensory root of the facial nerve (CN VII), through the *chorda tympani*, supplies the taste buds in the anterior two-thirds of the tongue; the posterior third is innervated by the glossopharyngeal nerve (CN IX).

The Larynx

The larynx is immediately behind and below the oral cavity; the epiglottic tip is often visible through the mouth. Because the larynx is on the anterior wall of the pharynx with the sloping plane of its rim facing posteriorly, it is easily viewed by a laryngeal mirror held behind it (Fig. 7–11). The laryngeal apparatus may be visualized as three parallel stacked incomplete rings, one atop the other, held together by ligaments. Topmost is the arched *hyoid bone*, which opens posteriorly; suspended below are the arched *thyroid cartilage*, which also opens posteriorly and the cricoid cartilage, which is a complete ring affixed to the tracheal rings

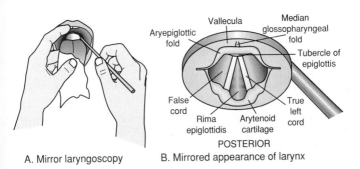

A. Mirror laryngoscopy   B. Mirrored appearance of larynx

Fig. 7–11 *Mirror Laryngoscopy. A. Hand and instrument position for Laryngoscopy. B. Appearance of the Larynx in the mirror. This is the appearance with the cords abducted.*

below. Although these structures are practically subcutaneous and palpable in the neck, their openings are posterior and well protected.

The ability to phonate depends on the shape, position, and action of the two *arytenoid cartilages* (Fig. 7–12). Each is a three-sided pyramid with a triangular base. The base is slightly concave to glide on a convex joint surface on the posterior

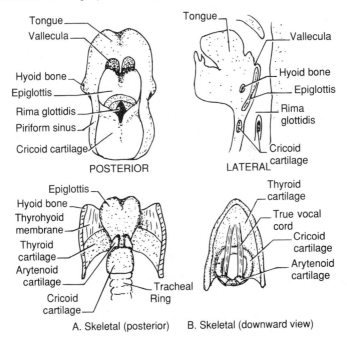

A. Skeletal (posterior)   B. Skeletal (downward view)

Fig. 7–12 *Anatomy of the Larynx. The larynx faces posteriorly; it is seen with the mirror behind the plane of the vocal cords. The arytenoid cartilages are small pyramids perched on the cricoid cartilage, to which they are connected by true joints. The arytenoid cartilages twist on their bases to vary vocal cord tension.*

rim of the cricoid cartilage, the *cricoarytenoid joint*, which is surrounded by a capsule. The two pyramids stand erect on either side of the midline of the cricoid. Muscles pull on the various faces of the pyramids, causing their bases to rotate in the joints. The apex of each pyramid is surmounted by a horizontal crescent of small cartilages and ligaments pointing medially toward its opposite and curving anteriorly. From the curve of each crescent, a tough fibroelastic band, the true *vocal cord* (vocal fold), extends forward to the midline of the thyroid cartilage. The two vocal cords thus form an opening into the trachea, the *rima glottidis*. When open, the rima is an isosceles triangle, with apex anterior beneath the epiglottis and base posterior, formed by the tissue bridge between the two arytenoid crescents. Rotation of the arytenoids brings the legs of the triangle together posteriorly to approximate the cords over their entire length, closing the airway.

Lateral, parallel to, and above the true cords is a pair of tissue folds, the *false vocal cords* (ventricular folds). A membrane covers the epiglottis and continues around posteriorly to envelop the crescents of the arytenoids, forming the *aryepiglottic folds*. Because the larynx protrudes slightly from the anterior pharyngeal wall, several pockets are formed: two *valleculae* between the epiglottis and the base of the tongue, and two *piriform sinuses*, one on either side of the cricoid. Most of the intrinsic muscles of the larynx are supplied by fibers of the *recurrent laryngeal nerve*, a branch of the vagus nerve (CN X).

The Salivary Glands

Parotid Gland

This is the largest of the salivary glands. Normally, it is not palpable as a distinct structure, but its location and extent must be known to recognize parotid enlargement (Fig. 7–13). A *superficial portion* lies subcutaneously extending from the zygomatic arch superiorly to the angle of the mandible inferiorly and from the external auditory canal posteriorly to the midportion of the masseter muscle anteriorly. A *tail portion* wraps around the angle and horizontal ramus of the

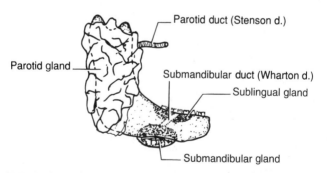

Parotid duct (Stenson d.)

Parotid gland

Submandibular duct (Wharton d.)

Sublingual gland

Submandibular gland

Fig. 7–13 *Anatomic Relations of the Salivary Glands to the Mandible.* *Note that the parotid gland lies on the lateral surface of the mandibular ramus, curling behind its posterior margin. The submaxillary gland is on the medial surface of the mandible with its lower margin protruding below the bone. The sublingual gland is behind the medial mandibular surface near its superior margin. Using the jaw for a landmark, the glands can be located accurately by palpation.*

mandible in the upper neck, and a *deep lobe* extends from the tail medial to the stylomandibular ligament and styloid muscles. The *parotid* (*Stensen*) *duct* is approximately 5 cm long and runs forward, horizontally on the superficial surface of the masseter muscle, approximately one fingerbreadth below the zygomatic arch, in a line drawn from the inferior border of the concha of the ear to the commissure of the lips. At the muscle's anterior border, it pierces the buccinator muscle to reach its orifice in a papilla on the buccal mucosa opposite the upper second molar.

Submandibular (formerly Submaxillary) Glands

Approximately the size of a walnut, the gland lies medial to the inner surface of the mandible; its lower portion can be palpated from beneath the inferior mandibular border somewhat anterior to the angle of the jaw. Bimanual palpation, with a gloved finger in the floor of the mouth and the opposite hand under the jaw, reveals the finely lobulated glandular architecture. The *submandibular* (*Wharton*) *duct* is approximately 5 cm long; it courses upward and forward to the floor of the mouth, where its orifice is crowned by the *caruncula sublingualis*, beside the lingual frenulum.

Sublingual Glands

The smallest of the glands, it lies beneath the floor of the mouth, near the symphysis mentis. It empties through several short ducts, some with orifices in the plica sublingualis, some entering the submandibular duct.

The Thyroid Gland

Knowledge of thyroid embryology is necessary to understand thyroid disorders. A median diverticulum, evaginating from the ventral pharyngeal wall (the future *foramen cecum* in the tongue), goes downward and backward in front of the trachea as a tubular duct (the *thyroglossal duct*), bifurcating and further dividing into cords that later fuse to form the thyroid isthmus and lateral lobes. Normally, the thyroglossal duct is obliterated, but remnants may persist in the adult to form thyroglossal sinuses or cysts. At the duct's superior end, a normally functioning lingual thyroid gland may form. Inferiorly, ductal tissue frequently forms a *pyramidal lobe* arising from the isthmus or a lateral lobe, usually the left. The pyramidal lobe may ascend in front of the thyroid cartilage as high as the hyoid bone. Occasionally, a normal glandular component, such as the isthmus or lateral lobe, may fail to develop. Rarely, the lingual growth may be the only active thyroid tissue in the body.

The thyroid is the largest endocrine gland. It consists of two lateral lobes whose upper halves lie on either side of the projecting prow of the thyroid cartilage; the lower halves are at the sides of the trachea (Fig. 7–14). A flat band of isthmus passes in front of the upper tracheal rings, joining the lateral lobes at their lower thirds. The major outline of the gland is trapezoidal, with a parallel top and bottom, and with the sides converging downward. The normal adult gland weighs approximately 25 to 30 g; it is slightly larger in the female. Each lateral lobe is an irregular cone approximately 5 cm long; the greatest diameter is approximately 3 cm, the thickness approximately 2 cm. The right lobe is, normally, one-fourth larger than the left. The lateral posterior borders touch the common carotid

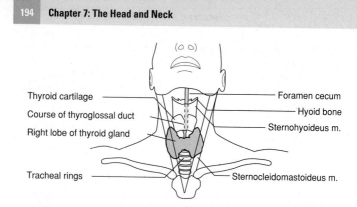

Fig. 7–14 *Anatomic Relations of the Thyroid Gland, Anterior View.* *The blue structures are the thyroid gland and the course of the obliterated thyroglossal duct.*

arteries. Usually, on the posterior lateral surfaces are the *parathyroid glands.* The *recurrent laryngeal nerves* lie close to the medial deep surface. Each lobe is covered anteriorly by the respective sternocleidomastoideus, while the isthmus lies on the tracheal rings and is practically subcutaneous. Pairs of *superior and inferior thyroid arteries* supply an exceedingly vascular parenchyma. The gland is firmly fixed to the trachea and larynx, so that it ascends with them during swallowing; this movement distinguishes thyroid structures from other masses in the neck. The thyroid actually lies in the upper anterior mediastinum. Enlargement by downward growth extends behind the sternum, a retrosternal goiter. The *thymus gland* also occupies the anterior mediastinum. Thus, a tumor of the anterior mediastinum may arise from either gland.

Physical Examination of the Head and Neck

Examination of the Scalp, Face, and Skull

Examination is by inspection and palpation. *Inspect* for asymmetry of the skull, ears, eyes, nose, mouth, jaw, and cheeks. Use a tongue blade in the sagittal plane from the midline of the glabella to the midline of the lips to detect nasal deformity. Observe the position of the ears, viewing from the front. Note any masses or deformities. Inspect the skin of the scalp by displacing the hair sequentially to reveal the roots. Inspect for actinic changes and lesions on the sun-exposed skin, especially the helix of the ear, the temples above the zygoma, the forehead, cheeks, and lips. Gently *palpate* the skull for irregularities. Run a fingertip around the orbital rim and along the zygoma on each side. Palpate the ramus, angle, and arch of the mandible.

Examination of the Ears, Hearing, and Labyrinthine Function

Pinna

Inspect the pinna for size, shape, and color. Note discharges from the meatus. Palpate the consistency of the cartilages and any swellings. Assess for pain with movement of the pinna and tragus.

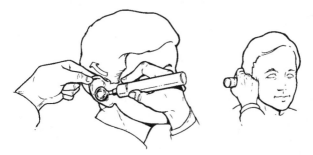

Fig. 7–15 *Use of the Otoscope.* Insert the ear speculum by pulling the upper edge of the pinna upward and backward to straighten the cartilaginous meatus so that it coincides with the axis of the bony canal.

External Acoustic Meatus

Prepare the canal for inspection by taking time to clean it properly. Remove liquid material with a cotton applicator. Remove solids through an ear speculum with either a cotton applicator or a cerumen spoon under direct vision. Use a speculum attached to a lighted otoscope or a speculum and a headlamp. Select the largest speculum that will fit the cartilaginous canal. Tip the head toward the opposite shoulder to bring the canal horizontal. Insert the speculum while retracting the pinna upward and backward for adults so that the flexible cartilaginous canal aligns with the axis of the bony canal; use downward traction for infants and young children (Fig. 7–15). The lining epithelium of the bony canal is very sensitive, so use gentle manipulation.

Tympanic Membrane and Middle Ear

When a beam of light shines on the TM, it reflects a brilliant wedge of light, the *light reflex*, whose apex is at the center or umbo with its legs extending radially in the anterior inferior quadrant of the membrane, approximately at a right angle to the manubrium. Examine the normal landmarks of the drumhead: the *manubrium of the malleus* that forms a smooth ridge from the umbo or center and runs radially upward and forward toward the circumference and ends in the knob of the *short process*; the two *malleolar folds*, diverging from the knob to the periphery; the *shadow of the incus*, often showing through the membrane in the upper posterior quadrant; and, finally, look carefully around the entire circumference of the annulus for perforations just inside its border. Note the color and sheen of the membrane, which is, normally, shiny and pearly gray. Serum in the middle ear colors it *amber or yellow* and air bubbles may be seen; pus shows as a *chalky white* membrane; blood appears *blue*. Note changes in the *definition of the manubrium*; a bulging membrane makes the landmarks indistinct or completely obscures them completely. Inadequate auditory (Eustachian) tube function produces *retraction* of the membrane sharpening the outline of the manubrium and mallear folds. With either bulging or retraction the wedge of the light reflex will be distorted or absent. When the incus is visible through the membrane, a normal middle ear is fairly certain.

Rough Quantitative Test for Hearing Loss

Difficulty understanding spoken questions during history taking may alert you to hearing loss.

Whisper test. Test with the whispered voice at the patient's side approximately 60 cm (2 ft) from her ear. Cover the far ear and whisper test numbers that the patient should repeat or whisper questions that cannot be answered yes or no. Test with loud, medium, and soft tones. Alternatively, use the same intensity for all tests and find the maximal distance from the ear at which the whisper may be understood.

Tuning fork. Hearing acuity may also be tested with the vibrations of a tuning fork. A fork with a frequency from 256 to 1024 cycles per second is preferred; the 128-cycle fork for testing vibratory sense is too low-pitched.

Distinguishing Between Neurosensory and Conductive Hearing Loss

Use a tuning fork with frequencies of 256 to 1024 cycles per second. Set the fork in motion by gently tapping the base of the other hand.

The Weber test (Fig. 7–16A). Place the handle of the vibrating fork against the midline of the skull and ask the patient whether the sound is louder in one ear than in the other. With normal neurosensory hearing and no conductive loss, the sounds are equal in both ears (see page 223).

The Rinne test (Fig. 7–16B). Test each ear sequentially. First, press the handle of a vibrating fork against the mastoid process (*bone conduction*) and then place the tines near the ear canal (*air conduction*). Ask, if it was louder behind the ear or at the ear canal. When air conduction is louder than bone conduction, the test is arbitrarily said to be *Rinne-positive*, a normal result. The test is *Rinne-negative* when bone conduction is louder than air conduction. Have the patient indicate when they can no longer detect the sound by air conduction; see if you can hear the vibrating fork to compare their hearing to yours (see page 223).

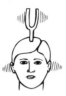

A. Weber test

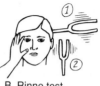

B. Rinne test

Fig. 7–16 *Tests of Hearing Perception and Conduction. A. Weber test:* the vibrating tuning fork is on the midline of the skull. Lateralization of the sound to one ear indicates a conductive loss on the same side, or a perceptive loss on the other side. *B. Rinne test:* the handle of the tuning fork is first placed against the mastoid process then near the external ear. Each time the patient indicates when the sound ceases. Normally, air conduction persists twice as long as bone conduction.

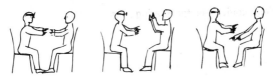

Fig. 7–17 *Past Pointing Test for Labyrinthine Disorders.*

Labyrinthine Test for Positional Nystagmus: Dix-Hallpike Maneuver

Have the patient sit on the examination table and inspect the eyes carefully for spontaneous nystagmus. Then, keeping the eyes open, have the patient lie supine with the head extending beyond the end of the table, the chin elevated approximately 30 degrees and the head turned 45 degrees to the right. Observe the eyes for 30 seconds looking for nystagmus. Return the patient to the sitting position. After a short rest, repeat the test with the head turning to the left. Have the patient sit up and inspect the eyes for 30 seconds. A positive test induces nystagmus, often accompanied by intense nausea. The slow component of the nystagmus is in the direction of the endolymph flow; *the nystagmus is named for its fast component.*

Labyrinthine Test for Past Pointing

Have the patient sit facing you, pointing his forefingers toward you with his eyes closed (Fig. 7–17). Place your forefingers lightly under his and hold them there. Ask the patient to raise his arms and hands, and then return his fingers to yours. Normally, this maneuver can be performed accurately. Past pointing indicates either loss of positional sense or labyrinthine stimulation (see page 223).

Labyrinthine Test for Falling: Romberg Test

Have the patient stand with the feet close together (heel and toe) (Fig. 7–18). Assure the patient that you will not let him fall, and be prepared to catch him

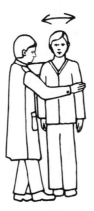

Fig. 7–18 *Falling Test for Labyrinthine Disorders (Romberg Sign).* Normally, the patient will waver somewhat, but not fall. With labyrinthine stimulation, the patient tends to fall in the direction of the flow of endolymph. Falling may also indicate loss of positional sense as in cerebellar deficits.

should he fall. Have the patient close his eyes and observe him for several seconds. Normally, patients will be steady, even with gentle, forewarned, pushes on the trunk. Falling during the test is the *Romberg sign.*

Examination of the Eyes, Visual Fields and Visual Acuity

Remote Eye Examination

Examine the palpebral fissures and position of the globe.   From a distance, note the width and symmetry of the palpebral fissures (normal, increased, or diminished). Look for protrusion or recession of one or both globes by inspecting the eyes from the front, from the profile, and from above (looking downward over the forehead), or from below (looking up over the cheekbones). Accurate measurement of the distance between the anterior surface of the cornea and the outer edge of the bony orbit can be made with a Hertel exophthalmometer, which requires some practice but can be used to document suspected proptosis (protrusion) of an eye. Individual variation is great, and there are familial and racial trends toward proptosis. The best evidence of pathologic exophthalmos lies in a series of accurate measurements showing progressive anterior displacement.

Inspect for inflammation.   Inspect for redness and or swelling: Is it in one or both eyes? Does it involve the eyelid and/or the ocular surface?

Test for lid lag, lid retraction, and scleral show.   Use your finger or a penlight as a target. Start in the midline above eye level, approximately 50 cm (20 in) away, moving the target slowly and repeatedly up and down in the midline (Fig. 7–19). A *lag* is indicated by the upper lid lagging, often in a ratcheting pattern, behind the upper limbus, allowing the white sclera to appear between lid margin and limbus. Lid *retraction* is the dynamic elevation of the upper lid on gaze at an object, and scleral *show* a more constant exposure of the upper sclera. The inferior sclera may be seen below the limbus in normal individuals depending on the anatomy of their orbit and midfacial architecture.

Tests for Strabismus (Heterotropia)

Be sure that the patient has useful vision in each eye.

Cover-uncover test.   Ask the patient to fixate on an object at the end of the room, or at a near target such as the examiner's nose. First, cover the patient's left eye with your right hand (Fig. 7–20). Watch the uncovered right eye to see if it moves to take up fixation. Uncover the left eye and allow the patient to look with both

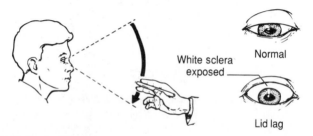

Normal

White sclera exposed

Lid lag

Fig. 7–19 *Test for Lid Lag.*

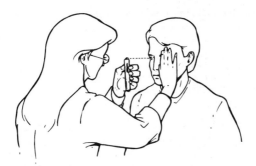

Fig. 7–20 *Testing for Strabismus.*

eyes. Then cover the right eye and watch the uncovered left eye to see if it moves to fixation. If there is fixation movement, the patient has *heterotropia* (strabismus, squint). A constant misalignment of this type is known as *manifest deviation* or *tropia.*

Alternate cover test. While the patient is holding visual fixation, alternately and repeatedly swing to cover each eye in sequence. If the eyes start to alternately move to pick up fixation when they are uncovered, but they did not have a manifest deviation by the first cover/uncover test, then they were initially aligned by the central nervous system ability to fuse the image, but have a *latent deviation* uncovered by breaking that fusion. This latent misalignment is also known as a *phoria.* This is also demonstrated by having the patient fix on the object with both eyes; cover one eye for a few seconds, then uncover it while observing to see if it moves to reestablish fixation. If there is fixation movement, the eye has heterophoria.

Naming the deviation. If the eye swings inward to pick up fixation, it was initially deviated outward (*exotropia* or *exophoria*). If the eye swings outward, it was initially deviated inward (*esotropia, esophoria*).

To determine if the heterotropia is comitant or incomitant, ask the patient to follow your penlight in the six cardinal directions of gaze outlined below. If the eyes move equally without restriction, the deviation is *comitant.* If one eye over-shoots and the other fails to look the entire distance in one or more directions, the deviation is *incomitant,* and may represent either a paralytic or restrictive misalignment. A *paralytic misalignment* is pathological and could represent ischemia (stroke) or compression (tumor); *restrictive misalignments* can be caused by scarring or by fibrosis, such as seen in thyroid eye disease.

Test extraocular movements. Ask the patient to indicate if they see double as you test the six cardinal positions of gaze. Have the patient follow your finger to the right, right and up, right and down, to the left, left and up, left and down, and then return to the primary position (see Fig. 14–16, page 714). When testing horizontally, acting muscles hold the stimulus with the long dimension vertically; for testing vertically acting muscles, hold it horizontally. This allows the patient to more easily see a doubled image. Finally, test convergence by holding the target in the midline and at eye level, approximately 50 cm (20 in) from the face, gradually moving the target toward the bridge of the nose; note the near point at which convergence fails, normally, 50 to 75 mm (2 to 3 in).

Tests for Gross Visual Fields Defects: Confrontation Methods

Use one or a combination of the following tests to detect visual field defects. Finger, face, and hand confrontation readily detect temporal field cuts. *To detect nasal field cuts, you must test each eye independently.*

Finger confrontation.   Fingers are presented in each quadrant on both sides of the vertical midline in each quadrant while the gaze is kept straight ahead. The patient should be looking at a focal point; it is convenient to use the examiners nose. This allows the examiner to use their visual field as a control. The patient is asked to sum the number of fingers seen. Because it is difficult to differentiate three fingers from four, it is best to use 1, 2, or 5 fingers. This testing tells whether there is an absolute defect in one quadrant. You can increase the sensitivity by decreasing the presentation time and increasing the distance from the patient.

Face and hand confrontation.   The patient looks at the examiner's face first with one eye and then the other, and is asked if the face is clear with each eye and if the images are the same. A lack of clarity in one eye or a difference between the eyes suggests a field defect. With *hand confrontation,* the patient fixes on the examiner's nose and the examiners hands are held on either side of the vertical midline first above then below the plane of gaze. The patient is asked if the hands appear the same. A cloudy or a faded-color appearing hand represents a relative and subtle defect along the vertical plane.

Color confrontation.   This test is traditionally done with red caps of mydriatic bottles. (1) *Color comparison* about the vertical midline is performed as hand comparison above. This is a very sensitive test for relative hemianopic defects, (2) For *central scotoma testing* of each eye, the subject is asked to cover the opposite eye and fix their vision on one red cap while the other is held in their nasal visual field. Ask which cap is redder or brighter. If the peripheral cap is brighter when in fact they are the same color, there is a central scotoma. Do not hold the peripheral cap in the temporal field as a cecocentral defect may confound interpretation; likewise, you might place the cap in the patient's blind spot.

Kinetic boundary test (Fig. 7–21).   Have the patient cover her left eye with her hand. Place your face in front of the patient's and at the same eye level, with your nose approximately 1 m (40 in) from the unmasked eye. Ask the patient to fix constantly on your eye. Cover your own right eye; fix your left eye on the patient's unmasked eye. Hold your left hand off to the side in the midplane between your faces. With a flicking finger or penlight for a target, bring it slowly toward the midline between you (Fig. 7–21). Ask the patient to indicate when the target first appears and compare that with your own experience. Also, test vertical and oblique runs. Test the nasal field with your right hand. Test the second eye similarly. This technique is more time consuming and less sensitive and specific than the first three; it is not recommended [Pandit RJ, Gales K, Griffiths PG. Effectiveness of testing visual fields by confrontation. *Lancet.* 2001;358:1339–1340].

Techniques for uncooperative patients.   In obtunded adults, watch for eye movements to novel targets or a blink in response to a threat and movement

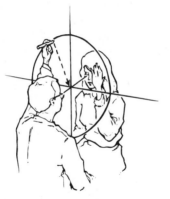

Fig. 7–21 Test for Tunnel Vision. *The patient fixes on the examiner's left eye. The examiner imagines a line of sight extending between the patient's open eye and the examiner's own eye; the two can be termed the opposing eyes. The examiner imagines radii that are perpendicular to the line of sight and center at a point equidistant between the two opposing eyes. A target on any point of such a radius will be equidistant between the opposing eyes at all locations. The examiner slowly moves a flicking finger or a penlight target along a radius from the periphery toward the center until the patient indicates that she can see it. Simultaneously, the examiner checks his view of the target.*

toward the head in each field. If the movement pushes air over the cornea, it will stimulate a corneal reflex that can be misinterpreted as a visual response.

Close External Examination of the Eyes

Eyelids.   Look for swelling about the lids, above, below, and near the canthi. Note inversion or eversion of the lid margins. Examine the lid margins for scaling, normal secretions, exudate, papules, or pustules. Look for lashes turned inward (*trichiasis*). Press on the lacrimal sac; if fluid can be expressed through the punctum, the tear duct is obstructed.

Bulbar conjunctiva and sclera.   Gently retract the lids with the thumb and forefinger. Note the color of the sclera, any pigment deposits, vascular engorgement, or vascular pterygium (which must be distinguished from the avascular pinguecula).

Palpebral conjunctiva.   *To evert the lower lid*   (Fig. 7–22A) place the thumb tip on the loose skin beneath the margin and slide the skin down, pressing it gently into the orbit) and ask the patient to look up. Look for congestion, discharge, and other lesions. If indicated, *evert the upper lid*   (Fig. 7–22B). Face the patient asking her to look downward and keep both eyes open to prevent elevation that accompanies lid closure. Pinch the lashes of the upper lid and pull it gently downward and away from the globe. Press the tip of an applicator against the upper lid just above the tarsal plate. Using this as a fulcrum, pull the eyelid quickly upward so that the tarsal plate everts. After the lid has been everted, stabilize it with the fingers of one hand. Have the patient glance upward to return the lid to its normal position.

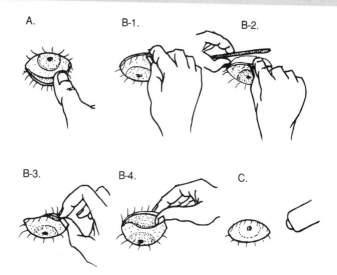

Fig. 7–22 *Examination of the Eyelids. A. Eversion of the lower lid. B. Eversion of the upper lid:* tell the patient to look downward and proceed with four steps: (1) with the right thumb and forefinger, grasp a few cilia of the upper lid and pull the lid away from the globe; (2) lay an applicator along the crease made by the superior edge of the tarsal plate and the soft adjacent tissue; (3) quickly fold the lid over the applicator so the tarsal plate turns over and its upper edge faces downward; and (4) replace the right thumb and finger by the corresponding left ones to hold the lid. *C. Testing pupillary reaction to light.*

Cornea.   Shine light from a penlight obliquely on the cornea to search for scars, abrasions, or ulcers. The corneal light reflex should look smooth and regular as you play the light over the surface. Abrasions are readily demonstrated by fluorescein staining. Place the tip of a moistened fluorescein strip in the inferior fornix. After removing it, ask the patient to blink. Observe with a blue light; corneal abrasions appear green. The cornea may also be examined with a lens.

Iris, pupils and lens.   Note the clarity of the iris, whether it appears distinct or muddy. Look for new vessels and deposits. Note the size, shape, and equality of the pupils. Test **pupillary reaction to light** by having the patient fix on a distant object (>3 m [10 ft] away). Shine a penlight into the right pupil from the side (Fig. 7–22C) while observing the *direct pupillary reaction*; remove the light and repeat the process on the left eye. Now swing the light back to the right eye but continue to observe the left pupil. In a normal eye, as the flashlight is swung toward the right eye from the left, there is a minimal dilatation followed by constriction of the left pupil, the normal *consensual reaction*. Repeat the latter process this time observing the right pupil for the normal dilation followed by constriction as the light is moved back to the left eye. This is the swinging light test for a *relative afferent pupillary defect* (page 242). Test pupillary reaction to near point by having the patient fix on her own finger as it is gradually brought closer to her nose. Shine the penlight obliquely through the lens to discover deposits on the surface and opacities in the matrix such as cataracts.

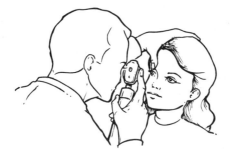

Fig. 7–23 *Ophthalmoscopic Examination.*

Schirmer test for lack of tears (see Fig. 7–41D, page 238). A thin strip of filter paper is folded over the lower eyelid without anesthetic. Wetting of less than 10 mm of the paper, after 5 minutes, indicates keratoconjunctivitis sicca.

Ophthalmoscopic examination. Ophthalmoscopic examination requires considerable practice in order to obtain useful information. Examine the right eye observing with your right eye and using your right hand to manipulate the ophthalmoscope; examine the left eye using your left eye with the ophthalmoscope in your left hand (Fig. 7–23). Undilated examination of the right eye is described. Grasp the instrument with your right hand, your forefinger on the disk of lenses. Rest your left hand on the patient's forehead so that your thumb can pull up the upper lid slightly to uncover the pupil and prevent excessive blinking. Ask the patient to fix her eyes straight ahead on a distant object.

The media. Place the $+8$ or $+10$ diopter lens in the sight hole, bring it close to your eye or glasses, and move forward to approximately 30 cm (12 in) in front of the patient's eye. Shine the light into her pupil to see the red retinal reflex. A dull red or black reflex is produced by diffuse dense opacities. Look for black spots showing against the red; these are the shadows of opacities in the lens or vitreous made by the light reflected from the retina. Move forward or backward until the spots are clearly focused. While watching the opacities, ask the patient to elevate the eyes slightly; if the spots move upward, they are on the cornea or anterior part of the lens; little movement occurs when the location is near the lenticular center; downward movement indicates a location in the posterior lens or vitreous. Vitreous opacities appear more distinct when viewed obliquely with the white optic disk as a background.

The fundus (Plate 11). Hold the instrument approximately 5 cm (2 in) from the patient's eye with your forehead near or touching your hand on the patient's forehead. The left hand rests on the forehead with the thumb gently retracting and holding the upper lid to prevent excessive blinking. Adjust the lenses to find the optimal focus to view the retina; the setting is governed by the refractive error and the degree of accommodation in both patient and examiner. In the absence of both factors, the best view should be obtained at zero. Minus lenses are required to correct for involuntary accommodation. When a cataract has been extracted without intraocular lens replacement, approximately $+10$ is needed for correction. High astigmatism cannot be corrected with the spherical lenses of the instrument, so examine the fundi through the patient's glasses. When the correct setting is found, examine the following regions (see Plate 11 and Fig. 7–44A, page 245).

Optic Disk: The optic disc lies 10 degrees into the nasal retina and slightly inferior to the visual axis. Therefore, angle the ophthalmoscope 10 degrees nasally from the line of sight to be in the vicinity of the optic disc. Note the shape and color of the optic disk. The shape is round or oval vertically. Most of the disk is red-orange, the color imparted by the capillaries around the nerve fibers. The *physiologic cup* is a pale area in the center of the disk devoid of nerve fibers; it forms a depression whose base is the nonvascular *lamina cribrosa*. The size and shape of the cup vary greatly in normal eyes. It is measured by the **cup-to-disk ratio**. If the cup is not circular, the vertical ratio is used. The site of ingress and egress of vessels, called the *vessel funnel*, also lacks nerve fibers, so it is pale and white. The borders of the disk may merge gradually into the surrounding retina, or they may be sharply demarcated by a white scleral ring. Outside the ring, on the temporal side, a crescent of pigment may occur.

Retinal Vessels: The arteries are bright red with a central stripe, the *light reflex.* Note the width of the reflex stripe. Normally, the veins are wider than the arteries in a ratio of approximately 4:3; they are darker red and lack a stripe. The vessel branching pattern shows great individual variation. As they emerge from the disk, the afferent vessels are true arteries; branches beyond the second bifurcation, approximately 1 disk diameter from the disk margin, are arterioles. Look for sheathing of the arteries. Observe the veins carefully at the arteriovenous crossings for nicking, deviation, humping, tapering, sausaging, or banking. Retinal veins, normally, pulsate; arteries in the retina do not.

Retina: The amount of pigmentation corresponds to the patient's complexion and race. The retina is thinner in the nasal periphery and therefore paler. Note areas of white or pigment from scarring. Look for hemorrhages and exudates. Express the size of abnormalities in disk diameters. Measure depression or elevation by the diopters of correction required to focus on an arterial reflex in the area.

Macula: The macula is slightly below the horizontal plane of the disk and from 2 to 3 disk diameters to the temporal side of its margin. Examination of the macula is usually fleeting because illumination of this region produces discomfort; examine it last. In the center of the macula, the *fovea* appears as a small darker-red area, set apart from visible vessels. In its center appears a small darker spot, the *foveola*, whose center gives off a speck of reflected light.

Bedside tests for visual acuity. Gross tests for visual acuity can be made without special equipment. Test a single eye at a time. Show the patient a newspaper or magazine, testing first with the fine print. If this is not perceived, show the larger letters. If the patient fails on large letters, hold up several fingers 1 m (3 ft) away and ask the patient to count them. If the patient cannot count them, determine if the patient can see movements of the hand. Failing this, flash a light beam into the eye, asking the patient to indicate when it appears. Test whether the patient can perceive the direction of the light source.

When gross visual acuity is fair, more accurate tests can be made with the standard *Snellen charts.* Be sure there is adequate illumination and the appropriate distance to the chart. Determine the smallest line of letters the patient can read without error with each eye, and then with both eyes together. Express the reading as a ratio of the distance at which the test is conducted and the distance at which the line of letters should be read by a normal eye. The distance is expressed in feet or meters; 20/20 feet and 6/6 meters are normal. If the patient could only read the line for 40 feet, her acuity is expressed as 20/40.

It should always be noted whether the patient's optical correction (glasses or contact lens) were used. If the visual acuity is abnormal, the potential acuity from an improved optical correction using lenses can be estimated by using the *pinhole test*. To perform this, a 1-mm hole (or series of holes) is made in a note card. The patient is then asked to read a Snellen chart through the pinhole. The patient then selects only those rays of light that are in focus. A close approximation to the patient's best-corrected visual acuity can then be recorded.

Tests for color vision.   Ask the patient to identify the colors of objects immediately available. For more precise testing, use a book of Ishihara plates. Remember that color vision is a mixture of red, blue, and green.

Slit-lamp microscopy.   Slit-lamp examination requires special equipment and is reserved for an experienced ophthalmologist. A powerful light is focused in a narrow slit upon the various layers of the cornea, the anterior chamber, the lens, and the anterior third of the vitreous chamber, while the objects are examined through a corneal microscope. Accurate inspection of opacities and minute foci of inflammation can be made.

Examination of the Nose and Sinuses
Routine Nasal Examination

Inspect the nasal profile, contour and symmetry. Test the patency of each naris by closing the other while the patient inhales with the mouth closed. *Transilluminate* the nasal septum: push the nasal tip upward while a penlight in the other illuminates one naris (Fig. 7–24A); view the transilluminated septum through the opposite nares for deviations, perforations, and masses. Palpate the cheeks and supraorbital ridges over the maxillary and frontal sinuses for tenderness.

Detailed Nasal Examination

If abnormalities are found on the screening exam, a more thorough exam is required.

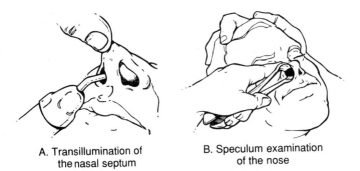

A. Transillumination of
the nasal septum

B. Speculum examination
of the nose

Fig. 7–24 *Examination of the Nasal septum and Nares. A. Transillumination of the nasal septum. B. Speculum examination of the nose.*

Examination with the nasal speculum.   Examine the anterior nasal chambers with a nasal speculum and a head mirror or head lamp. Hold the speculum in the left hand (Fig. 7–24B); the right hand is free to position the head or hold instruments. Insert the closed blades approximately 1 cm into the vestibule; open the blades vertically, in the plane of the septum, with the left forefinger anchoring the ala nasi against the superior blade to avoid pressure on the septum. Reposition the speculum and the patient's head to see each structure. Examine the *vestibule* for folliculitis and fissures. Note the color of the *mucosa* and any swelling. Inspect the nasal septum for deviation, ulcer, or hemorrhage. Examine the *inferior turbinate* on the lateral wall for swelling, increased redness, pallor, or blueness. Identify the *middle turbinate*; inspect the *middle meatus* for purulent discharge from frontal, maxillary, and anterior ethmoid sinuses.

Examination of the nasopharynx using the postnasal mirror.   A head mirror or headlamp is required for illumination. Warm a No. 0 (small) postnasal mirror in warm water; touch it to your hand to check its temperature. Depress the tongue as described for the oropharyngeal examination, inserting the blade from the corner of the mouth (Fig. 7–25A). Hold the mirror like a pencil, steadying your hand against the patient's cheek. Insert the mirror from the side opposite the tongue blade; keep the mirror upright, avoiding contact with tongue, palate, and

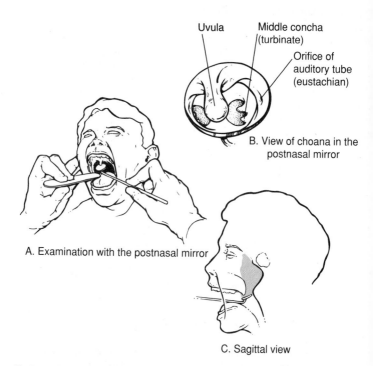

Uvula

Middle concha (turbinate)

Orifice of auditory tube (eustachian)

B. View of choana in the postnasal mirror

A. Examination with the postnasal mirror

C. Sagittal view

Fig. 7–25 *Examination of the Nasopharynx. A. Examination with the postnasal mirror. In the drawing, all deep spaces are heavily stippled. B. View of the choana in the postnasal mirror. C. Sagittal view.*

uvula. Position it behind the uvula near to the posterior pharyngeal wall. Turn the mirror upward, focus the light on it, and adjust it to view the *choana* (Figs. 7–25B and C). Locate the posterior end of the *nasal septum*, the *vomer*, in the midline. Identify the *middle meatus*; pus draining posteriorly from this region comes only from the maxillary sinus. The *inferior meatus* is not well visualized posteriorly. The orifices of the *auditory* (*Eustachian*) tubes are behind and lateral to the middle meatus. The orifice appears pale or yellow and is approximately 5 mm in diameter. The tubes are closed except during swallowing or yawning. Look for the *pharyngeal tonsil* (*adenoids*) hanging from the roof into the fossa, and for inflammation, exudate, polyps, and neoplasms in the nasopharynx, uvula, and soft palate. If available, a fiberoptic instrument will simplify your examination.

Transillumination of the maxillary sinuses.   In a fully darkened room press a cool light against the each maxilla while observing the hard palate through the mouth for transmitted light. Asymmetry of transillumination is most significant.

Transillumination of the frontal sinuses.   Place the light under the nasal half of the supraorbital ridge shielding the orbit up to the eyebrow. Look for bright areas in the forehead.

Examination of the Lips, Mouth, Teeth, Tongue, and Pharynx

Inspect using a tongue blade and penlight. Use of headlamp or mirror frees one hand to hold instruments. Completely inspect the oral cavity before beginning palpation.

Lips

Look for congenital and acquired defects. Note the lip color and look for angular stomatitis, rhagades, ulcers, granulomas, and neoplasms. Have the patient attempt to whistle to reveal weakness of the facial nerve (CN VII). Inspect the inner surface of the lips by retracting them with a tongue blade while the teeth are approximated.

Teeth

Note the absence of teeth and the presence of caries, discoloration, fillings, and bridges. Notice abnormal dental shape, such as notching. Tap each tooth with a probe for tenderness.

Gums

Have the patient remove any dental appliances. Look for retraction of the gingival margins, pus in the margins, gum inflammation, spongy or bleeding gums, lead or bismuth lines, or localized gingival swelling.

Breath

Smell the breath for acetone, ammonia, or fetor.

Tongue

Have the patient protrude his tongue. Assess its size and note deviation from the midline or restricted protrusion. Examine the dorsal surface coat for color,

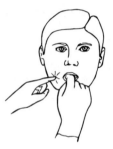

Fig. 7–26 *Palpation of the Roof of the Tongue.*

thickness, and adhesiveness. Have the patient raise the tip to the roof of the mouth; inspect the undersurface, including *frenulum* and *carunculae sublingualis.*

Palpation of the Roof of the Tongue

Palpate the accessible portions of a tongue that is painful or has restricted motion for deep-seated masses. Have the tongue inside the teeth when palpating to relax the muscles. Palpate the sublingual salivary glands and the submandibular ducts for calculi. If the patient gags readily, spray the throat with a topical anesthetic; otherwise, proceed without anesthesia. While wearing gloves, have the patient open his mouth wide. To avoid having your fingers bitten, push a fold of the patient's cheek between their teeth. Insert your forefinger to the back of the mouth and palpate the roof of the tongue, the valleculae, and the tonsillar fossae (Fig. 7–26).

Examination of a lingual ulcer.   Dry the ulcer gently with a cotton sponge and then inspect it carefully. Palpate the surrounding and underlying tissue with gloved fingers. The pain from lingual lesions may be referred to the ear.

Buccal Mucosa

Retract the cheek with the tongue blade. Look for melanin deposits, vesicles, petechiae, *Candida*, Koplik spots, ulcers, neoplasms. Examine the orifice of the parotid duct opposite the upper second molar.

Oropharynx

Hold a tongue blade with the thumb underneath and the index finger and long finger on top. Have the patient relax the tongue tip behind the lower incisors. Press the midpoint of the lingual dorsum downward and forward with the tip of the blade by depressing the middle with the two fingers while the thumb pushes upward on the end (Fig. 7–27A). Steady the left hand with the ring and little fingers on the patient's cheek. The patient should breathe steadily through the nose keeping the mouth open. Pressing farther back causes gagging while pressing anteriorly causes posterior bulging. An optimal view may require several placements of the blade transversely at the midpoint. Test for vagal nerve (CN X) paralysis by noting whether the uvula is drawn upward in the midline when the patient says "e-e-e".

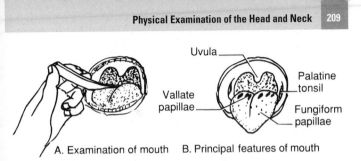

Uvula

Palatine tonsil

Vallate papillae

Fungiform papillae

A. Examination of mouth B. Principal features of mouth

Fig. 7–27 *Examination of the Oral Cavity. A. Use of the tongue blade. B. Principal anatomic features seen in the oral cavity.*

Tonsils

Look for hyperplasia, ulcers, membrane, masses, and small, submerged tonsils.

Examination of the Larynx

Mirror Laryngoscopy

Use a head mirror or head lamp so both hands are free. To use a mirror, seat the patient in a chair with a bright light source immediately behind and to the side of the patient's head. Reflect this light with your head mirror; practice is required. Have the patient sit erect with the chin somewhat forward, both feet on the floor and knees together. Seat yourself in front of the patient with your knees outside the patient's knees. Explain exactly what you are about to do and have the patient concentrate on breathing softly and regularly through the mouth (Fig. 7–11A, page 191). Have the tongue protrude maximally over the lower teeth; with your left hand, wrap a piece of gauze over the tongue, grasp the wrapped portion between thumb and middle finger, bracing your hand against the patient's upper teeth with the forefinger; pull the tongue gently to the side. Hold a No. 5 (large) laryngeal mirror like a pencil at the midpoint of the handle. Warm the mirror in warm water to avoid condensation; check its temperature on your wrist. Brace your fourth and fifth fingers against the patient's cheek; insert the mirror from the side, with the face of the mirror downward and parallel to the tongue surface. Move it posteriorly until its back rests against the anterior surface of the uvula. Press the uvula and soft palate steadily upward; to prevent gagging, avoid touching the back of the tongue. Have the patient breathe steadily while you inspect the larynx. While still viewing the vocal cords, ask the patient to say "e-e-e" or "he-e-e" in a high-pitched voice. Sing along with him in the desired pitch and for the proper duration. When looking in the mirror, remember that upward is anterior, downward is posterior. Examine the *vallate papillae, lingual tonsils, valleculae,* and *epiglottis* (Fig. 7–11B, page 191). Then look at the *false cords, true vocal cords, arytenoids,* and *piriform sinuses.* Finally, observe the true vocal cords during quiet respiration when the rima is tent-shaped. During phonation, watch the cords meet in the midline.

K, L, M Test for Dysarthria

To parse cranial nerve deficits causing dysarthria, ask your patient to say: "Ka, Ka, Ka" (gutturals, CN IX and CN X); "La, La, La" (linguals, CN XII); and "Me, Me, Me" (labials, CN VII).

Examination of the Salivary Glands
Parotid Gland

When fullness is present anterior to the tragus, ascertain whether it is continuous with the inferior mass, as in parotid swelling, or discontinuous, as in swelling of a preauricular lymph node. Swelling from the parotid gland is seen in front of the tragus and earlobe and behind the lower ear, pushing the pinna outward. Have the patient clench his teeth to tense the masseter muscle; palpate against the hard muscle to determine extent, consistency, and tenderness of the mass. Feel for swelling behind the mandibular ramus, which is always present in parotid enlargement. Palpate for calculus in the parotid duct. The normal duct is thick enough to be felt when rolled against the tensed masseter. Inspect the orifice of the parotid duct; while watching the orifice, press the cheek looking for discharge from the duct. With a gloved finger, palpate the orifice and posteriorly for calculus or other mass.

Submandibular (Submaxillary) Gland

Note a swelling under the mandible and slightly anterior to the angle of the jaw. When no mass is present but there is a history of a mass appearing after meals, have the patient sip some lemon juice and watch for the development of a swelling; the appearance of a mass or the enlarging of a preexisting swelling is diagnostic of ductal obstruction. Also compare the appearance of the ductal orifice with its homologue. Using bimanual palpation, with gloved finger in the floor of the mouth, feel for calculus or a mass; look for the drainage when the mass is pressed in the submandibular triangle. To test for the secretion of saliva, place dry cotton under the tongue, have the patient sip lemon juice and then remove the swab and watch for salivary flow from each orifice.

Examination of the Temporomandibular Joint

Palpate over the temporomandibular joint (TMJ), anterior to the tragus, while the patient opens and closes the mouth, feeling for clicking or crepitus (Fig. 7–28). Corresponding noises may be heard by placing the bell of the stethoscope over the joint during movement. To elicit joint tenderness, face the patient and place the tips of your forefingers behind the tragi in each external acoustic meatus. Pull forward while the patient opens her mouth.

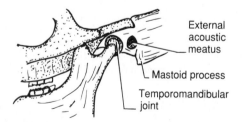

External
acoustic
meatus

Mastoid process

Temporomandibular
joint

Fig. 7–28 *Anatomy of the TMJ.* *Note the nearness of the joint to the external acoustic meatus, so the joint may be palpated by a finger in the meatus (see Fig. 7–66).*

Examination of the Neck

Examination of Cervical Muscles and Bones

If cervical fracture is suspected, and in trauma cases, immobilize the patient and obtain X-rays before trying to elicit physical signs. Have the patient's neck and shoulders uncovered. Face the patient looking for any swellings, especially in the sternocleidomastoideus and the cervical spine. Note any asymmetry of shoulder height and clavicles or fixed posture of the neck. Note the extent of movement and pain elicited by cervical flexion, extension, lateral bending, and rotation. Palpate the cervical vertebrae and muscles for tenderness, tightness and masses. See if massage of muscles brings relief.

Examination of the Thyroid Gland

The normal adult thyroid is often not palpable. In a thin neck, the normal isthmus may be felt as a band of tissue that just obliterates the surface outlines of the tracheal rings. A *goiter* is any enlarged thyroid gland.

Inspection.   Have the patient seated in a good cross-light. Inspect the lower half of the neck in the anterior triangles. Have the patient swallow looking for an ascending mass in the midline or behind the sternocleidomastoid. If the patient is obese or has a short neck, tilt the patient's neck back, and have them support their occiput with their clasped hands; ask the patient to swallow while in this posture.

Palpation from behind.   Have the patient seated in a chair and stand behind her. Instruct the patient to lower her chin to relax her neck muscles. Place your thumbs in back of the patient's neck, curling your fingers anteriorly so long and ring finger tips just touch while resting over the upper tracheal rings (Fig. 7–29A). Have the patient hold some water in her mouth and swallow on demand. Run the fingers up and down the tracheal rings, feeling for any tissue on their anterior surface; if found, it is likely to be a hyperplastic thyroid isthmus. Palpate systematically the lower poles of both lateral lobes. During the examination, shift the inclination of the patient's head to relax the neck muscles, and have the patient swallow to test

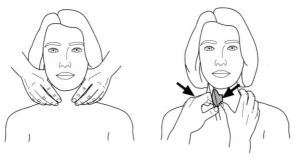

A. Palpation of the thyroid
from behind

B. Palpation of the thyroid
from in front

Fig. 7–29 *Palpation of the Thyroid Gland and Adjacent Structures. A. Palpation from behind. B. Frontal palpation of the thyroid gland.*

the adherence of palpated masses to the trachea. Palpate the anterior surface of each lateral lobe through the sternocleidomastoid with the patient's head slightly inclined toward the side being examined. Occasionally, the thyroid is more easily felt when the neck is dorsiflexed.

Palpation from the front.   Place the fingers of one hand behind the neck with the on the base of the thyroid cartilage (Fig. 7–29B) pushing the trachea gently away from the midline. The fingers of the other hand palpate behind the opposite sternocleidomastoid to feel the posterior aspect of the lateral lobe while the thumb palpates the anterior surface medial to the muscle. Having the patient swallow or depress the chin may further assist in the examination. Palpate the other lateral lobe in the same manner with the tasks of the two hands reversed.

Auscultation of a goiter.   Use the bell of the stethoscope to auscultate a goiter for a bruit.

Examination of the Lymph Nodes

See Chapter 5, page 93 ff.

Examination of the Vascular System

See Chapter 8, page 324 ff.

Head and Neck Symptoms

General Symptoms

> **KEY SYMPTOM   Headache**

See Chapter 14, page 731 ff.

Skull, Scalp, and Face Symptoms

> **KEY SYMPTOM   Blushing and Flushing**

Transient dilation of the superficial blood vessels of the head, face, and neck occurs with emotional, pharmacologic, or physical stimulation. Flushing is a normal response to exercise, hot environments, and ingestion of vasoactive substances such as capsaicin in hot peppers or alcohol. Flushing is common in patients with rosacea or carcinoid syndrome and in women at the menopause. *Blushing* is a term usually reserved for flushing associated with embarrassment or self-consciousness.

> **KEY SYMPTOM   Pain in the Face**

Facial pain is usually well localized, indicating the structure involved. In some cases, it may present a difficult diagnostic problem. *CLINICAL OCCURRENCE:*   An anatomic approach to identifying the cause is useful. Sort the likely causes by the structure involved: *Nerves*   trigeminal neuralgia, postherpetic neuralgia;

Blood Vessels temporal arteritis, cavernous sinus thrombosis; ***Teeth*** peri-apical abscess, periodontitis, unerupted teeth; ***Bones*** sinusitis, osteomyelitis; ***Joints*** temporomandibular arthritis; ***Salivary Glands*** parotitis.

KEY SYNDROME   Facial Pain—Trigeminal Neuralgia (Tic Douloureux)

Compression of the CN V by an artery as it exits the brainstem is a common cause. A nonpainful stimulus provokes a paroxysm of "hot" lancinating pain, always unilateral, and initially limited to one division of the trigeminal nerve (CN V). The intense pain causes grimacing, hence the French term *tic.* Each patient has a unique, adequate stimulus in the trigger area: a light touch, chewing, sneezing, a draft, or a tickling of the skin. The second, maxillary, division is most commonly involved with pain in the maxilla, upper teeth and lip and lower eyelid. Uncommonly, the third, mandibular, division is involved with pain in the lower teeth and lip, the oral portion of the tongue and the external acoustic meatus. The ophthalmic branch is rarely affected. There are no motor or sensory changes. **DDX:** The initial stage of herpes zoster may suggest tic douloureux.

KEY DISEASE   Facial Pain—Herpes Zoster

Sharp burning pain occurs unilaterally in the distribution of one trigeminal nerve branch 2 to 3 days before vesicles appear. Persistent pain after resolution of the skin lesions is postherpetic neuralgia.

KEY SYNDROME   Facial Pain—Acute Suppurative Sinusitis, Orbital Cellulitis

See page 289.

KEY SYMPTOM   Spasms of the Jaw Muscles—Trismus

See page 220.

KEY SYMPTOM   Pain With Chewing—Masseter Claudication

Ischemia of the masseter and/or temporalis muscles is induced by chewing. Pain occurs with chewing, especially tough meats and is relieved by rest. The patient may have altered their diet to avoid the symptom. Giant cell arteritis should be suspected.

KEY SYNDROME   TMJ Pain

Symptoms include pain, which may be felt in the ear or temple, clicking, and occasionally locking. Trauma is associated with injury and crepitation. See, also, Syndromes, page 281.

KEY SYMPTOM   Numb Chin Syndrome

Involvement of the mental or inferior alveolar nerve causes numbness in the chin. Patients present with a complaint of numbness of the chin; no other symptoms or signs may be present. If a thorough oral examination does not identify a local cause of nerve injury, a search for neoplastic disease is indicated.

Ear Symptoms

> **KEY SYMPTOM** Tinnitus

Ringing in the ears or tinnitus is sufficiently distressing that it brings the patient to the physician [Lockwood AH, Salvi RJ, Burkard RF. Tinnitus. *N Engl J Med.* 2002;347:904–910]. Unilateral tinnitus may be the first symptom of an acoustic neuroma. *CLINICAL OCCURRENCE:* *Outer Ear* cerumen, foreign body or polyp in the external meatus; *Middle Ear* inflammation, otosclerosis, polychondritis; *Inner Ear* Meniere disease, syphilis, fevers, suppuration of the labyrinth, basilar skull fracture, acoustic neuroma, trauma; *Drugs* quinine, salicylates, aminoglycoside antibiotics.

> **KEY SYMPTOM** Temporary Altered Hearing—Eustachian Tube Block

The patient experiences mild intermittent pain, a feeling of fullness in the ear and altered hearing. The patient may hear a popping sound on swallowing or yawning. Inspection of the eardrum shows it to be retracted (see Fig. 7–30B, page 222).

> **KEY SYMPTOM** Earache

The middle ear arises from the first and second pharyngeal pouches. Pain may arise from inflammation of structures in the ear or be referred from other pharyngeal sites, including the thyroid. Although the cause of acute pain in the ear is usually readily discovered, chronic earache may offer considerable challenge to diagnosis. *CLINICAL OCCURRENCE:* *Auricle* trauma, hematoma, frostbite, burn, epithelioma, perichondritis, gout, eczema, impetigo, insect bites, carcinoma, herpes zoster; *Meatus* external otitis, malignant external otitis, carbuncle, meatitis, eczema, hard cerumen, foreign body, injury, epithelioma, carcinoma, insect invasion, herpes zoster, trigeminal neuralgia (CN V3); *Middle Ear* acute otitis media, acute mastoiditis, cholesteatoma, malignant disease; *Referred Pain* (through CN V, IX, and X and the second and third cervical nerves) unerupted lower third molar, carious teeth, arthritis of TMJ, tonsillitis, carcinoma or sarcoma of pharynx, ulcer of epiglottis or larynx, cervical lymphadenitis, subacute thyroiditis, trigeminal neuralgia.

> **KEY SYMPTOM** Dizziness and Vertigo

See page 286 ff.

Eye Symptoms

> **KEY SYMPTOM** Double Vision—Diplopia

Perception of two visual images results from abnormalities of refraction or, less commonly, nonconjugative gaze. A careful history should determine the pattern of the symptom (e.g., vertical or horizontal), precipitating activities, the field of vision where the diplopia is apparent, and the position of the head or gaze that relieves the diplopia. If the patient reports monocular diplopia or diplopia when one eye is covered, the cause is nearly always refractive. Binocular diplopia results from impairment of the CN III, IV, and/or VI, damage to or weakness of the extraocular muscles, or displacement of the globe. Careful physical examination should be able to differentiate between these causes. Important diagnostic considerations are myasthenia gravis, Graves' ophthalmopathy, and ophthalmoplegias.

KEY SYMPTOM   Dry Eyes

See page 283, Keratoconjunctivitis sicca.

KEY SYMPTOM   Blurred Vision

Loss of sharp focus of light on the retina occurs with inability of the eye to accommodate the shape of the lens to near or far vision, or scattering of light as a result of opacities in the cornea, lens, or vitreous. The history is the key to identifying the problem. Pain in the eye suggests inflammation of one of the structures (keratitis, iritis and uveitis) or acute angle closure glaucoma. Abnormality of the oils in the tear film is a frequent cause of visual aberration. Use of topical and systemic drugs, especially anticholinergics, results in decreased accommodation and dilation of the pupil. Loss of vision in one eye may also be described as "blurred vision," meaning the vision is less distinct than normal with loss of binocular sight. The pinhole test (see page 205) can be used to determine, if the blurred vision is refractive [Shingleton GJ, O'Donoghue MW. Blurred vision. *N Engl J Med.* 2000;343:556–562].

KEY SYMPTOM   Pain in the Eye

Pain in the eye results from inflammation, infection, trauma, and increased intraocular pressure. Inspect the lids, conjunctivae, and sclera for lesions. Careful examination of the cornea, anterior chamber, iris, and retina are mandatory. Always assess visual acuity in each eye. Optimal examination requires an ophthalmologist.

✔ **CLINICAL OCCURRENCE:**   *Idiopathic*   cluster headache;   *Inflammatory/ Immune*   hordeolum (sty), chalazion, interstitial keratitis, iritis, iridocyclitis, episcleritis, scleritis, band keratopathy, optic neuritis;   *Infectious*   infective keratitis (herpes simplex, zoster and others), sinusitis (ethmoid, frontal, sphenoid); *Mechanical/Trauma*   foreign body, corneal abrasion, entropion, glaucoma, eyestrain.

KEY SYMPTOM   Visual Loss

Injury or impairment to any portion of the visual pathways can lead to visual loss. Acute loss of vision is a medial emergency (see page 284). Chronic progressive loss of vision is common with diseases of the cornea, lens, or retina. Standard tests of visual acuity will quantitate the degree of impairment and formal visual field testing is required. Referral to an ophthalmologist is indicated.

Nose Symptoms

> **KEY SYMPTOM** Loss of Smell: Anosmia

See page 254.

> **KEY SYMPTOM** Abnormal Smell or Taste—Dysgeusia

This is a common complaint in patients who have loss of smell (*anosmia*). If it is paroxysmal and associated with behavioral symptoms, it suggests complex partial seizures.

Lip, Mouth, Tongue, Teeth, and Pharynx Symptoms

> **KEY SYMPTOM** Soreness of Tongue or Mouth

Pain or tenderness in the tongue or mouth is a presenting symptom for a number of disorders. Inspection and palpation assist in the differential diagnosis [Drage LA, Rogers RS. Clinical assessment and outcome in 70 patients with complaints of burning or sore mouth symptoms. *Mayo Clin Proc.* 1999;74:223–228].

✔ *CLINICAL OCCURRENCE:* **No Lesions** tobacco smoking, early glossitis from all causes, menopausal symptom, heavy metal poisoning; **Deep Lesions** calculus in duct of submaxillary or sublingual gland, foreign body, myositis of lingual muscles, trichinosis, periostitis of hyoid bone, neoplasm of lingual muscles; **Localized Superficial Lesions** biting the tongue, trauma to lingual frenulum, dental ulcer, injury while under anesthesia, foreign body (e.g., fish bone), epithelioma or carcinoma, ranula, tuberculous ulcer, herpes, Vincent stomatitis, leukoplakia, *Candida*; **Generalized Disease** pellagra, riboflavin deficiency, scurvy, pernicious anemia, atrophic glossitis, leukemia, exanthematous disorders, collagen diseases, pemphigus, cicatricial pemphigoid, lichen planus, heavy-metal poisoning, phenytoin, uremia, cancer chemotherapy, drug sensitivity; systemic fungal infections, for example, histoplasmosis; **Irradiation** Therapeutic irradiation for head and neck malignancy causes temporary or permanent loss of saliva production. Within 2 to 4 weeks of the beginning of treatment, and lasting 6 or more weeks, patients experience increasing dryness and generalized soreness of the mouth and throat.

> **KEY SYMPTOM** Difficult or Painful Swallowing—Dysphagia and Odynophagia

A disorder in swallowing is termed *dysphagia*. With *oropharyngeal dysphagia* the patient describes difficulty initiating a swallow or choking and coughing with swallowing. With *esophageal dysphagia*, the patient experiences a sense of obstruction at a definite level when fluid or a bolus of food is swallowed. *Neurogenic dysphagia* may be accompanied by regurgitation through the nose. Some varieties of dysphagia may cause localized pain (*odynophagia*); others are painless. Deglutition involves muscles in both the oropharynx and the esophagus. Pain from the oropharynx is accurately localized, but esophageal pain is dispersed in the thoracic six-dermatome band, presenting as chest pain (see page 333 and Chapter 9 pages 467 and 491).

✔ *DYSPHAGIA AND ODYNOPHAGIA—CLINICAL OCCURRENCE:* **Oropharynx** *Painful dysphagia from intrinsic lesions:* glossitis, tonsillitis, stomatitis, pharyngitis, laryngitis, lingual ulcer, carcinoma, pemphigus, erythema multiforme, Ludwig angina, mumps, bee sting of the tongue, angioneurotic edema, candidiasis, sometimes Plummer-Vinson syndrome; *Painful dysphagia from local extrinsic lesions:* cervical adenitis, subacute thyroiditis, carotid arteritis, infected thyroglossal cysts or sinuses, pharyngeal cysts or sinuses, carotid body tumor, spur in cervical spine, pericarditis; *Painful dysphagia from systemic conditions:* rabies, tetanus; *Painless dysphagia from intrinsic lesions:* cleft palate, flexion of the neck from cervical osteoporosis, xerostomia in Sjögren syndrome, and magnesium deficiency; *Painless dysphagia from neurogenic lesions:* CN-IX or CN-X damage, globus hystericus, postdiphtheritic paralysis, bulbar paralysis, West Nile virus, myasthenia gravis, amyotrophic lateral sclerosis, Wilson disease, syphilis, parkinsonism, botulism, poisoning (lead, alcohol, fluoride); **Esophagus** *Painful dysphagia from intrinsic lesions (see Pain in the Chest, page 273⋯):* foreign body, carcinoma, esophagitis, diverticulum, hiatal hernia; *Painless dysphagia from intrinsic lesions:* achalasia, congenital stricture, stricture, scleroderma, dermatomyositis; Sjögren syndrome, amyloidosis, thyrotoxicosis; *Painless dysphagia from extrinsic lesions:* aortic aneurysm, aberrant right subclavian artery (see page 291), vertebral spurs, enlarged left atrium.

Larynx Symptoms

> **KEY SYMPTOM** **Hoarseness**

See page 272.

Salivary Gland Symptoms

> **KEY SYMPTOM** **Dry Mouth—Xerostomia**

See page 296.

Neck Symptoms

> **KEY SYMPTOM** **Pain in the Neck**

Pain in the neck is a common complaint whose cause is often readily diagnosed by a careful history, palpation of the neck, and examination of the oropharynx. Posttraumatic or postural cervical strain is the most common cause of pain in the neck. Each anatomic structure should be palpated systematically. Increased pain with specific movements may be helpful in localizing the source of pain.

✔ *NECK PAIN—CLINICAL OCCURRENCE:* **Neck Pain Increased by Swallowing** *Pharynx:* pharyngitis, Ludwig angina, inflamed thyroglossal duct or cyst; *Tonsils:* tonsillitis, neoplasm; *Tongue:* ulcers, neoplasm; *Larynx:* laryngitis, neoplasm, ulcer, foreign body; *Esophagus:* inflamed diverticulum, esophagitis; *Thyroid:* suppurative or subacute thyroiditis, hemorrhage; *Carotid Artery:* carotodynia, carotid body tumor; *Salivary Glands:* mumps, suppurative parotitis; **Neck Pain Increased by Chewing** *Mandible:* fracture, osteomyelitis, periodontitis; *Salivary Glands:* mumps, suppurative parotitis; **Neck Pain Increased**

by Movements of the Head *Sternocleidomastoideus:* torticollis, hematoma; *Nuchal Muscles:* viral myalgia, muscle tension; *Cervical Spine:* herniated intervertebral disk, spinal arthritis, meningitis, meningismus, craniovertebral junction abnormalities; **Neck Pain Increased by Shoulder Movement** *Superior Thoracic Aperture:* cervical rib, scalenus anticus syndrome, costoclavicular syndrome; **Neck Pain Not Increased by Movement** *Skin and Subcutaneous Tissues:* furuncle, carbuncle, erysipelas; *Lymph Nodes:* acute adenitis. *Branchial Cleft Remnants:* inflamed pharyngeal cyst; *Salivary Glands:* duct calculus; *Subclavian Artery:* aneurysm; *Nervous System:* poliomyelitis, West Nile virus, herpes zoster, epidural abscess, spinal cord neoplasm. *Spinal Vertebrae:* herniated intervertebral disk, metastatic carcinoma; *Referred Pain:* Pancoast syndrome, angina pectoris, and other conditions in the six-dermatome band.

> **KEY SYNDROME**   **Carotodynia**

The patient complains of constant or throbbing pain in the anterior lateral neck intensified by swallowing. It may radiate to the mandible or ear. Symptoms frequently follow a viral pharyngitis with fever. Some patients have profound lassitude. Several relapses may occur within a few months. The carotid bulb is exquisitely tender and may seem enlarged with exaggerated pulsations; the common carotid may be tender as well. Carotid compression causes radiation of pain along the branches of the external carotid to the jaw, ear, and temple (*Fay sign*). One or both common carotid arteries may be involved. The pharynx and larynx are normal or slightly hyperemic and edematous. The diagnosis is made by demonstrating tenderness of the carotid artery.

> **KEY SYMPTOM**   **Neck Fullness—Tracheal Displacement from Goiter**

Many patients with a small goiter complain of a sense of constriction or fullness in the neck. See page 279ff.

Head and Neck Signs

Scalp, Face, Skull, and Jaw Signs

> **KEY SIGN**   **Scalp Wounds**

Because the scalp is extremely vascular, scalp wounds bleed profusely. Wounds do not gape unless the galea aponeurotica is lacerated. If gaping is noted, an open skill fracture should be suspected.

> **KEY SIGN**   **Fluctuant Scalp Masses—Hematoma, Abscess, Depressed Fracture**

When blood or pus accumulates in the skin or subcutaneous layer of the scalp, it is sharply localized and the mass readily slides over the skull. A boggy, fluctuant mass in the entire adult scalp results from blood or pus in the loose connective tissue under the aponeurosis; the same finding in a young child may also be evidence of parietal bone fracture. A fluctuant mass bounded by the skull suture lines indicates subperiosteal blood or pus or a depressed fracture. A hematoma under the periosteum usually has a soft center that is plastic, while the edges are firm and feel much like a depressed fracture.

Scalp cellulitis. The scalp is tender, soft, and boggy. The infection extends rapidly, causing edema of the eyelids and pinnae; the regional lymph nodes are tender and swollen.

Scalp mass—sebaceous cyst (WEN). A common lesion, it is either single or multiple. Because it arises from the skin, it slides easily over the skull. The mass is firm, nontender and often hemispheric. When infected, it bleeds easily and may be mistaken for a squamous cell carcinoma.

Scalp mass—lipoma: In the subcutaneous layer it feels smooth and soft; the finger slides around its edges. When it occurs beneath the pericranium, its movement is strictly limited, but the finger can detect a smooth, rounded border.

KEY SIGN Swelling of the Cheek

Parotid enlargement. See page 275.

Preauricular abscess. Suppuration of the preauricular lymph node produces an abscess that may ulcerate. The swelling is localized, tender and sometimes warm. The source of infection is in the side of the face, pinna, anterior wall of the external acoustic meatus, anterior third of the scalp, eyebrows, or eyelids.

Masseter muscle hypertrophy: Either one or both masseter muscles may undergo spontaneous hypertrophy producing swelling of the face that must be distinguished from parotid gland swelling. If the entire mass hardens when the patient clench his teeth, it is muscular.

Redness of the cheeks: Erythema, scaling, pustules, and tenderness in a malar distribution may be due to sunburn, cellulitis, rosacea, seborrheic dermatitis, discoid or systemic lupus erythematosus (SLE) or acne vulgaris.

Forehead wrinkles: Absence of normal transverse furrowing with upward gaze is a sign of hyperthyroidism. Deep wrinkling, with longitudinal furrowing and prominence of intervening tissue is the *bulldog skin* in pachydermatosis. Unilateral loss of wrinkling results from facial nerve (CN VII) paralysis.

KEY SIGN Enlarged Adult Skull—Paget Disease

See page 682. In addition to bone pain, the patient may complain that his hats have become too small. The calvarium is large compared with the facial bones. A bruit is sometimes heard in the skull.

KEY SIGN Mastoid Pain and Tenderness—Mastoiditis

See page 285.

Skull Masses—Neoplasms: An *osteoma* frequently occurs in the outer table of the skull, producing a hard, sessile bony eminence. Hard or soft masses in the cranial bones may be a *pericranial sarcoma*, carcinomatous metastasis, lymphomas, leukemia, or multiple myeloma.

> **KEY SIGN   Limited Jaw Opening—Trismus**

Trismus is the forceful closing of the jaws from spasm of the masticatory muscles. Trismus is common with tetanus, but it has many other causes. Failure of the mouth to open from other causes is far more common.   *CLINICAL OCCURRENCE: Local Disorders*   impacted third molar, TMJ arthritis, malignant external otitis, lymphadenitis, trigeminal neuralgia, scleroderma, dermatomyositis;   *Disorders with Widespread Muscle Spasm*   trichinosis, rabies, tetany, tetanus, strychnine poisoning, typhoid fever, cholera, septicemia;   *Cerebral Disorders*   encephalitis, epilepsy (transient), catalepsy, hysteria, malingering.

> **KEY SIGN   Inability to Close the Jaw—TMJ Dislocation**

Because the TMJ is a shallow biconcave surface, it can easily partially sublux or completely dislocate. After a yawn or an upward blow on the chin with the mouth wide open, the jaw cannot be closed. The mandible protrudes and the lower teeth override the upper. There is a depression or pit anterior to the tragus that is more obvious when bilateral; in unilateral dislocation, the pretragal depression occurs only on the affected side. No movement of the mandibular head is felt when palpating through the external acoustic meatus on the affected side.

Ear Signs

External Ear Signs

> **KEY SIGN   Earlobe Crease**

A visible crease extending at least one-third of the distance from tragus to posterior pinna has been associated with a higher rate of cardiac events in patients admitted to the hospital with suspected coronary heart disease [Elliott WJ, Powell LH. Diagonal earlobe creases and prognosis in patients with suspected coronary artery disease. *Am J Med.* 1996;100:205–211].

Darwin Tubercle: A developmental eminence in the upper third of the posterior helix, this condition is harmless. It must be distinguished from acquired nodules, such as tophi.

Other Nodules: These may be basal cell carcinomas, rheumatoid nodules, or leprosy. Calcification of the cartilage is a rare complication of Addison disease. The nodule is not usually tender.

> **KEY SIGN   Earlobe Nodule: Gouty Tophus**

In long-standing gout, accumulations of sodium urate crystals may occur in the helix and antihelix; they also occur in the olecranon bursa, the tendon sheaths, and the aponeuroses of the extremities. The nodules are painless, hard, and irregular. They may open discharging chalky contents.

> **KEY SIGN   Hematoma**

Trauma or a hemostatic defect results in blood accumulating between the cartilage and perichondrium. There is a tender, blue, doughy mass, usually without spontaneous pain. Prompt incision and drainage avoids suppuration or cauliflower ear.

> **KEY SYNDROME**   **Recurring Inflammation—Relapsing Polychondritis**

There is inflammation and degeneration of cartilage especially of the pinna, nasal septum, laryngeal cartilages, tracheal and bronchial rings; joint cartilages may be affected. The ear is painful, swollen, and reddened, except over the lobule. Hoarseness indicates laryngeal involvement; blindness may result from involvement of the sclerae, and tinnitus and deafness from middle ear involvement. Rarely, degeneration of the aortic or mitral valve ring produces valvular regurgitation or aortic aneurysm.

Dermoid cyst: A favorite site is just behind the pinna. This lesion is soft and slightly fluctuant.

> **KEY SIGN**   **Pinna Neoplasms**

Squamous cell carcinoma is more common than basal cell carcinoma on the pinna. Any small crusted, ulcerated, or indurated lesion that fails to heal promptly should be biopsied.

External Acoustic Meatus Signs

> **KEY SIGN**   **Cerumen Impaction**

The wax of Native Americans and East Asians is often dry and flakey, and more yellow than amber. Excessive wax production or a narrow meatus leads to impacted cerumen and partial or complete obstruction of the canal. When obstruction is complete, partial deafness results. Tinnitus or dizziness may occur. A partial obstruction may suddenly become complete when water enters the meatus during bathing or swimming. The obstructing wax is easily seen in the external meatus.

> **KEY SIGN**   **Discharge from the Ear—Otorrhea**

Discharge from the Ear has many causes. The type of discharge suggests the diagnosis: *Yellow Discharge* melting cerumen; *Serous Discharge* eczema, early ruptured acute otitis media; *Bloody Discharge*   trauma of the external canal or longitudinal temporal bone fracture causing TM and external canal laceration; *Purulent Discharge*   chronic external otitis, perforation of acute suppurative otitis media, chronic suppurative or tuberculous otitis media with or without cholesteatoma.

> **KEY SIGN**   **External Otitis**

See page 284.

> **KEY SIGN**   **Dermatitis**

Seborrheic dermatitis commonly causes scaling and pruritus of the choana and meatus. Medicated eardrops can cause contact dermatitis.

> **KEY SIGN**   **Carcinoma**

Either squamous cell or basal cell carcinoma can involve the meatal epithelium. Pain and discharge are the presenting symptoms. In advanced stages, deafness and facial paralysis may occur.

Foreign body: Children often place objects in their ears. A purulent discharge from the canal or an earache may be the first indication.

Polyps: A bulbous, reddened, pedunculated mass arises from the wall or the middle ear. Gently moving the mass with forceps may indicate its origin. They cause a foul purulent discharge.

Exostoses and chondromas: Exostoses form nodules in the osseous canal near the TM. They rarely produce obstruction, although the TM may be partially obscured. A single bony osteoma may occur. Rarely, chondromas arise from the cartilaginous canal, usually without obstruction.

Furuncle: A red, tender prominence with or without a pustule forms in the cartilaginous canal producing extreme pain.

Vesicles: Pain in the ear with vesicles in the canal and facial weakness is due to herpes zoster of CN VII (Ramsey-Hunt Syndrome), Chapter 14, page 715.

Tympanic Membrane (TM) Signs

> **KEY SIGN** **Retracted TM**

See Otitis Media with Effusion, page 285.

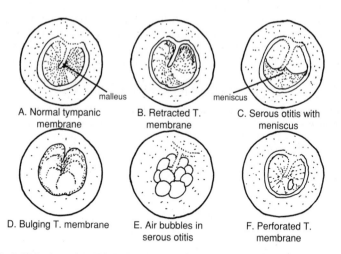

A. Normal tympanic membrane

B. Retracted T. membrane

C. Serous otitis with meniscus

D. Bulging T. membrane

E. Air bubbles in serous otitis

F. Perforated T. membrane

Fig. 7–30 *Lesions of the TM. A. Normal:* The normal TM is slanted downward and forward; its surface glistens and contains a brilliant triangle, the light reflex, with its apex at the center, or umbo, and its base at the annuals. The handle of the malleus makes an impression on the disk from the umbo upward and forward. *B. The retracted eardrum:* The light reflex is bent and the malleus stands out in sharper relief than normally. *C. Serous middle ear fluid:* Hairline menisci curve from the handle of the malleus to the annulus. *D. Bulging drumhead:* The curves in the membrane abscure the normal landmarks of the malleus and distort the light reflex. *E. Serous fluid mixed with air:* Bubbles may be seen through the drumhead. *F. Perforations* of the membrane appear as oval holes with a dark shadow behind.

KEY SIGN   Red or Bulging TM

See Acute Suppurative Otitis Media, page 285.

KEY SIGN   Vesicles on the TM

Infection with *Mycoplasma pneumoniae* causes severe ear pain and an inflamed TM with often hemorrhagic vesicles (bullous myringitis).

KEY SIGN   Perforated TM

A healed suppurative middle ear infection has eroded through the TM leaving an oval hole through which the middle ear cavity is seen. Other than some decrease in auditory acuity, chronic perforations are asymptomatic.

Hearing Signs

KEY SIGN   Lateralizing Weber Test—Ipsilateral Conductive Hearing Loss or Contralateral Neurosensory Loss

When neurosensory hearing is intact bilaterally, the sound will lateralize to the side of conductive loss, which loses the masking effect of background noises. Neurosensory loss on one side results in a *louder* sound on the opposite side. Therefore, lateralization of sound to the right ear means conductive loss on the right or perceptive loss on the left.

KEY SIGN   Bone Conduction Greater Than Air Conduction (Rinne-Negative Test)—Conductive Hearing Loss

When amplification of sound by the TM and ossicles is impaired, direct transmission of vibrations through bone to the cochlea is louder than sound transmitted through air. Conductive hearing loss results from obstruction of the auditory canal, damage to the TM, middle ear fluid and destruction or ankylosis of the ossicles.

Balance and Position Signs

KEY SIGN   Positive Past Pointing Test

Deviation to the right or left of the target fingers, past pointing, indicates either labyrinthine stimulation or loss of positional sense. The flow of endolymph is in the same direction as the past pointing.

KEY SIGN   Romberg Sign

Stable standing with the eyes closed requires normal labyrinthine function, position sense, cerebellar function and muscular strength. Persistent labyrinthine stimulation or loss of position sense leads to unsteadiness, elevation of the arms for balance or falling. With labyrinthine stimulation, the patient will fall in the same direction as the flow of endolymph. Inability to maintain balance with the eyes open suggests abnormalities of the labyrinth, cerebellum or sight.

Eye Signs
Lid Signs

> **KEY SIGN** **Lacrimation**

Lacrimation usually refers to any condition resulting in tears, although strict usage indicates an overproduction. *Epiphora* means an overflow of tears from any cause. **CLINICAL OCCURRENCE:** **Increased Secretion** weeping from emotion, irritation from foreign body, corneal ulcer, conjunctivitis, coryza, measles, hay fever, poisoning (iodide, bromide, arsenic); **Lacrimal Duct Obstruction** congenital, cicatrix, eyelid edema, lacrimal calculus, dacryocystitis; **Separation of the Puncta from the Globe** facial paralysis, aging, chronic marginal blepharitis, ectropion, proptosis.

> **KEY SIGN** **Widened Palpebral Fissures**

The fissures are widened by lid retraction (contraction of Mueller muscle) or protrusion of the globe. With eyes in the primary position the upper lid covers the limbus and a white scleral strip usually shows between limbus and lower lid. Widening of the palpebral fissure uncovers the upper border of the limbus to expose white sclera superiorly. When there is no actual proptosis, widened fissures produce the optical illusion of global protrusion. A few normal persons have widened palpebral fissures.

> **KEY SIGN** **Exophthalmos (Ocular Proptosis)**

Proptosis is proven by measurement (see page 198). Unilateral proptosis is recognized by comparing the two eyes. If both eyes seem equally prominent, inspect them in profile (Fig. 7–31). Unilateral proptosis suggests orbital tumor or inflammation. When the globe is displaced medially, disease of the lacrimal gland should be suspected; upward displacement suggests disease in the maxillary sinus; lateral displacement can occur from a lesion in the ethmoid or sphenoid sinus. Graves' disease is the most common cause of bilateral proptosis. **CLINICAL OCCURRENCE:** **Unilateral Exophthalmos** Graves' disease, mucocele, orbital cellulitis and abscess, cavernous sinus thrombosis, orbital periostitis, myxedema, orbital fracture, hemangioma, orbital neoplasm, arteriovenous aneurysm, fungal infection, histiocytosis; **Bilateral Exophthalmos** Graves' disease, myxedema, acromegaly, cavernous sinus thrombosis, empyema of the nasal accessory sinuses, lymphoma, leukemia, histiocytosis.

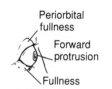
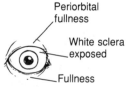

Fig. 7–31 *Exophthalmos (proptosis).*

KEY SIGN   Lid Lag—Hyperthyroidism

Thyrotoxicosis increases sympathetic stimulation producing contraction of Mueller muscle in the upper lid. Lid lag indicates increased tone even without widened fissures in the primary position. Usually the finding is bilateral; occasionally one fissure is much wider than the other.   *Other Lid Signs in Hyperthyroidism*   Stellwag Sign: infrequent blinking; Rosenbach Sign: tremor of the closed eyelids; Mean Sign: global lag during elevation; Griffith Sign: lag of the lower lids during elevation of the globes; Boston Sign: jerking of the lagging lid; Joffroy Sign: absence of forehead wrinkling with upward gaze, the head being tilted down.

KEY SIGN   Narrowed Palpebral Fissures—Enophthalmos

The globe is recessed in the orbit. When bilateral, it is usually caused by decreased orbital fat or congenital microphthalmos. Unilateral enophthalmos is caused by trauma or inflammation. Enophthalmos has been described as a sign of *Horner syndrome*; actually, the accompanying droop of the eyelid merely produces an optical illusion of globe recession.

KEY SIGN   Failure of Lid Closure—Paralysis of Orbicularis Muscle

The facial nerve (CN VII) supplies the orbicularis oculi muscle. Damage to CN VII, as in Bell palsy, causes partial or complete paralysis of the orbicularis. When complete, both upper and lower lids remain retracted so the eye is unprotected and tears drain onto the face. *Bell phenomenon* occurs: the globes elevate during attempted closure of the lids. Failure of lid closure is also present in severe grades of exophthalmos.

KEY SIGN   Failure of Lid Opening—Ptosis of the Lid

The congenital form is usually bilateral from paralysis of or failure to develop the levator palpebrae superioris. The acute acquired condition usually results from disease of the oculomotor nerve (CN III). In the congenital form, the eyelid will show lid lag as the child looks down. With CN III lesion paralysis of other eye muscles may be present.   *CLINICAL OCCURRENCE:*   Supranuclear lesions (e.g., encephalitis), Horner syndrome, paralysis of the levator muscle, levator dehiscence, thinning of levator tendon (the lid droops, but has normal excursion, 15–18 mm).

KEY SIGN   Horner's Syndrome

Lesions anywhere along the three neurons of the sympathetic chain blocks sympathetic innervation of the eye and face. The complete syndrome has ptosis, miosis, and anhydrosis on the affected side. The ptosis is incomplete, distinguishing it from paralysis of the levator muscle.

Blepharospasm: Frequent spasmodic lid closure, either unilateral or bilateral, may progress to the point that it interferes with function. It is a form of focal dystonia. Unilateral disease may follow Bell palsy.

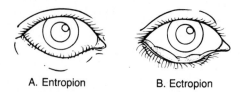

A. Entropion   B. Ectropion

Fig. 7–32 *Pathologic Inversion and Eversion of the Eyelids.*

> **KEY SIGN** Epicanthal Fold—Down Syndrome

See page 282.

> **KEY SIGN** Shortened Palpebral Fissures—Fetal Alcohol Syndrome

The combination of shortened palpebral fissures, epicanthic folds, shortened nose with anteverted nostrils, hypoplastic upper lip with thinned vermilion and flattened or absent philtrum, together with mental retardation, are stigmata of fetal alcohol syndrome.

> **KEY SIGN** Lid Inversion—Entropion

Structural changes or muscular contraction turns the eyelashes inward to impinge upon the globe. **Spastic entropion** occurs only in the lower lid and is caused by increased tone of the orbicularis oculi; the lid turns in only when forcibly closed (Fig. 7–32A). **Cicatricial entropion** occurs in either lid from contracture of scar tissue, as in trachoma. Irritation from the inverted eyelashes may produce *blepharospasm.*

> **KEY SIGN** Lid Eversion—Ectropion

The lid turns outward (Fig. 7–32B). Both lids may be affected by **spastic** or **cicatricial ectropion**, but **paralytic ectropion** involves only the lower lid. Senile atrophy of tissues sometimes results in ectropion rather than entropion.

> **KEY SIGN** Violaceous Lids

Heliotrope or violaceous discoloration of the periorbital skin occurs in dermatomyositis and after chronic quinacrine ingestion.

Lid Erythema: Generalized reddening of the lids is nonspecific. Erythema of the nasal half of the upper lid suggests inflammation of the frontal sinus. Disease of the lacrimal sac can cause erythema of the medial lower lid. Hyperemia of the temporal upper lid should suggest dacryoadenitis. The lid is frequently red over sty.

Lid Cyanosis: Blueness of the eyelid occurs from thrombosis of the orbital veins, orbital tumors, and arteriovenous malformations in the orbit.

> **KEY SIGN** Lid Hemorrhage

Trauma to the lids may result in extravasation of blood into the surrounding tissue, colloquially known as a "black eye." Palpebral hematoma can occur from nasal

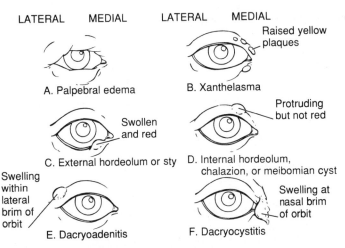

LATERAL   MEDIAL   LATERAL   MEDIAL

A. Palpebral edema

B. Xanthelasma — Raised yellow plaques

C. External hordeolum or sty — Swollen and red

D. Internal hordeolum, chalazion, or meibomian cyst — Protruding but not red

E. Dacryoadenitis — Swelling within lateral brim of orbit

F. Dacryocystitis — Swelling at nasal brim of orbit

Fig. 7–33 *Lesions of the External Eye.* (See text for descriptions of each condition.)

fracture. The appearance of hematoma many hours after head trauma suggests a skull fracture; the greater the time interval, the more remote the fracture site. Fractures of the basilar skull may produce hematoma of the lid several days later. Involvement of both eyes is called *raccoon sign.*

KEY SIGN   Lid Edema

Noninflammatory edema is frequent in acute nephritis, but uncommon in chronic nephritis and cardiac failure (Fig. 7–33A). Lid edema occurs early in the course of both myxedema and Graves' ophthalmopathy. Palpebral edema is frequent in angioedema and trichinosis. Contact dermatitis frequently involves the lids; the patient may not react to an allergen on the hands, but when transferred to the lids swelling occurs. Local infections cause inflammatory edema of the eyelids, which is readily identified by finding redness, warmth, and pain. More serious causes are thrombosis of the intracranial sagittal sinus or cavernous sinus.

KEY SIGN   Yellow Lid Plaques—Xanthelasma

Xanthelasma are raised yellow, painless and nonpruritic plaques on the upper and lower lids near the inner canthi (Fig. 7–33B). They grow slowly and may disappear spontaneously. These xanthoma are frequently associated with hyper-cholesterolemia.

KEY SIGN   Lid Scaling and Redness—Blepharitis

Seborrheic blepharitis is an oily inflammation of the lid margins that produces greasy flakes of dried secretion on the eyelashes and reddening of the lid margins. When ulceration of the lid margin occurs, it is usually *staphylococcal blepharitis.* *Angular blepharitis* is a specific disease caused by the diplococcus of Morax-Axenfeld, in which the margins near the temporal canthi are inflamed.

> **KEY SIGN** **External Hordeolum (Sty)**

When a sebaceous gland of an eyelash hair follicle becomes inflamed, a pustule forms on the lid margin (Fig. 7–33C). It may be surrounded by hyperemia and swelling. Many rupture and heal spontaneously.

> **KEY SIGN** **Internal Hordeolum and Meibomian Cyst (Chalazion)**

Acute inflammation of a meibomian (tarsal) gland is termed an internal hordeolum or internal sty. A granuloma of the gland is known as a chalazion or meibomian cyst (Fig. 7–33D). These internal sebaceous gland lesions produce localized swelling that frequently causes a protrusion on the lid. Lid eversion shows hyperemia, a localized cyst or enlarged gland.

> **KEY SIGN** **Dacryoadenitis**

Obstruction of the lacrimal duct produces acute inflammation of the lacrimal gland. This causes pain and tenderness within the temporal edge of the orbit; it must be distinguished from orbital cellulitis and hordeolum of the upper lid (Fig. 7–33E).

> **KEY SIGN** **Dacryocystitis**

Nasolacrimal duct obstruction leads to inflammation and infection. Patients present with pain and an overflow of tears onto the cheek (*epiphora*). Symptoms are increased by irritants such as wind, dust, or smoke. Tenderness, swelling, and redness beside the nose, near the medial canthus (Fig. 7–33F) are present. The swelling is anterior to the eyelid, distinguishing it from hordeolum. Fluid can be expressed with pressure on the duct. Conjunctivitis, blepharitis and lid edema may be present.

Eye Movement Signs

> **KEY SIGN** **Nystagmus**

One or both eyes cannot maintain fixation so the eyes drift slowly to one side returning back to the original position by a quick correcting movement. This is the normal eye movement to maintain fixation when the head is in motion. It can result from damage to the labyrinth, its cerebellar connections, or the cerebellum; there is instability when the patient stands with eyes open. Jerk nystagmus is named after the direction of the quick component. It may be horizontal, vertical, rotatory, oblique, or mixed. When both eyes participate, the nystagmus is *associated*; movement of one eye only is *dissociated*. Fewer than 40 jerks per minute is "slow"; more than 100 jerks per minute is "fast". Amplitudes <1 mm are *fine*; amplitudes >3 mm are *coarse*. **DDX:** Ocular instabilities resembling nystagmus include ocular flutter, opsoclonus, and ocular bobbing.

There are several varieties of nystagmus:

Congenital Nystagmus. is characterized by unsystematic wandering movements, with various frequencies and amplitudes.

End-Position Nystagmus. Nystagmus occurs only with fixation far to the side, so it is always in the direction of fixation (Fig. 7–34A).

A. End-position nystagmus

B. Nystagmus in primary position

Fig. 7–34 Nystagmus. *A slow drift of the eyes away from the position of fixation (indicated by the broken arrow) is corrected by a quick movement back (solid arrow). The direction of the nystagmus is named from the quick component. Nystagmus from the primary position is more likely to be of serious import than that from the end position.*

Labyrinthine end-position nystagmus usually occurs in disease of the semicircular canals; it is horizontal-rotatory and is initiated by fixation in the end position, but it persists for some time after the primary position has been resumed.

Fixation nystagmus occurs in many normal persons when they are required to fix to one side or the other; it is horizontal or horizontal-rotatory, moderate to coarse.

Muscle-paretic nystagmus presents as a dissociated movement of an eye with a paretic muscle when visual fixation is directed in the direction of action of the paretic muscle and the muscle attempts to maintain fixation.

Gaze-paretic nystagmus appears in paralysis of conjugate movements. Both eyes show more nystagmus to one end position than to the other.

Primary Position Nystagmus occurs with fixation in the primary position or at a point away from the direction of the quick component (Fig. 7–34B).

Peripheral labyrinthine nystagmus is horizontal-rotatory, with medium frequency and amplitude, commonly seen in Ménière syndrome, benign paroxysmal positional vertigo, labyrinthitis, perilymphatic or labyrinthine fistula, and vestibular neuritis.

Central nystagmus may be horizontal, rotatory, vertical, or mixed, usually in the direction of the diseased side. Commonly, it is found in multiple sclerosis, encephalitis, brain tumors, and transient or permanent vascular insufficiency states involving the vestibular nuclei or the medial longitudinal fasciculus.

Vertical nystagmus usually indicates a lesion in the midbrain.

Three types of nystagmus identify more localized lesions.

Convergence-retraction nystagmus occurs in the dorsal midbrain syndrome with lid retraction (Collier sign), limited up-gaze and light-near dissociation.

Seesaw nystagmus, found in parasellar lesions, is characterized by rising and intorting of one eye while the other falls and extorts.

Downbeat nystagmus typically signifies lesions at the foramen magnum such as the Arnold-Chiari malformation, but may be seen with other disorders, including magnesium depletion, Wernicke encephalopathy and lithium intoxication.

Saccadic Intrusions: Saccadic movements are rapid start-stop movements as opposed to the normal smooth pursuit movements when the eyes are fixed on a moving object. Voluntary eye movements are saccadic; you cannot move your eyes smoothly without fixing on a moving object. When saccadic eye movements occur inappropriately they suggest cerebellar disease. The quick component of nystagmus is a saccadic movement.

Ocular Flutter is the arrhythmic and rapid movement of the eyes horizontally. When both horizontal and vertical components exist, it is termed *opsoclonus.*

These conditions are associated with vascular, immune, neoplastic and paraneoplastic processes.

Ocular Bobbing is the intermittent, conjugate, rapid, downward movement of the eyes followed by a slow return to primary position and is often seen in comatose patients with pontine lesions.

Abnormalities of Gaze

> **KEY SIGN   Comitant Strabismus (Nonparalytic Heterophoria)—Constant Squint Angle**

The muscles are normal; the disorder probably results from abnormal innervation in the nuclei of the cranial nerves, because the squint angle disappears during general anesthesia. The word *comitant*, when applied to strabismus, indicates that the angle between the two optic axes, the *squint angle*, remains constant in all positions assumed by the globes, no matter which eye fixates. Neither eye has limited motion (Fig. 7–35A). Because comitant strabismus occurs in the very young, children learn to suppress the image from one eye and do not have diplopia. In most cases, the optic axes converge, which is termed *comitant convergent strabismus* or **esotropia**. When hypermetropia causes excessive convergence, the condition is called *accommodative squint*. Occasionally the optic axes diverge, which is termed comitant divergent strabismus or **exotropia**.

> **KEY SIGN   Varying Squint Angle—Noncomitant Strabismus (Paralytic Heterotropia)**

This is caused by paralysis of one or more eye muscles: *ophthalmoplegia*. The squint angle changes with the direction of fixation. As opposed to comitant strabismus, the motions of the paralyzed eye are limited. The head is moved to limit the action of the paralyzed muscle in order to avoid diplopia. The squint angle is greatest when the unaffected eye is fixed on the visual field requiring the action of the paralyzed muscle, *secondary deviation*. When paralysis is acquired during maturity, diplopia occurs at the onset, frequently accompanied by vertigo.

To avoid confusion, only paralyses of the right eye are used as examples. In the figures, only the deficient eye movements are illustrated; all others are normal.

Right Lateral Rectus Paralysis (Fig. 7–35B): In the primary position, the optic axes may be parallel, or the right eye may converge slightly. The right eye cannot move laterally. The lateral rectus muscles are the most frequent site of isolated paralysis. The abducens nerve (CN VI) may be damaged by ischemia, inflammation or in infectious diseases, periostitis of the orbit, fracture of the petrous portion of the temporal bone, aneurysm of the carotid artery within the cavernous sinus, and lesions of the posterior pons near the midline.

Right Medial Rectus Paralysis (Fig. 7–35C): In the primary position, the right eye deviates laterally; it cannot move medially. The head is turned to the left to avoid diplopia.

Right Superior Rectus Paralysis (Fig. 7–35D): In the primary position, the right eye deviates downward; it cannot move upward to the right. The squint angle and the diplopia increase with fixation of the left eye upward to the right.

Right Inferior Rectus Paralysis (Fig. 7–35E): In the primary position, the right eye deviates upward; it cannot move down to the right. With the left eye

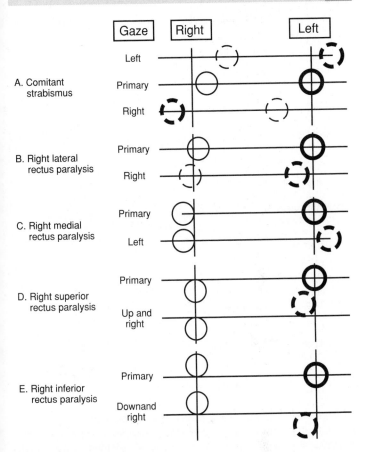

Fig. 7–35 *Strabismus (Squint).* This term refers to disorders in which the optic axes are not parallel. The diagrams illustrate positions of the patient's eyes as they appear to the observer. The unbroken circles connected by the unbroken lines show pairs in the primary position with the normal or fixing eye represented in heavier lines. Pairs with broken lines are in secondary positions with the heavier lines for the fixing eye. **A. Comitant strabismus:** the squint angle between the two optic axes is constant in all positions regardless of which eye fixates. **B. Right lateral rectus paralysis:** the right eye is unable to move laterally. **C. Right medial rectus paralysis:** right eye is lateral in the primary position; it fails to move medially. **D. Right superior rectus paralysis:** the right eye is slightly depressed in primary position and fails to move farther upward. **E. Right inferior rectus paralysis:** the right eye is elevated slightly in primary position; it cannot move downward.

fixed downward and to the right, the squint angle and the degree of diplopia increase.

Right Superior Oblique Paralysis (Fig. 7–36A): In the primary position, the right eye deviates upward; movement is limited down and to the left. The squint angle is increased when the left eye is fixed downward and to the left. Most

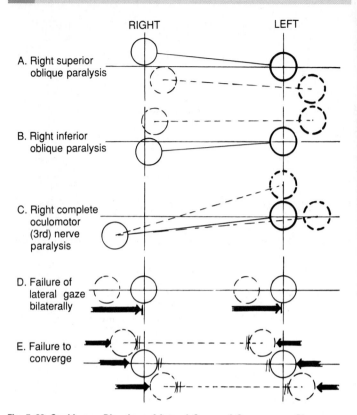

RIGHT   LEFT

A. Right superior oblique paralysis

B. Right inferior oblique paralysis

C. Right complete oculomotor (3rd) nerve paralysis

D. Failure of lateral gaze bilaterally

E. Failure to converge

Fig. 7–36 Strabismus: Disorders of Lateral Gaze and Convergence. Diagrams constructed as in Fig. 7–35. **A. Right superior oblique paralysis:** in primary position, right eye slightly elevated and can only be slightly depressed. **B. Right inferior oblique paralysis:** the right eye is slightly depressed in primary position; it can be elevated only slightly. **C. Right complete oculomotor nerve paralysis:** the right eye is fixed in depressed and lateral position. **D. Failure of lateral gaze:** both eyes cannot be moved beyond the median to the left or right, as the case may be. **E. Failure of convergence:** in no position can the two eyes converge.

characteristic is the tilt of the head toward the left shoulder to compensate for the pronounced extorsion (*ocular torticollis*). This position results in the normal intorsion of the left eye correcting the torsional diplopia. If the head is tilted to the right side, the right eye rotates upward.

Right Inferior Oblique Paralysis (Fig. 7–36B): In the primary position, the right eye deviates downward; its movement is limited upward and to the left. The squint angle increases when the left eye is fixed upward to the left.

Paralysis of Two or More Ocular Muscles: Only the oculomotor nerve (CN III) supplies more than a single muscle, so partial ophthalmoplegia only involves CN III. Unilateral total ophthalmoplegia is caused by involvement of all the nerves in the superior orbital fissure or the cavernous sinus; a bilateral lesion could result only from a focus in the base of the brain.

Varying Squint Angle—Complete Right Oculomotor (CN III) Nerve Paralysis (Fig. 7–36B): This produces paralysis of the levator, the superior, medial, and inferior recti, and the inferior oblique muscles and the pupillary sphincter. Only the superior oblique and the lateral rectus muscles are functioning. In the primary position, the right eye is deviated downward and outward to the right. Motion to the left and upward is absent. The squint angle and the degree of diplopia are increased when the left eye is fixed to the left. Ptosis is present from paralysis of the levator. The most frequent causes are an aneurysm in the circle of Willis and acute diabetic neuropathy; the latter usually spares the pupil.

> **KEY SIGN** **Internuclear Ophthalmoplegia**

Internuclear ophthalmoplegia is caused by lesions of the medial longitudinal fasciculus interconnecting the nuclei of CN III, IV and VI to coordinate conjugate eye movements. There is failure of adduction in horizontal lateral gaze, but convergence is normal. Common causes are multiple sclerosis or stroke.

> **KEY SIGN** **Conjugate Failure of Lateral Gaze**

A disturbance in the frontopontine pathway is the cause (Fig. 7–36D). When the lesion is on the right, there is constant conjugate deviation to the right; the patient turns the head to the left to fixate in front. The optic axes are parallel in all positions, so there is no diplopia. Neither eye can move to the left of the midline. In partial failure of lateral gaze, the patient can *will* the gaze to the left, but cannot fix it, so there is bilateral nystagmus to the left. **DDX:** This is distinguished from combined paralysis of the left lateral rectus and the right medial rectus by retention of convergence.

> **KEY SIGN** **Conjugate Failure of Vertical Gaze**

This is a supranuclear disorder thought to be in the rostral midbrain. The patient is unable to gaze upward as the eyes cannot move above the horizontal so the head tilts backward. There is no diplopia. When failure is incomplete, there is slight upward movement with upward nystagmus. Rarely, upward failure is combined with downward failure, or failure of downward gaze may be present alone. **DDX:** Bilateral paralyses of the superior recti and the inferior obliques (innervated by CN III) produce similar findings, but vertical gaze palsy is distinguished by retention of the normal *Bell phenomenon*: reflex elevation of the globes when the lids close. This reflex is mediated by fibers between the nuclei of CN III and CN VII in the medial longitudinal fasciculus; CN III supplies the superior rectus and the inferior oblique, CN VII serves the orbicularis. Persistence of the reflex proves the intactness of both nuclei, so the lesion must be supranuclear.

> **KEY SIGN** **Failure of Convergence**

A lesion in the frontopontine pathway is responsible. All movements are normal except convergence (Fig. 7–36E). Normal abduction of both globes to the right and left proves the medial recti to be normal.

KEY SYNDROME   Transient Weakness of Ocular Muscles—Myasthenia Gravis

See Chapter 14, page 759. **DDX:** Diplopia is important in distinguishing myasthenia from other ocular mobility disorders that also worsen with muscle fatigue.

KEY SIGN   Restriction of Motion

Movement of the globe may be restricted in all directions by orbital tumor or the increase in orbital contents with Graves' disease.

Visual Field Signs

KEY SIGN   Bilateral Visual Field Defects—Hemianopsia (Hemianopia)

Hemianopsi means half (hemi) is not seen (anopsia). By definition, hemianopsia involves nerves projecting from both eyes, thus it must be caused by a lesion in the optic chiasm, the optic tracts, or the brain. The optic nerves carry all the nerve fibers from the ipsilateral retina. At the optic chiasm the fibers from the nasal retinas cross the midline (decussate) joining the fibers of the lateral retina from the opposite side to form the optic tracts. The right optic tract carries all fibers to the right side of the brain, projecting the left visual field (Fig. 7–37). The left side of the brain receives the right nasal and left temporal retinal fibers, projecting the right visual field of each eye.

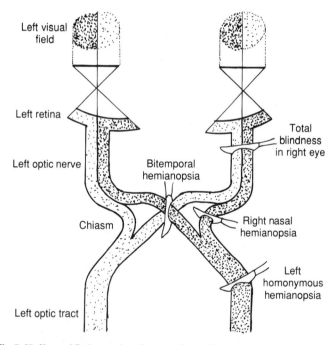

Fig. 7–37 Nneural Pathways from Retina to Brain. The cutting knives indicate points of lesions and the resulting visual defects.

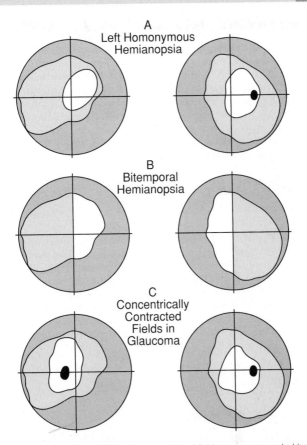

Fig. 7–38 *Pathologic Visual Fields.* *The normal visual field areas are gray and white in the blue background. Those areas obscured by pathologic conditions are gray, leaving white open areas that remain visible.*

Homonymous Hemianopsia: The same side of each *field* contains a defect (Fig. 7–38A). A left homonymous hemianopsia can be caused by a lesion in the right optic tract or the right side of the brain. With a tract lesion, the pupillary reflex is lost if light is only projected from the blind hemifield; the pupil reacts when the lesion is posterior to the geniculate body in the optic radiations or occipital lobe. Transient homonymous hemianopsia may occur with migraine.

Crossed Hemianopsia: Signals from both temporal or both nasal retinae are blocked, so the defect is *bitemporal or binasal.* A lesion of the decussating fibers in the chiasm causes *bitemporal hemianopsia* (Fig. 7–38B) by injuring the fibers from both nasal retinae, commonly a pituitary macroadenoma. *Binasal hemianopsia* is uncommon because it requires injury to both lateral halves of the optic nerves or tracts. When only a quadrant of each field is lost, it is termed *quadrantanopsia.*

> **KEY SIGN** **Monocular Field Defects—Optic Nerve or Retina**

Monocular visual field loss can occur from disease isolated to that eye. This would include disease of the retina or optic nerve. The optic nerve may be damaged to variable degrees from ischemia (giant cell arteritis, Anterior Ischemic Optic Neuropathy (AION), page 246), increased intraocular pressure (glaucoma), demyelinating disease (optic neuritis), trauma, and increased intracranial pressure. Destructive lesions of the retina also result in monocular field defects. Retinal ischemia from emboli, arteritis, or stenosis of the ipsilateral internal carotid artery may produce transient monocular blindness (amaurosis fugax). Retinal ischemia also results from ophthalmic artery or vein occlusion.

> **KEY SIGN** **Glaucoma**

See page 283ff.

Monocular Visual Loss—Amblyopia: Monocular loss of vision in an otherwise normal eye occurs in the first few years of life during visual development due to one of three causes: malalignment of the optic axes (strabismus), large differences in refractive error between the two eyes (anisometropia), or deprivation of vision in one eye which may result from bilateral severe refractive errors. Amblyopia causes preventable visual loss in approximately 3% of the population; early childhood screening, recognition, and treatment can help to prevent and in some cases restore visual acuity [Holmes JM, Clarke MP. Amblyopia. *Lancet.* 2006;367:1343–1351].

Conjunctiva Signs

> **KEY SIGN** **Subconjunctival Vessels**

The scleral vessels may be prominent in normal individuals. They run in from the sides (Fig. 7–39A).

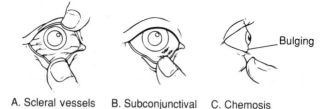

A. Scleral vessels   B. Subconjunctival   C. Chemosis
                         hemorrhage

Fig. 7–39 *Vascular Disorders of the External Eye. A. Scleral vessels:* These are the most prominebt vessels seen normally. *B. Subconjucatival hemorrhage:* Bright-red superficial blotches show through the sclera. They appear suddenly and painlessly. *C. Chemosis:* The conjuctival edima may be demonstrated by pressing the lower lid against the globe, producing a bulge in the boggy global conjunctiva above the point of compression.

KEY SIGN Subconjunctival Hemorrhage

Bleeding under the conjunctiva is obvious (Fig. 7–39B) and harmless. It may be induced by coughing, sneezing, weight lifting, or defecation; frequently, the cause is not apparent.

KEY SIGN Conjunctival Injection

Mild diffuse capillary hyperemia of the scleral and palpebral conjunctivae, without hemorrhage, is common in the coryza phase of respiratory infections or from exposure to direct sunlight or environmental irritants. It may be mildly uncomfortable. Significant pruritis, pain or discharge should suggests another disorder such as allergic conjuctivitis

KEY SIGN Conjunctival Edema—Chemosis

Usually associated with edema of the lids, the conjunctiva is swollen and transparent. The edema may be demonstrated by looking at the globe in profile while pressing the lower lid against the bulbar conjunctiva; the edge of the lid pushes up a wave of edematous bulbar conjunctiva (Fig. 7–39C). It is frequent in Graves' ophthalmopathy.

KEY SIGN Hyperemia of the Globe and Ciliary Flush

Bulbar conjunctival injection is dilation of the radial conjunctival vessels and their branches running from the fornices toward the center of the cornea (Fig. 7–40A). When the deeper, netlike episcleral vessels dilate they produce a more violaceous injection, particularly noted as ciliary flush at the corneal limbus (Fig. 7–40B). Suffusion in the conjunctiva blanches with pressure; the ciliary flush does not blanch. Ciliary flush indicates inflammation of the uveal tract (see page 283).

KEY SIGN Conjunctivitis

Inflammation of the conjunctiva, with or without infection, is conjunctivitis. The patient may complain of awakening with eyelids stuck shut and a gritty or burning sensation with excessive lacrimation. There is marked redness of

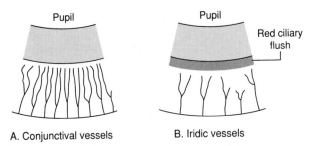

Fig. 7–40 Hyperemia and Congestion of the Globe. A. Hyperemic scleral vessels are superficial, coursing radially from the periphery to the limbus in tortuous branches. **B. Iritis:** the vessels of the iris are deeper; when congested, individual vessels are not visible, but they produce a pink or red band around the limbus, the ciliary flush.

the eye(s) from hyperemia of the palpebral and peripheral global conjunctival vessels. There are many causes; consider viral and bacterial infections, foreign-body reaction, allergies, and blepharitis. **DDX:** Awakening with the lids stuck together by purulent discharge increases the probability for bacterial infection; itching suggests a nonbacterial etiology.

KEY SIGN   Hyperemic Conjunctiva with Calcification

These lesions occur when the serum calcium-phosphorus product exceeds 70 in renal failure and sarcoidosis. *Conjunctival Lesions:* The segments from limbus to canthus at 7 to 10 o'clock and at 2 to 5 o'clock show hyperemic reddening, calcified plaques, and pingueculae. The eyes are painful or feel gritty. The affected areas contain calcium deposits, visible to the unaided eye or through the slit lamp. *Corneal Lesions:* These are called *band keratopathy*. White material is visible in the limbal arcs at 2 to 5 o'clock and 7 to 10 o'clock. The slit lamp reveals calcium deposits. It is in hypercalcemia and in renal disease with conjunctival calcification.

KEY SIGN   Pterygium

Chronic irritation from wind and dust is thought to stimulate the growth of the pinguecula, resulting in the extension of a vascular membrane over the limbus toward the center of the cornea, called a pterygium. This is a raised, subconjunctival fatty structure, growing in a horizontal band toward and over the pupil (Fig. 7–41A); vision may be obstructed. It has a firm attachment to the bulbar surface and is strictly in horizontal; it is usually bilateral. A *pseudopterygium* is a band of scar tissue that may extend in any direction and adhere only partially to the bulbar conjunctiva, so a probe may be passed beneath it.

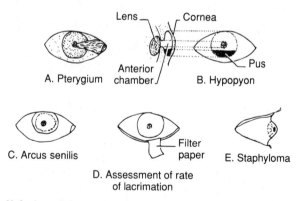

Fig. 7–41 *Lesions of the Cornea and Iris. A. Pterygium:* *this abnormal growth of the pinguecula appears as a raised, subconjunctival fatty structure, growing in a horizontal band toward a position over the pupil. **B. Hypopyon:** a collection of pus in the lowest part of the anterior chamber between the cornea and the iris. **C. Arcus senilis:** a gray, opaque, circular band in the cornea, separated from the limbus by a narrow, clear zone. **D. Assessment of lacrimation:** the schirmer test, see page 203. **E. Staphyloma:** anterior protrusion of the cornea or sclera.*

Pigmented Pingueculae: Brownish pigmentation of the pingueculae is as one of the few signs of Gaucher disease; others are hepatosplenomegaly, thrombocytopenic purpura, and patchy brown pigmentation on the face and legs.

Cornea Signs

> ### KEY SIGN   Hypopyon

Inflammation in the iris or anterior chamber produces a purulent discharge in the anterior chamber. The opaque fluid settles to the dependent portion of the chamber where it is seen as a fluid level behind the cornea (Fig. 7–41B). Iritis is a common cause.

> ### KEY SIGN   Lusterless Cornea—Superficial Keratitis

Corneal inflammation or drying causes epithelial loss. There is loss of the normal corneal luster with grayness of the anterior stroma. A ciliary flush is often present. Fluorescein staining demonstrates ulceration or denuded epithelium. A corneal ulcer is extremely painful and causes miosis and photophobia. *Disruption of the epithelium demands urgent expert therapy, because visual loss can occur rapidly.* **CLINICAL OCCURRENCE:**   There are many causes of superficial keratitis including contact lens-related ulcers, infected abrasions, herpes simplex and zoster, corneal exposure, trigeminal nerve (CN V) injury, amiodarone deposits and spread of infection from the conjunctiva.

Cloudy Cornea—Interstitial Keratitis: The prototype is congenital syphilis, in which interstitial keratitis, deafness, and notched teeth constitute the **Hutchinson triad.** During the early stages of inflammation, between ages 5 and 15 years, a faint opacity begins in the central zone of the cornea together with a faint ciliary flush. Usually, pain and lacrimation occur as well. Later, the cornea becomes diffusely clouded, so the iris may be obscured. Blood vessels grow into the cornea. After the acute stage, there is more or less permanent corneal opacity. Acquired syphilis and tuberculosis occasionally cause this lesion.

> ### KEY SIGN   Arcus Senilis

A gray opaque band in the cornea, 1.0- to 1.5-mm wide, is separated from the limbus by a narrow clear zone (Fig. 7–41C). Early on only a segment of the circumference is involved; later the circle is completed. It is present to some degree in most persons older than 60 years of age; it is bilateral. If seen before age 40, hyperlipidemia should be suspected.

> ### KEY SIGN   Keratoconjunctivitis Sicca—Sjögren Syndrome

Lymphocytic infiltration of exocrine glands (lacrimal and salivary) reduces tear flow producing dry inflamed eyes. Sjögren syndrome is likely if persistent dry eyes, dry mouth, and a positive Schirmer test (page 282 and Fig. 7–41D) are present without obvious cause. Similar findings can be seen with HIV infection and sarcoidosis.

> **KEY SIGN** **Kayser-Fleischer Ring—Wilson Disease**

A 2-mm wide golden-brown circular band is seen in the peripheral cornea near the limbus. The ring is formed by copper deposited in Descemet's membrane, the basement membrane of the cornea endothelium. This deposit begins superiorly, spreads inferiorly; it accompanies the neurologic manifestations of Wilson disease. A slit lamp and gonioscopy are often required to see the ring.

Central Corneal Opacity: This results from trauma or infection and is seen in 75% of patients with Hurler syndrome.

Dots in the Cornea—Fanconi Syndrome: Cystine crystals are deposited throughout the stroma with no accompanying inflammatory reaction.

Sclera Signs

> **KEY SIGN** **Yellow Sclera—Icterus and Fat**

In obstructive jaundice (page 470), conjugated bilirubin infiltrates all body tissues and fluids; it colors the sclera evenly. The conjunctiva of the fornices is usually a deeper yellow because it is thicker. Deposits of fat beneath the conjunctiva commonly impart a yellow color to the periphery, leaving the perilimbal area relatively white. It is more obvious with advancing age and in patients with anemia.

> **KEY SIGN** **Red Sclera—Scleritis and Episcleritis**

Inflammation of the sclera and/or Tenon capsule can produce loss of scleral integrity. *Scleritis* may be diffuse or nodular and frequently associated with autoimmune diseases. The patient will have severe, deep, boring pain. In sunlight, the lesion will have a violaceous, red-purple appearance. Suppurative scleritis is rare and usually metastatic. Tuberculosis, sarcoidosis, and syphilis cause a granulomatous scleritis with localized scleral elevation and nodule formation. Scleral thinning may be nonnecrotizing (*scleromalacia perforans*) or necrotizing with acute inflammation surrounding an area of ischemia which may ulcerate. *Episcleritis* is a much milder form of inflammation involving Tenon capsule, and appears clinically as a diffuse or nodular violaceous injection (Plate 14).

Blue Sclera—Osteogenesis Imperfecta: Light reflecting off the pigmented choroid appears blue through the thinned sclera. This finding is classic for osteogenesis imperfecta; it may be mimicked by minocycline deposits, scleral thinning after scleritis, or age related calcification of the horizontal rectus muscle insertions.

Brown Sclera—Melanin or Homogentisic Acid: Patches of melanin are commonly seen on the conjunctiva of dark complexioned people, especially blacks. In alkaptonuria with ochronosis wedge-shaped areas of brown homogentisic acid color the sclera near the attachments of the ocular muscles extending their apices toward the limbus.

Scleral Protrusion—Staphyloma: Scleral injury or increased intraocular pressure leads to a protrusion from the surface of the globe. An anterior staphyloma forms near the cornea creating a characteristic profile (Fig. 7–41E); a posterior staphyloma cannot be seen.

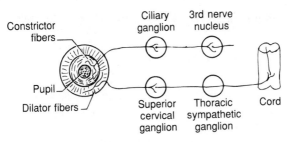

Fig. 7–42 *Innervation of the Pupillary Muscles.*

Pupil Signs

> **KEY SIGN   Normal Pupillary Reaction**

The sphincter contracts the pupil through parasympathetic stimulation; the dilator widens the pupil by sympathetic stimuli. The sphincter pupillae is a circular muscle embedded in the iris near the pupillary margin. It is innervated by parasympathetic fibers from the Edinger-Westphal nucleus near the oculomotor nerve (CN III) nucleus (Fig. 7–42). The fibers enter the orbit in the third nerve and accompany its motor branch to the inferior oblique muscle, whence the parasympathetic fibers synapse in the ciliary ganglion; from there, other fibers enter the eye through the short ciliary nerves. The dilator pupillae is arranged radially in the peripheral two-thirds of the iris. It receives sympathetic fibers arising in the cortex, descending to the hypothalamus and ciliospinal center; postsynaptic fibers go to the cervical sympathetic chain and ascend to the superior cervical ganglion. They synapse with third-order neurons that run to the carotid plexus, and then to the first division of the trigeminal nerve (CN V) into the eye. Pupillary size fluctuates from changes in tone. Exaggerated wavering is termed *hippus*, or *physiologic pupillary unrest*; it is of little clinical significance. *Mydriasis* is dilatation; miosis is pupillary constriction. Bright light causes constriction, accompanied by a consensual reaction in the unexposed eye. In older persons, the pupils may react sluggishly to light; the reaction is hastened after several stimulations. Near point miosis, associated with lens accommodation, occurs when the eye is fixed on a near object. The pupils of patients with Cheyne-Stokes respirations may dilate during the phase of hyperventilation and constrict with apnea.

> **KEY SIGN   Unequal Pupils—Anisocoria**

Unequal pupils occur from either constriction or dilation of one pupil. Anisocoria is often unimportant, and beware the artificial eye. To determine whether one pupil is too small or the other too large, measure them in bright and dim light. If one pupil cannot contract the discrepancy is exaggerated in bright light. If one pupil cannot dilate, the difference is greater in darkness. *Physiologic anisocoria* is a normal finding in twenty percent of patients; it manifests as a constant difference in pupillary diameter in light and dark.   ***CLINICAL OCCURRENCE:***   Miosis of one pupil with a large size disparity suggests damage to the sympathetic nerves (Horner Syndrome), iris sphincter inflammation (iritis), or use of a miotic drug (e.g., pilocarpine). Dilatation of one pupil can result from parasympathetic nerve damage (CN III paralysis from posterior communicating artery aneurysm), iris ischemia from acute, severe increase in intraocular pressure (angle closure glaucoma), damage to the ciliary ganglion (Adie's tonic pupil), or a mydriatic drug (e.g., atropine), An artificial eye will be painted with a pupil midway between constricted and dilated so will also manifest anisocoria.

KEY SIGN   Relative Afferent Pupillary Defect (Marcus-Gunn Pupil)

There is an asymmetric decrease in light detection by the retina or in signal transmission through the optic nerve and tract to the geniculate ganglia and Edinger-Westphal nuclei. Both pupils constrict less when light is directed into the pupil or the affected eye than when light is directed into the unaffected eye as detected by the swinging light test (page 202).

KEY SIGN   Argyll Robertson Pupil

There is no agreement on the site of the lesion in the nervous system. The classic signs are severely miotic pupils with weak or absent contraction to light that do not improve with dark adaptation, but have normal or exaggerated contraction to near point ("accommodation"). The pupils may be irregular and unequal pupils in size. The fully developed Argyll Robertson pupil is almost pathognomonic of tabes dorsalis or taboparesis.

KEY SIGN   Tonic Pupil (Adie Pupil)

Adie's tonic pupil is in the differential diagnosis of anisocoria due to a dilated pupil. The reaction to light and near focus are present but extremely sluggish and have a prolonged latent period prior to onset of constriction. The response to light may be absent, with a full but tonic response to near point focus. Classically there are sectoral or vermiform movements of both the pupillary border and the related sector of iris stroma, demonstrating the partial parasympathetic denervation of the pupil. It is usually unilateral, but may be bilateral. **DDX:** Tonic pupil is most frequently encountered in young women with normal-sized pupils, in contrast to the requisite miosis in the Argyll Robertson pupil; whatever the degree of reaction in the Argyll Robertson pupil, its reaction is prompt.

KEY SIGN   Unreactive Pupil—Pupillary Paralysis (Internal Ophthalmoplegia)

The pupil lacks the ability to constrict from either light or accommodation. It is generally dilated, never miotic. *CLINICAL OCCURRENCE:*   Topical mydriatics are most common; less-common causes are syphilitic meningitis, vasculitis, viral encephalitis, diphtheria or tetanus toxin, lead poisoning, midbrain lesions, bilateral CN III lesions, Adie pupils, iris dysfunction from trauma, and systemic anticholinergic medications (e.g., scopolamine patches, benztropine mesylate).

KEY SIGN   Unilateral Miosis—Horner Syndrome

This is caused by a lesion of the sympathetic pathway. In the complete syndrome it is accompanied by ptosis and anhydrosis on the affected side. See Chapter 14, page 763.

Lens Signs

> **KEY SIGN   Cataract**

Discoloration or disruption of the layers of the lens produce focal or diffuse opacities that can obstruct and/or scatter light before it reaches the retina. Because nearly all adults have some opacity of the lenses, a clinical definition of cataract implies interference with vision [Asbell PA, Dualan I, Mindel J, et al. Age-related cataract. *Lancet*. 2005;365:599–609]. Some cataracts are seen by shining a light beam obliquely through the lens (*focal illumination*), by ophthalmoscopic inspection against the red retinal reflex with 0 diopter magnification from approximately 40 cm (15.7 in), or by using +10 diopter magnification with close inspection (*direct illumination*). Many can only be identified with the slit lamp. Centrally placed cataracts can be seen without pupillary dilatation; those in the periphery are only visualized with dilation. *This discussion is limited to cataracts detectable without mydriatics or the slit lamp.*

Anterior and Posterior Polar Cataract. A small congenital white plaque can be seen in the center of the pupil. It results from a congenital defect in the anterior or posterior capsule.

Nuclear Cataract. Diffuse yellow to brown discoloration occurs first in the central portion of the lens then gradually becomes diffuse discoloration throughout the lens. There is a black spot centrally against the red retinal reflex.

Cortical Cataract. Wedge-shaped anterior or posterior cortical opacities, arranged radially and extending in from the periphery, appear gray with the penlight and black against the red retinal reflex (Plate 16).

Secondary Cataract. Fibrosis of the posterior capsule is a common occurrence after cataract surgery as the peripheral lens epithelial cells migrate across the capsular bag left to support the intraocular lens implant. "Secondary Cataract" is more correctly known as an opacified posterior capsule. It appears as dense folds of tissue and clusters of clear vesicles.

Diabetic Cataract. Older diabetic patients have an increased tendency to develop nuclear or cortical cataracts with no distinctive character. Juvenile diabetic patients acquire a distinctive snowflake cataract containing chalky white deposits; the entire lens subsequently becomes milky.

Posterior Subcapsular Cataract. This lesion is commonly seen after long-term use of corticosteroids, with diabetes, and after trauma or uveitis (Plate 17).

> **KEY SIGN   Lens Subluxation and Dislocation**

Rupture of the zonula ciliaris (zonule of Zinn) permits the lens to move from its fixed position behind the pupil. Slight displacement, with the lens still backing the pupillary aperture, is termed *subluxation* (Fig. 7–43A); it is manifest by tremulousness of the iris (*iridodonesis*), when the eye moves horizontally. Viewed through the ophthalmoscope, the equator of the lens may show as a dark, curved line crossing the pupillary aperture; a double image of the retina with different

A. Subluxation   B. Dislocation

Fig. 7–43 *Displacement of the Lens. A. Subluxation. B. Anterior chamber dislocation.*

magnifications may be seen, one through the lens, the other without the lens. When the lens is displaced completely it is a dislocation; when it enters the anterior chamber (Fig. 7–43B), it is easily seen. Lenticular displacement is usually caused by trauma. Nontraumatic dislocation occurs in several hereditary conditions including Marfan disease, homocystinuria and hereditary spherophakia.

> **KEY SIGN**   **Intraocular Pressure Changes**

Increased tension occurs in glaucoma; decreased tension is seen with myotonic dystrophy, globe rupture and extreme dehydration. Accurate assessment is made by measurement of pressure with the tonometer.

Retina Signs

The following article provides a good review of retinal diseases with pathophysiology and photographs of many retinal signs [D'Amico DJ. Diseases of the retina. *N Engl J Med.* 1994;331:95–106].

> **KEY SIGN**   **Increased Cup-to-Disk Ratio—Glaucoma**

See page 283, and Plate 17.

> **KEY SIGN**   **Myelinated Nerve Fibers**

Myelination of the optic nerve fibers usually ends at the lamina cribrosa; infrequently myelin sheaths are maintained into the retinal nerve fiber layer (Fig. 7–44B). Semi-opaque white patches emerge from the optic disk spreading into one or two retinal quadrants. The disk margin appears frayed and the underlying vessels are partially or completely obscured. It may appear to be a serious lesion, but it is a normal variation of no clinical significance. Patches of myelinated nerves may occur remote from the disc.

> **KEY SIGN**   **Disk Pallor—Optic Atrophy**

Damage to the optic nerve (compression, ischemia, inflammation, or increased intracranial pressure) leads to atrophy of the nerve fibers and loss of normal vascularity (Fig. 7–44C and Plate 18). The disk is pale pink, yellow, or white, the margins may be less distinct and the physiologic cup and lamina cribrosa are variably seen. The emerging vessels may be surrounded by perivascular glial sheathing, seen as white lines. **DDX:** Pigmented high water marks around the nerve or residual exudate in the peripapillary retina may indicate previous disc edema, suggesting increased intracranial pressure producing the optic atrophy. It is important to recognize that an atrophic nerve can no longer swell, so cannot be used to monitor the presence of papilledema. A common cause of incidentally found optic atrophy is brain tumor, thus all optic atrophy should be evaluated promptly by an ophthalmologist. In optic atrophy from chorioretinitis, the disk may have a yellow cast, and the surrounding retina may contain hemorrhages, areas of atrophy, and pigment. The distinction between optic atrophy resulting from intrinsic optic nerve lesions versus increased intracranial pressure cannot be made reliably by the physical findings; interestingly, disc pallor does not occur in glaucoma until very late in its course. *CLINICAL OCCURRENCE:*   Intrinsic optic nerve lesions: multiple sclerosis, syphilis; increased intracranial pressure:

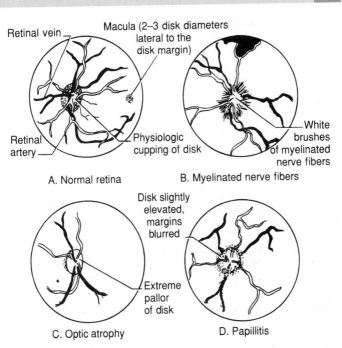

Fig. 7–44 *Retinal Abnormalities I. A. Normal left retina:* the background of the retina is red-orange; it contains a variable amount of black pigments, depending on race and complexion. Diverging blood vessels emerge from the optic disk to spread over the retina, usually in pairs of an artery and a vein. The veins are solid and dark red, and they may pulsate normally. The arteries are brighter red, contain central white stripes, and are pulseless. The width of an artery is usually approximately four-fifths that of the adjacent vein. The optic disk is lighter red, with sharp borders, often outlined by a strip of black pigment in the adjacent retina. The physiologic cup is white or pale yellow. The macula lies in the horizontal plane of the disk and from 2 to 3 disk diameters to the temporal side. The macular area is pale red with a central white or shining dot. *B. Myelinated nerve fibers:* white brushes of myelinated nerves emerge from the disk, obscuring segments of vessels and disk margins. *C. Optic atrophy:* the disk is chalk-white with sharply defined borders. The blood vessels are normal. *D. Papillitis:* the disk is hyperemic and its borders are blurred.

idiopathic intracranial hypertension, brain tumors; optic nerve compression without increased intracranial pressure.

> **KEY SIGN   Disk Edema—Papillitis, Optic Neuritis**

When optic neuritis involves the portion of the optic nerve within the globe, papillitis, with loss of vision, is produced (Fig. 7–26D) with disk edema indistinguishable from papilledema. Visual loss occurs early in optic neuritis and usually later with papilledema. The disk is hyperemic and its margins may be indistinct from edema in the peripapillary nerve fiber layer. The disk surface may be elevated above the surrounding retina (a + 1 or + 2 lens correction is required to focus on the disk) [Balcer LJ. Optic neuritis. *N Engl J Med.* 2006;354:1273–1280]. **CLINICAL OCCURRENCE:** ocular inflammation (e.g., uveitis, retinitis, sympathetic ophthalmia), intrinsic inflammation of the optic nerve (e.g., demyelinating optic neuritis in multiple sclerosis), intracranial inflammation (e.g., meningitis, venous sinus thrombosis), infections (e.g., syphilis, tuberculosis, influenza, measles, malaria, mumps), and intoxications (e.g., methyl alcohol).

► **KEY SYNDROME** Anterior Ischemic Optic Neuropathy (AION)

Infarction of the optic nerve head results from inadequate perfusion of the posterior ciliary arteries. AION occurs in two forms, the arteritic, related to giant cell arteritis, and the nonarteritic, which occurs in patients with vasculopathies such as hypertension or diabetes mellitus and intercurrent hypotension. The onset is usually sudden and painless, with profound visual loss, typically altitudinal, involving the upper and lower field. The optic nerve appears edematous, with scant hemorrhage and more pallor than typical for papilledema. **DDX:** In a patient of age >55 years, it is imperative to search for giant cell arteritis. The nonarteritic form is commonly accompanied by a small to absent optic cup in the uninvolved eye and often a period of systemic hypotension.

► **KEY SIGN** Papilledema

Increased intracranial pressure causes the cerebrospinal fluid (CSF) to compress the optic nerve within its sheath resulting in axoplasmic flow stasis and ischemia (Fig. 7–45A). Early papilledema causes a C-shaped halo of nerve fiber layer edema that surrounds the disc with a gap temporally (Plate 19). With more advanced papilledema, the halo becomes circumferential; next there is obscuration of major vessels as they leave the disc; and later there is obscuration of vessels on the optic disc. The emerging vessels bend sharply in passing over the elevated disk edge (Plate 20). Macular retinal edema creates traction folds (*choroidal folds*), seen as white lines radiating from the macula (Fig. 7–45B). Patients with papilledema

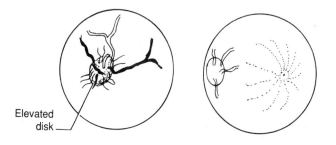

Elevated disk —

A. Papilledema, choked disk   B. Star figure of macula

Fig. 7–45 *Rretinal Abnormalities II. A. Papilledema (choked disk):* the disk surface is elevated, the nasal borders blurred. The vessels curve downward over the borders. The veins are distended and pulseless. Both arteries and veins in the disk may be obscured by the swollen structure. *B. Star figure of the macula:* edema throws the retina into traction folds that radiate from the macula as white lines.

will have an enlarged physiologic blind spot documented with formal visual field testing. **DDX:** In contrast to papillitis, central vision is unimpaired, but, like glaucoma, there is usually peripheral visual loss. ***CLINICAL OCCURRENCE:*** The principal causes are brain tumor, and idiopathic intracranial hypertension. Less common causes are hydrocephalus, malignant hypertension, subarachnoid hemorrhage, meningitis, and salicylate poisoning.

> **KEY SIGN   Pseudopapilledema—Drusen Bodies**

These are granular deposits in the optic disk that cause pseudopapilledema. The distinctions between early papilledema and drusen bodies are reported as follows: drusen cause obvious irregular, lumpy, bumpy elevation of the disk; drusen are pink or yellow, the surface of papilledema is hyperemic; drusen cause the nerve fiber layer to glisten and often show a halo of feathery reflections, whereas the layer in papilledema is dull; drusen are in the disk center; in papilledema, the vessels show absence of venous pulsation and the light reflexes are dulled; drusen make the disk outline irregular and are more frequent in small, hypermetropic eyes.

> **KEY SIGN   Venous Engorgement**

Distention of the retinal veins suggests retinal vein occlusion, polycythemia vera, cyanotic congenital heart disease, leukemia, and macroglobulinemia.

> **KEY SIGN   Retinal Hemorrhage**

Hemorrhage may occur in any layer of the retina. The shape of the hemorrhage frequently reveals its depth. A large, deep hemorrhage in the choriocapillaris produces a dark, elevated area that looks like a melanotic tumor (Fig. 7–46A); you should suspect a *subretinal vascular membrane* seen in association with macular degeneration. A smaller, more superficial hemorrhage appears as a round red spot, with blurred margins, called a *blot hemorrhage* (Fig. 7–46B). *Microaneurysms* are also round red spots, but their borders are sharp, they are not reabsorbed like hemorrhages, and they may occur in clusters about vascular sprigs (Fig. 7–46C). *Flame-shaped hemorrhages* occur in the nerve fiber layer of the retina; they are

A. Deep retinal hemorrhage   B. blot hemorrhages   C. retinal microaneurysms

   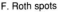

D. Flame hemorrhages   E. Subhyaloid hemorrhages   F. Roth spots

Fig. 7–46 *Hemorrhages and Similar Lesions in the Retina.*

red and striated (Fig. 7–46D and Plate 23). In the *subhyaloid or preretinal hemorrhage,* a pool of blood accumulates between the retina and the hyaloid membrane forming a boat-shaped hemorrhage appearing as a turned-up half-moon; the straight upper border is a fluid level (Fig. 7–46E). A small hemorrhagic spot with a central white area is called a *Roth spot,* (Fig. 7–46F) classically seen in subacute bacterial endocarditis and leukemia. **CLINICAL OCCURRENCE:** Many conditions produce retinal hemorrhages, examples are hypertension, diabetes mellitus, papilledema, retinal vein occlusion, SBE, HIV, SLE, Takayasu arteritis, macroglobulinemia, thiamine deficiency, leukemia, polycythemia, sickle cell disease and sarcoidosis.

Diabetic Retinopathy: Diabetic retinopathy often leads to blindness from damage to the macular region. Microaneurysms occurring around the macula need to be distinguished from blot hemorrhages. With advanced diabetic retinopathy there are white or yellow waxy exudates having distinct, often serrated, borders (Plate 24). The exudates gradually coalesce to form a broken circle around the macula. *Neovascularization* of the disk or neovascularization elsewhere in the retina is an ominous sign requiring laser phototherapy (Plates 25 and 26). The signs of atherosclerosis and hypertension are sometimes superimposed [Frank RN. Diabetic retinopathy. *N Engl J Med.* 2004;350: 48–58]. **DDX:** Although microaneurysms around the macula are characteristic of diabetes, retinal microvasculopathy with cotton-wool spots, intraretinal hemorrhages, and microaneurysms occurs in radiation retinopathy and in some patients with HIV-AIDS.

➤ **KEY SIGN**   **Arterial Occlusion**

Sudden loss of vision occurs when the central retinal artery is occluded, usually from thrombosis or embolism. Early the retina is very pale from ischemic edema; the arteries are extremely narrowed, and the smaller ones are invisible (Fig. 7–47A and Pate 21). Although the veins are full, they are pulseless. The lack of circulation

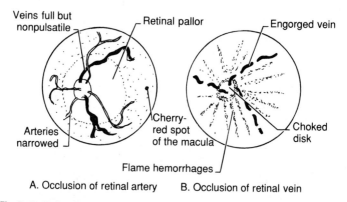

A. Occlusion of retinal artery   B. Occlusion of retinal vein

Fig. 7–47 *Retinal Vascular Occlusions. A. Retinal artery occlusion:* the retinal background is white and the arteries are much narrowed. The veins are pulseless. ***B. Retinal vein occlusion:*** the affected veins are engorged and tortuous. Hemorrhages occur near the veins.

is demonstrated by the absence of induced pulsation in either artery or vein with pressure on the eyeball. Retinal edema initially causes macular pallor that is less dense over the fovea due to an anatomical lack of the nerve fiber layer at this location. The fovea appears as a *cherry red spot* due to visualization of the choroidal blood flow within the macular edema; this finding will disappear as the edema resolves over weeks. Occlusion of a branch artery causes findings limited to its distribution area. ***CLINICAL OCCURRENCE:*** Common causes are vascular disease, cardiac valve disease or vegetations, rheumatic fever, and vasculitis, most commonly temporal arteritis. Rarely, it is a complication of SLE, sickle cell disease, cryoglobulinemia, syphilis or thromboangiitis obliterans.

> **KEY SIGN** **Venous Occlusion**

Central retinal vein thrombosis is followed by engorgement and tortuosity of all visible veins (Fig. 7–47B). Significant nerve fiber layer and blot hemorrhages appear throughout the retina. Edema of the macula and disk is commonly present. Occlusion of a branch of the central vein produces findings limited to its drainage area. ***CLINICAL OCCURRENCE:*** Venous occlusive disease is most associated with hypertension, as the stiffened arterioles will compress the more compliant retinal veins as they cross in their common sheath. Hypercoagulable states can also cause venous occlusion from sluggish blood flow, and can be seen in polycythemia, multiple myeloma, macroglobulinemia, and leukemia. In sickle cell disease, multiple venous thromboses may be accompanied by neovascularization.

> **KEY SIGN** **Arteriolar Sclerosis**

The retinal changes do not necessarily parallel atherosclerotic disease elsewhere in the body.

Arterial Stripe. Normal retinal arteries show a central bright stripe from light reflecting off the curved blood column. Increases in mural thickness cause widening of the stripe and brightening of the reflex. In moderate disease, the walls look like burnished copper (copper-wire reflex); in advanced disease, the entire width of the artery reflects as a white stripe (silver-wire reflex).

Vessel Sheaths. Normal vessel walls are invisible. Mural thickening with lipid infiltration produces a milky white streak on either side of the blood column called pipestem sheathing.

Arteriovenous Crossings. As the arterial and arteriolar walls become denser and less compliant arteriovenous crossing signs are produced (Fig. 7–48A). Arteriovenous nicking (Fig. 7–48B) occurs when the thickened arterial sheath obscures a short segment of the more compliant vein, seen as a notch on either side of the artery at their crossing. *Deviation of the vein is* produced when the stiffened artery causes the vein to assume a 90 degrees crossing angle (Fig. 7–48C), the normal angle is acute). When an overlying vein is elevated by the thickened artery, it is called *humping* (Fig. 7–48D). *Tapering of the veins* results if the artery compresses the vein (Fig. 7–48E). When venous flow is partially obstructed, the vein dilates upstream from the artery, called *banking* (Fig. 7–48F), which may induce a retinal vein occlusion.

The degree of involvement of the retinal vessels by the arteriolar sclerotic process has been variously scored. Table 7–2 represents the Kirkendall and Armstrong modification of the Scheie classification.

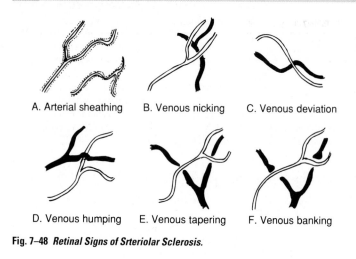

A. Arterial sheathing   B. Venous nicking   C. Venous deviation

D. Venous humping   E. Venous tapering   F. Venous banking

Fig. 7–48 *Retinal Signs of Srteriolar Sclerosis.*

> **KEY SIGN** **Hypertensive Retinopathy**

Arterial hypertension produces distinctive retinal signs that often coexist with the signs of arteriolar sclerosis (Plates 22 and 23). For example, the appearance of a retina may be classified as "grade 3 arteriolosclerosis, grade 4 hypertension." The signs attributed to hypertension may also be graded by using the classification of Kirkendall and Armstrong (Table 7–3) [Wong, T, Mitchell P. The eye in hypertension. *Lancet.* 2007;369:425–435]. Most ophthalmologists will simply describe the retinal and vascular finding without the use of these grading scales.

> **KEY SIGN** **Retinal Spots**

Many different disease and pathogenic process leave there marks in the retina: scars, deposits, pigmentation, etc. In addition, active retinal disease and systemic diseases with retinal manifestations can appear as unifocal or multifocal spots against the normal retina. Careful retinal examination of patients with confusing

Table 7–2 **Grades of Retinal Arteriolar Sclerosis**

Grade 1	Thickening of vessels with slight depression of veins at arteriolar-venular (AV) crossings.
Grade 2	Definitive AV crossing changes and moderate local sclerosis.
Grade 3	Venule beneath the arteriole is invisible; severe local sclerosis and segmentation.
Grade 4	To the preceding signs are added venous obstruction and arteriolar obliteration.

Kirkendall WM, Armstrong ML. Vascular changes in the eye of the treated and untreated patient with hypertension. *Am J Cardiol.* 1962;9:663.

Table 7–3   Grades of Retinal Hypertension

	Signs
Grade 1	Narrowing in terminal branches of vessels.
Grade 2	General narrowing of vessels with severe local constriction.
Grade 3	To the preceding signs are added striate hemorrhages and soft exudates.
Grade 4	Papilledema is added to the preceding signs.

systemic disease may assist in diagnosis. The clinician's first task is to distinguish active disease from the tracks of past events.

Cholesterol Emboli: Ulcerated atherosclerotic plaque in the aorta or carotid artery shed cholesterol crystals that become lodged at the bifurcations of retinal vessels. Patients may be asymptomatic or present with transient monocular visual loss, amaurosis fugax, or transient ischemic neurologic attacks (TIA) in a carotid distribution. Finding cholesterol emboli proves plaque rupture with embolization. It is difficult, if not impossible, to differentiate cholesterol emboli from calcific emboli from diseased heart valves.

Cotton-Wool Patches: Thickening and swelling of the terminal retinal nerve fibers results from ischemic infarcts. Gray to white areas with ill-defined fluffy borders occur within the posterior pole of the retina (Plate 22). They are often accompanied by microaneurysms that may rupture producing small striate hemorrhages known as flame hemorrhages. ***CLINICAL OCCURRENCE:*** Hypertension, diabetes, SLE, HIV, central retinal vein occlusion, papilledema.

Hard Exudates: This is lipid deposition from leaking capillaries left behind as a high water mark after the retinal pigment epithelium resorbs the associated serous fluid. Distinct from the superficial cotton-wool patches, these are small white spots with sharply defined edges. They are deeper than the superficial retinal vessels.

Pigmented Spots: Old inflammation or scarring may appear as a pigmented region of the retina.

Talc Deposits: White or yellow spots are seen in the retinae of intravenous drug users who have injected ground-up tablets containing talc.

▶ **Cytomegalovirus (Cmv) Retinitis:** Advanced immunosuppression from HIV infection is frequently accompanied by cytomegalovirus infection of the retina. Patients describe visual loss, blurring, floaters, and flashes of light. Look for whitening of the retina, cotton-wool spots, and intraretinal hemorrhages. Although less common, consider varicella zoster infection, toxoplasmosis, and syphilis [ET Cunningham, TP Margolis. Ocular manifestations of HIV infection. *N Engl J Med.* 1998;339:236–244]. CMV retinitis has become less common with the advent of highly active antiviral therapy.

▶ ***Candida* Endophthalmitis:** Systemic Candida infection associated with immunosuppression and indwelling venous catheters can be difficult to diagnose. Patients have fever, but blood cultures are often negative. Small white patches on the retina may be the only sign of disease. With advancing disease, there is pain, visual disturbance and large white globular lesions invading the vitreous are seen.

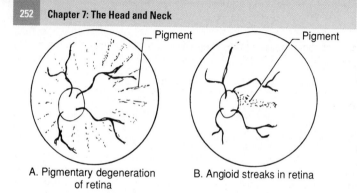

A. Pigmentary degeneration   B. Angioid streaks in retina
of retina

Fig. 7–49 *Retinal Pigmentation.*

Macular Degeneration: Although vision is much reduced, the only visible sign may be a few spots of pigment near the macula and blurring of the macular borders. In other cases, subretinal hemorrhages, patches of retinal atrophy, yellow drusen, and pigmented areas may be seen.

Retinitis Pigmentosa: Inherited singly or as a component of several syndromes, retinitis pigmentosa is manifest by arteriolar narrowing, waxy pallor of the optic disc, and perivascular retinal pigmentation. Night blindness is the earliest symptom; later, all types of vision are greatly impaired as the retinal degeneration progresses from the periphery to the posterior retina. Spidery strands of pigmented spots form a girdle about the global equator (Fig. 7–49A).

Angioid Streaks: These probably represent elastic tissue degeneration. Broad lines of pigment radiate from the optic disk, branching like blood vessels (Fig. 7–49B). They occur in Paget disease and in pseudoxanthoma elasticum.

> **KEY SIGN** **Retinal Detachment**

Retinal detachments may be symptomatic or asymptomatic. Patients complain of flashing lights followed by floaters and then a curtain crossing their vision. The earliest sign is elevation of a retinal area so that it is out of focus with the surrounding structures. The arteries and veins in the separated membrane appear elevated (Fig. 7–50). When widely separated, the retinal sheet is gray and frequently folded. Underlying inflammation may produce

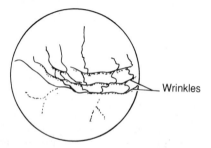

Wrinkles

Fig. 7–50 *Retinal Detachment.*

areas of choroiditis and vitreous opacities. A torn edge may be encountered, often shaped like a horseshoe. The cause of detachment is often undetermined (idiopathic).

Nose and Sinus Signs

> **KEY SIGN** **Epistaxis (Nosebleed)**

In the anterior nose, the most common site of bleeding is Kiesselbach plexus, a vascular network in the anterior nasal septum. Posteriorly, hemorrhage occurs frequently at the back third of the inferior meatus; vessels in the region are large and belong to the external carotid artery system. In some cases, there are multiple oozing points in the mucosa. Nosebleed can be a spontaneous and trivial occurrence or a sign of serious local or generalized disease. Hemorrhage from the external nares is obvious, but bleeding from the choana must be distinguished from hemoptysis and even hematemesis. The first problem is to ascertain the bleeding site and judge whether trauma or some predisposing disease is present. Inquire about trauma, predisposing local or systemic disease, and the amount of blood lost. Seat the patient in a chair and seat yourself in front of the patient. Observe universal precautions: use gloves, gown, and face protection to avoid blood contamination. Remove the clots by suction or have the patient clear the nose by blowing. Inspect the anterior nasal chambers, especially the septum. If hemorrhage is so profuse as to obscure the site, advance the sucker tip backward in small increments, clearing the blood at each step, until a point is reached where the passage immediately fills after clearing; this is the bleeding site. Blood-tinged fluid suggests a CSF leak. Consult textbooks for methods of arresting hemorrhage.

✔ *EPISTAXIS—CLINICAL OCCURRENCE:* *Local Causes* coughing, sneezing, nose picking, fractures, lacerations, foreign bodies, adenoid growth, nasopharyngeal fibroma, angioma, rhinitis sicca. *Generalized Causes: Congenital* hereditary telangiectasia; *Inflammatory/Immune* Wegener granulomatosis, lethal midline granuloma; *Infectious* viral rhinitis, typhoid fever, scarlet fever, influenza, measles, infectious mononucleosis, diphtheria, pertussis, psittacosis, Rocky Mountain spotted fever, erysipelas, mucosal leishmaniasis; *Metabolic/Toxic* pernicious anemia, aspirin, scurvy; *Mechanical/Trauma* (see local causes) changes in atmospheric pressure (mountain climbing, caisson disease, flying) exertion; *Neoplastic* nasopharyngeal carcinoma, squamous cell carcinomas, leukemia; *Vascular:* coagulopathy, cirrhosis, uremia, hemophilia, von Willebrand disease, thrombocytopenia; *Elevated Arterial Pressure* hypertension, aortic coarctation; *Elevated Venous Pressure* cor pulmonale, congestive heart failure, superior vena cava syndrome.

Nasal and maxilla fracture. Nasal fractures are usually simple or comminuted; seldom are they compound. A blow from the side displaces both nasal bones to the opposite side, producing an S-shaped curve in the dorsum nasi. The septum may be fractured with or without nasal bone fracture. Frontal blows depress the nasal bones. Palpation along the inferior border of the orbit may disclose an irregularity indicating fracture of the maxilla; a fragment may displace downward into the sinus. Malocclusion of the teeth indicates backward displacement of the maxilla. Fracture of the zygoma produces flattening of the cheek.

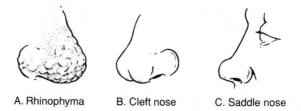

A. Rhinophyma   B. Cleft nose   C. Saddle nose

Fig. 7–51 *External Nasal Deformities. A. Rhinophyma. B. Cleft nose. C. Saddle nose:* *note the sinking of the dorsum with relative prominence of the lower third.*

> **KEY SIGN   Anosmia**

Lesions of CN I, often shearing of the nerve ending passing through the cribriform plate, or nasal obstruction produce loss of smell. Anosmia is invariably accompanied by a perceived change in the taste of food, which seems bland and unpalatable. The most common identified cause is closed head trauma.

Congenital nasal deformities.   Disturbances in development of the nose are myriad, but they are so obvious as to pose little problem in diagnosis. Perhaps the most common is cleft nose from incomplete fusion at the tip and dorsum.

> **KEY SIGN   Acquired Nasal Deformities**

Acquired deformities are commonly the result of trauma, infection, or neoplasms. *Rhinophyma* is an erythematous bulbous enlargement of the distal two-thirds of the nose from multiple sebaceous adenomas. It may follow long-standing rosacea (Fig. 7–51A, B). *Saddle nose* is distinguished by the sunken bridge (Fig. 7–51B) that results from loss of cartilage; common causes are septal hematoma or abscess. Rarely, it can follow relapsing polychondritis, Wegener granulomatosis, or congenital or acquired syphilis. A crooked nose results from fracture.

> **KEY SIGN   Vestibule Folliculitis**

Mild inflammation around the hair follicles is evident on inspection.

> **KEY SIGN   Vestibule Furunculosis**

A small superficial abscess forms in the skin or mucous membrane. Easily seen from the exterior, the lesion is typical of all furuncles. The area is extremely tender, swollen, and reddened. Swelling may involve the nasal tip, alae nasi, and upper lip (Fig. 7–52A). Avoid instrumentation or other trauma to pyogenic lesions within the triangle anterior to a line from the corners of the mouth to the glabella; this may cause spread of the infection directly to the cavernous sinus.

Fissure: Fissures often develop at the mucocutaneous junction. They become overlaid with crusts that cover tender surfaces.

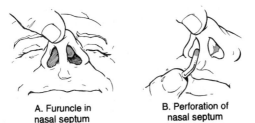

A. Furuncle in
nasal septum

B. Perforation of
nasal septum

Fig. 7–52 *Lesions in the Nasal Vestibule.* ***A. Furuncle:*** *avoid trauma that might spread infection to the cavernous sinus.* ***B. Perforation of nasal septum:*** *transillumination of the septum discloses a hole.*

KEY SIGN   Deviated Septum

In the adult, the nasal septum is seldom precisely a midline structure. The cartilaginous and bony septum may deviate as a hump, spur, or shelf to encroach on one nasal chamber, occasionally causing obstruction. Columnar dislocation of the septum may occur.

KEY SIGN   Perforated Septum

The cartilaginous portion is usually involved. Perforation is commonly caused by chronic infection, repeated trauma in picking off crusts, as a result of nasal or transphenoidal pituitary surgery or cocaine abuse. Perforation is readily demonstrated by looking in one naris while a light shines in the other (Fig. 7–52B).

KEY SIGN   Septal Hematoma

Even slight trauma to the nose may produce bleeding under the mucoperichondrium, usually causing bilateral hematomas. Nasal obstruction necessitates breathing through the mouth. The hematoma is seen as a violaceous, compressible, obstructive mass. The columella may be widened; the nasal tip pales from stretching of the skin. Pressure on the anterior ethmoidal nerve by the hematoma may cause anesthesia of the tip. Long-standing hematomas interfere with the blood supply of the septum, causing slow necrosis of the cartilage and a saddle nose deformity.

KEY SIGN   Septal Abscess

The septum swells into both nasal chambers, and the mucosa is edematous. Infection of a septal hematoma invariably results in loss of cartilage; it must be immediately incised, drained, and treated with appropriate antibiotics. There is risk of progression through the angular veins to produce cavernous sinus thrombosis.

Foreign body.   Children frequently put objects into the nose that remain for long periods and produce foul, purulent unilateral discharge.

Neoplasm. Sinus carcinomas cause obstruction, bloodstained discharge, and constant, boring pain. They invade bone: in the orbit, they may cause ocular disturbances; in the maxillary antral floor, upper teeth may become loose, a denture may no longer fit properly, or bulging and softness of the hard palate is seen.

➤ | **KEY SIGN**   **Cerebrospinal Rhinorrhea**

A traumatic fistula occurs between the subarachnoid space and the nasal cavity. A unilateral discharge of clear spinal fluid occurs after head injury or surgery. The fluid may be blood-tinged, but is easily distinguished from nosebleed. Jugular vein compression vein increases the flow. If spinal fluid is suspected, the specimen should be tested for beta$_2$-transferrin. There is substantial risk for meningitis; recurrent meningitis should lead to a search for CSF leak.

| **KEY SIGN**   **Nasal Discharge—Acute Suppurative Sinusitis**

See page 289.

| **KEY SIGN**   **Nasal Discharge—Chronic Suppurative Sinusitis**

See page 290.

| **KEY SIGN**   **Sinusitis and Periorbital Edema—Periorbital Abscess**

See page 281.

| **KEY SIGN**   **Sinusitis and Periorbital Edema—Orbital Cellulitis**

See page 282.

| **KEY SIGN**   **Sinusitis and Ocular Palsies—Cavernous Sinus Thrombosis**

See page 290 and Fig. 7–53A.

| **KEY SIGN**   **Nasal Polyps**

Nasal polyps are sessile or pedunculated mucosal overgrowths developing after recurrent episodes of mucosal edema. They are frequently seen in long-standing

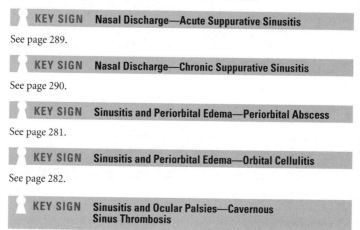

A. Cavernous sinus thrombosis   B. Nasal polyps

Fig. 7–53 *Lesions About the Nose. **A. Cavernous sinus thrombosis:** Early there is paralysis of a single ocular muscle, with the development of edema and proptosis (shown). **B. Nasal polyps:** The parasagittal section shows the lateral wall with three polyps emerging from the middle meatus.*

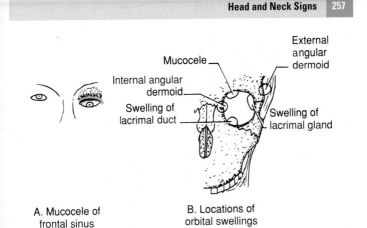

A. Mucocele of frontal sinus

B. Locations of orbital swellings

Fig. 7–54 *Some Masses About the Orbit. A. Mucocele of frontal sinus.* *An example of a mucocele, this occurring in the floor of the supraorbital ridge and presenting medially.* **B. *Locations of masses about the eye.***

allergic rhinitis, aspirin-sensitive asthma, and cystic fibrosis. Polyps are commonly multiple, most frequently protruding from the middle meatus as smooth, pale, spheric mucosal masses (Fig. 7–53B). Polyps may enlarge to obstruct the air passages; they frequently recur after removal. **DDX:** they are mobile and insensitive, distinguishing them from swollen turbinates.

KEY SIGN   Periorbital Masses—Mucocele and Pyocele

Permanent obstruction of the frontal or ethmoid sinus orifices causes mucus, normally, secreted by their mucosae to accumulate. The resulting sac, or mucocele, slowly enlarges; the pent-up mucus exerts pressure on the surrounding structures and erodes bone, behaving like a neoplasm. The sac may eventually erode through the floor of the frontal sinus or the lateral ethmoid wall producing a painless swelling beneath the supraorbital ridge, medial to the ocular globe (Fig. 7–54). The painless mass feels rubbery and slightly compressible. The globe is pushed downward and laterally, causing diplopia; proptosis may also occur. Upward and medial motions of the eye are restricted. Intranasal examination may be negative. An infected mucocele is termed a pyocele. **DDX:** Swelling from the mucocele occurs above the inner canthus; dacryocystitis forms a swelling below the canthus.

Benign neoplasms.   Benign *papillomas* are often found in the vestibule. Slow-growing, benign neoplasms of the sinuses are usually *osteomas* or *chondromas*. They grow slowly and cause no symptoms until air passages or a sinus orifice is obstructed.

KEY DISEASE   Midline Granuloma

The cause is unknown, but some classify it as one of the angiocentric immuno-proliferative lesions. The inflammation is attended by granuloma formation. It is most common in fifth and sixth decades, with a slight preference for women. Symptoms include sneezing, nasal stiffness, obstruction, and pain. Signs are rhinorrhea, nasal congestion, and paranasal sinusitis progressing to inflammation and ulcerations of the nasal septum, palate, and nasal ali. Advanced disease is indicated by destruction of midfacial structures including pharynx, mouth, sinuses, and eyes with death from cachexia, pneumonia, meningitis, or hemorrhage. Indolent ulceration and mutilation suggest the diagnosis. **DDX:** Unlike Wegener granulomatosis, here there is no systemic involvement or primary vasculitis.

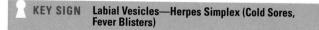

KEY DISEASE   Wegener's Granulomatosis

This is one of the systemic necrotizing vasculitides (see Chapter 8, page 413).

Lip Mouth, Teeth, Tongue and Pharynx Signs
Breath Signs

KEY SIGN   Breath Odor

Breath odor is an important diagnostic sign. There is great variation in olfactory acuteness and description of odors is meaningless, so experience is necessary. A foul breath odor, *fetor oris,* is common in infection (dental, tonsillar) atrophic rhinitis, putrefaction of food (achalasia, esophageal diverticula, pyloric obstruction), and infected sputum (bronchiectasis, lung abscess). *Acetone* on the breath indicates ketonemia in diabetic or starvation acidosis. In some patients with uremia, *ammonia* is detected. A curious *musty odor* occasionally is smelled in patients with severe liver disease. When a person has inhaled or swallowed *volatile hydrocarbons,* the odor is detectable in the exhaled air (natural gas is odorless). *Alcohol* on the breath indicates recent ingestion, but medical illness, trauma, or the ingestion of other drugs must be excluded as comorbid conditions. A few patients in coma have no alcohol odor on the breath while the aspirated gastric contents smell strongly of alcohol. The chronic alcoholic may smell of *acetaldehyde* instead of alcohol. The odor of *paraldehyde* should be recognized. When *garlic* is eaten, the methyl mercaptan causing its odor is excreted from the lungs for more than 24 hours.

Lip Signs

Cleft lip: In the embryo, incomplete fusion of the frontonasal process with the two maxillary processes leaves a persistent cleft in one or both sides of the upper lip. Cleft lip is sometimes accompanied by cleft palate.

Labial enlargement: The lips may appear large in cretinism, myxedema, acromegaly, and collagen injections.

KEY SIGN   Labial Vesicles—Herpes Simplex (Cold Sores, Fever Blisters)

Latent herpes simplex virus is reactivated producing local inflammation when the carrier develops another infectious disease, has local trauma, or is exposed to sunlight. Groups of vesicles containing clear fluid are surrounded by areas of erythema. Frequently, they occur on the lips. The lesions may burn or smart.

> **KEY SIGN** **Cheilosis (Angular Stomatitis)**

Maculopapular and vesicular lesions are grouped on the skin at the corners of the mouth and the mucocutaneous junction (Fig. 7–55A). Irritation of the skin leads to crusting and fissuring. Often accompanying profuse salivation from any cause, it is specifically associated with riboflavin deficiency or ill-fitting dentures; secondary *Candida* infection is common (*perlèche*). The entire labial surface may be inflamed from overexposure to sunlight, *actinic cheilosis*.

> **KEY SIGN** **Carbuncle**

Painful localized swelling with erythema and increased skin warmth suggests early cellulitis or carbuncle. When it occurs on the upper lip, it may be exceedingly dangerous, because the veins drain into the cavernous sinus.

> **KEY SIGN** **Carcinoma of the Lip**

Early, the lesion is indurated and discoid; later, it becomes warty and crusted, forming a shallow ulcer that slowly extends. The ulcerated border is elevated, sometimes pearly (Fig. 7–55B). Regional lymph nodes are involved late. It is more frequent in men and 95% of the cases are on the lower lip. Biopsy all the ulcers that are more than 2 weeks old.

> **KEY SIGN** **Lip Chancre**

The initial lesion of syphilis occurs at the inoculation site. The lip is the most common extragenital site of primary syphilitic chancre; usually the upper lip is involved. The lesion is discoid, without sharply defined borders and can be moved over the underlying tissues. It soon ulcerates to exude a clear fluid teeming with Treponema pallidum. The regional lymph nodes are involved early and feel larger and softer carcinomatous nodes. Serologic tests for syphilis are frequently negative while the chancre is present.

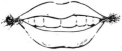

A. Cheilosis

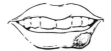

B. Epidermoid carcinoma of lip

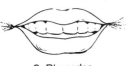

C. Rhagades

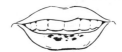

D. Labial pigmentation of intestinal polyposis (Peutz-Jeghers syndrome)

Fig. 7–55 *Some Lip Lesions. A. Cheilosis. B. Epidermoid carcinoma of lip:* notice the sharply demarcated elevated edges with the ulcerating base, typically located at the mucocutaneous junction. **C. Rhagades. D. Signs of Peutz-Jeghers syndrome.**

Molluscum Contagiosum: A nodular growth in the lip may ulcerate to discharge caseous material. The ulcer border may be elevated. The lesion is caused by Molluscipoxvirus. The resemblance to carcinoma may be striking, so biopsy may be required.

Rhagades: The white radial scars about the angles of the mouth are stigmata of previous syphilitic lesions (Fig. 7–55C).

> ### KEY SIGN Actinic Keratosis

A dry, flat, light-colored precancerous growth occurs on the lip and produces scaling; it bleeds easily.

> ### KEY SIGN Labial Pigmentation—Peutz-Jeghers Syndrome

Multiple pigmented brown to black spots on the lips resemble freckles (Fig. 7–55D); freckles are uncommon on the mucosa. This autosomal dominant syndrome is associated with intestinal polyposis and an increased risk for gastrointestinal cancer.

> ### KEY SIGN Labial Telangiectasias—Hereditary Hemorrhagic Telangiectasia

The first and most obvious lesions may occur on the buccal mucosa, tongue and lips. See page 150.

Oral Mucosa and Palate Signs

> ### KEY SIGN Xerostomia, Sjögren Syndrome

See page 282.

> ### KEY SIGN Buccal Pigmentation—Addison Disease

Small patches of pigment in the buccal mucosa are common in blacks and other darkly pigmented races. In whites, however, dappled brown pigment in the lining of the cheek strongly suggests Addison disease or Peutz-Jeghers syndrome.

Retention Cyst: An obstructed mucous gland produces a blue-domed translucent cyst anywhere on the buccal surface.

Mucosal Sebaceous Cysts (Fordyce Spots): The lip, cheek, and tongue mucosa show isolated white or yellow, sometimes slightly raised, spots <1 mm in diameter. Often a bit of white sebum may be expressed from the lesion. They are painless and harmless.

> ### KEY SIGN Koplik Spots (Measles)

Koplik spots are the earliest diagnostic sign of the measles; they are pathognomonic. One or 2 days before the exanthem appears, small white spots appear opposite the molars, and sometimes elsewhere, on the buccal mucosa (Fig. 7–56A). Each is surrounded by a narrow red areola.

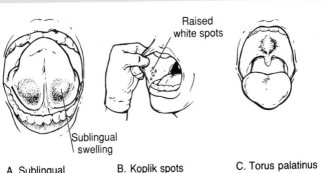

A. Sublingual   B. Koplik spots   C. Torus palatinus
dermoid cyst

Fig. 7–56 *Some Lesions of the Oral Cavity. A. Sublingual dermoid cyst. B. Koplik spots. C. Torus palatinus.*

> **KEY SIGN**   **Lichen Planus**

The lesions are thin, bluish-white, spiderweb lines resembling leukoplakia. Circumscribed areas of flattened papules on the flexor surfaces of the wrists and the middle of the shins strengthen the diagnosis of lichen planus (page 158).

> **KEY SIGN**   **Leukoplakia**

This often occurs at the site of chronic irritation from ill-fitting dentures or smokeless tobacco; it is precancerous. Tobacco and alcohol are cocarcinogens. The first lesion is a whitened hyperkeratotic plaque. On the tongue, one or more areas on the dorsal surface show obliteration of the papillae with thin white lesions that are wrinkled and sometimes pearly. Early lesions coalesce; as they persist and enlarge, they become chalk-white and thick and are palpably more firm than the adjacent mucosa. Biopsy is indicated.

> **KEY SIGN**   **Thrush, Candidiasis**

Infection of the oral mucosa with *Candida* spp. occurs in patients who are diabetic, immunosuppressed (e.g., HIV, immunosuppressant drugs) or have received broad spectrum antibiotics. The lesions may be painless or cause mouth soreness. Examination reveals white plaques that are easily removed with a tongue blade. Less commonly, the mucosa is erythematous and thin, without the white plaques. Pain with swallowing suggests concomitant *Candida* esophagitis.

> **KEY SIGN**   **Buccal Telangiectasias—Hereditary**
> **Hemorrhagic Telangiectasia**

The first and most obvious lesions may occur on the buccal mucosa, tongue and lips. See page 150.

> **KEY SIGN**   **Oral Vesicles, Blisters and Ulcers**

Several diseases result in oral vesicles or bullae, often with multiple ulcerations. The major mechanisms of disease are infection and immune mediated processes. Larger ulcers result from tissue destruction due to infectious, neoplastic or metabolic causes.

Herpes Simplex: Primary infection with herpes simplex often causes severe stomatitis with painful vesicles that rupture to form shallow ulcers, which heal slowly.

Herpangina: Infection with coxsackievirus 16 results in fever and sore throat. On examination, there are small vesicles or whitish papules on the soft palate.

Lichen Planus: Painful chronic ulcers may be surrounded by the characteristic lacy white mucosal lines.

KEY SIGN   Cicatricial Pemphigoid

Autoantibodies directed against hemidesmosomes in the basal layer of the mucosa and skin lead to separation of the epithelial layers with blister formation. Pain is mild to moderate. The incidence increases with age; oral lesions may be accompanied by skin lesions (page 169). The course is chronic and recurrent. It must be distinguished from Pemphigus Vulgaris (page 168).

KEY SIGN   Stevens-Johnson Syndrome

This is a severe allergic reaction with generalized involvement of the skin and mucous membranes. The most common cause is medication exposure. Early recognition, withdrawal of the offending agent, and supportive therapy may be life saving.

KEY SIGN   Aphthous Ulcer (Canker Sore)

A few small vesicles appear in crops on the tip and sides of the tongue and on the labial and buccal mucosa. After vesicle has ruptured, the lesion is a small, round, painful ulcer with a white floor, yellow margins and surrounding narrow erythematous areola. The cause is unknown. Recurrent or persistent aphthous ulcers are seen in Crohn disease and Behçet syndrome [Scully C. Aphthous Ulceration. *N Engl J Med.* 2006;355:165–172].

KEY SIGN   Mucous Patches (Condyloma Latum)

This is the common lesion of secondary syphilis, occurring on the tongue and the buccal and labial mucosa regardless of the site of the primary lesion. The patches are round or oval, 5 to 10 mm in diameter, slightly raised, and covered by gray membrane. They may ulcerate slightly. They feel indurated and are painless. Regional lymphadenopathy is common.

Osteonecrosis: Ionizing irradiation, especially of the mandible, leads to suppression of bone turnover and acute or delayed necrosis of bone with ulceration of the overlying mucosa. Bisphosphonate therapy (especially intravenous bisphosphonates for malignant hypercalcemia and myeloma) also suppresses bone turnover and is associated with bone necrosis and ulceration of the overlying mucosa. Patients present with one or more slowly progressive often painful ulcerations exposing underlying bone. A history of irradiation or bisphosphonate use is essential for making the diagnosis. Formerly, exposures to white phosphorus in the munitions industry caused a similar syndrome known as *phossy jaw* [Woo SB, Hellstein JW, Kalmar JR. Bisphosphonates and osteonecrosis of the jaws. *Ann Intern Med.* 2006;144:753–761].

> **KEY SIGN** **Cancer Chemotherapy—Mucositis**

The bone marrow and oral and intestinal mucosa are the most rapidly proliferating tissues in the body. Cytotoxic chemotherapy transiently stops proliferation and leads to impaired mucosal repair. Mouth ulcers commonly occur 5 to 10 days after intermittent bolus cytotoxic chemotherapy. They can occur anytime in the course of chronic oral therapy with alkylating agents or antimetabolites.

> **KEY SIGN** **Behçet's Syndrome**

See page 416.

Disseminated histoplasmosis. A persistent oral ulcer can be the presenting sign of disseminated histoplasmosis. Diagnosis is made by biopsy.

Reddened parotid duct orifice—mumps: The parotid (Stensen) duct orifice, opposite the upper second molar, may become reddened in mumps or other acute parotitis.

Bony palatine protuberance—torus. This is a common anatomic variation; a bony knob or ridge occurs in the midline of the hard palate. It is harmless.

Palatine mass—mixed tumor of ectopic aalivary gland: This occurs in the soft or hard palate. Unless noticed accidentally, it is silent until ulceration causes pain. It may invade the base of the skull.

Arched palate: There are many causes for high-arched palate. It is common in Marfan and Turner syndromes.

Cleft palate: A midline opening in the hard palate results from congenital failure of fusion of the maxillary processes. It is usually associated with cleft lip but also occurs in isolation. Its severity varies from a complete cleft of the entire soft and hard palate, including the alveolar ridge, to a partial cleft of the soft palate alone.

Bifid uvula: This results from incomplete cleft of the soft palate and may be accompanied by disoriented palatal muscles. Test for elevation of the uvula; deviation of the uvula and asymmetry of the soft palate suggest muscular abnormality.

Teeth and Gum Signs

Wide interdental spaces. This may occur congenitally or be acquired as the jaw enlarges in acromegaly.

Caries. Usually the presence of cavities in the teeth is obvious. Decreased saliva production following irradiation or with sicca syndrome is associated with an increased risk for caries.

Loss of enamel. Loss of dental enamel results from erosion by regurgitated acidic stomach contents in patients with bulimia nervosa and by acid water in swimming pools with excessive chlorination.

Fluoride pits. Opaque chalk-white spots, 1 to 2 mm in diameter, are seen scattered on the surface of multiple teeth. This is a harmless condition found exposure to large amounts of fluoride in the water during childhood.

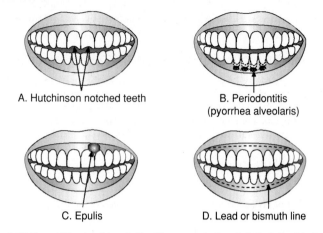

A. Hutchinson notched teeth

B. Periodontitis
(pyorrhea alveolaris)

C. Epulis

D. Lead or bismuth line

Fig. 7–57 *Dental Abnormalities. A. Hutchinson notched teeth. B. Periodontitis:* in the drawing, some of the lower teeth are involved: the gums are retracted and pus is exuding from behind the gingival margins. *C. Epulis:* it is sessile, lighter in color than the gums. *D. Lead or bismuth line in the gums.*

> **KEY SIGN** **Notched Teeth—Hutchinson Teeth**

This results from congenital syphilis. The permanent upper central incisors are misshapen (Fig. 7–57A). They are smaller than normal and peg-topped, resembling the frustum of a cone; the tips are notched. Notching is one component of the Hutchinson triad, together with interstitial keratitis and labyrinthine deafness.

Periapical abscess: An abscess forms at the root tip within the bone. The inflammation produces a very painful increase in intraosseous pressure. An abscess in an alveolus is suspected when toothache pain is accentuated by tapping the tooth with a tongue blade or probe. Tender swelling occurs in the adjacent gum and a draining sinus tract may form.

> **KEY SIGN** **Bleeding Gums**

Gum bleeding signals local gum lesions or generalized disorders of the blood vessels or hemostasis. The patient may complain of bleeding accompanying brushing, or may notice blood in expectorated phlegm. Other signs of a systemic vascular or hemostatic process should prompt direct questioning about bleeding from the gums because many patients do not consider this abnormal.

Gum recession. In older persons, the gingival margins may recede to expose the rough, lusterless cementum, proximal to the enamel border.

> **KEY SIGN** **Periodontitis**

Adherent dental plaque produces gum inflammation leading to recession and erosion of the dental ligament. The receding gums are inflamed with deep pockets (>3 mm) between gum and tooth. The teeth may be loose and the roots are exposed (Fig. 7–57B). The breath is often foul and the gums bleed easily. A particularly virulent form is come with methamphetamine abuse ("meth mouth").

> ▶ **KEY SIGN** **Necrotizing Ulcerative Stomatitis (Trench Mouth, Vincent Stomatitis)**

Inflammation of the gums and adjoining mucosa is attributed to a symbiotic infection with *Borrelia vincentii* and *Fusobacterium plauti-vincenti*. The infection may remain localized in the gums or it may extend to involve pharyngeal structures, including bone. It produces punched-out ulcers on the gums covered with a gray-yellow membrane that sometimes resembles diphtheria.

> ▶ **KEY SIGN** **Swollen Gums—Scurvy**

The gums are deep red or purple; they become swollen, tender, spongy and bleed easily. There is a general bleeding tendency with subperiosteal hemorrhages and purpura.

> ▶ **KEY SIGN** **Gingival Hyperplasia**

The gum volume increases, occasionally covering the teeth. Phenytoin is the most common cause [Meraw SJ, Sheridan PJ. Medically induced gingival hyperplasia. *Mayo Clin Proc.* 1998;73:1196–1199]. Gum infiltration with monocytes in monocytic leukemia produces a similar appearance.

Epulis. A fibrous tumor of the gum, it arises from the alveolar periosteum and emerges between the teeth. It appears as a nontender sessile mass (Fig. 7–57C), lighter in color than the gum; rarely, it is pedunculated. A similar tumor, but bright red, is a fibroangiomatous epulis.

Mass in gums—granuloma: A granuloma may occur in the gums spontaneously, or it may result from an ill-fitting denture. It is firm, pink, and nontender; it may break down to form an ulcer.

Blue gums—lead and bismuth lines: With chronic exposure to lead (occupational) or bismuth (therapeutic), the heavy metals may be deposited in the gums forming a blue line approximately 1 mm from the gingival margin. The metallic deposit appears as a solid line to the unaided eye (Fig. 7–58D). Insert a corner of white paper behind the gingival border to see the line more clearly. Viewing through a magnifying lens shows the line to be composed of small, discrete dots. Because the lead sulfide is formed only in the presence of bacterial infection, the deposit does not occur when the teeth are absent. Chronic quinacrine ingestion colors the gums diffusely blue or purple.

Tongue Signs

Dry tongue without longitudinal furrows. The lingual surface may be dry from mouth breathing or lack of saliva (xerostomia) from Sjögren syndrome or irradiation. The tongue volume remains normal, so no longitudinal furrows develop.

> ▶ **KEY SIGN** **Dry Tongue with Longitudinal Furrows**

Longitudinal furrows develop in the lingual surface from reduction of tongue volume. This is a reliable sign of severe volume depletion. This degree of volume depletion is always accompanied by loss of skin turgor.

> **KEY SIGN   Tongue Enlargement**

The tongue is enlarged in Down syndrome, cretinism, and adult myxedema. It increases in size during development of acromegaly and amyloidosis. Transient swelling occurs with glossitis, stomatitis, and cellulitis of the neck. Occlusions of the lymphatics by carcinoma and obstruction of the superior vena cava often produce enlargement. It may be the site of transient angioedema or abscess. Hematoma results from trauma; look for bite marks on the lateral aspects of the tongue.

Tremor: Increased sympathetic activity is associated with fine tremor. A fine tremor of the tongue is often present in hyperthyroidism. A coarser tremor is frequently seen in anxious persons; it also occurs in alcoholism and drug withdrawal; it may accompany any debilitating disease.

> **KEY SIGN   Fasciculation**

Denervation leads to spontaneous firing of motor units. It is a sign of denervation in bulbar poliomyelitis, West Nile virus encephalitis and amyotrophic lateral sclerosis.

Shortened frenulum (Tongue-Tied).   The frenulum is congenitally short. This limits protrusion and prevents the patient from placing the tip of the tongue in the roof of the mouth, impairing articulation of lingual consonants.

> **KEY SIGN   Limited Lingual Protrusion—Carcinoma**

Infiltration of the lingual muscles with neoplasm may limit protrusion of the tongue. Inspection usually reveals an ulcerated, whitish lesion that is hard on palpation compared with the surrounding muscle. A firm, nontender nodule in the base of the tongue may not be visually impressive, but it can represent squamous carcinoma. Palpation of the tongue discloses the buried neoplasm.

Unilateral carcinoma.   A unilateral neoplasm may hinder muscle action on that side; the deviation is toward the side of the lesion. Palpation discloses the mass.

> **KEY SIGN   Lingual Deviation—Paralysis of the Hypoglossal Nerve (CN XII)**

The tongue protrudes by tensing the two lateral muscle bundles; paralysis of one bundle causes the tongue to deviate to the paralyzed side (Fig. 7–58). With longstanding lesions, the two halves of the tongue are of unequal size because of muscle atrophy. Absence of a palpable mass excludes infiltration with carcinoma.

Geographic tongue.   The normal lingual coat is interrupted by circular areas of smooth red epithelium without papillae, surrounded by light-yellow rings of piled-up cells (Fig. 7–59B). The patches heal in a few days and are succeeded by new ones in other areas. This is a harmless condition of unknown cause.

Hairy tongue.   The appearance is caused by hyperplasia of the filiform papillae entangled with an overgrowth of mycelial threads of *Aspergillus niger* or *Candida albicans*. Patients are asymptomatic. The distal two-thirds of the dorsum looks as if it were growing short hairs, usually black (Fig. 7–59C) but occasionally green,

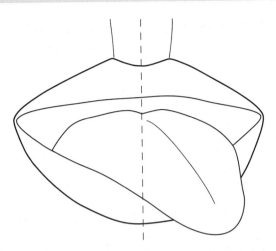

Fig. 7–58 *Paralysis of the Left Side of the Tongue. Deviation is toward the paralyzed side.*

either from the fungus or because of chewing gum containing chlorophyll. It is seen in debilitated patients and with fungal overgrowth after antibiotics.

Congenital furrows (Scrotal Tongue):   The median sulcus is deepened, the dorsal surface is interrupted by deep transverse furrows that are not inflamed (Fig. 7–59A). This is a harmless condition, frequently inherited. It must be distinguished from the longitudinal furrowing in syphilitic glossitis.

Lingual fissures—syphilitic and herpetic glossitis: The furrows of syphilitic glossitis are mainly longitudinal and deeper than the congenital type. The intervening epithelium is desquamated (Fig. 7–59D). A similar lesion with painful inflamed tongue and longitudinal fissures has been described with herpes infection in HIV-infected patients.

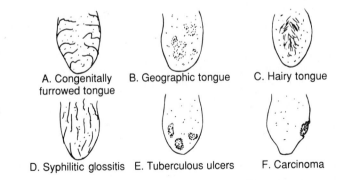

A. Congenitally furrowed tongue   B. Geographic tongue   C. Hairy tongue

D. Syphilitic glossitis   E. Tuberculous ulcers   F. Carcinoma

Fig. 7–59 *Tongue Surface Patterns. A. Congenitally furrowed tongue. B. Geographic tongue. C. Black hairy tongue. D. Syphilitic glossitis. E. Tuberculous ulcers. F. Carcinoma: a typical location of carcinoma of the tongue is on the lateral edge.*

> **KEY SIGN** Hairy Leukoplakia

Epithelial hyperplasia results from Epstein-Barr virus infection in patients with HIV infection. The sides of the tongue have elongated "hairy" filiform papillae.

> **KEY SIGN** Smooth Tongue—Glossitis

There are many causes of tongue inflammation. It is important to think of nutritional, hormonal and infectious disorders. The very high turnover rate of cells in the oral mucosa and tongue, combined with the extreme sensitivity of the tongue explains the susceptibility of these tissues to nutritional deficiencies and the prominent symptoms.

Atrophic Glossitis. Nutritional deficiency results in impaired mucosal proliferation. The patient may complain of tongue dryness, intermittent burning and paresthesias of taste. The tongue becomes smaller, its surface slick and glistening, and the mucosa thins. In the advanced stages, there is considerable pain and swelling. The color is pink, red or blue-red with atrophied hyperemic papillae appearing as small punctate red dots. *CLINICAL OCCURRENCE: Deficiency of Vitamin B*$_{12}$ pernicious anemia, postgastrectomy syndrome, blind intestinal loop, extreme vegetarian diets, infestation with fish tapeworm (Diphyllobothrium latum); *Folic Acid Deficiency* megaloblastic anemia of pregnancy, chronic liver disease; *Other Causes* iron deficiency anemia, idiopathic gastritis, mixed B-complex deficiency, unknown causes.

Pellagra. Deficiency of niacin (nicotinic acid and nicotinamide) results from a poor diet. In the early stages, the patient complains of tongue burning with hot or spicy foods, but the tongue appears normal. Later, the burning is constant; *D*iarrhea, *D*elirium, and *D*ermatitis may appear (the three Ds). The tongue becomes reddened at the tip and borders; later the erythema spreads and the tongue swells. The surface is denuded presenting a fiery-red mucosa with ulcerations and indentations from the teeth. After treatment, the tongue is pallid and atrophied.

Magenta Cobblestone Tongue—Riboflavin Deficiency: Riboflavin deficiency is a result of dietary insufficiency. Burning of the tongue is relatively mild; more discomfort is caused by the lesions of the lips and eyes. Swollen hyperemic fungiform and filiform papillae produce rows of reddened elevations that suggest the name cobblestone tongue. Edema at the bases of the papillae modifies the color to magenta, in contrast to the fiery red of the pellagrous tongue, in which the epithelium is denuded. Cheilosis and angular stomatitis are common, beginning as a painless gray papule at one or both corners of the mouth. The papule enlarges and ulcerates to produce indolent fissures with piled-up yellow crusts, leaving permanent scars. Similar lesions may occur at the ocular canthi and the nasolabial folds; the sebaceous glands in the nose become hyperplastic. Superficial keratitis and conjunctival injection are common.

Nonspecific Glossitis. Localized infections of the pharynx may also involve the tongue, producing redness and swelling. The tongue may burn and feel tender.

Strawberry Tongue (Raspberry Tongue). In streptococcal or staphylococcal infection with release of exotoxins (e.g., scarlet fever, toxic shock syndrome), the lingual papillae become swollen and reddened. According to Osler, the name *strawberry tongue* was given to the stage in which the inflamed and hyperplastic papillae show through the white coat. Later, the epithelium desquamates, carrying away the coat and leaving a fiery-red, denuded surface surmounted by hyperplastic papillae; this has also been termed a strawberry tongue, but others prefer the more accurately descriptive term *raspberry tongue*. During the desquamated period, the sense of taste is diminished.

Menopausal Glossitis: This is ascribed to estrogen deficiency. Intense burning of the tongue and slight atrophy of the lingual mucosa often occurs at menopause or in other estrogen deficiency states. The symptoms and signs improve with estrogens administration.

KEY SIGN Leukoplakia

See *Buccal Leukoplakia*, page 261. In the early stages, the areas are thin and white, often wrinkled or pearly; they obliterate the papillae. Later, the lesions coalesce, thicken, and become chalk white. In advanced stages, they look like dried, cracked white paint.

KEY SIGN Dental Ulcer

The ulcer results from irritation of a projecting tooth or an ill-fitting denture. These are always on the sides or undersurface of the tongue. Frequently, the ulcer is elongated; its base is sloughing, and its borders erythematous. The ulcer margin may be elevated and surrounded by induration, suggesting carcinoma. Removal of the irritating surface should result in a trend toward healing in a few weeks. Lacking improvement, biopsy is indicated.

KEY SIGN Carcinoma

Tobacco and alcohol are cocarcinogens for oropharyngeal squamous cell carcinoma. Pain while drinking acidic or alcoholic beverages should arouse suspicion. Carcinoma is usually seen on the sides, base, and undersurface of the tongue (Fig. 7–59E). It presents as an ulcerating mass with rolled and everted margins. Palpation discloses a discrete firm mass with surrounding induration. It is not tender unless ulcerated. If the patient complains of discomfort, dysphagia, or inability to protrude the tongue, yet no lesions are visible, palpate the root of the tongue. Also feel the submental, submandibular, and deep cervical lymph nodes.

KEY SIGN Sublingual Mass—Carcinoma

The patient often notices a carcinoma in the floor of the mouth. Ulceration produces pain and tongue motion may also cause discomfort. Secondary infection is common. It may begin as a leukoplakic area. Ulceration and a palpably discrete mass suggest carcinoma. Fixation to the mandible and metastases to submental or anterior jugular lymph nodes occur early.

Sublingual mass—ranula: This is any cystic distention of the sublingual or submandibular salivary ducts, usually caused by obstruction at the orifice. Hippocrates used the Greek word for "little frog" to describe this lesion, because it looks like a frog's belly. When the tongue is raised, a translucent mass is seen beside the frenulum linguae. The swelling may extend to the other side behind the frenulum. Bimanual palpation can often track the mass to the submandibular gland. Transillumination may show the submandibular duct traversing the upper part of the cyst.

Sublingual Varices—Caviar Lesions. With aging the superficial sublingual veins may develop varicosities resembling a mass of purple caviar under the tongue (see Fig. 6–16A, page 151). They are of no clinical significance.

Sublingual Mass—Dermoid Cyst: This is an opaque fluctuant cyst; when superficial, it may appear white. It may occur behind the frenulum or beside it (see Fig. 7–56A). Bimanual palpation allows assessment of size and demonstrates fluctuation.

> **KEY SIGN** **Posterior Lingual Mass—Lingual Thyroid**

A lingual thyroid presents as a round, smooth, red, nontender mass at the base of the tongue, near the foramen cecum; it does not ulcerate. It arises from thyroglossal duct remnants. It may be the only site of functioning thyroid tissue.

Pharyngeal Signs

Oropharyngeal soft tissue hypertrophy: Enlargement of the base of the tongue and narrowing of the pharynx by soft tissue hypertrophy combine to compromise the airway especially during sleep in the supine position when the tongue is relaxed. The extent of visualization of the normal oropharyngeal structures with the patient sitting and the tongue relaxed in the floor of the mouth predicts both the ease of tracheal intubation and the risk of upper airway obstruction during sleep. The modified Mallampati score is based upon visualization of the complete tonsillar bed, base of the uvula, and soft palate; loss of visualization proceeds sequentially. A score of 1 means all of the structures are visualized; 2 means the full tonsillar bed is not seen; 3 means the base of the uvula is not seen; and 4 means the soft palate is not seen. Scores of 3 and 4 indicate high-risk patients.

> **KEY SIGN** **Tonsillar Enlargement—Hyperplasia**

The normal adult tonsils seldom protrude beyond the faucial pillars; the tonsils are larger in children, shrinking at puberty. For adequate examination, take a tongue blade in each hand; depress the tongue with one and retract the anterior faucial pillar laterally with the other to disclose the anterior tonsillar surface. Normally, the color of the tonsil matches the surrounding mucosa; its surface is interrupted with deep clefts or crypts; these may contain white or yellow debris which is not a sign of infection. Hyperplasia is usually attributed to chronic infection, but it may be associated with obesity, hyperthyroidism, or lymphoma. Hyperplasia is usually bilateral.

Tonsillar Exudate: Bacterial and viral pharyngeal infections can produce a purulent exudate on the tonsils which may spread to the lateral and posterior pharyngeal walls. The most common causes are viral infections, including acute mononucleosis (EB virus) and Group A Streptococcal pharyngitis (see page 292 for a complete discussion).

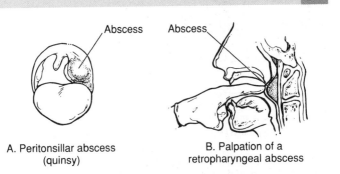

A. Peritonsillar abscess
(quinsy)

B. Palpation of a
retropharyngeal abscess

Fig. 7–60 *Lesions of the Oral Cavity. A. Peritonsillar abscess (quinsy). B. Palpation of a retropharyngeal abscess:* the sagittal section shows the relation of the abscess to the palpating finger. The gloved finger feels a boggy indentable mass as it presses gently against the anterior surfaces of the vertebral bodies.

Tonsillar carcinoma. Human papilloma virus, especially type 16, causes more than half of tonsillar cancers. The patient may complain of earache from referred pain. The breath is foul with a bleeding ulceration. Palpation of the tonsil discloses characteristic induration.

Peritonsillar abscess (Quinsy). Pyogenic infection of the tonsil spreads into the peritonsillar and pharyngeal spaces. The affected side is very painful and edematous. Mouth opening is always limited and may be difficult because of muscle spasm (trismus). An anterior abscess between the tonsil and the anterior faucial pillar is easily seen; the swelling also displaces the uvula to the opposite side (Fig. 7–60A). The adjacent soft palate is edematous and bulging. When the abscess is posterior to the tonsil, earache accompanies the sore throat and the tonsil is pushed forward and much of the swelling is hidden from direct vision. Surgical drainage is necessary.

> **KEY SIGN** **Retropharyngeal Abscess**

An accumulation of pus occurs in the space between the pharynx and the prevertebral fascia. If the swelling is in the oropharynx, it may be seen directly through the mouth, with the tongue depressed, as an anterior swelling of the posterior pharyngeal wall. In the nasopharynx, or opposite the larynx, it is never directly visible. This should be suspected when nose breathing is impaired (often attributed to adenoids) or with laryngeal respiratory distress or swallowing difficulty. Gentle palpation (Fig. 7–60B) discloses a unilateral soft swelling. It usually occurs in children younger than 5 years old. Urgent surgical drainage is necessary to avoid airway obstruction.

> **KEY SIGN** **Uvula Edema**

Localized edema of the uvula may result from allergic or nonallergic angioedema; it has occurred with thrombosis of an internal jugular vein containing a central venous line. Edema of the uvula together with bronchitis, asthma, and rhinopharyngitis, suggests inhalational injury, often from recreational drug use (e.g., recent heavy smoking of marijuana, crack cocaine, hashish).

Larynx and Trachea Signs

> **KEY SIGN**   **Stridor**

Narrowing of the extrathoracic airway is worsened as the transtracheal pressure increases during inspiration due to decreased intratracheal and constant atmospheric pressures. Inhalation is accompanied by a high-pitched sound that has the same pitch and intensity throughout inspiration. It indicates a high degree of airway obstruction and is almost always accompanied by significant dyspnea. It is caused by mass lesions, such as carcinoma, which restrict vocal cord mobility or reduce the size of the glottic aperture, by bilateral vocal cord paralysis, which limits the effective glottic opening, or a swollen epiglottis in acute epiglottitis or inhalation injury.

> **KEY SIGN**   **Laryngeal Edema**

The usual signs of laryngeal obstruction are present, ranging through hoarseness, dyspnea, and stridor. Inspection through the mirror is diagnostic. Glistening, swollen mucosa may be seen on the vocal cords, the arytenoid prominences, and the epiglottis (Fig. 7–61A). The membranes may not be reddened, depending on the cause.   **CLINICAL OCCURRENCE:**   Acute laryngitis, lymphatic obstruction by neoplasm or abscess, trauma to the larynx from instrumentation, radiation, anaphylaxis, angioedema, and myxedema.

KEY SIGN   **Hoarseness**

Paralysis of a cord, or edema, infiltration, or masses on the vocal cords, changes their vibratory response to airflow. More than any other sign, hoarseness focuses attention directly on the larynx. A multitude of disorders cause hoarseness.

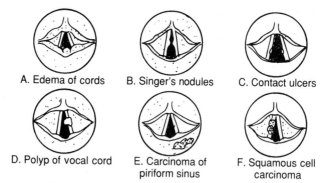

A. Edema of cords   B. Singer's nodules   C. Contact ulcers

D. Polyp of vocal cord   E. Carcinoma of piriform sinus   F. Squamous cell carcinoma

Fig. 7–61 *Laryngeal Lesions in the Mirror. A. Laryngeal edema:* *the mucosa on the vocal cords, arytenoid prominences, and epiglottis is swollen and glistening.* ***B. Singer's nodules:*** *apposing swellings on the free margins of the vocal cords at a distance one-third posteriorly in their extent.* ***C. Contact ulcers*** *apposed on the free margins of the cords at their junctions with the arytenoid cartilages.* ***D. Laryngeal polyp*** *on the free margin of the left cord.* ***E. Laryngeal carcinoma*** *in the left piriform sinus.* ***F. Squamous cell carcinoma*** *along the anterior half of the right cord.*

✔ *HOARSENESS—CLINICAL OCCURRENCE:* **Recent Onset** *Overuse* shouting, cheering; *Infections* upper respiratory infections, chlamydia, diphtheria, measles; *Drugs* anticholinergic drugs, strychnine (laryngeal spasm), aspirin aspiration (chemical burn), potassium iodide and uremia (cord edema); *Angioedema* insect bites, drug allergy, angiotensin-converting enzyme inhibitors, hereditary angioedema; *Foreign Body* food aspiration, after endotracheal intubation; *Laryngeal Spasm* croup, tetany, tetanus; *Burns* inhalation of irritant gases, swallowing of hot or caustic liquids. **Chronic Course** *Occupational Overuse* in the clergy, orators, singers, teachers; *Foreign Body* food aspiration, prolonged endotracheal intubation; *Lack of Mucus* Sjögren syndrome; *Chronic Vocal Cord Inflammation* nonspecific chronic laryngitis, gastroesophageal reflux, alcoholism, gout, tobacco smoking; *Edema of Cords* myxedema, chronic nephritis; *Surface Lesions of Cords* keratosis, pachyderma, herpes, leukoplakia, pemphigus; *Ulcers of Cords* tuberculosis, syphilis, leprosy, SLE, typhoid fever, trauma, contact ulcer; *Neoplasm of Cords* vocal nodules, sessile or pedunculated polyp, vocal process granuloma, vallecula cyst, leukoplakia, carcinoma in situ, epidermoid carcinoma, papilloma, angioma; *Innervation of Cords* compression of recurrent laryngeal nerve by aortic aneurysm, large left atrium of the heart, mediastinal neoplasm, mediastinal lymphadenopathy, retrosternal goiter, injury during thyroidectomy; *Weakness of Cord Muscles* debilitating diseases, severe anemia, myasthenia gravis, myxedema, hyperthyroidism, normal aging process; *Laryngeal Bones and Cartilages* perichondritis of cricoid or arytenoids, ankylosis of cricoarytenoid joints (rheumatoid arthritis); *Compression of Larynx* retropharyngeal abscess, tuberculosis of cervical vertebrae, neoplasm of pharynx, large goiters, actinomycosis; *Neck Irradiation.*

Vocal Cord Paralysis. The vocal cords are innervated by the recurrent laryngeal nerves, which are susceptible to injury in the neck and chest inferior to the larynx. In unilateral cord paralysis, the affected cord may be immobilized near the midline or slightly more laterally in the paramedian position. In the latter case, vocal cord approximation is poor and the voice is husky. During phonation, laryngoscopy shows the normal cord crossing the midline to meet the abducted immobile cord. In bilateral cord paralysis, the cords are usually fixed near the midline, so the voice is normal but dyspnea is extreme and inspiratory stridor with strenuous exertion is pronounced. *CLINICAL OCCURRENCE:* Following thyroidectomy, aneurysm of the left aortic arch (left cord), mitral stenosis with enlarged left atrium (left cord), and mediastinal tumor.

Ankylosis Of Cricoarytenoid Joint. Inflammatory or traumatic arthritis limits motion at the cricoarytenoid joint. Hoarseness and voice weakness are common and there is limited or absent motion of the true cords, resembling paralysis. Passive mobility, tested by an otolaryngologist, is absent in ankylosing, but present with paralysis. If the joints are not completely immobilized, crepitus over the larynx may be heard with the stethoscope. It may be so insidious that dyspnea is not recognized. Causes are rheumatoid arthritis and prolonged contact with an esophageal feeding tube.

Polypoid Corditis: The entire free margins of the true cords are loose and sagging. Hoarseness results from imperfect approximation of the edematous cords. Causal factors include voice strain, irritation from alcohol and tobacco, and upper respiratory allergy or infection.

Vocal Nodules (Singer's Nodules). With voice overuse, apposing 1 to 3 mm nodules form on the free margins of the true cords at the junction of the anterior one-third and the posterior two-thirds (Fig. 7–61B). The early lesions appear red; fibrosis later turns them white.

Laryngeal Contact Ulcer. Apposing ulcers occur on the free edges of both vocal cords at their junctions with the arytenoid cartilages. The irregular borders of the ulcers cause hoarseness (Fig. 7–61C). They usually result from overuse trauma or instrumentation, for example, intubation. Granulation tissue may develop on one or both ulcers and become sizable enough to cause airway embarrassment.

> **KEY SIGN** Leukoplakia

This results from chronic irritation, such as smoking tobacco, and may progress to invasive carcinoma A superficial nonulcerative white membrane appears on one or both vocal cords. Hoarseness may occur but pain is absent.

> **KEY SIGN** Laryngeal Neoplasm

Tumors in the larynx may be benign or malignant, pedunculated or sessile, localized or infiltrative. Infiltrative lesions are malignant; localized masses must be biopsied for diagnosis (Figs. 7–61E and F).

Salivary Gland Signs

> **KEY SIGN** Xerostomia

Dry mouth is caused by mouth breathing, obstruction of the salivary gland ducts, irradiation, and Sjögren syndrome. **DDX:** Dry eyes and salivary gland enlargement accompany Sjögren syndrome (page 282).

> **KEY SIGN** Sialorrhea (Ptyalism)

Sialorrhea implies excessive production of saliva, but the diagnosis is frequently extended to any condition in which saliva seems overabundant, from rapid secretion, inability to swallow, production of saliva that is more viscid and more difficult to swallow, or failure of the lips to contain the saliva. **CLINICAL OCCURRENCE:** The most common cause is poor neuromuscular control of the lips, tongue and perioral soft tissues. Other causes are drugs, intoxicants, and local inflammation stimulating salivary secretion. **Drugs:** mercury, copper, arsenic, antimony, iodide, bromide, potassium chlorate, pilocarpine, aconite, cantharides, carbidopa-levodopa. **Stomatitis:** aphthous ulcers, septic ulcers, suppurative lesions, periodontal disease, chemical burns. **Specific Oral Infections:** diphtheria, syphilis, tuberculosis. **Single Oral Lesions:** alveolar abscess, epulis, salivary calculus. **Reflex Salivation:** Gastric dilatation, gastric ulcer or carcinoma, acute gastritis, pancreatitis, hepatic disease.

> **KEY SIGN** Enlarged Salivary Glands

Salivary glands enlargement can be an indication of local or systemic disease. Painless enlargement of a single gland suggests tumor or ductal obstruction.

Pain in an enlarged gland is more likely with acute viral or suppurative bacterial infection, whereas painless enlargement is characteristic of indolent mycobacterial and fungal infections. Generalized salivary gland enlargement suggests a systemic disease involving the salivary glands either primarily or secondarily or a condition of excessive salivary stimulation (e.g., bulimia). *CLINICAL OCCURRENCE:* Sjogren syndrome, sarcoidosis, diabetes mellitus, amyloidosis, neoplasm (primary salivary gland tumors, lymphoma, Warthin tumor), bulimia, chronic alcohol consumption, metal sensitivity (lead, iodide, copper), infections: bacterial (staph, gonorrhea, syphilis, trachoma, actinomycosis); viral (mumps, EBV, hepatitis C, HIV); mycobacterial (tuberculosis); fungal (histoplasmosis).

Painless Bilateral Parotid Enlargement. Parotid enlargement is associated with a great diversity of conditions: its mechanism is unknown. *CLINICAL OCCURRENCE:* *Endocrine* diabetes mellitus, pregnancy, lactation, hyperthyroidism; *Idiopathic* fatty salivary gland atrophy; *Inflammatory/Immune* Sjögren syndrome, sarcoidosis, amyloidosis; *Metabolic/Toxic* malnutrition (cirrhosis, kwashiorkor, pellagra, vitamin A deficiency), poisoning (iodine, mercury, lead), drugs (e.g., thiouracil, isoproterenol, sulfisoxazole), obesity, starch ingestion; *Neoplastic* lymphocytic leukemia, lymphoma, salivary gland tumors; *Psychosocial* bulimia nervosa, stress.

Acute Nonsuppurative Parotitis: There is brawny induration of the parotid region, with swelling in front of the tragus, and behind the mandible and earlobe, pushing it outward. The skin is warm and there is pain and exquisite tenderness; fever is common. The pain is accentuated by opening the mouth or chewing. The duct orifice may be red, occasionally with a discharge of pus. One or both sides may be involved. Mumps is the classic cause; occasionally bacterial infection is responsible. Allergy to iodine can cause the same symptoms.

Acute Suppurative Parotitis: Acute bacterial parotid infection is seen in debilitated, immunosuppressed or previously irradiated patients. The gland is swollen, tender, and painful; induration and pitting edema are often present. Local inflammation is accompanied by high fever. The duct orifice discharges pus. Multiple abscesses may form, although fluctuation may be difficult to detect.

Chronic Suppurative Parotitis: Repeated episodes of ductal obstruction may produce chronic inflammation in the gland without fever or pain.

Neck Signs

> **KEY SIGN**   **Stiff Neck**

Pain and limitation of neck motion direct attention to the muscles, bones, and joints of the neck. The history is the best starting place for diagnosis. **DDX:** Be sure that mental status is normal and there are no signs of meningeal inflammation (page 730) before evaluating for other causes.

✔ *STIFF NECK—CLINICAL OCCURRENCE:* *Congenital* torticollis, syringomyelia, Chiari syndromes; *Idiopathic* fibromyalgia, myofascial pain syndrome, stiff-man syndrome; *Inflammatory/Immune* osteomyelitis, epidural abscess, tuberculosis, RA, ankylosing spondylitis, polymyalgia rheumatica;

Infectious pharyngitis, laryngitis, prevertebral or retropharyngeal abscess, cervical lymphadenitis, meningitis; *Metabolic/Toxic* strychnine, hypercalcemia, tetanus; *Mechanical/Trauma* acquired torticollis, trauma to cervical vertebrae (fracture, dislocation, subluxation, disk herniation), muscles and soft tissues (e.g., whiplash), cervical spondylitis, spinal stenosis; *Neoplastic* thyroid cancer, lymphoma, oropharyngeal carcinoma, metastatic carcinoma; *Neurologic* Parkinson disease; *Psychosocial* malingering, pending litigation secondary to injury.

KEY SYNDROME Torticollis (Wryneck)

The congenital type is attributed to hematoma or partial rupture of the muscle at birth resulting in unilateral muscle shortening. Dystonic reactions to phenothiazine drugs may cause it. The head may be tipped to one side. The dystonic sternocleidomastoideus may be more prominent than the other. If tipping is present but the muscles are not prominent, ask the patient to straighten his head; this will cause the sternal head of one muscle to tense more than the other. If the torticollis is of long-standing, the face, and even the skull, may be asymmetrical. DDX: The head tilt of torticollis must be distinguished from a head posture assumed to correct for vertical squint or ocular muscle palsy, *ocular torticollis* (page 232). To demonstrate the latter, slowly but firmly straighten the neck with your hands while watching the eyes for the appearance of squint. Asymmetrical erosion of the occipital condyle from rheumatoid arthritis or neoplastic disease may result in cranial settling in a tilted position.

Lateral Deviation of the Head—Hematoma of the Sternocleidomastoideus: A mass can be felt in the belly of the muscle; it is usually a hematoma.

KEY SIGN Meningitis

The neck is held stiffly in slight or extreme dorsiflexion from pain and reflex muscle spasm. Forceful anteflexion of the neck results in involuntary flexing of the hips, knees, and ankles, *Brudzinski sign*, an indication of meningeal irritation. See Chapter 14, page 735.

KEY SIGN Septic Thrombophlebitis of the Internal Jugular Vein (Lemierre's Syndrome)

Local infection in the face or oropharynx leads to septic thrombophlebitis of the internal jugular vein. This is a medical and surgical emergency, so early recognition is mandatory. The patient is systemically ill with fever, chills, and signs of septicemia. Septic emboli to the lungs may result in multiple pulmonary abscesses [Chirinos JA, Lichstein DM, Tamiriz LJ. The evolution of Lemierre syndrome. *Medicine (Baltimore)*. 2002;81:458–465; Bliss SJ, Flanders SA, Saint S. A pain in the neck. *N Engl J Med*. 2004;350:1037–1042].

Nongoitrous Cervical Masses and Fistulas

After the thyroid gland has been excluded by inspection and palpation as the site of a cervical mass, consider the other neck structures.

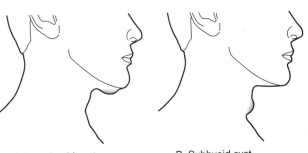

A. Suprahyoid cyst   B. Subhyoid cyst

Fig. 7–62 _Thyroglossal Cysts and Sinuses._ _A. Suprahyoid cyst_: *this is above the hyoid bone.* **_B. Subhyoid cyst._**

> **KEY SIGN** **Midline Cervical Mass—Thyroglossal Cysts and Fistulas**

Cysts arise from midline remnants of the thyroglossal duct (see Fig. 7–14, page 194). A thyroglossal cyst may appear at any time in life. A few of the cysts are translucent. A fistula results from drainage of an inflamed cyst or the incomplete excision of a thyroglossal remnant; the sinus tract opening will be in or near the midline. Cysts at various levels present specific challenges in diagnosis:

Suprahyoid Level (Fig. 7–62A). A thyroglossal cyst immediately above the hyoid bone must be distinguished from a sublingual dermoid cyst, which may be visible under the tongue as a white, opaque body shining through the mucosa.

Subhyoid Level (see Fig. 7–62B). The cyst is in the midline between the hyoid bone and the thyroid cartilage. Sometimes swallowing causes the mass to hide temporarily under the hyoid; ask your patient to dorsiflex her neck and open her mouth, causing the cyst to reappear.

Thyroid Cartilage Level. At this level a thyroglossal cyst may deviate from the midline, usually to the left; the forward pressure of the prow-like thyroid cartilage pushes it aside. To distinguish the mass from an enlarged lymph node, have the patient protrude her tongue maximally. If the mass is connected with the structures of the thyroglossal duct, this maneuver gives it an upward tug.

Cricoid Cartilage Level. A thyroglossal cyst in this region must be distinguished from a mass of the thyroid pyramidal lobe. The cyst tugs upward with protrusion of the tongue.

Pyramidal lobe of thyroid: See the preceding discussion on thyroglossal cyst at the cricoid level. The pyramidal lobe may extend from the isthmus of the thyroid to the hyoid bone (Fig. 7–63A); true to its name, its base on the isthmus is usually wider and can be felt as an isthmic projection. It may be palpable in Hashimoto thyroiditis.

Mass in suprasternal notch—dermoid cyst: Frequently, a nonpulsatile fluctuant mass in the suprasternal notch (*Burns space*) proves to be a dermoid cyst. The mass does not adhere to the trachea, nor does it move upward with tongue protrusion. The cyst may be confused with a tuberculous abscess.

Mass in the suprasternal notch—tuberculous abscess: This has the same physical characteristics as a dermoid cyst, except that it is slightly less fluctuant. It may

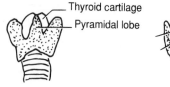

A. Pyramidal lobe of thyroid gland   B. Delphian nodes

Fig. 7–63 *Thyroid-Associated Masses. A. Pyramidal lobe of thyroid gland. B. Delphian nodes.*

arise from an abscess in the lung apex or by drainage from the deep cervical chain of lymph nodes.

Pulsatile mass in the suprasternal notch—aorta or innominate artery. Occasionally, elongation of the aortic arch or the innominate artery causes the vessel to bow upward into the suprasternal notch. This is not necessarily evidence of aneurysmal dilatation.

> **KEY SIGN** **Lateral Cervical Masses**

Intermittent or persistent cystic feeling masses in the lateral neck compartments usually arise from normal structures that have become or are intermittently distended. The history, exact location and characteristics of the mass can usually identify the probably etiology. Solid masses in these locations frequently arise in the lymph nodes and suggest neoplasms, usually malignant (see page 99). A fluctuant lymph node mass suggests infection, suppurative bacteria if acute and tuberculosis if chronic.

Branchial cyst. Remnants of the embryonic branchial clefts undergo cystic enlargement. The cyst usually appears in adults. Commonly, there is a single cystic mass just anterior but deep to the upper third of the sternocleidomastoid. The mass feels slightly soft and resilient; intercurrent inflammation makes it tender and firm. Aspirated fluid appears to be pus, but if it is spread on a watch glass, oil droplets may be seen floating on the surface.

Branchial Fistula: In the same location as the branchial cyst, the fistula may be either congenital or have developed from an inflamed cyst. Probing of the tract usually discloses a blind end in the lateral pharyngeal wall. Fistulas become intermittently infected.

Hygroma: The mass is formed by many cysts of occluded lymphatic channels. The soft, irregular, and partially compressible mass is usually present from childhood. It occupies the upper third of the anterior cervical triangle, but may extend downward or under the jaw. It is readily distinguished from all other cysts by its brilliant translucence. Its size may vary from time to time and it may become inflamed.

Carotid body (Glomus) tumor: This arises from the chromaffin tissue of the carotid body; it can be familial or sporadic. It appears in middle life and grows very slowly. The mass can be palpated near the bifurcation of the common carotid artery (Fig. 7–64A). Usually shaped like a potato (*potato tumor*), it is freely movable laterally, but cannot be moved in the long axis of the artery. Although growing

A. Tumor of carotid body

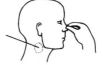
B. Intermittent cervical pouches

Fig. 7–64 *Single Tumors of the Lateral Neck II. A. Carotid body tumor. B. Laryngocele.*

in the carotid sheath, it does not always transmit arterial pulsations. Early it may feel cystic; later it becomes hard. Pressure on the tumor sometimes produces slowing of the heart rate and dizziness. Occasionally, the tumor produces vasoactive amines, and palpation can produce pupillary dilatation and hypertension, a useful diagnostic sign. In 20% of cases, regional extension eventually occurs upward along the carotid sheath.

Zenker's diverticulum (Pharyngeal Pouch): A pharyngeal diverticulum occurs proximal to the cricopharyngeus muscle. The patient complains of gurgling in the neck, especially during swallowing. Regurgitation of food is common during eating or when lying on the side. An intermittent swelling may be seen in the side of the neck, usually the left. If not apparent, the swelling may be induced by swallowing water. Pressure on the distended pouch causes regurgitation of old food.

Laryngocele: Herniation of a laryngeal diverticulum through the lateral thyrohyoid membrane causes an intermittent neck swelling (Fig. 7–64B). Blowing the nose will often induce an air-filled swelling that is resonant to percussion. Usually the condition occurs from chronic severe coughing or sustained blowing on a musical instrument.

Cavernous hemangioma: As in other parts of the body, the swelling is soft, compression partially empties the cavity of blood and refilling is slow. A faint blue color under the skin may be discerned.

Thyroid Signs

> **KEY SIGN** **Tracheal Displacement from Goiter**

A large or strategically located goiter may cause tracheal compression or displacement or both (Fig. 7–65). Patients may complain of tightness or pressure

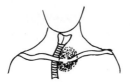

Tracheal displacement
by retrosternal goiter

Fig. 7–65 *Tracheal Displacement:* the retrosternal goiter on the patient's left compresses the trachea transversely pushing it to the right. The tracheal deviation can be demonstrated by palpation.

in the throat; rarely is stridor the presenting complaint. *Tracheal Compression:* The trachea is most vulnerable at the thoracic inlet, especially in small patients with short necks; usually the trachea is narrowed transversely. Small degrees of compression are not apparent from history or physical examination. With severe narrowing, slight pressure on the lateral thyroid lobes produces stridor (Kocher test). *Tracheal Displacement:* Lateral tracheal deviation in the neck is evident when the midpoint of the tracheal rings is not centered in the suprasternal notch.

KEY SIGN Tender Thyroid—Subacute Thyroiditis and Acute Suppurative Thyroiditis

See page 300.

KEY SIGN Thyroid Bruit

As the thyroid undergoes hyperplasia the increased blood flow produces a *thyroid bruit*. A thyroid bruit may be confused with a carotid bruit; the latter radiates to the angle of the jaw. DDX: An aortic murmur originates at the base of the heart and can be followed into the neck from below. A venous hum has a different pitch and is abolished by light compression of the jugular vein. This bruit suggests Graves' disease.

KEY SIGN Thyroid Enlargement: Goiter

See page 297ff.

KEY SYMPTOM Thyroid Nodules

See page 299.

KEY SIGN Enlarged Delphian Lymph Nodes

A few lymph nodes are regularly present in the thyrohyoid membrane; when enlarged, they are termed the Delphian nodes because they may indicate metastases from thyroid carcinoma. Enlargement of the Delphian nodes indicates either subacute thyroiditis or thyroid cancer (Fig. 7–63B).

Head and Neck Syndromes

Scalp, Face, Skull, and Jaw Syndromes

KEY SYNDROME Headache

For a full discussion of headache see Chapter 14, page 731ff. Discussed below are regional causes of headache related to extracranial disease.

Fever: Many febrile illnesses are associated with headache. The location varies; the pain may be slight or severe, throbbing or steady. The cause of pain is thought to be distention of the cranial arteries.

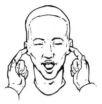

Fig. 7–66 *Palpation of the TMJ*. Place the tips of your index fingers in each external acoustic meatus and have the patient open and close his mouth. Clicking or crepitation is felt with TMJ arthritis; the joint will be tender if rheumatoid arthritis is the cause.

Giant Cell Arteritis, Temporal Arteritis: See Chapter 8, page 414. Temporal headache and scalp tenderness results from ischemia in the temporal artery distribution. The headaches are constant and relatively severe. Scalp tenderness is often present; exquisite scalp sensitivity is nearly diagnostic. Search for nodularity and/or decreased pulsations in the temporal artery.

Occipital Neuritis: Entrapment of the occipital nerve radiates pain in its distribution. Shooting sharp pain over the ear and posterior scalp suggests occipital neuritis.

Paranasal Sinusitis: See page 289ff.

Ice Cream Headache: Application of cold to the palate triggers intense pain felt in the medial orbital area. This common problem is precipitated by eating very cold foods, classically ice cream. It lasts 20 to 120 seconds, during which time the pain is intense. It may be more common in people with migraine.

KEY SYNDROME   TMJ Pain

See also page 213. Pain in front of the ear either episodic or constant, but worsened with eating and accompanied by clicking or grating sensations is typical for TMJ disease (Fig. 7–66). Common causes are trauma and being edentulous with loss of the correct spacing between the mandible and maxilla for chewing, placing abnormal forces on the TMJ. Other diseases that occasionally affect the TMJ are RA, rheumatic fever, SLE, gout, Sjögren syndrome, and Familial Mediterranean Fever. **DDX:** Pain in the side of the head with chewing suggests giant cell arteritis with claudication of the masticators; the mechanical symptoms distinguish TMJ. Tenderness in this location is distinguishes RA from rheumatic fever.

Displaced Cartilage: The patient may hear a snap in the ear after which an annoying click occurs each time the mouth is opened; the click can be palpated in the auditory meatus anteriorly. Occasionally, the joint locks, with sudden pain in the ear radiating to the pinna and the skin above, accompanied by salivation from stimulation of the auriculotemporal nerve. Pain persists until the cartilage is reduced.

KEY SYNDROME   Periorbital Abscess

In suppurative ethmoid sinusitis, pus may extend through the lateral wall of the sinus to form an abscess between the ethmoid plate and the periosteum lining the orbit. This is accompanied by fever, pain on eye movement, and edema between the inner canthus and the bridge of the nose. The edematous region is tender and may extend to involve most of both lids. The pus may push the ocular globe slightly downward and laterally. No chemosis is present. Surgical drainage is essential.

► **KEY SYNDROME   Orbital Cellulitis**

A periorbital abscess may extend to produce a diffuse cellulitis of the orbital tissue. Invasion may be heralded by a chill, high fever, and dull pain in the eye. The eyelids become edematous, particularly near the inner canthus. Chemosis develops. Ultimately, the eye becomes fixed. The patient appears very ill and requires the immediate surgical care.

Eye Syndromes

KEY SYNDROME   Sjögren Syndrome—Keratoconjunctivitis Sicca

There is lymphocytic infiltration of the salivary and lacrimal glands with loss of exocrine function. This is an autoimmune disorder first described as kerato-conjunctivitis sicca, xerostomia in patients with rheumatoid arthritis. Primary Sjögren syndrome is a relatively common disorder with symptoms of fatigue, dry mouth, eyes, and other mucosal surfaces, arthralgias and arthritis, and nephritis. Both central and peripheral neurologic symptoms may be present. Other autoimmune diseases, in addition to rheumatoid arthritis, may accompany the syndrome. There is an increased risk of non-Hodgkin lymphomas [Fox R. Sjogren's syndrome. *Lancet.* 2005;366:321–331].

KEY DISEASE   Graves' Ophthalmopathy

Deposition of mucopolysaccharides and fibrotic degeneration of the extraocular muscles and orbital fat leads to forward displacement of the globe and impaired extraocular motions. Acquired bilateral exophthalmos is most commonly associated with Graves' disease. In Graves' disease, the proptosis occurs independently of the abnormalities of thyroid function; the patient may be hyperthyroid, euthyroid, or hypothyroid. The proptosis is often permanent, although acute infiltration and edema may be treated and resolve. Accompanying signs may be lid edema, periorbital swelling, lid lag, lid retraction, and scleral show (page 224). Patients may present with diplopia due to asymmetric muscle involvement. At onset, the proptosis may be unilateral, raising concern for other intraorbital pathology.

KEY SYNDROME   Down Syndrome

The four ocular signs of Down syndrome (trisomy 21) are an epicanthic fold persisting after the age of 10 years; unilateral or bilateral slanting eyes in which the lateral canthus is elevated more than 2 mm above a line through the medial canthi; *Brushfield spots*, accumulations of lighter-colored tissues in the concentric band of the outer third of the iris; and hypoplasia of the iris, showing as darker discolorations of the iris.

KEY SYNDROME   Uveal Tract Inflammation—Uveitis (Iritis, Iridocyclitis, and Choroiditis)

Inflammation of the uveal tract, the vascular layer of the eye, may involve only the iris (iritis), extend to the ciliary body (iridocyclitis), or involve the choroid (choroiditis) or retina (retinitis). Iritis is characterized by ciliary flush and miosis, accompanied by deep pain, photophobia, blurring, and lacrimation. The inflamed iris may become adherent to the anterior lenticular surface, forming *posterior synechiae*, manifest by irregularities in the pupil. Cast-off cells in the anterior chamber form a sterile *hypopyon* (see Fig. 7–41B, page 238). Deposits of yellow or white dots of aggregated inflammatory and pigmented cells known as keratic precipitates occur on the posterior surface of the cornea. Uveitis is most commonly idiopathic, but result from trauma, infection, allergy, sarcoidosis, collagen vascular diseases, and autoimmune conditions such as ankylosing spondylitis.

KEY SYNDROME   Patients with Red Eye

A red eye may result from benign self-limited conditions or be an indication of serious sight-threatening eye disease. **DDX:** Generalized redness of the bulbar and tarsal conjunctivae with minimal discharge and no visual loss is usually a viral conjunctivitis or blepharitis. Localized redness and swelling of a lid suggests hordeolum or chalazion. Severe photophobia, ciliary flush, visual loss, elevated intraocular pressure, corneal haze, acute proptosis and acute scleritis require urgent evaluation by an ophthalmologist. ***CLINICAL OCCURRENCE:*** ***Benign Disorders*** environmental irritation, allergic and viral conjunctivitis, external hordeolum (sty), internal hordeolum (chalazion), and blepharitis; ***Serious Disorders*** (urgent care of an ophthalmologist required): acute keratitis (herpes simplex, bacterial, trauma, foreign body), gonococcal and chlamydial conjunctivitis, acute glaucoma, acute iridocyclitis, uveitis, and acute scleritis.

KEY SYNDROME   Glaucoma

Increased intraocular pressure produces ischemic damage to the nerve fibers at the optic disk. A progressive increase in cup-to-disk ratio discovered by sequential observations, suggests increasing intraocular pressure (Plate 17). Early damage leads to nasal steps and arcuate defects. Later, there is generalized constriction of the visual field from destruction of the optic nerve by increased intraocular pressure or vasculopathy of the nerve head (see Fig. 7–38C, page 235) [Coleman AL. Gaucoma. *Lancet.* 1999;354:1803–1810]. Visual fields must be examined with automated perimetry to detect early visual field loss. Pupillary dilation is often present.

Narrow Angle Glaucoma. Obstruction to aqueous drainage from the anterior chamber results from narrowing of the chamber angle and increased production of aqueous. Acute symptoms are extreme ocular pain with nausea and vomiting and loss of vision. Chronic symptoms include halos around lights, tunnel vision, ocular pain, and headache. Chemosis, corneal edema, ciliary flush, and a fixed dilated pupil are seen on examination.

Open Angle Glaucoma. There is increased secretion of aqueous and obstruction to outflow with normal chamber angles. This is the most common type of glaucoma. It occurs in older persons who may see colored halos around lights and experience insidious, painless blindness.

> ### KEY SYNDROME   Sudden Visual Loss

This always requires the urgent care of an ophthalmologist. Visual loss is usually monocular resulting from retinal detachment, vitreous hemorrhage, retinal artery occlusion (embolus, thrombus, and vasculitis), optic nerve compression or anterior ischemic optic neuritis (AION, arteritic and nonarteritic). Transient visual loss in one eye for 5 to 15 minutes (*amaurosis fugax*) usually results from embolic occlusion of the retinal artery. On funduscopic examination, refractile cholesterol emboli may be seen at the retinal artery bifurcations. Loss of vision in a single visual field (right or left hemianopsia) indicates a lesion between the optic chiasm and the visual cortex. Patients are often unaware of this visual field loss. Sudden bilateral visual loss with nystagmus and/or confusion suggests thiamine deficiency in patients with nutritional deficiency or increased metabolic demands.

Ear Syndromes

KEY SYNDROME   Acute External Otitis

A variety of organisms can cause the inflammation, but the usual *offender is Pseudomonas aeruginosa*, or, less commonly, streptococci, staphylococci, or *Proteus vulgaris.* This may result from an increased pH in the canal ("swimmer's ear"). Pain may be mild or severe; it is accentuated by movement of the tragus or pinna. The epithelium appears either pale or red; it may swell to close the canal and impair hearing; the tragus may also swell. An aural discharge often results. Fever is not uncommon. Tender, palpable lymph nodes may appear in front of the tragus, behind the pinna, or in the anterior cervical triangle.

KEY SYNDROME   Chronic External Otitis

Bacteria and fungi are the chief causative agents, although the condition may accompany a chronic dermatitis, such as seborrhea or psoriasis. Instead of pain, pruritus is the chief symptom. Aural discharge may be present. The epithelium of the pinna and the meatus is thickened and red; it is abnormally insensitive to the pain during instrumentation.

> ### KEY SYNDROME   Malignant (Necrotizing) External Otitis

Pseudomonas aeruginosa invades the soft tissues, cartilage, and bone in patients with diabetes mellitus. Although some patients have minimal clinical findings, others may experience pain, discharge, and fever with swelling and tenderness of the tissues around the ear. Examination of the auditory canal may reveal edema, redness, granulation tissue, and pus obscuring the TM. The process can advance to osteomyelitis of the mastoid, temporal bone and the base of the skull, involving the seventh and other cranial nerves and presenting with a facial palsy. An otolaryngology consult must be obtained.

Middle Ear Glomus Tumor: Fibrovascular tumors arise from the glomus bodies in the jugular bulb or the middle ear mucosa. They present with pulsatile tinnitus in the involved ear, or sometimes the glomus jugulare type is associated with paralysis of CN IX and CN XI, which pass through the jugular foramen. Glomus tumors appear as red masses behind the TM. Identical tumors arise from the carotid artery bifurcation. Rarely, the tumors are multiple, malignant or secrete vasoactive amines. If biopsied, they bleed profusely. Familial forms occur.

KEY SYNDROME Acute Otitis Media with Effusion (Serous Otitis Media)

Obstruction of the Eustachian tube prevents middle ear aeration. Resorption of trapped air produces a negative pressure, leading to inward displacement of the TM from atmospheric pressure. Decreased middle ear pressure leads to effusion. Initially, the TM is retracted around the malleus, making it more distinct and curving the light reflex (Fig. 7–30B). Later, serous amber fluid may be seen behind the membrane (Fig. 7–30C); a fluid meniscus appears as a fine black line and sometimes air bubbles are visible (Fig. 7–30E). The cause is usually an upper respiratory infection [Rovers MM, Schilder AGM, et al. Otitis media. *Lancet*. 2004;363:465–473].

KEY SYNDROME Acute Suppurative Otitis Media

Bacteria from the nasopharynx (*Streptococcus pneumonia, Haemophilus influenza, Moraxella catarrhalis*) enter the middle ear via the Eustachian tube; fluid in the chamber favors purulent infection. Throbbing earache, frequently with fever and hearing loss, is the complaint. The TM bulges obliterating the normal landmarks (Fig. 7–30D); its surface is bright red and lusterless. Perforation is marked by rapid relief of pain and the appearance of pus in the canal. If the infection has extended into the mastoid air cells, pressure on the mastoid process may elicit pain. Fever and constitutional symptoms are more prominent in children than adults. **DDX:** Movement of the pinna and tragus do not cause pain, unlike acute external otitis.

KEY SYNDROME Acute Mastoiditis

The mastoid air cells communicate with the middle ear. Usually, infection of the mastoid cells results from inadequate treatment of acute suppurative otitis media. The symptoms of otitis gradually increase. There is low-grade fever. The eardrum is lusterless and edematous. Deep bone pain can be elicited by percussion on the mastoid process. Imaging confirms the diagnosis by showing clouding of the mastoid air cells and bony destruction, which is evident radiographically after 2 to 3 weeks of suppuration. Extension can cause a subperiosteal abscess of the mastoid process. Less commonly, erosion of bone damages the facial nerve (CN VII), with facial paralysis. Extension through the inner table can cause meningitis, epidural abscess, or abscess of the temporal lobe or cerebellum. Infection of the internal ear can produce labyrinthitis.

KEY SYNDROME Chronic Suppurative Otitis Media

By definition, the condition is associated with a permanent perforation of the eardrum. A marginal perforation of the annulus is graver than a central defect. The chief symptom is painless aural discharge. Hearing is always impaired. The amount of discharge may wax and wane, but recurrence is invariable. Painless discharge accompanying an upper respiratory infection suggests previously existing perforation. Occurrence of pain or vertigo indicates development of a complication, such as subdural irritation, brain abscess, or labyrinthine involvement.

Cholesteatoma. In chronic suppurative otitis media with a deep retraction pocket in the attic or posterior superior quadrant of the eardrum, the squamous epithelium of the meatus may grow into the attic of the tympanic cavity. Desquamation produces a caseous mass of cells, keratin, and debris, which becomes infected, and slowly enlarges, extending into the mastoid antrum. The mass may ultimately erode bone. Patients may have fullness in ear, pain, headache and hearing loss. Signs include chronic foul-smelling suppurative discharge from middle ear, hearing loss, and a pearly gray mass visible with the otoscope.

KEY SYNDROME   Hearing Loss

Sensorineural loss (nerve deafness) results from disorders of the cochlea or the acoustic nerve (CN VIII). Conductive loss occurs from failure in transmission of sound vibrations to the neurosensory apparatus. Some causes of sensorineural loss are hereditary deafness, congenital deafness, trauma, infections, drug toxicity, and aging (*presbycusis*). Unilateral hearing loss with unilateral tinnitus may be the first symptoms of an acoustic neuroma. Conductive loss occurs with obstruction of the external acoustic meatus, disorders of the eardrum and middle ear, and overgrowth of bone with fixation of the stapes (*otosclerosis*). Effective screening for hearing loss involves asking the patient (and family members) whether hearing loss is present; affirmative or equivocal responses should have the whispered voice test performed [Bagai A, Thavendiranathan P, Detsky AS. Does this patient have hearing impairment? *JAMA.* 2006;295;416–428].

KEY SYNDROME   Dizziness

Symptoms described as dizziness may arise from problems in the inner ear, CN VIII, or vestibular nucleus; from loss of proprioception from peripheral neuropathy or visual impairment; from autonomic dysfunction or intravascular volume depletion; and from anxiety and other psychiatric disorders. This is a very common complaint and must be approached with a careful history *without ever suggesting relevant descriptive terms (spinning, lightheaded, unsteady, etc.) to the patient. You must have them, in their own words, describe the symptoms without using the word dizzy.* From the description given, you should try to sort the patient into one of four general categories, those with true vertigo (a hallucination of motion), orthostatic lightheadedness and hypotension, postural unsteadiness due to sensory abnormalities or weakness, and the last group for whom no clear physiologic explanation is suggested.

🖋 *DIZZINESS—CLINICAL OCCURRENCE:* **Endocrine** hypothyroidism, pregnancy, hypoparathyroidism, aldosteronoma; **Idiopathic** multisystem atrophy; **Inflammatory/Immune** vestibular neuritis; **Infectious** meningitis, encephalitis, brain abscess, syphilis; **Metabolic/Toxic nutritional:** pellagra, alcoholism, vitamin B_{12} deficiency, cerebral hypoxia, fluid and electrolyte disturbances; **Mechanical/Trauma ears:** utricular trauma from skull fracture, otosclerosis, leaks from tears in the oval or round windows, perilymph fistula; **eyes:** muscle imbalance, refractive errors, glaucoma; **Neoplastic** brain tumors (primary, metastatic); **Neurologic** migraine, absence seizures, peripheral neuropathy; **Psychosocial** panic attack, generalized anxiety disorder; **Vascular** hypotension, orthostatic hypotension.

KEY SYNDROME Vertigo

Persistent stimulation of the semicircular canals or vestibular nucleus when the head is at rest gives a hallucination of motion. When the eyes open, the patient's surroundings seem to be whirling or spinning about. With the eyes closed, the patient continues to feel in motion. Severe vertigo is accompanied by nausea and vomiting. The first task of the clinician is to distinguish between positional vertigo, which is common, and usually benign and spontaneous vertigo unrelated to position. Next, distinguish peripheral (labyrinth, CN-VIII) from central (brainstem) causes. Nausea and vomiting are more common with peripheral lesions. The patient can stand and walk with peripheral lesions despite severe discomfort; with central lesions, they may be completely unable to stand without falling. Also, peripheral vertigo tends to improve with fixation of the eyes; this leads to improvement of the vertigo with time. Both are less likely with central vertigo. Change of direction of the nystagmus with alteration of gaze suggests a central etiology. The Fukuda stepping test helps identify peripheral vestibular dysfunction. Have the patient stand upright with the eyes closed and the arms outstretched. Ask them to march in place: rotation of >30 degrees is a positive test indicating asymmetric inner ear function. [Froehling DA, Silverman MD, Mohr DN, Beatty CW. The rational clinical examination. Does this dizzy patient have a serious form of vertigo? *JAMA.* 1994;271:385–388; Baloh RW. Vertigo. *Lancet.* 1998;352:1841–1846]. **CLINICAL OCCURRENCE:** **Peripheral Labyrinthine System** serous labyrinthitis, perilymph fistula, labyrinthine fistula, viral labyrinthitis, otosclerosis, otitis media with effusion, benign paroxysmal positional vertigo, Ménière disease, motion sickness, cholesteatoma, temporal bone fracture, postural vertigo; **Central Labyrinthine System** migraine, vertebrobasilar insufficiency, brainstem or cerebellar hemorrhage or infarction, thrombosis of the posteroinferior cerebellar artery, infarction of the lateral medulla (Wallenberg syndrome), cerebellopontine angle tumors, intra-axial tumors (pons, cerebellum, medulla), craniovertebral abnormalities causing cervicomedullary junctional compression, multiple sclerosis, encephalitis, meningitis, intracranial abscess (temporal lobe, cerebellum, epidural, subdural), trauma; **CN-VIII** infections (acute meningitis, tuberculous meningitis, basilar syphilitic meningitis), trauma, tumors.

Acute Labyrinthitis (Vestibular Neuritis). This is the most frequent cause of vertigo. The patient gradually develops a sense of whirling that reaches a climax in 24 to 48 hours. During the height of the symptoms, nausea and vomiting may occur. The patient seeks comfort in the horizontal position; raising the head may induce vertigo. The patient is incapacitated for several days. The symptoms gradually subside, and they disappear in 3 to 6 weeks. There is no accompanying tinnitus or hearing loss.

Benign Paroxysmal Positional Vertigo (BPPV). Dislodged calcium deposits (otoliths), usually in the posterior labyrinth, move in response to gravity eliciting a feeling of motion. This is most common in older individuals and may occur after head trauma or acute labyrinthitis. The onset is sudden, often when rolling over in bed or arising in the morning. There is no headache or fever. There is often intense nausea and inability to stand. Symptoms are minimized by avoiding any head motion. Dix-Hallpike maneuver produces mixed vertical and rotational nystagmus, after a 1- to 2-second(s) latent period, with fast components toward the dependent ear and upwards toward the forehead [Furman JM, Cass SP. Benign paroxysmal positional vertigo. *N Engl J Med.* 1999;341:1590–1596]. The nystagmus may be accompanied by profound symptoms of vertigo and nausea. Canilith repositioning is curative, but recurrences are not uncommon [Froehling DA, Bowen JM, Mohr DN, et al. The canalith repositioning procedure for the treatment of benign paroxysmal positional vertigo: A randomized controlled trial.' *Mayo Clin Proc.* 2000;75:695–700].

Labyrinthine Hydrops (Ménière Disease). Swelling of endolymphatic labyrinthine spaces with degeneration of the organ of Corti occurs with unknown cause. Symptoms are characterized by sudden attacks of whirling vertigo, tinnitus, and neurosensory hearing loss; there are intervals of complete freedom from vertigo, but the hearing loss and the tinnitus persist. An attack lasts hours but not days. Hearing loss predominates on one side and is fluctuating, but slowly progressive. Tinnitus also fluctuates, accentuating before an attack. The disease is self-limited. The cause of the hydrops is unknown. Labyrinthine tests are normal or hypoactive on the involved side.

Vascular Disease: Transient vertigo may be caused by vascular spasm or obstruction with transient low flow states. More severe and prolonged symptoms occur from thrombosis or dissection of a brainstem artery. There is sudden vertigo with nystagmus, loud tinnitus, and sudden deafness. Partial recovery is usual in 3 to 4 weeks.

Trauma: Skull fracture through the inner ear, concussion, or a loud noise may induce symptoms similar to a stroke. Tinnitus and hearing loss are present. Labyrinthine tests show delay and hypoactivity on the affected side.

Damage To CN VIII Or Brainstem Nuclei: Lesions, at either level; produce vertigo and nystagmus. Disorders of the eighth nerve (e.g., acoustic neuroma) are accompanied by hearing loss; this is absent with lesions of the brainstem except when other cranial nerves are also damaged.

Nose and Sinus Syndromes

KEY SYNDROME Rhinosinusitis

Infection, allergic inflammation or irritation of the respiratory epithelium lining the nose and paranasal sinuses leads to hyperemia, edema, increased mucous production and exudation of inflammatory cells. Patients experience congestion, nasal and postnasal discharge, sneezing, facial pressure and sometimes fever. Diagnosis depends upon an accurate history noting time of year, exposures and current infectious disease activity in the home and community. **DDX:** Sore throat and fever are not seen with rhinovirus infections. Fever, purulent or bloody discharge, or pain in the upper teeth beginning several days after onset of a cold suggests suppurative sinusitis. Sneezing and itchy eyes suggest allergic rhinosinusitis with allergic conjunctivitis.

Acute rhinitis. Rhinoviruses, and many others, infect the mucous membranes of the nose and sinuses causing inflammation and increased nasal secretions.

Beginning with a watery discharge (*rhinorrhea*) and sneezing, the nasal secretion ultimately becomes purulent, possibly accompanied by fever and malaise. Nasal obstruction occurs from edema of the mucosa. A sore throat is not part of the picture. Severe local pain suggests a complication, such as bacterial sinusitis.

Chronic Rhinitis. Chronic bilateral rhinorrhea suggests chronic environmental irritants (dust, smoke, perfume, dry or cold air), allergic rhinitis (seasonal or perennial), rhinitis medicamentosa or vasomotor rhinitis.

Atrophic Rhinitis. The complains of nasal discomfort or "stuffiness." The membranes appear dry, smooth, and shiny; they are studded with crusts. A foul odor (*ozena*) may be present. The cause is unknown.

The Common Cold. Rhinoviruses, and many others, infect the mucous membranes of the nose and sinuses causing inflammation and increased nasal secretions. The onset is abrupt with a watery discharge (*rhinorrhea*) and sneezing, often with malaise and mild myalgia, but without fever. Nasal obstruction occurs from edema of the mucosa. A sore throat is not part of the picture. The sinuses are involved in 75% of patients. Symptoms last 3 to 10 days and most people have 4 to 6 such infections per year. Severe local pain suggests a complication, such as bacterial sinusitis.

Allergic Rhinosinusitis. IgE-mediated mast cell degranulation follows exposure to specific allergens to which the patient has been sensitized by previous exposure. Itching of the nose and eyes, rhinorrhea, and lacrimation are accompanied by sneezing. Headache is common. The membranes are typically pale, swollen, and edematous; occasionally they are dull red or purplish. Allergic rhinitis may be seasonal or perennial. Common allergens are pollens, molds, animal danders, house dust mite and cockroach antigens. Symptoms are associated with seasonal exposure to pollens (trees in the spring; grasses in the summer; ragweed in the fall) or to antigens associated with a specific environment. Perennial allergic rhinitis suggests exposure to environmental antigens such as house dust mite and animal danders (usually cats) in the home.

Vasomotor Rhinitis Nonallergic mucosal edema and rhinorrhea are associated with vasodilation of the nasal vessels and increased mucous production. It is associated with environmental, hormonal, and pharmacologic exposures. Environmental irritants such as smoke, perfumes, strong odors, and cold air trigger increased mucous production and mucosal edema. Pregnancy and therapeutic estrogens and progestins have been associated. Chronic vasomotor rhinitis seems to result from an over reaction of the nasal and pharyngeal mucosa to environmental exposures.

Rhinitis Medicamentosa. Topical vasoconstrictors use for more than a few days leads to rebound hyperemia on withdrawal, triggering more medication use. The appearance is similar to allergic rhinitis. A history of using nasal vasoconstrictors and the absence of eosinophils in nasal secretions suggest the diagnosis.

> **KEY SYNDROME** **Suppurative Paranasal Sinusitis**

Most viral upper respiratory infections are accompanied by inflammation of the sinuses. Obstruction of the narrow sinus orifices leads to mucous accumulation which becomes secondarily infected by bacteria (*Streptococcus pneumoniae,*

Haemophilus influenzae, Moraxella spp.) leading to suppurative sinusitis. The maxillary sinus with its dependent antrum and superiorly positioned orifice is at particular risk. Severe pain in the face occurring 7 to 14 days after signs and symptoms of an acute upper respiratory infection suggests complicating acute suppurative bacterial sinusitis. Pain and pressure without fever earlier in the course of illness suggests sinus obstruction requiring decongestants [Williams JW, Simel DL. The rational clinical examination. Does this patient have sinusitis? Diagnosing acute sinusitis by history and physical exam. *JAMA*. 1993;270:1242–1246; Engels EA, Terrin N, Barza M, Lau J. Meta-analysis of diagnostic tests for acute sinusitis. *J Clin Epidemiol*. 2000;53:852–862; Piccirillo JF. Acute bacterial sinusitis. *N Engl J Med*. 2004;351:902–910]. Extension of infection beyond the sinus into surrounding soft tissue and bone is a serious complication; the symptoms and signs are specific to the sinus involved.

Maxillary Sinusitis causes dull throbbing pain in the cheek and the ipsilateral upper teeth. Thumb pressure discloses localized tenderness on the maxilla. Examination discloses a reddened, edematous mucosa and swollen turbinates. A purulent blood-tinged discharge may be seen. Pus in the posterior middle meatus may be seen in the nasopharyngeal mirror. **DDX:** Pain in the teeth with maxillary sinusitis must be distinguished from inflammation about a tooth; in the latter case, only one tooth is painful and may be tender when tapped with a probe.

Frontal Sinusitis produces pain in the forehead above the supraorbital ridge; pressure in this region elicits tenderness. Edema of the eyelids on the affected side is infrequent.

Ethmoid Sinusitis pain is medial to the eye and seems deep in the head or orbit; there is no localizing tenderness, although lid edema is common.

Sphenoid Sinusitis generates pain either behind the eye, in the occiput or in the vertex of the skull; no tenderness is produced.

Transillumination may reveal an opaque maxillary or frontal sinus; plain films may show clouding of the sinus or a fluid level. CT imaging is definitive. *There is no pain associated with chronic inflammation or infection of the paranasal sinuses.* **DDX:** Many patients with a history of recurrent "sinus headaches" actually have migraine; nasal and sinus symptoms are commonly seen with migraine as well as cluster headaches. Persistent and progressive symptoms should raise consideration of more serious diseases such as Wegener granulomatosis, nasopharyngeal carcinoma, and lethal midline granuloma.

Chronic Suppurative Sinusitis. When a purulent nasal discharge persists for more than 3 weeks, subacute or chronic sinusitis should be suspected. Pain over the sinuses is not a prominent symptom, and tenderness is frequently absent. Examination after instillation of a vasoconstrictor may disclose the source of the pus. Transillumination of the sinuses may assist in localization. The diagnosis of sinusitis is confirmed by CT. **DDX:** Chronic sinusitis resistant to medical therapy should suggest the possibility of common variable immunodeficiency. The finding of chronic suppurative sinusitis, especially with unusual organisms (e.g., fungi like *Aspergillus* spp. or Mucor spp.), warrants a search for other immunodeficiency.

► **KEY SYNDROME** **Sinusitis and Ocular Palsies—Cavernous Sinus Thrombosis**

Usually infection spreads from the nose through the angular vein to the cavernous sinus, where septic thrombosis occurs. This is the most feared complication of

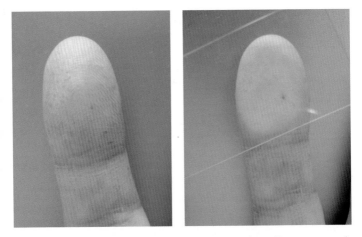

Plate 1. Petechia Confirmed by Diascopy. Several red vascular markings are seen on the index fingertip. Diascopy discloses that the lesions do not blanch and are therefore extravasated blood.

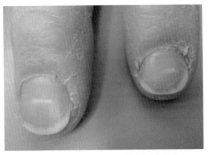

Plate 2. Mees Lines. White transverse lines form in the nails at the time of an acute illness. With very severe illness grooves appear called Beau's lines.

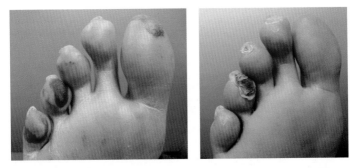

Plate 3. Atheroemboli (Blue Toes Syndrome). *Left:* Multiple sharply demarcated hemorrhagic blisters with surrounding erythema and edema. The foot is intensely painful. *Right:* The same foot six weeks later.

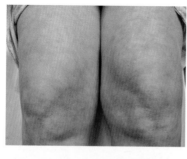

Plate 4. Livedo Reticularis. The net-like pattern of dilated cutaneous veins is readily apparent on both thighs.

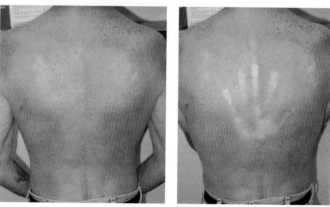

Plate 5. Erythroderma. There is diffuse, generalized cutaneous capillary dilation which blanches with hand pressure. This patient's erythroderma is due to systemic lupus erythematosus.

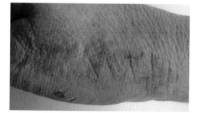

Plate 6. Contact Dermatitis. This lesion on the side of the thumb resulted from latex allergy in a nurse. The skin is erythematous, itchy, thickened and fissured (lichenoid) due to scratching.

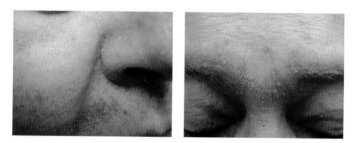

Plate 7. Seborrheic Dermatitis. Erythema and scaling in the nasolabial fold, eyebrows and glabella.

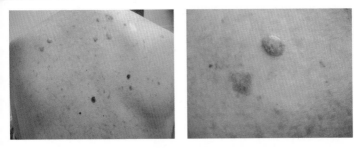

Plate 8. Seborrheic Keratoses and Lipoma. *Left:* Multiple "stuck on" lesions on the upper back with great variation in color. A subcutaneous lipoma is faintly visible superior and medial to the upper border of the right scapular spine. *Right:* Close up of two seborrheic keratoses showing variation in coloration and degree of elevation.

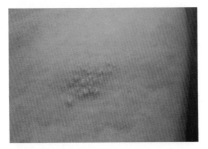

Plate 9. Herpes Simplex. A painful crop of vesicles and pustules has erupted on a well demarcated erythematous base in this patient's left groin.

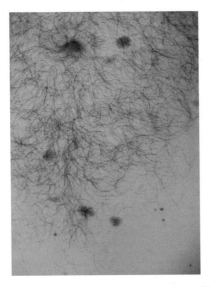

Plate 10. Cutaneous Nevi (Moles). Several benign nevi on the chest with different patterns of pigmentation.

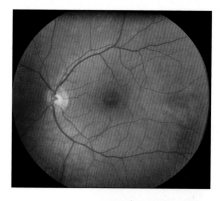

Plate 11. Normal Fundus. Normal left retinal vessels, macula, periphery and disc (Courtesy of Brice Critser, CRA).

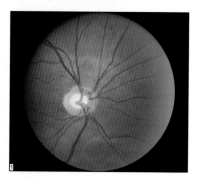

Plate 12. Physiologic Cupping. This right disc has an enlarged cup-to-disk ratio of approximately 0.5. The nerve rim is symmetrical top, bottom, nasal, and temporal. Physiologic cupping is confirmed by evaluation of intraocular pressure, formal visual fields, and the appearance of the optic nerve over time.

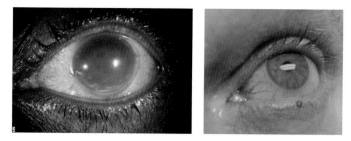

Plate 13. Uveitis. *Left:* This African American patient has severe uveitis from sarcoidosis. The episcleral vessels are dilated, the corneal endothelium is covered with inflammatory precipitates, and the iris is indistinct due to the anterior chamber cellular reaction. There is a mixed hypopyon (layered white blood cells) and hyphema (hemorrhage) within the inferior anterior chamber. The pupil has scarred in places to the lens by posterior synechiae, which causes the irregular appearance of the pupil. *Right:* This man with spondyloarthritis presented with bloody diarrhea and a red painful eye. He was diagnosed with ulcerative colitis complicated by spondyloarthropathy and uveitis. Note the ciliary flush.

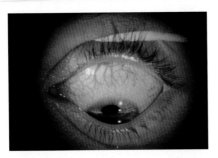

Plate 14. Episcleritis. Because the episcleral vessels lie below the conjunctival vessels, the dilated episcleral arterioles in episcleritis and uveitis has a violet hue.

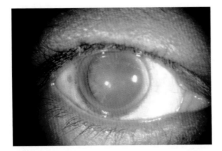

Plate 15. Cortical Cataract. This African American patient has characteristic anterior cortical spokes of the milky cortical cataract overlying a milder nuclear cataract.

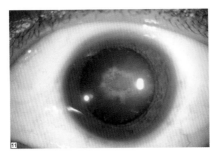

Plate 16. Posterior Subcapsular Cataract. This cataract is just inside the posterior lens capsule. The melanosis of the sclera is a normal variant in African Americans.

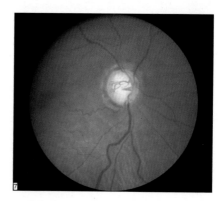

Plate 17. Glaucoma: Optic Atrophy. The right eye of this darkly pigmented patient shows a deeply excavated cup with a cup-to-disk ratio of 0.7–0.8. There is a large notch in inferior rim of the optic nerve (arrow), thinning of the rim elsewhere, and a disc hemorrhage nasally all consistent with advanced glaucoma. The remaining rim is pink. The cribriform plate can be seen in the base of the cup superiorly. Note the normal variation in the choroidal pattern of dark pigment and choroidal vessels.

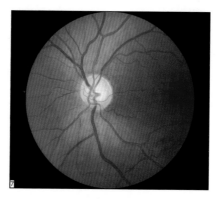

Plate 18. Optic Atrophy. This left optic nerve demonstrates pallor of the rim, making the distinction of the cup difficult. There is a small area of pink rim superonasally, but the remainder of the rim is atrophic. (Photo courtesy of Andrew Lee, MD)

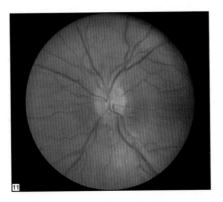

Plate 19. Disc Edema, Early. This left optic nerve head (disc) is hyperemic and the nerve fiber layer shows some edema, obscuring the details of the disc margin. There is a hemorrhage inferiorly on the disc head, dilation of some smaller disc vessels, and obscuration of some of the vessels as they cross within the edematous nerve fiber layer. (Photo courtesy of Andrew Lee, MD)

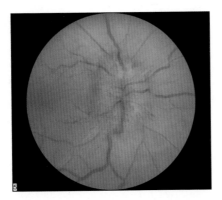

Plate 20. Disc Edema, Late. This right eye shows marked disc edema with hyperemia, nerve fiber layer edema obscuring the disc margins and disc vessels, and small flame hemorrhages. The disc is elevated, evidenced by the different focal plane of the disc head and the retina. The retinal veins are engorged and tortuous, and there is dilation of the smaller vessels on the disc head. (Photo Courtesy of Andrew Lee, MD)

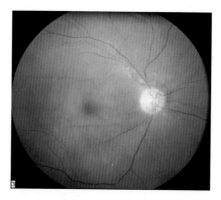

Plate 21. Central Retinal Artery Occlusion (CRAO). This right eye shows a CRAO from cholesterol emboli, fragments of which are lodged in the superior and inferior temporal arteries (Hollenhorst plaques). There is diffuse macular edema, a central cherry red spot, and thready residual arterial flow.

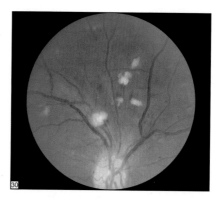

Plate 22. Hypertensive Retinopathy: Cotton Wool Spots and Arteriolar Changes. The superior aspect of this right eye and has multiple cotton wool spots (nerve fiber layer infarctions). There is increased arteriolar light reflex, arteriolar narrowing, and arteriovenous crossing changes consistent with hypertensive retinopathy.

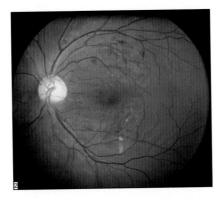

Plate 23. Hypertensive Retinopathy: Flame Hemorrhages. The left eye of this poorly controlled, hypertensive African American patient has a darkly pigmented choroid, a normal variant, which darkens the entire photograph. There are multiple flame hemorrhages within the plane of the nerve fiber layer. There are several cotton wool spots (nerve fiber layer infarctions). The nerve pallor is an artifact, but the enlarged cup-disc ratio of 0.6-0.7 suggests glaucoma.

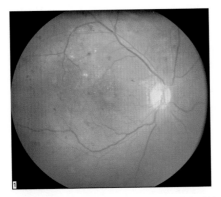

Plate 24. Diabetic Retinopathy: Non-Proliferative Retinopathy. This right eye shows diffuse, scattered dot and blot hemorrhages and microaneurysms. There is a small flame hemorrhage in the inferior macula. There is evidence of old superior macular focal photocoagulation for diabetic macular edema, as well as peripheral panretinal photocoagulation (PRP) for proliferative diabetic retinopathy (small, dull grey spots). There is recurrent neovascularization of the disc superotemporally. The central macula is dull and the landmarks indistinct suggesting persistent macular edema. The arterial caliber is narrow and the reflex increased, and there are several areas of arteriovenous nicking along the superior temporal arcade suggesting coexisting hypertension.

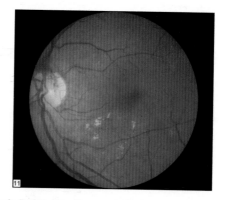

Plate 25. Diabetic Retinopathy: Neovascularization of the Disc (NVD). This left eye shows a superior area of NVD, as well as scattered and inferior macular exudate around background microaneurysms and dot-blot hemorrhages. The disc pallor is an artifact due to manipulating this photo to better demonstrate the diabetic findings.

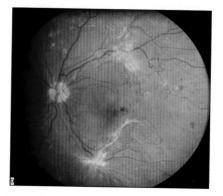

Plate 26. Diabetic Retinopathy: Proliferative Neovascularization. This left eye shows multifocal areas of proliferative fibrovascular diabetic neovascularization elsewhere (NVE), with traction between the superior and inferior vascular arcades. There are multiple omega loops in the veins, with venous beading and irregularity. There are several vessels on the disc head suspicious for neovascularization of the disc (NVD), and evidence peripherally of old incomplete pan retinal photocoagulation. There are multiple areas of dot blot hemorrhages and microaneurysms.

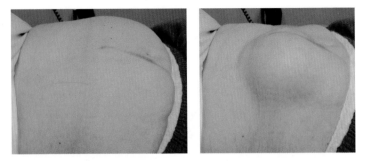

Plate 27. Abdominal Wall Hernia. This hernia is not evident when the patient is at rest on the exam table. Straining forces the abdominal contents into the hernia as the abdominal wall muscles contract.

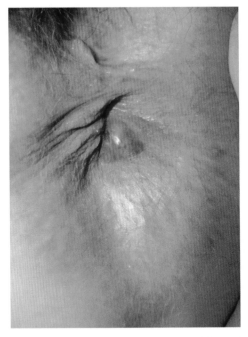

Plate 28. Hemorrhoid. External Hemorrhoid with a small skin break that resulted in bleeding.

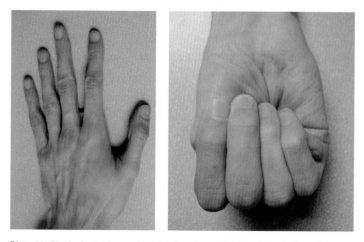

Plate 29. Marfan's Syndrome: Arachnodactyly and Positive Thumb Sign. These are signs of Marfan's syndrome. The long thin fingers are notable and the tip of the thumb extends beyond the fifth finger when bent into the palm of the hand.

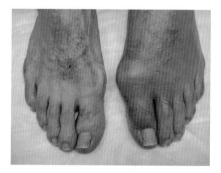

Plate 30. Podagra: Gout. The left first MTP joint is swollen and exquisitely tender; the entire forefoot is erythematous and warm. Note also the bunions (L > R).

nasal infections because it can cause blindness or death. There are sudden chills, high fever and deep in the eyes; the patient becomes prostrate and may rapidly become comatose. Early, there is ocular palsy involving the oculomotor (CN III), trochlear nerve (CN IV) or abducens nerve (CN VI) in the cavernous sinus. Both eyes are involved fairly early, with immobilization of the globes, periorbital edema, and chemosis. Death may occur within 2 or 3 days. **DDX:** Selective ocular palsy occurs early in cavernous sinus thrombosis, whereas orbital abscess produces complete immobilization of the globe gradually, without preliminary disorder of a single nerve. Bilaterality strongly suggests cavernous sinus thrombosis.

Oral Syndromes (Lips, Mouth, Tongue, Teeth, and Pharynx)

KEY SYNDROME   Difficulty Swallowing—Dysphagia

Swallowing is a complex voluntary and reflex event requiring normal sensory and neuromuscular function of the tongue, mouth, and pharynx. Impairment of any of these structures can produce difficulty swallowing. Careful patient observation during attempts to swallow thin and thickened liquids, soft foods and solid boluses will help to identify the site and nature of the problem. Speech therapists should assist with the evaluation and videofluoroscopy. See also page 216, and Chapter 9, pages 467 and 491.

CLINICAL OCCURRENCE: **Congenital** cerebral palsy, mental retardation; **Endocrine** hypothyroidism; **Inflammatory/Immune** amyloidosis, Sjögren syndrome, scleroderma; **Infectious** tonsillitis, quinsy, mononucleosis, epiglottitis, mumps, retropharyngeal abscess, chancre, gumma, actinomycosis, oral and esophageal herpes simplex and *Candida*; **Mechanical/Trauma** fractures, dislocation of the jaw, TMJ ankylosis, irradiation; **Neoplastic** sarcoma of the jaw, carcinoma; **Neurologic** stroke, bulbar paralysis, pseudobulbar paralysis, bilateral facial nerve palsy, myasthenia gravis, palsy of the hypoglossal nerve, diphtheritic palsy, Parkinson disease, rabies, botulism; **Psychosocial** hysteria.

KEY SYNDROME   Aberrant Right Subclavian Artery (Dysphagia Lusoria)

The right subclavian artery arises anomalously from the descending aorta distal to the left subclavian artery (Fig. 7–67). It crosses left to right and upward, either posterior to the esophagus, between the esophagus and trachea, or rarely anterior to the trachea, to reach the right axilla. In the first two positions, it puts pressure on the esophagus. Symptom onset is in adolescence or early adulthood with difficulty swallowing solid food. An esophagram shows a pressure notch in the esophagus.

KEY SYNDROME   Acute Pharyngitis

The chief problem is to distinguish treatable bacterial pharyngitis from viral infections. The clinician relies on antigen detection and cultures from the throat to make a specific diagnosis when this is felt necessary [Bisno AL. Acute pharyngitis. *N Engl J Med*. 2001;344:205–211].

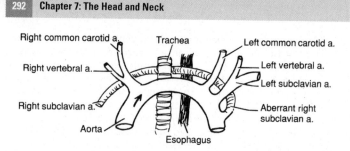

Fig. 7–67 *Aberrant Right Subclavian Artery.* *The right subclavian artery arises in the descending aorta, distal to the origin of the left subclavian artery. It crosses the midline either behind the esophagus, between the esophagus and the trachea, or anterior to the trachea. In either of the first two patterns, the artery may compress the esophagus producing difficulty in swallowing, "dysphagia lusoria." A transverse compression band in the esophagram suggests the diagnosis.*

Viral Pharyngitis. Pharyngeal inflammation accompanies many viral infections; the most common are Ebstein-Barr virus (EBV), respiratory syncytial virus (RSV), parainfluenza, influenza, adenovirus, and coxsackievirus. The patient complains of sore throat, often with mild rhinorrhea and hoarseness. In influenza, the patient is febrile and usually complains of malaise, myalgia, and often a moderately sore throat and rhinorrhea. Inspection of the oral cavity discloses only swelling of lymphoid tissue in the mucosa of the posterior oropharyngeal wall, seen as elevated oval islands (Fig. 7–68). The mucosa may be dull red and the faucial pillars slightly edematous. Herpes simplex may produce painful ulcers of the posterior pharynx, soft palate, buccal mucosa, or tongue, with punched out edges surrounded by a rim of erythema. A pale, boggy mucosa of the posterior pharynx caused by adenovirus may accompany the scratchy sore throat preceding the coryza of a cold.

Streptococcal or Staphylococcal Pharyngitis. The onset is often sudden; pain in the throat is severe; the temperature may rise to 39.5°C (103°F) or higher. The pharyngeal mucosa is bright red, swollen, and edematous, especially in the fauces and uvula; it is studded with white or yellow follicles. When the tonsils

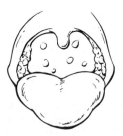

Fig. 7–68 *Granular Pharyngitis in Viral Infections.* *Elevated islands of lymphoid tissue are seen in the oropharyngeal mucosa. The mucosa is only slightly reddened; seldom is there any edema or exudate.*

infarction is indicated by the onset of shock, jaundice, or right-sided heart failure. Pulmonary hypertension is marked by the increasing loudness of P2 and the appearance of a palpable precordial RV thrust. Sudden death is not uncommon. Occasionally, pulmonary embolism may be accompanied by board-like rigidity of the abdomen, usually in the upper quadrant beneath the lung involved with the embolism. This is involuntary muscle spasm, so the region is not tender. Its occurrence is confusing because it tends to focus attention upon the abdomen. The evaluation for pulmonary emboli is controversial, but the clinician must have a high index of suspicion and pursue the diagnosis aggressively since recurrent emboli may be fatal. Chronic recurrent pulmonary emboli lead to pulmonary hypertension [Fedullo PF, Auger WR, Kerr KM, Rubin LJ. Chronic thromboembolic pulmonary hypertension. *N Engl J Med.* 2001;345:1465–1472]. **DDX:** Sudden onset of pain in the chest or dyspnea, tachypnea, or unexplained sinus tachycardia in a patient with a predisposing condition should raise the question of pulmonary embolism with or without infarction. The symptoms and signs may suggest asthma, bronchopneumonia, pleurisy, pericarditis, spontaneous pneumothorax, myocardial infarction, acute pancreatitis, or perforated peptic ulcer [Chunilal SD, Eikelboom JW, Attia J, et al. Does this patient have pulmonary embolism? *JAMA.* 2003;290:2849–2858].

> **KEY SYNDROME   Sleep-Disordered Breathing—Obstructive and Central Sleep Apnea**

Sleep-disordered breathing results from either mechanical obstruction by redundant, lax oropharyngeal soft tissues (*obstructive sleep apnea*) or from decreased medullary respiratory drive (*central sleep apnea*). Hypoventilation and hypoxia at night produce frequent arousals, disrupting effective sleep. Patients are often, but not always, obese. They have daytime hypersomnolence and irritability, and frequently have morning headaches and hypertension; snoring is prominent, but may not have been noted by the patient. History from the bed partner is critical. In severe disease, pulmonary hypertension develops as a consequence of severe hypoxia, leading to signs of right heart failure. Findings of enlargement of the base of the tongue and oropharyngeal soft tissue thickening by Mallampati score of 3 or 4 (Chapter 7, page 270) or neck circumference >43 cm (17 inches) in men or >40.5 cm (16 inches) in women are associated with an increased risk for obstructive sleep apnea.

> **KEY SYNDROME   Chronic Cough**

Chronic nonproductive cough results from chronic upper or lower airway, or esophageal irritation. Patients present with complaints of chronic irritating cough, with normal physical findings. The most common causes, accounting for 90% of cases, are chronic postnasal drip, unsuspected asthma, and gastroesophageal reflux. Specific evaluation for each entity is required. Angiotensin-converting enzyme inhibitors also cause chronic cough, which may begin months after starting the medication.

> **KEY SYNDROME   Pleural Effusion**

See page 352.

KEY DISEASE Lung Cancer

Most primary lung cancers result from cigarette smoking or exposure to ionizing radiation. Patients present with symptoms and signs related to the chest (cough, hemoptysis, dyspnea, pneumonia, pleural effusion), regional symptoms (lymphadenopathy, SVC syndrome, brain mass) or systemic symptoms (weight loss, weakness, hypercalcemia, hyponatremia). Endobronchial lesions may present as recurrent or slowly resolving pneumonia or atelectasis. *Bronchioloalveolar cell carcinoma* presents with cough, hypoxia and diffuse infiltrates, often mistaken for an infection. Early detection strategies are controversial. Superior sulcus tumors (neoplasms in the pulmonary apex, the upper mediastinum, or the superior thoracic aperture) produce *Pancoast syndrome* in which there is severe pain in the neck or shoulder or down the arm [Arcasoy SM, Jett JR. Superior pulmonary sulcus tumors and Pancoast's syndrome. *N Engl J Med.* 1997:337:1370–1376].

➤ KEY SYNDROME Pulmonary Edema

Pulmonary interstitial edema leading to alveolar flooding is caused by LV failure, mitral regurgitation or acute lung injury. An acute increase in LV end-diastolic pressure is transmitted across the mitral valve to the left atrium and pulmonary veins. The increased hydrostatic pressure in the pulmonary capillaries causes transudation of fluid into the pulmonary interstitium and subsequently the alveoli. Increased fluid in the lung leads to decreased pulmonary compliance, shortness of breath, and cough. As the alveoli are flooded, hypoxia and extreme respiratory distress ensue. Intense dyspnea is accompanied by crackles, rhonchi and gurgles throughout the lungs. Breathing is labored, with cyanosis and frothy sputum, often pink, occasionally bloody. Percussion is resonant and auscultation reveals bubbling crackles and sometimes wheezes. **DDX:** In chronic heart failure, the condition is often relapsing and the diagnosis fairly obvious. It may occur suddenly with acute myocardial infarction, especially with papillary muscle rupture and flail mitral valve. Occasionally, paroxysmal nocturnal dyspnea in cardiac patients may closely resemble asthma with a prolonged expiratory phase and wheezing.

✔ ***PULMONARY EDEMA—CLINICAL OCCURRENCE:*** ***Idiopathic*** high altitude; ***Inflammatory/Immune*** mismatched blood transfusion, hypertransfusion syndrome, SLE; ***Metabolic/Toxic*** acute lung injury (inhalation of noxious gases, aspiration, radiation, hemorrhagic pancreatitis, sepsis, drugs, fresh water drowning, etc.), intravenous heroin, snakebite; ***Mechanical/Trauma*** LV failure-systolic and diastolic dysfunction (myocardial infarction, cardiomyopathies, tachy- and bradyarrhythmias), mitral stenosis, mitral and aortic insufficiency (especially acute), pulmonary embolism; ***Neoplastic*** bronchioloalveolar cell carcinoma (not pulmonary edema, but may appear similar radiographically), lymphangitic carcinoma or lymphoma; ***Neurologic*** postictal, head trauma, subarachnoid hemorrhage; ***Vascular*** severe hypertension, intravascular volume overload (crystalloid, colloid, transfusions, kidney failure).

KEY SYNDROME Interstitial Lung Disease

Inflammation with cellular infiltration, interstitial edema, and/or collagen deposition leads to thickening of the alveolar walls and septa, decreased lung compliance, reduced lung volume, and impaired gas exchange. Inflammation may involve the entire alveolus; granuloma formation is characteristic of some diseases and is diagnostically important. Patients usually present with chronic cough and dyspnea, with little or no sputum production. A thorough occupational and avocational exposure history is critical to the identification of respiratory irritant, toxins, and allergens. Physical examination shows resonant percussion, decreased breath sounds, and crackles of varying intensity, often at end inspiration and usually most prominent at the bases. X-ray films show increased interstitial markings, with or without alveolar signs [Gong MN, Mark EJ. Case records of the Massachusetts General Hospital. Case 40-2002. *N Engl J Med*. 2002;347:2149–2157]. High-resolution CT may be diagnostic with characteristic patterns for specific entities [Gross TJ, Hunninghake GW. Idiopathic pulmonary fibrosis. *N Engl J Med*. 2001;345:517–525; Collard HR, King TE Jr. Demystifying idiopathic interstitial pneumonia. *Arch Intern Med*. 2003;163:17–29].

INTERSTITIAL LUNG DISEASE—CLINICAL OCCURRENCE: *Inhaled Toxic Substances* asbestosis, fumes and gases, aspiration pneumonia; with granulomas—hypersensitivity pneumonitis (organic dusts, e.g., farmer's lung), inorganic dusts (beryllium, silica); *Lung Injury* after acute respiratory distress syndrome, radiation; *Connective-Tissue Diseases* SLE, RA, ankylosing spondylitis, systemic sclerosis, CREST (calcinosis cutis, Raynaud phenomenon, esophageal motility disorder, sclerodactyly, and telangiectasia) syndrome, Sjögren syndrome, polymyositis-dermatomyositis; *Pulmonary Hemorrhage Syndromes* Goodpasture, idiopathic pulmonary hemosiderosis; *Congenital Diseases* tuberous sclerosis, neurofibromatosis, Niemann-Pick disease, Gaucher disease; *Miscellaneous* drugs (antibiotics, amiodarone, gold, bleomycin and other chemotherapy agents), eosinophilic pneumonia, lymphangioleiomyomatosis, amyloidosis, graft-versus-host disease, with gastrointestinal or liver disease (Crohn disease, ulcerative colitis, primary biliary cirrhosis, chronic active hepatitis); *Idiopathic Interstitial Pneumonia* idiopathic interstitial pneumonia (usual interstitial pneumonia), desquamative interstitial pneumonia, respiratory bronchiolitis-associated interstitial lung disease, acute interstitial pneumonia, cryptogenic organizing pneumonia, nonspecific interstitial pneumonia.

KEY SYNDROME Hypersensitivity Pneumonitis

Exposure to organic dusts in the work or home environment elicits a chronic inflammatory response in the lung which may progress to irreversible fibrosis. Careful history is the key to diagnosis. Patients present with cough, shortness of breath, and increasing dyspnea, often with airflow obstruction on exposure to the agent. Examination may be normal or show crackles and wheezes.

KEY SYNDROME Pulmonary-Renal Syndromes

Antibodies to glomerular basement membrane and pulmonary capillaries (Goodpasture), or vasculitis involving the lung and glomeruli (Wegener's granulomatosis), injure glomeruli injury and cause pulmonary inflammation and/or hemorrhage. Goodpasture syndrome often presents acutely with dyspnea, hemoptysis, and cough. Wegener's may be either acute or subacute. Limited forms of both occur. Prompt diagnosis and treatment is required to preserve renal function.

KEY SYNDROME   Sarcoidosis

Noncaseating granulomatous inflammation involves many organs singly or in combination. The cause is unknown. The lungs and hilar and mediastinal lymph nodes are most commonly affected. Patients may be asymptomatic or present with nonproductive cough and dyspnea accompanied by fever, malaise, weight loss, and night sweats. Lung examination may be normal or show crackles; hepatosplenomegaly, lymphadenopathy, uveitis, cutaneous plaques and salivary gland enlargement may be present.

KEY SYNDROME   Hepatopulmonary Syndrome

Pulmonary arteriovenous shunts enlarge with standing leading to decreased oxygen saturation (*orthodeoxia*) and shortness of breath. The cause appears to be circulating vasodilators usually metabolized by the liver. Patients all have advanced liver disease with portal hypertension and portosystemic shunting, with or without cirrhosis. They complain of shortness of breath and weakness with standing and may become visibly cyanotic in the upright position. Symptoms are often relieved by sitting and always by lying down; patients may become unable to sit or stand for any length of time. Physical examination shows stigmata of chronic liver disease including spider angiomata and ascites; cyanosis may be present in the upright position. Diagnosis is by bubble contrast echocardiography which shows appearance of contrast in the left atrium in more than 3 and less than seven cardiac cycles [Lange PA, Stoller JK. The hepatopulmonary syndrome. *Ann Intern Med.* 1995;122:521–529].

► KEY SYNDROME   Tracheal or Bronchial Obstruction

Complete obstruction of the trachea is incompatible with life. Partial tracheal obstruction by a foreign body, neoplasm or other plug produces forceful prolonged inspiratory effort with retraction of the intercostal spaces, suprasternal notch, supraclavicular fossae, and epigastrium. A low-pitched rhonchus, or stridor, may be heard over the chest and at the opened mouth during inspiration and expiration. In a ball-valve obstruction, the rhonchus occurs only during inspiration or expiration. An isolated wheeze suggests a localized bronchial obstruction by bronchial adenoma, carcinoma, or foreign body. Bagpipe sign is another indication of partial bronchial obstruction. While listening to the chest, have the patient cut short a forced expiration; an expiratory sound continues after the patient's effort has ceased. If the obstructive rhonchus is heard on both sides of the chest, the affected side is the one with the palpable rhonchus. In obstruction of a large bronchus, there is a pendular movement of the trachea toward the affected side during inspiration and away from it with expiration. Movement of a foreign body may cause an audible slap with coughing or breathing. Slow development of bronchial obstruction may be asymptomatic; sudden obstruction causes severe dyspnea. Higher-pitched rhonchi arise from smaller bronchi. **CLINICAL OCCURRENCE:**   Aspirated foreign bodies, intraluminal neoplasms (benign [bronchial adenoma, amyloidoma] or malignant [primary lung cancer]), relapsing polychondritis, extrinsic compression from mediastinal masses (retrosternal goiter, neoplasms, teratoma), laryngeal mass or paralysis, tracheomalacia following prolonged endotracheal intubation.

Chronic Obstructive Pulmonary Diseases

Airflow obstruction in expiration is the hallmark of asthma and chronic obstructive lung disease (COPD). The obstruction is fully reversible, at least initially, in asthma and may be either fixed or partially reversible in COPD. Expiratory airflow obstruction leads to air trapping (increased residual volume) and a sustained inspiratory position of the chest (flat diaphragm, horizontal ribs, increased anterior-posterior diameter, hyperresonance) which increases the work of breathing and decreases the inspiratory capacity. The combination of history, physical signs, chest radiographic features and results of pulmonary function testing allow differentiation of the different syndromes [Straus SE, McAlister FA, Sackett DL, et al. The accuracy of patient history, wheezing, and laryngeal measurements in diagnosing obstructive airway disease. *JAMA*. 2000;283:1853–1857; Holleman DR Jr, Simel DL. The rational clinical examination. Does the clinical examination predict airflow limitation? *JAMA*. 1995;273:313–319].

> **KEY SYNDROME   Asthma**

Asthma is an acquired syndrome of increased airway responsiveness to allergic and nonallergic stimuli, airway inflammation, bronchospasm, hyperplasia of mucous-producing cells, and bronchial smooth muscle hypertrophy. Airway obstruction leads to air trapping and lung hyperinflation. Asymptomatic patients may have active airway inflammation. Between attacks, the patient is well and the chest findings are normal. An asthma flair frequently begins with nonproductive cough and progressive dyspnea. Nocturnal awaking with attacks of coughing and chest tightness is common. Sitting and leaning over a table or chair back improves the dyspnea. The respiratory rate does not increase, but inspiration is short while expiration is prolonged and labored; the patient is often anxious. As air trapping increases, the chest becomes hyperresonant, the diaphragm flattens and the thorax maintains the inspiratory position. The costal margins only diverge slightly, or they may actually converge during inspiration. In severe asthma attacks, the sternocleidomastoid and platysma muscles tense and the alae nasi flare with each inspiratory effort. Wheezing becomes less prominent as the attack worsens. Auscultation discloses decreased air movement, wheezes, and coarse crackles. Localized absence of breath sounds suggests bronchial plugging. As the attack subsides, clear tenacious sputum is raised, and breathing gradually becomes less labored. Asthma can occur without wheezing. The only sign that consistently identifies severe asthma is use of the accessory muscles of respiration. Clinical history and bedside or home airflow measurements are useful for assessment of severity (Table 8–1) and planning management. **DDX:** Asthma can be confused with other

Table 8–1   Asthma Clinical Severity Classification

| Asthma Severity | Symptoms | | FEV_1; *Peak expiratory flow variability* |
	Day	Night	
Mild Intermittent	2 or less days/week	2 or less nights/month	≥ 80; *<20%*
Mild Persistent	>2 days/week	>2 nights/month	≥ 80; *20–30%*
Moderate Persistent	Daily	> 1 night/week	60–79%; *>30%*
Severe Persistent	Continual	Frequent	<60%; *>30%*

Table 8–2 Gold Criteria for COPD Severity

Stage	Severity	FEV$_1$ (% predicted)	FEV$_1$/FVC
I	Mild	≥ 80	<0.7
II	Moderate	< 80	<0.7
III	Severe	< 50	<0.7
IV	Very severe	<30 or < 50 with respiratory failure or right heart failure	<0.7

conditions. Wheezing occurs in acute bronchitis, without the labored respiration. When wheezing is limited to a single region, bronchial obstruction from foreign body or neoplasm should be considered. The sudden occurrence of LV failure or mitral regurgitation may closely simulate asthma: there are wheezes and crackles, and labored breathing may limit heart auscultation. Vocal cord dysfunction (i.e., paradoxical closure of the cords during inspiration) may be identified by examination of the glottis during an attack; it is suggested when the wheezes are loudest over the neck. The symptoms and signs of asthma are often relieved in a few minutes by inhaled bronchodilators; reversible airway obstruction can be demonstrated with pulmonary function testing.

KEY SYNDROME Emphysema

Smoking leads to the destruction of alveolar walls with loss of alveolar surface area and decreased elastic recoil produces collapse with expiration. Patients present with progressive dyspnea, often accompanied by gradual weight loss. They often exhale with pursed-lips, especially with exertion. The chest is hyperresonant with decreased breath sounds and prolonged expiration (page 354). Wheezes and crackles are uncommon unless infection supervenes. Physical findings are poorly correlated with the severity of airflow obstruction or abnormalities of gas exchange. Early detection of obstructive airways disease in patients with symptoms or risk factors is best accomplished by spirometry. The Gold clinical staging system is now used to classify patients, see Table 8–2.

KEY SYNDROME Chronic Bronchitis

Chronic inflammation and secondary infection of the airways results from chronic exposure to tobacco smoke. Airways obstruction is prominent and hypoxia common. Patients present with chronic cough with >60 mL/d of sputum (chronic bronchitis with or without bronchiectasis) and progressive dyspnea. Lung examination shows diminished breath sounds and prolongation of expiration; wheezing and inspiratory crackles may be present. Physical finding are poorly correlated with the severity of airflow obstruction or abnormalities of gas exchange.

Bronchiectasis. Severe acute or chronic pulmonary infections result in multiple chronically infected dilatations of the smaller bronchi. Cough with purulent sputum and occasionally hemoptysis or recurrent pneumonia is the presenting symptom. Sputum is copious and purulent. A resonant chest with coarse basilar crackles suggests bronchiectasis. Clubbing may be present. Chronic infection with nontuberculous mycobacteria is common. High-resolution CT imaging is diagnostic [Barker AF. Bronchiectasis. *N Engl J Med.* 2002;346:1383–1393].

Churg-Strauss disease: See page 415.

Lymphomatoid granulomatosis.   A variegated array of lymph cells, atypical lymphocytoid, plasmacytoid, and reticuloendothelial cells invade various tissues and vessels. Nodules of various sizes occur in the lungs, skin, kidneys, and central nervous system; the spleen, lymph nodes, and bone marrow are usually spared. In contrast with Wegener granulomatosis, the lung is always involved but the upper respiratory tract is seldom involved. Transition to malignant lymphoma is common.

Cardiovascular Syndromes
Fourfold Diagnosis of Heart Disease

Proper assessment of patients with heart disease requires a fourfold description: the etiology, anatomic abnormalities, physiologic disorders and functional capacity. A formal statement of the diagnosis is as follows: "rheumatic heart disease, inactive; mitral stenosis, right ventricular hypertrophy and dilatation, pulmonary congestion; atrial fibrillation; functional class II."

Etiologic diagnosis.   Common etiologies are congenital, infectious, rheumatic, hypertensive, and ischemic.

Anatomic diagnosis.   Abnormalities of the aorta and pulmonary arteries, coronary arteries, endocardium and valves, myocardium and pericardium are listed. Congenital anatomic abnormalities are listed as either cyanotic or noncyanotic (i.e., with or without significant right-to-left shunt).

Physiologic diagnosis.   Disturbances in cardiac rhythm and conduction, myocardial, systolic or diastolic dysfunction, and clinical syndrome (e.g., anginal syndrome, CHF, cardiac tamponade) are listed.

Functional cardiac diagnosis.   Two commonly used functional classification systems are:

New York Heart Association (for classification of angina or dyspnea)
Class I (No Incapacity). Although the patient has heart disease, the functional capacity is not sufficiently impaired to produce symptoms.
Class II (Slight Limitation). The patient is comfortable at rest and with mild exertion. Symptoms occur only with more strenuous activity.
Class III (Incapacity with Slight Exertion). The patient is comfortable at rest but dyspnea, fatigue, palpitation, or angina appears with slight exertion.
Class IV (Incapacity with Rest). The slightest exertion invariably produces symptoms, and symptoms frequently occur at rest.

Canadian Cardiovascular Society (use restricted to patients with angina)
Class I. No angina with ordinary activity but angina occurs with strenuous or rapid or prolonged exertion.
Class II. Slight limitation of ordinary activity (e.g., walking more than two level blocks or climbing more than one flight of stairs at a normal pace).
Class III. Marked limitation of ordinary activity (walking one to two blocks on the level and climbing one flight of stairs).

Class IV. Inability to carry on any physical activity without angina; angina may also be present at rest.

More recently a new classification has been created for chronic heart failure [ACC/AHA guideline update for the diagnosis and management of chronic heart failure in the adult. *J Am Coll Cardiol.* 2005;46:1116–1143 or *Circulation.* 2005;112:1825–1852].

Stage A: Patients at high risk for heart failure but without structural heart disease or symptoms of heart failure

Stage B: Patients with structural heart disease but without signs or symptoms of heart failure.

Stage C: Patients with structural heart disease with *prior or current* symptoms of heart disease.

Stage D: Patients with refractory heart failure (symptoms at rest despite maximal medical therapy) requiring specialized intervention.

Patients once assigned to a given heart failure stage cannot be reclassified to an earlier stage, e.g., reverting back from Stage C to Stage B. This is in contrast to the New York Heart Association and Canadian Cardiovascular Society classifications where patients may move from any class to another as symptoms change.

Six-Dermatome Pain Syndromes

See Six-Dermatome Pain, page 333.

Myocardial Ischemia Six-Dermatome Pain Syndromes

KEY SYNDROME   Angina Pectoris

Angina is caused by a reversible increase in local myocardial oxygen demand exceeding supply. Angina may result from inadequate oxygen supply, excessive demand, or a combination of both. Abnormalities of oxygen delivery can be best remembered by rearrangement of the Fick equation: $MVO_2 =$ (coronary blood flow) × (myocardial arteriovenous oxygen difference). Because the arteriovenous oxygen difference is nearly maximal at rest, decreased oxygen delivery is most likely due to decreased coronary flow. Flow is directly proportional to the pressure driving blood through the coronary arteries, the aortic diastolic pressure, and inversely proportional to the coronary artery flow resistance. The most common cause of impaired oxygen delivery is coronary artery obstruction caused by atherosclerotic narrowing. Cold or exertion induced vasospasm may be superimposed. Increased myocardial oxygen demand is caused by increases in heart rate, myocardial contractility, ventricular systolic pressure, and/or ventricular cavity radius. The increase in oxygen demand occurs whether or not there is a change in cardiac output or stroke volume. Angina pectoris is a deep, steady pain or discomfort lasting 1 to 10 minutes in the six-dermatome region and often accompanied by shortness of breath, anxiety and diaphoresis. It is classically precipitated by exercise or anxiety and relieved by rest. Other precipitants are related to the cause of increased myocardial oxygen demand: clinically important examples of increased rate work are sinus tachycardia and atrial or ventricular tachycardias; digitalis, other inotropic agents and anxiety increase contractility; hypertension and aortic stenosis increase systolic LV pressure; and aortic regurgitation and systolic heart failure increase LV radius. Stable angina is reproducible, does not awaken the patient at night, or occur at rest without significant provocation [Chun AA, McGee SR. Bedside diagnosis of CAD: A systematic review. *Am J Med.* 2004;117:334–343]. **PQRST:** *Provocation* Stable angina has several classic provocations. (1) *Exertion.* An important characteristic of exertional angina is the lag period before the pain begins, and again, before it subsides with rest. Exertional pain without a lag period suggests another etiology; (2) *Postprandial.* Exertion after a heavy meal is especially an issue; (3) *Intense emotion.* Fear, anxiety and sexual desire increase heart rate, blood pressure and contractility; (4) *Cold.* Peripheral vasoconstriction and increased blood pressure and heart rate may play a role; (5) *Positive inotropic or chronotropic drug effects.* Caffeine, amphetamines and cocaine increase the heart rate and blood pressure; (6) *Anemia.* Oxygen delivery is reduced when the hemoglobin is less than 10 g/dL. *Palliation* Rest, a warm environment, nitroglycerin, and the Valsalva maneuver each may relieve an angina attack. ***Complete relief of pain or other discomfort in the six-dermatome band after the administration of nitroglycerin is strongly suggestive of angina pectoris but it is not diagnostic.*** The pain of esophageal spasm may also respond to nitroglycerin. If headache or flushing occurs without pain relief, stable angina is unlikely. **Quality** Angina is usually described as crushing, aching, or a sense of tightness or pressure, frequently illustrated by clenching the fist over the sternum, the *Levine sign.* **Region-Radiation** The pain may occur anywhere in the six-dermatome band. Often it is most intense behind the sternum or in the precordium, radiating upward into the neck or throat, or down the medial aspect of either arm. Ischemia in the right coronary artery distribution may radiate to the interscapular region of the back. Less frequently, the pain is felt in the spine or right shoulder and arm. The rare patient complains of pain in the limbs or neck exclusively, denying chest pain. **Severity** Pain may be mild, moderate, or severe and sometimes causing a sense of impending death. **Timing** The pain is continuous, not fleeting or lancinating usually lasting from 1 to 10 minutes. **Physical Signs**. No physical findings may be present. S4 frequently occur during angina because of decreased compliance of the ischemic ventricle. Less commonly, an S3 may appear. If papillary muscle ischemia occurs, an apical systolic mitral insufficiency murmur may be heard. A precordial bulge or apical thrust due to LV dyskinesia may be palpated. **DDX:** Anginal attacks are brief (<10 minutes), which usually excludes myocardial infarction, dissecting aneurysm, pulmonary embolism, and neoplasm. Atherosclerotic CAD is the most common cause, but less common causes of reduced coronary flow include vasculitis, aortic regurgitation, LV hypertrophy, anemia and hypoxemia. Pain with swallowing and a sensation of food sticking suggest an esophageal source. The supine position often initiates gastroesophageal reflux pain, "heartburn." Pain from cholecystitis often occurs after meals but without concurrent exertion; epigastric and/or right upper quadrant tenderness support gallbladder disease. When walking induces pains in the shoulder girdle or spine, as well as the chest, and there is no lag period, musculoskeletal pain is favored. Angina is now clinically classified as follows:

TYPICAL (OR DEFINITE) ANGINA: (1) substernal chest discomfort with the characteristic quality and duration that is (2) provoked by exertion or emotional stress and (3) relieved by rest or nitroglycerin.

ATYPICAL (OR POSSIBLE) ANGINA: meets two of the three characteristics listed above.

NONCARDIAC CHEST PAIN: meets one or none of the typical angina characteristics.

Variant Angina Pectoris (Prinzmetal Angina): Coronary artery spasm with ST-segment elevations occurs with or without angiographically detectable coronary narrowing. The pain quality and location resemble classic angina, but it occurs at rest. The pain recurs in cycles, often at the same time each day. ST segments on ECG are transiently elevated during pain suggesting myocardial injury. Pain is relieved promptly by nitroglycerin. Migraine and Raynaud phenomenon occur more commonly in patients with variant angina.

> **KEY SYNDROME** — Acute Coronary Syndromes: Unstable Angina and Myocardial Infarction

There is almost always disruption of the endothelium overlying an atherosclerotic coronary plaque, exposing the plaque contents to platelets and procoagulants, initiating formation of a platelet plug, a fibrin clot, and release of vasoconstrictor substances resulting in intermittent or fixed arterial obstruction. Myocardial necrosis occurs with prolonged severe ischemia. Lesser degrees of ischemia result in unstable angina syndromes and myocardial hibernation (decreased contractile function without pain or necrosis). Less-common causes of acute coronary syndromes are coronary artery embolism and vasculitis. The transition from severe ischemia to infarction is gradual and depends upon the collateral coronary flow to the ischemic area, the contractile state of the myocardium, and the previous history of that myocardium. There is evidence that myocardium subjected to repeated episodes of ischemia (stable angina) is relatively less susceptible to infarction.

➤ **Unstable Angina:** Patients present with classic anginal pain that is new in onset, worsening in severity (more easily provoked and/or more difficult to relieve, lasting >15 minutes), occurring at rest or awakening the patient from sleep, but *is not associated with evidence of myocardial necrosis.* These syndromes are best described as unstable angina with a detailed description of the unstable pattern, for example, prolonged pain, occurring at rest, and increasing frequency. A substantial number of patients, although a minority, will develop an acute myocardial infarction if untreated.

The **TIMI Risk Score** is used to estimate risk for rapid evolution to acute ST-elevation myocardial infarction in patients with unstable angina and non-ST-elevation acute MI. Give 1 point each for age ≥65 years, ≥3 traditional risk factors (CAD family history, hypertension, hypercholesterolemia, diabetes, current smoker), known ≥50% coronary stenosis, ST-segment changes, ≥2 anginal episodes in the preceding 24 hours, aspirin use in the last 7 days and elevated CK or troponin. Scores of 0–2 are low risk, 3–4 intermediate risk and ≥5 are high risk.

➤ **Acute Myocardial Infarction (MI).** MI occurs most commonly from the early morning hours to midday. The pain is usually not induced by exertion, nor does it remit with rest. The discomfort is identical to angina pectoris in its quality, location, intensity, and constancy, but it lasts from 20 minutes to several hours. In some cases, the pain quickly increases to an intensity seldom experienced with angina; this may be sustained for hours, after which the pain subsides to a dull ache that can last for days. The patient often complains of shortness of breath that may be related to increased LV end diastolic pressure, depressed systolic function or mitral insufficiency due to papillary muscle dysfunction. Nausea and vomiting are common, particularly with inferior wall infarction. A sympathetic response is triggered with sweating, pallor, and cold moist skin. The heart rate may be slow, normal, or accelerated; similarly, blood pressure may be low, normal, or quite elevated. An S4 may be heard; the heart sounds often become muted. Crackles may appear at the lung bases. Cardiac rhythms requiring immediate therapy may occur at any time. A pericardial friction rub appears in approximately 15% > 24 hours after onset of the MI. Occasionally, myocardial infarction is painless and the diagnosis is suggested by the associated symptoms and signs. Large infarcts produce rapid progression to shock, cardiac failure, and death. **DDX:** Simple angina is excluded by the longer pain duration and unresponsiveness to nitroglycerin. Three potentially life-threatening disorders may closely mimic the pain and presentation of MI: massive, central pulmonary embolism (PE) (page 392), acute dissection of the thoracic aorta (page 405) and acute pericarditis (page 404). The clear lung fields by physical examination and chest X-ray in the setting of marked dyspnea and hypotension suggests PE rather than MI. Pain from dissection may be more excruciating and reach peak intensity more rapidly than MI. Prominent pain in the back makes dissection more likely, however, pain radiation to the back occurs with MI and may be absent with dissection. Development of an aortic diastolic murmur transmitted, down the right sternal border, and/or asymmetrical pulses or blood pressures between extremities, suggests supports dissection. The pain of acute pericarditis may be severe and resemble MI; the pain may be intensified by reclining, breathing or swallowing. Adding potential confusion is the fact that pericarditis can be a sequel of MI [Panju AA, Hemmelgarn BR, Guyatt GH, Simel DL. The rational clinical examination. Is this patient having a myocardial infarction? *JAMA.* 1998;280:1256–1263; Goldman L, Kirtane AJ. Triage of patients with acute chest pain and possible cardiac ischemia: The elusive search for diagnostic perfection. *Ann Intern Med.* 2003;139:987–995].

Current recommended terminology for myocardial infarction (necrosis documented by elevated cardiac biomarkers such as troponin) is based on the EKG interpretation. Those presenting with ST elevations are termed *ST elevation infarctions.* Most of these will go on to form Q waves, so that the infarction is then also called a *Q-wave myocardial infarction.* If no Q forms, the term non-Q-wave myocardial infarction is then applied. If no ST elevation occurs, the term *non-ST elevation myocardial infarction* is applied. Most of these do not form Q waves, and the term *non-Q-wave myocardial infarction* is then also applied. If a Q wave does appear, then the infarction is also labeled as a Q-wave infarction.

Inflammatory Six-Dermatome Pain Syndromes

KEY SIGN Postcardiotomy Syndrome

Several weeks after myocardial infarction, cardiac surgery, or penetrating and nonpenetrating heart injury, a hypersensitivity reaction to antigen derived from injured myocardium occurs. The syndrome is characterized by fever, pericarditis, pleuritis, pericardial or pleural effusions, and pneumonitis. Recurrences are common, usually with decreasing severity. The symptoms often respond dramatically to anti-inflammatory drugs. Recurrent myocardial infarction should be considered when the syndrome occurs in patients with ischemic heart disease. The appearance of a pericardial friction rub with the pain and absence of new Q waves or ST-segment depressions on the ECG help distinguish the syndrome from recurrent MI.

> **KEY SIGN** **Acute Pericarditis**

The visceral pericardium and the inner surface of the parietal pericardium are anesthetic (Fig. 8–44), but the outer surface of the lower parietal pericardium is pain sensitive. Closely enveloping the anterior and lateral pericardium is the sensitive parietal pleura explaining pleural involvement from pericarditis. Inflammation of the esophagus and phrenic nerves due to their close proximity causes dysphagia and phrenic pain. All these structures are innervated by fibers from the vagus and six-dermatome band. Phrenic nerve sensory fibers from the central diaphragm can be irritated in the lower pericardium causing neck pain at the superior border of the trapezius. **Symptoms** Deep constant or pleuritic pain occurs in the six-dermatome band or the phrenic distribution, often with a pericardial friction rub or ECG signs. The location and quality of pain often resembles that of myocardial infarction, but it is usually accentuated by breathing or coughing, worse in recumbency, and lessened while sitting and leaning forward. It may be intensified by swallowing. Pleuritic pain referred to the shoulder, particularly the left trapezius ridge, is quite suggestive of pericarditis (see Fig. 8–43, page 389). The pain may last for hours; it is not relieved by nitroglycerin. Rarely, the pain is throbbing and synchronous with the heartbeat. **Signs** The onset of pain may be followed by fever. A transient pericardial friction rub is often heard. **ECG** Widespread elevation of the ST segments followed by inversion of T waves, when present, is fairly diagnostic. The ECG signs of pericarditis must be differentiated from the injury currents of infarction and from early repolarization changes that

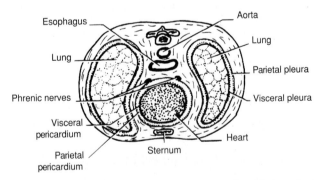

Fig. 8–44 Pleuropericardial Relationships. *A transverse section of the lower thorax with anesthetic serosal surfaces represented by heavy beaded lines and pain-sensitive surfaces by lighter beaded lines. Note the proximity of the phrenic nerves and esophagus to the parietal pericardium, so pericarditis can produce pain in the phrenic nerve distribution or pain on swallowing.*

represent a normal variant. **DDX:** Pericarditis may result from almost any infectious agent, malignancy, rheumatic fever, collagen vascular diseases, trauma, uremia, or following myocardial infarction or radiation to the chest. Until a pericardial friction rub appears or ECG signs develop, the steady pain suggests myocardial infarction, dissecting aneurysm, pulmonary infarction, cholecystitis, or peptic ulcer. Pain on swallowing may suggest an esophageal lesion. The pleural pain must be distinguished from that of pleurisy, subphrenic abscess, and splenic infarction [Spodick DH. Acute pericarditis: Current concepts and practice. *JAMA.* 2003;289:1150–1153].

Mediastinal and Vascular Six-Dermatome Pain Syndromes

➤ **KEY SYNDROME** Aortic Dissection

Cystic medial necrosis and intramural hemorrhage lead to intimal rupture, or intimal tears may be the primary event. The intimal tear occurs most commonly in the lateral wall of the proximal ascending aorta, or, less commonly, just distal to the ligamentum arteriosum in the descending aorta. Luminal blood penetrates the weakened media producing a hematoma that splits the vessel wall. Distal progression sequentially occludes the mouths of aortic branches causing ischemia in the affected parts. A second intimal tear may occur distally providing egress from the false lumen; thus the aorta may consist of two concentric tubes, a double-barreled aorta. There is progressive diminution of pulses in the aortic branches and loss of specific nerve functions. **Symptoms** In 80% of cases, the onset is sudden, with excruciating pain that is felt in the precordium and/or the interscapular region, and that may shift successively to the lower back, abdomen, hips, and thighs. The pain often suggests myocardial infarction. In some, the onset is gradual often without chest pain. **Signs** Blood pressure is usually sustained, in contrast to hypotension in MI. Hypotension and collapse occur with rupture into the pericardium or left pleural space. **Proximal Progression:** When the hematoma extends proximally from a tear in the aortic arch, it may: (1) distort the aortic valve ring separating the commissures and causing aortic regurgitation, the murmur often transmits down the right sternal border; (2) occlude the coronary ostia and cause an MI; (3) produce hemopericardium with a pericardial rub and cardiac tamponade; or (4) swell the base of the aorta, causing a pulsating sternoclavicular joint. This sign distinguishes dissection from myocardial infarction. **Distal Progression:** When the hematoma extends away from the heart, progression is indicated by sequential asymmetrical decrease or loss of arterial pulses in aortic branches and signs of nervous system injury in these regions. Carotid occlusion causes cerebral ischemia with localizing neurologic signs. Obstruction of the spinal arteries is indicated by paraplegia and anesthesia. Renal artery occlusion with infarction causes pain simulating renal colic. Aortic dissection may be rapidly fatal [Klompas M. The rational clinical examination. Does this patient have an acute thoracic aortic dissection? *JAMA.* 2002;287:2262–2272]. **Chest X-ray** Widening of the aorta, an enlarged aortic knob or separation of calcified intimal plaques from the outer border of the aortic wall all suggest dissection. Imaging studies should be performed urgently when dissection is suspected. **DDX:** Most commonly, dissection occurs in association with cystic medial necrosis of the aorta, especially in patients with Marfan and Ehlers-Danlos syndromes. It occurs with less frequency in patients with hypertension, advancing age, during labor, and after penetrating or blunt trauma. Dissection may occur in a thoracic aortic aneurysm afflicted with aortitis from bacteria, syphilis, or giant cell arteritis.

➤ **Leakage and Rupture of Aortic Aneurysm:** Expansion of aneurysms is usually painless, but breach of the wall with leakage of blood into the surrounding tissue is accompanied by the sudden onset of severe pain at the site of leakage or radiating into the body wall at that spinal segment. The pain is often accompanied by restlessness, diaphoresis and tachycardia. The specific pain pattern reflects the site of leakage. Urgent evaluation and surgery is life saving. Complete rupture presents as sudden severe pain followed shortly by refractory hypotension and death.

> **KEY SYNDROME** Mediastinal Tumors

Although mediastinal lesions rarely cause chest pain, they are considered here because of their location in the six-dermatome band. Most mediastinal masses attract attention by compression of normal structures or are found incidentally on chest X-ray. Physical signs suggesting mediastinal tumors are dyspnea from retrosternal goiter, hoarseness and brassy cough from compression of the recurrent laryngeal nerve, *Horner syndrome* (unilateral ptosis, miosis, and anhidrosis) from involvement of the superior cervical ganglion, edema of the arms and neck with cyanosis from obstruction of the SVC and chylous pleural effusion. Lymph nodes are enlarged in Hodgkin disease, non-Hodgkin lymphoma, carcinoma, germ cell tumors or tuberculosis. Other locations of neoplastic tissue are retrosternal goiter, thymoma, and teratoma (dermoid cyst). When a dermoid forms a tracheal fistula, it may produce the elegant sign of coughing hair, or *trichoptysis*.

> **KEY SYNDROME** Mediastinal Emphysema

See page 345 and Esophageal Rupture, below.

Gastrointestinal Six-Dermatome Pain Syndromes

> **KEY SYNDROME** Spontaneous Esophageal Rupture (Boerhaave Syndrome)

Forceful vomiting is suddenly accompanied by pain in the chest or upper abdomen and severe dyspnea. Subcutaneous emphysema may appear in the supraclavicular fossae along with a crunching sound in the precordium indicating mediastinal emphysema (*Hamman sign*). Chest X-ray shows air in the mediastinum. DDX: The symptoms are common to MI, perforated peptic ulcer, cholecystitis, pancreatitis, esophagitis, hepatitis, nonperforating ulcer, and pneumonia. The demonstration of mediastinal emphysema excludes all the foregoing in favor of ruptured esophagus.

Esophageal Discomfort: See Chapter 9, page 491.

> **KEY SYNDROME** Six-Dermatome Pain with Dysphagia

See Chapter 9, page 491.

KEY SYNDROME Subphrenic Diseases

Although lesions below the diaphragm usually produce abdominal pain, frequent exceptions make it imperative to consider subphrenic disorders with six-dermatome band pain. It is dangerous to the patient and embarrassing to the physician to overlook this possibility. Subphrenic abscess, acute cholecystitis, peptic ulcer, acute pancreatitis, and splenic infarction need to be considered.

Pulmonary Six-Dermatome Pain Syndromes

KEY SYNDROME Pulmonary Artery Embolism and Pulmonary Infarction

See page 392.

KEY SYNDROME Pneumothorax

See pages 390.

Other Cardiovascular Syndromes

KEY SYNDROME Pulmonary Edema

See page 394.

KEY SYNDROME Cardiac Dilatation

Dilatation of heart chambers is caused by either poor systolic function or chronic volume overload. The dilated heart of trained athletes accommodates a larger stroke volume maintaining a high cardiac output at relatively low heart rates, thereby minimizing myocardial oxygen demand. Heart enlargement detectable by physical examination (apical impulse and borders of cardiac dullness) or chest radiograph implies dilatation of a cardiac chamber. The elongated fibers of the dilated heart with depressed contractility produce a weak apical impulse, which may be more diffuse than normal. Displacement of the apical impulse to the left with a normal right heart border suggests LV dilation. **DDX:** Pericardial effusions will enlarge the heart silhouette and borders of dullness, but the apical impulse is usually undetectable and the heart sounds are diminished. **CLINICAL OCCURRENCE:** **LV Dilation** aortic insufficiency, mitral insufficiency, ischemic cardiomyopathy, after myocardial infarction, dilated cardiomyopathy, viral myocarditis; **Right Ventricular Dilation** pulmonic insufficiency, tricuspid insufficiency, ASD with left-to-right shunt, right ventricular infarction, pulmonary hypertension with right ventricular failure.

KEY SYNDROME Cardiac Hypertrophy

Hypertrophy occurs with or without dilation because of pressure and/or volume overload or hypertrophic cardiomyopathy. Hypertrophied LV myocardium produces a more powerful apical impulse than normal. Enlargement of the chamber on physical examination is not present without concomitant dilation (Fig. 8–45). A palpable thrust along the left sternal edge, over the right ventricle, may be

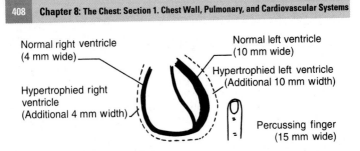

Fig. 8–45 *Contribution of Myocardial Hypertrophy to the Area of Cardiac Dullness.* *Without dilatation of the chambers, concentric hypertrophy of the cardiac muscle to twice its normal thickness and weight cannot cause enough increase in an area of cardiac dullness to exceed the width of the percussing finger. Therefore, increase in the area of dullness must be attributed to dilatation when pericardial effusion is excluded.*

produced by right ventricular hypertrophy. **CLINICAL OCCURRENCE:** *LV Hypertrophy* valvular aortic stenosis, mitral or aortic insufficiency, hypertension, hypertrophic cardiomyopathy; *Right Ventricular Hypertrophy* pulmonic stenosis, ASD, pulmonary hypertension, hypertrophic cardiomyopathy.

KEY SYNDROME Congestive Heart Failure (CHF)

Classically, decreased LV contractility leads to increased left ventricular end-diastolic pressure and LV dilation, maintaining higher stroke volume at the expense left atrial hypertension and dilation and distention of the pulmonary veins. Decreased cardiac output with renal hypoperfusion leads to retention of salt and water, weight gain, and edema. The ventricular ejection fraction is low when systolic function is impaired but not when congestion is principally caused by diastolic dysfunction, that is, decreased diastolic compliance. Symptoms and signs are attributable to decreased cardiac output and volume expansion with pulmonary and peripheral vascular congestion. Early symptoms of LV failure are pulmonary congestion with dyspnea, orthopnea, nocturia, and cough. Crackles are heard in the lung bases. Retrograde congestion causes right-ventricular failure with elevated CVP, indicated by engorged jugular veins [Butman SM, Ewy GA, Standen JR, et al. Bedside cardiovascular examination in patients with severe chronic heart failure: Importance of rest or inducible jugular venous distension. *J Am Coll Cardiol.* 1993;22:968–974; Dosh SA. Diagnosis of heart failure in adults. *Am Fam Physician.* 2004;70:2145–2152]. Even before the increase in CVP, a hepatojugular reflux sign can be demonstrated. Frequently an S3 develops [Drazner MH, Rame JE, Stevenson LW, Dries DL. Prognostic importance of elevated jugular venous pressure and a third heart sound in patients with heart failure. *N Engl J Med.* 2001;345:574–581; Marcus GM, Gerber IL, et a l. Association between phonocardiographic third and fourth heart sounds and objective measures of left ventricular function. *JAMA.* 2005;293:2238–2244; Badgett RG, Lucey CR, Mulrow CD. The rational clinical examination. Can the clinical examination diagnose left-sided heart failure in adults? *JAMA.* 1997;277:1712–1719; Wang CS, Fitz Gerald JM, Schulzer M, et al. Does this dyspneic patient in the emergency department have congestive heart failure? *JAMA.* 2005;294:1944–1956]. Arterial pressure response to the Valsalva maneuver correlates inversely with the left ventricular filling pressure; absence of the normal "overshoot" of systolic pressure arrhythmias. All health care personnel should be trained in basic cardiopulmonary resuscitation, and nurses and physicians should be trained in Advanced Cardiac Life Support.

Pericardial Syndromes

Acute Pericarditis: See page 404.

Postpericardiotomy Syndrome: See page 403.

Pericardial effusion. Fluid accumulates within the pericardial sac due to infection, inflammation, malignancy or transudation. Slowly accumulating fluid distends the pericardium compressing surrounding lung; rapidly accumulating fluid is more likely to compress the heart chambers producing tamponade. Symptoms may be absent or will reflect the etiology (e.g., pain and fever with pericarditis, weakness, nausea and anorexia with uremia) or the hemodynamic consequences (e.g., shortness of breath and fatigue with tamponade). Signs include absent precordial impulse, decreased intensity and muffling or heart sounds, and low voltage ECG; a rub may be present. Ewart's sign is dullness at the left scapular due to compression atelectasis of the left lower lobe from large effusions.

✔ **PERICARDIAL EFFUSION—CLINICAL OCCURRENCE:** *Congenital* Familial Mediterranean Fever, familial pericarditis; *Endocrine* hypothyroidism; *Idiopathic* sarcoidosis; *Inflammatory/Immune* rheumatic fever, SLE, RA, ankylosing spondylitis, scleroderma, Wegner's, drug reactions; *Infectious* bacterial, viral, tuberculosis, fungal, Whipple's; *Metabolic/Toxic* drug induced, uremia; *Mechanical/Trauma* trauma, post-pericardiotomy, post-irradiation; *Neoplastic* metastatic carcinoma, especially lung and breast, lymphoma; *Vascular* myocardial infarction, aortic dissection with rupture into the pericardium, chylopericardium, vasculitis.

| KEY SYNDROME | Constrictive Pericarditis |

Progressive pericardial fibrosis leads to restricted diastolic filling and cardiac output. Symptoms are shortness of breath and fatigue. Signs are those of right heart failure: jugular venous distention, dependent edema, ascites, and hepatic congestion. The initial pericardial injury is caused by pericarditis (viral, tuberculosis, neoplasm), cardiac surgery, mediastinal irradiation, and uremia [Wang ZJ, Bhore TM. Undercover and overlooked. *N Engl J Med*. 2004;351:1014–10]. DDX: It must be distinguished from restrictive cardiomyopathies and right ventricular failure.

| KEY SYNDROME | Pericardial Tamponade |

For massive accumulation of fluid within the relatively noncompliant pericardial space leads to compression of the heart chambers, impairing diastolic filling of the atria and ventricles. Cardiac output falls and CVP is elevated. Patients complain of shortness of breath and fatigue that may rapidly progress to hypotension and circulatory failure due to decreased cardiac output. The key signs are an elevated CVP with clear lung fields, no stigmata of chronic ventricular failure, and a drop in systolic blood pressure during inspiration of mm Hg (paradoxical pulse, page 384 and Fig. 8–42). Pulsus paradoxus is found in the presence of aortic insufficiency, left or right ventricular

following release the Valsalva and failure of the BP to drop during the breath hold suggest increasing LV filling pressure [Felker GM, Cuculich PS, Gheorghiade M. The Valsalva maneuver: A bedside "biomarker" for heart failure. *Am J Med*. 2006;119:117–122]. With biventricular failure, the liver becomes large, tender, and painful. Chronic congestive hepatomegaly may produce capsular and parenchymal fibrosis without tenderness. Edema fluid accumulates as right-sided or bilateral hydrothorax, ascites, and pitting edema of the ankles, legs, genitals, and abdomen. The lips, ears, and nail beds may be cyanotic. Impaired cerebral circulation may result in confusion and periodic breathing. Physical examination findings have independent prognostic value [Marantz PR, Tobin JN, Wassertheil-Smoller S, et al. Prognosis in ischemic heart disease. Can you tell as much at the bedside as in the nuclear laboratory? *Arch Intern Med*. 1992;152:2433–2437]. **DDX:** Portal hypertension may present similarly except that the patient does not have orthopnea or elevated jugular venous pressure. Metastasis from carcinoma may produce fluid in the abdominal and thoracic cavities with a distribution similar to that in cardiac failure [Jessup M, Brozena S. Heart failure. *N Engl J Med*. 2003;348:2007–2018]. **CLINICAL OCCURRENCE:** The most common cause is chronic ischemic CAD. Dilated cardiomyopathy (pregnancy and postpartum, alcohol, hemochromatosis, idiopathic, secondary to viral infections) is also common, especially in younger patients. Diastolic heart failure is common in long-standing hypertension with LVH and hypertrophic cardiomyopathies. Restrictive cardiomyopathy may result from amyloidosis, hemochromatosis, sarcoidosis and other infiltrative diseases.

Right Ventricular Failure and Cor Pulmonale: Right ventricular failure occurs because of damage to the myocardium, volume overload, and/or pressure overload of the right ventricle. The right and left ventricles function together; so LV failure also may be accompanied by some of right ventricular function. When the CVP exceeds 22 cm, the liver enlarges; above 25 cm, there are ascites, edema, and orthopnea. The venous pressure is always high with RV failure, but it falls before other signs of failure resolve. The most frequent cause of right ventricular failure is advanced ischemic heart disease. Right ventricular failure caused by primary pulmonary disease is called *cor pulmonale*. It occurs as a consequence of pulmonary hypertension resulting from hypoxia induced vasoconstriction or obliteration of the pulmonary vascular bed. **CLINICAL OCCURRENCE:** *Impaired Myocardial Function* ischemic heart disease (especially right ventricular infarction), hypertrophic and dilated cardiomyopathies, endomyocardial fibrosis (e.g., drugs, carcinoid syndrome), restrictive myocardial disease (e.g., amyloidosis); *Volume Overload* TR, ASD with left-to-right shunt, pulmonic insufficiency; *Pressure Overload* primary pulmonary hypertension, secondary pulmonary hypertension—cor pulmonale (hypoxia caused by emphysema, cystic fibrosis, interstitial pulmonary diseases, pneumoconioses, hypersensitivity pneumonitis, pulmonary fibrosis, etc.), pulmonary embolus, pulmonic stenosis, Eisenmenger complex, mitral stenosis, pulmonary veno-occlusive disease.

| KEY SYNDROME | Restrictive Cardiomyopathy |

Cardiac output is limited by impedance to ventricular filling as a result of decreased myocardial compliance leading to elevated ventricular end-diastolic pressure. Systolic function is preserved. Patients present with dyspnea exacerbated by exertion and intermittent pulmonary congestion. Signs of right ventricular failure with edema, elevated CVP, and ascites may predominate. The heart is not enlarged. S4 gallops are common. Causes are ventricular diastolic dysfunction, infiltrative disease of the heart (amyloid, sarcoid, hemochromatosis), and endomyocardial fibroelastosis. **DDX:** This must be distinguished from hypertrophic cardiomyopathy and constrictive pericarditis.

KEY SYNDROME   Hypertrophic Cardiomyopathy

Inherited defects of myocardial contractile proteins lead to progressive hypertrophy, disorganization of myocardial architecture, impaired diastolic relaxation, ventricular conduction abnormalities and dysrhythmias. Asymmetric septal hypertrophy may produce dynamic obstruction to LV outflow during early systole. A family history of sudden death is common. Patients present with dyspnea, angina, and presyncopal symptoms. The carotid upstrokes are brisk and may show a bisferiens pattern. S4 gallop is common. A characteristic murmur, augmented with Valsalva, is heard when outflow obstruction is present (see page 376). Presentation without a family history may represent spontaneous mutations. Echocardiography is diagnostic.

KEY SYNDROME   Infective Endocarditis

Infection of the heart valves leads to formation of fibrin-platelet vegetations harboring the infective agent. Low virulence organisms (e.g., viridans streptococci, HACEK organisms) present with subacute disease; high virulence organisms (e.g., *Staphylococcus aureus*, fungi) present with acute symptoms and rapid valvular destruction with or without systemic emboli.   ***Subacute Bacterial Endocarditis***   Patients present with a subacute or chronic illness with fever, weight loss, arthralgia, myalgias, and signs of immune complex disease.   ***Acute Endocarditis***   Patients have fever and rigors and often a history of injection drug use. Peripheral emboli with organ infarction and metastatic infection are common. Systemic illness with diffuse manifestations, especially with a new insufficiency murmur, should always trigger an evaluation for endocarditis. The Duke criteria are sensitive and specific for the diagnosis [Durack DT, Lukas AS, Bright DK. New criteria for diagnosis of infective endocarditis. *Am J Med.* 1994;96:200–209].

KEY SYNDROME   Nonbacterial Thrombotic Endocarditis (NBTE)

NBTE results from inflammation of the endocardium with sterile vegetations. Multiple large emboli suggest *marantic endocarditis* associated with occult neoplasms, most often a mucin-secreting adenocarcinoma. Libman-Sacks lesions occur on the valves and endocardium with SLE and antiphospholipid syndrome. The latter patients may be asymptomatic, have peripheral emboli to the brain and elsewhere, or present with progressive valvular stenosis or regurgitation.

KEY SYNDROME   Valvular Heart Disease

These clinical conditions are discussed with their physical findings under the sections Cardiovascular Signs, page 361 and Auscultation of Heart Murmurs, page 372ff.

Valvular Aortic Stenosis: See page 372.
Aortic Regurgitation: See page 378.
Valvular Pulmonic Stenosis: See page 374.
Pulmonary Insufficiency: See page 379.
Tricuspid Stenosis: See page 379.
Tricuspid Regurgitation: See page 376.
Mitral Valve Stenosis: See page 380.
Mitral Regurgitation: See page 370.
Mitral Valve Prolapse: See page 377.

KEY SYNDROME   Congenital Heart Disease

Many patients with congenital heart disease are surviving well into adult life. clinicians should be familiar with the more common syndromes. ASDs and sm VSDs may be asymptomatic for decades and elude diagnosis well into adult li

Atrial Septal Defect: See page 374.
Ventricular Septal Defect: See page 376.
Patent Ductus Arteriosus: See page 381.
Coarctation of Aorta: See pages 374 and 421.
Eisenmenger Syndrome: Due to intra or extra-cardiac left-to-right shunting of blood between the pulmonary and arterial circulation, chronic volume and/or pressure overload occurs on the right ventricle and pulmonary arteries which respond with hypertrophy and fibromuscular hyperplasia, respectively, leading to severe pulmonary hypertension and eventual reversal of the original flow into a right-to-left shunt with peripheral hypoxemia and cyanosis. This should be suspected when valvular signs are coupled with cyanosis, decreased oxygen saturation not relieved with 100% oxygen, right-to-left shunt, clubbing of the fingers and/or toes and polycythemia. Imaging is required to determine the underlying anatomy and flows.
Tetralogy of Fallot: The components of the tetralogy are a VSD, obstruction to right ventricular outflow (usually infundibular pulmonic stenosis), a overriding aorta, and right ventricular hypertrophy (see Fig. 8–41D, r 375).
Ebstein Anomaly: There is congenital tricuspid valve deformity with s cusps; a portion of the valve originates below the AV ring, produc ized" portion of the right ventricle. TR is present but not a prom dysrhythmias are common.

KEY SYNDROME   Sudden Cardiac Death—Cardia

Cardiac arrest demands immediate treatment for any 25% of patients, sudden cardiac death is the first sym most are subsequently found to have severe disease pertrophic cardiomyopathy (especially in young emboli, right ventricular dysplasia, Brugada sy anomalous coronary artery anatomy. Public basic cardiopulmonary resuscitation. Increa present in public places for use by trained in following release the Valsalva and failure of the BP to drop during the breath hold suggest increasing LV filling pressure [Felker GM, Cuculich PS, Gheorghiade M. The Valsalva maneuver: A bedside "biomarker" for heart failure. *Am J Med.* 2006;119:117–122]. With biventricular failure, the liver becomes large, tender, and painful. Chronic congestive hepatomegaly may produce capsular and parenchymal fibrosis without tenderness. Edema fluid accumulates as right-sided or bilateral hydrothorax, ascites, and pitting edema of the ankles, legs, genitals, and abdomen. The lips, ears, and nail beds may be cyanotic. Impaired cerebral circulation may result in confusion and periodic breathing. Physical examination findings have independent prognostic value [Marantz PR, Tobin JN, Wassertheil-Smoller S, et al. Prognosis in ischemic heart disease. Can you tell as much at the bedside as in the nuclear laboratory? *Arch Intern Med.* 1992;152:2433–2437]. **DDX:** Portal hypertension may present similarly except that the patient does not have orthopnea or elevated jugular venous pressure. Metastasis from carcinoma may produce fluid in the abdominal and thoracic cavities with a distribution similar to that in cardiac failure [Jessup M, Brozena S. Heart failure. *N Engl J Med.* 2003;348:2007–2018]. **CLINICAL OCCURRENCE:** The most common cause is chronic ischemic CAD. Dilated cardiomyopathy (pregnancy and postpartum, alcohol, hemochromatosis, idiopathic, secondary to viral infections) is also common, especially in younger patients. Diastolic heart failure is common in long-standing hypertension with LVH and hypertrophic cardiomyopathies. Restrictive cardiomyopathy may result from amyloidosis, hemochromatosis, sarcoidosis and other infiltrative diseases.

Right Ventricular Failure and Cor Pulmonale: Right ventricular failure occurs because of damage to the myocardium, volume overload, and/or pressure overload of the right ventricle. The right and left ventricles function together; so LV failure also may be accompanied by some of right ventricular function. When the CVP exceeds 22 cm, the liver enlarges; above 25 cm, there are ascites, edema, and orthopnea. The venous pressure is always high with RV failure, but it falls before other signs of failure resolve. The most frequent cause of right ventricular failure is advanced ischemic heart disease. Right ventricular failure caused by primary pulmonary disease is called *cor pulmonale*. It occurs as a consequence of pulmonary hypertension resulting from hypoxia induced vasoconstriction or obliteration of the pulmonary vascular bed. **CLINICAL OCCURRENCE:** **Impaired Myocardial Function** ischemic heart disease (especially right ventricular infarction), hypertrophic and dilated cardiomyopathies, endomyocardial fibrosis (e.g., drugs, carcinoid syndrome), restrictive myocardial disease (e.g., amyloidosis); **Volume Overload** TR, ASD with left-to-right shunt, pulmonic insufficiency; **Pressure Overload** primary pulmonary hypertension, secondary pulmonary hypertension—cor pulmonale (hypoxia caused by emphysema, cystic fibrosis, interstitial pulmonary diseases, pneumoconioses, hypersensitivity pneumonitis, pulmonary fibrosis, etc.), pulmonary embolus, pulmonic stenosis, Eisenmenger complex, mitral stenosis, pulmonary veno-occlusive disease.

KEY SYNDROME **Restrictive Cardiomyopathy**

Cardiac output is limited by impedance to ventricular filling as a result of decreased myocardial compliance leading to elevated ventricular end-diastolic pressure. Systolic function is preserved. Patients present with dyspnea exacerbated by exertion and intermittent pulmonary congestion. Signs of right ventricular failure with edema, elevated CVP, and ascites may predominate. The heart is not enlarged. S4 gallops are common. Causes are ventricular diastolic dysfunction, infiltrative disease of the heart (amyloid, sarcoid, hemochromatosis), and endomyocardial fibroelastosis. **DDX:** This must be distinguished from hypertrophic cardiomyopathy and constrictive pericarditis.

KEY SYNDROME   Hypertrophic Cardiomyopathy

Inherited defects of myocardial contractile proteins lead to progressive hypertrophy, disorganization of myocardial architecture, impaired diastolic relaxation, ventricular conduction abnormalities and dysrhythmias. Asymmetric septal hypertrophy may produce dynamic obstruction to LV outflow during early systole. A family history of sudden death is common. Patients present with dyspnea, angina, and presyncopal symptoms. The carotid upstrokes are brisk and may show a bisferiens pattern. S4 gallop is common. A characteristic murmur, augmented with Valsalva, is heard when outflow obstruction is present (see page 376). Presentation without a family history may represent spontaneous mutations. Echocardiography is diagnostic.

KEY SYNDROME   Infective Endocarditis

Infection of the heart valves leads to formation of fibrin-platelet vegetations harboring the infective agent. Low virulence organisms (e.g., viridans streptococci, HACEK organisms) present with subacute disease; high virulence organisms (e.g., *Staphylococcus aureus*, fungi) present with acute symptoms and rapid valvular destruction with or without systemic emboli.   ***Subacute Bacterial Endocarditis***   Patients present with a subacute or chronic illness with fever, weight loss, arthralgia, myalgias, and signs of immune complex disease.   ***Acute Endocarditis***   Patients have fever and rigors and often a history of injection drug use. Peripheral emboli with organ infarction and metastatic infection are common. Systemic illness with diffuse manifestations, especially with a new insufficiency murmur, should always trigger an evaluation for endocarditis. The Duke criteria are sensitive and specific for the diagnosis [Durack DT, Lukas AS, Bright DK. New criteria for diagnosis of infective endocarditis. *Am J Med.* 1994;96:200–209].

KEY SYNDROME   Nonbacterial Thrombotic Endocarditis (NBTE)

NBTE results from inflammation of the endocardium with sterile vegetations. Multiple large emboli suggest *marantic endocarditis* associated with occult neoplasms, most often a mucin-secreting adenocarcinoma. Libman-Sacks lesions occur on the valves and endocardium with SLE and antiphospholipid syndrome. The latter patients may be asymptomatic, have peripheral emboli to the brain and elsewhere, or present with progressive valvular stenosis or regurgitation.

KEY SYNDROME   Valvular Heart Disease

These clinical conditions are discussed with their physical findings under the sections Cardiovascular Signs, page 361 and Auscultation of Heart Murmurs, page 372ff.

Valvular Aortic Stenosis: See page 372.

Aortic Regurgitation: See page 378.

Valvular Pulmonic Stenosis: See page 374.

Pulmonary Insufficiency: See page 379.

Tricuspid Stenosis: See page 379.

Tricuspid Regurgitation: See page 376.

Mitral Valve Stenosis: See page 380.

Mitral Regurgitation: See page 370.

Mitral Valve Prolapse: See page 377.

KEY SYNDROME   Congenital Heart Disease

Many patients with congenital heart disease are surviving well into adult life. All clinicians should be familiar with the more common syndromes. ASDs and small VSDs may be asymptomatic for decades and elude diagnosis well into adult life.

Atrial Septal Defect: See page 374.

Ventricular Septal Defect: See page 376.

Patent Ductus Arteriosus: See page 381.

Coarctation of Aorta: See pages 374 and 421.

Eisenmenger Syndrome: Due to intra or extra-cardiac left-to-right shunting of blood between the pulmonary and arterial circulation, chronic volume and/or pressure overload occurs on the right ventricle and pulmonary arteries which respond with hypertrophy and fibromuscular hyperplasia, respectively, leading to severe pulmonary hypertension and eventual reversal of the original flow into a right-to-left shunt with peripheral hypoxemia and cyanosis. This should be suspected when valvular signs are coupled with cyanosis, decreased oxygen saturation not relieved with 100% oxygen, right-to-left shunt, clubbing of the fingers and/or toes and polycythemia. Imaging is required to determine the underlying anatomy and flows.

Tetralogy of Fallot: The components of the tetralogy are a VSD, obstruction to right ventricular outflow (usually infundibular pulmonic stenosis), an overriding aorta, and right ventricular hypertrophy (see Fig. 8–41D, page 375).

Ebstein Anomaly: There is congenital tricuspid valve deformity with small thin cusps; a portion of the valve originates below the AV ring, producing "atrialized" portion of the right ventricle. TR is present but not a prominent feature; dysrhythmias are common.

KEY SYNDROME   Sudden Cardiac Death—Cardiac Arrest

Cardiac arrest demands immediate treatment for any chance of survival. For 25% of patients, sudden cardiac death is the first symptom of CAD, even though most are subsequently found to have severe disease. Less-common causes are hypertrophic cardiomyopathy (especially in young male athletes), coronary artery emboli, right ventricular dysplasia, Brugada syndrome, long QT syndrome, and anomalous coronary artery anatomy. Public education seeks to teach all adults in basic cardiopulmonary resuscitation. Increasingly, automated defibrillators are present in public places for use by trained individuals to reverse fatal ventricular arrhythmias. All health care personnel should be trained in basic cardiopulmonary resuscitation, and nurses and physicians should be trained in Advanced Cardiac Life Support.

Pericardial Syndromes

Acute Pericarditis: See page 404.

Postpericardiotomy Syndrome: See page 403.

Pericardial effusion. Fluid accumulates within the pericardial sac due to infection, inflammation, malignancy or transudation. Slowly accumulating fluid distends the pericardium compressing surrounding lung; rapidly accumulating fluid is more likely to compress the heart chambers producing tamponade. Symptoms may be absent or will reflect the etiology (e.g., pain and fever with pericarditis; weakness, nausea and anorexia with uremia) or the hemodynamic consequences (e.g., shortness of breath and fatigue with tamponade). Signs include absent precordial impulse, decreased intensity and muffling or heart sounds, and low voltage ECG; a rub may be present. Ewart's sign is dullness at the left scapular tip due to compression atelectasis of the left lower lobe from large effusions.

✒ *PERICARDIAL EFFUSION—CLINICAL OCCURRENCE:* **Congenital** Familial Mediterranean Fever, familial pericarditis; **Endocrine** hypothyroidism; **Idiopathic** sarcoidosis; **Inflammatory/Immune** rheumatic fever, SLE, RA, ankylosing spondylitis, scleroderma, Wegner's, drug reactions; **Infectious** bacterial, viral, tuberculosis, fungal, Whipple's; **Metabolic/Toxic** drug induced, uremia; **Mechanical/Trauma** trauma, post-pericardiotomy, post-irradiation; **Neoplastic** metastatic carcinoma, especially lung and breast, lymphoma; **Vascular** myocardial infarction, aortic dissection with rupture into the pericardium, chylopericardium, vasculitis.

> **KEY SYNDROME** **Constrictive Pericarditis**

Progressive pericardial fibrosis leads to restricted diastolic filling and cardiac output. Symptoms are shortness of breath and fatigue. Signs are those of right heart failure: jugular venous distention, dependent edema, ascites, and hepatic congestion. The initial pericardial injury is caused by pericarditis (viral, tuberculous, neoplasm), cardiac surgery, mediastinal irradiation, and uremia [Wang A, Bashore TM. Undercover and overlooked. *N Engl J Med.* 2004;351:1014–1019].
DDX: It must be distinguished from restrictive cardiomyopathies and right ventricular failure.

> **KEY SYNDROME** **Pericardial Tamponade**

Rapid or massive accumulation of fluid within the relatively noncompliant pericardial space leads to compression of the heart chambers, impairing diastolic filling of the atria and ventricles. Cardiac output falls and CVP is elevated. Patients complain of shortness of breath and fatigue that may rapidly progress to hypotension and circulatory failure due to decreased cardiac output. The key physical signs are an elevated CVP with clear lung fields, no stigmata of chronic right ventricular failure, and a drop in systolic blood pressure during inspiration of >10 mm Hg (paradoxical pulse, page 384 and Fig. 8–42). Pulsus paradoxus may not be found in the presence of aortic insufficiency, left or right ventricular hypertrophy or pulmonary hypertension. The heart size is usually normal by examination and chest X-ray. Any time it is suspected, tamponade must be urgently evaluated by echocardiography. **DDX:** Conditions easily confused with tamponade are acute PE, right ventricular infarction, constrictive pericarditis and restrictive cardiomyopathy.

Disorders of the Arterial and Venous Circulations

KEY SYNDROME Vasculitis

Large vessel vasculitides are of unknown etiology. Vasculitis of medium-sized arteries may be associated with infection (polyarteritis nodosa with hepatitis B and C) or specific immunologic markers (Wegener with c-ANCA). Small-vessel vasculitides are associated with immune complex deposition in the vessel walls. In some cases the association with a specific infection is strong (e.g., mixed cryoglobulinemia and chronic hepatitis C infection), while in others there is a strong association with serologic markers (e.g., microscopic polyangiitis and p-ANCA). Each involves inflammation of the vessel wall leading to vascular obstruction and end-organ damage. The current working classification for vasculitis syndromes has proven helpful in selecting appropriate treatment for patients. Vasculitides are classified by the size of the involved vessel, Table 8–3 [Jennette JC, Falk RJ, Andrassay K, et al. Nomenclature of systemic vasculitides: Proposal of an

Table 8–3 Systemic Vasculitis Syndromes

Size of the vessel	Specific diseases
Large arteries	Giant cell arteritis Takayasu arteritis Primary central nervous system vasculitis
Medium arteries*	Polyarteritis nodosa Kawasaki disease Churg-Straus syndrome Wegener granulomatosis

Small vessels	Leukocytoclastic vasculitis
	  (e.g., Henoch-Schonlein purpura,
	  cryoglobulinemia, infections, drugs)
	Microscopic polyangiitis
	Urticarial vasculitis
	Systemic rheumatic syndromes

Pseudovasculitis[†]	Antiphospholipid syndrome
	Embolic phenomena (atrial myxomas,
	  cholesterol, nonbacterial thrombotic
	  endocarditis/Libman-Sacks endocarditis)
	Bacterial endocarditis
	Endovascular lymphoma

*May involve small vessels as well.
[†]May involve vessels of any size.
From Coblyn JS, McCluskey RT. Case 3-2003: Case records of the Massachusetts General Hospital. A 36-year-old man with renal failure, hypertension, and neurologic abnormalities. *N Engl J Med.* 2003;348:333–342.

international consensus conference. *Arthritis Rheum.* 1994;37:187–192]. The clinical manifestations depend upon the size and distribution of the vessels involved. Symptoms and signs are related to local ischemia and systemic inflammation. Skin involvement is usually manifest as palpable purpura with or without skin infarction. Involvement of arteries to other organs is manifest as signs of specific organ dysfunction, for example, renal failure, transient ischemic attacks, stroke, and pneumonitis. The pattern of involvement suggests the size of the vessel and the specific vasculitis syndrome [Weyand CM, Goronzy JJ. Medium- and large-vessel vasculitis. *N Engl J Med.* 2003;349:160–169; Jennette JC, Falk RJ. Small-vessel vasculitis. *N Engl J Med.* 1997;337:1512–1523; McCluskey P, Powell R. The eye in systemic inflammatory diseases. *Lancet.* 2004;364:2125–2133; Kathiresan S, Kelsey PB, Steere AC, et al. Case 14-2005: A 38-year-old man with fever and blurred vision. *N Engl J Med.* 2005;352:2003–2012].

Giant Cell Arteritis (GCA), Temporal Arteritis: The cause is unknown. Histologic examination shows patchy medial necrosis of temporal artery segments, with diffuse mononuclear infiltration and giant cells throughout the vessel walls (giant cell arteritis). Thromboses are frequent. GCA affects major branches of the proximal aorta, especially the external carotid. Patients over age 50 present with fever and weight loss and may have headache, jaw claudication, or scalp tenderness. Visual symptoms forebode irreversible visual loss from inflammation of the retinal and ophthalmic arteries. The headache is severe, persistent, and throbbing. *Polymyalgia rheumatica* (see page 681) may antedate other manifestations or occur simultaneously. Systemic symptoms (fever, profound weakness, weight loss, malaise, and prostration) are common and may be the only manifestations of disease. Physical signs are few, but scalp tenderness and tortuous, tender, or nodular temporal arteries may be identified. The overlying skin is often red and swollen. Vision is often impaired and ophthalmoplegia may occur, temporarily or permanently. The retina may be normal or show evidence of retinal ischemia. Prompt diagnosis and treatment may prevent loss of vision. The typical ophthalmic finding is anterior ischemic optic neuropathy (AION, page 246). The disk appears pale and swollen because of closure of the posterior ciliary arteries that supply the nerve head. Aortic aneurysms (thoracic and abdominal) and dissection occur with increased frequency [Salvarani C, Cantini F, Boiardi L, Hunder GG. Polymyalgia rheumatica and giant cell arteritis. *N Engl J Med.* 2002;347:261–271].

Takayasu Aortitis: There is inflammation of the aorta and its major branches producing markedly reduced flow and thrombosis in the involved vessels. Patients are usually young women presenting with arterial ischemic symptoms. A characteristic triad of signs is (1) absent pulses in upper extremity or neck vessels (pulseless disease), (2) carotid sinus sensitivity with head movement inducing syncope, and (3) ocular disorders, such as cataract and retinal defects.

Polyarteritis Nodosa: Small and intermediate muscular arteries have transmural inflammation and necrosis, sometimes extending to adjacent veins and arterioles. Involvement is segmental with a predilection for arterial bifurcations and branch points. Vascular occlusion leads to tissue ischemia and necrosis. Aneurysms up to 1 cm in diameter are frequent. Symptoms include fever, weight loss, malaise, and pain in viscera and muscles. Skin lesions are common, especially on the legs, and subcutaneous nodules may be palpable along the course of vessels or nerves. Frequently involved organs are the kidneys (renal failure, hypertension), gastrointestinal tract (visceral infarction), heart (myocardial infarction, pericarditis), liver (acute to chronic hepatitis), peripheral nerves (mononeuritis multiplex), skin (subcutaneous nodules on superficial vessels, palpable purpura, livedo reticularis), joints and muscles (myalgias, arthralgias, arthritis). The lungs are rarely involved [Stone JH. Polyartertitis nodosa. *JAMA*. 2002;288:1632–1639; Coblyn JS, McCluskey RT. Case records of the Massachusetts General Hospital. Case 3-2003. A 36-year-old man with renal failure, hypertension, and neurologic abnormalities. *N Engl J Med*. 2003;348:333–342].

➤ **Wegener's Granulomatosis:** The cause is unknown. Inflammation of small arteries and veins is associated with granuloma formation; neutrophil anti-cytoplasmic antibody (c-ANCA) to proteinase 3 is highly specific. Patients present with fever, malaise and signs of upper airway disease (sinusitis, obstructive and/or destructive symptoms and signs), pulmonary involvement and/or progressive renal failure. Other organ systems, including the skin, may be involved. Disease may be limited to the upper airway. It is most common in the fourth and fifth decades. Facial pain and epistaxis are caused by erosion of the nose (resulting in saddle deformity), sinuses, palate or nasopharynx. The lungs may have infiltrates, nodules, and cavitations; the kidney lesion is a rapidly progressive glomerulonephritis.

Churg-Strauss Syndrome (Allergic Angiitis and Granulomatosis): The cause is unknown. Eosinophilia is associated with nodular lung infiltrates and asthma; systemic symptoms and signs mimic polyarteritis nodosa. Patients present with signs and symptoms of asthma in association with eosinophilia and persistent slowly evolving abnormalities on the chest radiographs. It may appear on reduction of corticosteroid treatment or introduction of leukotriene inhibitor therapy for asthma [Wolf M, Rose H, Smith RN. Case 28-2005: A 42-year-old man with weight loss, weakness, and a rash. *N Engl J Med*. 2005;353:1148–1157].

➤ **Microscopic Polyangiitis:** The cause is unknown, but immune complexes and complement are not present in the vessel walls (pauci-immune vasculitis). There is a high prevalence of anti-cytoplasmic antibodies to myeloperoxidase, (p-ANCA); granuloma formation does not occur. Patients are systemically ill with fever, malaise, dyspnea, nonproductive cough, arthralgias and myalgias. Acute rapidly progressive glomerulonephritis is very common and pulmonary hemorrhage may be fatal. It is clinically indistinguishable from Wegener granulomatosis, except for the absence of airway involvement.

Leukocytoclastic Vasculitis: Immune complexes lodge in the walls of the terminal arteriole and venules inciting an inflammatory response that may lead to vessel occlusion with local tissue infarction. This common vasculitis most frequently affects the skin, particularly on the lower legs. The physical finding is purpura which is often palpable. The lesions come in crops that clear over days without scarring. Systemic symptoms (fever, malaise) and involvement of visceral organs including the kidneys (glomerulonephritis), lungs, gut, and rarely the heart and central nervous system can occur. Precipitating events include infection, drugs, malignancies and primary inflammatory disorders. Several distinct syndromes are identified, but overlap is frequent. **DDX:** This vasculitis must be distinguished from other causes of vasculopathy that may present similarly including disseminated fungal (e.g., histoplasmosis), viral (e.g., Rocky Mountain spotted fever) and bacterial infections (e.g., meningococcemia, gonococcemia), atheroembolism, scurvy and thrombocytopenia.

Secondary Vasculitis: This describes leukocytoclastic vasculitis occurring in association with another primary disease or condition that incites formation of immune complexes. Commonly encountered causes are infections (endocarditis, HIV, EBV, etc.), primary inflammatory diseases (e.g., SLE, RA, Sjögren syndrome and polymyositis-dermatomyositis), and drugs (see below).

Idiopathic Cutaneous Vasculitis: This applies to immune-complex vasculitis limited to the skin and without any identifiable inciting event or exposure. It may be recurrent and the crops of purpura may be preceded by a burning sensation. Other skin signs that may accompany the purpura include urticaria, bullae and erythematous macules. The lesions may itch.

Drug-Induced Vasculitis: Many drugs, especially the penicillins and sulfonamides, are associated with immune-complex mediated, typically cutaneous and/or urticarial, vasculitis. A p-ANCA positive small vessel vasculitis clinically identical to microscopic polyangiitis has been described with use of propylthiouracil and hydralazine. Drug induced TTP-HUS (page 148) is a vasculopathy that may be confused with vasculitis.

Henoch-Schönlein Purpura (Anaphylactoid Purpura): This is thought to represent a postinfectious condition. There is IgA deposition and inflammation in the small vessels of the skin, gastrointestinal tract, and kidneys. Patients, usually children or young adults, present with palpable purpura on the abdomen, buttocks and lower extremities, abdominal pain, fever, and heme-positive stools. Proteinuria and hematuria indicate glomerulitis. Nausea, vomiting, arthralgias, and myalgias are common. Urticaria may be present. The condition resolves spontaneously within a few days.

Behçet Syndrome: This is a vasculitis of unknown cause characterized by the triad of relapsing iridocyclitis, oral aphthous ulcerations, and genital ulcers. The great majority of cases have come from Greece, Cyprus, Turkey, the Middle East, and Japan, but an increasing number of cases are reported in the US. There is a high incidence of erythema nodosum and arthritis. A characteristic sign is *pathergy*, formation of sterile pustules at needle puncture sites in the skin. Many patients have thrombophlebitis, neurologic disorders, or intestinal involvement. The disease is chronic with relapses and remissions [Sakane T, Takeno M, Suzuki N, et al. Behçet's Disease. *N Engl J Med.* 1999;341:1284–1291].

> **KEY SYNDROME**   Arteriovenous Fistula: Acquired

Communication between an artery and adjacent vein may be induced surgically to facilitate venous access or be caused by a stab or gunshot wound, diagnostic catheterization, or erosion from neoplasm or infectious arteritis. Hemorrhage after the inciting trauma is profuse but easily controlled. A thrill and bruit may develop some hours later. After the wound has healed, signs of chronic circulatory disturbance develop. Although fistulas may occur in many parts of the body, the greatest variety of signs are evident when an extremity is involved (Fig. 8–46). Venous congestion is manifest by dilated veins and changes of stasis dermatitis.

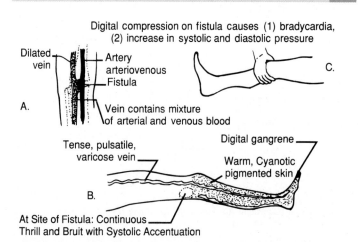

Fig. 8–46 *Signs of Arteriovenous Fistula.* A fistula between the popliteal artery and vein is represented. **A.** Shows the communication between artery and vein behind the knee joint. **B.** The lesion is in the left leg. The superficial veins are greatly dilated from blood under arterial pressure; they are tense to the touch and sometimes pulsatile. Distal to the fistula, the skin is warm from the arterial blood in the veins, cyanotic, and pigmented from hemostasis. Distal gangrene may occur. At the site of the leak a thrill and bruit may be felt. These are continuous throughout the cardiac cycle, with systolic accentuation. The arterial pulse pressure is greater than normal if the orifice of the fistula is large enough. **C.** Closure of the fistula by digital compression produces slowing of the heart rate (Branham bradycardiac sign) and augmentation of both systolic and diastolic arterial pressures in the general circulation.

Arterial hypoperfusion produces gangrene of the distal parts. If injury occurs before the epiphyses have closed, hypertrophy of the extremity may occur. A thrill and bruit are present throughout the cardiac cycle, with systolic accentuation. The skin temperature is increased distal to the fistula. Paradoxically, these signs assure that an arteriovenous shunt established surgically to facilitate venous access has remained patent. When the shunt is large, the dilated superficial veins become tense, venous pressure approaches arterial diastolic pressure, venous flow velocity increases, the RV dilates, arterial diastolic pressure falls and cardiac failure may result. External compression, temporarily closing the fistula, produces a sharp slowing of the heart rate, called the *Branham bradycardiac sign.* Shunts deep in the abdomen or thorax give only the bruit and the remote effects on venous and arterial pressure for diagnostic signs.

Congenital Arteriovenous Fistula: Cutaneous birthmarks are found in one-half of the cases, so arteriovenous fistula should be considered when one sees port-wine spots, blue-red cavernous hemangiomas, or diffuse hemangiomas. Frequently, congenital fistulas are quite small, so the signs associated with the acquired type are not evident: thrills and bruits may be absent and the bradycardiac sign of Branham is less pronounced. The affected limb may

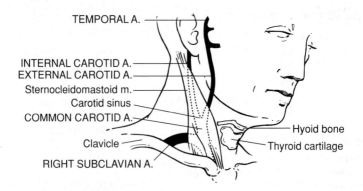

Fig. 8–47 *Large Superficial Arteries of the Head and Neck.* *The accessible arterial segments are diagrammed in solid black; inaccessible parts are stippled. The temporal artery courses anterior to the ear and upward to the temporal bone. The carotid arteries are deep to the anterior margin of the sternocleidomastoid muscle. The carotid sinus, at the bifurcation of the common carotid, is located by being level with the upper margin of the thyroid cartilage. A short segment of the subclavian artery is often palpable in the supraclavicular fossa.*

be hypertrophied, and it may exhibit increased sweating and hypertrichosis. There is no history of trauma.

Disorders of Circulation in the Head, Neck, and Trunk

The large arteries and veins in the head, neck, and trunk are less accessible to inspection and palpation than those in the extremities (Figs. 8–47 and 8–48A). Vascular disorders in these regions frequently must be inferred from combinations of physical signs.

Carotid Artery Disease: The carotid arteries supply blood to the head and brain. The external carotid system supplies the extracranial tissues; vascular symptoms and signs in its territory are unusual except for frequent involvement in giant cell (temporal) arteritis producing jaw claudication and scalp tenderness. The internal carotid system supplies the brain and eye and is frequently involved with atherosclerotic occlusive disease and atheroembolic events such as amaurosis fugax. The most common sites for atherosclerotic obstruction are the carotid bifurcation, the carotid siphon and the middle cerebral artery. Disease of the carotid bifurcation at the angle of the jaw is frequently accompanied by a bruit audible in the neck. Carotid bruits with ipsilateral cerebral symptoms carry a high risk for stroke within hours or days; bruits without symptoms must also be evaluated to assess the severity of obstruction.

Vertebral Artery Disease: The vertebral arteries are not accessible to direct examination. They join to form the basilar artery in the posterior fossa and collateralize the cerebral circulation via the posterior cerebral and posterior communicating arteries. Vertebral occlusive disease occurs due to atherosclerosis or dissection giving symptoms of brainstem ischemia (e.g., vertigo, dysarthria, dysequilibrium).

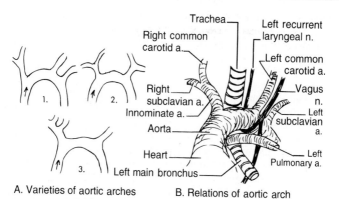

A. Varieties of aortic arches   B. Relations of aortic arch

Fig. 8–48 *The Aortic Arch. A.* Aortic Arch Variations. The normal pattern 1. is only slightly more common than the other two; it has a right innominate artery, branching into the subclavian and common carotid. There is no left innominate artery; the left subclavian and common carotid originate from the aorta itself. There may be both a right and left innominate 2. or the right innominate may give off the left common carotid 3. in addition to the right carotid and subclavian. *B.* Anatomic Relations of a Dilated Aortic Arch. Aneurysm of the aortic arch or dilatation of the left atrium may compress the left recurrent laryngeal nerve against the vertebrae or the left main bronchus to produce paralysis of the left vocal cord, resulting in hoarseness or a brassy cough. Expansion of the arch downward impinges upon the left main bronchus so the trachea is depressed with each pulse wave, giving a physical sign called the tracheal tug.

Aneurysmal arterial dilatation may be congenital or result from cystic medial necrosis, atherosclerosis, hypertension, vasculitis, or infection. The forms of aneurysms *are fusiform, saccular,* and *dissecting.* Aneurysms may consume platelets and clotting factors lowering their concentrations in the blood. Similar physical signs are produced by fusiform and saccular dilatations, but the dissection of an artery presents an entirely different clinical picture (see page 405). If pain accompanies an aneurysm, consider a penetrating aortic ulcer, leakage of the aneurysm or dissection of the arterial wall.

Thoracic aneurysms. The cause of thoracic aneurysms is multifactorial. Breakdown of structural proteins in the aortic media and adventitia plays a central role. The process also leads to smooth muscle necrosis and development of cystic spaces filled with mucoid material (cystic medial necrosis). Predisposing factors include genetic abnormalities (e.g., Marfan syndrome), hypertension, pregnancy, inflammation (e.g., giant cell arteritis, syphilis) and possibly atherosclerosis. Thoracic aneurysms are classified by their proximal extent, regardless of distal extension, into those involving the ascending aorta and those only involving the aorta distal to the left subclavian artery. The signs and symptoms are related to compression or distortion of adjacent structures and pain related to medial dissection or sudden dilation without dissection. Dissection may occur prior to aneurysmal dilatation. *Ascending Aortic Aneurysms* can produce aortic regurgitation from either dilation of the ascending aorta or dissection extending proximally to the valve ring and leaflets. The murmur characteristically transmits down the right sternal border rather than the left. A palpable thrust may develop in the right second or third intercostal spaces. The width of retromanubrial dullness is increased. Erosion of ribs and protrusion of a pulsatile mass may occur. Compression signs include hoarseness (recurrent laryngeal nerve traction), and cough, wheezing, or hemoptysis (compression and/or erosion of bronchi). Acute "six-dermatome" chest pain may result from dissection or myocardial ischemia from dissection of coronary ostia (usually the right). Proximal dissection can rupture into the pericardium, producing acute tamponade. *Aneurysms of the Aortic Arch* Retrosternal pain is frequent, radiating to the left scapula, left shoulder, or left neck. Dilatation of the arch can compress the left recurrent laryngeal nerve against the trachea or the left main bronchus causing hoarseness and a brassy cough (Fig. 8–48B). Obstruction or dissection of the left subclavian artery causes delay and diminution of pulse volume and reduction of blood pressure by more than 20 mm in the left arm. The dilated aortic arch can depress the left main bronchus producing a pulsating tracheal tug with each beat: grasp the cricoid cartilage lightly with the thumb and forefinger to feel the trachea dip with each pulse (Fig. 8–48B). *Aneurysms of the Descending Aorta* These are frequently silent and discovered incidentally. They may erode vertebral bodies causing back pain radiating around the chest via the intercostal nerves. With dissection, the spinal arteries may be occluded producing paraplegia. Pain from dissection of descending thoracic aneurysms is similar to pain from acute MI or ascending aorta dissection, except that the vast majority has pain in the back with or without anterior chest pain.

Abdominal aortic aneurysm (AAA). AAA involves all three layers of the aorta; the risk of rupture is directly related to the diameter of the aneurysm. Atherosclerosis is uniformly present in the aorta and often widespread. These are the most common aortic aneurysms. AAA is uncommon in individuals younger than 60 years of age, but increases in prevalence with each decade thereafter. Major risk factors are atherosclerosis, cigarette smoking, and male sex. Family clustering has been noted. Estimate the width of the aneurysm by locating the pulsatile mass just cephalad to the umbilicus, placing the fingers on the lateral walls. Pulsatile expansion is demonstrated by lateral as well as anteroposterior movement; this does not occur with a solid mass anterior to the aorta transmitting pulsations. Imaging is required for reliable tracking of aneurysm size over time. The presence or absence of abdominal or femoral bruits has no predictive value for the presence or absence of AAA. Pain in the mid to lower abdomen and appearance of a pulsatile epigastric mass suggest recent expansion or leaking of the aneurysm; rapid enlargement in size may, however, be asymptomatic. Rupture is associated with severe pain felt in the abdomen, back, and/or inguinal areas, accompanied by hypotension. The sensitivity of abdominal palpation for the detection of AAA depends upon the size of the aneurysm and the body habitus of the patient. Aneurysms >5 cm in diameter have a high risk of rupture and should be considered for elective surgery; physical examination is only approximately 75% sensitive for detecting aneurysms of this size. Diagnostic imaging is the preferred method of detection, and male smokers between 65 and 73 years of age should be considered for screening [Arnell TD, de Virgilio C, Donayre C, et al. Abdominal aortic aneurysm screening in elderly males with atherosclerosis: The value of physical exam. *Am Surg.* 1996;62:

861–864; Rink HA, Lederle FA, Roth CS, et al. The accuracy of physical examination to detect abdominal aortic aneurysm. *Arch Intern Med.* 2000;160:833–836; Lederle FA, Simel DL. The rational clinical examination. Does this patient have abdominal aortic aneurysm? *JAMA.* 1997;281:77–82; Lin PH, Lumsden AB. Small aortic aneurysms. *N Engl J Med.* 2003;348:19; Ashton HA, Buxton MJ, Day NE, et al. The Multicentre Aneurysm Screening Study (MASS) into the effect of abdominal aortic aneurysm screening on mortality in men: A randomised controlled trial. *Lancet.* 2002;360:1531–1539]. Aneurysms of the iliac arteries are not rare and may rupture. They are identified as pulsatile masses in the lower quadrants of the abdomen on deep palpation [van der Wliet JA, Boll APM. Abdominal aortic aneurysm. *Lancet.* 1997;349:863–866].

➤ **Dissecting aortic aneurysm:** See page 405.

Mycotic Aneurysms: These are saccular aneurysms caused by weakening of the arterial walls from infectious processes other than syphilis. Mural involvement may develop as an extension of localized suppuration, actinomycosis, or tuberculosis. More frequently, an embolic arteritis occurs in the course of subacute bacterial endocarditis or septicemia. Mycotic aneurysms usually involve vessels subject to bending and lightly protected by overlying muscles, for example, the axillary, brachial, femoral, and popliteal arteries.

KEY SYNDROME Coarctation of the Aorta

A congenital aortic arch stricture occurs just proximal or distal to the insertion of the ductus arteriosus into the aorta (preductal or postductal). The most common constriction is distal to the left subclavian artery takeoff. Almost invariably, the adult type has a closed ductus. Perfusion of tissues distal to the coarctation is maintained via high resistance collaterals in the chest wall perfused at the cost of sustained central arterial hypertension. The collateral arterial circulation is via the left internal mammary artery and other branches of the left subclavian to the left intercostal arteries (excepting the first two), the musculophrenic and the superior epigastric arteries (Fig. 8–49). In most cases the collateral circulation is sufficient for the patient to remain asymptomatic into adulthood. Hypertension develops in the upper limbs with slight hypotension and a dampened pulse wave in the legs. A coincident bicuspid aortic valve is common so aortic systolic (often with an early systolic ejection sound) and/or diastolic murmurs may be heard. **The Murmur** The murmur of the coarctation itself is heard best in the interscapular area posteriorly. The site of constriction is remote from the precordium, so the murmur is faint, if heard at all, on the anterior chest. When a murmur is audible anteriorly, it is usually a brief early systolic ejection murmur caused by an associated bicuspid aortic valve. This murmur is faint and maximal in either the left or right second interspace. A continuous bruit can sometimes be heard over the sternum from the dilated internal mammary arteries. **Arterial Pulses** The pulse waves in the distal aorta and its branches are dampened; this is most easily detected by palpating the femoral arteries. If the femoral pulses have good volume, coarctation is suggested when there is a peak pulse lag between the femoral and radial arteries. The collateral circulation through the dilated intercostal arteries may be palpated in the posterior intercostal spaces (which is diagnostic). Notching in the inferior rib margins posteriorly is visible on chest

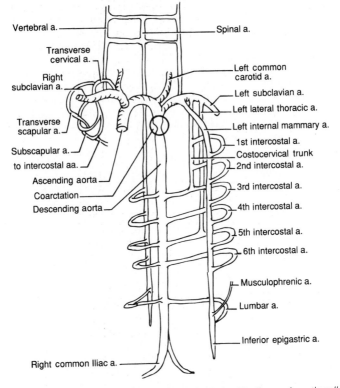

Fig. 8–49 *Coarctation of the Aorta: Collateral Circulation.* The diagram shows the collateral channels causing dilatation of the intercostal arteries from the costocervical trunk and the internal mammary artery. The circulation around the scapula is augmented by blood through the transverse cervical artery. The pulse volume in the arms is normal; in the femoral arteries it is diminished. The dilated scapular and intercostal arteries may be palpated in the back.

X-ray. Hypertension in young adults should suggest the possibility of coarctation; it is common in patients with the gonadal dysgenesis (Turner syndrome).

Aberrant right subclavian artery (Dysphagia Lusoria): See Chapter 7, page 291.

Subclavian steal syndrome. Patients have atherosclerotic subclavian artery stenosis proximal to the vertebral artery origin. Retrograde flow occurs in the ipsilateral vertebral artery inducing brainstem ischemia with neurologic signs (Fig. 8–50). A bruit can be heard in the supraclavicular fossa, occasionally with a thrill. The arterial pulse volume and blood pressure are diminished in the affected arm. Symptoms and signs of cerebral ischemia are intermittent or continuous, ranging from vague dizziness to vertigo, slurring of speech and hemiparesis. The neurologic signs and symptoms can be induced by exercising the affected arm.

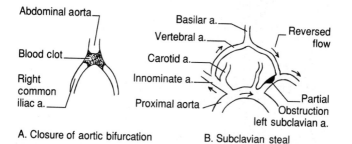

A. Closure of aortic bifurcation   B. Subclavian steal

Fig. 8–50 *Two Syndromes of Large Artery Obstruction. A. Obstruction at the aortic bifurcation (Leriche syndrome):* A short thrombus closes the lower part of the abdominal aorta and extends a variable distance down the common iliac arteries. The accessible segments of the femoral, popliteal, dorsalis pedis, and posterior tibial arteries are pulseless. Pain in the legs and intermittent claudication are the common symptoms. **B. Subclavian steal syndrome:** The most common site of narrowing is the left subclavian artery, although other sites have also been reported.

KEY SYNDROME   **Thoracic Outlet Syndromes—Subclavian and Brachial Plexus Compression**

The roots of C5-T1 form the brachial plexus in the lateral neck, between the Scalenus medius and S. anticus. The subclavian artery exits the rib cage over the first rib. Artery and nerves run together over the first and second rib and under the clavicle and pectoralis minor into the upper arm. These syndromes result from the compression of nerves and vessels as they course between muscles and bones while making their exit from the neck and chest respectively (Fig. 8–51A). The symptoms arise from brachial plexus compression and are largely sensory (paresthesias); the signs are those of positional arterial obstruction. Therefore, the patient presents with subjective neurologic symptoms and the clinician evaluates for signs of arterial compression.

Scalenus Anticus Syndrome: There is intermittent or constant pain and/or paresthesia in the ulnar aspect of the arm and hand, sometimes associated with weakness and wasting. **Adson Test** Have the patient sit with the palms on the knees, chin high and turned to the side being examined. Examine the radial pulse while they hold the breath in deep inspiration. A positive test is a dampening or obliteration of the radial pulse that disappears when the chin turns forward, still holding the breath. *CLINICAL OCCURRENCE:* Muscular hypertrophy or edema may occur after unusually vigorous arm use or in those with unusual occupations, such as weight lifters. Muscle spasm may result from poor posture, anomalous first rib, or cervical rib.

Cervical Rib: In addition to producing spasm of the scalenus anticus muscle (Scalenus Anticus Syndrome, above), a cervical rib may directly compress the subclavian artery dampening the radial pulse in any position (Fig. 8–51B). Occasionally, the extra rib is palpable in the supraclavicular fossa. The rib may also compress the brachial plexus to produce pain or paresthesias in the hand.

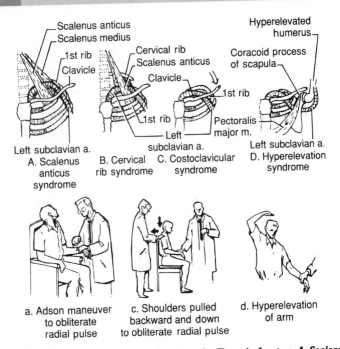

Fig. 8–51 *Compression Syndromes of the Superior Thoracic Aperture. A. Scalenus anticus syndrome:* The scalenus anticus muscle has attachments to the transverse processes of the cervical vertebrae above and below to the first rib. Posteriorly and behind the subclavian artery, the scalenus medius attaches to the same bones. Hypertrophy of the bellies of the two muscles causes compression of the artery between them, with motions such as turning the head to the ipsilateral side. This is tested by the Adson maneuver (a), where the patient sits with chin raised, head rotated to the left, and chest held in the inspiratory position. A positive test is marked by diminution or disappearance of the left radial pulse. The other side is tested similarly. *B. Cervical rib syndrome:* The diagram shows a cervical rib compressing the left scalenus anticus muscle and indirectly the subclavian artery. This may produce diminution in the radial pulse or a peripheral neuritis of parts of the brachial plexus. *C. Costoclavicular syndrome:* The geometry of the aperture may be such that rotation of the clavicles downward and backward compresses the subclavian arteries against the first rib. This is tested (c) by having the patient seated in a chair and the examiner standing behind him. The physician pushes the shoulders downward and backward while an assistant feels for diminution of the radial pulses. *D. Hyperelevation of the arm:* The geometry of the thorax in some persons is such that hyperelevation of the arm causes the coracoid process of the scapula to impinge and compress the subclavian artery. This is tested by (d) demonstrating that the radial pulse is lost with hyperelevation.

Costoclavicular Syndrome: There is intermittent or constant pain and/or paresthesia in the ulnar aspect of the arm and hand. Have the patient stand with elbows flexed at 90 degrees; then elevate the elbows, maintaining 90 degrees of abduction, to 45 degrees, 90 degrees, and 135 degrees (the last position places the hands on the head). Palpate the radial pulse and auscultate beneath the midportion of the clavicle at each position. Patients with costoclavicular syndrome have pulse obliteration in at least one position; a palpable pulse with a subclavicular systolic bruit indicates partial obstruction. The **Costoclavicular Maneuver** tests for clavicular compression of the subclavian artery on the first rib. The patient sits while his radial pulses are palpated by an assistant. Stand behind the patient forcing his shoulders down and back narrowing the thoracic outlet (Fig. 8–51C). The pulse volumes are diminished if compression is sufficient to cause symptoms. This test is specific but not sensitive. *CLINICAL OCCURRENCE:* Situations in which the shoulders are forced downward and backward, such as walking with a heavy backpack carried on the shoulders.

Ischemia from Arm Elevation: In some persons, elevation of the arm causes compression of the subclavian artery by the coracoid process of the scapula (Fig. 8–51D). The patient complains of intermittent or constant numbness and tingling in one or both hands or arms. Patients often sleep on their backs with the hands behind or over the head. Another precipitant is working with the arms elevated, such as painting ceilings. *Hyperabduction Test* Have the patient lift the hand to the top of the head then open and close his hand several times noting whether the radial pulse is diminished or abolished.

➤ **KEY SYNDROME** **SVC Obstruction—SVC Syndrome**

The principal signs are edema and cyanosis of the head, neck, and both arms, edema of the face, both arms, and the upper third of the thoracic wall, with venous engorgement without the pulsations normally transmitted from the right atrium (Fig. 8–52). The neck is enlarged by nonpitting edema (*Stokes collar*) and collateral veins may be visible on the chest and abdominal wall. *CLINICAL OCCURRENCE:* Mediastinal neoplasm; cervical or retrosternal goiter; thoracic aortic aneurysm; chronic mediastinitis; thrombosis from an indwelling intravenous catheter.

KEY SYNDROME **IVC Obstruction**

IVC occlusion retards venous drainage from the lower extremities and pelvis leading to development of collateral veins in the hemorrhoidal complex and abdominal wall. Renal vein thrombosis causes acute renal failure. *Acute IVC Obstruction* may be asymptomatic until lower extremity edema develops. Symmetrical rapidly progressive edema of both legs without evidence of heart or kidney disease suggests mechanical IVC obstruction. *Chronic IVC Obstruction* is suggested by dilated superficial collateral veins with cephalad flow on the abdomen. Visible collaterals may appear within a week of obstruction, the veins attaining maximal size in 3 months. To localize the obstruction, consider the vena cava in three segments (Fig. 8–52). *Lower Segment (below the renal veins):* The collaterals are distributed over thighs, groins, lower abdomen, and flanks. Leg edema, initially pitting, develops fibrosis with chronic venous stasis dermatitis. Pelvic congestion produces low back pain and genital edema. *Middle Segment (above the renal veins and below the hepatic vein):* The venous collaterals are large intra-abdominal veins without abdominal wall collaterals. Occlusion of the renal veins produces nephrotic syndrome. Gastrointestinal manifestations include nausea, vomiting, diarrhea and abdominal pain; malabsorption may develop. *Upper Segment (above the hepatic veins):* Venous Collaterals form a prominent periumbilical

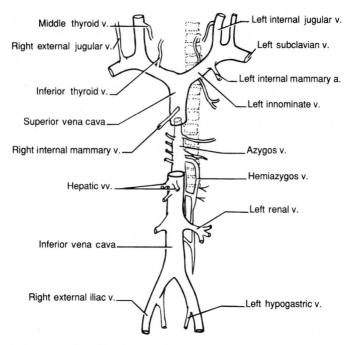

Middle thyroid v.
Right external jugular v.
Inferior thyroid v.
Superior vena cava
Right internal mammary v.
Hepatic vv.
Inferior vena cava
Right external iliac v.

Left internal jugular v.
Left subclavian v.
Left internal mammary a.
Left innominate v.
Azygos v.
Hemiazygos v.
Left renal v.
Left hypogastric v.

Fig. 8–52 *Superior and Inferior Venae Cavae.*

plexus and large veins appear over the anterior abdomen. ***Budd-Chiari syndrome*** develops with hepatosplenomegaly, ascites, jaundice, and elevated transaminases. ***CLINICAL OCCURRENCE:*** *Intraluminal* thrombosis, embolism, neoplastic invasion or extension from renal cell carcinoma; *Intramural* rare benign or malignant neoplasms; *External Pressure* hepatomegaly, lymphadenopathy, aortic aneurysm, surgical ligation, pregnancy.

Disorders of Large Limb Arteries

Arterial disorders are either nonocclusive or occlusive, and occlusion may be partial or complete. Four mechanisms cause arterial circulatory deficit: (1) extrinsic compression; (2) vasospasm; (3) luminal obstruction (intimal thickening, thrombus, embolus); or (4) arteriopathy (vasculitis, fibromuscular dysplasia). Temporary arterial compression is often related to extremity positioning, demonstrated by assuming the position. Transient vasospasm is recognized by the sharp border between ischemic and normal tissue. Intimal proliferation is inferred when the blood flow is diminished but still present. Complete occlusion is usually caused by embolism or thrombosis. Thrombosis is often the result of gradual, usually atherosclerotic, narrowing allowing development of collaterals; symptoms are gradual in onset and relatively mild. Sudden embolic or thrombotic occlusion causes severe pain and a cold white part. Arteriopathy such as vasculitis is usually inferred from the total clinical picture.

When an acute arterial occlusion is suspected, first determine the most distal site with adequate flow by noting the presence or absence of pulses along the vessel; the vessel walls are palpated for signs of intrinsic disease. Urgent vascular imaging with Doppler ultrasound, MR angiography, or contrast angiography is required.

Atherosclerosis. Atherosclerosis is characterized by medial degeneration and fibrosis, together with occlusive proliferation of the intima. Arterial narrowing results from progressive intimal thickening, plaque formation with accumulation of cholesterol rich lipid deposits, foam cells and smooth muscle proliferation. Rupture of intimal plaques lead to formation of thrombi. Arterial segments lengthen and, when the ends of a segment are anchored, the elongated vessel buckles producing visible and palpable tortuosity. The disease may be diffuse or focal, often occurring at arterial bifurcations. In patients age >45, atherosclerosis is the most likely cause of major arterial obstruction. Patients with diabetes mellitus have an increased risk inversely related to glycemic control. Hyperhomocysteinemia, congenital or acquired (folic acid and B_{12} deficiency), also increases risk for atherosclerosis and thromboembolic events. Atheromatous plaques may be felt in the walls of accessible arteries; the vessels may be noncompressible and feel thick. Noninvasive vascular examination with Doppler ultrasonography and plethysmography are required for accurate diagnosis; angiography with contrast or MRA is anatomically definitive.

Acute Arterial Obstruction: Occlusion of arteries to the organs of the head, thorax, and abdomen present with symptoms referable to those organs: stroke, acute MI, PE, mesenteric, renal, or splenic infarction.

➤ **KEY SYNDROME** **Acute Extremity Artery Obstruction—Embolism and Arterial Thrombosis**

This is most common in the legs, but can occur in the arms. The patient experiences sudden excruciating pain followed by numbness and weakness. Occasionally, anesthesia and weakness precede the pain which appears more gradually. The distal extremity is pulseless and becomes pallid, the skin becoming cool. Venous pooling causes the skin distally to gradually become cyanotic while mottling occurs proximally; the cyanosis diminishes with limb elevation. Occasionally, the pain may be quite mild. Thrombosis is more likely when there are signs of diffuse vascular disease or a history of claudication. Embolism is likely with atrial fibrillation. *CLINICAL OCCURRENCE:* *Thrombosis* atherosclerosis; thromboangiitis obliterans; vasculitis; sludging from polycythemia, hemoconcentration, cryoglobulinemia, and hyperglobulinemia; infection; trauma; antiphospholipid syndrome *Embolism* atrial fibrillation, mitral stenosis, endocarditis (infectious, NBTE) left atrial myxoma, LV mural thrombus following MI, atheroembolism.

KEY SYNDROME **Chronic Extremity Peripheral Vascular Disease**

This is most common in the legs but may involve the arms. The patient complains of claudication and coldness progressing to continuous and/or night pain. Assess the ABI; see page 331. Arterial insufficiency can cause: *skin* pigmentation, pallor, purplish discoloration that fades with elevation, coldness, warm areas of

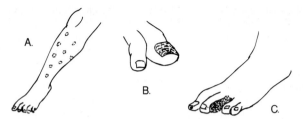

Fig. 8–53 *Swellings of the Knee and Their Diagnosis. A. Knee effusion. B. Signs of knee effusion. C. Charot Knee.*

collateral circulation, local hair loss, and malnutrition of toenails, ulceration, or gangrene (see Figs. 8–24 and 8–53). Pulses are weak or absent. Muscular atrophy may be present. Popliteal artery occlusion leads to collateral circulation in the branches of the geniculate artery, producing cold feet with especially warm knees or anteromedial lower thigh. ABI of < 0.9 is associated with an increased risk of cardiovascular morbidity and mortality. ABI <0.5 is more strongly associated with decreased physical activity and absence of sustained walking than are symptoms of claudication [McDermott MM, Greenland P, et al. The ankle brachial index is associated with leg function and physical activity: the walking and leg circulation study. *Ann Intern Med.* 2002;136:873–883].

Pulseless Femoral Artery: (Fig. 8–50A, page 423). After examining the abdomen, always palpate the femoral arteries. When a femoral pulse is diminished or absent, palpate the iliac pulses up to and including the aortic bifurcation, 2 cm below and slightly to the left of the umbilicus. The iliac arteries run in a line between the bifurcation and the midpoint of the inguinal ligament; the upper third represents the common iliac, the lower two-thirds marks the external iliacs. These vessels may not be palpable in normal persons, but asymmetric findings are significant. Bilateral decreased or absent femoral pulses suggests coarctation of the aorta, distal aortic thrombosis (*Leriche syndrome*), or dissecting aortic aneurysm; unilateral absence suggests thrombosis of the common iliac artery. The significance of an absent or diminished femoral pulse must be judged by the presence or absence of the distal pulses.

KEY SYNDROME   **Thromboangiitis Obliterans (Buerger Disease)**

Beginning as an acute segmental panarteritis involving all three layers of medium-sized arteries, intimal granulation tissue ultimately causes arterial obstruction, producing tissue ischemia and necrosis. Thromboangiitis is a condition of young male smokers, usually between 20 and 40, an earlier appearance than atherosclerosis. It is often associated with superficial migrating thrombophlebitis. **DDX:** No physical signs distinguish Buerger disease from atherosclerosis. The distribution of affected vessels may differ from atherosclerosis: thromboangiitis has a predilection for the radial, ulnar, and digital arteries, in addition affecting the lower extremities [Olin JW. Thromboangiitis obliterans (Buerger's disease). *N Engl J Med.* 2000;343:864–869]. Approximately 7% of Japanese patients are nonsmokers [Naito AT, Minamino T, Tateno K, et al. Steroid-responsive thromboangiitis obliterans. *Lancet.* 2004;364:1098].

KEY SYNDROME   Raynaud Disease and Phenomenon

Intense spasm of the digital arteries and dermal vessels produces initial pallor, followed over minutes by capillary dilatation and filling with deoxygenated venous blood, producing a phase of cyanosis. Relaxation of arterial spasm flushes the capillaries with arterial blood producing the warm red phase of vasodilation. Approximately 80% of the patients are young women. Attacks are induced by cold exposure or emotional stress. The onset is sudden, either unilateral or bilateral, most commonly affecting the fingers and involving the toes in half the cases. One to four fingers may be affected, rarely the thumbs. Episodes last up to 60 minutes, the terminal digits become chalk-white, numb and sweaty; the pallor is succeeded by intense cyanosis and pain. Sometimes either pallor or cyanosis is absent. During spontaneous recovery, or after warm water immersion, projections of hyperemia replace cyanosis until the digit becomes brilliant red. Hyperemia is accompanied by tingling, throbbing, and edema. After many attacks, trophic changes may appear in the nails and adjacent skin and small areas of gangrene may develop on the fingertips and toes. The term *Raynaud disease* is used when there is no associated disease and *Raynaud phenomenon* when it is associated with another condition, for example, scleroderma, vibratory trauma, SLE, polyarteritis, peripheral neuropathy, thromboangiitis obliterans, atherosclerosis. Raynaud phenomenon occurs more frequently in patients with migraine (26%) than in persons without migraine (6%). There is also an increased prevalence of chest pain and migraine in patients with Raynaud disease [O'Keeffe SJ, Taspatsaris NP, Beethan WP Jr. Increased prevalence of migraine and chest pain in patients with primary Raynaud disease. *Ann Intern Med.* 1992;116:(12) (pt 1):985–989]. **DDX:** Always inspect the nailbed capillaries (page); abnormal capillaries are highly suggestive of scleroderma. The sequence of pallor, cyanosis, and redness is diagnostic when induced by exposure to cold. It should not be confused with the vascular changes of complex regional pain syndromes [Wigley FM. Raynaud's phenomenon. *N Engl J Med.* 2002;347:1001–1008].

KEY SYNDROME   Acrocyanosis

Excessive arteriolar constriction is ascribed to increased sympathetic tone, although humoral factors may contribute. This is a benign painless condition in which the skin of the hands and feet is persistently cold, cyanotic and moist. It is most common in young women. The skin is uniformly cyanotic, which worsens on cold exposure. The cyanosis is abolished with elevation and sleep.

KEY SYNDROME   Digital Gangrene

Gangrene of the finger and toe tips can be caused by any disease or condition impairing peripheral perfusion. *CLINICAL OCCURRENCE:* Scleroderma, pneumatic hammer disease, atherosclerosis, thromboangiitis obliterans, cold agglutination disease, cryoglobulinemia, atheroemboli, sepsis, meningococcemia, vasopressor medications, antiphospholipid syndrome, warfarin skin necrosis (protein C deficiency), ergotism, chronic renal failure.

Ergotism: An intense constriction of the peripheral blood vessels is caused by the ingestion of ergot; some individuals are particularly sensitive. Ergot may be taken as a drug or eaten with dietary grain contaminated by a fungus. The first symptom is often burning pain in the extremities (*St. Anthony fire*) with loss of arterial pulses in the hands or feet; headache, weakness, nausea, vomiting, visual disturbances, and angina pectoris may occur. Cold skin and mottled cyanosis of the extremities follows. Finally, symmetrical gangrene involves the fingers and toes, sometimes extending proximally.

Cavernous hemangioma. Congenital cavernous hemangiomas may occur anywhere in the body. The limb is circumferentially enlarged and dilated, purplish, blood-filled, readily compressible sinuses raise the skin surface. This is distinguished from varicosities by the distribution, which does not correspond to the large limb veins. With leg involvement, standing may pool enough blood to cause orthostatic hypotension. Massive cavernous hemangiomas (Kasabach-Merritt syndrome) trap platelets producing thrombocytopenia, purpura, and bleeding.

Aneurysms in the arms and neck. The subclavian, axillary, and brachial arteries are most commonly affected; the carotids are rarely involved. Trauma to the vessel wall is the most common cause; rarely, the vessels are involved by mycotic, necrotizing, or atherosclerotic aneurysms. The dilatations may be readily palpated.

Aneurysms in the legs. The most common sites are the femoral artery in the Scarpa triangle and the popliteal artery in its fossa. Atherosclerosis is the most common cause. The lesions are readily palpable.

Disorders of the Major Extremity Veins

> **KEY SYNDROME** **Deep Vein Thrombosis (DVT)**

See Pulmonary Embolism, page 392. Intraluminal thrombus forms with or without an inciting event, usually in association with a lower extremity venous valve. The thrombus may propagate proximally or distally; it may partially or completely occlude flow. Absence of inflammation facilitates dislodgment of the thrombus. Leg veins are the most common identified source of pulmonary embolism. Hip and knee surgery have particularly high incidence of associated DVT. This term is usually applied to thrombosis of the deep veins of the legs. Deep venous thrombosis requires timely diagnosis to initiate appropriate therapy, the goals of which are to prevent pulmonary embolus and diminish damage to the venous valves, which predisposes to future thrombosis and stasis damage to the skin. The history and physical examination can separate patients into low, intermediate and high risk categories (Table 8–4); all patients in whom DVT is suspected should undergo further testing [Anand SS, Wells PS, Hunt S, et al. The rational clinical examination. Does this patient have deep vein thrombosis? *JAMA*. 1998;279:1094–1099; Kearon C, Julian JA, Newman TE, et al. Noninvasive diagnosis of deep venous thrombosis. *Ann Intern Med*. 1998;128:663–677; Miron MJ, Perrier A, Bounameaux H. Clinical assessment of suspected deep vein thrombosis: Comparison between a score and empirical assessment. *J Intern Med*. 2000;247:249–254]. Diagnostic algorithms are constantly changing, so consult current protocols. Early diagnosis can be lifesaving. *Symptoms* Often, tightness or a sense of fullness is noted in the leg which is aggravated by standing and walking. *Signs* DVT may be accompanied by cutaneous *cyanosis* of the dependent foot and lower leg. Pitting edema of the foot, ankle, or leg that does not resolve overnight, and venous engorgement on the feet persisting with the legs elevated to 45 degrees, suggest venous obstruction. Leg pain following the course of the thrombosed vein may be

Table 8–4   Wells Criteria for Deep Venous Thrombosis Risk Stratification

Clinical feature	Score
Current cancer or within the last 6 months	1
Paralysis, significant limb weakness or immobilization of one or both legs	1
Bedridden for >3 days or surgery within 4 weeks	1
Localized tenderness along the deep veins	1
Entire leg swollen	1
Calf circumference >3 cm compared to the asymptomatic leg, 10 cm below the tibial tuberosity	1
Pitting edema greater in the symptomatic leg	1
Collateral (nonvaricose) superficial veins in the symptomatic leg	1
Alternative diagnosis as likely or more likely the dvt	2

Summary Pretest Risk Estimation Score Observed Prevalence of DVT:

Low	0 or less	3%
Moderate	1–2	17%
High	3 or more	75%

Adapted from Wells PS, Anderson DR, et al. Value of assessment of pretest probability of deep-vein thrombosis in clinical management. *Lancet.* 1997;350:1795–1798.

induced by sneezing or coughing; the pain disappears when the vein is compressed proximal to the obstruction (*Louvel sign*). Palpation may detect tenderness of vein segments. *Homan Sign* With the knee in flexion, the examiner forcefully dorsiflexes the ankle; calf or popliteal pain occurs in approximately 35% of the patients with DVT. Homan sign is neither sensitive nor specific for DVT.

Thrombophlebitis: As the name implies, thrombosis and inflammation of the venous walls are associated; inflammation may either precede or follow clot formation. In addition to the signs and symptoms described above, pain and inflammation are prominent features. When acute, the veins are painful and tender and the overlying skin is red and hot. Adjacent muscles may cramp. Fever and leukocytosis are common. Often there is elevated skin temperature overlying the inflamed vein. Acute femoral vein thrombophlebitis may present with excruciating pain, massive leg edema, and pallor from arterial spasm (*phlegmasia alba dolens*). The signs can suggest arterial embolism, but the pallor is less intense, there is more cyanosis, the femoral vein is tender, and anesthesia is absent; arterial pulses can usually be demonstrated by ultrasound. When the entire venous drainage of an extremity is obstructed, there is extreme pain, massive edema, and deep cyanosis of the entire limb (*phlegmasia cerulea dolens*). Arterial and venous imaging is indicated.

Post-Phlebitic Syndrome: This is the sequelae to DVT in a proximal leg vein in up to 50% of patients. Pain and tenderness are slight and the skin is normal to cool. The leg is swollen, initially with edema, but, if untreated, with nonpitting fibrosis of the subcutaneous tissues and skin. Varicose veins may or may not be prominent. Venous stasis dermatitis is common. Severe cases can be disabling [Prandoni P, Lensing AWA, Prins MH, et al. Below-Knee elastic compression stockings to prevent the post-thrombotic syndrome. *Ann Intern*

Med. 2004;141:249–256]. ***CLINICAL OCCURRENCE: Congenital***   Congenital thrombophilia is suggested by DVT at a young age, at an unusual sites (upper extremity, mesenteric vessels, etc.), a history of recurrent thromboses or emboli, a family history of DVT, or DVT with minimal trauma or minor surgery. Identified etiologies include resistance to activated protein C, factor V Leiden mutation, protein C deficiency, protein S deficiency, dysfibrinogenemia, homocystinuria, antithrombin III deficiency, and sickle cell disease.   ***Acquired*** Antiphospholipid syndrome (lupus-like anticoagulant, anticardiolipin antibodies), heparin-induced thrombocytopenia and thrombosis (HITT syndrome), leg fractures, limb surgery, trauma, prolonged inactivity (bed rest, international air travel, automobile travel), infection, cancer (especially mucin producing adenocarcinomas), hyperhomocysteinemia, estrogen-containing medications, pregnancy, obesity, venous stasis and insufficiency, diabetes mellitus, polycythemia vera, idiopathic thrombocythemia, and paroxysmal nocturnal hemoglobinuria. Recurrent deep venous thrombosis may precede the diagnosis of cancer.

KEY SIGN   Superficial Thrombophlebitis

Thrombosis and inflammation of superficial veins occurs either alone, or extending from the deep veins. The patient complains of tender red nodules or cords under the skin. Often there is a history of recent trauma, although it may be incidental. Superficial thrombophlebitis may mask the coincidental occurrence of deep vein disease. Superficial thrombophlebitis is a very rare cause of life-threatening pulmonary embolus. Underlying DVT should be investigated. **DDX:** Lymphangitis and other skin and soft-tissue infections can be confused with superficial thrombophlebitis, but the firm palpable venous cords are diagnostic, unless secondary to the infection.

Migratory Superficial Thrombophlebitis: Successive episodes of thrombophlebitis involve different veins in widely separated parts of the body. In a single episode, a segment of vein becomes tender, reddened, and indurated. Involution begins in a few days and the adjacent tissues become successively blue and yellow, often resolving with some pigmentation of the skin. Veins of the extremities are most commonly involved, but the subcutaneous veins of the abdomen and thorax may be affected. Although the lesions do not cause serious discomfort, this complex should prompt a search for an underlying disease.   ***CLINICAL OCCURRENCE:***   Antiphospholipid syndrome, thromboangiitis obliterans, Behçet syndrome, pancreatic carcinoma, and thrombophilic hematologic disorders, especially paroxysmal nocturnal hemoglobinuria.

KEY SYNDROME   Venous Stasis

See Stasis Dermatitis, page 155. Venous stasis results from vein occlusion or incompetence of the valves. Occlusion is caused by external compression of the walls or from plugging of the lumina by fibrosis, thrombi, or neoplasms growing in the vessel lumen. Dilation of vessels exacerbates stasis. Dilated superficial veins drain poorly into smaller communicating veins. Dilatation of deeper veins leads to incompetence of their valves. Decreased capillary flow produces poor skin nutrition, inflammation, and fibrosis. Signs of venous stasis are

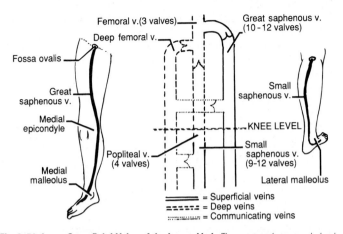

Fig. 8–54 *Large Superficial Veins of the Lower Limb.* *The great saphenous vein begins on the medial aspect of the foot, courses backward under the medial malleolus, up the medial aspect of the calf, behind the medial epicondyle, and then obliquely across the anterior thigh to the femoral vein as it enters the femoral canal beneath the inguinal ligament. The* ***small saphenous vein*** *begins on the lateral side of the foot, curves backward beneath the lateral malleolus, and then upward on the posterior surface of the calf to enter the popliteal fossa and join with the popliteal vein. The middle figure diagrams the communications between the superficial veins (heavy solid lines) and the deep veins (broken lines) and the communicating vessels (dotted lines).*

pitting edema, stasis pigmentation (hemosiderin), erythema, fibrosis and de-creased elasticity of the skin and ulceration. The pumping action of voluntary muscles is inhibited by bed rest and by immobilizing an extremity [Bergan JJ, Schmid-Schonbein GW, Smith PD, et al. Chronic venous disease. *N Engl J Med.* 2006;355:488–498].

KEY SYNDROME   Varicose Veins

Varicose veins are grossly dilated subcutaneous veins, often filling by retrograde flow from the deep veins due to incompetent valves in the perforating and deep veins; the are most common in leg (Fig. 8–54). Primary varicosities develop spon-taneously; secondary varicosities result from proximal obstruction, e.g., preg-nancy, trauma, thrombophlebitis. When unilateral, extrinsic compression or an arteriovenous fistula should be considered. An arteriovenous fistula produces pulsation in the dilated veins.

KEY SYNDROME   Thrombosis of the Axillary Vein

This usually follows trauma or intensive use of the arm in hyperabduction, such as throwing. The entire arm swells and aches. The tissues are firm and there is no pitting edema. The superficial veins at the superior thoracic aperture may be dilated. Poor collateral circulation produces cyanosis of the skin. Axillary vein thromboses are less likely to lead to lethal pulmonary emboli than deep venous thromboses in the legs, but it does occur. **DDX:** In chronic cases, it must be distinguished from lymphedema. Both conditions produce solid, non-pitting swelling, but venous obstruction causes some cyanosis of the skin; the skin is pallid in lymphedema. Lymphedema of the arm is common after radical mastectomy.

SECTION 2

THE BREASTS

Breast Physiology

The Female Breast

The breast is a highly complex, specialized skin-related gland. The mammary glands are undeveloped in children and men. In women, ovarian estrogen production at puberty initiates development which reaches maturity in the childbearing years. Luteal progesterone secretion at onset of ovulation results in alveolar development. Other hormones, including prolactin, adrenocorticotropic hormone, corticosteroids, growth hormone, thyroxine, and androgens play facultative roles in breast development and milk production. The mature breast is conical or hemispheric, containing 15 to 20 subdivided lobes, arranged radially, each with a separate excretory lactiferous tubule and nipple orifice. Considerable fat surrounds the glands, so discrete lobes are not ordinarily palpable. Vertical fibrous bands (Cooper ligaments) pass from the pectoralis fascia through the breast parenchyma to the skin, suspending the breast on the chest wall. A fascial cleft separates the deep surface of the breast from the thoracic wall, permitting some mobility.

The adult breast has four major components: stroma, ductal epithelium, glandular acini, and the myoepithelium, each influenced by a variety of hormonal signals. The breast glands respond to pituitary and ovarian hormones. Follicular estrogens stimulate minimal mitotic activity, while luteal progesterone provokes significant cell division and the breasts increase in size. If conception takes place, estrogens, progesterone and prolactin cause extensive alveolar and ductal proliferation. With parturition, the epithelium becomes actively secretory, as the release of prolactin inhibition by progesterone causes milk to be released.

The Male Breast

The undeveloped male breast is more easily examined than the woman's. Unfortunately, examination is frequently neglected and recognition of serious disease is delayed. Men have residual breast anlage that can respond to hormones at any time from adolescence to old age. Breast development occurs secondary to abnormal hormone production, including hyperthyroidism, prolactin-secreting adenomas, acromegaly, tumors of the testes and adrenals, and a variety of drugs

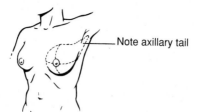
Note axillary tail

Fig. 8–55 *Quadrants of the Breast.* *The hemisphere of the breast is divided into quadrants by imaginary vertical and horizontal lines intersecting at the nipple. The quadrants are named upper medial, upper lateral, lower medial, and lower lateral. Popularly, these quadrants are also named, respectively, upper inner, upper outer, lower inner, and lower outer. Note the protrusion of the upper lateral quadrant, called the axillary tail, in which breast tissue extends to the axilla.*

including, of course, estrogens. It is not infrequently observed in alcoholic males, as liver disease leads to increased-circulating estrogenic hormones.

Superficial Anatomy of the Breasts

The breast has a circular area of contact, from the second to the sixth or seventh ribs, on the pectoral fascia and an axillary tail projecting laterally and superiorly along the axillary and serratus anterior fascia (Fig. 8–55) that is important in evaluating axillary masses.

The nipple, lying slightly below and lateral to the center of the breast, has pigmented skin, roughened with papillae containing the orifices of the lactiferous tubules, that extends onto the surface of the breast as the areola. The color of the nipple and areola varies from pink to brown, depending on the individual's complexion and parity. Both darken and the areola enlarges after the second month of pregnancy. The sebaceous glands of Montgomery (areolar glands) are small elevations on the areolar surface whose secretions protect the nipples during nursing. Areolar stimulation causes contraction of the subcutaneous radial and circular muscle fibers producing nipple erection.

Physical Examination of the Breasts

The American Cancer Society and other groups provide guidelines for periodic physical examination and mammography for breast cancer screening of women. The male breast must also be examined since breast cancer, and other conditions causing enlargement of breast tissue, occur in men and are easily identified, if examination is performed.

The breasts are usually inspected, including transillumination of masses, and palpated with the patient sitting and supine. If the patient complains of a breast lump or a possible mass is detected, more extensive examination is required. The breasts may engorge before menses and during pregnancy, making examination more painful and less accurate. The best time for breast examination is 5 to 7 days after onset of menses.

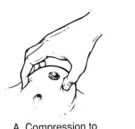 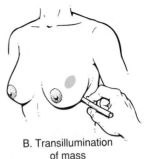

A. Compression to
show dimpling

B. Transillumination
of mass

Fig. 8–56 *Further Breast Examination. A. Breast compression to accent dimpling:* Dimpling is a sign of shortening of the suspensory ligaments of the breast from neoplasm or inflammation. *B. Transillumination:* The density of a mass may, on occasion, be ascertained by transillumination of the breast; transparency probably means a cyst full of fluid; other masses are opaque.

Breast Examination

The patient is examined sequentially both sitting and supine. Be certain to examine the creases under and between the breasts. If the patient has noted a lump, ask her to point it out; always palpate the opposite breast first. Palpate in all four quadrants of both breasts by compressing breast tissue between the pads of the three middle fingers and the chest wall (Jatoi I. Screening clinical breast examination. Surgical Clinics of North America 2003;83:789–801). Feel carefully for increased heat, tenderness, and masses. If a mass is found, ascertain its location, size, mobility, and consistency. Grasp the mass between thumb and forefinger moving it back and forth transversely, then up and down, testing for fixation to the underlying fascia. Repeat this test after tensing the pectoralis muscle (see below). Gently pinch the overlying skin to reveal dimpling, which indicates fixation of the mass to the skin (Fig. 8–56A). Transilluminate the mass, determining whether it is opaque or translucent (Fig. 8–56B). Finish with palpation of the regional lymph nodes (see page 100ff). The total time to complete a thorough breast examination should be approximately 6 to 10 minutes.

Patient sitting with arms down (Fig. 8–57A). With the patient sitting and disrobed to the waist, compare the size and shape of the breasts; the left may normally be slightly larger. Look for bulging or flattening of the lateral contour, nipple placement and retraction, skin dimpling or unilateral dilated superficial veins, or peau d'orange skin changes.

Patient sitting with arms raised (Fig. 8–57B). Have the patient raise her arms overhead; look for a shift in the relative position of the nipples, dimpling, or bulging.

Patient sitting with hands pressing hips (Fig. 8–57C). Pressing the hands downward on the hips may bring out dimpling by putting tension on the breast ligaments arising from the pectoralis major fascia. For a mass in the axillary tail, tense the serratus anterior muscle by having the patient press her hand downward on your shoulder.

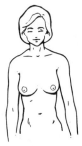
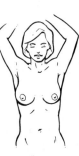
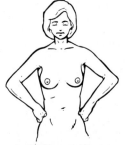

A. Patient standing with arms down

B. standing with arms elevated

C. Pushing on hips to tense pectoral muscles

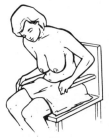

D. Bent forward so breasts hang free

E. Breasts palpated against pectoral muscles

Fig. 8–57 *Patient Positions for Breast Examination.* The patient is stripped to the waist and sits facing the examiner. *A.* The patient stands with arms at sides; the examiner looks for elevation of the level of a nipple, dimpling, bulging, and peau d'orange. *B.* When the patient raises her arms, dimpling and elevation of the nipple are accentuated when there is a mass fixed to the pectoral fascia. *C.* The patient pushes her hands down against her hips to flex and tense the pectoralis major muscles; the examiner moves the mass to determine fixation to the underlying fascia. *D.* When the breasts are large and pendulous, the patient is asked to lean forward, so the breasts hang free from the chest wall; retraction and masses become more evident. *E.* In the supine position, the examiner presses the breasts against the chest wall with the flat of his hand; the normal nodosity from the lobules is less prominent and significant masses are more distinctly felt.

Patient sitting with trunk bent forward (Fig. 8–57D). When the breasts are large and pendulous, having the patient lean forward, so the breasts hang free from the chest wall, may facilitate inspection and palpation between the flats of both hands.

Patient supine (Fig. 8–57E). The vast majority of breast masses are detected in this position and proper technique is critically important. The entire breast from the second to sixth rib and from the left sternal border to the midaxillary line must be palpated against the chest wall. Palpate with the pads of the three middle fingers, rotating the fingers in small circular motions and moving in vertical overlapping passes from rostral to caudal and then back caudal to rostral in the next pass. The pressure of the fingers should be varied from light to medium to deep. The lateral half of the breast is best palpated with the patient rolled onto the contralateral hip and the medial half with the patient supine, both with the ipsilateral hand behind the head [Barton MB, Harris R, Fletcher SW. Does this patient have breast cancer? The screening clinical breast examination: Should it be done? How? *JAMA*. 1999;282:1270–1280].

Nipple Examination

Inspect the anterior trunk for supernumerary nipples. Look for fissures, scaling, excoriation, retraction or deformity of the nipple; recent deformities suggest acquired disease. Nipple discharge may be detected by gently compressing the nipple and areola between the thumb and forefinger; this has not proven to be productive for cancer screening. Palpate the periphery of the areola for tenderness, nodules or cords.

The total time to complete a thorough breast examination should be approximately 6 to 10 minutes. An additional portion of the examination should include palpation of the axillary and supraclavicular fossae, searching for lymphadenopathy.

Breast Symptoms

KEY SYMPTOM   Pain in the Breast

The patient with pain or a lump in the breast often fears cancer. Most women will, at some time, experience breast discomfort significant enough to seek a physician's advice [Barton MB, Elmore JG, Fletcher SW. Breast symptoms among women enrolled in a health maintenance organization: Frequency, evolution, and outcome. *Ann Intern Med*. 1999;130:651–657]. Mastodynia, chronic breast pain without evident pathology, is common. *CLINICAL OCCURRENCE:*   Common causes of breast pain are engorgement during the luteal phase of the menstrual cycle, pregnancy, hematoma, cysts, mastitis and abscess, galactocele and nipple disorders including fissures, inflammation, and epithelioma.

Breast Signs

KEY SIGN   Breast Masses

Masses in the breast may arise from cystic changes, benign proliferation of ductal or acinar tissue, infection, inflammation or fibrosis of the breast stroma, and neoplastic change in the ductal epithelium (ductal carcinoma) or the acinar tissues (lobular neoplasia). Masses in the breast, as elsewhere, must be accurately described noting their location (use the nipple as the center of a clock face: state the o'clock position and the radial distance from the nipple), size, shape, consistency (hard, firm, fluctuant, soft), texture (smooth, irregular), mobility (mobile, fixed to the breast tissue, pectoral fascia or skin) and the presence of tenderness. Always thoroughly examine the regional lymph nodes (axillary, infraclavicular and supraclavicular) for lymphadenopathy. Masses identified by the patient or clinician should never be ignored or be assumed to be benign; the patient's age and breast cancer risk factors should not deter evaluation of a breast mass.

 All masses that persist through one complete menstrual cycle and all masses in postmenopausal women require evaluation by a clinician experienced in the diagnosis and management of diseases of the breast and breast cancer. A normal mammogram or nonvisualization of a palpable mass by ultrasonography does not exclude cancer.

See page 441 for a discussion of common breast masses.

KEY SIGN   Breast Tenderness

During the luteal phase of the menstrual cycle, and with pregnancy and lactation, the breasts undergo glandular proliferation and become larger and more engorged. These changes are associated with increased tenderness. Many women of child-bearing years have persistent tenderness that may vary with the menstrual cycle, but never resolve completely (*mastodynia*). The breasts may be more firm and lobular on examination, but distinct masses are not felt. The finding is normal and not a cause of concern.   ***CLINICAL OCCURRENCE:***   Common causes of breast pain are engorgement during the luteal phase of the menstrual cycle, pregnancy, hematoma, cysts, mastitis and abscess, galactocele and nipple disorders including fissures, inflammation, and epithelioma.

KEY SIGN   Cysts

Cystic change in the breast creates single or multiple tender fluid-filled cysts. The patient complains of tenderness that fluctuates with the menstrual cycle. Examination discloses one or more smooth, usually mobile tender tense masses that may be fluctuant or firm. Ultrasonography or needle aspiration confirms the presence of a cyst.

Supernumerary nipples (polythelia) and breasts (polymastia).   Extra nipples occur frequently in both sexes as minor errors in development; rarely they are associated with glandular tissue to form a complete breast. Supernumerary nipples are smaller than normal and often mistaken for moles; close examination usually discloses a miniature nipple and areola. Most occur in the mammary or milk line on the thorax and abdomen; rarely, they are found in the axilla or on the shoulder, flank, groin, or thigh. The only significant issue is to distinguish them from moles.

Inverted bipples.   A common, harmless developmental anomaly results in the nipple having a crater-like depression. Nipple retraction appearing after maturity suggests underlying neoplastic or inflammatory disease.

Nipple fissures.   Breaks in the skin are usually caused by local infection; their presence may indicate an unsuspected abscess.

Duct fistula.   A chronic draining wound close to the nipple and areola may herald a fistulous tract between an underlying duct and the skin.

KEY SIGN   Skin or Nipple Retraction

Acquired nipple retraction and skin dimpling are due to shortening of the suspensory ligaments of the breast, and/or fixation of the breast to the underlying pectoral fascia, by tumor or inflammation. Always examine for skin and nipple retraction and limited mobility of the breast on the chest wall. If present, carefully examine for an underlying mass and regional lymphadenopathy. Although this can result from previous mastitis, it should only be assumed so if the evolution from acute mastitis to fixation and retraction has been personally observed. Otherwise, this finding should be pursued as you would a breast mass.

> **KEY SIGN** **Nipple Discharge**

Abnormal secretions from the breast result from a large number of causes. It is important to determine if the secretion is spontaneous or induced. The former is usually of greater consequence than the latter [Fiorica JV. Nipple discharge. *Obstet Gynecol Clin North Am.* 1994;21:453–460].

Serous, Bloody, or Opalescent Discharge: This type of secretion may occur with benign or malignant lesions; benign causes are most common. Bilateral secretion without pregnancy is usually a result of hormonal influences. When unilateral discharge is present, a pathologic condition is more likely. If the cause is not evident from the history or physical examination, cytologic examination of the fluid or biopsy of the breast tissue may be necessary. *CLINICAL OCCURRENCE:* Common causes of breast discharge are intraductal papilloma, fibrocystic disease, and sclerosing adenosis. Less-common causes are chronic cystic mastitis, duct ectasia, galactocele, papillary cystadenoma, keratosis of nipple, fat necrosis, acute mastitis or abscess, tuberculosis, toxoplasmosis, and eczema of the nipple. Invasive cancers of the breast do not ordinarily cause discharges. Malignant lesions include ductal carcinoma, lobular carcinoma, sarcomas, and Paget disease of the nipple.

> **Scaling and Excoriation of the Nipple—Paget Disease:** A deep-seated invasive malignancy is present in half the cases, the cells of which have extended along the ductal system, lactiferous tubules and superficial lymphatics onto the nipple, areola and skin. Patients experience "tingling, itching, and burning." A scaling eczematoid lesion involves the nipple which becomes reddened and excoriated; complete destruction of the nipple may result. The process extends along the skin as well as in the ducts.

Abscess of the Areolar Gland: The sebaceous glands of Montgomery become inflamed, forming tender, palpable abscesses in the periphery of the areola. The abscess may become large and invade the breast unless drained. An underlying cancer with secondary infection should be considered.

Breast Syndromes

The Female Breast

> **KEY SYNDROME** **Galactorrhea**

Lactation depends on prolactin from the anterior pituitary and progesterone and estrogen from the ovaries and placenta. Milk ejection is initiated by mechanical stimulation sending afferent impulses to the hypothalamus, causing release of oxytocin from the posterior pituitary. Prolactin levels must be checked in patients with galactorrhea or amenorrhea. Pituitary prolactinomas cause elevated prolactin levels leading to galactorrhea and suppression of ovulation. Many physiologic states, clinical disorders, and drugs may be associated with the secretion of milk.

✔ *GALACTORRHEA—CLINICAL OCCURRENCE: Endocrine* pregnancy, adolescence, hypothyroidism, hyperthyroidism; *Idiopathic* uterine atrophy with amenorrhea and lactation (Frommel disease); *Inflammatory/Immune* mastitis; *Infectious* herpes zoster, post-encephalitis; *Metabolic/Toxic* drugs (phenothiazines, reserpine, methyldopa, oral contraceptive, tricyclic antidepressants, antihistamines, opiates); *Mechanical/Trauma* mechanical stimulation of the nipples, suckling, trauma to the chest wall, thoracoplasty, pneumonectomy, mammoplasty, irradiation; *Neoplastic* pituitary prolactinoma.

> **KEY SYNDROME** **Breast Mass**

Breast masses arise from benign and malignant neoplastic change in the ductal or acinar epithelium, cystic changes, duct obstruction, infection, bleeding and infiltration by abnormal cells or accumulation of intra- or extracellular substances, especially fibrosis. Some masses retain hormonal control; many do not. The most important distinction is between benign and malignant lesions. Cysts are overwhelmingly benign and aspiration of nonbloody fluid with disappearance of the mass is diagnostic. Smooth regular borders and tenderness are suggestive of adenofibroma as opposed to malignancy. Tenderness is not common with cancer; it is more characteristic of inflammatory breast disease with or without infection. The only way to assure benignity is histologic confirmation on aspiration cytology or biopsy. *Benign Masses Fibrocystic breast disease* is a term is used in the professional and lay literature to describe a broad spectrum of benign pathologic conditions of the female breast. The specific pathologic diagnosis depends on the preponderance of one component over others. If the pathology is confined to stromal proliferation, fibroadenoma, virginal hypertrophy of the breast, and intracanalicular fibroadenoma may be diagnosed. When an abnormal ductal system predominates, micro or macrocystic disease, cystic mastitis, sclerosing adenosis, intraductal papilloma, and ductal ectasia involving the lactiferous sinus are terms that are used to describe the changes. If the main source of changes is in the terminal ductule and glandular elements, lobular hyperplasia is identified. Finally, hyperplasia of the myoepithelium leads to a diagnosis of myoepithelial hyperplasia of Reclus. *Premalignant and Malignant Masses* Malignant neoplasms usually arise from the ductal epithelium and have a strong genetic contribution (BRCA-1, BRCA-2). The finding of *atypical ductal hyperplasia* is associated with an increased risk of subsequent *in situ or invasive ductal carcinoma*. Neoplasia of the acinar lobules is called *lobular neoplasia*. It is usually noninvasive, but is associated with an increased risk for *invasive ductal carcinoma*. *Malignant lymphoma* may involve the lymph nodes and other tissues of the breast. For the patient and clinician, it is essential to remember that the primary distinctions are between malignant and nonmalignant conditions and invasive and noninvasive malignancies. Biopsy of discrete, dominant lesions is necessary for correct diagnosis. Only the pathologist can make a histologic diagnosis. Neither the surgeon nor the radiologist can speak with the certainty of the pathologist. Normal or nondiagnostic mammography must not prevent biopsy of a clinically suspicious mass. *The only virtue in diagnosing a benign breast condition lies in excluding malignancy.* The evaluation of breast masses and their management is constantly

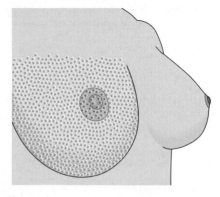

Fig. 8–58 *Peau d'Orange.* *Cutaneous edema of the breast is indicated by skin that is indented deeply with holes, the accentuated orifices of the sweat glands. This gives the appearance of an orange skin or a pig's skin.*

evolving. Expert consultation is advised and many specialty breast clinics exist for just this purpose.

Carcinoma of the Breast: There may be a dominant nontender mass in the breast [Barton MB, Harris R, Fletcher SW. The rational clinical examination. Does this patient have breast cancer? The screening clinical breast exam: Should it be done? How? *JAMA.* 1999;282:1270–1280]. Suspensory ligament infiltration causes retraction revealed by dimpling, nipple deviation and fixation to the pectoral muscles. Flattening of the nipple and a bloody or clear discharge indicates disease in the lactiferous tubules. Lymphatic obstruction produces edema of the skin, manifest by peau d'orange (Fig. 8–58). Lymphatic spread is marked by regional lymphadenopathy. A solitary breast mass mandates a diagnostic biopsy. Occasionally, the presenting sign is a bloody discharge, enlarged lymph axillary nodes, or dermal inflammation without a mass. **DDX:** The incidence of cancer in women <30 years of age is 1%, and there is a steady rise with increasing age; it is now estimated that 1 in 9 or 10 women will eventually develop breast cancer. The median age at which the various pathologic breast abnormalities appear in women is known, and on that basis, probabilities are estimated. The data in Table 8–5 is from patients operated on at New York Medical College-Flower Fifth Avenue Hospitals during the period 1960–1975.

Inflammatory Breast Carcinoma: Breast cancer can present as an acute inflammatory disease, especially in the lactating breast. The signs are similar to those of acute mastitis except that the entire breast is swollen and there is early

Table 8–5　Relationship of Breast Abnormalities and Age

Diagnosis	Age range (median)
Fibrocystic disease	20–49 (30)
Fibroadenoma	15–39 (20)
Intraductal papilloma and ductal ectasia	35–55 (40)
Carcinoma	40–71 (54)

involvement of the axillary lymph nodes (see page 440). **DDX:** In contrast acute mastitis the inflammation is usually limited to a single breast quadrant and lymphadenopathy is uncommon.

Fluctuant Breast Mass—Cyst, Lipoma, Abscess: Cysts are very common and must be distinguished from other fluctuant masses, for example, lipomas and abscesses. Fluctuation is demonstrated by holding the edges of the mass tightly to the chest wall with one hand and pressing its center with the fingers of the other hand. Abscess is often quite tender and has erythema; true lipomas are exceedingly rare, accounting for less than 1% of all breast lesions. Transillumination suggests a cyst; ultrasound or aspiration confirms the diagnosis.

Fibroadenoma: This is usually found in a young woman with large breasts. The ovoid or lobulated nodule is firm, elastic, or rubbery in consistency. It may be the size of a pinhead or quite large. The mass is nontender and freely movable, causing it to slip easily in the breast tissue. The mass must be distinguished from dysplasia, carcinoma, and cystosarcoma phyllodes.

Fat Necrosis: Breast trauma may produce a hematoma and fat necrosis resulting in a scar that adheres to the surrounding tissue and causes retraction. The findings may suggest carcinoma. A history of trauma should not weigh too heavily in the diagnosis because a common inclination of patients is to attribute neoplastic masses to some remote traumatic incident. Even though this lesion is inconsequential, excisional biopsy may be necessary.

Diabetic Fibrous Breast Disease: Some women with type 1 diabetes develop diabetic fibrous breast disease presenting as one or more painless hard mobile irregular breast masses; histology shows intralobular and perilobular B-lymphocyte inflammatory nodules with fibrosis in the breast fat [Zimmerli L, Yurtsever H, et al A diabetic breast lump. *Lancet.* 2000;357:1670].

Acute Mastitis: The breast is flushed, tender, hot, swollen, and indurated, frequently accompanied by chills, fever, and sweating. Usually a single breast quadrant is involved. Often the inflammation proceeds to abscess formation. In approximately two-thirds of the cases, the disease occurs during lactation. Inflammatory carcinoma must be considered, especially in the presence of nontender axillary lymphadenopathy.

Abscess: Usually this is the sequel of acute mastitis. There is a localized, hot, exquisitely tender and painful fluctuant mass frequently accompanied by chills and fever with leukocytosis.

Chronic Breast Abscess: Pus may become enclosed by a thick wall of fibrous tissue, presenting a nontender, irregular, firm mass requiring biopsy to distinguish from carcinoma.

Juvenile Mastitis: A tender unilateral firm mass with signs of inflammation occurs beneath the nipple in young boys and in women between 20 and 30 years of age. The condition is benign and resolves in a few weeks.

The Male Breast

> **KEY DISEASE** **Carcinoma of the Male Breast**

Approximately 1% to 2% of carcinomas of the breast occur in men; there is an increased risk with the BRCA2 mutation. The mass is apparent early because of the paucity of breast tissue. The lesion begins as a painless induration with retraction of the nipple and fixation to the skin and deep tissues. The mass does not transilluminate. It must be distinguished from gynecomastia. Fine-needle aspiration biopsy or excision should is diagnostic. Mammography in the male is usually not helpful.

KEY SYNDROME   Gynecomastia

Breast development is controlled by circulating estrogens. Increased estrogen levels associated with puberty, liver disease, drugs, and endocrine abnormalities can lead to proliferation of breast tissue in men. Gynecomastia is defined as a transient or permanent noninflammatory enlargement of the male breast [Braunstein GD. Gynecomastia. *N Engl J Med* 1993;328:490–495]. Physical examination reveals a finely lobulated often tender subareolar mass that is mobile on the chest wall. Increased sensitivity of the nipple is frequently noted by the patient. The mass may be small and unilateral, or gynecomastia can develop bilaterally to the dimensions of the female breast. Hard masses or those with fixation to the skin or chest wall must be excised to exclude carcinoma. ***CLINICAL OCCURRENCE:*** The idiopathic type frequently appears at puberty and is usually unilateral. Hormonal stimulation causes bilateral enlargement, for example, administration of estrogens, after castration, Cushing syndrome, and in testicular choriocarcinoma. Enlargement of the breasts may also occur in cirrhosis of the liver, probably from incomplete hepatic destruction of estrogen. Refeeding gynecomastia occurs when patients with severe malnutrition are given food. Gynecomastia may occur in association with leukemia, lymphoma, pulmonary carcinoma, familial lumbosacral syringomyelia, and Graves' disease. Among the drugs occasionally causing gynecomastia are digitalis, isoniazid, spironolactone, phenothiazine, and diazepam.

Acute Mastitis in the Male Breast.   This usually occurs from trauma. The signs are similar to the condition in women. Irritation and chafing of the nipple and breast occur in active sports, like jogging and similar activities.

Juvenile Mastitis: See above, page 443.

CHAPTER 9

The Abdomen, Perineum, Anus, and Rectosigmoid

Abdominal symptoms are common. Mastery of the abdominal examination is essential since judgments based primarily on history and physical examination are the basis for differential diagnosis and selection of laboratory and imaging studies to confirm a diagnosis. An accurate and thorough history is essential to delineate the specific characteristics and sequence of the patient's symptoms. Frequent repetition of the abdominal exam and correlation with the patient's symptoms are essential. Correct assessment of abdominal findings requires familiarity with anatomic pathology and pathophysiology. Surgeons must excel in abdominal examination because their findings influence the decision to operate.

In the supine position, the abdominal cavity is a shallow oval basin with a rigid W-shaped bottom of vertebral column and back muscles. Heavy flank muscles constitute the long sides and the diaphragm and pelvic floor muscles close either end. The brim is formed by the lower rib margins at one end, and the pubes and ilia at the other. The cover is formed by the flat muscles and fascia of the anterior abdominal wall, reinforced by two parallel bands of rectus muscles attached to the ends of the basin.

The abdominal viscera are solid or hollow. The solid viscera are the liver, spleen, kidneys, adrenals, pancreas, ovaries, and uterus. Most of these organs retain their characteristic shapes and positions as they enlarge. Many are clustered under the protecting eaves of the lower ribs. The hollow viscera are the stomach, small intestines, colon, gallbladder, bile ducts, fallopian tubes, ureters, and urinary bladder. They are normally not palpable, unless distended by gas, fluid or solid masses.

Two systems have been used to describe abdominal topography (Fig. 9–1). Most physicians prefer the simpler division into quadrants by an axial and a transverse line through the umbilicus; we use that plan here.

Major Systems and Their Physiology

Alimentary System

The alimentary system is responsible for converting ingested foodstuffs into biologically available nutrients and fuels, and for eliminating solid wastes while maintaining a barrier to an enormous variety of microorganisms, parasites, and toxic molecules. This is a complex process involving ingestion, mastication, bulk transport, storage, mechanical disruption, mixing, and digestion of ingested food and absorption of nutrients coordinated with production, storage, transport, and

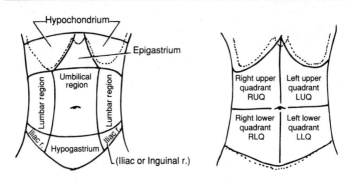

Fig. 9–1 *Topographic Divisions of the Abdomen.* On the left are the regions of the abdomen as defined in the Basle Nomina Anatomica terminology. Most of the nine regions are small, so that enlarged viscera and other structures occupy more than one. On the right is a simpler plan with four regions; it is preferred by most clinicians and is employed in this book. Many occasions arise when the quadrant scheme needs supplementing by reference to the epigastrium, the flanks, or the suprapubic region.

carefully timed release of digestive enzymes and bile acids. The alimentary system starts at the mouth and ends at the anus. The oral cavity and pharynx, were discussed previously. Most of the alimentary system is located in the abdomen, extending from the gastroesophageal junction at or near the diaphragmatic hiatus to the anus. Normal motility and digestion are dependent upon coordination of muscular and secretory functions via local and systemic neural and endocrine mechanisms. The bowel is a muscular tube suspended by a mobile mesentery (stomach, small intestine, cecum, transverse and sigmoid colon) or anchored to the posterior abdominal wall (duodenum, ascending and descending colon) or pelvic floor (rectum). It is susceptible to intraluminal obstruction at narrow points (gastroesophageal junction, pylorus, ileocecal valve), to extraluminal obstruction by compression anywhere in its course, and to twisting or kinking when suspended on a mesentery (especially the small bowel, cecum, and sigmoid). Disruption of this system by local or systemic disease results in symptoms and signs referred to the abdomen. Symptoms include changes in appetite and interest in food, changes in abdominal sensations, including pain, and alterations in stool character and frequency. Physical signs are reflective of changes in overall nutrition, abnormal abdominal contour, evidence of altered intestinal motility or obstruction, solid-organ enlargement, increased peritoneal fluid, and localized mass or tenderness.

Hepatobiliary and Pancreatic System

The hepatobiliary-pancreatic system arises from condensation of mesenchymal tissues around embryonic evaginations of the gut (biliary and pancreatic ducts). The pancreas produces bicarbonate and digestive enzymes (amylase, lipase, and proteinases), which are released in response to ingestion of specific foodstuffs and changes in duodenal contents. It also contains the endocrine islets of Langerhans, which release insulin, glucagon, and somatostatin in response to changes in the blood glucose level and a variety of other stimuli. The liver receives venous blood from the gut, pancreas, and spleen via the portal vein, and percolates it from the portal triads through a radial array of sinusoids to the central vein. From the central vein, blood passes to the heart via the hepatic vein and inferior vena cava (IVC). Hepatocytes perform three general functions: (1) they remove toxic molecules derived from the intestinal contents and systemic metabolism, process them, and release them back into the circulation or secrete them with the bile; (2) they synthesize many of the molecules necessary for maintenance of systemic homeostasis including albumin, coagulation factors, lipoproteins, and transport molecules; and (3) they synthesize and secrete the bile salts that are necessary for digestion and absorption of fats. Kupffer cells are found within the sinusoids. They are phagocytic antigen-presenting cells that clear bacteria from the portal circulation and release cytokines, which enter the systemic circulation. Symptoms related to the hepatobiliary-pancreatic system are changes in general and specific food interest, pain or discomfort associated with the ingestion of food, and maldigestion with changes in bowel function, stool consistency, and frequency. Physical signs relate to (1) changes in the size, consistency, and shape of the liver; (2) to localized pain and masses; and (3) to local and systemic changes caused by alterations in hepatobiliary-pancreatic function, such as jaundice, weight loss, bleeding, and ascites.

Spleen and Lymphatics

See Chapter 5, page 92ff for a discussion of the lymph nodes.

The spleen is the largest lymphatic organ. It has a complex sinusoidal structure that serves several functions. Arterial blood is distributed into sinusoids where senescent red blood cells, intracellular inclusions, and membrane abnormalities are removed. The spleen is important in the generation of specific humoral immune responses to encapsulated bacteria and their removal from the blood. The abdominal organs are rich in lymphatics. The lymphatic capillaries drain into regional lymph nodes located at the hila of solid organs and in the mesentery of the bowel. These drain into the periaortic nodes, which also receive lymph from the lower extremities and pelvis. The periaortic nodes drain cephalad toward the thoracic duct. Few specific symptoms arise from alterations in these organs. Enlargement of the spleen will be felt as upper abdominal fullness, and retroperitoneal lymph node enlargement can present as flank and back pressure or pain. Fever, weight loss, and sweats may be the only symptoms of intraabdominal lymphoma. Moderate splenomegaly can be detected by physical examination, but intraabdominal lymph nodes are rarely palpable.

Kidneys, Ureters, and Bladder

See the discussion of urogenital function in Chapter 10. The kidneys are located in the retroperitoneum deep to the lower ribs (Fig. 9–2). The ureters course in the retroperitoneum along, then over, the psoas muscle, over the pelvic brim, and into the pelvis, where they enter the bladder. Symptoms referred to the abdomen arise mostly from obstruction of the renal pelvis or ureter, giving rise to deep, poorly localized visceral pain in the abdomen, flank, pelvis, or testicles. Symptoms referred to the back and flanks include fullness and pain because of kidney enlargement or invasion of adjacent structures by inflammatory, infectious, or neoplastic masses. Physical signs are palpable enlargement of the kidney or bladder, or pain on deep palpation over these structures.

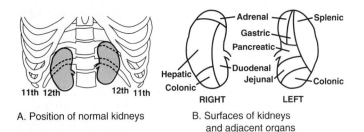

A. Position of normal kidneys

B. Surfaces of kidneys and adjacent organs

Fig. 9–2 *Anatomic Relations of the Normal Kidneys. A. The position of the normal kidneys* as viewed from the anterior surface of the abdomen. Note that the right kidney is lying in front of the twelfth rib, while the slightly higher left kidney is in front of the eleventh and twelfth ribs. *B. The anterior surfaces of both kidneys*, showing the regions touched by overlying viscera.

Superficial Anatomy of the Abdomen and Perineum

The Abdomen

It is mandatory to have a thorough mental picture of the location and relative relationships of all abdominal organs, the bowel mesentery and its attachment to the posterior abdominal wall, and the arterial, venous, and lymphatic vascular supply of each organ. Next, it is necessary to anchor this picture to the superficial landmarks used during the physical examination: the spine, ribs and costal margins, umbilicus, rectus muscle, inguinal ligament, ilia, and pubes. Lastly, you must accurately associate this picture with the images presented by plain X-ray films, ultrasonography, computed tomography (CT), and MRI images. This is neither simple nor intuitive. The only way to become expert is to repeatedly study textbooks of gross anatomy, review the details of imaging studies with your radiologist, and validate your picture by attending autopsies, reviewing gross dissections, and observing surgical procedures.

The Anus

Fig. 9–3 depicts the structure of the anal canal. It is 2.5 to 4 cm long in the adult and is surrounded by two concentric layers of striated muscle—the voluntary external sphincter and the involuntary internal sphincter. A small band of the external sphincter overrides the distal end of the internal sphincter and thus is felt first by the entering finger. The name of the external sphincter refers to its position surrounding the internal sphincter, rather than to its more distal position in the anal canal. The mucocutaneous junction may be inspected without a speculum by everting the anal mucosa.

The Rectum

The rectum is the terminal 12 cm of the colon. It begins at the rectosigmoid junction and ends at the entrance to the anal canal. Near its distal end, it dilates to form the rectal ampulla. In the rectum are found semilunar transverse folds,

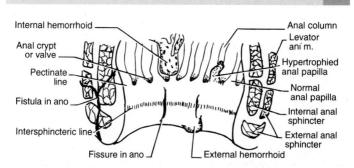

Fig. 9–3 *Anatomy of the Anal Canal: Interior and Cross-Section.* *The anal columns (columns of Morgagni) descend vertically from the rectum and end in anal papillae that fuse to form the pectinate or dentate line; behind are the anal valves (crypts of Morgagni). The cut walls show the internal anal sphincter surrounded by the external sphincter that extends distally. The junction between the edges of the two sphincters forms the intersphincteric line. Internal hemorrhoids arise proximal to the pectinate line, external hemorrhoids distally. Two anal fissures are shown, one distal to a resulting hypertrophied papilla. A fistula (black and irregular) drains from an abscess in a rectal crypt (or valve) to the skin near the anus.*

the valves of Houston, which are inconstant in number and position. Because the combined length of the anal canal and the rectum is approximately 16 cm, the examining finger cannot reach the entire length. The upper two-thirds of the rectum is covered by peritoneum. In men, the anterior peritoneal reflection extends downward as the rectovesical pouch to within 7.5 cm of the anal orifice, so it is potentially accessible to the examining finger. In women, the rectouterine pouch extends downward anteriorly to within 5.5 cm of the anal orifice.

The Sigmoid and Descending Colon

The descending colon starts at the splenic flexure and descends in the retroperitoneum to the left iliac fossa, where it becomes the sigmoid colon at the iliac flexure. The sigmoid colon, suspended on its mesentery, extends from the iliac flexure to the rectum. In the pelvis, the sigmoid runs transversely from the left ileum toward the right side of the pelvis, then, doubling on itself, it passes leftward toward the midline, and then downward to meet the rectum at the level of the third sacral vertebra, frequently forming a crude S, from which the name is derived.

Physical Examination of the Abdomen

The abdomen is examined in the following sequence: inspection, auscultation, percussion, and palpation. Ensure a warm room and adequate covering so that the patient does not chill and tense the abdominal wall. The patient should lie supine with a pillow under the head. A pillow under the knees, to support passive hip and knee flexion, may add additional comfort and relax the abdominal wall muscles. When orthopnea is present, raise the backrest to support the trunk. Patients with kyphosis require more elevation of the head and shoulders. Drape

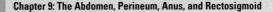

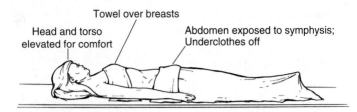

Towel over breasts

Head and torso elevated for comfort

Abdomen exposed to symphysis; Underclothes off

Fig. 9–4 *Draping for Abdominal Examination.* The patient lies supine on the examining table with a sheet or blanket covering the lower extremities up to the pubes. For women, the breasts are covered with a folded towel or gown. A small pillow supports the head. To further relax the abdominal muscles, a pillow can be placed to support the knees in slight flexion.

the abdomen with a sheet or blanket, covering the lower limbs up to the pubes (Fig. 9–4). Cover a woman's breasts with a folded towel or gown. Examination is best performed from the patient's right side.

The Abdomen

Inspection

Do not slight this step because of an urge to start palpating. Effort and discipline are required to inspect properly, thoroughly, and unhurriedly (Fig. 9–5). Arrange a single source of light to shine across the abdomen toward you, or, alternatively, have the light shine lengthwise over the patient. Inspect the abdomen sequentially for contour, distention, scars, engorged veins, visible peristalsis, and masses. Additional inspection from the foot of the table can reveal asymmetry of the abdomen and thorax.

The distended abdomen. Experience with hundreds of examinations is necessary to learn the normal range of abdominal contour and what constitutes abnormal abdominal contours and distention. Distention may be caused by several simultaneous conditions, so be thorough and consider all potential contributing conditions.

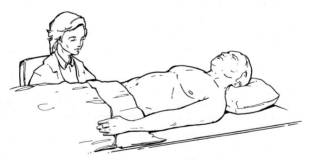

Fig. 9–5 *Abdominal Inspection.* The patient is supine with a single source of light shining across from feet to head, or across the abdomen toward the examiner. The examiner should sit in a chair at the right of the patient with her head only slightly higher than the abdomen. In this manner, the physician can concentrate on the abdomen for several minutes, if needed.

Auscultation

Peristaltic Sounds. Only by auscultating as part of *every* abdominal examination can you learn to distinguish normal from abnormal peristaltic sounds and correlate the variety of abnormal sounds with different types of abdominal pathology. Auscultate the abdomen before palpation alters bowel activity. Listen with the bell of the stethoscope in all four quadrants and the midline. If bowel sounds are not audible, sit and listen for at least 5 minutes. Occasional weak tinkles are not evidence of good peristaltic activity. High-pitched tinkling sounds and rushes may be heard in partial obstruction. ***Abdominal Murmurs.*** A murmur indicates turbulent blood flow in a dilated, constricted, or tortuous artery.

Percussion

Percussion of the abdomen is performed as in percussion elsewhere (Chapter 3, page 3pff). Dullness over the liver in the right upper quadrant (RUQ) and a hollow tympanic note over the stomach in the left upper quadrant (LUQ) and lower chest should be expected. The remainder of the abdomen usually gives a flat percussion note. Gas in the abdomen or bowel increases the area of tympany. Enlargement of the spleen is suggested by percussion dullness in the LUQ over the lower ribs (*Traube space*); bladder distention produces dullness in the suprapubic area. Pain elicited by percussion, especially pain remote to the immediate site of percussion suggests peritoneal inflammation (rebound). Gentle *fist percussion* performed with the heel of the hand on the ribs overlying the liver, spleen, and kidneys (Fig. 9–6) is useful to identify pain caused by stretching or inflammation of the capsules surrounding these organs. ***Percussion and Palpation for Costovertebral Angle Tenderness:*** This is elicited by palpation with one finger or thumb. The finger is pressed in a radial direction into the soft tissues enclosed by the costovertebral angle between the spine and the twelfth rib (see Fig. 9–2). Alternatively, the ulnar side of the fist may be used to strike the same point to cause jarring of the surrounding tissues in the area of the kidney.

If the patient complains of abdominal pain, start with maneuvers that cause movement of peritoneal surfaces without contact by the examiner; pain implies peritoneal inflammation. First, ask the patient to point to the area of maximum

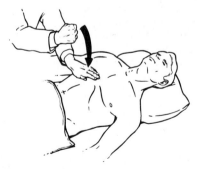

Fig. 9–6 *Fist Percussion Over the Liver.* The palm of the left hand is applied anteriorly to the lower ribs of the right hemithorax. The back of the applied hand is struck lightly with the fist of the right hand.

tenderness. Then ask her to suck in her abdomen while indicating any areas of discomfort. Next, position your hand approximately 15 cm over the abdomen and ask her to push her stomach out toward your hand, again while indicating any areas of discomfort. Finally, ask her to cough.

Palpation

The anterior abdominal wall muscles resist palpation proportionally to their strength and tone. To minimize resistance, be gentle and reassuring, explaining what you are doing while starting with deliberately gentle techniques. As a last resort, the examiner may press hard on the lower sternum with the left hand while palpating the abdomen with the right. When the patient attempts inspiration against this pressure, she must relax her abdominal muscles.

Posture of the patient. Although usually performed with the patient supine, palpation with the patient on either side or in the knee-elbow posture can reveal masses not otherwise discernible. The standing position is mandatory to identify some hernias.

Light abdominal palpation. Before attempting deep palpation, always palpate the entire abdomen lightly searching for edges, regions of tenderness or increased resistance, and, sometimes, masses that cannot be felt when pushing harder. Place the entire palm and approximated fingers on abdomen pressing the fingertips gently to a depth of approximately 1 cm (Fig. 9–7A). Sweep the entire hand gently over the surface, beginning at the pubes and working upward to the costal margins. Be attentive that a huge liver or spleen is not missed because the low edge is not felt. Examine symptomatic areas last. As you palpate watch the patient's face for evidence of discomfort. *Ticklishness.* Ticklishness causes tense muscles impairing evaluation of underlying tenderness or masses. Use pressure of the stethoscope to elicit tenderness. Additionally, have the patient follow your motions with her fingers on yours (Fig. 9–7C); the patient is not ticklish to their own touch which is now mimicked.

Deep abdominal palpation. Pursue previous findings and search for unsuspected deep tenderness and masses. Continue to watch the patient's face as you palpate with the approximated fingertips pressed ever more deeply; the palm may just touch the abdomen. The fingertips are placed so most tactile sensations are received on the pads. In addition to downward pressure, the fingers should move slowly, laterally, and longitudinally, 4 or 5 cm, causing the abdominal wall to glide over the underlying structures (Fig. 9–7E). For *single-handed palpation*, one hand is used for the examination. When the muscular resistance is strong, *reinforced palpation* is employed. The fingers of the one hand press on the distal phalangeal joints of the other; one hand produces the pressure while the other receives the tactile sensations with its muscles and tendons relaxed (Fig. 9–7B). When a mass is small, its thickness is determined by grasping it between the thumb, middle, and index fingers; when large, bimanual palpation is employed by placing a hand on each side of the mass. When ascites is present, *ballottement* is useful. The fingers are thrust rapidly and sequentially more deeply into the abdomen in the region of the suspected mass. The mass may tap the tips of the examining fingers (Fig. 9–8).

Attributes of masses. When you feel a mass in the abdomen, you must decide which anatomic structure is involved and the nature of the pathologic process. Nearly all masses arise from previously normal tissues. Many inferences may be

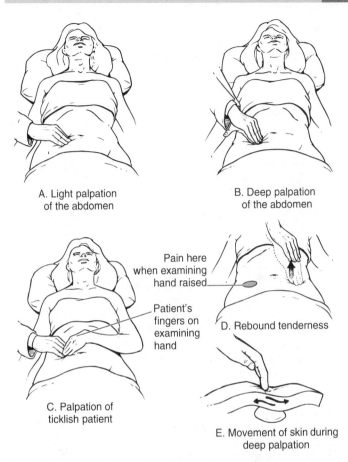

A. Light palpation
of the abdomen

B. Deep palpation
of the abdomen

Pain here
when examining
hand raised

Patient's
fingers on
examining
hand

D. Rebound tenderness

C. Palpation of
ticklish patient

E. Movement of skin during
deep palpation

Fig. 9–7 *Abdominal Palpation. A. Light palpation:* *Care should be taken to avoid digging into the wall with the tips of the fingers.* ***B. Deep palpation. C. Palpation of the ticklish abdomen. D. Rebound tenderness:*** *The hand is slowly pushed deep into the abdomen remote from the suspected tenderness, and then abruptly withdrawn. Pain in the affected region results from rebound of the tissue, usually a sign of peritoneal irritation.* ***E. Exploration during Palpation:*** *When palpating the abdomen, especially deeply, the hand is moved in a special manner. The fingers remain relatively fixed to a place on the skin, and the wall of the abdomen is carried with the fingers in a slow gentle to-and-fro motion to distinguish underlying masses and surfaces. The fingers do not glide over the skin but carry the skin with them.*

drawn from the characteristics of a mass. A complete description of the mass must be obtained; omission of any attribute may lead to erroneous conclusions. *Location.* The location of an abdominal mass suggests the organs to be considered; for example, a mass in the LUQ may be spleen, left kidney, stomach, or colon. *Size.* This gives insight into the pathologic process, its extent and change over time. *Shape.* Some organs have a characteristic shape; for example, kidney,

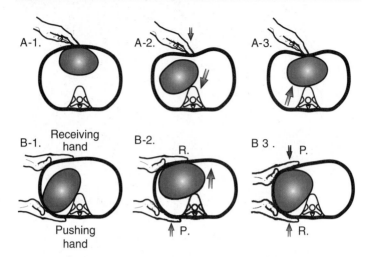

Fig. 9–8 *Ballottement of Abdominal Masses.* *The term ballottement is applied to two somewhat different maneuvers.* **A. One hand ballottement:** *The approximated fingers are abruptly plunged into the abdomen and held there; a freely movable mass will rebound upward and be felt with the fingers. This is most commonly employed to feel a large liver obscured by free fluid in the abdominal cavity.* **B. Bimanual ballottement. B1-2:** *This is used to determine the size of a large mass in the abdomen. One hand (P) pushes the posterior abdominal wall, while the receiving hand (R) palpates the anterior abdomen.* **B3:** *The receiving hand is now in the flank, the pushing hand compresses the mass to get an estimate of its thickness.*

spleen, and liver. ***Consistency.*** The pathologic process may be inferred from the resistance of the mass to pressure; for example, carcinoma may be stony hard, lymphoma rubbery, and abscess soft and fluctuant. ***Surface.*** A smooth surface implies a diffuse homogeneous process, while a nodular surface suggests metastases, granulomas, or irregular fibrosis. ***Tenderness.*** This may be caused by an inflammatory process (infectious or sterile), distention of a solid organ capsule (e.g., liver) or viscus, or ischemia. ***Mobility.*** Abdominal viscera suspended by long mesenteries permit them to move. Movement with diaphragmatic respiration suggests association with the liver or spleen or a mobile abdominal organ rather than a retroperitoneal location. ***Pulsatility.*** This implies vascular, usually major arterial, association with the mass. Aneurysmal dilation of the aorta or one of its major branches must be assumed until excluded by imaging. Solid masses and tense cysts can transmit normal aortic pulsations, simulating aneurysms.

Palpation of the LUQ. Normally, no organs are palpable in this region. The normal spleen lies posterior laterally under the left diaphragm with its surface separated from the chest wall by the lung during deep inspiration. In this position, it is not palpable (Fig. 9–9). Its long axis lies parallel to the tenth rib in the midaxillary line. Because of its oblique orientation, the width determines the vertical extent of the area of splenic dullness in the midaxilla. Percussion of this area (*Traube space*) is a desirable routine. Extension of the area of splenic dullness to obliterate the tympany over the gastric air bubble may be caused by fluid in

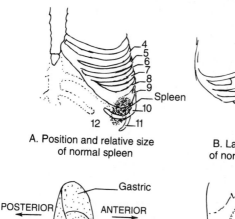

A. Position and relative size
of normal spleen

B. Lateral view
of normal spleen

POSTERIOR

Renal

Gastric

ANTERIOR

Pancreatic

Colonic

C. Surfaces of spleen

D. Directions of splenic
enlargement

Fig. 9–9 *Anatomic Relations of the Normal and Enlarged Spleen. A. Position of the normal spleen, anterior view:* The area of splenic dullness is in the left posterior axilla and usually does not exceed a vertical distance of more than 8 or 9 cm. *B. Normal spleen, left lateral view:* The spleen lies obliquely with its long axis along the tenth rib, its long borders coinciding with the ninth and eleventh ribs. *C. Anterior surface of the spleen:* The regions touching other viscera are indicated. *D. Splenic enlargement:* The directions in which the spleen enlarges are indicated by the dotted lines; the long axis of enlargement points downward and obliquely toward the symphysis pubis.

the stomach or feces in the colon, but finding it should prompt the examiner to search more carefully for a large spleen [Barkun AN, Camus M, Green L, et al. The bedside assessment of splenic enlargement. *Am J Med.* 1991;91:512–518]. To feel for a moderately enlarged spleen or left kidney, stand at the right side of the supine patient and use *bimanual palpation,* with the right hand palpating under the costal margin while the left hand lifts gently from the back and the patient inspires deeply (Fig. 9–10). To begin, lay the palm of the right hand on

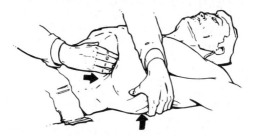

Fig. 9–10 *Bimanual Palpation of the LUQ.*

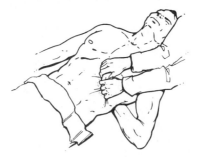

Fig. 9–11 *Palpation of the Spleen, Middleton method.*

the abdominal wall in the LUQ and place the tips of the approximated index and middle fingers 4 to 5 cm inferior to the rib margin in the anterior axillary line. Place the palm of the left hand on the left midaxillary region of the thorax, with the fingers curling posteriorly to support the thoracic wall at the eleventh and twelfth ribs. Ask the patient to take a slow deep breath. During inspiration, bring the two hands closer together by lifting the posterior wall with the left hand while gently, but firmly, pushing the approximated fingers of the right hand posteriorly and upward behind the costal margin. When the movement of both hands coincides with the rhythm of inspiration, the descending margin of an enlarged spleen will touch the palpating fingertips. Repeat the procedure with the patient lying partially on his right side. The spleen is superficial; the left kidney is deep and closer to the midline. Greatly enlarged spleens may be felt without bimanual palpation. The two-handed method is also employed with a type of ballottement (see Fig. 9–8). Place the hands in the position previously described; lift the posterior chest wall with the left hand, but let the right hand passively receive the impulse from the mass that is pushed forward. In the *Middleton method* for palpating the spleen, the patient lies with his left fist beneath the left thorax (Fig. 9–11). Stand on the patient's left side, facing the patient's feet, and curl your fingers over the left costal margin so that your fingertips are pointing cephalad under the ribs. Feel for the splenic tip during a deep inspiration.

Palpation of the RUQ. The liver, gallbladder, hepatic flexure of the colon, and right kidney are the organs in this region. *Bimanual palpation* is used to detect a normal or mildly enlarged liver. The right hand with fingers together is placed on the abdominal wall below the right rib margin. The supinated left hand is placed under the right lower thorax and the right thorax is lifted in the direction of the arrow in Fig. 9–12. As the patient inspires deeply, the right hand is moved upward and inward, then as the height of inspiration is approached, the fingertips are lifted towards the costal margin catching the liver edge from below. To avoid missing the edge of an enlarged liver, start palpation in the right lower quadrant (RLQ) and move cephalad. An enlarged right kidney is felt as a fixed mass deep to the liver.

Palpation of the lower quadrants. Palpation of the right and left lower quadrants is straightforward. There are normally no palpable organs here, except for stool in the colon. Remember that the spine and posterior sacral prominence are easily palpable in thin individuals and should not be confused with masses. *Psoas*

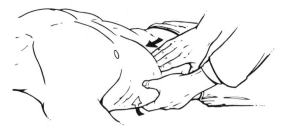

Fig. 9–12 *Bimanual Palpation of the RUQ.*

and obturator signs should be performed in patients with abdominal pain (Fig. 9–13). To elicit the psoas sign, lay the patient supine or on their side and put the hip through a full range of motion in flexion and extension. Pain suggests inflammation of the psoas muscle or the overlying peritoneum. Repeat on the opposite side. The *obturator sign* is elicited with the patient supine, and the hip and knee flexed to 90 degrees. Put the hip through a full range of internal and external rotation; deep pelvic pain suggests inflammation of the obturator muscle or pelvic peritoneum.

Examination of the abdomen and pelvis per rectum and vagina.   (See below for the rectal examination; Chapter 11, page 544, for the description of the female pelvic examination; Chapter 12, pages 570, for the description of the male rectal examination.) A chaparone must be present during these examinations. Digital palpation via the rectum and vagina serves three purposes: (1) to detect intrinsic disease of the rectum and vagina; (2) to gain information about adjacent structures of the male and female genitourinary tract; and (3) to examine the lower part of the peritoneal cavity. Because the peritoneal cavity extends into the pelvis, masses in the lower abdomen should be palpated from below the pelvic brim as well as from above (Figs. 9–14 and 9–15). *Errors in the diagnosis of abdominal conditions are notoriously common because these examinations have not been*

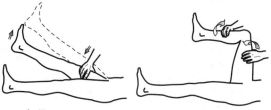

A. Iliopsoas test   B. Obturator test

Fig. 9–13 *Tests for Irritation of the Iliopsoas and Obturator Muscles.* *Abscesses in the pelvis may be localized by demonstrating irritation of the more lateral iliopsoas or the medial obturator internus muscles.* ***A. Iliopsoas test:*** *The supine patient keeps his knee extended and is asked to flex the thigh against the resistance of the examiner's hand. Pain in the pelvis indicates irritation of the iliopsoas.* ***B. Obturator test.*** *The supine patient flexes the right thigh to 90 degrees. The examiner moves the hip in internal and external rotation. Pelvic pain indicates an inflamed muscle. Examine from the side of the limb being tested.*

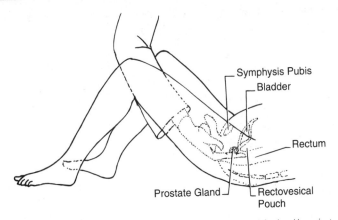

Fig. 9–14 *Palpation of the Male Abdomen per Rectum.* *The examining hand is supinated. Anteriorly, the finger pad feels the prostate gland and seminal vesicles. Superiorly on the anterior rectal surface, the fingertip reaches the location of the rectovesical pouch of the peritoneum. Normally, this pouch is not palpable; in the presence of pus or a tender mass it may be perceived. Cancer cells may settle in this pouch from the abdominal cavity, producing a hard, nontender, transverse ridge, called a rectal shelf or Blumer shelf.*

performed. Post-voiding vaginal examination is part of the abdominal examination for symptomatic women, even when speculum examination cannot be performed. The lithotomy position is preferred for both vaginal and rectal examinations because masses will tend to fall upon the examining finger. With the patient lying supine, flex the thighs and knees while the feet rest on the bed or

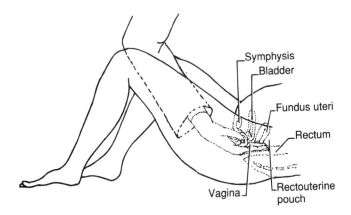

Fig. 9–15 *Palpation of the Female Abdomen per Rectum.* *The finger pad feels the cervix uteri and the fundus uteri through the anterior rectal wall. Passing the finger inward, superior to the cervix, the fingertip reaches the location of the rectouterine pouch (Douglas pouch). Normally, this is not palpable; a tender mass is evidence of pus. See legend of Fig. 9–14 for Blumer shelf.*

in stirrups. Wear gloves and lubricate the exploring fingers, the index finger for a rectal examination, the index and long fingers for the vagina. Palpate the vagina first, then the rectum. For bimanual palpation, palpate between the fingers of the left hand pressing into the suprapubic region of the abdominal wall and the finger in the rectum. When the examination is complete, provide tissues for the patient to clean themselves.

Examination for abdominal hernias.   (See pages 521.) Hernias are protrusions of abdominal contents through a weak point in the abdominal wall. In most cases, the hernia has a peritoneal sac, which may contain bowel, stomach, omentum, urinary bladder, colon, or even liver. Start with inspection. If the patient suspects a problem, have him demonstrate his observation. Many hernias are encountered unexpectedly; a bulge may be seen at rest, or it may appear or be felt by the examining finger during maneuvers that increase intraabdominal pressure, for example, when the patient coughs or performs a Valsalva maneuver. Palpate the abdominal wall defect and its contents. Omentum feels soft and nodular, whereas bowel is smooth and fluctuant. Gas in herniated bowel may cause peristaltic sounds or crepitation. If the hernia can be pushed back into the abdomen, it is *reducible*; if not, it is *irreducible* or *incarcerated*.

Zieman inguinal examination.   See Chapter 12, page 569

Examination of the Perineum, Anus, Rectum, and Distal Colon

The patient may be examined in several positions (Fig. 9–16). The left lateral prone (Sims) and bent-over-table positions permit adequate inspection of the perianal region, palpation of the anal canal and rectum, followed by inspection of the anal and rectal mucosa using an anuscope. These positions are inadequate for bimanual palpation of the peritoneal contents through the rectum (see above). Examination in the lithotomy position is facilitated by having the buttocks raised on a pillow; this position can be used if inspection of the anal canal is not required. The knee-chest or knee-elbow position is uncomfortable for the patient and should be reserved for special conditions such as the evacuation of gaseous colon distention.

Inspection of the perineum.   Whatever position is selected for the patient, the buttocks should be spread wide apart. Inspect the skin of the perineum and

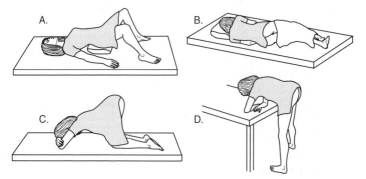

Fig. 9–16 *Positions of the Patient for Rectal Examination. A. Modified lithotomy position. B. Left lateral prone position (Sims position). C. The knee-chest position. D. Bent over the table.*

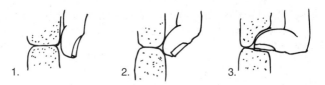

Fig. 9–17 *Insertion of the Gloved Finger into the Anus. 1.* *The pad of the gloved index finger is placed gently over the orifice, until the external sphincter is felt to relax.* ***2.*** *and* ***3.*** *Rotate the tip of the finger into the axis of the canal and insert gently. The entire procedure should be slow and gentle.*

perianal region for signs of local inflammation, sinuses, fistulas, excoriations, hemorrhoids, masses, and cutaneous lesions.

Examination of the Anus

Anal palpation. Ask the patient to breathe normally and explain each step of the procedure as you go along. After gloving both hands, palpate the perineum gently around the orifices of sinuses and fistulas feeling for subcutaneous cords that indicate the direction of tracks. Palpate any bulges in the perineal and perianal tissue for warmth, tenderness and consistency. Palpate carefully between the anus and the ischial tuberosities, the site of ischiorectal abscesses. Next, lubricate the gloved examining finger, place the pad of the finger on the anal sphincter, and exert gentle pressure, directed inward and somewhat anteriorly, until the sphincter relaxes, admitting the tip of the finger (Fig. 9–17). When inserting a finger or instrument it is important to remember that the anal canal slants anteriorly, so the axis of entry should point toward the umbilicus. Gradually insert the finger as far as possible while palpating the walls and estimating sphincter tone and the length of the anal canal. Proper examination is not painful unless a fissure in ano or a thrombosed hemorrhoid is present. To identify the abscess causing a fistula, use bidigital palpation between the index finger in the canal and the thumb on the skin of the perineum. *Be sure that there is a clear indication before performing a rectal examination on a patient with neutropenia.*

Anoscopy. The anal canal is not routinely inspected; it can only be viewed with a speculum. Anocopy is indicated when symptoms or external signs suggest pathology in the canal. The anoscope is a tube with a cone-tipped obturator. Plastic disposable anoscopes allow some visualization through their walls. The patient is placed in the left lateral, the knee-chest, or standing position (see Fig. 9–16). A good light must be available. After palpation has demonstrated no obstruction, the anoscope is well lubricated with the obturator in place; then the tip and tube are gently inserted, aiming toward the umbilicus. Once the anoscope is fully inserted, the obturator is removed and the rectal mucosa and walls of the anal canal are inspected as the tube is slowly withdrawn.

Examination of the Rectum

There are three parts to the rectal examination: (1) palpation of the contents of the lower peritoneal cavity (see above), (2) palpation of adjacent internal urogenital organs (see Chapters 11 and 12), and (3) examination of the rectum itself.

Rectal palpation. This is a continuation of palpation of the anal canal; the finger is merely pushed beyond the rectoanal junction, and the walls of the ampulla are felt. After entering the rectum in the male, the finger sequentially palpates on the anterior wall, the prostate gland, the seminal vesicles, and the rectovesical pouch. Posteriorly is the hollow of the sacrum and the coccyx. The lateral walls are also examined. On the anterior wall of the female, one encounters, in sequence, the uterine cervix, the uterine fundus (if retroverted), and the rectouterine pouch. The rectal wall is palpated for masses and narrowing of the lumen.

Examination of the Sigmoid Colon

The rectosigmoid and descending colon are accessible to inspection through the sigmoidoscope. The flexible sigmoidoscope has replaced rigid instruments, which restricted inspection to approximately 25 cm (Fig. 9–18). The flexible sigmoidoscope gives the examiner a wide field of view and can usually be advanced without anesthesia to the splenic flexure. Sigmoidoscopic examination is an exceedingly useful aid in diagnosing colonic disease. Because the sigmoidoscopy is employed without anesthesia, it should be considered part of the examination of the abdomen. Specific indications for sigmoidoscopy are beyond the scope of this text. Please refer to appropriate texts for techniques of examination and interpretation of findings at sigmoidoscopy.

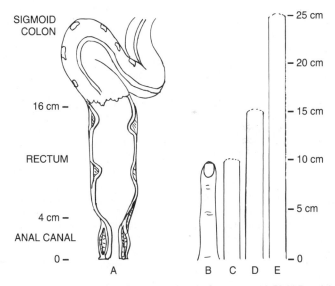

Fig. 9–18 *Comparison of Lengths of Rectosigmoid Segments with Rigid Examining Instruments. All lengths are drawn to scale.* ***A.*** ***The rectosigmoid is shown with the anal canal of 4 cm,*** *the rectum and valves of Houston of 12 cm, and the lower part of the sigmoid colon, whose total length is 40 cm.* ***B.*** *An average index finger, 10 cm long and 22 mm in diameter.* ***C.*** *A typical anoscope, 9 cm, with an added 1 cm of curved obturator.* ***D.*** *A proctoscope of 15 cm.* ***E.*** *Rigid sigmoidoscope of 25 cm. The fiberoptic flexible instruments are considerably longer.*

Abdominal, Perineal and Anorectal Symptoms

General Symptoms

> **KEY SYMPTOM** Six-Dermatome Pain—Esophageal Discomfort

See Six Dermatome Pain, Chapter 8, page 333, and page 400.

> **KEY SYMPTOM** Acute Abdominal Pain

See also page 493ff. It is important to understand the physiology of pain specific to each organ and site in the abdomen. For instance, distention of the bowel produces pain, whereas mechanical laceration does not. In general, pain arising in the viscera and transmitted in the vagal visceral afferent nerves and sympathetic afferent nerves give sensations of deep, boring, poorly localized pain that is frequently accompanied by autonomic features such as nausea, vomiting, and diaphoresis. Pain transmitted via the spinal somatic afferent nerves innervating the body wall and peritoneum is generally described as sharp and well localized to the anatomic site of the inflammation or injury. This is a complex subject, the details of which are beyond the scope of this book, but knowledge of the innervation of each abdominal organ (somatic versus visceral, vagus, and/or sympathetic) will help the examiner understand the nature and pattern of the patient's pain history. Severe, acute abdominal pain can herald a variety of disorders from the benign to the immanently life-threatening; this is known in surgical slang as *the acute abdomen.* The specific diagnosis must be pursued with a sense of urgency, since early surgical intervention may be lifesaving in some disorders (abdominal aortic aneurysm [AAA], bowel infarction, appendicitis) and contraindicated in others (acute intermittent porphyria [AIP], sickle cell crisis). Accurate diagnosis relies greatly on history and physical examination. Some assistance is obtained from imaging examinations, while laboratory tests are less useful. A careful history and personally repeated examinations over a few hours, be it day or night, are mandatory. Of particular importance are the locations of the pain and tenderness (Fig. 9–19), any change in location, and their variations in quality during the period of observation. Relatively few findings may distinguish several conditions. For example, the patient with intraabdominal visceral pain may walk about, but if peritonitis supevenes, the patient will hold very still and guard the abdomen. Usually, acute pain brings the patient to the physician within a few hours of onset. Acute processes or acute complications of chronic diseases are most likely. Pain increased with walking, jumping, sneezing, or coughing is equivalent to the jar test (page 481) and suggests the presence of peritoneal inflammation [Spiro HM. An internist's approach to acute abdominal pain. *Med Clin North Am.* 1993;77:963–972]. A pregnancy test must be obtained in all women of childbearing age with acute abdominal pain.

✔ *ACUTE ABDOMINAL PAIN—CLINICAL OCCURRENCE:* *Congenital* Meckel diverticulum, sickle cell crisis, pancreas divisum, angioedema; familial Mediterranean fever, AIP, and variegate porphyria; *Endocrine* gastrinoma, adrenal insufficiency; *Idiopathic* diverticulosis, endometriosis; *Inflammatory/Immune* pancreatitis, gastritis, esophagitis, autoimmune hepatitis, peritonitis, serositis, mesenteric lymphadenitis, systemic lupus erythematosus (SLE), vasculitis, inflammatory bowel disease (Crohn disease, ulcerative colitis); *Infection* typhoid

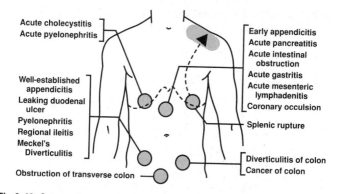

Fig. 9–19 *Common Locations of Acute Abdominal Pain.* *In general, the painful spot is also tender, but not always. Note especially that the pain of acute appendicitis is in the epigastrium early and later in the RLQ. Pain in the spleen commonly radiates to the top of the left shoulder. These pains are ordinarily constant, in contrast to the intermittent pain of colic.*

fever and enteritis; *Clostridium difficile* enterocolitis; viral gastroenteritis; visceral larval migrans; varicella-zoster virus; cytomegalovirus; viral autoimmune hepatitis; tuberculous peritonitis and lymphadenitis; purulent peritonitis (spontaneous or secondary to perforation or penetration); **Metabolic/Toxic** familial Mediterranean fever, AIP, and variegate porphyria, ingestions, heavy metal poisoning (lead, cadmium, arsenic, mercury), nonsteroidal antiinflammatory drug gastroduodenitis, macrolide antibiotics; **Mechanical/Trauma** fracture of a solid organ, perforation of bowel, bladder, or gallbladder, obstruction of the cystic, common bile, pancreatic ducts, ureter, ureteropelvic junction, or bowel by stones, masses, parasites, or bezoars; volvulus or strangulation of bowel in internal or abdominal wall hernias; penetrating and blunt trauma; **Neoplastic** mass effect of tumors pressing on other structures or causing traction on bowel or mesentery, hemorrhage into tumor, ischemia and necrosis of tumor, erosion into or metastasis to blood vessels, nerves or adjacent organs; **Neurologic** herpes zoster; diabetic radiculopathy, mononeuritis multiplex, abdominal cutaneous nerve entrapment, transverse myelitis; **Psychosocial** history of physical, emotional or sexual abuse in childhood or as an adult; poisoning, substance abuse with drug seeking, drug withdrawal; **Vascular** AAA, aortic dissection, ischemic bowel, infarction of bowel or solid organs, vasculitis, mesenteric venous thrombosis or emboli (bland, septic, or atheroembolic), Henoch Schönlein purpura, strangulation of hernias, rectus sheath hemorrhage, retroperitoneal hemorrhage.

KEY SYMPTOM Chronic and Recurrent Abdominal Pain

Chronic pain is physiologically distinct from acute pain. The role of conditioning in the spinal cord and thalamus in the setting of chronic pain are under study, as is the decreased threshold to the perception of pain with visceral stimulation in some individuals with chronic abdominal pain. The pattern of pain and associated symptoms will help to make inferences about the possible pathophysiology, while the location of the pain suggests the organs involved. Pain that is vague in onset but steadily worsens over time suggests a progressive, anatomically advancing obstructive lesion or mass effect. Intermittent pain separated by periods free of pain suggests painful smooth-muscle contraction or dynamic obstruction, recurrent inflammation or ulceration, and relapsing infection. Careful history is required to identify precipitating factors (e.g., meals and type of food), timing (e.g., relation to menstrual cycle, starting new medications), and previous surgeries, symptoms, or illnesses that could help explain the current problem (e.g., adhesions from surgery or irradiation, trauma, infections, and travel). It is important to recognize that nonspecific abdominal and pelvic pain is a common symptom in persons with histories of current or previous abuse. An empathetic, nonjudgmental history with specific questions relating to current safety, sexual practices, sexual abuse, and physical or emotional abuse is essential. Up to 30% of women presenting to a physician in the ambulatory setting have a history of abuse, and and one-third of these have been abused within the last 12 months. The link between abuse and abdominal pain is not clear; it is clear that many thousands of dollars are frequently wasted on fruitless undirected laboratory and imaging investigations when an explanation can be found with a few minutes of history and physical examination. If the history and physical examination do not suggest specific leads for further investigation, a barrage of laboratory and imaging tests are extremely unlikely to be helpful. There is a tendency to project pain inward to intraabdominal structures when it actually arises from the abdominal wall. Make the effort to think of disorders of the abdominal wall; this will avoid many unnecessary studies.

📖 *CHRONIC ABDOMINAL PAIN—CLINICAL OCCURRENCE:* **Congenital** malrotation, familial pancreatitis, pancreas divisum, polycystic kidney disease, porphyrias, familial Mediterranean fever, sickle cell anemia, Meckel diverticulum, cystic fibrosis, hereditary angioedema; **Endocrine** adrenal insufficiency, hypothyroidism; **Idiopathic** diverticulosis, diverticulitis, gastroesophageal reflux disease, gastritis, pancreatitis, ovarian cysts, arthritis of axial skeleton, AAA, gastric ulcer, endometriosis; **Inflammatory/Immune** ulcerative colitis, Crohn disease, gastritis, chronic pancreatitis, autoimmune hepatitis, chronic cholecystitis, sclerosing cholangitis, primary biliary cirrhosis, pancreatic pseudocyst, celiac disease, adhesions, peritonitis, SLE, sarcoidosis, retroperitoneal and mesenteric fibrosis; **Infectious** Whipple disease, viral hepatitis (B, C), tuberculosis, *Giardia*, duodenal and gastric ulcers, diverticulitis, chronic malaria, schistosomiasis, visceral larval migrans, leishmaniasis, hookworm, roundworms, bartonellosis (peliosis hepatitis), HIV, syphilis with tabes; **Metabolic/Toxic** heavy metal poisoning, porphyrias, ketoacidosis, uremia, nonsteroidal antiinflammatory drug gastropathy and gastric ulcer; **Mechanical/Trauma** partial bowel obstruction and strictures, cholelithiasis, nephrolithiasis, pancreatic duct stricture, sphincter of Oddi spasm and stricture, biliary stricture, dumping syndromes; adhesions; ureteral obstruction, ureteropelvic junction obstruction, chronic hydrosalpinx; **Neoplastic** splenic and retroperitoneal lymphoma, primary carcinomas of the esophagus, stomach, colon, pancreas, liver, bile ducts, gallbladder, ovary; metastatic cancer to the liver (especially from pancreas, colon, lung, breast, pancreatic islets, carcinoid), spleen (lymphoma), retroperitoneal lymph nodes (cervix, testis, lymphoma, melanoma, bladder), and peritoneal surface (especially ovary); **Neurologic** postspinal cord injury, postherpetic neuralgia, diabetic radiculopathy, diabetic autonomic neuropathy, abdominal cutaneous nerve entrapment; **Psychosocial** history of domestic, sexual, or child abuse, substance abuse, opiate withdrawal; **Vascular** intestinal ischemia, vasculitis, atheroemboli, abdominal aortic or iliac aneurysm.

KEY SYMPTOM   Nausea and Vomiting

Nausea is an unpleasant sensation referred to the stomach and suggesting that vomiting is imminent. Vomiting is an involuntary integrated movement of pharyngeal and thoracoabdominal smooth and voluntary muscles to expel stomach contents. Nausea and vomiting are triggered by cortical (emotional), gastrointestinal (GI), vestibular, and chemical (via the central nervous system [CNS] chemoreceptor trigger zone) stimuli, and vomiting is coordinated by the brainstem. The violence and discomfort of nausea and vomiting often make them a presenting complaint. Vomiting is usually preceded by nausea. The history should include inciting events and exposures, the nature of the vomitus and its relationship to meals. *Variants of Vomiting: Projectile Vomiting*   is a particularly forceful type associated with increased intracranial pressure and lacking antecedent nausea.   *Retching*   involves all movements of vomiting except that gastric contents are not expelled.

✔ *CLINICAL OCCURRENCE: Congenital*   pyloric   stenosis;   *Endocrine* adrenal insufficiency, pregnancy;   *Idiopathic*   pyloric stricture, gastroparesis, other GI motility disorders (e.g., scleroderma, pseudoobstruction), Ménière disease, glaucoma;   *Inflammatory/Immune*   numerous disorders of the alimentary canal, biliary system, and pancreas, for example, hepatitis, pancreatitis, peritonitis;   *Infection*   viral gastroenteritis, CNS infections, peptic ulcer (*Helicobacter pylori*);   *Metabolic/Toxic*   bacterial food poisoning; opiates, ipecac, chemotherapy agents, macrolide antibiotics, chemical toxins, many more; uremia, hepatic failure, ketoacidosis;   *Mechanical/Trauma*   upper GI obstruction;   *Neoplastic*   brain tumors, primary or metastatic;   *Neurologic* autonomic reflexes associated with visceral stimulation, for example, myocardial infarction, ureteral stone, biliary colic, postvagotomy, head injury with concussion, intracranial mass;   *Psychosocial*   offensive tastes, odors, and sights; severe pain; psychogenic;   *Vascular*   myocardial infarction, superior mesenteric ischemia (arterial or venous), migraine.

KEY SYMPTOM   Abdominal Bloating

See Distended Abdomen, page 472. The sensation of bloating can be caused by increased gaseous distention of the bowel, increased sensitivity to normal bowel gas, enlargement of abdominal or pelvic organs, ascites, or masses. Patients often try to induce burping, during which they swallow more gas. Smoking and chewing gum are other causes of swallowed gas. Patients with the irritable bowel syndrome have pain and complaints of distention at volumes of intestinal gas not sensed by others.

KEY SYMPTOM   Belching, Flatus, and Sensible Peristalsis

See *Tympanites,* page 480, and Bloating Syndromes, page 504.

Site-Attributable Symptoms
Abdominal Wall Symptoms

KEY SYMPTOM   Abdominal Wall Pain

Injury to the muscles, nerves, skin, and soft tissues of the abdominal wall, and referral of pain from the bones, nerve roots, and soft tissues of the spine, commonly present as complaints of abdominal pain. Well-localized (finger-tip precise) pain suggests somatic pain in the body wall. Band-like pain described as wrapping around the body suggests neuropathic pain, sclerotomal pain from bone lesions or myotomal pain originating in the muscles, tendons or ligaments at that segmental level. Pain exacerbated by specific motions and tenderness to palpation support this diagnosis.

✔ **CLINICAL OCCURRENCE:** *Congenital* urachus abnormalities; *Idiopathic* xiphodynia; *Inflammatory/Immune* suture abscess, mononeuritis, polyneuritis, diabetic polyradiculopathy and amyotrophy, myositis; *Infectious* abscess, herpes zoster, pyomyositis; *Metabolic/Toxic* diabetic neuropathy; *Mechanical/Trauma* abdominal cutaneous nerve entrapment (rectus abdominis nerve entrapment syndrome), abdominal wall hernia, abdominal wall muscle tear, rib cartilage injury, rib tip syndrome, spinal disc herniation, burns, retention sutures, foreign bodies; *Neoplastic* desmoid tumors, lipoma, sarcoma, metastases; *Neurologic* complex regional pain syndrome, postherpetic neuralgia, mononeuritis multiplex, diabetic amyotrophy; *Psychosocial* abuse, somatization, malingering; *Vascular* vasculitis with mononeuropathy or polyneuropathy.

Esophagus, Stomach and Duodenum Symptoms

KEY SYMPTOM   Regurgitation

See Heartburn below. Regurgitation is reflux of esophageal and stomach contents back into the mouth or upper airway without active vomiting. It is passive and occurs under the influence of normal body positions and activities, suggesting loss of function of the normal esophageal sphincters or increased intraabdominal pressure. Unlike vomiting, regurgitation may not be volunteered by the patient as a major complaint; you must ask specifically. Particular attention should be paid to nocturnal regurgitation, with recumbency and after meals. Regurgitation of stomach contents while fasting produces a sour bitter taste (water brash or pyrosis), whereas regurgitation after eating will return food. Regurgitation of food more than 2 hours after eating suggests delayed gastric emptying or achalasia.

✔ **REGURGITATION—CLINICAL OCCURRENCE:** *Congenital* abnormal lower esophageal sphincter (LES) and upper esophageal sphincter tone; *Idiopathic* decreased LES tone with or without hiatal hernia, achalasia; *Infectious* Chaga's disease; *Inflammatory/Immune* esophagitis, scleroderma, CREST syndrome; *Metabolic/Toxic* alcohol, tobacco, caffeine, uremia; *Mechanical/Trauma* achalasia, gastric outlet and upper intestinal obstruction, gastroparesis; *Neoplastic* esophageal or gastric cardia cancer.

KEY SYMPTOM   Heartburn

Regurgitation of gastric acid or bile produces chemical imitation in the esophagus with or without esophagitis. Patients complain of burning retrosternal pain aggravated by alcohol, tobacco, caffeine and obesity, frequently occurring after meals. Symptoms increase with recumbancy and are decreased by antacids. Gastroesophageal reflux due to decreased LES tone is the most common cause.

KEY SYMPTOM Difficulty Swallowing—Dysphagia

See also Chapter 7, page 216 and 291. Swallowing is a complex neuromuscular act involving both striated muscles under conscious control and smooth muscle innervated by the autonomic system and the intestinal myenteric plexus. Abnormalities in voluntary motor function of the pharynx, smooth-muscle function, salivary function, or mechanical obstructions in the pharynx or esophagus lead to complaints of dysphagia. Have the patient indicate the level where they feel the difficulty. Ask if the problem is more with liquids or solids. **DDX:** Ask whether they have coughing or choking with swallowing, which indicates a pharyngeal or laryngeal problem. If they regurgitate food after meals, it may indicate esophageal obstruction by mass or achalasia. If pain is present (*odynophagia*), then infection, neoplasm, or erosive disease is likely.

Dysphagia lusoria (aberrant right subclavian artery): See Chapter 7, page 291. Pain is rarely present, with dysphagia the only symptom. The esophagram shows a transverse band of indentation produced by the anomalous right subclavian artery arising from the descending aorta.

KEY SYMPTOM Pain with Swallowing—Odynophagia

See Six-Dermatome Pain with Dysphagia in Syndromes, page 406.

➤ KEY SYMPTOM Hematemesis

Bloody emesis indicates recent or active bleeding in the nose, oral cavity, pharynx, esophagus, stomach, duodenum, or, less frequently, the tracheobronchial tree. Bright red blood is arterial whereas dark blood is either venous or has been in the stomach for some time. Exposure to gastric acid and pepsin give blood a brown "coffee grounds" appearance. Ask the patient to estimate the volume of blood lost. Patients frequently overestimate the amount, especially if mixed with water, as in a sink or toilet bowel. Occasionally, the patient has difficulty in distinguishing between hematemesis and hemoptysis (coughing up blood), especially when coughing induces vomiting. Hematemesis following prolonged and violent retching or vomiting is characteristic of a linear tear of the mucosa at the esophagogastric junction (*Mallory-Weiss tear*). If a bleeding site is not evident in the nose, mouth, or pharynx, upper endoscopy should be performed for diagnosis and possible therapy.

✔ **HEMATEMESIS—CLINICAL OCCURRENCE:** *Congenital* hereditary hemorrhagic telangiectasia (Osler-Weber-Rendu), Dieulafoy lesion; *Endocrine* gastrinoma (Zollinger-Ellison syndrome), hyperparathyroidism; *Idiopathic* peptic ulcer, duodenal diverticulum, gastritis; *Inflammatory/Immune* gastritis, esophagitis; *Infectious* H. pylori ulcers; *Metabolic/Toxic* NSAID (nonsteroidal antiinflammatory drug) gastropathy; *Mechanical/Trauma* Mallory-Weiss tear, portal hypertension (esophageal and gastric varices), foreign bodies, gallstone erosion; *Neoplastic* cancer of the esophagus, stomach, and pancreas; *Psychosocial* factitious; *Vascular* arteriovenous malformations, gastric antral vascular ectasia, esophageal and gastric varices, portal gastropathy, thrombocytosis, coagulation defects.

Small Intestine and Colon

> **KEY SYMPTOM** Diarrhea

See Syndromes page 505.

> **KEY SYMPTOM** Constipation

See Syndromes page 511.

> **KEY SYMPTOM** Fecal Incontinence

Loss of bowel control can result from severe diarrhea of any cause, rectal inflammation, damage to the anal sphincters, or loss of normal sensory, autonomic, or voluntary muscle function. Vaginal delivery commonly injures the anal sphincter and pelvic nerves accounting for the large female predominance of this problem [Sultan AH, Kamm MA, Hudson CN, et al. Anal-sphincter disruption during vaginal delivery. *N Engl J Med.* 1993;329:1905–1911]. Fecal and urinary incontinence are most common in women, especially those in institutions [Wald A. Fecal Incontinence in adults. *N Engl J Med.* 2007:356:1648–1655]. Evaluation of mental status, vaginal speculum and bimanual examination, and neurologic examination, including anal sensation and sphincter tone and strength during rectal examination, are necessary. Look for dementia, a flaccid anal sphincter, rectocele, rectal prolapse, impacted feces, mass, and neurologic deficit of the sacral nerves [Madoff RD, Parker SC, Varma MG, et al. Faecal incontinence in adults. *Lancet.* 2004;364:621–632]. Further evaluation requires specialty consultation [Rudolph W, Galandiuk S. A practical guide to the diagnosis and management of fecal incontinence. *Mayo Clin Proc.* 2002;77:271–275; Hirsh T, Lembo T. Diagnosis and management of fecal incontinence in elderly patients. *Am Fam Physician.* 1996;54:1559–1564,1569–1570].

✔ *FECAL INCONTINENCE—CLINICAL OCCURRENCE:* ***Congenital*** cerebral palsy, mental retardation, meningomyelocele; ***Endocrine*** hyperthyroidism; ***Idiopathic*** amyloidosis; ***Inflammatory/Immune*** ulcerative colitis, Crohn disease, ulcerative proctitis, microscopic colitis, amyloidosis; ***Infectious*** herpes simplex, gonorrhea or cytomegalovirus proctitis, dysentery syndrome caused by bacterial infection, infectious diarrhea, perirectal abscess; ***Metabolic/Toxic*** drugs, especially cathartics, laxative abuse; ***Mechanical/Trauma*** fissure, fistula, fecal impaction, pelvic floor relaxation, rectal prolapse, rectocele; ***Neoplastic*** anal or rectal carcinoma, metastatic invasion of the sacral plexus or spinal cord; ***Neurologic*** dementia, cauda equina syndrome, transverse myelitis, sacral plexopathy, weakness or immobility, peripheral neuropathy including diabetes, postherpetic neuralgia; ***Psychosocial*** malingering, psychosis; ***Vascular*** ischemic colon, stroke.

> **KEY SYMPTOM** Pruritus Ani

Although pruritus is a symptom, the signs of chronic itching are evident in the perianal skin containing excoriations and thickening (*lichenification*). Patients may have a maddening, uncontrollable desire to scratch, but relief is very short-lived. Pinworms are common in children and in adults with young children.

When the involved skin is moist, the etiology may be infection with bacteria or fungi (*Candida*). Poor hygiene, contact allergies, irritation from bathroom tissue, and perianal dermatitis of unknown cause are also common.

> **KEY SYMPTOM   Pain with Bowel Movements**

See Anal Fissure, page 485.

Pelvic Symptoms

> **KEY SYMPTOM   Pain in the Perineum**

Perineal pain accompanies many disorders in the pelvis and can involve somatic or sacral sympathetic afferents. Take a history and perform a thorough physical examination looking for any pathology involving the rectum, anus, scrotum and its contents, vagina, pelvic floor muscles, pelvic bones, and perineal skin.

✔ *CLINICAL OCCURRENCE:*   *Inflammatory/Immune*   eczema, nonbacterial prostatitis, Bartholin gland inflammation;   *Infectious*   intertrigo, candidiasis, condyloma, vaginitis, cervicitis, urethritis, cystitis, prostatitis, epididymitis;   *Mechanical/Trauma*   thrombosed hemorrhoids, fissure in ano, fistula in ano, anal ulcer, cystocele, rectocele, testicular torsion or trauma, proctalgia fugax;   *Neoplastic*   anal, rectal, bladder, prostate, vaginal, cervical, uterine cancer; intramedullary tumors.

> **KEY SYMPTOM   Pelvic Pain**

See Abdominal Pain, pages 462ff, 492ff, 499–502; and Pelvic Pain, Chapter 11, page 548.

Stool Symptoms

> **KEY SYMPTOM   Blood in the Feces**

Blood in the bowel eventually passes in the feces. Its appearance depends on the volume of blood, the site of bleeding and the transit time in the GI tract. Partially digested blood, depending upon quantity, rate, and site of bleeding can take on any character from bright blood through black loose stools to frank melena. Small amounts of blood loss insufficient to change the color or character of the stool is occult bleeding. The stool guaiac test is a screening test for the presence of blood in the stool. Readings are either positive or negative. The test is not designed to quantify the amount of blood detected. Therefore, terms such as "weak positive" and "strong positive" should not be used. Numerous foods, such as red meats and horseradish root, will give false-positive stool guaiac tests. Newer immunologic bedside tests defect only human hemoglobin so are easier to use and more specific.

▶ **Black Tarry Stools—Melena:** Fifty to sixty milliliters of blood in the stomach produces a black, sticky (tarry) stool because of the effect of gastric acid and digestive enzymes. Black, but not tarry, stools also occur with ingestion of iron and bismuth and some fruits (e.g., black cherries and blueberries) or leafy green vegetables (e.g., spinach and collard greens). Difficulty cleaning the anus after a stool because of the sticky quality of the stool is characteristic of melena and not present with other causes of black stools. Melena may have a slight reddish hue and an acrid-sweet odor similar to creosote.

Bloody red stools—hematochezia: Blood unchanged by passage through the gut usually has entered the bowel in the colon, or passed very quickly through the gut. Because blood in the bowel is cathartic, large bleeds stimulate rapid passage. History and physical examination should try to determine whether the blood is mixed in the stool or on the outside of an otherwise normal stool. Blood mixed in the stool suggests bleeding onto a semiformed stool in the colon, whereas blood on the outside suggests a source near the anus.

✔ **GI BLEEDING—CLINICAL OCCURRENCE:**   *Congenital*   congenital polyps and hamartomas; hereditary hemorrhagic telangiectasia; pseudoxanthoma elasticum; von Willebrand disease; hemophilia; Meckel diverticulum, Dieulafoy lesion;   *Idiopathic*   arteriovenous malformations, colonic diverticulosis, duodenal diverticulum;   *Inflammatory/Immune*   immune thrombocytopenia, ulcerative colitis, Crohn disease, gastritis;   *Infectious*   see Acute Bloody Diarrhea, page 507, *C. difficile* colitis, typhoid enteritis, leptospirosis, Herpes simplex esophagitis and proctitis, parasites;   *Metabolic/Toxic*   vitamin K deficiency, scurvy, heavy metal poisoning, nonsteroidal antiinflammatory drugs;   *Mechanical/Trauma*   Mallory-Weiss tear, ulcers, intussusception, anal fissure, anal fistula, fecal impaction, epistaxis, swallowed blood;   *Neoplastic*   polyps or cancer anywhere in the GI tract, cancer invading the bowel wall, for example, pancreatic cancer, gastrinoma (Zollinger-Ellison syndrome);   *Psychosocial*   factitious;   *Vascular*   thrombocytopenia, arteriovenous malformations, ischemic bowel, erosion of AAA into the gut, gastric antral vascular ectasia, esophageal varices, gastric varices, portal gastropathy, hemorrhoids.

> **KEY SYMPTOM**   **Red Stools with Negative Guaiac Test**

Passage of red pigments from ingested fruits and vegetables. The patient often presents with a complaint of blood in the stool. This should always be confirmed by a positive guaiac test. When negative, history will often identify ingestion of beets or certain fruits, usually in large quantity.

Abdominal, Perineal and Anorectal Signs

Abdominal Signs
Inspection

> **KEY SIGN**   **Jaundice**

Jaundice refers to the staining of tissues and fluids by bilirubin. Yellow skin is also caused by carotene and rare chemical toxins, conditions that must be distinguished from jaundice. Although jaundice merely means "yellow," medical use reserves the term for bilirubin staining. Bilirubin stains all tissues, but jaundice is most intense in the face, trunk, and sclerae. Jaundice is usually visible when the concentration of conjugated bilirubin exceeds 3 mg/dL in serum. Jaundice is less visible in artificial light than daylight. When the jaundice is of long standing, the deep yellow may acquire a green hue.

Normal Bile Pigment Cycle. When senescent erythrocytes are destroyed in the spleen and other reticuloendothelial tissues, hemoglobin is metabolized to unconjugated bilirubin, iron, and globin. Unconjugated bilirubin is insoluble in water and circulates bound to albumin, hence it cannot be filtered by the kidneys. The liver takes up the unconjugated bilirubin, combines it with glucuronic acid to form water-soluble conjugated bilirubin, excretes it into the gut with the bile, where bacterial enzymes convert it to urobilinogen. Most urobilinogen is lost in the feces, but small amounts are reabsorbed by the intestine and reexcreted, some in the bile (enterohepatic circulation) and some in the urine. Excess water-soluble conjugated bilirubin in the blood is filtered by the kidneys and excreted in the urine. Jaundice occurs when there is a marked increase in production of unconjugated bilirubin, with impairment of hepatocellular uptake, conjugation or excretion of bilirubin, or obstruction of the intra- or extrahepatic bile ducts.

Scleral Color. Bilirubin is distributed uniformly throughout the sclera, in contrast to the yellow subscleral fat that collects in the periphery, farthest from the limbus. Carotene does not stain the sclerae, but it accumulates in the skin of the forehead, around the alae nasi, and in the palms and soles.

Pruritus. Itching leading to cutaneous excoriation often accompanies obstructive jaundice and biliary cirrhosis; it may become excruciating. The intensity of the itching is usually proportional to the bilirubin concentration and the duration of jaundice.

Urine color. Conjugated, but not unconjugated, bilirubin is excreted in the urine. High concentrations of conjugated bilirubin in the urine impart a dark-yellow to brown color. Shaking a specimen produces yellow foam because the bile salts lower the surface tension of water. Jaundice without darkening of the urine suggests unconjugated bilirubinemia.

Acholic Feces. In complete biliary obstruction or with severe hepatocellular loss, the stools are malodorous and appear white or gray, that is, clay colored.

Unconjugated hyperbilirubinemia. This is usually caused by hemolysis producing unconjugated bilirubin at a rate exceeding the maximal rate of liver uptake, conjugation and excretion. The stools are normal in color. The increase in bilirubin excretion into the gut leads to an increase in urinary urobilinogen. The urine contains no bilirubin because only water-soluble conjugated bilirubin is excreted in the urine. Tests for intrinsic liver disorders are negative. Less often, unconjugated bilirubinemia is caused by diminished hepatic uptake or a defect in hepatic conjugation. *CLINICAL OCCURRENCE: **Increased Production:** Hemolysis of normal red cells* autoimmune hemolytic anemia, transfusion hemolysis, hemolysis from chemicals, drugs, or infections; *Red cell defects* sickle cell disease, thalassemia, glucose-6-phosphate dehydrogenase (G-6-PD) deficiency, pyruvate kinase deficiency, paroxysmal nocturnal hemoglobinuria; *Ineffective erythropoiesis* thalassemia major, folate, and vitamin B_{12} deficiency; *Miscellaneous* absorption of hematoma, pulmonary infarction. ***Deficient Hepatic Uptake:*** sepsis, fasting, hypotension, and drugs. ***Deficient Hepatic Conjugation:*** *Congenital* Gilbert syndrome, Crigler-Najjar syndromes; *Acquired:* advanced hepatocellular disease, sepsis, competitive inhibition by drugs metabolized to glucuronides.

Conjugated hyperbilirubinemia. This results from impaired excretion of conjugated bilirubin from the hepatocyte into the bile canaliculi or obstruction of the biliary flow through the canaliculi, intrahepatic, and extrahepatic bile ducts to the duodenum. The feces may be acholic in which case the urine lacks urobilino-gen but contains bilirubin. The serum alkaline phosphatase is elevated out of proportion to the transaminases. Clinically, it is important to distinguish mechanical extrahepatic obstruction from intrahepatic obstruction that results from either mechanical obstruction or altered hepatocyte and canalicular function (*cholestasis*). In most cases of extrahepatic obstructive jaundice, dilatation of the bile ducts can be detected by ultrasonography. **CLINICAL OCCURRENCE:** **Intrahepatic Cholestasis:** **Congenital** Dubin-Johnson syndrome, Rotor syndrome; **Acquired** hepatocellular disease, drugs (especially sex steroids), sepsis, hypotension, primary biliary cirrhosis. **Extrahepatic Obstruction:** **Intrinsic** gallstones, biliary sludge, biliary carcinoma, sclerosing cholangitis, stricture, parasites; **Extrinsic** pancreatic carcinoma, portahepatis lymphadenopathy, pancreatitis, pancreatic pseudocyst.

Mixed hyperbilirubinemia. This results from a combination of hepatocellular and biliary tract injury. This is common in advanced hepatobiliary disease of almost any etiology, as these diseases are complex dynamic processes whose clinical and biochemical patterns evolve over time. The clinician should attempt to distinguish the primary etiology of hepatobiliary injury from the secondary consequences (e.g., cirrhosis or pigment stones). More than one process may be present, for example, alcohol, viral hepatitis, and drug effects. The diagnosis is made on the basis of a careful history supported by serologic testing and liver biopsy. The plasma will contain both conjugated and unconjugated bilirubin; the serum transaminase level will depend upon the degree of active hepatocellular injury and the remaining hepatocyte mass; the alkaline phosphatase is variably elevated. The stools may be acholic.

KEY SIGN   Distended Abdomen

The abdomen becomes distended by the accumulation of normal or abnormal fluids or tissue (Fig. 9–20). These can be categorized as adipose tissue (obesity), gas (tympanites), peritoneal fluid (ascites), organomegaly of solid organs caused by tissue hypertrophy or cysts (e.g., hepatomegaly, splenomegaly, polycystic kidneys, ovarian cysts, fibroids), obstruction of hollow organs (stomach, small and large intestine, bladder, gallbladder), neoplasms (benign or malignant), and pregnancy. See Abdominal Distention, page 504, Tympanites, page 480 and Ascites page 473.

Obesity: Abdominal obesity results from excessive caloric intake and/or redistribution of adipose tissue caused by hormonal factors, especially glucocorticoids. Obesity causes a uniformly rounded abdomen with an increase in girth (see Fig. 9–20). The umbilicus is buried deeply in the wall because it is adherent to the peritoneum. Excess fat is usually evident in other parts of the body, although men disproportionately deposit fat into the abdominal viscera and mesentery. Estimate the thickness of the panniculus by grasping a double layer between thumb and index finger; measure in centimeters half the thickness of the resulting fold at the base. The girth of the belly also reflects fat in the mesentery, omentum, and retroperitoneum. Because generalized obesity is obvious, the problem usually is to determine if any other causes of abdominal distention are present.

Pregnancy: See Fig. 9–20. In pregnancy, the uterus can resemble a large ovarian cyst. The breasts are engorged, fetal movements and parts may be felt,

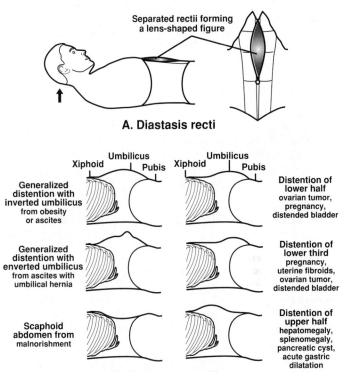

Separated rectii forming
a lens-shaped figure

A. Diastasis recti

| | Umbilicus | Umbilicus | |
| Xiphoid | Pubis | Xiphoid | Pubis | |

Generalized distention with inverted umbilicus from obesity or ascites

Distention of lower half ovarian tumor, pregnancy, distended bladder

Generalized distention with enverted umbilicus from ascites with umbilical hernia

Distention of lower third pregnancy, uterine fibroids, ovarian tumor, distended bladder

Scaphoid abdomen from malnorishment

Distention of upper half hepatomegaly, splenomegaly, pancreatic cyst, acute gastric dilatation

B. Abdominal profiles

Fig. 9–20 *Visible Abdominal Signs. A. Diastasis Recti:* *This is abnormal separation of the abdominal rectus muscles. It is frequently not detected when the patient is supine unless the patient's head is raised from the pillow so that the abdominal muscles are tensed.* **B. *Abdominal profiles:*** *Careful inspection from the side may give the first clue to abnormality, directing attention to a specific region and prompting search for more signs.*

the cervix is softened, and the fetal heart should be audible. With a molar pregnancy, there will be no signs of a fetus.

Feces: An accumulation of large amounts of feces, as in megacolon, may cause distention. Chronic abuse of laxatives, disorders of the myenteric plexus, advanced age, and use of anticholinergic drugs are frequent causes. A history of chronic constipation or laxative use is common. A review of the patient's medication history is essential. The plastic nature of the masses can often be palpated through the abdominal wall and rectal examination may show stool in the vault. Tympanites is usually absent.

KEY SIGN Ascites

Ascites results from an increased accumulation of peritoneal fluid by any one or more of several mechanisms: transudation of fluid from the surface of the liver as

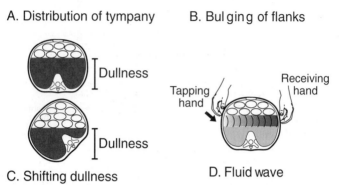

A. Distribution of tympany   B. Bulging of flanks

C. Shifting dullness   D. Fluid wave

Fig. 9–21 *Signs of Ascites. A. Distribution of Tympany:* *In the supine position, free fluid causes the gas-filled gut to float, so an area of tympany forms at the top of the bulging wall.* ***B. Bulging flanks:*** *The weight of free fluid pushes the flanks outward so they bulge toward the table or the bed; fat in the mesentery also will cause this when the abdominal muscles are weak.* ***C. Shifting dullness:*** *The dependent fluid causes an area of dullness in the lowest part; this shifts to remain lowest with changes in position of the body.* ***D. Fluid wave:*** *A wave in the fluid, elicited by tapping one side of the abdomen, is transmitted to the receiving hand laid on the opposite side; the wave takes perceptible time to cross the abdomen.*

a result of increased portal venous pressure (portal hypertension); obstruction of the normal lymphatic drainage of the peritoneum, or decreased plasma oncotic pressure; increased production of peritoneal fluid from peritoneal carcinomatosis or inflammation, usually infectious. Each of these mechanisms produces a recognizable clinical pattern discernible by history and physical examination. Unless distorted by surgical scars, diastasis recti, or hernia, the profile of the fluid-filled abdomen describes a single curve from xiphoid process to pubes (see Fig. 9–20B). The umbilicus is sometimes everted.

Four signs are characteristic of free fluid: (1) *Bulging flanks* in the supine position are produced by the weight of the fluid pressing on the sidewalls (Fig. 9–21B). (2) An area of *tympany* at the top of the abdominal curve is caused by gas-filled, mobile intestines floating to the uppermost surface of the fluid, regardless of the position of the patient (Fig. 9–21A). (3) Free fluid produces *shifting dullness*. With the patient supine, percuss the level of dullness in the flanks and mark it on the skin. Then turn the patient on one side for a minute and percuss the new level of dullness; considerable shift indicates the presence of fluid (Fig. 9–21C). (4) A *fluid wave* can be demonstrated by tapping a flank sharply with one hand while the other receives the impulse against the opposite flank. There is a perceptible time lag between the tap and reception of the impulse (Fig. 9–21D). Fat in the mesentery produces a similar wave, so the fat must be blocked by having the patient or an assistant press the ulnar surface of their hand into the midline of the abdomen. A wave passing this block is usually caused by free fluid. These signs will not detect less than 500 mL of peritoneal fluid [Williams JW, Simel DL. The rational clinical examination. Does this patient have ascites? How to divine fluid in the abdomen. *JAMA.* 1992;267:2645–2648].

Ascites—An Approach to Differential Diagnosis: Listed below is a useful physiologic approach to the differential diagnosis of ascites based upon an assessment of the likely mechanism of ascitic fluid accumulation:

Increased Central Venous Pressure: Right ventricular failure from any cause, pulmonary hypertension (primary or secondary), constrictive pericarditis, tricuspid stenosis, or obstruction. *Hepatic Vein Obstruction:* Budd-Chiari syndrome, thrombosis, proximal IVC obstruction or thrombosis. *Obstruction of the Hepatic Sinusoids and Intrahepatic Portal Veins:* cirrhosis from any cause, primary biliary cirrhosis, amyloidosis, schistosomiasis, neoplastic infiltration. *Obstruction of the Portal Vein:* portal vein thrombosis, pylephlebitis, extrinsic compression by lymph nodes or masses in the portahepatis. *Peritoneal Irritation:* acute or chronic peritonitis, neoplastic implants (especially ovarian cancer), tuberculosis. *Decreased Oncotic Pressure:* nephrotic syndrome, hepatocellular dysfunction, repeated large volume paracentesis, protein-losing enteropathy, malnutrition. *Obstruction of the Thoracic Duct or Lymphatics (Chylous Ascites):* lymphoma, metastatic neoplasm, trauma, surgical injury, trauma to thorax or abdomen, tuberculosis, filariasis, intestinal lymphangiectasia. *Miscellaneous:* myxedema, benign ovarian adenoma with ascites and hydrothorax (Meigs syndrome), starvation edema, and wet beriberi (thiamine deficiency and hypoproteinemia are only contributing factors).

KEY SIGN   Ovarian Cyst

Large ovarian cysts can fill much of the abdominal cavity and must be distinguished from ascites. Because they are thin-walled and filled with fluid, they can evert the umbilicus and produce a fluid wave and shifting dullness. The pelvic examination is not diagnostic. Three signs help identify these cysts (Fig. 9–22): (1) careful inspection of the abdominal profile reveals two curves instead of one (Fig. 9–22A and Fig. 9–20B); (2) when a ruler is pressed transversely across the abdomen, the pulsations of the abdominal aorta are not transmitted with free fluid. If the fluid is enclosed in a tight cyst, the aortic pulsation will move the ruler (*the ruler test*) (Fig. 9–22B); (3) in the supine position the tympanitic intestines are pushed superiorly by the cyst, so the lower abdomen may be dull (Fig. 9–22C).

KEY SIGN   Depressed Abdomen—Scaphoid Abdomen

In extreme malnutrition, the abdominal wall sinks inward toward the vertebral column, forming a depression, pointed superiorly by the costal angle and inferiorly by the wings of the ilia. This has the shape of an ancient Greek boat called a skaphe (see Fig. 9–20B). The abdominal contents are more visible and more readily felt than normal. Be careful not to overestimate the size and significance of structures that are unfamiliar because they are normally not palpable.

KEY SIGN   Cutaneous Scars and Striae

See Chapter 6, The Skin, page 133.

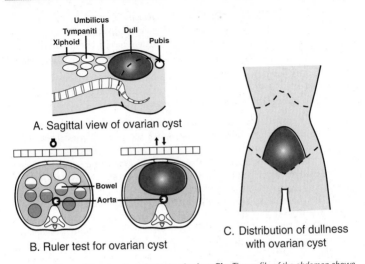

A. Sagittal view of ovarian cyst

B. Ruler test for ovarian cyst

C. Distribution of dullness with ovarian cyst

Fig. 9–22 *Signs of Ovarian Cyst. A. Abdominal profile:* *The profile of the abdomen shows a curve more pronounced in the lower half. The gas-filled intestines, producing tympany, fill the superior half of the cavity, instead of floating to the top. B. The ruler test. C. Distribution of dullness.*

> **KEY SIGN**   **Engorged Veins**

Ordinarily, the veins in the abdominal wall are scarcely seen unless the skin and subcutaneous fat are thin. Distention of the abdominal wall veins occurs when collateral flow through the abdominal and thoracic wall veins increases as a result of obstruction to normal venous drainage. Because the venous system normally has a low pressure (<30 cm H_2O) it is easily obstructed by extrinsic compression; the low flow velocities in veins also increases the risk of thrombosis. Obstruction of venous drainage from the abdominal viscera is most common (see the discussion of Portal Hypertension, page 488). Obstruction of the IVC distal to the hepatic vein, iliac veins, the femoral veins, the superior vena cava, the brachiocephalic, and subclavian veins can each lead to collateralization on the chest and abdominal wall. Because the abdominal wall veins do not have valves, flow can be in either direction. The direction of flow is away from the site obstruction. Engorged veins are often visible through a normal abdominal wall. Above the umbilicus, the venous flow is normally cephalad; below the navel, it is caudad. The direction of flow can be determined by identifying the direction of most rapid refilling of an empty venous segment (Fig. 9–23). Obstruction of the IVC causes a cephalad flow in the lower abdomen (*flow reversal*). Portal obstruction causes an increase in normal cephalad flow in the upper abdomen and caudad flow in the lower abdomen. Obstruction of the superior vena cava causes caudad flow in the upper abdomen (reversal). Very rarely, engorged veins form a knot around the umbilicus called *caput medusae*. The pattern of distended veins on the abdomen, chest and extremities together with the direction of flow can accurately predict the site of venous obstruction. The differential diagnosis will be developed on the basis of the patient's history, the site(s) of venous obstruction,

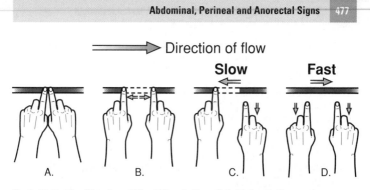

Fig. 9–23 *Testing Direction of Blood Flow in Superficial Veins. A.* The examiner presses the blood from the veins with his index fingers in apposition. *B.* The index fingers are slid apart, milking the blood from the intervening segment of vein. *C.* The pressure upon one end of the segment is then released to observe the time of refilling from that direction. *D.* The procedure is repeated and the other end released first. The flow of blood is in the direction of the faster flow.

and the other physical findings. ***CLINICAL OCCURRENCE:*** *Mechanical/Trauma* extrinsic compression from mass lesions (superior vena cava, IVC, and their major tributaries), obliteration of hepatic sinusoids (portal hypertension), strictures caused by traumatic or iatrogenic injury (surgery, instrumentation, or irradiation); *Vascular* thrombosis caused by intravenous catheters or pacemakers (subclavian, jugular, brachiocephalic, femoral), spontaneous thrombosis from congenital or acquired thrombophilia (any vein, superficial or deep).

KEY SIGN   Visible Peristalsis

When the abdominal wall is thin, normal contractions of the stomach and intestines may be visible as slow undulations under the skin. Visible peristaltic waves through a wall of normal thickness usually reflect increased amplitude and strength of peristalsis. Peristaltic waves in the stomach or small bowel sometimes can be seen in the upper abdomen. They usually appear as oblique ridges in the wall that begin near the LUQ and gradually move downward and rightward. Occasionally parallel ridges form a "ladder" pattern. The waves are slow; to see them, watch the abdomen for several minutes. Sit beside the bed with your eyes near the level of the abdominal profile. Abnormally, powerful waves indicate obstruction of a tubular viscus. *Borborygmus*, intestinal rumblings heard without a stethoscope, in conjunction with visible peristalsis and pain are most suggestive of pyloric obstruction or obstruction of small or large bowel, either partial or complete.

KEY SIGN   Visible Pulsations

Normally, the abdominal aorta causes a slight pulsation in the epigastrium. The amplitude is increased with widened pulse pressure, tortuous aorta, or aneurysm. The pulse may be transmitted to the surface with increased facility by a solid mass overlying the aorta. Aortic tortuosity may be distinguished from dilatation by palpation. Feeling a pulsatile mass raises the question of aneurysm or a solid structure adjacent to the aorta. An aneurysm is expansile laterally as well as anteroposteriorly. A murmur near the mass suggests aneurysm. Ultrasonography or CT are diagnostic.

Diastasis recti. This occurs when the two abdominal rectus muscles lack their normal fibrous attachment in the midline. With the supine abdomen relaxed, no abnormality may be noted. When the patient raises his head from the pillow, the abdominal recti tense; revealing the separation. This may be visible or evident only on palpation (see Fig. 9–20A).

Everted umbilicus. Without a hernia, this is a sign of increased intraabdominal pressure from fluid or masses in the cavity.

Umbilical fistula. This may discharge (1) urine through a patent urachus, (2) pus from a urachal cyst or tract or an abscess in the abdominal cavity, or (3) feces from a connection with the colon.

Umbilical calculus. In persons with poor hygiene, a hard mass of dirt and desquamated epithelium may accumulate in the umbilical cavity and cause inflammation.

Bluish umbilicus (cullen sign). A faintly blue coloration may occur as the result of retroperitoneal bleeding from any cause.

> **KEY SIGN** **Ecchymoses on Abdomen and Flanks (Grey Turner Sign)**

This results from dissection of blood along the extraperitoneal tissue planes to the skin surface. Nontraumatic ecchymoses may occur in the skin of the lower abdomen, groin, and flanks as a result of massive retroperitoneal hemorrhage. The color may be blue-red, blue-purple, or green-brown, depending on the degree of degradation of the hemoglobin. First associated with hemorrhagic pancreatitis, it with retroperitoneal hemorrhage from any cause.

Auscultation

> **KEY SIGN** **Decreased or Absent Peristaltic Sounds**

Absence of bowel sounds is a sign of ileus, which can have many causes, but is most often metabolic in the absence of peritonitis. Listen for at least 5 minutes by the clock before accepting a total absence of bowel sounds. Occasional weak tinkles are not evidence of good peristaltic activity. High-pitched tinkling sounds and rushes may be heard in partial obstruction. Except in intestinal pseudoobstruction, ileus is never a primary problem, but the sign of a metabolic/toxic, inflammatory, or infectious process.

✔ *DECREASED BOWEL SOUNDS—CLINICAL OCCURRENCE:* **Endocrine** myxedema; **Idiopathic** intestinal pseudoobstruction; **Infectious** peritonitis; **Metabolic/Toxic** electrolyte abnormalities: hypokalemia, hypomagnesemia, hypocalcemia; uremia; drugs: opiates, anticholinergics; **Mechanical/Trauma** advanced intestinal obstruction; **Neurologic** spinal cord injury; **Vascular** mesenteric ischemia.

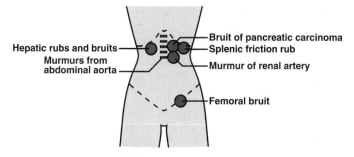

Fig. 9–24 *Abdominal Bruits and Rubs.* Blue shading indicates the optimum areas for the auscultation of these abdominal sounds.

KEY SIGN Increased Peristaltic Sounds

Increased peristalsis indicates irritation of the bowel usually as a result of luminal toxins, irritants, or early obstruction. Correlation of the ausculatory findings with the patient's history and other findings on physical examination will readily differentiate between diarrheal illness or obstruction.

Succussion splash. The combination of air and fluid in the normal stomach produces audible splashes with movement or palpation. A very loud splash and distention suggests gastric dilatation often due to gastroparesis or outlet obstruction.

KEY SIGN Peritoneal Friction Rub

Its presence indicates peritoneal inflammation (Fig. 9–24). Like its pleural counterpart, this sound resembles two pieces of leather rubbing together. It may be elicited with breathing, movement, peristalsis, or palpation. *CLINICAL OCCUR-RENCE:* *Infectious* liver or splenic abscess, perihepatitis (Fitz-Hugh-Curtis syndrome); *Mechanical/Trauma* after liver biopsy; *Neoplastic* hepatocellular carcinoma, liver metastases, peritoneal mesothelioma; *Vascular* splenic infarction.

KEY SIGN Abdominal Bruits

Bruits imply arterial flow through a narrowed or tortuous artery (generally systolic only), or large volume flow from high to low pressure as in an arteriovenous malformation (both systolic and diastolic). Hepatocellular carcinoma frequently produces a harsh arterial bruit that is either systolic or continuous with systolic accentuation. Rarely, a venous hum may be audible over a hemangioma in the liver or in the dilated periumbilical circulation with a patent umbilical vein (Cruveilhier-Baumgarten syndrome). A continuous systolic-diastolic bruit may occur from an arteriovenous fistula in renal vessels. Renal artery stenosis is found in approximately two-thirds of patients with systolic renal artery bruits. These murmurs are soft, medium- or low-pitched, and most commonly heard just above and to the left of the umbilicus (see Fig. 9–24) [Turnbull JM. The rational clinical examination. Is listening for abdominal bruits useful in the evaluation of hypertension? *JAMA.* 1995;274:1399–1401].

Percussion

> **KEY SIGN** Tympanitic Percussion—Tympanites

Tympanites is the presence of excessive gas within the bowel or free in the peritoneal cavity. Tympanites is synonymous with intestinal obstruction and ileus, conditions in which the flow of intestinal contents is diminished, reversed, or arrested. The physical signs are abdominal distention and a large area of tympany. The abdominal profile describes a single curve (see Fig. 9–20B). Tympanites is not necessarily seen in intestinal obstruction proximal the ligament of Treitz, since the gut is too short to contain much air and is mechanically fixed in the retroperitoneum. Gastric distention from such a proximal obstruction results initially in distention of the left upper abdomen and localized LUQ tympany; if prolonged the distended stomach may reach down to the pelvic brim. The causes of obstruction are either mechanical (intraluminal mass, extraluminal compression, intussusception, volvulus), or nonmechanical (decreased bowel motility, which can be diffuse or segmental). Mechanical obstruction commonly produces vomiting and colicky pain. These symptoms are lacking in nonmechanical obstruction, although anorexia and nausea are common. Both types of obstruction may occur sequentially or together. Voluntary or involuntary muscle spasm of the abdominal wall may be present, especially with perforation. Learn to recognize the following clinical patterns: noisy tympanites with colic and vomiting; silent tympanites without colic or vomiting; tympanites with normal bowel sounds and no vomiting (see Obstruction Syndromes, page 513).

Tympanitic Percussion—Intraluminal Gas: Increased gas in the intestinal lumen is common, but less so than symptomatic complaints of excessive gas. Aerophagia is common and has many causes, including chewing gum, ingestion of carbonated beverages, and inducing eructation.

✔ **INTRALUMINAL GAS—CLINICAL OCCURRENCE:** *Congenital* lactase deficiency, fructose malabsorption; *Idiopathic* intestinal pseudoobstruction, lactase deficiency; *Inflammatory/Immune* megacolon from ulcerative colitis or Crohn disease; *Infectious* bacterial overgrowth in the small bowel; *Metabolic/Toxic* toxic megacolon, lactase deficiency, artificial sweateners; *Mechanical/Trauma* volvulus, ileus, endoscopic procedures, air contrast barium enema, aerophagia, carbonated beverage ingestion, bowel obstruction; *Neurologic* ileus from spinal cord injury; *Psychosocial* factitious disorders; *Vascular* ileus from ischemia.

Tympanitic Percussion—Pneumoperitoneum: A small amount of gas in the peritoneal cavity cannot be identified by physical examination. With a larger quantity, the area of tympany is expanded. Pain and peritonitis may be absent, depending on the presence of contaminants; gut motility is normal if peritonitis is absent.

✔ **PNEUMOPERITONEUM—CLINICAL OCCURRENCE:** *Idiopathic* ruptured diverticulum, perforated ulcer, pneumocystoides; *Inflammatory/Immune* perforated megacolon; *Infectious* typhoid fever with perforation; ruptured diverticular abscess; *Mechanical/Trauma* perforating abdominal wounds, perforating ingested foreign bodies, volvulus with perforation, postparacentesis, postlaparoscopy, perforated diverticulum, posthysterosalpingogram, peritoneal dialysis; **Neoplastic** perforated colon cancer; **Vascular** ischemic bowel with perforation.

> ### KEY SIGN   Abdominal Pain with Percussion

Percussion sends a wave of movement through the free wall of the abdomen and peritoneal surfaces. Pain induced by percussion, especially when referred to areas remote from the point of percussion suggests peritoneal inflammation. See Rebound Tenderness, below.

> ### KEY SIGN   Costovertebral Tenderness

Tenderness in this region indicates inflammation of the kidney or the paranephric region, as in pyelonephritis.

Palpation

> ### KEY SIGN   Rebound Tenderness (Blumberg Sign)

The inflamed peritoneum is painful when disturbed by direct pressure or movement, especially when two inflamed peritoneal surfaces slide over one another. Because the peritoneum has somatic sensory afferents, the site of pain is well localized. Press the fingertips gently into the abdomen, then suddenly withdraw them (see Fig. 9–7D). Pain worsened after withdrawal is rebound tenderness. The pain may occur at the site of pressure or remote from it. If a site of inflammation is suspected, do your first maneuvers in the other quadrants. An alternate and less-painful method is the use of light percussion. Rebound tenderness is a reliable sign of peritoneal inflammation. Another test for peritoneal irritation is to vigorously move the patient's pelvis from side to side with your hands.

Jar Tenderness (Markle Sign). The finding of jar tenderness may prove superior to rebound tenderness as a localizing sign of peritoneal irritation, especially in the pelvis. The sign is produced by the heel-drop test. With the examiner demonstrating, the patient stands on the floor with straightened knees, rises on the toes, then drops on the heels. The location and severity of pain is noted. False-positive signs are uncommon. This sign may be elicited when firm abdominal muscles prevent the deep palpation necessary to elicit rebound tenderness. Abdominal pain on running or walking is an equivalent finding.

✔ **REBOUND TENDERNESS—CLINICAL OCCURRENCE: Congenital** familial Mediterranean fever, acute intermittent and variegate porphyria; **Endocrine** ectopic or tubal pregnancy; **Inflammatory/Immune** peritonitis of any cause, appendicitis; cholecystitis, regional enteritis (Crohn disease) familial Mediterranean fever, acute intermittent and variegate porphyria; **Infectious** pelvic inflammatory disease, intraabdominal abscess; diverticulitis; **Mechanical/Trauma** intraabdominal bleeding; **Vascular** infarction of abdominal organs.

> ### KEY SIGN   Direct Tenderness

Tenderness may be caused by inflammation of the abdominal wall, the peritoneum, or a viscus. A solid organ may be tender when its capsule is distended. Palpate the abdomen in the area of tenderness while the patient raise their head off the pillow or feet off the table. If the tenderness diminishes, an intraabdominal process is more likely. If the tenderness is unchanged or worsens, a disorder of the abdominal wall is more likely.

> **KEY SIGN**   **Cutaneous Hyperesthesia and Allodynia**

See Chapter 14, page 725. In acute appendicitis, an area of hyperesthesia is frequently found in the RLQ; it precedes perforation.

> **KEY SIGN**   **Subcutaneous Crepitus**

See Chapter 6, page 134.

> **KEY SIGN**   **Resistance to Palpation—Voluntary Rigidity of Muscle**

Increased abdominal wall muscle tone can result from an unrelaxed posture, a cold room or examining hands, and anxiety. The rigidity interferes with effective deep palpation. It is distinguished from involuntary rigidity by being abolished with suitable maneuvers (see page 452).

➤ > **KEY SIGN**   **Resistance to Palpation—Involuntary Rigidity of Muscle**

Reflex muscle spasm is caused by peritoneal irritation. Persistence of rigidity despite relaxing maneuvers suggest it to be involuntary. Pain is elicited when the patient attempts a sit-up without using the arms. Involuntarily rigid muscles are not necessarily tender and must be distinguished from abdominal wall masses. Rigidity of this type may be unilateral, while voluntary rigidity is symmetrical. When asymmetry is suspected, compare right to left in upper and lower quadrants by placing your hands symmetrically on the patient's abdomen and evaluating muscle tenseness on each side.

Subphrenic Abscess: Pus may collect in the spaces under either diaphragm secondary to suppurative lesions in the liver or spleen or elsewhere in the abdomen, such as a perforated appendix. The patient has unexplained fever or anorexia; there may be no symptoms to direct attention to the subphrenic region. Learn to suspect abscesses under the diaphragm and search for the local signs. Elevation of either hemidiaphragm may be demonstrated by percussion and confirmed by X-ray. Pleural effusion, evidenced by percussion dullness, decreased breath sounds, and decreased fremitus, may occur on the affected side. Gas under the right diaphragm should be suspected when percussion over the normal area of hepatic dullness in the right chest yields tympany. Further localization in the involved subphrenic spaces may be obtained by palpation for tenderness and edema in specific locations, as follows (Fig. 9–25). *Right Anterior Superior Space:* under the right costal margin in front of the liver, between the sixth and tenth right intercostal spaces anteriorly. *Right Anterior Inferior Space:* below the right anterior costal margin behind the liver. *Left Anterior Superior Space:* under the left costal margin anteriorly, between the sixth and tenth left interspaces in the midclavicular line. *Left Anterior Inferior Space:* under the left costal margin in the midaxillary line. *Left Posterior Inferior Space:* over the left twelfth rib.

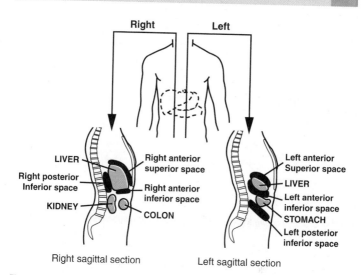

Right **Left**

LIVER

Right posterior
Inferior space

KIDNEY

Right anterior
superior space

Right anterior
inferior space

COLON

Left anterior
Superior space

LIVER

Left anterior
inferior space

STOMACH

Left posterior
inferior space

Right sagittal section   Left sagittal section

Fig. 9–25 Locations of Subphrenic Abscesses. *The loci are in the right midclavicular line, behind the costal margin, and the LUQ. Posteriorly, the region of the right kidney should be examined.*

> **KEY SIGN   Resistance to Palpation—Abdominal Masses**

See Abdominal Masses, page 515. If sufficiently large or close to the abdominal wall, masses cause increased resistance to light palpation. Note the pattern of resistance, and whether it corresponds to abdominal muscles or resembles the shape of a viscus. When a mass is demonstrated, determine whether it is in the wall or in the abdominal cavity. Failure to consider an intramural location results in the erroneous conclusion that all masses are intraabdominal. Intramural masses are palpable when the abdominal muscles are tensed; masses in the cavity are shielded from palpation in this situation (Fig. 9–26). Light palpation can determine only the presence of a mass and its location; further information must be sought by deep palpation and other procedures. Note all the characteristics of the mass: location, size, shape, consistency, surface, tenderness, and mobility (page 451). **DDX:** A frequently misdiagnosed mass is hematoma of the rectus muscle.

> **KEY SIGN   Shallow Abdominal Cavity**

Enlargement of the paraaortic and/or mesenteric lymph nodes (retroperitoneal lymphadenopathy) fills the retroperitoneal space. The hyperplastic nodes are covered with fascia and abdominal viscera, so the floor of the abdominal cavity seems more accessible than normal; discrete nodes cannot be felt. With deep palpation the abdominal cavity is shallower than normal, but without definite masses (Fig. 9–27). The retroperitoneal nodes are best visualized by CT or MRI; lymphoma, metastatic germ cell tumors, and granulomatous diseases are most common. The massively enlarged kidneys in polycystic kidney disease will also produce this finding.

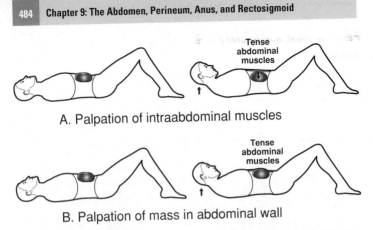

Fig. 9–26 *Distinguishing Between Intramural and Intraabdominal Masses.* Palpate the mass while the patient raises his head from the pillow. When the abdominal muscles tense, the intraabdominal mass moves away from the palpating hand, while the intramural mass remains accessible.

> **KEY SIGN** **Abdominal Wall Mass—Nodular Umbilicus (Sister Mary Joseph Nodule)**

Abdominal carcinoma, especially gastric, may metastasize to the navel [Moll S. Images in clinical medicine. Sister Joseph's node in carcinoma of the cecum. *N Engl J Med.* 1996;335:1568].

> **KEY SIGN** **Pulseless Femoral Artery (Leriche Syndrome)**

Always palpate the femoral arteries during examination of the abdomen. See page 428 for further discussion.

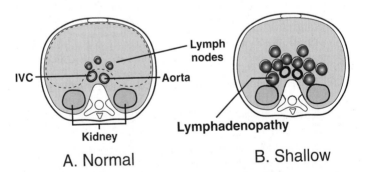

Fig. 9–27 *Shallow Abdominal Cavity. A. Normal small paraaortic lymph nodes are not palpable. B. Massive enlargement of prevertebral and preaortic lymph nodes cannot be distinguished from other retroperitoneal masses by palpation.* These conditions merely give an impression that the abdomen is shallower than normal. IVC = inferior vena cava.

Perineal, Anal, and Rectal Signs

Inspection

Pruritus ani: See symptoms page 468.

Prolapsed rectal polyp.   When pedunculated, polyps in the lower rectum may prolapse from the anus as spherical masses.

> **KEY SIGN   Hemorrhoids**

Large submucosal hemorrhoidal veins are normal anal cushions. They may dilate in normal people to form hemorrhoids; they are more common and severe with portal hypertension or obstruction of the IVC. *Internal Hemorrhoids* (see Fig. 9–3) are irregular globular masses which arise above the pectinate line so are covered with rectal mucosa; they may prolapse into the anal canal (Fig. 9–28C). *External Hemorrhoids* arise below the pectinate line and are covered with skin. When thrombosed; they are purple-red, firm, and very painful (Fig. 9–28B and Plate 28). With edema of the overlying skin, they may be white.

> **KEY SIGN   Fistula in Ano**

Most fistulae in ano arise from abscesses in the anal crypts (crypts of Morgagni) and track to the perianal skin. Look for a small sinus track opening in the perianal skin (see Fig. 9–28D). The internal orifices of the tracks are found just above the pectinate line (see Fig. 9–3A page, 449); fistulas should not be probed from the exterior. Gentle palpation around the orifice of the fistula may reveal the course of the track as a subcutaneous cord. The origin may be inferred from the location of the fistula on the perineum (Fig. 9–29A). **DDX:** Chronic lesions stimulate hypertrophy of an anal papilla (*sentinel pile*). Multiple fistulas suggest Crohn disease or tuberculous proctitis.

> **KEY SIGN   Fissure in Ano**

The extreme pain associated with fissures results from anal sphincter spasm. If the patient presents with pain, do not attempt a digital examination before

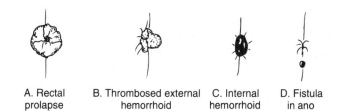

| A. Rectal prolapse | B. Thrombosed external hemorrhoid | C. Internal hemorrhoid | D. Fistula in ano |

Fig. 9–28 *Some External Anal Findings. A.* *Rectal Prolapse appears as a red doughnut of most rectal mucosa protruding through the anus. **B.** Thrombosed External Hemorrhoids are semispheric masses of erythematous skin at the mucocutaneous junction with the anus. **C.** Internal Hemorrhoids are mucosal masses sometimes seen through the retracted anus. **D.** Fistulous Opening in the skin is accompanied by a papule of hypertrophied skin on the margin of the orifice.*

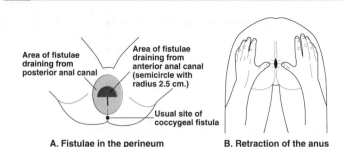

A. Fistulae in the perineum **B. Retraction of the anus**

Fig. 9–29 *Examination of the Perineum.* *A. Fistulae in the perineum:* The dark blue semicircular area anterior to the anus, with a radius of 2.5 cm, indicates the location of fistulae sinuses that drain from the anterior surface of the anal canal (Salmon's law). Anal fistulae draining to the skin in the light blue area arise in abscesses from the posterior surface of the canal. A coccygeal fistula (pilonidal) is usually in the midline, near coccyx or sacrum. *B. Retraction of the anus:* This is a method of stretching the anal orifice to inspect for fissure in ano, external hemorrhoids, or prolapsing internal hemorrhoids or polyps.

inspecting the mucosa by retracting the skin on both sides and looking for the fissure posteriorly (Fig. 9–29B). It is an extreme unkindness to the patient to attempt further examination without giving either local anesthetics or analgesics. The fissure is a slit-like separation of the superficial anal mucosa, suggesting a longitudinal tear, rarely becoming an ulcerating crater.

Sentinel pile. Various authors seem to apply this term to two structures. More commonly, it refers to a hyperplastic tag of skin frequently found external to a fissure in ano, resembling an external hemorrhoidal tag; it is also called a *fibrous anal polyp*. The name has been applied to a hypertrophied anal papilla internal to a fissure in ano (see Fig. 9–3). This lesion arises from the pectinate line, while an internal hemorrhoid arises above it.

KEY SIGN Rectal Prolapse

When the patient strains, as if to defecate, the rectal mucosa may evert below the sphincter (Fig. 9–28). When symptoms suggest prolapse, but the procedure fails to demonstrate it, have the patient squat and strain in the position for defecation. The prolapse may be either mucosal or complete; in the latter case, the sphincters are included.

Palpation

KEY SIGN Anal Stricture

A congenital stricture is occasionally encountered as a narrow crescentic fold at the rectal entrance to the anal canal. A fibrous stricture in the same region is usually the result of surgery for internal hemorrhoids. A sharply delimited stricture is usually the result of radiation therapy.

Carcinoma of the Anus: Squamous cell carcinoma of the anal skin is related to human papillomavirus infection and is most common in homosexual men practicing anal-receptive intercourse; its incidence is greatly increased in HIV-infected men. The tumor presents as an exophytic or ulcerating mass narrowing the anal canal.

Carcinoma of the Rectum: Cancer may cause plateau-like, nodular, annular, or cauliflower mass in the rectum. Endoscopic visualization and biopsy are essential.

Fibrosis of Anal Sphincter Muscles: The entire canal is narrowed so the finger feels encased in a rigid tube. This is caused by fibrosis of the anal muscles, frequently producing fecal impaction.

> **KEY SIGN** **Tight Sphincter—Apprehension**

The most common cause of a tight anal sphincter is apprehension. Preliminary reassurance should be combined with a gentle and slow examination. When you feel the sphincter tighten, stop advancing your finger until the sphincter is felt to relax, then advance a little further. Even though the procedure may be uncomfortable, it should not be painful.

> **KEY SIGN** **Tight Sphincter—Fissure in Ano**

When the sphincter is in spasm that cannot be relaxed by gentleness, suspect a fissure.

> **KEY SIGN** **Relaxed Sphincter—Lacerated Anal Muscles**

Damage to the anal sphincter is the result of childbirth or of sphincter injury during surgery. When the anus is retracted by pulling the skin from each side, a dimple is visible in the posterior part of the anal ring. The sphincter feels weak when the finger is inserted. Ultrasonography of the sphincter will reveal the defect.

Relaxed anal sphincter—atony of the muscles. Damage to the peripheral and central sensory and motor control of the sphincters can produce decreased tone. The finding should prompt a careful neurologic examination.

Rectal polyps. Some polyps can be palpated, especially if sessile. Because they are soft and, if pedunculated, mobile, they are easily missed.

Coccygeal tenderness. When a patient complains of pain in the region of the coccyx exacerbated by sitting or defecation, you should test for tenderness in the sacrococcygeal joint during digital rectal examination: place the index finger in the rectum on the anterior surface of the coccyx and press the posterior surface of the bone with the thumb on the skin outside. The bone is moved anteriorly and posteriorly to elicit pain in the joint. The coccyx may be displaced from previous injury.

> **KEY SIGN** **Fecal Impaction**

The symptoms may be vague. The patient may complain of constipation or obstipation; but sometimes there is diarrhea, the fecal stream passing around the impaction to produce incontinence. The debilitated or postoperative patient may be merely restless or have fever or anorexia. Barium suspensions administered for X-ray examination commonly cause impaction. The rectum is filled with hard, dry masses of feces. These must be removed by breaking up and extracting the pieces with the examining finger.

> **KEY SIGN** Coccygeal Sinus (Pilonidal Sinus)

A congenital track extends from the coccyx or sacrum to the perineum, where it drains to the exterior, usually in the midline posterior to the anus (Fig. 9–29). The sinus is lined with epithelium and hairs, hence the alternate name pilonidal. When blocked, it may form a tender dimple or bulge just below the coccyx or on one side, usually the left.

Ischiorectal abscess. Abscess forms within the pelvic floor muscles and tissue spaces between the rectum and the ischium, often associated with neutorpenia. Because it is deep-seated there may be no signs on inspection. Tenderness on deep palpation between the anus and ischial tuberosity identifies the site.

Anal intermuscular abscess. Abscesses between the muscles of the anus cause agonizing pain during defecation and discomfort during sitting. In high abscesses, a tender mass is felt just above the anorectal junction. Low abscesses are most frequently found with bidigital palpation near the distal end of the anal canal.

Abdominal, Perineal and Anorectal Syndromes

GI, Hepatobiliary and Pancreatic Syndromes

Obstruction of the portal and hepatic veins. When occlusion occurs rapidly, symptoms of hepatic and/or mesenteric vascular congestion (pain, anorexia, diarrhea) occur before signs of portal hypertension. Slowly developing obstruction presents as ascites or signs from vessels forming the portosystemic shunts.

> **KEY SYNDROME** Chronic Portal Vein Obstruction—Portal Hypertension

Any obstruction to the blood flow in the portal vein, the liver (presinusoidal, sinusoidal, postsinusoidal) or the hepatic vein produces portal hypertension. Increased pressure in the portal system (Fig. 9–30) produces splenic congestion with splenomegaly, development of venous collaterals about the esophagus, the rectum, and the abdominal wall, and the development of ascites because of increased hydrostatic pressure in the liver capsule and mesenteric veins. Look for splenomegaly, visible collateral veins, and ascites. Collaterals veins can be seen in the anus, the abdominal wall, the esophagus and proximal stomach. Hemorrhoids may be portal collaterals, but their occurrence from local causes is so common that their presence is rarely diagnostic. Dilatation of the paraumbilical vein can produce a venous rosette around the navel, a *caput medusae,* but it is

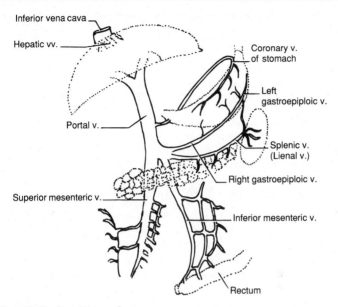

Fig. 9–30 *The Portal Venous System.*

rare. The common demonstrable collaterals are dilated superficial veins in the abdominal wall between the umbilicus and the lower thorax containing blood flowing upward, in the normal direction. When the veins are greatly dilated; a venous hum with systolic accentuation may be heard below the xiphoid process, over the epigastric surface of the liver, or around the navel. Formerly, this hum was attributed to a patent umbilical vein in the *Cruveilhier-Baumgarten syndrome;* now it is recognized as coming from varices in the falciform ligament. Dilated veins in the lower esophagus and gastric cardia produce esophageal varices and portal gastropathy visible during endoscopy. Ascites is painless and may be mild, moderate, or severe. **DDX:** Portal obstruction with ascites and edema of the ankles may be mistaken for right heart failure. Both conditions may produce pleural effusions, hepatomegaly, ascites, and ankle edema. Engorged neck veins and orthopnea are frequent with heart failure but absent with portal hypertension. **CLINICAL OCCURRENCE:** Thrombosis of the hepatic veins, cirrhosis of the liver, intrahepatic tumors and cysts, granulomatous diseases of the liver, portal vein thrombosis, septic thrombosis of the portal vein.

Acute Portal Vein Thrombosis: Occlusion occurs after surgical manipulation of the portal vein, septic thrombophlebitis of the portal vein (*pylephlebitis*), trauma, polycythemia vera, neoplastic invasion of the vein lumen, or prolonged debilitating illness. At the onset, there is abdominal pain and tenderness, abdominal distention, ileus, diarrhea, and vomiting. Ascites and splenomegaly rapidly follow. Infarctions of the upper GI tract may occur. Clinical suspicion should lead to imaging studies [Cohen J, Edelman RR, Chopra S. Portal vein thrombosis: A review. *Am J Med.* 1992;92: 173–181].

KEY SYNDROME   Acute Hepatic Vein Thrombosis: Budd-Chiari Syndrome

Hepatic vein thrombosis results in hepatic sinusoidal congestion, obstruction to portal flow through the liver, and development of signs of portal hypertension. Acute distention of the liver capsule produces pain. The onset may be abrupt, with pain in the abdomen and vomiting. The liver is tender and enlarges rapidly. Mild jaundice may be present. Ascites rapidly accumulates. Shock may ensue, with death in a few days. Obstruction of the IVC at or above the confluence with the hepatic vein will produce similar symptoms and additional signs related to the lower exptremities. If the initial stage is survived, the chronic findings may appear [Menon KVN, Shah V, Kamath PS. The Budd-Chiari syndrome. *N Engl J Med.* 2004;350:578–585; Chung RT, Iafrate AJ, Amrein PC, et al. Case 15-2006: A 46-year-old woman with sudden onset of abdominal distention]. *CLINICAL OC-CURRENCE:* cirrhosis, acute or subacute liver disease due to abscess, malignancy or trauma, polycythemia vera, paroxysmal nocturanal hemoglobinuria, myelo-proliferative disorders and thrombophilic disorders including oral contraceptive use.

Chronic Hepatic Vein Occlusion. This the late phase of the Budd-Chiari syndrome. Portal hypertension and ascites are present, together with hepatomegaly, and secondary hepatocellular failure. Sudden onset and lack of alcohol intake or hepatitis suggests the correct diagnosis.

Acute Abdominal Pain Syndromes

The abdomen contains the following paired organs: kidneys, ureters, adrenals, iliac and renal arteries and veins, and ovaries. A disease or syndrome associated with abdominal pain arising in one of these organs may occur with either right or left lateralization. We will only discuss it as it presents on one side.

KEY SYNDROME   Acute Abdominal Pain

See General Symptoms, page 462.

KEY SYNDROME   Six-Dermatome Pain

For a discussion of the six-dermatome pain pathophysiology and differential diagnosis, see Chapter 8, page 333 and Fig. 8–27, page 334.

KEY SYNDROME   Six-Dermatome Pain—Esophageal Discomfort

Esophageal spasm consists of uncoordinated contractions of the esophagus and is often associated with dysphagia (a sensation of food sticking retrosternally). Hypertensive or nutcracker esophagus consists of coordinated but prolonged high-pressure contractions (probably with decreased compliance of the esophageal muscle). In achalasia, the LES fails to relax, causing dysphagia and retrosternal chest pain. Esophageal spasm consists of uncoordinated contractions of the esophagus and is often associated with dysphagia (a sensation of food sticking retrosternally). Disorders of esophageal motility often cause chest discomfort identical in character and location to that found with angina or myocardial infarction. Gastroesophageal reflux may cause pyrosis (heartburn), a burning or constricting lower retrosternal discomfort. The key to distinguishing angina from esophageal spasm is a careful history. For example, association with dysphagia or meals or the ingestion of cold liquids in the absence of exercise, precipitation by reclining or bending over, or relief with antacids all favor esophageal origin. Because nitroglycerin relaxes smooth muscle, whether in arteries, veins, or esophagus, it may relieve discomfort from both disorders. An ECG recorded during intense pain is useful; a normal tracing favors esophageal pain, although it does not exclude cardiac ischemia. *The presence of a hiatal hernia has no diagnostic significance in the differential diagnosis of chest pain.*

KEY SYNDROME   Esophageal Pain and Dysphagia

Mechanical disruption of normal swallowing and activation of esophageal nociceptors leads to this combination of findings. Sone of the more frequent causes are discussed below:

Esophageal Laceration—Mallory-Weiss Tear: Esophageal laceration occurs near the esophagogastric junction following severe retching and vomiting. Hematemesis occurs after retching and vomiting. Bleeding is usually self-limited.

Acute Esophagitis: There is retrosternal pain intensified by swallowing. This occurs after prolonged vomiting, nasogastric tubes, pill esophagitis, esophageal burns from corrosive substances, acute infections (herpes simplex, *Candida spp.*, cytomegalovirus), and reflux of acid or bile.

Chronic Esophagitis: Pain and dysphagia persists for weeks or months. The inflammation may be complicated by ulceration and/or intestinal metaplasia (Barrett esophagus), a premalignant lesion. Progressive fibrosis may produce esophageal stricture. Acid reflux is the most common cause. Irradiation, infections (HIV, *Candida,* herpes, and cytomegalovirus) are less common.

Esophageal Achalasia: Unremitting forceful contraction of the LES results in functional obstruction at the gastroesophageal junction with proximal dilation of the esophagus. Symptoms include weight loss, dysphagia and regurgitation of food, saliva, and esophageal secretions. Chest pain may be present; cough, especially after meals or with recumbency, suggests aspiration.

Zenker's Diverticulum: This is a pulsion diverticulum in the posterior hypopharynx protruding downward between spine and esophagus. It fills with food, causing dysphagia and regurgitation of putrefied food. Occasionally, there is retrosternal pain. The esophagram visualizes the pouch.

Plummer-Vinson Syndrome: This occurs with severe iron deficiency. A postcricoid esophageal web demonstrated by esophagram explains the dysphagia in some; no anatomic basis for dysphagia is identified in many patients.

Esophageal Cancer: Adenocarcinomas at or just above the gastroesophageal juction are increasing in frequency; squamous cell carcinomas predominate more proximally. Dysphagia usually precedes pain by weeks or months. The pain sometimes radiates to the neck or back. Chronic esophagitis with metaplasia (Barrett esophagus) substantially increases the risk for developing adenocarcinoma. [Spechler SJ. Barrett's esophagus. *N Engl J Med.* 2002;346:836–842].

Foreign Body: Swallowed rigid objects may lodge at the level of the aortic arch or diaphragm, causing pain and dysphagia.

➤ **KEY SYNDROME   Acute Abdominal Pain—Acute Peritonitis**

Acute inflammation of the peritoneum due to infection and/or sterile chemical irritaions produces physiologic changes leading to an intense inflammatory response and profound loss of intravasuclar fluid into the peritoneal space (systemic inflammatory response syndrome). The syndrome may be complicated by bleeding and bacterial infection (sepsis) resulting from the inciting event. Common causes are penetrating trauma, rupture of the bowel and bowel infarction. Three stages of symptoms may be seen: (1) *Stage of Prostration (Primary Shock)*. The patient experiences a sudden, excruciating pain in the epigastrium and frequently collapses. Soon the pain spreads over the entire abdomen. The patient is anxious, pale, and diaphoretic. The respiratory movements are shallow because of pain with diaphragmatic breathing. Retching or vomiting occurs. Hypothermia and hypotension are common. This initial stage may last from a few minutes to several hours, (2) *Stage of Reaction (Masked Peritonitis)*. This stage is a brief respite for the patient, but it may deceive the inexperienced physician. Although the blood pressure rises and the skin becomes warmer, the generalized abdominal pain and tenderness persist, although lessened in intensity. The patient moves cautiously because of pain; the thighs are flexed for comfort. Board-like involuntary rigidity results from contraction of abdominal muscles and shallow respiratory movements. The pelvic peritoneum is tender when examined rectally. Free fluid may rarely be demonstrated in the abdominal cavity. Gas under the diaphragm may be suggested by a diminished area of liver dullness in the RUQ, and (3) *Stage of Frank Peritonitis*. The classic signs of advanced peritonitis appear. Ileus distends the abdomen, vomiting resumes and persists with increased violence, and the temperature again declines to subnormal levels. The entire abdomen is tender, but rigidity may lessen in the late stage. Dehydration and pain produce the classic *facies hippocratica*, with hollow features and anxious expression. An expidited team approach to the evaluation and management of suspected peritonitis is essential to minimize morbidity and mortality through rapid diagnosis and combined medical and surgical treatments.

➤ **Spontaneous Bacterial Peritonitis:** Portal hypertension producing ascites with a low serum albumin ascites gradient is transudative and relatively low in immunoglobulins. Seeding of bacteria from the gut leads to persistant infection with minimal localizing symptoms. Patients have advanced liver disease and may present with fever or confusion without abdominal pain or tenderness. If the serum albumin ascites gradient is <2.1 and there are >250 PMNs/mm^3 in the ascites fluid, treatment should be started pending culture results.

➤ **Acute Abdominal Pain—Rupture of Solid Organs:** Blunt trauma to the lower thorax, back, and abdomen may fracture kidneys, liver, or spleen. The fracture and hemorrhage may be contained by the surrounding capsule. Rupture of the capsule resulting in severe hemorrhage may occur acutely or be delayed by hours or days. Upper quadrant and flank pain are present and tenderness may be present anteriorly or posteriorly. Renal fracture results in gross hematuria unless the ureter is obstructed. Fracture of solid organs must be sought emergently; CT scan is the diagnostic method of choice.

➤ **Acute abdominal pain—volvulus.** Volvulus most commonly occurs in the sigmoid colon (90%) or the cecum (10%) where the gut is suspended by a lengthy mesentery. Twisting causes vascular compromise, distention of the involved segment, and formation of a closed loop, leading to ischemic perforation. Early diagnosis and treatment are imperative. A vague, tender mass may be felt, but frequently the only findings are a distended bowel that produces tympany, pain, violent peristalsis, and vomiting. A bird beak cutoff is noted in the colonic gas on noncontrast X-rays. Colonoscopy may be both diagnostic and therapeutic.

➤ **KEY SYNDROME** Abdominal Pain and Pallor

Abdominal pain accompanied by pallor is an ominous presentation requiring expeditious evaluation. Of greatest concern is major hemorrhage from rupture of a major vessel or organ. Intense sympathetic activation, even without hemorrhage, may cause pallor and diaphoresis.

➤ **KEY SYNDROME** Ruptured Ectopic Pregnancy

See Chapter 11, page 558 and 566.

➤ **Corpus luteum hemorrhage:** See Chapter 11, page 559.

➤ **Ruptured aortic or iliac aneurysm:** See page 420.

➤ **Peptic Ulcer With Hemorrhage:** Erosion of an ulcer into a major vessel can lead to life-threatening hemorrhage. Although bleeding may be proceeded by the typical symptoms of ulcer disease, it is not uncommon, especially for nonsteroidal antiinflammatory drug-induced ulcers, to present with painless hemorrhage and/or perforation. Blood should be sought in the stools and a nasogastric aspirate.

Hemorrhagic Pancreatitis: Pancreatic inflammation erodes blood vessels in the retroperitoneum, leading to hemorrhage into the necrotic pancreas and dissection of hemorrhage into the retroperitoneal spaces. See page 494 for complete discussion.

KEY SYNDROME Acute Epigastric Pain

Visceral pain arising in the intestine from the stomach to the transverse colon is carried by the vagus nerve and projects to the epigastrium. In addition, somatic pain from the upper abdominal peritoneum and retroperitoneal structures will be well localized to the epigastrium.

➤ **Early acute appendicitis:** See Acute RLQ Pain—Appendicitis, page 499.

➤ **Perforated Peptic Ulcer:** Perforation causes leakage of acid, digestive enzymes, blood, bacteria, and bowel contents into the peritoneal cavity, lesser sac, or retroperitoneum. With free perforation, sterile peritonitis is followed by purulent peritonitis, septicemia, shock, and death. There may be a history of epigastric pain occurring 3 or 4 hours after meals and relieved by food or antacids. Occasionally, there are no antecedent symptoms, particularly in elderly patients taking nonsteroidal antiinflammatory drugs. The patient describes sudden, excruciating pain in the epigastrium that spreads over the entire abdomen; sometimes it intensifies in the suprapubic region because of the downward flow of gastric contents (Fig. 9–31). Without prompt diagnosis and treatment, generalized peritonitis will supervene (see page 492).

Limited Perforation of Peptic Ulcer: When the perforation is into a closed space, the released gastric contents are walled off to produce a local abscess. The

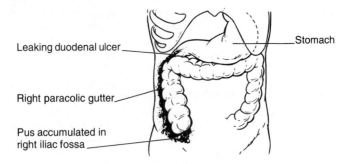

Fig. 9–31 *Iliac Abscess from a Leaking Duodenal Ulcer.* *The drainage of a duodenal ulcer is down the right paracolic gutter into the right iliac fossa, as indicated by stippling.*

stage of prostration is mild, with the pain limited to the epigastrium or flank. The abscess may form in the subphrenic space or lesser peritoneal sac.

Acute Gastritis: Inflammation of the gastric mucosa can occur as a result of infection, chemical irritation, autoimmune injury, or drug-induced injury. Frequently, the cause is unknown. Symptoms of gastritis are anorexia, nausea, and vomiting, sometimes with hematemesis, and epigastric pain with or without tenderness. Upper endoscopy is diagnostic revealing mucosal inflammation, erosions, and submucosal hemorrhage. Common causes are ingestion of aspirin, nonsteroidal antiinflammatory drugs, alcohol, or contaminated food, uremia, infection with *H. pylori*, cytomegalovirus, herpes simplex, or enteroviruses, and autoimmune gastritis.

Acute Pancreatitis: Autodigestion of the pancrease from release of pancreatic enzymes into the parenchyma as a consequence of ductal obstruction, inflammation, ischemia or trauma incites an intense sterile inflammatory response. Dissection of the expanding inflammatory mass within the retroperitoneum and occasional decompression intraperitoneally lead hypotension and shock. Secondary infection of necrotic tissue is common after the first few days. Without warning, the patient develops excruciating epigastric pain often with radiation to the back or flank. Irritation of the left hemidiaphragm causes pain radiation to the left shoulder via the phrenic nerve afferents. Occasionally, the pain spreads over the entire abdomen (generalized peritonitis) or primarily to the RLQ. The pain is knife-like with a boring quality, going directly through to the back. Because pain is aggravated when supine, the patient may assume a sitting or fetal position, leaning forward or curled up. Retching and vomiting are severe. The symptoms are more intense and prolonged than in perforation of the stomach and shock can occur. There is often a disparity between the severity of the symptoms and the paucity of abdominal findings since the process is confined to the retroperitoneum. Epigastric tenderness is always present, but muscle rigidity is usually absent; when present, it is confined to the epigastrium. Occasionally, one can feel a tender transverse mass deep in the epigastrium. Two or 3 days after onset, blue or green ecchymoses occasionally appear in the flank (*Turner sign*) or the umbilicus (*Cullen sign*) from extravasation of hemolyzed blood. Late complications include pseudocysts that are an accumulation of blood, necrotic debris, and fluid in the retroperitoneum; they are rarely palpable.

Acute pancreatitis may be an isolated episode or an acute exacerbation of chronic, relapsing pancreatitis. Common causes of acute pancreatitis are alcohol and gallstones. Other causes include hypertriglyceridemia, pancreatic ductal obstruction and stricture, pancreas divisum, perforated peptic ulcer, ampulla of Vater dysfunction, mumps, and drugs.

➤ **Occlusion of Mesenteric Vessels:** The superior mesenteric artery or vein is most commonly involved, by either embolism or thrombosis. Arterial occlusion is more likely to produce the typical clinical picture; venous thrombosis is often atypical. Predisposing conditions for venous thrombosis include thrombophilic states. The onset is sudden with acute agonizing pain between the xiphoid and the umbilicus; slight if any relief is afforded by narcotics. This presentation in an individual with rheumatic or atherosclerotic heart disease suggests the possibility of an arterial embolism. A history of recurrent postprandial abdominal pain suggestive of abdominal angina is reported in up to 50% of those with arterial thrombosis. Usually, there are few localizing signs, but occasionally, a tender mass is palpable in the epigastrium. These events are soon followed by the signs of intestinal obstruction: abdominal distention, ileus, and vomiting. Blood may be passed per rectum. There is a severe metabolic acidosis as endotoxemia and shock supervene. Common causes are atherosclerosis, thrombophilia, atheroembolism, fibromuscular dysplasia, acute bacterial or fungal endocarditis, embolism of mural cardiac thrombus, nonbacterial thrombotic (marantic) endocarditis and thrombophilic states including paroxysmal nocturnal hemoglobinuria. [Kumar S, Sarr MG, Kamath PS. Mesenteric vein thrombosis. *N Engl J Med.* 2001;345:1683–1688].

➤ **Aortic Dissection:** See Chapter 8, page 407. Dissections extending into the abdominal aorta may produce abdominal and back pain, pain in the groins, and occlusion of the abdominal branches of the aorta leading to ischemia of the downstream tissues. In some instances, abdominal pain is the initial complaint. The pain is usually in the epigastrium, causing intense involuntary rigidity of the abdominal muscles and so severe that narcotics do not provide relief. The blood pressure is not affected early. Branches of the abdominal aorta may be progressively occluded, and ischemia of the spinal cord may cause paraplegia. A disparity in the pulses may be the most important clue to the diagnosis. Occasionally, dissection is slow and symptomless. Causes to consider are hypertensive vascular disease, giant cell arteritis, arteriosclerosis, Marfan syndrome, and pseudoxanthoma elasticum.

➤ **Leak and Rupture of AAA:** AAA is often painless until it begins to rupture with leakage of blood into the adventitia and retroperitoneal space. Pain is moderate to severe, usually well localized, and often accompanied by nausea. Pain may radiate to one or both groins. Pain in the back and flank may dominate the presentation. Gentle palpation and urgent diagnosis are necessary [Lederle FA, Simel DL. The rational clinical examination. Does this patient have abdominal aortic aneurysm? *JAMA.* 1999;281:77–82].

> **KEY SYNDROME** Acute RUQ Pain

The liver, gallbladder, duodenum, head of the pancreas, right kidney, and pleural reflections of the right lung are the leading causes of pain located in the RUQ. Failure to consider pneumonia with pleural involvement or myocardial infarction

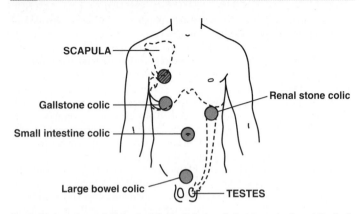

Fig. 9–32 *Locations of Abdominal Colic.* *Colic is a distinct type of pain, notable for its paroxysmal occurrence, severity and crescendo-decrescendo cycling. It occurs when a hollow viscus is obstructed; pain results from smooth-muscle contractions trying to overcome the obstruction. Note the radiation of gallstone colic from the RUQ to the angle of the right scapula posteriorly. The colic of renal calculus frequently radiates to the testis on the same side.*

in the differential diagnosis of acute RUQ abdominal pain has led to inappropriate surgical exploration of the abdomen.

Cholelithiasis with Biliary Colic: Gallstones are made predominantly of cholesterol, bile pigments, or a mixture. They rarely cause symptoms unless a stone perforates the gallbladder wall or obstructs the cystic duct, the common bile duct, or the pancreatic duct, producing colic because of forceful peristaltic contraction against the impacted stone. An attack of biliary colic may be uncomplicated, or it may be associated with acute cholecystitis, obstructive jaundice, or gallstone pancreatitis. Onset of biliary colic is sudden, with pain in the epigastrium or RUQ that radiates to the inferior border of the right scapula (Fig. 9–32). The pain is severe, recurring in cyclic paroxysms, and is associated with nausea and vomiting. During the attack, the RUQ is rigid. Calcified gallstones can be seen on plain X-ray films, but ultrasonography is the preferred diagnostic examination. Gallstones are common in patients with hemolytic anemias and in certain racial groups, for example, Native Americans. Stones are more prevalent with obesity, female sex, multiparity, diabetes, and some drugs.

Acute Cholecystitis: Obstruction of the cystic duct, usually by gallstone impaction, results in distention and sterile inflammation of the gallbladder wall. *Acalculous cholecystitis* is a complication of surgical or medical illness, with progressive gallbladder enlargement, ischemia, and rupture; it has a high mortality. The onset is acute or subacute, the pain is poorly localized, may radiate to top of the right shoulder and is frequently preceded by episodes of more mild RUQ postprandial pain. Nausea and anorexia are usual, and vomiting, although less common, may be severe. Tenderness over the gallbladder at the inferior margin of the liver is constant. When the tips of the fingers are held under the right costal margin and the patient is asked to inspire, there is inspiratory arrest (*Murphy sign*). Fist percussion over the liver produces pain, but this sign also occurs in acute hepatitis. The abdominal muscles do not become rigid unless peritonitis is present. In some patients, the gallbladder is palpable as an exquisitely tender globular mass behind the lower border of the liver [Trowbridge RL, Rutkowski NK, Shojania KG. The rational clinical examination. Does this patient have cholecystitis? *JAMA.* 2003;289:80–86]. Rarely, the distended gallbladder in cholecystitis reaches the RLQ. Moderate fever is usually present, but high fever or chills suggest *ascending cholangitis* or *suppurative cholecystitis.* Ultrasonography demonstrates a thickened, edematous gallbladder wall with sludge or stones in the lumen. The most common cause is gallstone disease, including microlithiasis with sludge. Uncommonly, parasites, bacterial infection, and primary biliary cancer can precipitate attacks. The diagnosis may be confirmed with a radionuclide scan showing obstruction of the cystic duct. False-positive radionucleotide studies may occur in hospitalized patients who have been fasting for many days, because the fluid-filled gallbladder is distended and does not easily contract.

➤ **Acalculous Cholecystitis—Hydrops of the Gallbladder:** Dilation of the gall bladder with poor muscular contactions produces a tense, thin edematous wall that occasionally ruptures. This is an infrequent but serious complication of other serious medical and surgical illnesses. It is either asymptomatic or accompanied by epigastric pain, nausea, and vomiting. There is fever and RUQ abdominal tenderness, and a palpable tender RUQ mass may be appreciated.

➤ **Acute RUQ Pain—Rupture of the Gallbladder, Bile Peritonitis:** Bile is extremely irritating to the peritoneum, producing a severe chemical peritonitis. Perforation of the gallbladder from erosion of a stone, infection, or ischemic necrosis are most common. The initial picture may be that of acute cholecystitis or gallstone colic, but the RUQ pain gradually spreads throughout the abdomen with signs of generalized peritonitis progressing to prostration and shock. Bile leak following cholecystectomy produces the same picture.

Leaking Duodenal Ulcer: A small duodenal perforation causes limited retroperitoneal leakage of duodenal contents into the right abdominal gutter leading to localized inflammation. The presentation is pain, tenderness, and rigidity in the RUQ; pain may radiate through to the back. A history of peptic ulcer disease may be present. There is tenderness in the midline of the epigastrium, but no peritoneal signs. The gastric and duodenal contents can track down into the RLQ and lead to pain and a mass in the RLQ (see Fig. 9–31).

Ureteral Colic: Acute ureteral obstruction induces vigorous peristaltic ureteral smooth muscle contractions that are intensely painful, but localize poorly and can radiate to similarly innervated regions, for example, the testicle, vulva, or groin. Proximal obstructions radiate pain to the flank (see Fig. 9–32). Patients are restless, frequently changing position seeking comfort. Anorexia is constant, nausea and vomiting can be severe. Microscopic hematuria is expected and sometimes gross hematuria occurs. A calcium-containing stone may be seen on plain X-ray films. **DDX:** Patients with peritonitis, pancreatitis and leaking aneurysms prefer to hold still, not move.

Pyelonephritis: Infection in the kidney produces inflammation and swelling, which distends the capsule, producing pain. Acute pyelonephritis produces upper quadrant and flank pain that is initially poorly localized and exacerbated by fist percussion over the kidney at the costovertebral angle posteriorly. The pain may be severe and accompanied by nausea. In the RUQ, the tenderness is deeper and less severe than with acute cholecystitis. Urinalysis and culture are diagnostic in most cases. Pyelonephritis results from ascending infection from a cystitis, or septic emboli. In women with recurrent infections or men with a first infection, suspect congenital or acquired anatomic abnormalities in the urinary tract (stones, tumor, diverticulum, etc.).

➤ **Renal or Perirenal Abscess:** Progressive necrotizing infection occurs, especially in the setting of infection complicating obstruction. Spread to the perinephritic space can lead to tracking into the pelvis. The patient Ies abdominal pain radiating into the groin with costovertebral angle tenderness and fever. If the cortex, but not the medulla, has been seeded by bacteremia, pyuria may be absent.

Acute hepatitis: Acute inflammation of the liver results from infections, alcohol, or drugs producing hepatocyte injury and secondary inflammation. Pain results when acute parenchymal swelling creates distention of the Glisson capsule. Fever, malaise, and anorexia are usually present. Smokers may lose their taste for cigarettes. If palpable, the entire liver is tender, the edge blunt and smooth. Fist percussion over the liver produces a dull aching pain. Jaundice appears after several days.

Pleurisy: Right lower lobe pneumonia can present primarily with pain referred to the RUQ. The patient has pain in the RUQ, but there are no findings on abdominal examination. Deep breathing may accentuate the pain, so the patient takes shallow breaths. A pleural rub and signs of pneumonia should be sought. A chest X-ray is mandatory in the evaluation of any patient with upper abdominal pain.

KEY SYNDROME   Acute LUQ Pain

The spleen, stomach, left kidney, splenic flexure of the colon, and pleural reflections of the left lung base are the most likely sources of LUQ pain.

Splenic Infarction: The spleen is highly vascular, and the sinusoidal structure creates a low redox environment that is susceptible to ischemic injury. Severe, sharp pain develops in the LUQ accompanied with splinting of the abdominal muscles. Frequently the pain radiates to the top of the left shoulder. Fever and leukocytosis may be present. A splenic friction rub may develop. A CT scan will identify splenic infarction. Infarction results from emboli (e.g., endocarditis), vasculitis, or in situ vascular occlusion (as with sickle cell disease). Splenomegaly from hematologic disorders, such as polycythemia vera, chronic myelocytic leukemia, or myelofibrosis may also lead to infarction.

➤ **Ruptured Spleen:** Rarely, the spleen ruptures spontaneously or with minimal trauma when it is enlarged from infectious mononucleosis, sepsis, or infarction. Large, soft spleens have been ruptured during palpation. Intense pain occurs in the LUQ, radiating to the top of the left shoulder (*Kehr sign*). The pain may be accentuated by elevating the foot of the bed, increasing contact between peritoneal blood and the diaphragm. Abdominal CT scan is diagnostic.

Pyelonephritis, ureteral colic and perinephric abscess: See discussion on pages 497.

Pleurisy: See RUQ pain above.

KEY SYNDROME   Acute RLQ Pain

The RLQ is the usual anatomic site of the cecum, appendix, and terminal ilium, each of which is the site of unique inflammatory disorders.

➤ **Acute Appendicitis:** Obstruction of the appendix leads sequentially to appendiceal inflammation, transmural inflammation involving the peritoneum, ischemia, perforation of the wall, and localized or generalized peritonitis. Appendicitis usually results from impaction of fecal material or foreign matter in the appendiceal lumen. Less commonly, carcinoid tumors, vasculitis, or lymphoma may be implicated. Initial pain is mediated by vagal afferents, is poorly localized, accompanied by nausea and vomiting, and referred to the epigastrium. Local peritonitis is sensed by peritoneal somatic afferent nerves, is sharper, and locates to the appendix, commonly the RLQ; generalized peritonitis is diffuse sharp and accompanied by generalized abdominal and systemic signs. Epigastric pain is usually the first in a predictable sequence of symptoms and signs. The pain is poorly localized in the midline between the xiphoid and the umbilicus, is not accompanied by tenderness in the same area, but nausea or vomiting may occur. As the pain worsens, it shifts to the RLQ accompanied by fever and leukocytosis. Until this localization occurs, the diagnosis of appendicitis cannot be made, and often it is not even considered. If the patient presents a different sequence of events, the diagnosis of appendicitis should be questioned. Deep tenderness is first demonstrated just below the midpoint of a line between the anterior superior iliac spine and the umbilicus, where the appendix is typically located. When the appendix lies behind the ileum or ascends behind the cecum, the deep RLQ tenderness is less. When it is in the true pelvis, the RLQ is not tender, but rectal palpation may elicit tenderness in the peritoneal pouches [Paulson EK, Kalady MF, Pappas TN. Suspected appendicitis. *N Engl J Med.* 2003;348:236–242; Wagner JM, MKinney P, Carpenter JL. Does this patient have appendicitis. *JAMA.* 1996;276:1589–1594].

➤ **Acute Appendicitis with Perforation:** When the appendix ruptures, pain may transiently decrease, only to accentuate again over the next couple of hours. Generalized peritonitis may occur, or the perforation may be contained to form a local abscess identified as a tender mass. This finding may also be caused by edema and inflammation of the cecum without abscess, a phlegmon. Other signs depend on the location of the appendix.

Extrapelvic Appendix. When perforation is retrocecal, the back muscles are inflamed with tenderness below the twelfth rib on the right. If the appendix is lateral to the cecum, a mass may be felt, guarded by intense involuntary rigidity of the abdominal muscles. Irritation of the psoas muscle causes the patient to flex the right thigh or hold it rigidly extended. The iliopsoas test elicits pain when the supine patient tries to flex the thigh against resistance (see Fig. 9–13A, page 460). When the appendix is medial and behind the ileum, an abscess may involve the right ureter, causing pain on urination and white cells in the urine.

Intrapelvic Appendix. When the appendix lies within the true pelvis, diffuse suprapubic pain occurs. There is no rigidity of the abdominal muscles. Irritation of the bladder and rectum produces painful urination and tenesmus. A key diagnostic sign is palpation of a tender mass in the peritoneal pouch by rectal examination. The abscess may lie in contact with the obturator muscle;

the obturator test produces suprapubic pain by flexing the thigh and rotating the femur internally and externally (see Fig. 9–13B). Typhlitis, Crohn disease, pelvic inflammatory disease, ovarian disease, and ectopic pregnancy are frequently in the differential.

➤ **Typhlitis (Neutropenic Enterocolitis, Cecitis):** Neutropenia of any cause, particularly following chemotherapy for malignancy, especially acute leukemia, is associated with acute inflammation of the cecum, progressing rapidly to ischemia with bloody diarrhea and perforation. Aerobic gram-negative bacteria play a role and bacteremia is common. Symptoms and signs are similar to acute appendicitis, although the patient may be more toxic initially. CT reveals thickening of the cecal wall.

Terminal ileitis (Crohn disease, regional enteritis): See page 508.

➤ **Perforated Duodenal Ulcer:** See page 493. A perforated ulcer drains down the right paracolic gutter into the right iliac fossa (see Fig. 9–31, page 498). RLQ pain, tenderness, and rigidity may be pronounced, suggesting acute appendicitis. Some pain and tenderness are likely to persist in the epigastrium, directing attention to the possibility of peptic ulcer and a search for prior symptoms.

KEY SYNDROME Acute LLQ Pain

The left lower quadrant is filled with colon; consequently, most LLQ pain will be caused by colonic disorders.

Diverticulitis: Diverticulosis is common and usually asymptomatic. Obstruction of a diverticulum by feces can lead to local inflammation, abscess, and perforation (diverticulitis). LLQ pain and tenderness may be accompanied by muscular guarding. With a pelvic location, diverticulitis cannot be clinically distinguished from pelvic appendicitis. Known diverticulosis, a history of prior diverticulitis or appendectomy suggest diverticulitis. Clinical differentiation between perforation from a right-sided diverticulum or colonic neoplasm and a ruptured appendix is exceedingly difficult. CT scan is the preferred diagnostic modality.

KEY SYNDROME Acute Suprapubic Pain

Acute suprapubic pain is most often the result of pathology in the pelvis. Visceral pain from the pelvic organs is poorly localized until the process involves the peritoneum.

➤ **Rupture of the Urinary Bladder:** When the bladder is full of urine, blunt abdominal trauma may cause it to burst; pelvic fractures can directly lacerate the bladder. Perforation may be into the peritoneal cavity or retroperitoneum. Deceleration injuries from motor vehicle accidents, especially with improperly worn lap seat belts, may include injury to the urinary bladder, bowel, mesentery, and intraabdominal vessels. Leakage of urine into the peritoneal cavity produces mild peritonitis with pain and tenderness in the suprapubic region. The usual bladder fullness cannot be felt above the prostate in the rectal examination or through the vagina in the female. When the rupture is retroperitoneal, urine extravasation dissects to the perineum, producing palpable bogginess about the rectum and vagina on rectal examination. Scrotal swelling may occur, but it is not as consistent or considerable as from extravasation of urine from a severed ureter.

➤ **Acute salpingitis (pelvic inflammatory disease):** See Chapter 11, page 557.

➤ **KEY SYNDROME** Ovarian Torsion

An ovarian cyst or mass increases the risk for twisting of the ovary on its mesentery producing strangulation. Sudden pelvic pain accompanied by vomiting and tenderness over the mass suggests a twisted pedicle.

➤ **KEY SYNDROME** Ectopic Pregnancy

See Chapter 11, page 558.

Chronic Abdominal Pain Syndromes

KEY SYNDROME Chronic Abdominal Pain

See page 466. Pain is the presenting symptom for many chronic abdominal disorders. Chronic disease of a viscus usually produces pain in the same location as that from acute processes (see Fig. 9–19, page 463), but chronic pain is usually less severe.

Diabetic Radiculopathy (Diabetic Amyotrophy): Acute abdominal and/or thoracic pain accompanies ischemic or inflammatory radiculopathy of one or more thoracic and/or lumbar nerves. Pain and allodynia in the dermatomes and weakness of the muscles supplied by affected nerves are demonstrable by careful clinical examination. The acuity and severity of the pain is often mistaken for an acute intraabdominal event. The pain persists, relieved only by narcotics, for 6–24 months or longer. It is unrelated to the duration or control of the diabetes, and usually resolves over 8 to 16 months. EMG is diagnostic.

Abdominal Angina (Visceral Ischemia, Intestinal Ischemia): Increased intestinal oxygen consumption required for digestion and absorption of food following a meal exceeds the supply available because of obstruction of the mesenteric arteries. The bowel perfused by inferior mesenteric artery is most vulnerable because of limited collaterals. Visceral ischemia is characterized by the triad of postprandial pain, anorexia from fear of eating, and weight loss. Usually the pain is in the upper abdomen or the periumbilical region; sometimes it radiates to the back. It is typically intermittent, often coming on 30 minutes after eating, and persisting from 20 minutes to 3 hours, but many persons notice no relationship between the pain and the meals. Diarrhea, occasionally bloody, is fairly frequent. Sometimes a short systolic bruit is audible in the epigastrium or the umbilical regions. Similar symptoms are seen with mesenteric vein occlusions; in addition, these patients develop gastric and esophageal varices.

Carcinoma of the Pancreas: Pain may occur as a result of acute or chronic pancreatitis, or invasion of the retroperitoneal structures and nerves of the celiac plexus. Retroperitoneal invasion causes constant, dull, poorly localized pain in the midepigastrium, flank, or back. When the head of the pancreas is involved, early, painless, persistent jaundice is the rule. As the tumor enlarges, the nearly universal triad of pain, weight loss, and jaundice is seen. The first sign of pancreatic carcinoma may be superficial migrating thrombophlebitis, recurrent deep vein thromboses (*Trouseau syndrome*) or nonbacterial thrombotic endocarditis (*marantic endocarditis*).

> **KEY SYNDROME**   Recurrent Abdominal Pain

Recurrent pain suggests an intermittent mechanical problem, a partially treated inflammatory disorder, or an episodic metabolic/toxic syndrome.

✔ RECURRENT ABDOMINAL PAIN—CLINICAL OCCURRENCE: *Congenital* porphyria, sickle cell disease, familial Mediterranean fever, other familial fever syndromes; *Idiopathic* chronic pancreatitis, sphincter of Oddi dysfunction; endometriosis; *Infection* chronic hepatitis, schistosomiasis, *H. pylori* ulcers and gastritis; *Inflammatory/Immune* SLE, autoimmune gastritis; *Metabolic/Toxic* lead poisoning; *Mechanical/Trauma* biliary colic, ureteral colic, adhesions, and partial bowel obstruction; *Neoplastic* partial bowel obstruction from luminal masses; *Psychosocial* domestic, sexual, and child abuse; *Vascular* mesenteric ischemia.

> **KEY SYNDROME**   Abdominal Wall Pain Syndromes

Specific signs to be looked for are point tenderness (*trigger points*) not abolished by contraction of the abdominal muscles; sensitivity to touch from clothing (*hyperesthesia* or *allodynia*); abdominal wall defects, with or without hernia; masses; surgical and varicella-zoster scars; and weakness or asymmetry of the abdominal wall. Injection of trigger points with local anesthetic frequently answers the diagnostic question without further testing [Suleiman S, Johnston DE. The abdominal wall: an overlooked source of pain. *Am Fam Physician.* 2001;64:431–438]. Be sure, to fully examine the spine for evidence of problems referring pain to the abdomen.

Abdominal Cutaneous Nerve Entrapment (Rectus Abdominis Nerve Entrapment Syndrome): Anterior cutaneous nerve branches from T7 to L1 may be entrapped as they pass through the rectus sheath. Entrapment may occur from overuse of the rectus muscles or weight gain by putting increased traction on the nerve. The pain usually occurs laterally to the entrapment site and is increased when the patient tenses the rectus muscles. Pressure over the exit site in the fascia, felt as a small fascial defect, reproduces the pain. The pain is relieved by injection of local anesthetic into the trigger point.

Pain and Paramedial Mass—Hematoma of Rectus Abdominis Muscle: The epigastric artery and vein run vertically within the rectus sheath; hemorrhage within the sheath above the arcuate line is confined to the sheath, but dissects into the lateral abdominal wall below the arcuate line. It is often mistaken for such an intraabdominal mass. If one considers it, the diagnosis is easy; the mass remains palpable when the abdominal wall is tensed, a maneuver that obscures intraabdominal masses (see Fig. 9–26, page 483). The mass may be tender and painful. The diagnosis is readily proved by ultrasonography or CT. The usual setting is trauma; either direct or as a result of coughing, paracentesis, and operative injury, especially in a debilitated or anticoagulated patient.

> **KEY SYNDROME** Chronic Epigastric Pain

See the discussion of Acute Epigastric Pain, page 493.

Xiphisternal Arthritis: The patient complains of epigastric or retrosternal pain that radiates around to the back. Palpation elicits tenderness in the xiphoid-sternal joint that reproduces the complaint. Injection of lidocaine into the joint gives complete relief. When the xiphoid cartilage is not palpated, the pain may be mistaken for that of angina pectoris, peptic ulcer, hiatal hernia, biliary colic, or chronic pancreatitis.

Peptic Ulcer: Peptic ulcer is caused by infection with *H. pylori*, nonsteroidal antiinflammatory drugs, or gastrin-secreting islet cell tumor (Zollinger-Ellison syndrome). Ulcer pain results from gastric acid irritation of exposed nerves. Epigastric pain occurs predictably 1 to 4 hours postprandially, and is relieved by food, H_2 blockers, and antacids. The symptoms are similar regardless of whether the ulcer is gastric, pyloric, duodenal, or stomal (anastomotic, marginal). Ulcer pain is aggravated by fasting, drinking alcohol, or coffee. The pain is described as gnawing, aching, burning, or hunger and is felt in the epigastrium near the xiphoid, sometimes radiating to the back. The pain varies from mild discomfort to severe and may awaken the patient from sleep. Untreated, ulcer symptoms may recur with periods of pain lasting from a few days to several months. Frequently there is moderate tenderness localized to the epigastrium. Diagnosis is by endoscopy.

Pyloric obstruction: Usually obstruction results from scarring of the pylorus from peptic ulceration. Pain is not an invariable accompaniment; if present, it ranges from vague discomfort to colicky epigastric pain, usually soon after eating. Emesis of undigested food eaten many hours or days before may be observed. Palpation of the abdomen may elicit a succussion splash. Occasionally, the condition is practically symptomless and is found incidentally on abdominal X-ray. When gastric retention is demonstrated, fixed outlet obstruction must be distinguished from gastroparesis and acute pylorospasm that will subside with treatment of peptic ulcer.

Postgastrectomy Syndrome: Loss of gastric storage capacity and pyloric sphincter function from subtotal gastrectomy often results in the uncontrolled dumping of hypertonic gastric contents into the small intestine. The large fluid shifts into the small bowel and the increased intestinal motility contribute to the symptoms. Gastric stapling procedures create a defunctionalized pouch which can develop inflammation (*pouchitis*) and the small remnant stomach can be a source of postprandial discomfort. *Early Dumping Syndrome* occurs shortly after eating; the patient experiences epigastric discomfort (not pain), weakness, sweating, nausea (but not vomiting), tachycardia, palpitation, and a feeling of epigastric fullness. Reclining may relieve the symptoms. Foods with high osmotic loads exacerbate the symptoms. *Late Dumping Syndrome* occurs more than 2 hours after eating with symptoms of sweating, trembling, weakness, hunger, nausea, vomiting, and, rarely, syncope.

Chronic Pancreatitis: See page 510.

Gastric Carcinoma: Pain is usually preceded by anorexia, loss of weight, and weakness. The pain may be a steady, unremitting ache in the epigastrium, sometimes radiating to the back, or it may resemble that of peptic ulcer.

> **KEY SYNDROME**   Chronic RUQ Pain

See the discussion of RUQ Pain, page 495.

Chronic Cholecystitis with or Without Cholelithiasis: See page 496. The RUQ pain varies from continual, ill-defined distress to recurring attacks of biliary colic with paroxysms of colicky pain radiating to the right scapula. Tenderness is localized to the right lower margin of the liver. Fist percussion tenderness is usually present during the attack and for several days afterward.

Hepatocellular Carcinoma: Hepatocellular carcinoma arises in a cirrhotic liver, particularly following chronic viral hepatitis B and C. Abdominal pain is the most common symptom. A hard, nodular, localized mass in the liver with centrifugal extension may be detected by palpation, sometimes with an overlying peritoneal friction rub. A bruit may be heard.

Metastatic Carcinoma: Hematogenous metastases via the portal vein are frequent in colon, and pancreatic cancer. Metastases from lung and breast cancer are also common. Poorly localized upper abdominal pain or discomfort may be the presenting symptom. Seldom does the patient have abdominal distention or mass. The diagnosis is suggested by palpation of a mass in the liver. The liver is often stony hard. When a single discrete hepatic mass is felt, hepatocellular carcinoma or abscess should be suspected. A peritoneal friction rub or a bruit may rarely be present.

Bloating and Distention Syndromes

These common complaints can be the presenting signs for mechanical or functional bowel obstruction and abnormalities of digestion. Often, the sensations described by the patient are not matched by any physical finding of abdominal distention or obstruction. The syndrome of visceral hyperalgesia may underlie this presentation.

> **KEY SYNDROME**   Gastric Distention

Gastroparesis with gastric distention can result from reflex loss of gastric tone following abdominal surgery or upper intestinal inflammation, autonomic neuropathy as in diabetes, vagotomy, or with the decreased bowel motility associated with chronic illness and bed rest. In acute distention, the patient, often bedridden from some other disorder, becomes acutely more ill with vomiting, distention of the upper abdomen, and hypotension. The greatly dilated stomach fills the epigastrium, rarely reaching to the pelvis, is tympanitic and may have a succussion splash. Visible peristalsis may be present initially, while later, peristaltic sounds are weak or absent, indicating ileus. Nasogastric suction yields a large volume of fluid and the distention resolves. The major provocative factors are pain, abdominal trauma, and immobilization; postoperative cases are common. Less dramatic and more chronic gastroparesis is frequent and more difficult to diagnose. Difficult to control glucose in diabetics (because of the irregular gastric emptying) or presentation with nausea and emesis of undigested food several hours after meals should suggest the diagnosis. Many conditions may precipitate this syndrome, but gastroparesis associated with diabetes mellitus is the most frequent cause. Other causes of visceral autonomic neuropathy should be considered [Bityutskiy LP, Soykan I, McCallum RW. Viral gastroparesis: A subgroup of idiopathic gastroparesis—Clinical characteristics and long-term outcomes. *Am J Gastroenterol.* 1997;92:1501–1504].

Ascites: See page 473.

Irritable bowel syndrome: See page 512.

Lactose and fructose intolerance: See page 508.

Diarrhea Syndromes

Diarrhea. Diarrhea is defined as >200 g of stool per day on a Western low-residue diet. It is also used to describe watery or loose stools, and some patients will use the term to describe increased stool frequency. Increased volume of fecal output accompanied by increased water loss in the stools has several general pathophysiologic causes. Osmotic diarrhea results from ingestion of non-absorbable osmotically active solutes that draw water into the bowel and retain it there. Secretory diarrhea results when the normal secretions into the bowel are increased (e.g., Zollinger-Ellison syndrome) or the bowel abnormally secretes fluid into the lumen (e.g., cholera). Inflammatory/immune diarrhea results from inflammation of the bowel wall leading to exudation of fluid, proteins and cells into the lumen, usually combined with increased motility and decreased absorption from the same injury. Increased bowel motility from any cause will decrease the time available for absorption of solutes (small intestine) or water (colon) leading to diarrhea. Malabsorption and maldigestion result in diarrhea, the former from loss of effective absorptive surface (e.g., celiac disease), the latter from inadequate digestion of ingested food (e.g., pancreatic insufficiency). Short bowel syndrome results in loss of absorptive surface from surgical resection or fistulas and from bile acid malabsorption producing colonic irritation. First, determine exactly what the patient means by diarrhea, and decide if the diarrhea is acute, chronic, or recurrent. Second, obtain a detailed description of the stools, their frequency and pattern. Ask specifically about nocturnal diarrhea, which is always pathologic. Third, focus the history on exposures, such as travel and drugs, previous surgery, dietary habits, contact with others with a similar illness, and associated symptoms such as anorexia, nausea, vomiting, fever, weight loss, or abdominal pain. You should have a good working hypothesis as to the pathophysiologic mechanism of the diarrhea on completion of the history. On physical examination, look for fever and signs of weight loss or volume depletion, increased bowel motility (borborygmi), and abdominal tenderness. For suspected viral diarrhea, laboratory evaluation is usually not required. If you suspect a bacterial or protozoal etiology, stool culture and tests for bacterial and protozoal antigens are necessary [Thielman NM, Guerrant RL Acute infectious diarrhea. *N Engl J Med.* 2004;350:38–47]. You should always inspect a typical stool yourself. Diarrhea in persons infected with HIV is a complex clinical problem with multiple infectious and noninfectious causes. Consultation with a specialist in HIV-related diseases is recommended. **Patterns:** Recognition of several relatively distinct diarrheal syndromes can be helpful in forming a concise differential diagnosis: acute diarrhea; dysentery syndrome; diarrhea with maldigestion/malabsorption; steatorrhea; diarrhea with weight loss; diarrhea with bloody stools.

> **KEY SYNDROME** Acute Nonbloody Diarrhea

Diarrhea lasting less than 2 weeks, and not preceded by a history of recurrent or relapsing diarrhea, qualifies as acute diarrhea. Infectious and toxic causes are by far the most common. *CLINICAL OCCURRENCE:* *Infectious* enteroviruses, Rotavirus, noroviruses (e.g. Norwalk agent), enterotoxigenic *Escherichia coli*, *Salmonella, Shigella, Campylobacter spp., Giardia, Cryptosporidium,* microspora, amebiasis, *C. difficile, Vibrio cholerae*; *Metabolic/Toxic* food poisoning (*Bacillus cereus*, staphylococcal, *Clostridium perfringens*), antibiotic-associated diarrhea, alcohol, osmotic laxatives, sugar-free candy and foods, drug withdrawal; *Vascular* ischemic colitis [Bartlett JG. Antibiotic-associated diarrhea. *N Engl J Med.* 2002;346:334–339].

Traveler's Diarrhea: Travelers ingest the colonic flora of their host country via contaminated food and water. Within 1 week of arrival in a tropical, under-developed area, temperate zone travelers may experience watery diarrhea, abdominal cramping, and anorexia which is self-limited to 1 to 5 days. The most common organism is enterotoxigenic *E. coli*, while *Shigella, Salmonella, Campylobacter, V. cholerae, Giardia, Cryptosporidium,* and viruses are also causes.

Viral Gastroenteritis: Infection of the bowel epithelium with loss of absorptive function. Systemic signs vary from none to mild (Norwalk) to severe (rotavirus). This common epidemic illness has sudden onset of nausea, vomiting, and explosive diarrhea, with or without abdominal cramps. Myalgia, malaise, and anorexia, usually without fever, are common. The diarrhea and vomiting subside within 48 hours; lassitude may persist for several days. The stools consist of water and fecal remnants; blood, pus, and mucus are absent. Common causes are rotavirus, noroviruses, adenovirus, caliciviruses, enterovirus, and coronavirus. Specific diagnosis is not required.

► **Cholera:** Cholera toxin inhibits gut Na^+ absorption and activates Cl^- excretion, producing severe secretory diarrhea. Waterborne infection with *V. cholerae* is locally endemic in some countries, and epidemic and pandemic disease occurs. There is sudden abdominal cramping, vomiting, and voluminous watery stools containing flecks of mucus ("rice-water stools") progressing to dehydration, electrolyte imbalances, prostration, shock, and death.

Food Intolerance: Local and systemic allergic response to specific food allergens. Food allergens cause nausea, vomiting, abdominal cramping, and diarrhea. Angioedema can occur. Identification of the allergen in first episodes can be difficult. Shellfish, peanuts, cow's milk, and cereals are common culprits.

Food Poisoning: Usually, preformed bacterial exotoxins in contaminated food are ingested. *B. cereus* also causes a longer incubation diarrhea probably from exotoxin production in the gut. Severe cramping abdominal pain, nausea, vomiting, diarrhea, and prostration begin 1 to 6 hours after a meal. The symptoms resolve within hours. Frequently large groups of diners are affected. The type of food is a clue to the etiology: potato salad, mayonnaise, and cream pastries—*Staphylococcus aureus*; meat, poultry, legumes—*C. perfringens;* fried rice—*B. cereus.*

Acute Illness after dining—Chinese restaurant syndrome. This has been attributed to monosodium glutamate, a seasoning used in Asian cooking. It is characterized by severe headache, burning sensations, and feelings of pressure about the face starting 10 to 20 minutes after eating,. Occasionally, chest pain, prostration, gastric distress, and pain in the axillae, neck, and shoulders develop.

> ### KEY SYNDROME   Acute Bloody Diarrhea

Acute diarrhea with blood indicates that the mucosa of the bowel, usually the colon, is being compromised. Infections that invade the mucosa or that cause toxic epithelial necrosis are most likely. Chronic inflammatory bowel diseases can present as diarrhea initially, or with relapse. Patients present with abdominal pain and tenesmus (*dysentery syndrome*) or without pain. Fever and leukocytosis suggest an enteroinvasive organism with the risk of systemic spread or local complications. Painless bleeding in otherwise healthy individuals suggests bleeding from a structural abnormality (Meckel diverticulum, diverticulosis, polyp, or cancer).

✔ *ACUTE BLOODY DIARRHEA—CLINICAL OCCURRENCE:*   *Congenital*   Meckel diverticulum; *Inflammatory/Immune*   ulcerative colitis, Crohn disease; *Infectious*   bacteria (*Campylobacter jejuni*, *Salmonella* spp., *Shigella* spp., enterohemorrhagic *E. coli* [0157:H7]), protozoa (*Entamoeba histolytica*, *Balantidium coli*), cytomegalovirus; *Metabolic/Toxic*   heavy-metal poisoning (arsenic, mercury, cadmium, copper, iron); *Mechanical/Trauma*   rectal foreign body; *Neoplastic*   villous adenoma with malignant change; *Vascular*   ischemic colitis.

Dysentery: Dysentery is an infectious diarrhea syndrome in which the stools contain pus and blood, indicating intestinal inflammation, often with invasion and ulceration, leading to painful defecation. Bloody stools with mucous, fever, and tenesmus are distinct from simple gastroenteritis. Stool culture and examination for ova and parasites is required; sigmoidoscopy may be useful. Common etiologies are bacterial (*C. jejuni*, *Salmonella* spp., *Shigella* spp., enterohemorrhagic *E. coli* including 0157:H7) and protozoa (*E. histolytica*, *B. coli*, strongyloidiasis).

Amebiasis: Colon infection with *E. histolytica* occurs after ingestion of contaminated water, leading to ulcerations of the colon and terminal ilium and liver abscess. Onset may be acute and fulminant with cramping abdominal pain, bloody diarrhea, and tenesmus; examination reveals fever, diffuse abdominal tenderness, dehydration, and weight loss. Subacute infection is manifest by milder abdominal cramps, diarrheal stools containing mucus or blood, often alternating with intervals of normal function; examination may show fever and RLQ tenderness. Liver abscess is marked by spiking fevers, prostration and RUQ pain with mildly abnormal liver function tests.

Ulcerative Colitis: See Chronic Constant Diarrhea—Ulcerative Colitis, page 515. Although a chronic disease, its onset may be sudden, resembling acute dysentery.

➤ **Poisoning with Heavy Metals or Drugs:** The heavy metals (such as arsenic, cadmium, copper, or mercury) may be ingested accidentally or with suicidal or homicidal intent. Nausea, vomiting, cramping abdominal pains, and bloody diarrhea begin soon after ingestion.

KEY SYNDROME Chronic Intermittent Diarrhea

Diarrhea lasting more than 2 weeks is chronic and is less likely to be infectious. Intermittent diarrhea implies a disease with a relapsing-remittent course (e.g., Crohn disease) or an interaction of the host and the environment, particularly the diet (e.g., lactase deficiency). Most of the causes of chronic persistent diarrhea can present as chronic intermittent diarrhea.

Irritable bowel syndrome: See page 512.

Lactase Deficiency (Lactose Intolerance): Deficiency of small bowel mucosal lactase in many blacks, Asians, and a few caucasians leads to incomplete digestion of lactose, the disaccharide in milk. The lactose is then fermented by colonic bacteria, producing gas and diarrhea. Eating milk products produces a watery diarrhea, gas, and often abdominal cramps. Patients are often unaware of the association because of the ubiquitous presence of milk products in the diet. Avoidance of milk products leads to prompt resolution and is the treatment of choice. Malabsorption of other disaccharides, such as sorbitol, used in sugarless candies, and fructose, may cause a similar picture.

Fructose Intolerance: Some individuals are unable to absorb fructose in the quantities ingested, especially those who consume large amounts of soft drinks sweetened with high fructose corn syrup. The unabsorbed fructose creates an osmotic diarrhea and increased intestinal gas when fermented by colonic bacteria. Symptoms and signs are identical to lactose intolerance.

Regional Enteritis (Crohn Disease, Terminal Ileitis): Transmural granulomatous inflammation of the small and large intestine with perianal and enteroenteral fistula formation interferes with gut motility and absorption while producing chronic inflammation and blood loss. Attacks RLQ colicky pain occur, commonly accompanied by diarrhea. Weight loss may be severe. Perforations, strictures, and fistulas are common complications including perianal fistulas and anal stricture. Colon involvement is segmental with skip areas. Extraintestinal manifestations (oligoarthritis, spondylitis, pyoderma gangrenosum) may be the presenting complaint. Barium in the small bowel may show strictures, fistulas, loss of mucosal detail, and tubular thickening of the submucosa. Diagnosis is by endoscopic biopsy with gross and microscopic examination of resected tissue. Infections need to be considered including *Yersinia, Salmonella, Shigella,* tuberculosis, amebiasis, and cytomegalovirus. **DDX:** The first attack of ileitis may be clinically indistinguishable from acute appendicitis although diarrhea usually precedes the attack and a RLQ mass may be appreciated early in the course. If similar prior episodes have occurred, the probability is strong for chronic ileitis with an exacerbation [Podolsky DK. Inflammatory bowel disease. *N Engl J Med.* 2002;347:417–429].

Ulcerative Colitis: See page 509.

KEY SYNDROME Chronic Constant Diarrhea

Chronic constant diarrhea suggests an unremitting underlying structural or functional process involving digestion, absorption, bowel motility, or metabolism. The history (age of onset, exacerbating or palliative maneuvers), comorbid conditions, and characteristics of the stools are critical to a parsimonious differential diagnosis [Donowitz M, Kokke FT, Saidi R. Evaluation of patients with chronic diarrhea. *N Engl J Med.* 1995;332:725–729].

✔ *CHRONIC DIARRHEA—CLINICAL OCCURRENCE:* **Congenital** cystic fibrosis, lactase deficiency, celiac disease; **Endocrine** hyperthyroidism, adrenal insufficiency, carcinoid syndrome, pheochromocytoma; **Idiopathic** irritable bowel syndrome, chronic pancreatitis, diverticulitis; **Inflammatory/Immune** ulcerative colitis, Crohn disease, microscopic colitis, mastocytosis, chronic pancreatitis, celiac disease, amyloidosis; **Infectious** *Giardia*, HIV/AIDS and opportunistic infections, microsporidiosis, cyclosporiasis, Whipple disease, small bowel bacterial overgrowth, intestinal parasites; **Metabolic/Toxic** hyperthyroidism, lactase deficiency, drugs (metformin, proton pump inhibitors, misoprostol, colchicine, digitalis, antacids), bile salt-induced, laxative abuse, nonsteroidal antiinflammatory drugs, alcohol; **Mechanical/Trauma** short-bowel syndrome, enterocolic fistulas, radiation enteritis; **Neoplastic** mastocytosis, villous adenoma, pancreatic islet cell tumors (producing vasoactive intestinal peptide, gastrin, glucagon, etc.), small-bowel lymphoma; **Neurologic** autonomic neuropathies; **Psychosocial** laxative abuse; **Vascular** vasculitis.

Ulcerative Colitis: There is intense confluent chronic mucosal inflammation and ulceration with crypt abscess formation beginning at the rectum and extending proximally. The mucosa is red, edematous, and friable, with the slightest touch causing bleeding; often the entire rectosigmoid is covered by purulent exudate obscuring the multiple ulcers. The clinical picture varies from acute dysentery, with fever, abdominal pain, tenesmus, bloody diarrhea, and weight loss, to mild abdominal discomfort with mostly formed stools and little blood. Inflammation is always present in the rectum and extends proximally in continuity. The extent of the disease varies from rectal involvement only to pancolitis. In long-standing disease, the lumen is contracted and irregular because of pseudopolyp formation. The terminal ileum may be inflamed and dilated, in contrast to the constriction found in regional enteritis. The diagnosis is made by endoscopic inspection and biopsy. Disease duration greater than 10 years and pancolitis, but not the severity of symptoms, are associated with an increased risk for colon cancer. Ulcerative colitis must be distinguished from Crohn colitis, ischemic colitis, amebiasis, and bacillary infections [Podolsky DK. Inflammatory bowel disease. *N Engl J Med.* 2002;347:417–429].

Amyloidosis: Deposition of amyloid proteins in the bowel progressively impairs motility and absorptive capacity. Amyloidosis is classified by the specific amyloid protein (e.g., immunoglobulin light chains-AL, amyloid A protein-AA) and the presence of specific associated diseases, predominately hematologic cancer (e.g., multiple myeloma, chronic lymphatic leukemia) or chronic inflammatory disease (e.g., regional enteritis and ulcerative colitis). Amyloidosis may produce a chronic diarrhea, hypomotility, obstructive symptoms, ulceration, hemorrhage, and a protein-losing enteropathy.

Zollinger-Ellison Syndrome: A gastrinoma usually in the pancreas or duodenum produces high levels of gastrin stimulating excessive HCl secretion in the stomach, leading to diarrhea and ulcers in esophagus, duodenum, and jejunum. There are recurrent attacks of epigastric pain, nausea, vomiting, and diarrhea. Malabsorption and weight loss may occur. The diagnosis is suspected when finding severe ulcer disease, absence of *H. pylori*, and diarrhea.

Carcinoid Syndrome: Hepatic metastases from a carcinoid tumor of the GI tract produce large amounts of serotonin. Symptoms include intermittent flushing of skin, recurrent diarrhea, nausea and vomiting, and abdominal pain. Intermittent migratory flushing of face and neck occur with rapid color changes between red, white, and violet. Right-sided heart failure may develop from endomyocardial fibrosis with tricuspid insufficiency [Kulke MH, Mayer RJ. Carcinoid tumors. *N Engl J Med.* 1999:340:858–868].

KEY SYNDROME   **Chronic Diarrhea and Malabsorption (Maldigestion-Malabsorption Syndrome)**

Maldigestion results from failure to deliver sufficient pancreatic enzymes and bile salts into the duodenum, inadequate mixing of luminal contents, or insufficient time in the small bowel for digestion to occur. Malabsorbtion results from damage to the small-bowel epithelium or bypass or loss of absorptive surface area. Steatorrhea occurs when triglycerides are not digested or absorbed because of a lack of micelle formation or insufficient pancreatic lipase secretion. Fat appears in the stool as triglycerides. Steatorrhea is suggested when the stools are frothy, greasy, and foul smelling. Weight loss is common despite a good appetite. Fat-soluble vitamins (A, D, E, and K) are malabsorbed and deficiency syndromes of each may be present or be the presenting complaint. Microscopic stool examination shows fat globules when stained with Sudan III.

Small Bowel Bacterial Overgrowth (Blind Loop Syndrome): Decreased small intestinal motility leading to stasis, loss of protective gastric acid and decreased ileocecal valve function increase the risk of bacterial overgrowth, the blind- or stagnant-loop syndrome. Bacteria consume nutrients, including vitamins, leading to malnutrition and vitamin deficiency, particularly vitamin B_{12}. The patient presents with diarrhea, abdominal bloating and flatus, steatorrhea, weight loss, macrocytic anemia, and sometimes feculent belching. Because the bacterial overgrowth is responsible for the malabsorption, a short course of antibiotics should lead to demonstrable improvement. Common antecedent conditions include surgically created blind pouches, enteroenterostomies, a long afferent loop, strictures, fistulous communications, and small bowel diverticula. Tapeworms can produce a similar picture.

Chronic Pancreatitis and Pancreatic Insufficiency: Chronic pancreatitis results from alcohol, drugs, or ductal strictures. Chronic pancreatitis is characterized by episodes of abdominal pain and loose, fatty stools. The stools are soft, frothy, and malodorous; they frequently float on water. There are repeated attacks of pain which are identical with those of acute pancreatitis. Extensive loss of pancreatic tissue leads to inadequate endocrine and exocrine function producing diabetes and steatorrhea. When present, pancreatic calcification is diagnostic. Alcohol abuse and mild forms of cystic fibrosis are common causes. A palpable pancreatic pseudocyst may develop.

Celiac Disease (Gluten-Sensitive Enteropathy, Nontropical Sprue): In persons with specific HLA-DQ2 alleles, ingestion of gluten (gliadin) from wheat flour induces chronic mucosal and submucosal inflammation, which produces characteristic flattening of the villi and chronic malabsorption. Patients present with fatigue, cramping, diarrhea, steatorrhea, and weight loss without anorexia. A family history may be present and dietary modifications may already have been made by the patient. The stools are soft, frothy, and malodorous from unabsorbed fat. Patients may present with unexplained iron deficiency, hypocalcemia, neuropathy, dermatitis herpetiformis, or weight loss without complaints of diarrhea [Farrell RJ, Kelly CP. Celiac sprue. *N Engl J Med*. 2002;346:180–188].

Whipple Disease: Invasion of the intestinal mucosa and lamina propria with *Tropheryma whippelii* produces foamy macrophages filled with glycoprotein leading to lymphatic obstruction and malabsorption. Dissemination produces arthritis, lymphadenopathy, and an indolent meningitis. This can occur at any age, most commonly in the fourth and fifth decades in white men. Migratory polyarthralgias and polyarthritis may precede the intestinal symptoms of abdominal cramping and episodic diarrhea of fatty, foul-smelling stools and weight loss. There is generalized malaise and weakness with cough and dyspnea. The fever is intermittent and may be accompanied by hypotension, edema, lymphadenopathy, and emaciation. CNS infection causes slowly progressive chronic meningitis.

Giardiasis: *Giardia* organisms adhere to the brush-border of enterocytes in the duodenum and upper small bowel, impairing absorption of nutrients, leading to diarrhea and weight loss. A travel history and exposure to surface water potentially contaminated by livestock and wildlife is useful. Stool antigen testing is available.

Cystic Fibrosis: An autosomal recessive disease usually diagnosed in childhood. Patients with mild disease may present in adult life with pancreatic insufficiency, rhinosinusitis and recurrent pulmonary symptoms.

Enteroenteric Fistula: A fistula between the proximal and distal bowel produces diarrhea with undigested food in the feces and/or fecal emesis. The diarrhea may be intermittent and results, in part, from bacteria overgrowth in the proximal gut. The malabsorption of nutrients, fluids and electrolytes causes weight loss, hypoproteinemia, and dehydration. Fecal belching and vomiting suggests gastrocolic fistula.

Constipation Syndromes

Constipation.   Bowel motility is under autonomic control and requires an intact myenteric plexus. Multiple factors, including luminal contents, drugs, emotional state, physical activity level, and acquired habits (bowel training), affect the frequency of stooling and the character of the stool. Defecation requires a coordinated sequence of involuntary and voluntry muscular contrations and relaxations; failure of the proper sequencing of these events will prevent effective defecation. Each of these factors must be investigated in the evaluation of constipation, and several may be operative at one time. First, determine by history of the patient's baseline bowel movement pattern, the onset of the current difficulty, and any therapeutic interventions they have undertaken. Patients and physician use the term "constipation" to mean any combination of infrequent stools, hard desiccated stools, or stools that are difficult to pass for whatever reason. Many people do very well with two or three evacuations a week. Patients often describe the gradual development of a sensation of abdominal fullness. Acute or subacute constipation developing on a lifelong history of normal bowel movements requires investigation; chronic constipation of years' duration may indicate an underlying disorder of the bowel wall, a gut motility problem or poorly coordinated defecation (often failure to relax the voluntary sphicter during rectal contraction, *dyssynergy*) [Prather CM, Ortiz-Camacho CP. Evaluation and treatment of constipation and fecal impaction in adults. *Mayo Clin Proc*. 1998;73:881–887].

✔ **CONSTIPATION—CLINICAL OCCURRENCE:** *Congenital* Hirschsprung disease; *Endocrine* hypothyroidism, hyperparathyroidism, pregnancy; *Idiopathic* intestinal pseudoobstruction; diverticulosis, diverticulitis; *Inflammatory/Immune* scleroderma (progressive systemic sclerosis), amyloidosis; *Infectious* Chagas disease, toxic megacolon; *Metabolic/Toxic* drugs, including opiates, anticholinergics, tricyclic antidepressants, and many others; hypokalemia, hypomagnesemia, hypocalcemia; *Mechanical/Trauma* excessive fiber intake, mechanical obstruction by stricture or mass, irradiation, anal fissure; *Neoplastic* colon polyps, colon and anal cancers; *Neurologic* spinal cord injury, sacral plexus lesions, multiple sclerosis, Parkinson disease, irritable bowel syndrome; *Psychosocial* eating disorders, substance abuse (opiates), depression, dyssynergistic defecation; *Vascular* stroke.

Intestinal Obstruction: See page 513.

Fecal Impaction: There may be no discomfort or the patient may complain of constipation, tenesmus, or inability to defecate. Diarrhea is frequently the complaint because of liquid stool passes around the impacted mass. A digital examination of the rectum reveals hard fecal masses that must be removed manually. Common inciting factors are immobilization, bedrest, dehydration, anticholinergic medications, dementia, and barium for GI contrast X-rays.

Irritable Bowel Syndrome: This common cause of constipation is characterized by periods of constipation alternating with bouts of diarrhea. Either symptom may be the main complaint. The triad of symptoms is long-standing intermittent constipation, scybalous stools, and abdominal pain relieved by defecation. The cause is uncertain, although many patients have increased sensitivity to visceral discomfort (*visceral hyperalgesia*) [Talley NJ, Spiller R. Irritable bowel syndrome: A little understood organic bowel disease? *Lancet.* 2002;360:555–564; Horwitz BJ, Fisher RS. The irritable bowel syndrome. *N Engl J Med.* 2001;344:1846–1850].

Laxative Abuse, Atonic Colon: Chronic use of stimulant laxatives leads to loss of normal colonic reflexes and sensation producing an adynamic, dilated colon dependant upon more laxatives use for defecation. The patient has a long history of constipation, fancied or real. The stools may be alternately voluminous and scanty. Palpation of the abdomen often reveals large fecal masses; stool may be felt in the rectum.

Dyssynergistic Defecation: Normal defecation requires contraction of the colonic and rectal smooth muscle with simultaneous relaxation of the internal (involuntary) and external (voluntary) sphincters. Failure of this coordinated process often leads to attempts to defecate against closed anal sphincter producing constipation. Patients complain of difficulty defecating and having to strain excessively even with soft stools. On examination, they may be unable to voluntarily relax the external sphincter on command.

Megacolon: Lifelong constipation with occasional passage of an enormous formed stool suggests megacolon. Causes are congenital (Hirschsprung disease) or acquired defects in the intrinsic myenteric innervation of the colon, for example, idiopathic intestinal pseudoobstruction, and Chaga disease.

Drug Effects: Many drugs slow bowel motility, including opiates, anticholinergic drugs, antihistamines, chronic laxative use, and overuse of bulk laxatives. Pill bezoars have been described. Medication history with particular inquiry into the use of laxatives and enemas is key. Ophthalmologic medications are systemically absorbed and can effect gut function.

Bowel Obstruction Syndromes

> **KEY SYNDROME**   **Noisy Tympanites with Colic and Vomiting—Mechanical Obstruction**

This pattern suggests localized bowel obstruction causing an increased force of peristaltic contraction proximal to the obstruction, producing colic and proximal bowel distension by retained luminal contents leading to decompression by vomiting. Mechanical obstruction is probable. Tympanites is present when the obstruction is distal to the mid jejunum. Increased peristalsis proximal to an obstruction is indicated by frequent, loud peristaltic sounds (*borborygmi*) accompanied by cramping, colicky pain. With partial obstructions, high-pitched high-pressure-to-low-pressure sounds ("rushes") accompanying the pain may be appreciated. Vomiting appears earlier and is more intense the more proximal the obstruction. Distal obstruction may result in feculent emesis which classically indicates colonic obstruction in a person with an incompetent ileocecal valve or a cologastric or coloenteric fistula [Bohner H, Yang Q, Franke C, et al. Simple data from history and physical examination help to exclude bowel obstruction and to avoid radiographic studies in patients with acute abdominal pain. *Eur J Surg.* 1998;164:777–784].

Acute intestinal obstruction.   Colicky pain is almost invariably present from the onset. In general, the more proximal the obstruction, the more severe the symptoms.   *Proximal Small Intestine.*   Epigastric pain is intense and vomiting is early and severe. If the vomitus contains bile, the obstruction is beyond the second portion of the duodenum. Abdominal distention appears late, and then is limited to the epigastrium.   *Distal Small Intestine.*   Symptoms are less severe, vomiting is delayed, but the vomitus may have become feculent. Diffuse abdominal distention gradually develops.   *Colon.*   The colon narrows distally, especially in the descending and sigmoid regions, making them most susceptible to obstruction by mass or luminal narrowing. The pain is less than from obstruction of the small intestine. Vomiting is late and may be fecal. Constipation is invariable, but the bowel must first empty its contents below the obstruction, delaying recognition. An empty rectal ampulla, void of gas, is strong presumptive evidence of colonic obstruction.

✔ *MECHANICAL BOWEL OBSTRUCTION—CLINICAL OCCURRENCE:*   **Inflammatory/Immune**   Crohn disease, diverticulitis with stricture;   **Infectious**   parasites, diverticular abscess;   **Mechanical/Trauma**   adhesions (most common), gallstone impaction, bezoars, foreign body, pyloric stenosis, volvulus, hernias (internal and abdominal wall), intussusception, external compression from intraabdominal cysts and neoplasms;   **Neoplastic**   benign and malignant tumors.

Bezoars: These are concretions of hair (*trichobezoar*), plant fibers (*phytobezoar*), or medicines (aluminum hydroxide gel or polystyrene sodium sulfonate) formed in the GI tract. They may present with obstructive symptoms when they lodge at the pylorus (gastric outlet obstruction) or ileocecal valve (small-bowel obstruction). They may cause mechanical erosion of the bowel wall, leading to ulceration with bleeding and pain.

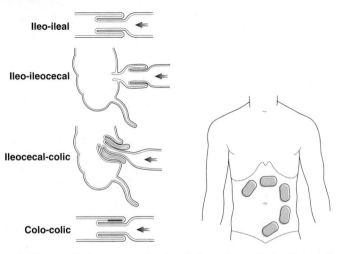

Ileo-ileal

Ileo-ileocecal

Ileocecal-colic

Colo-colic

A. Types of intussusception　　**B. Location of intussusception**

Fig. 9–33 *Intussusception.* *This is the prolapse of one segment of intestine into an adjoining segment. **A. The four types of intussusception:** The enfolding of the lumen is in the direction of fecal flow, as shown by the arrows. In the intracolic type, the stippling indicates a neoplasm that is usually the cause of the telescoping. **B. Locations:** The usual sites of palpable masses are shown as sausage-shaped outlines; these are usually in the colon.*

Strangulated Hernias: See page 521.

Intussusception: Intussusception is the invagination of bowel into the lumen of adjacent bowel. The enfolded portion always points down the fecal stream. There are four types: ileum into ileum, ileum into ileocecal valve, ileocecal valve into colon, and colon into colon (Fig. 9–33). This is the most common cause of intestinal obstruction in infants. It is frequently preceded by a viral infection in children; in adults, neoplasm in the intestinal wall is usually the cause. In addition to obstructive symptoms, mucus, and sometimes blood, are passed from the rectum. The pathognomonic sign is an oblong mass in the right or upper mid-abdomen and absence of bowel in the RLQ (*Dance sign*) [Case records of the Massachusetts General Hospital. Case 26-2002. *N Engl J Med.* 2002;347:601–606].

Colon Cancer: This is the second most common cause of intestinal obstruction in persons older than 50 years of age. Gradually increasing constipation culminates in the onset of low intestinal obstruction. Right colon obstruction distends the cecum, which forms a painful, rounded mass in the RLQ. Distal cancers cause gradual distention of the sigmoid and/or descending colon which is readily palpated in the LLQ.

Volvulus: See page 492.

> **KEY SYNDROME** Silent Tympanites without Colic or Vomiting—Ileus

This pattern suggests a diffuse decrease in bowel motility and muscular tone, producing a silent abdomen with distended bowel. Diffuse ileus without mechanical obstruction is probable. Abdominal tympany is always present and the peristaltic sounds are diminished or absent. When present, abdominal pain is mild and colic is absent; vomiting is uncommon, but anorexia and nausea are to be expected.

✔ *ILEUS—CLINICAL OCCURRENCE:* *Inflammatory/Immune* Sterile peritonitis: perforated viscus—HCl and gastric contents from perforated stomach or duodenum, bile peritonitis, ruptured bladder; miscellaneous: enzymes released by acute pancreatitis, ruptured ovarian cyst, blood (e.g., bleeding from follicular cyst), recurrent serositis syndromes (e.g., SLE, familial Mediterranean fever, familial Hibernian fever), inflammatory bowel disease (ulcerative colitis, Crohn disease), toxic megacolon; *Infectious* infectious peritonitis (spontaneous bacterial peritonitis in cirrhosis, perforated bowel, perforating neoplasm, ruptured colonic diverticulum or diverticular abscess, tuberculosis, penetrating abdominal trauma, surgical wound dehiscence), *C. difficile* colitis, amebic colitis, typhoid fever, *Giardia,* Whipple disease; *Metabolic/Toxic* hypokalemia, hypothyroidism, acidemia or alkalemia, diabetic ketoacidosis, uremia, heavy metal poisoning, porphyria, toxic megacolon or any major metabolic disorder, drugs (opiates, anticholinergics, vinca alkaloids, ganglionic blocking agents); *Mechanical/Trauma* manipulation of the gut (abdominal surgical procedures, trauma to the abdomen), adhesions, tumors, volvulus, intussusception, parasites; *Neurologic* trauma to the axial skeleton, spinal cord injury, compression fracture, herpes zoster, urinary retention, fecal impaction, aerophagia; *Vascular* Mesenteric arterial embolism or thrombosis, mesenteric venous thrombosis, hypotension, ischemic bowel.

Abdominal Masses

Rectus sheath hematoma: See page 502.

KEY SYNDROME   Visceral Enlargement

Solid organs can enlarge by several mechanisms: an expanded cell mass (either normal or abnormal, e.g. neoplastic infiltration, inflammatory cells, infection), intra or extracellular deposition of material (fat, amyloid, mucopolysaccharides, etc.), vascular congestion, or cystic change. The liver, spleen, adrenals and kidneys are the parenchymal organs susceptible to enlargement. A careful history and physical examination will identify the specific enlarged organs(s). The pattern and history suggest the mechanism of enlargement and when combined with a judicious selection of laboratory and imaging studies, the probable pathophysiology can be identified.

✔ *ENLARGED VISCERA—CLINICAL OCCURRENCE:* *Congenital* horseshoe kidney; infiltration by cells of the reticuloendothelial system (e.g., lipopolysaccharidases); *Idiopathic* single or multiple cysts; *Inflammatory/Immune* infiltration by cells of the reticuloendothelial system (e.g., histiocytosis syndromes), granulomatous diseases (sarcoid), deposition of extracellular proteins (amyloidosis); *Infectious* granulomatous diseases (fungal infections, tuberculosis), chronic infection and parasitosis (amebiasis, hydatid disease); *Metabolic/Toxic* hypertrophy of normal tissue as a consequence of increased functional demands (e.g., splenomegaly in hemolytic anemias), accumulation of intracellular inclusions (steatosis, glycogen storage diseases and lipopolysaccharidases); *Mechanical/Trauma* obstruction of normal effluent systems (hydronephrosis, hepatic vein obstruction), enlargement of fluid-containing hollow organs as a consequence of outflow obstruction (e.g., urinary retention and gallbladder hydrops); *Neoplastic* primary neoplasms, infiltration by metastatic neoplasm either diffusely or focally, extramedullary hematopoiesis; *Vascular* renal and hepatic vein obstruction.

Enlarged Kidney: See page 447 and Fig. 9–2, page 448 for a description of the anatomic relationships of the kidneys. When the kidney enlarges, it is contained posteriorly by the psoas and the twelfth rib, and the overriding liver and spleen prevent extension superiorly. Therefore, the enlarged kidney pushes forward and downward into a position similar to that of an enlarged spleen or liver only deeper. Palpable renal masses extend posteriorly farther than the spleen. The kidney always lacks the sharp edge the spleen and liver may present. A lobulation of the kidney may be mistaken for the splenic notch. The surface of an enlarged kidney is more often irregular than the spleen. Renal masses do not move with deep inspiratory effort because, unlike the spleen and liver, they are fixed in the retroperitoneum. *Clinical Occurrence: Congenital:* polycystic kidney disease, horseshoe kidney, compensatory hypertrophy opposite absent kidney; *Idiopathic:* cysts; *Inflammatory/Immune:* amyloidosis; *Mechanical/Trauma:* hydronephrosis, hematoma; *Neoplastic:* renal cell carcinoma and renal sarcoma, transitional cell carcinoma of renal pelvis and ureter.

Ptotic and Transplanted Kidney: The kidneys are only loosely constrained in their superior retroperitoneal location by the surrounding fascia, and inferior displacement is not rare. A displaced normal-sized kidney offers little difficulty in recognition by its shape and size, if it is considered. It may occur in the pelvis. Transplanted kidneys are placed in the pelvis where they are easily palpable above the inguinal ligament.

KEY SYNDROME   RUQ Mass

The liver, gallbladder, and right kidney are most likely to present as masses in the RUQ. Pancreatic pseudocysts may present here, as can colon masses.

Liver Enlargement: Hepatomegaly: The liver occupies the entire anterior RUQ behind the ribs while the left lobe extends to the left midclavicular line. It has convex and concave surfaces and the concave inferior plane is tipped backward and downward. Although the anterior-inferior extends across the midline, it is rarely felt. The liver is heavy while its suspension is relatively meager. The coronal ligaments attach it to the diaphragm posterior to the liver dome (Fig. 9–34). The diaphragm is assisted in supporting the liver's weight by negative intrathoracic pressure, the hilar vessels, and upward pressure from the abdominal viscera and abdominal wall muscles. There are two axes of liver rotation: a transverse axis near the attachment of the coronary ligaments and an anteroposterior axis near the hilum, to the left of the center of mass. Downward rotation through the transverse axis causes the liver to present more of its anterior surface below the costal margin (Fig. 9–34B). Downward rotation about the anteroposterior axis results in a tongue of liver appearing in the right flank (Fig. 9–34A). Rotation may be expected in any condition that lowers the dome of the diaphragm, decreases the normal amount of abdominal fat, or decreases abdominal muscle tone. The liver of many normal persons is readily palpable just below the costal margin. The

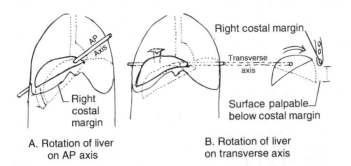

A. Rotation of liver on AP axis

B. Rotation of liver on transverse axis

Fig. 9–34 *Rotations of the Normal-Sized Liver Making it Palpable Beneath the Costal Margin. Normally, the liver is suspended by its coronary ligaments and the fixation to the prevertebral fascia by its hilar blood vessels, behind the right costal margin inaccessible to palpation. The muscles of the diaphragm could not hold a 1500-g liver, if they were not assisted by the negative intrapleural pressure, above; and the positive pressure of abdominal contents, below. Depression of the diaphragm or relaxation of the intraabdominal pressure permits the normal-sized liver to fall beneath the costal margin and become palpable (ptosis). With the diaphragm fixed, the liver may rotate on one or two axes to become palpable; depression of the diaphragm increases the amount of palpable surface permitted by rotation. A. The liver may rotate on an anteroposterior axis near its left side:* With this counterclockwise rotation the lower border appears below the costal margin, forming an angle with the costal margin. ***B. The normal-sized liver may rotate on a transverse axis:*** The edge presents below and approximately parallel to the costal margin. This is distinguished from enlargement of the liver only by the inward curve of the anterior surface.

margin should be roughly parallel to the costal margin rather than descending almost vertically in the flank (Fig. 9–34A). Liver size is estimated from the upper border of hepatic dullness to the lower border border determined by palpation or percussion. Only a tentative diagnosis of hepatomegaly is justified if the lower border is not definitely felt. A conclusion based solely on percussion is hazardous [Naylor CD. Physical examination of the liver. *JAMA.* 1994;271:1859–1865]. Many clinical diagnoses of hepatomegaly are not confirmed with imaging or autopsy because the rotation of the normal liver is not appreciated. The palpable surface should be examined for consistency and nodularity. Tenderness can be elicited by direct palpation or by fist percussion. Percussion tenderness occurs in acute cholecystitis and hepatitis. Palpate over the liver for friction rubs and auscultate for bruits. The coincidence of these two signs indicates a high probability of hepatic carcinoma.

✔ *HEPATOMEGALY—CLINICAL OCCURRENCE:* **Congenital** polycystic kidney disease, glycogen storage disease, lipopolysaccharidases, hemochromatosis; **Inflammatory/Immune** amyloidosis; **Infectious** liver abscess (bacterial or amebiasis), echinococcal cyst, viral hepatitis, schistosomiasis, leishmaniasis; **Metabolic/Toxic** steatosis, rickets; **Mechanical/Trauma** hematoma, CHF, tricuspid insufficiency, pulmonary hypertension, cor pulmonale, constrictive pericarditis, hepatic vein thrombosis; **Neoplastic** hepatocellular carcinoma, metastatic carcinoma (especially colon, pancreas, lung, breast), islet cell carcinoma and carcinoid, biliary carcinoma, histiocytosis syndromes, leukemic infiltration, lymphoma, myelofibrosis/extramedullary hematopoiesis; *Vascular* hemangioma, infarction, hematoma.

Pulsitile Liver: The liver may move with arterial pulsation. This may occur by transmission of the abdominal aortic pulse, or by retrograde flow of blood in the central veins during ventricular systole, leading to expansion and contraction of the liver parenchyma. Expansile pulsation is demonstrated by placing the hands on opposite sides of the liver and observing that the surfaces move apart in systole. Tricuspid insufficiency is the usual cause.

Steatosis and Steatohepatitis (Fatty Liver, Nash): Fat accumulates in hepatocytes in type 2 diabetes obesity, hypertriglyceridemia, and with older age, initially without inflammation. Inflammation (NASH) leading to fibrosis and cirrhosis occurs in some patients. The condition is asymptomatic until cirrhosis, portal hypertension and hepatic insufficiency appear. Transaminases may be elevated during the asymptomatic period of the disease [Clark JM, Diehl AM. Nonalcoholic fatty liver disease: An underrecognized cause of cryptogenic cirrhosis. *JAMA.* 2003;289:3000–3004; Angulo P. Nonalcoholic fatty liver disease. *N Engl J Med.* 2002;346:1221–1231].

Hemochromatosis: Homozygous or compound heterozygous recessive gene mutations result in excessive gut absorption of iron leading to iron accumulation in tissues and injury to the liver (cirrhosis), heart (failure), pancreas (diabetes mellitus), joints (arthritis), and pituitary (pituitary insufficiency). The penetrance of the disease is much higher in men; women are relatively protected during childbearing years by regular menstrual blood loss. Iron accumulation is asymptomatic. When organ damage occurs lassitude, weight loss, darkening of skin, joint pain, abdominal pain, and loss of libido may be seen. Signs are diffuse bronze pigmentation of skin (melanin), hepatomegaly, splenomegaly, spider angiomas, loss of body hair, edema, ascites, peripheral neuropathy, arthropathy, and testicular atrophy. Early diagnosis and therapeutic phlebotomy avoids organ damage. Iron overload as a result of hypertransfusion in refractory amenia produces a similar syndrome.

Enlarged Tender Gallbladder: See Cholecystitis, page 496.

Enlarged Nontender Gallbladder: Obstruction of the common bile duct can lead to progressive enlargement of the gallbladder. A palpable nontender gallbladder may also result from distention with stones, acalculous cholecystitis, and gallbladder hydrops, in which mucous cells continue to secrete in the face of obstruction of the cystic duct. Chronic cystic duct obstruction usually produces a contracted gallbladder. *Courvoisier* sign states that dilatation of the gallbladder occurs with carcinoma of the head of the pancreas but not with a common duct stone because of a scared gallbladder wall from chronic cholelithiasis in the latter, but not the former, condition. There are many exceptions. Carcinoma of the gallbladder produces a hard, irregular mass that is moderately tender.

Enlarged Right Kidney: The right kidney lies 1 or 2 cm lower than the left. In thin persons, the lower pole of the right kidney may be palpable while the left is not. Because the shapes of the kidney and liver are so dissimilar, there is usually no difficulty in distinguishing them with bimanual palpation. Rarely, a protruding renal mass may be confused with hydrops of the gallbladder or pancreatic pseudocyst. See page 516 for a discussion of renal enlargement.

KEY SYNDROME   Epigastric Masses

Smooth epigastric masses suggest enlargement or distention of the normal organs in this region, without infection, hemorrhage, or active inflammation; irregular masses suggest neoplasm or a polycystic organ; tender masses suggest hemorrhage, infection, and/or inflammation. Acute gastric dilatation produces a visible enlargement of the epigastrium and LUQ. A smooth mass in the epigastrium of a person not acutely ill suggests a pancreatic cyst or pseudocyst. If the mass pulsates, consider aortic aneurysm. The profile of the abdomen may offer a clue (see Fig. 9–20, page 473). Enlargement of the left lobe of the liver will also present in the epigastrium. Liver and retroperitoneal masses are immobile. Infections and neoplasms cause masses in the omentum, stomach, pancreas, left lobe of the liver, and transverse colon. A polycystic or horseshoe kidney sometimes presents as a midline epigastric mass. Periaortic lymph node enlargement may be palpable in lymphomas. Ultrasonography or CT are usually necessary for definition of the involved structure(s).

KEY SYNDROME   Left Upper Quadrant Mass: Splenomegaly

The enlarged spleen retains its characteristic shape with the splenic notch on the medial edge near the lower pole. Enlargement displaces the lower pole downward from behind the thoracic cage and along its oblique axis toward the left iliac fossa. The lower pole may reach the pelvis, rarely crossing the midline. Many acute infections produce a moderately enlarged soft spleen with blunted edges; chronic disorders cause firm or hard spleens and sharp edges. Tenderness indicates an inflamed peritoneum from infection or infarction. Although uncommon, the spleen can rupture from over-vigorous palpation, most often in infectious mononucleosis. **DDX:** The enlarged spleen and left kidney have the same general shape, but the kidney is deeper, rounded posteriorly, and never have a distinct edge. A medial border fissure might seem to identify spleen, but renal lobulation can closely mimic the splenic notch. Ultrasonography or CT may can make the distinction [Grover SA, Barkun AN, Sackett DL. The rational clinical examination. Does this patient have splenomegaly? *JAMA.* 1993;270:2218–2221; Tamayo SG, Rickman LS, Mathews WC, et al. Examiner dependence on physical diagnostic tests for the detection of splenomegaly: A prospective study with multiple observers. *J Gen Intern Med.* 1993;8:69–75].

✔ *SPLENOMEGALY—CLINICAL OCCURRENCE:* **Congenital** thalassemia minor and major, lipopolysaccharidases (Gaucher disease, Niemann-Pick disease); **Inflammatory/Immune** hemolytic anemia, SLE, RA, pernicious anemia, amyloidosis; **Infectious** acute and chronic malaria, typhoid fever, SBE, abscess, schistosomiasis, congenital syphilis, leishmaniasis; **Metabolic/Toxic** pernicious anemia; **Mechanical/Trauma** chronic CHF, portal hypertension, hematoma; **Neoplastic** ALL, lymphoma, CML, CLL; **Vascular** infarcts, vasculitis, hematoma.

KEY SYNDROME   RLQ Masses

Occasionally, the normal cecum can be felt as an indistinct soft mass, slightly tender, usually fluctuant or doughy. A firmer mass may be felt from involvement by tuberculous granuloma, pericecal or appendiceal abscess, Crohn disease involving the distal ileum, or carcinoma.

> **KEY SYNDROME**   **LLQ Masses**

Irregular plastic masses of feces may be palpated in sigmoid; they are occasionally mistaken for neoplasm until movement or disappearance is demonstrated in 1 or 2 days. A spastic sigmoid colon feels like a cord about the diameter of the little finger, lying vertically approximately 5 cm medial to the left superior anterior iliac spine; the cord can be rolled under the fingers and is slightly or moderately tender. A tender LLQ mass suggests diverticulitis complicated by phlegmon or abscess.

> **KEY SYNDROME**   **Suprapubic and Pelvic Masses**

Masses presenting in the suprapubic location most often arise from the pelvis. Pelvic and rectal examinations are necessary to define their extent and characteristics.

Pelvic masses arise from the colon, from the gravitational accumulation of neoplastic or inflammatory debris at the pelvic floor, or from infection or neoplastic change in the female or male pelvic organs.

Pregnancy: All women who have ever menstruated, but who have not gone through the menopause, and who present with a pelvic or suprapubic mass should be assumed to be pregnant until proven otherwise.

Distended Urinary Bladder: A chronically obstructed urinary bladder may reach the umbilicus, usually in the midline. The patient may have minimal urinary symptoms, or complain of incontinence (because of overflow). The mass is dull to percussion, fluctuant, painless, and disappears with catheterization. It is sometimes mistaken a neoplasm because of its size or when a diverticulum upsets its symmetry. It must be distinguished from ovarian cyst and pregnancy in the female.

Ovarian Cyst: The largest cysts simulate ascites; they are discussed elsewhere (pages 478 and 565). Those that extend just above the pelvic brim are in the midline and resemble a distended bladder. Often the cyst cannot be palpated vaginally because it is too high. Persistence of the fluctuant mass after catheterization suggests ovarian cyst gravid uterus or rectal sheath hematoma. Ultrasonography is diagnostic.

Uterine Fibroid: A markedly enlarged uterus with leiomyomas may be felt above the symphysis pubis as a hard, multinodular mass. Vaginal examination readily demonstrates that the masses move with the cervix and hence are attached to the uterine fundus.

Pelvic Abscess: Pelvic abscesses result from suppurative disease of pelvic organs, perforation of pelvic or abdominal organs, dissection of abdominal wall infections, and lymphatic extension of regional infections. Knowledge of the specific anatomy of the male and female pelvis is necessary for interpretation of the examination. In the male, a tender, rounded mass, felt through the anterior rectal wall, superior to the prostate gland, is likely to be a pelvic abscess in the rectovesical pouch. Similarly in the female, a mass felt through the anterior rectal wall, superior to the cervix uteri, is probably an abscess in the rectouterine pouch. These abscesses result from perforation of the appendix or a colonic diverticulum, salpingitis, or prostatitis.

Colon Cancer: A colon carcinoma on a long mesocolon may prolapse into the rectovesical or rectouterine pouch and be palpated as a firm mass.

Redundant Bowel: Occasionally, a loop of normal colon can be felt in the pelvic pouches. The mass is quite soft and freely movable; the sensation is distinctive and the mass will not be confused with cancer.

Rectal (Blumer) Shelf: Metastatic peritoneal seeding from a primary carcinoma high in the abdomen accumulates in the pelvis. A hard shelf in the rectovesical or rectouterine pouch is felt through the anterior rectal wall. Although usually caused by neoplasm, it can also occur from inflammation in female pelvic inflammatory disease and prostatic abscess in the male.

Mistatken Normal Structures: If a vaginal examination has not been performed, the unwary examiner may interpret the hard mass of the cervix felt through the anterior rectal wall as a neoplasm. When the uterus is retroverted, the normal fundus has been mistaken for cancer. A vaginal tampon or pessary may similarly mislead when felt through the rectal wall.

KEY SYNDROME Other Abdominal Masses

The masses previously described involve tissues more or less localized to a certain abdominal region. However, the gut may develop a localized lesion anywhere in its length, forming a palpable mass. **Volvulus** (page 496) is usually in the sigmoid colon or the cecum but may occur elsewhere. **Intussusception** (page 520) occurs primarily in children and is preceded by a viral syndrome. Intermittent colicky pain is common; the site is painful and tender. **Abscesses** may be present as palpable masses in any part of the peritoneal cavity. They should be suspected when a mass is palpated in a region normally devoid of solid organs. **Colon cancer** and inflammatory many associated with **Crohn disease** may be found virtually anywhere in the abdomen or pelvis. With the exception of intussusception, none of these conditions has distinctive physical findings.

Abdominal, Inguinal, and Other Hernias

➤ KEY SYNDROME Strangulated Hernia

Impingement on a hernial ring occludes the venous return of herniating gut or omentum. Swelling and edema prevent reduction and gradually increase the pressure until capillary and arterial flow are occluded; gangrene and perforation may quickly ensue (Fig. 9–35A). Usually, a known hernia becomes painful and tender. There is a tender, painful mass at the hernial site producing intestinal obstruction. Pinching and strangulation of only a partial circumference of the gut wall produces a *Richter hernia* (Fig. 9–36A). Strangulated bowel is painful, feels firm, but is usually not tender. Do not forcefully reduce a hernia because this may result in upture of strangulated gut or reduction en masse, where the sac accompanies the loop without relieving the strangulation.

KEY SYNDROME Incisional Hernia

When an operative scar is present on the abdomen, palpate for a defect in the abdominal wall, then have the patient perform the Valsalva maneuver or raise

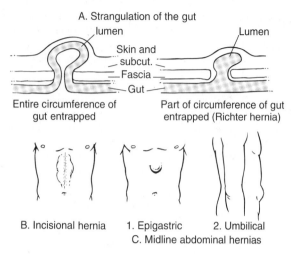

Fig. 9–35 **Some Hernias and Complications. A. Strangulation of the Gut:** *A loop of gut protrudes through a fascial and the edges of the opening impinge upon the blood supply of the entire circumference of the lumen. If only a part of the circumference of the gut is pinched in the opening, it is called a Richter hernia.* **B. Incisional hernia:** *A bulge near an operative scar usually indicates an incisional hernia. The lack of fascial support can be readily palpated.* **C. Midline abdominal hernias:** *In the adult-type umbilical hernia, the fascial ring is incomplete, so the bulge is superior to the umbilicus. An epigastric hernia is a small bulge of fat protruding from the deep layers through an opening in the linea alba. It may not be detected unless the patient is examined in the standing position and the examining finger is run down the linea alba.*

their head from the pillow. Herniation occurs adjacent to the scar (Fig. 9–35B and Plate 27).

KEY SYNDROME   Epigastric Hernia (Fatty Hernia of the Linea Alba)

The hernia consists of preperitoneal fat protruding outward between the fibers of the linea alba (Fig. 9–35C-1). The patient can have pain in the midline of the epigastrium. If a bulge cannot be seen, the patient should stand while the examiner runs a finger down the midline looking for a small nodule that is occasionally reducible. Usually this hernia does not have a peritoneal sac.

KEY SYNDROME   Umbilical Hernia

A defect in the abdominal fascia occurs normally where the umbilical vessels and urachus exit the abdomen into the umbilical cord. The navel may protrude when intraabdominal pressure is increased by standing or Valsalva maneuver. The congenital type is distinguished by protrusion through the umbilical scar; palpation of the ring reveals a complete fibrous collar continuous with the linea alba. In the adult type of hernia, the collar is lacking; the upper part of the hernia is covered only by skin (Fig. 9–35C-2). It is properly termed a *paraumbilical hernia*. These

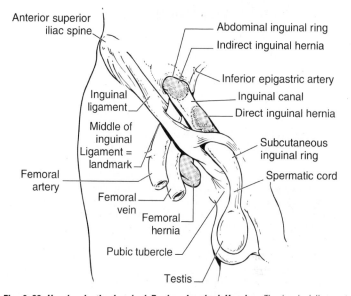

Fig. 9–36 *Hernias in the Inguinal Region. Inguinal Hernias:* *The inguinal ligament stretches from the anterior superior spine of the ilium to the pubic tubercle. The flattened tube of the inguinal canal lies just above and parallel to it, between the superficial and deep layers of abdominal muscles. The lateral end of the canal opens posteriorly into the abdominal cavity through the abdominal inguinal ring (internal ring). The internal ring is not palpable, but it is just above the midpoint of the inguinal ligament. The medial end of the canal opens anteriorly into the subcutaneous tissue through the subcutaneous inguinal ring (external ring). In the male, this is where the spermatic cord emerges from the abdominal muscles. A hernia is indirect when it enters the canal from the abdominal cavity through the abdominal inguinal ring; a hernia entering medial to this ring is direct. In small hernias, the relation of the bulge to the midpoint of the inguinal ligament is diagnostic of direct or indirect. If the hernia is large, palpation of the inguinal canal through the scrotum may determine its site of entrance into the canal. The direct hernia is represented as an anterior bulging of the posterior wall of the inguinal canal. **Femoral hernia:** The femoral artery and vein emerge from the abdomen beneath the midpoint of the inguinal ligament, where the artery is palpable. The impalpable femoral vein is immediately medial to it. The femoral canal lies medial to the vein, so the canal is approximately 2 cm medial to the pulsating artery. A bulge in the region of the femoral canal is produced by a femoral hernia, especially on coughing or straining. The diagram shows a femoral hernia protruding upward in front of the inguinal ligament, where it may be confused with an inguinal hernia. Careful palpation will demonstrate that the inguinal canal is empty.*

are soft except when chronic inflammation has caused thickening. Umbilical hernias are very common in infants and tend to resolve spontaneously by approximately 4 years of age. The adult type frequently develops during pregnancy, in long-standing ascites, or when intrathoracic pressure is repeatedly increased as in asthma, chronic bronchitis, and bronchiectasis.

KEY SYNDROME   Inguinal Hernias

See Physical Examination, Chapter 12, page 568.

Indirect Inguinal Hernia: The lateral end of the inguinal canal is the internal inguinal ring, lying just above the midpoint of the inguinal ligament. The spermatic cord of the male emerges through this ring from the abdominal cavity into the canal. The cord runs medially in the canal emerging from the subcutaneous (external) ring just lateral to the pubis, then drops over the brim of the bony pelvis into the scrotum. In the male, a hernia follows the course of the cord. From the abdominal cavity, it may enter the canal for only a slight distance, or it may descend to the bottom of the scrotal sac. In the female, the hernia follows a similar course in the canal that contains the round ligament, corresponding to the spermatic cord. In either sex, a small, indirect inguinal hernia may produce a bulge over the midpoint of the inguinal ligament, at the abdominal (internal) inguinal ring (Fig. 9–36). To palpate the male inguinal canal, place the fingertip at the most dependent part of the scrotum and invaginate the slack scrotal wall to insert the finger gently into the subcutaneous (external) inguinal ring (see Fig. 12–5, page 569). If the ring is sufficiently relaxed, guide the finger laterally and cephalad through the canal and have the patient cough or strain. A small hernia causes an impulse felt on the fingertip. A larger hernia may feel like a mass in the canal. In the female, palpation of the inguinal canal is usually unsatisfactory.

Direct Inguinal Hernia: A hernia through the posterior wall of the inguinal canal is termed direct. The site of the weakness is the *Hesselbach triangle*, bounded by the inferior epigastric artery, the lateral border of the rectus muscle and the inguinal ligament; thus, it lies nearly directly behind the subcutaneous (external) inguinal ring. A bulge is produced close to the pubic tubercle, just above the inguinal ligament; this is medial to the site of the bulge for an indirect hernia (Fig. 9–36). With the finger in the inguinal canal, coughing or straining causes an impulse to be felt not at the tip or end of the finger, but rather on the pad of the distal phalanx. A direct hernia seldom causes pain. It is always acquired and usually occurs in men.

Femoral Hernia: The femoral nerve, artery, and vein lie lateral to and just inferior to the midpoint of the inguinal ligament. Immediately medial to the vein is the femoral canal, a continuation of the femoral sheath, through which a hernia may bulge when intraabdominal pressure is increased (Fig. 9–36). Large femoral hernias become irreducible and may push upward in front of the inguinal ligament where they must be distinguished from inguinal hernias. When the neck of the hernial sac can be palpated just lateral to and below the pubic tubercle, a femoral hernia is demonstrated; the neck of an inguinal hernia's sac is found above the inguinal ligament.

Obturator Hernia: A peritoneal sac protrudes through the obturator foramen of the pelvis, causing a fullness or mass in the femoral triangle. The fullness is not sharply defined because the sac is covered by the pectineus muscle. This rare lesion occurs almost always in emaciated women, more than 60 years of age, with a history of weight loss. On the affected side, the thigh is usually held in semiflexion; all hip motion is painful. Pain extends down the medial thigh to the knee. Palpation through the rectum or vagina may reveal a soft, tender mass in the region of the obturator foramen. This condition must be distinguished from the far more common femoral hernia. The hernia is rarely diagnosed before it has caused intestinal obstruction. When only a portion of the circumference of the bowel is strangulated (*Richter type*) so obstruction does not occur, the presenting pain may occur late after perforation or sepsis has occurred. In almost half the cases of strangulation, the genicular branch of the obturator nerve is compressed, producing pain down the medial aspect of the thigh to the knee (*Romberg-Howship sign*).

KEY SYNDROME   **Mass Above the Inguinal Ligament—Spigelian Hernia**

A peritoneal sac with considerable extraperitoneal fat perforates the linea semilunaris to lie within the abdominal wall; it is covered only by skin, subcutaneous fat, and the aponeurosis of the external abdominal oblique muscle. Usually asymptomatic until it strangulates, it produces a tender mass within the abdominal wall approximately 3 to 5 cm above the inguinal ligament. This should be inspected and palpated while the patient stands.

Other Inguinal Masses

Among the structures to be considered when a mass is found in the groin are lymph nodes, lymphoma, hernia, varix, lipoma, ectopic testis, ectopic spleen, and inguinal endometriosis.

Inguinal Mass—Saphenous Vein Varix: A bulge just below the femoral canal may be caused by a varix of the saphenous vein; this fills upon standing and empties in the supine position; palpation of the filled varix yields a distinctive thrill.

Lymphadenopathy: Inflammation, infection, or neoplastic involvement of lymph nodes causes enlargement with or without tenderness. Inflammation and fluctuant swelling of inguinal lymph nodes in the area of the femoral vessels below the inguinal ligament is a so-called *bubo*. It occurs commonly in chancroid, syphilis, and lymphogranuloma venereum. Neoplastic enlargement is felt as nontender rubbery or hard, nonfluctuant nodes. See Chapter 5, page 101.

Perineal, Anal, and Rectal Syndromes

KEY SYNDROME   **Brief Intense Perineal Pain—Proctalgia Fugax**

The cause is unknown, but men are more often affected than women. The patient is awakened from sleep with intense, poorly localized pain in the perineum or rectum. The paroxysm reaches an agonizing maximum in 1 to 2 minutes, and then subsides rapidly and completely in approximately 5 minutes. During the pain, the patient may arise and walk about or attempt defecation. Relief has been reported from pressure on the perineum, nitroglycerin, or an enema of warm water. Occasionally, the paroxysm is initiated by straining at stool, prolonged sitting on a hard surface, or ejaculation.

KEY SYNDROME   **Fecal Incontinence**

See page 468.

Occult GI Blood Loss

> **KEY SIGN** **Normally Colored Stools with Positive Guaiac Test ("Occult Blood")**

Bleeding of small volume from any site in the alimentary tract or the upper respiratory tract may give a positive test for blood without coloring the stool. The source should be sought by endoscopy. Because colonic neoplasms may bleed intermittently or not at all, the stool guaiac test has a low sensitivity for detecting colon cancer and should be reserved for evaluating patients whose clinical circumstances provide a reason for testing [Gomez JA, Diehl AK. Admission stool guaiac test: Use and impact on patient management. *Am J Med.* 1992;92:603–606]. Most cases of occult GI blood loss are caused by duodenal ulcer, gastritis, malignancy, angiectasia, diverticulosis, or esophageal varices.

GI bleeding associated with dermal lesions. In some patients, GI blood loss is associated with dermal lesions having their counterparts in the GI tract.

Peutz-Jeghers Syndrome: Melanin spots on lips, buccal mucosa, and tongue suggest bleeding polypoid lesions in the small intestine.

Hereditary Hemorrhagic Telangiectasia (Rendu-Osler-Weber Disease): Telangiectases on the face, buccal mucosa, and extremities suggest similar lesions in the GI tract.

Blue Rubber-Bleb Nevus Syndrome: cavernous hemangiomas of the skin, especially on the trunk or extremities, suggest similar lesions of the small intestine.

Ehlers-Danlos Syndrome: Hyperelastic skin, hyperflexible joints, petechiae, and easy bleeding of the skin. They also may have intestinal hemorrhage from deficiency of factor IX.

Pseudoxanthoma Elastica: Lax elastic tissue of skin, eye, cardiovascular system, and GI tract. The skin contains small, soft yellow-orange papules running parallel to natural skin folds. Angioid streaks are seen in retina. Disintegration of arteries in the GI tract causes hemorrhages.

Neurofibromatosis (von Recklinghausen Disease): Café au lait pigmentation with sessile, pedunculated, or subcutaneous skin fibromas. Fibromas in GI tract may bleed.

Amyloidosis (Either Primary or Secondary): Wax-colored papules, nodules, or tumors about the face, lips, ears, and upper chest. Macroglossia may be seen. Deposits about blood vessels and in mucosa cause bleeding.

Malignant Atrophic Papulosis (Degos Disease): Vasculitis of the skin and mucosa. Small, red papules on the skin become umbilicated, with porcelain-white depressed centers and dry scale. The border disappears, leaving a white patch. Patients may have acute abdominal pain with vomiting and bleeding which can progress to peritonitis and gangrene.

Dermatomyositis: Nonpitting edema of the face, heliotrope discoloration of the eyelids, cutaneous erythematous rash and erythema over the extensor aspects of the interphalangeal joints. Skeletal muscles have local and general inflammation.

Schönlein-Henoch Purpura: Symmetrical purpura on the buttocks, extensor surfaces of the limbs, angioneurotic edema, GI pain with mucosal ulcers and bleeding.

Drug Eruptions: Aspirin causes macular and purpuric lesions of lower limbs. Erosive lesions cause bleeding from GI tract. Warfarin may cause petechiae, ecchymoses, and bleeding in the GI tract.

Scurvy: Perifollicular hemorrhages, ecchymoses of legs, bleeding gums, loose teeth, and GI bleeding.

Polycythemia Vera: Purplish red color of skin and mucosa with hemorrhages, spider nevi, rosacea, and peptic ulcer.

Kaposi Sarcoma: Endemic Kaposi sarcoma is usually on the feet with dark-blue nodules and plaques. HIV-associated Kaposi sarcoma frequently involves the mucous membranes of the mouth and GI and genitourinary tracts.

Mastocytosis: Brown-red macules on the skin with urticaria. Hepatic cirrhosis of with esophageal varices may occur.

ADDITIONAL READING

William Silen. *Cope's Early Diagnosis of the Acute Abdomen*, 21st Edition. New York, NY: Oxford University Press; 2005.

The Urinary System

Overview and Physiology of The Urinary System

The urinary system consists of the kidneys, collecting systems of the renal pelvis, ureters, urinary bladder, and urethra. Important sphincters are found at the ureterovesical junction, as the ureter passes obliquely through the bladder wall, and at the proximal urethra, as it passes through the urogenital septum. The urethral sphincter has an involuntary smooth muscle portion under parasympathetic and sympathetic control, and a voluntary striated muscle sphincter innervated via the lumbosacral plexus. The urinary system is designed to filter the blood at the glomerulus and to reabsorb and to secrete solutes and fluid across the renal tubules, and then to concentrate the urine in the medullary collecting ducts. The urine passes down the ureters to the bladder by gravity and peristaltic contractions. The bladder is a hollow muscular structure that actively relaxes with urinary distention keeping intravesical pressures low until capacity is reached. Further filling occurs by stretching of the bladder wall at rapidly increasing pressures. Continence is maintained by tonic contraction of the smooth muscle sphincter and active inhibition of detrusor muscle contraction as the bladder fills. Voiding is a complex process involving simultaneous, coordinated relaxation of the urethral sphincters and contraction of the previously relaxed detrusor muscle.

Anatomy of the Urinary System

The kidneys lie posteriorly, partially under the eleventh and twelfth ribs and lateral to L1–4 (see Fig. 9–2, page 448). They are enclosed in a tight capsule and lie retroperitoneally, surrounded by Gerota's fascia. The ureters course retroperitoneally, and descend over the psoas muscle and into the pelvis, where they run laterally and then anteriorly to enter the inferior portion of the bladder on either side of the midline. The bladder lies anteriorly in the pelvis behind and below the symphysis pubis. The urethra exits the bladder and runs through the urogenital diaphragm of the pelvic floor muscles to enter the male prostate and penis or the female perineum. In males, the proximal urethra is surrounded by the prostate gland and receives prostatic secretions from the prostate and seminal vesicles. In the female, the urethra is quite short. Only the urethral meatus is visible on physical examination and normally the deeper structures cannot be identified by palpation.

Physical Examination of the Urinary System

See also The Abdomen, Chapter 9; Chapter 11, The Female Genitalia and Reproductive System; and Chapter 12, The Male Genitalia and Reproductive System.

Determination of the postvoid residual urine volume. The adequacy of bladder emptying is measured by determining the volume of urine remaining in the bladder after a full voluntary voiding: the *residual volume*. First, have the patient empty his or her bladder completely. Residual volume can be estimated by ultrasonography devices or measured directly by passing a sterile urethral catheter into the bladder to collect the residual urine. The risk of infection increases sharply with residual volumes >100 cc.

Urinary System Symptoms

KEY SYMPTOM   Discolored Urine

See Urinary Signs—Discolored Urine, page 532.

KEY SYMPTOM   Urethral Discharge

See Urinary symptoms—Urethral Discharge, page 534 and Urethritis page 536 and Chapter 12, page 582.

KEY SYMPTOM   Renal Colic

See Abdominal Pain, pages 462 and 497. Vigorous contraction of visceral smooth muscle in the ureters against an obstruction is intensely painful. Obstructing stones in the renal pelvis, ureter, or bladder produce acute, colicky, often extremely intense pain, whose location is dependent upon the site of obstruction. Obstruction at the renal pelvis gives flank and upper abdominal pain. Ureteral obstruction produces pain in the upper abdomen, lower abdomen, pelvis, testicles, and perineum. Bladder outlet obstruction leads to pain in the pelvis. The diagnosis is supported by an acute onset, absence of systemic symptoms other than nausea and anorexia, a previous or family history of urolithiasis, and the presence of microscopic hematuria without pyuria.

KEY SYMPTOM   Frequent Urination without Polyuria

Although the average adult urinates approximately five or six times daily, frequency depends upon fluid balance, renal function, individual habits, and the presence or absence of irritation in the genitourinary tract. Frequent urination can be caused by increased total urinary volume (*polyuria*; see *Frequent Urination with Polyuria*, below), decreased bladder capacity, or increased stimulation of the micturition reflexes caused by irritation of the genitourinary tract. The history, physical examination, and measurement of 24-hour fluid intake and urine volume, volume of each voiding, and postvoid residual bladder volume will usually lead to the correct assessment.

✔ *URINARY FREQUENCY—CLINICAL OCCURRENCE:* **Congenital** small bladder capacity; ureterovesical reflux; urethral and meatal stricture; **Endocrine** atrophic vaginitis; ***Idiopathic*** benign prostatic hyperplasia, pelvic floor relaxation, cystocele, urethrocele; ***Inflammatory/Immune*** interstitial and chemical cystitis, prostatitis, appendicitis; ***Infectious*** bacterial and viral pyelitis, cystitis, urethritis, vaginitis, salpingitis; ***Metabolic/Toxic*** chemical cystitis, highly acidic urine; ***Mechanical/Traumatic*** pelvic floor relaxation, cystocele, urethrocele, bladder stone, extrinsic compression of the bladder or urethra, bladder wall fibrosis, urethral stricture, bladder neck obstruction; ***Neoplastic*** bladder cancer, prostate cancer, locally invasive cervical and rectal cancer; ***Neurologic*** spinal cord, cauda equina and sacral plexus lesions, autonomic neuropathy, detrusor instability; ***Psychosocial*** untrained bladder, voiding habits.

KEY SYMPTOM Frequent Urination with Polyuria

The adult male bladder holds approximately 500 mL whereas the adult female's bladder holds somewhat less. An average output of urine in 24 hours is 1200 to 1500 mL, but this volume is dependent upon the type and volume of fluid intake, sensible (vomiting, diarrhea) and insensible (sweating, respiratory) fluid losses, and the renal concentrating ability. Increased urinary volume (*polyuria*) can result from an increased osmotic load (e.g., diabetes mellitus), increased intake of fluids, medications, dietary exposures, and decreased renal concentrating ability. The history, physical examination, and urinalysis are able to establish the cause in most cases.

POLYURIA—CLINICAL OCCURRENCE: ***Congenital*** renal tubular defects (e.g., renal tubular acidosis type 1); ***Endocrine*** diabetes mellitus, central or renal diabetes insipidus; ***Idiopathic*** chronic renal failure of any cause; ***Inflammatory/Immune*** interstitial nephritis; ***Metabolic/Toxic*** diuretic use, hypercalcemia, hypokalemia; ***Mechanical/Traumatic*** postobstructive diuresis; ***Psychosocial*** excessive fluid intake, psychogenic polydipsia, alcohol and caffeine ingestion.

KEY SYMPTOM Nocturia

Urine production declines during sleep and sleep is usually not interrupted to urinate. Some people have habitual nocturia, which is aggravated by high fluid intakes, especially of caffeinated or alcoholic beverages taken in the evening. Nocturia also occurs with most disorders causing increased frequency of urination or polyuria. Edematous states (congestive heart failure, hepatic insufficiency, nephrotic syndrome, and chronic renal failure) are associated with nocturia caused by mobilization of dependent fluid from the lower extremities and abdomen during recumbency [Marinkovic SP, Gillen LM, Stanton SL. Managing nocturia. *BMJ.* 2004;328:1063–1066]. Reclining can also lead to loss of bladder support, particularly in women with pelvic floor relaxation or a history of hysterectomy, leading to increased frequency of urination at night.

KEY SYMPTOM Urinary Incontinence

Involuntary loss of urine by children at night is referred to *as enuresis.* Urinary incontinence in the adult should initiate an evaluation for a specific cause, most of which are treatable. See Urinary Syndromes—Incontinence, page 535, for further discussion.

KEY SYMPTOM Difficult Urination

Normal urination occurs with the effortless relaxation of the bladder sphincters coordinated with contraction of the detrusor muscle. Difficulty initiating or maintaining the urinary stream indicates an obstruction to flow or a decrease in detrusor strength. The patient may complain of hesitancy in starting the urinary stream, decreased force of urination, and/or dribbling at termination of urination. Occasionally, straining is required to maintain the stream.

✔ *CLINICAL OCCURRENCE:* *Idiopathic* prostatic hyperplasia, chronic sterile prostatitis; *Infectious* tabes dorsalis, prostatitis; *Mechanical/Traumatic* urethral stricture or valve, bladder neck obstruction, bladder stone or clot, pregnancy, hematoma; *Neoplastic* urethral carcinoma, prostate cancer, uterine fibroid, vaginal cancer, cervical cancer; *Neurologic* detrusor weakness, multiple sclerosis, spinal cord injury or epidural compression, myelitis, syringomyelia.

KEY SYMPTOM Painful Urination (Dysuria)

Inflammation of or breaks in the urethral epithelium (exposing the submucosa to the acidic urine) results in pain located in the penis or the female urethra with urination. This is usually the result of infection or trauma. Ask whether the pain is greater on initiation or on termination of voiding. Pain during urination occurs with urethral obstruction, urethritis, cystitis, vulvitis and meatal ulcers. Pain after urination is more typical of bladder calculus, cystitis, prostatitis and seminal vesiculitis.

Urinary System Signs

See also Abdominal Signs, Chapter 9; Chapter 11, Female Genital and Reproductive Signs; Chapter 12, Male Genital and Reproductive Signs.

KEY SYMPTOM Urinary Retention

See Urinary Syndromes—Urinary Retention, page 535.

➤ KEY SIGN Anuria and Oliguria

Obstruction of the bladder outlet is the most common cause of anuria and oliguria as measured by voided urine volumes. Decreased urine production measured in the bladder is a result of a profound decline in glomerular filtration due to a decrease in renal blood flow and/or intrarenal or ureteral obstruction. The process must involve both kidneys or obstruct both ureters. In *oliguria*, the 24-hour urinary output is between 50 and 400 mL (4–25 mL/h). The output is 0 to 50 mL in *anuria*. Even with dehydration, normal kidneys continue to excrete more than 500 mL daily. Therefore, oliguria and anuria indicate advanced degrees of renal dysfunction requiring immediate treatment. Acute renal failure may occur unexpectedly during the care of patients for another disorder. Usually patients do not complain of a lack of urine, thus delaying recognition. Often, the cause may be suspected from knowledge of the preexisting disease, but postrenal obstruction with hydronephrosis must always be excluded. *CLINICAL OCCURRENCE:* See Urinary Syndromes—Acute Renal Failure, page 536.

> **KEY SIGN   Discolored Urine**

Urine is normally clear and colored yellow because of urea. Dilution and concentration of the urine will change the intensity, but not the color, of the urine. A true color change results from the presence of colored substances in the urine, either filtered from the blood or arising in the urinary tract itself. Increased opacity of the urine arises with the precipitation of solutes or the addition of cellular material or mucous. A complaint of abnormal urine color requires further history. First, determine if the change is one of intensity of the normal yellow color or a true change in color. Also, determine if the change is persistent or episodic and whether there is an association with activities, intake of foods, medications, or other symptoms. Inspection and analysis of a freshly voided urine specimen to confirm the patient's observation should precede any further investigation. Note that patients will describe any red discoloration of the urine as blood, a conclusion you must avoid until it is proven [Nguyen JS, Marinopoulos SS, Ashar BH, et al. More than meets the eye. *N Engl J Med.* 2006;355:1048]. Often discoloration of the urine is discovered by someone handling specimens for examination.

✔ *DISCOLORED URINE—CLINICAL OCCURRENCE:*   *Colorless*   urine of low concentration from excessive fluid intake, chronic glomerulonephritis, diabetes mellitus, diabetes insipidus;   *Cloudy White*   phosphates in an alkaline urine (the cloud disappears with the addition of acid), epithelial cells from the lower genitourinary tract, bacteria, pus, chyle (when the urine is centrifuged, chyle remains homogeneously distributed; milk fat added for malingering floats to the top);   *Yellow*   Highly concentrated normal urine, tetracycline, pyridine;   *Orange*   urobilinogen, pyridium (antispasmodic that is orange in acid urine and red in alkaline urine), rhubarb (food and purgative), cathartics (senna aloes), anthracyclines;   *Red*   beets, blackberries, aniline dyes from candy, freshly voided hemoglobin or myoglobin, pyridine, porphyrin, phenolphthalein (a cathartic, red in alkaline urine, colorless in acid urine), cascara (cathartic), rifampin, doxorubicin;   *Blue-Green*   bilirubin (urine with yellow froth), methylene blue, *Pseudomonas* infection;   *Black-Brown*   highly concentrated normal urine, bilirubin (with yellow froth), acid hematin (hemoglobin standing in acid urine), methemoglobin, porphyrin, phenol (black in large quantities), cresol, homogentisic acid, tyrosine;   *Brown-Black After Standing*   porphyrin (changed from exposure to sunlight), melanin (changed from exposure to sunlight), homogentisic acid (changed from bacterial alkalinization of the urine).

Hematuria: Microscopic hematuria is defined as >3 erythrocytes per high-powered field on at least 2 out of 3 properly collected spun urine specimens; gross hematuria indicates sufficient red blood cells to discolor the urine. Dipstick identification of urinary heme suggests microscopic hematuria which must be confirmed by microscopic examination of the urine. Gross hematuria is frequently noticed by the male during micturition. Hematuria is distinguished from hemoglobinuria and myoglobinuria by finding erythrocytes in freshly voided urine collected within 1 hour after complete bladder emptying. In all three cases, chemical tests of the urine are positive for heme. Spectroscopic examination distinguishes myoglobin from hemoglobin, but it does not differentiate intracellular from extracellular hemoglobin. The pattern of gross hematuria observed by the patient may indicate the source of blood: *initial hematuria*—the urethra; *terminal hematuria*—a small hemorrhage from the trigone region of the bladder; *total hematuria*—hemorrhage from the kidney or profuse bleeding from the bladder; the presence of erythrocyte casts in the urine proves a renal source [Cohen RA, Brown RS. Microscopic hematuria. *N Engl J Med.* 2003;348:2330–2338].

In most instances, the occurrence of hematuria demands a complete investigation of the genitourinary tract, including upper tract imaging, urine cytology and cystoscopy. Bedside observations must suffice when instrumentation is contraindicated, as in urethral infection or hemorrhagic disorders.

✔ **HEMATURIA—CLINICAL OCCURRENCE:** *Congenital* hemophilia, sickle cell disease, polycystic kidney disease; *Endocrine* menstruation; *Idiopathic* bladder diverticulum, polyps, prostatic hyperplasia, endometriosis, uremia, thrombocytopenia; *Inflammatory/Immune* interstitial cystitis, fever, glomerulonephritis, polyarteritis, microscopic polyangiitis, Goodpasture syndrome, Wegener syndrome; *Infectious* urethritis, bacterial and viral (adenovirus 11) cystitis, prostatitis, pyelitis, schistosomiasis, malaria, yellow fever; *Metabolic/Toxic* chemical cystitis (e.g., cyclophosphamide or ifosfamide), analgesic nephropathy, anticoagulants, scurvy, vitamin K deficiency; *Mechanical/Traumatic* blunt or penetrating trauma, urethral stricture, instrumentation, postsurgical, decompression of a distended bladder, heavy exercise (e.g., marathon runners), foreign body, stones, rupture, radiation, medullary necrosis; *Neoplastic* kidney, ureter, bladder, prostate cancers; *Psychosocial* factitious; *Vascular* bladder and prostatic varices, renal infarction, vasculitis, arteriovenous malformation.

Hemoglobinuria: Hemoglobinuria is extracellular hemoglobin in the urine resulting from filtration of plasma free hemoglobin or lysis of red blood cells present in the urine. Sufficient concentrations produce a red color identical to myoglobinuria and hematuria. When hemoglobin enters the plasma by the intravascular hemolysis, it binds to plasma haptoglobin and the large hemoglobin-haptoglobin complex is not filtered by the normal glomerulus. When the binding capacity of haptoglobin is exceeded, free hemoglobin passes through the glomerular basement membrane and a freshly voided urine specimen usually contains hemoglobin casts. Their presence excludes the possibility that hemolysis occurred in the bladder. Hemoglobin gives positive chemical tests whether intracellular or extracellular, so hemoglobinuria must be distinguished from hematuria by the absence of erythrocytes in freshly voided urine. Although myoglobin (molecular weight [MW] 17 500) can be differentiated from hemoglobin (MW 68 000) by spectroscopic examination, look for a concomitant red coloration of the blood plasma, which suggests hemoglobinuria because the smaller myoglobin molecules are cleared more rapidly from the blood. Hematuria and hemoglobinuria from hemolysis in the bladder occur when the urine is so dilute as to hemolyze the erythrocytes (specific gravity less than 1.006). Transfusion of improperly stored or frozen blood results in the direct infusion of hemoglobin from the lyzed red blood cells.

✔ **HEMOGLOBINURIA—CLINICAL OCCURRENCE:** *Congenital* G-6-PD (glucose-6-phosphate dehydrogenase) deficiency; *Endocrine* pregnancy and the puerperium; *Idiopathic* paroxysmal nocturnal hemoglobinuria; *Inflammatory/Immune* major transfusion reaction, autoimmune hemolytic anemia, hapten-associated hemolysis (quinine, sulfonamides), high-titer cold-agglutinin disease; *Infectious* malaria, blackwater fever, typhus, gas gangrene, generalized anthrax, yellow fever; *Metabolic/Toxic* oxidant drugs or fava beans in persons with G-6-PD deficiency (sulfonamides, sulfones, primaquine), envenomation by snake or spider bites, infusion of outdated, frozen, or improperly stored blood; *Mechanical/Traumatic* march hemoglobinuria, mechanical heart valves, severe aortic and paraprosthetic mitral regurgitation, extracorporeal circulation, major burns, intravascular devices; *Psychosocial* injection of distilled water; *Vascular* microangiopathic hemolytic anemia-thrombotic thrombocytopenic purpura, hemolytic uremic syndrome, and malignant hypertension; renal infarction.

Myoglobinuria: Excretion of myoglobin released from damaged muscle colors the urine red and gives chemical tests for heme (see Hemoglobinuria above). Muscle pain and a history of crush injury or prolonged muscle ischemia are usual although loss of consciousness associated with severe injury may obscure the findings.

✔ MYOGLOBINURIA—CLINICAL OCCURRENCE: *Congenital* McArdle disease; *Inflammatory/Immune* autoimmune hemolytic anemia, transfusion of incompatible blood; *Metabolic/Toxic* severe hypokalemia, ingestion of quail (idiosyncratic), opiate and sedative abuse, Haff disease (an epidemic myoglobinuria encountered in Königsberg, Germany, caused by the ingestion of fish feeding in a lagoon polluted with industrial wastes); *Mechanical/Traumatic* crush injuries, compression injuries caused by prolonged immobilization or impaired consciousness, electrical shock, compartment syndromes, intravascular hemolysis.

Urethral Signs

KEY SIGN **Urethral Discharge**

Inflammation in the urethra and/or its exocrine glands distal to the urogenital septum leads to an increase in purulent secretions, which leak from the urethral orifice between times of urination. Men may complain specifically about discharge from the penis accompanied by staining of the underwear with pus or blood. Determine whether the discharge is clear or purulent, accompanied by painful and/or frequent urination and whether the patient has had any new sexual partners. Ask specifically about same-sex contacts and the use of condoms. In women, urethral discharge is confounded with vulvovaginitis. *CLINICAL OCCURRENCE:* Inflammatory/Immune Reiter syndrome, Behçet syndrome; Infectious *Chlamydia trachomatis, Neisseria gonorrhoeae, Ureaplasma urealyticum, Trichomonas vaginalis*, other sexually transmitted infections; *Mechanical/Traumatic* urethral catheter and foreign bodies.

Urinary System Syndromes

KEY SYNDROME **Hematuria**

See Urinary Signs—Hematuria, page 532.

KEY SYNDROME **Loin Pain-Hematuria Syndrome—IgA Nephropathy**

For unknown reasons, there are deposits of IgA in the mesangial region of the glomerulus. Patients present with painless hematuria or hematuria and loin pain, often following a mild viral infection. Progression is unpredictable, but a significant minority develops end-stage renal disease [Donanio JV, Grande JP. IgA nephropathy. *N Engl J Med.* 2002;347:738–748].

KEY SYNDROME **Urinary Incontinence**

Loss of bladder control results from abnormalities of genitourinary sensation and/or smooth muscle function (detrusor instability, overactive bladder, urge incontinence), inadequate sphincter function (stress incontinence), urinary retention leading to overflow incontinence, combinations of these (mixed incontinence), abnormalities of cognition, and inability to respond in a timely fashion to reach a toilet. Urinary incontinence in the adult should initiate an evaluation for a specific cause, most of which are treatable. The onset, pattern, precipitating factors, fluid intake, and measures taken by the patient to reduce the incontinence are essential historical information. A detailed review of all prescription and nonprescription medications and dietary supplements is mandatory. It is especially important to identify whether the patient feels an urge to void prior to the episode, whether coughing, sneezing or laughing precedes each episode and the volume of urine lost at each episode [Brown JS, Bradley CS, Subak LL, et al. The sensitivity and specificity of a simple test to distinguish between urge and stress urinary incontinence. *Ann Intern Med.* 2006:144:715–723]. Having the patient complete a bladder journal for at least 2 weeks, recording fluid intake (type and amount), urine volume and incontinent episodes, will greatly facilitate the evaluation.

✓ ***URINARY INCONTINENCE—CLINICAL OCCURRENCE:*** ***Idiopathic*** benign prostatic hyperplasia, cystocele urethrocele; ***Infectious*** cystitis, urethritis; ***Mechanical/Traumatic*** pelvic floor relaxation, sphincter injury from childbirth; ***Neoplastic*** prostate, bladder, cervix, and rectal cancers, especially with sacral plexus involvement; ***Neurologic*** spinal cord injury, epidural cord compression, cauda equina syndrome, stoke, dementia, autonomic and peripheral neuropathies, normal pressure hydrocephalus, multiple sclerosis, paralysis, muscular weakness and limited mobility.

KEY SYNDROME **Urinary Retention**

The bladder is unable to empty because of mechanical obstruction of bladder outflow and/or loss of detrusor strength. Rapid increase in bladder volume leads to high wall tension, whereas slow increases lead to increased bladder compliance and flaccidity of the wall. Retention is more common in men than in women. Acute urinary retention is usually painful, distinguishing it from painless anuria or oliguria. Seriously ill patients may be unable to communicate discomfort. Chronic retention develops gradually and is painless. The only symptoms may be frequent urination of small amounts or incontinence (overflow). The patient may have a sensation of fullness in the bladder, but this is often absent. Examination shows a suprapubic dullness and a rounded mass. Have the patient void, then measure the postvoid residual urine volume by catheterization or bladder ultrasonography.

✔ *URINARY RETENTION—CLINICAL OCCURRENCE:*   *Congenital*   urethral valves; *Inflammatory/Immune*   prostatitis (nonbacterial);   *Infectious*   prostatitis (bacterial) and prostate abscess;   *Mechanical/Traumatic*   prostate, hyperplasia, bladder stone, occluded catheter, urethral stricture or calculus, ruptured urethral;   *Neoplastic*   prostate and bladder cancer, locally invasive cervical or rectal cancer;   *Neurologic*   spinal cord injury, autonomic neuropathy, tabes dorsalis.

➤ **KEY SYNDROME   Acute Renal Failure**

Acute loss of renal function is classified as *prenal* (decreased effective renal blood flow), *renal* (glomerulonephritis, mesangial proliferation, tubular dysfunction, or interstitial inflammation), or *postrenal* (obstruction of the ureters or bladder). Patients do not ususally complain of lack of urine, which delays recognition. The physical examination, including assessment of intravascular volume, cardiac output, and the presence of severe liver disease, will identify prerenal causes. Obstruction must be excluded in all patients. Urinalysis helps to distinguish between glomerular causes (microscopic hematuria, red blood cell casts, proteinuria) and tubulointerstitial disease (cellular and granular casts, decreased concentrating ability, salt wasting). Medications commonly cause or contribute substantially to acute renal failure. Congenital solitary kidney or the prior nonfunctioning of one kidney may precipitate acute renal failure from unilateral events that would not normally be associated with a sudden and dramatic loss of renal function. The following clinical classification is more diagnostically useful than pathologic categorizations.

✔ *ACUTE RENAL FAILURE—CLINICAL OCCURRENCE:*   *Congenital*   sickle cell crisis;   *Endocrine*   hyperparathyroidism (severe hypercalcemia), thyroid storm; *Idiopathic*   advanced chronic renal failure of any cause;   *Inflammatory/Immune* vasculitis (see below), antibasement glomerular membrane disease (Goodpasture syndrome), systemic lupus erythematosus, progressive systemic sclerosis (scleroderma), serum sickness, retroperitoneal fibrosis;   *Infectious*   pyelonephritis, septicemia, hemorrhagic fevers, blackwater fever (malaria), bacterial endocarditis;   *Metabolic/Toxic*   *Medications:* antibiotics (aminoglycosides, amphotericin-B, sulfonamides), nonsteroidal antiinflammatory drugs, and hypersensitivity to any medication; *Toxins:* myoglobin, radiologic contrast material, heavy metals (mercury, bismuth, copper, uranium, arsenic), organic solvents (carbon tetrachloride), inorganic phosphorus, carbon monoxide, paraldehyde, ethylene glycol, heroin, biologics (mushrooms, rattlesnake venom), methemoglobinemia; *Blood Transfusion:* hemolysis from mishandled or incompatible blood;   *Mechanical/Traumatic*   *Major Trauma:* Hypovolemic shock, crush syndrome, burns, heat prostration, hematoma, ruptured kidneys, myoglobinemia; *Instrumentation:* retrograde pyelography and catheterization of ureters; *Postrenal Obstruction* (especially if one kidney is absent or poorly functioning): renal calculi, cysts, tumor or mass obstructing the ureters, obstruction by crystals of uric acid, oxalic acid, cystine, or calcium;   *Neoplastic*   lymphoma, extensive cervical cancer causing bilateral ureteral obstruction, tumor lysis syndrome;   *Vascular*   hypotension of any cause (sepsis, hemorrhage, obstetrical complications), postoperative (especially with major vascular procedures—aortic resection, cardiotomy, repair of injuries to blood vessels, etc.—or hemorrhage), vasculitis (polyarteritis nodosa, microscopic polyangiitis, Goodpasture syndrome, Wegener granulomatosis, hypersensitivity angiitis), or vasculopathy (hemolytic uremic

Table 10–1   Staging of Chronic Kidney Disease

Stage	Description	Glomerular Filtration Rate (mL/min per 1.73 m^2)
0	Increased risk	$\geq$90, but with risk factors for chronic kidney disease (e.g., hypertension, diabetes, etc.)
1	Kidney damage with normal or increased GFR	$\geq$90
2	Kidney damage with mildly decreased GFR	60–89
3	Moderately decreased GFR	30–59
4	Severely decreased GFR	15–29
5	Renal failure	<15 or dialysis

Adapted from Harrison's Principles of Internal Medicine, 16th ed.

syndrome, thrombotic thrombocytopenic purpura, malignant and accelerated hypertension, abdominal aortic dissection, atheroemboli).

KEY SYNDROME   Chronic Kidney Disease and Chronic Renal Failure

Chronic loss of renal function can occur from prerenal, renal, or postrenal causes. When functioning nephron mass falls below a critical level, progressive failure of the remaining nephrons results from the increased filtration required of them to maintain adequate solute clearance. This vicious cycle leads to end-stage kidney disease. Weakness, anorexia, fatigue, and nausea are common symptoms, while pruritus and dyspnea are late findings. The slow progression leads to adaptive metabolic and hemodynamic changes that may be apparent on physical examination. Hypertension, expansion of the extracellular fluid volume causing edema, muscle wasting, and anemia are common. Less frequently, pericarditis or soft-tissue calcifications may be found. Patients are now staged according to the categories listed in Table 10–1 [El Nahas AM, Bello AK. Chronic kidney disease: The global challenge. *Lancet.* 2005;365:331–340].

CHRONIC RENAL FAILURE—CLINICAL OCCURRENCE: *Note*: The causes of acute renal failure are not repeated here. **Congenital** polycystic kidney disease, Alport syndrome; **Endocrine** diabetes mellitus the metabolic syndrome; **Inflammatory/Immune** glomerulonephritis, systemic lupus erythematosus; **Infectious** chronic pyelonephritis, renal tuberculosis; **Metabolic/Toxic** nonsteroidal antiinflammatory drugs, acetaminophen; **Mechanical/Traumatic** bladder neck obstruction; **Vascular** hypertension, atherosclerotic renal artery stenosis, atheroemboli, vasculitis.

Polycystic Kidney Disease: An autosomal dominant defect of renal tubular development produces massive enlargement of the kidneys and progressive renal failure. Presenting symptoms are flank pain, nausea, malaise, renal colic, and hematuria. Hypertension is common and bilateral enlargement of the kidneys is often detected by palpation.

Uremia: Uremia is a clinical syndrome associated with advanced renal failure; it includes azotemia, although the symptoms do not necessarily parallel the degree of azotemia. Symptoms include increased fatigability, headache, anorexia, dyspnea, nausea and vomiting, diarrhea, hiccup, restlessness, and depression. Signs on physical examination include Cheyne-Stokes breathing, fetid breath, dehydration, pericardial friction rub, muscle twitching, delirium and coma.

Glomerulonephritis (Nephritic Syndrome): Inflammatory damage to the glomerular capillary endothelium, basement membrane, mesangium, and/or epithelial podocytes results in destruction of normal glomerular architecture. Proteinuria and hematuria with red blood cell casts result from loss of the integrity of the glomerulus. When the consequence of a systemic disease, the signs and symptoms of that disease will predominate. Primary renal diseases often present with oliguria, edema, severe hypertension, and electrolyte disorders accompanying end stage renal disease.

Nephrotic Syndrome: Damage to the glomerular basement membrane increases the filtration of low MW proteins, particularly albumin. When the capacity of the tubules to reabsorb this protein is exceeded, proteinuria occurs. Albuminuria of >3.5 g in a 24-hour collection or a urine protein/creatinine ratio of >3.5 are diagnostic; hypertension, edema, hypoalbuminemia, and elevated serum cholesterol are frequently present. Complications include protein malnutrition and increased risk of thrombosis, particularly in the renal vein. Creatinine and blood urea nitrogen may remain normal. Nephrotic syndrome may complicate many forms of glomerular injury and is particularly common in diabetic nephropathy.

KEY SYNDROME   Urolithiasis

Stones form either from solutes that accrete upon a nidus (usually calcium oxalate, but also uric acid) or as a result of chronic urinary tract infections with urea-splitting organisms (struvite stones). Microscopic or gross hematuria may be present intermittently, but most stones are asymptomatic until they lodge at a narrowing in the ureter or bladder outlet. Pain is the presenting symptom, the site depending upon the location of the impacted stone (See Renal Colic, page 529) [Moe OW. Kidney stones: Pathophysiology and medical management. *Lancet.* 2006;367:333–344].

KEY SYNDROME   Uroepithelial Cancer (Bladder, Ureters, Renal Pelvis)

The transitional cell epithelium becomes neoplastic under the influence of substances excreted in the urine. Risk factors include tobacco, industrial chemicals and certain chemotherapy agents (cyclophosphamide, ifosfamide). Hematuria, either gross or microscopic, is the only early sign. Advanced disease presents with direct extension to pelvic and retroperitoneal organs causing pain, fistulas, and obstructions.

Kidney Cancer: Most renal cancers arise from the epithelium and some have mutations of the von Hippel-Lindau gene, either inherited (von Hippel-Lindau syndrome) or acquired. Tobacco smoke is a major risk factor for acquired renal cell carcinoma. Renal cancers may invade the renal vein and inferior vena cava. They metastasize to the lungs and invade local retroperitoneal structures, including bone and CNS, causing pain. Microscopic hematuria may be present. Flank fullness or pressure may be a complaint prior to the onset of pain.

> **KEY SYNDROME** Urinary Tract Infection

Infection is usually by enteric organisms ascending from the urethral meatus. Metastatic infection most often affects the kidney. Sexually transmitted organisms predominate in the lower tract (urethra, urethral glands, and prostate). The presence of foreign bodies (catheters, stents, stones) or obstruction leads to persistent and complicated infections. Symptoms and signs depend upon the specific site of infection.

Urethritis And Urethral Syndrome: Infection is caused by sexually transmitted infections (with *Neisseria gonorrhoea*, *Chlamydia trachomatis*, genital mycoplasmas, or herpes simplex) or complicates prolonged catheterization. Burning dysuria and purulent discharge demonstrated by urethral stripping are nearly uniform. Untreated, progression to upper tract infection is possible. Dysuria, urgency, and frequency with negative cultures for bacteria and lack of response to antibiotics define the *urethral syndrome*. The etiology is poorly understood and may result from viral infection or sterile inflammation.

Cystitis: Ascending bladder infection is common in normal women because of urethral colonization with enteric (e.g. *Escherichia coli*) and vaginal flora and the short urethra. Cystitis in men suggests an anatomic, usually obstructing, abnormality. Residual urine volume >100 cc is associated with increased risk of infection. Inflammation of the bladder wall and trigone elicits urinary frequency, urgency, dysuria, and a sensation of incomplete voiding. Untreated, infection can ascend to the kidneys [Bent S, Nallamothu BK, Simel DL, et al. Does this woman have an acute uncomplicated urinary tract infection? *JAMA*. 2002;287:2701–2710].

Acute Pyelonephritis: Bacteria ascend from the bladder or, less commonly, reach the kidney via the bloodstream. Infection involves primarily the renal medulla and collecting system, but may extend to the cortex or perinephritic tissue with abscess formation. Symptoms are fever, chills, and flank pain. Physical examination reveals percussion tenderness at the costovertebral angle. Prompt diagnosis and treatment prevents bacteremia, urosepsis, and local suppurative complications.

Chronic Pyelonephritis: Chronic kidney infection is caused by nonpyogenic bacteria, including slowly growing, often intracellular organisms, such as tuberculosis and brucellosis. This is often asymptomatic until systemic symptoms (fever of unknown origin, anorexia, weight loss) occur. Sterile pyuria is the only sign. See Interstitial Nephritis below.

Vesicoureteral reflux. Incompetence of the ureterovesicle valve mechanism leads to reflux of urine from the bladder into the ureters, increasing ureteral and renal pelvis pressures, a functional obstruction. This is common is young children, especially girls, and during pregnancy. It is associated with recurrent infections in addition to producing pressure induced renal injury. It may be asymptomatic with only abnormalities on urinalysis (pyuria, cellular casts, and proteinuria) and declining renal function.

> **KEY SYNDROME** Interstitial Nephritis

Inflammation of the cortical and medullary renal interstitium (as distinct from the glomerular and vascular injury of glomerulonephritis) results in scarring, decreased tubular function, and progressive renal insufficiency. Injury may be acute (infection, drug induced) or chronic (toxins, drugs, infection, obstruction). This condition may be asymptomatic with abnormalities on urinalysis (pyuria, cellular casts, and proteinuria) and declining renal function the only findings.

✔ *INTERSTITIAL NEPHRITIS—CLINICAL OCCURRENCE:* *Congenital* polycystic kidney disease, medullary cystic and sponge kidney, sickle cell disease, vesicoureteral reflux; *Inflammatory/Immune* drug allergy (penicillins, sulfonamides, etc.), Sjögren syndrome, Goodpasture syndrome, transplant rejection; *Infectious* acute and chronic pyelonephritis, viral infection (Epstein-Barr virus, cytomegalovirus, HIV, hantavirus), brucellosis, yersinia, tuberculosis, leptospirosis, rickettsia, mycoplasma; *Metabolic/Toxic* drugs (nonsteroidal antiinflammatory drugs, diuretics, anticonvulsants, cyclosporin, and others), toxins (heavy metals, lithium, herbals, and others), hypercalcemia, hyperuricemia, prolonged hypokalemia; *Mechanical/Traumatic* chronic obstruction, ureterovesical reflux, radiation; *Neoplastic* multiple myeloma, lymphoma, leukemia; *Vascular* accompanying glomerulonephritis and vasculitis.

> **KEY SYNDROME** Interstitial Cystitis

A condition of unknown cause results in often painful inflammation of the bladder wall leading to fibrosis and decreased bladder capacity. This condition is most common in women who present with urinary frequency and bladder pain, but negative cultures for infection. Diagnosis is by exclusion of other causes of bladder pain with frequency and complete urologic evaluation.

The Female Genitalia and Reproductive System

Overview of Female Reproductive Physiology

Male and female external genitalia, arising from identical embryologic anlage, differentiate depending on the presence or absence of testosterone. Lack of the SRY gene (typically found on the Y chromosome) leads to development of ovaries, with subsequent maturation of female sex organs. The labia majora is a cognate of the scrotum and the clitoris and penis are similarly derived. Ambiguous genitalia occur when development and maturation occurs with a mixed genetic substrate or hormonal environment.

The female reproductive system consists of the ovaries on their suspensory ligaments, the Fallopian tubes, the uterine corpus and cervix, the vagina with its muscular wall, the vaginal and introital glands of Cowper and Bartholin, the labia minora and majora, and the clitoris with its covering prepuce.

The ovary cyclically matures one ovum within a follicle under the stimulation of follicle-stimulating hormone (FSH) from the pituitary. The developing follicle produces estrogen, which causes proliferation of the endometrium. When the serum estrogen level reaches a threshold, a luteinizing hormone (LH) surge is triggered from the pituitary, effecting ovulation and formation of the corpus luteum that secretes increased levels of progesterone, inducing transformation of the endometrium from its proliferative to its secretory phase. The released ovum is captured by the fimbriated end of the Fallopian tube down which it travels to the uterine corpus. If fertilized in the tube or uterine cavity, the ovum may implant into the receptive endometrium establishing a pregnancy. If not, implantation does not occur and the corpus luteum involutes. With the cessation of estrogen and progesterone production, the endometrium is sloughed as menstrual bleeding, FSH rises again to stimulate development of another follicle initiating another reproductive cycle. Implantation of a fertilized ovum leads to the development of the placenta, which secretes human chorionic gonadotropin, suppressing pituitary FSH and LH, leading to cessation of ovulation and menstruation.

Anatomy of the Female Genitalia and Reproductive System

The symphysis pubis is surmounted anteriorly by a fat pad, the mons pubis (Fig. 11–1). At puberty, the eminence becomes covered with hair that extends onto the skin of the abdomen to form a transverse borderline, the base of an inverted

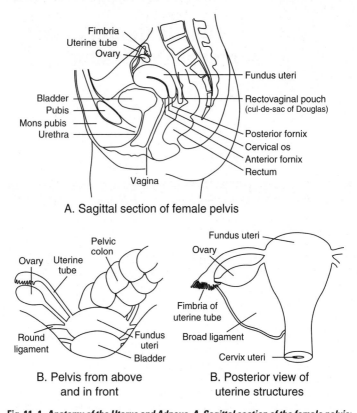

A. Sagittal section of female pelvis

B. Pelvis from above and in front

B. Posterior view of uterine structures

Fig. 11–1 *Anatomy of the Uterus and Adnexa. A. Sagittal section of the female pelvis:* Note the angle of the vagina with the vertical axis of the body, and the axis of the uterus perpendicular to the vaginal axis. The lips of the cervix uteri are shown to be in the same plane as the anterior vaginal wall, which is shorter than the posterior wall. The rectovaginal pouch (cul-de-sac of Douglas) lies anterior to the rectal wall; hence, it can be palpated during the rectal examination. The uterine fundus in the usual position is inaccessible to the rectal examining finger, but very close to palpation from the lower abdomen. *B. View of the pelvis from above and in front:* Note how the round ligament curves anteriorly and the uterine tubes curve posteriorly. *C. Posterior view of the uterus and broad Ligaments, Spread Out:* Note the suspension of the ovary near the fimbriated end of the uterine tube. The uterine tube forms the upper border of the broad ligament.

triangle called the *female escutcheon*. This hair distribution contrasts with that of the male escutcheon, which describes an upright triangle with the apex near the umbilicus.

The vulva. The vulva or pudendum is the female external genitalia (Fig. 11–2B). The *labia majora* are elevated ridges extending inferiorly and posteriorly from the mons pubis nearly to the anus. They contain fat, blood vessels, nerves,

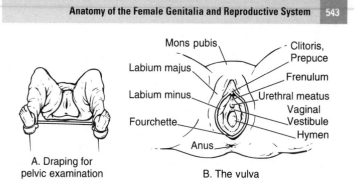

A. Draping for
pelvic examination

B. The vulva

Fig. 11–2 *Examination of the Vulva. A. Draping for pelvic examination:* The patient assumes the lithotomy position with feet in stirrups projecting from the end of the examining table. A sheet is spread over the patient so the two lower corners are wrapped about the thighs and legs. The middle of the lower edge of the sheet is slackly draped over the lower abdomen. *B. Topographic anatomy of the vulva:* The recessed vestibule contains a relatively small vaginal orifice, surrounded by one of the usual patterns of unruptured hymen. Bordering the vestibule are the two projecting folds of often deeply pigmented skin, the labia minora. Anteriorly, accessory folds of the labia form the prepuce that encloses the clitoris. Lateral to the labia minora are two parallel ridges of skin and fat that form the labium majus on either side of the labia minora.

and tissue that resemble the dartos tunic in the scrotum. Enclosed within the labia majora are two smaller skin folds, the *labia minora*, extending from the clitoris to unite in front of the anus by a transverse fold, the *fourchette*. The *clitoris* is the erectile homologue of the penis, composed of two small corpora cavernosa and surrounded superiorly by the prepuce and inferiorly by folds of the labia minora, the *frenulum*. The cleft posterior to the clitoris, between the two labia minora, is called the *vestibule*. It is pierced by the *urethral meatus*, approximately 2.5 cm posterior to the clitoris, and the *vaginal orifice*, immediately posterior to the meatus. The vaginal opening is a median slit, varying inversely with the size of the hymen. The *hymen* is a thin membrane covering part of the vaginal orifice. Commonly a perforate ring, widest posteriorly, the hymen may be cribriform, fringed, or even imperforate. After rupture, the hymenal remnants heal as irregular folds of mucosa. Two paired glands open onto the vestibular surface: just inferior to the urethra are the openings of the *paraurethral (Skene) glands*, and at the posterior edge of the vaginal orifice are found the openings of *the greater vestibular (Bartholin) glands*.

The vagina, uterus, and adnexa.   From its orifice, the *vagina* extends posteriorly into the pelvis (see Fig. 11–1). It is a collapsed tube with a posterior wall approximately 9 cm long and a shorter anterior vaginal wall (6–7.5 cm), which reflect onto the *uterine cervix* located most commonly at its anterior apex. The recess of the vagina behind the cervix is termed the *posterior fornix*; recesses on either side of the cervix are called *lateral fornices*. The vaginal mucosa is thrown into transverse rugae, separated by furrows of variable depths. Through the vagina, the nulliparous cervix appears as a smooth button with its face rounded and pierced by a hole or slit, the *cervical os*. The parous cervix may be somewhat irregular. The anterior and posterior lips of the os are usually in contact with the posterior vaginal wall. Dorsal to the posterior vaginal wall lies the *rectum*; ventral to the anterior vaginal wall are the *urethra* and *bladder*. The peritoneal cavity extends inferiorly behind the posterior fornix to form the *rectovaginal pouch* (cul-de-sac of Douglas); its lower part is interposed between the rectum and the cervix. The uterus is a muscular organ, shaped like an inverted pear flattened anteroposteriorly. From each side of the broad uterine fundus the *Fallopian tubes* extend for approximately 10 cm, curving laterally and posteriorly in the pelvis. The tubes, suspended by the *mesosalpinges*, form the upper borders of the *broad ligaments* that spread from the lateral margins of the uterus to the pelvic wall. The *uterus* with the two wings of broad ligament forms a transverse septum dividing the pelvis into an anterior and posterior fossa. On the posterior surface of the broad ligaments, the *ovaries* are suspended medial to and below the fimbriated ends of the Fallopian tubes by ligaments which attach to the uterus (*ovarian ligament*) and the pelvic wall (*suspensory ligament*).

Physical Examination of the Female Genitalia and Reproductive System

Inspection and palpation of the female pelvis can reveal many disorders of the reproductive organs, the lower urinary tract, and the lower abdomen. The pelvic examination is an extension of abdominal palpation and is mandatory for every female. Neglect of the pelvic examination often leads to serious errors in diagnosis. Routine Papanicolaou smear is effective in detecting early cervical cancer.

The Female Pelvic Examination

The pelvic examination should be at the end of the physical examination because it requires special positioning, equipment, and attendance of a female chaperone to assist. After emptying her bladder, the patient is placed in the lithotomy position on the examination table. Cover her body with a sheet, place her feet in stirrups attached to the table, and wrap the lower corners of the sheet around her legs, leaving considerable slack for the cloth to envelope the thighs and lower abdomen (Fig. 11–2A). When the patient is too weak to be examined on the table, have her assume the lithotomy position in bed elevating her pelvis on an inverted bedpan.

For a complete examination, the following sequence is suggested: (1) inspection of the vulva, (2) insertion of the vaginal speculum, (3) gathering of specimens for cytologic examination and bacteriologic tests, (4) inspection of the vaginal walls and cervix, (5) digital bimanual examination of the uterus and adnexa, (6) rectovaginal examination. Sit on a low stool within reach of a side table that holds specula, forceps, gauze, gloves, lubricating jelly, and the materials for making the Pap smear and cultures. Shine a bright light onto the perineum.

Inspection and Palpation of the Vulva (Fig. 11–2B). Observe the skin of the perineum for swelling, ulcers, and changes in color. Separate the labia with the gloved thumb and forefinger inspecting the clitoris, vestibule, urethral meatus and vaginal orifice. Palpate posteriorly and laterally to the hymen for enlargement of the Bartholin gland and for vestibular tenderness. Have the patient strain as if to defecate and look for bulging of the anterior or posterior vaginal wall through the introitus or leaking of urine.

Vaginal Speculum Examination (Fig. 11–3). Unlubricated vaginal speculum examination should precede digital examination because lubricating jelly

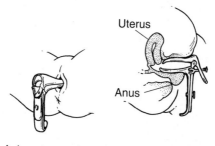

A. Insert speculum   B. Spread blades
of speculum

Fig. 11–3 *Using the Vaginal Speculum. The labia minora are retracted laterally with the gloved index and middle fingers. The closed blades of the vaginal speculum are inserted in the vagina with the widths of the blades almost horizontal. **A.** The closed blades of the speculum have been well inserted at a 30-degree to 45-degree angle posteriorly and the blades separated and locked open. **B.** A sagittal section shows the open blades of the speculum in proper position with the upper shorter blade lifting the vault of the vagina to expose the cervix uteri on the anterior vaginal wall.*

interferes with the Papanicolaou smear. Separating the vaginal walls by a speculum permits inspection of the vagina and cervix, and sample collection for cytologic and bacteriologic tests and for biopsies when indicted. Select a clean bivalve speculum of suitable size and ensure its proper temperature by immersing it in warm water.

With one hand grasp the handle and close the blades of the speculum while separating the labia minora at the level of the posterior fourchette with the other hand. Insert the closed blades into the vaginal orifice with slight downward pressure to avoid pinching the urethra against the symphysis pubis. When the speculum tips reach the upper vagina, separate the blades and illuminate the vaginal cavity with a suitable light. Move the speculum handle so the blade tips expose the cervix, then lock the blades open with the setscrew. If present, determine whether a discharge exudes from the cervical os or the vagina. When indicated, obtain a sample of discharge from the lateral and anterior vaginal walls for microscopic examination. If the cervical os is obscured by discharge, gently sponge it with a large, sterile cotton swab. Obtain specimens from the cervix for the *Pap test.* The cervical sample is obtained by gently scraping the cervix with a wooden spatula and turning a cytobrush in the cervical canal, or by using a special brush for liquid Pap preparation. When indicated, inoculate gonorrheal and chlamydial cultures from a swabbing of the cervical canal. Inspect the cervix for color, lacerations, ulcers, and new growths. Inspect the cervical os for size, shape, color, discharge, and polyps. Loosen the setscrew and *inspect the vaginal walls* by rotating the speculum to expose all the cavity. Look for abnormal redness or blueness of the mucosa and loss of rugation. Finally, carefully withdraw the speculum while inspecting the mucosa.

Bimanual pelvic examination. Always use the same hand for vaginal palpation. The invariable use of the same hand permits each hand to become accustomed

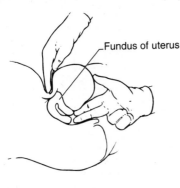

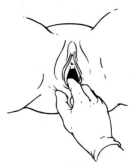

B. Palpating Bartholin's gland
(vulvovaginal gland)

A. Bimanual pelvic examination

Fig. 11–4 *Bimanual Pelvic Examination. A. Palpation of the Uterus: The index and middle fingers of the gloved right hand are inserted in the vagina with the tips of the fingers facing anteriorly and touching the cervix. The fingers of the left hand are pressed deep into the abdomen above the mons pubis, pushing the uterine fundus downward and forward toward the two vaginal fingers. The adnexa are examined similarly, except the vaginal fingers are placed to the side of the uterus and the abdominal fingers are pushed into the belly at a point 2 to 3 cm medial to the anterior superior iliac spine. Attempt to approximate the fingertips of the two examining hands. The abdominal fingers are pulled inferiorly to push the tube and ovary onto the tips of the vaginal fingers.* **B.** **Palpation of the greater vestibular gland (Bartholin gland***): The index finger is inserted in the vagina near the posterior introitus. The thumb is pressed outside on the labium majus and the finger and thumb are approximated.*

to its role. In the following directions, the right hand is arbitrarily assigned to the vagina and the left hand is employed to palpate the abdomen. When possible, use two fingers for vaginal examination.

Place the gloved right hand in the gynecologic position: index and middle fingers straight and close together, thumb widely abducted, fourth and fifth fingers folded into the palm. Lubricate the straight fingers; spread the labia with the left thumb and forefinger to avoid the discomfort of pulling pubic hair into the vagina. Insert the two lubricated fingers in the vaginal cavity with the finger pads facing the anterior vaginal wall (Fig. 11–4A). Examine each structure systematically forming a mental picture of your observations.

The *greater vestibular glands* (vulvovaginal glands or Bartholin glands) are examined with the forefinger inside the vagina and the thumb opposite and outside on the posterior part of the labium majus feeling the inner wall for abscess or tenderness (Fig. 11–4B). Evert that part of the vaginal mucosa to look for a red spot or pus marking the opening of an inflamed duct. The normal glands and ducts cannot be seen or felt. The *urethra* is palpated in the midline of the anterior vaginal wall near the introitus for tenderness or induration. The *base of bladder* is palpated in the midline of the anterior vaginal wall, halfway between the introitus and the cervix, for tenderness or induration produced by cystitis or neoplasm of the bladder. Palpate the *vaginal wall* for tenderness, induration (from scars, granulomas, or neoplasm), strictures, septa, and adhesions (not to be confused with the normal transverse rugae). Next, examine the *cervix* that normally feels like a button, with a convex face and a central depression, the consistency of the tip of the nose. Feel for nodules and ulcers and note any abnormality of shape, size, or consistency. Determine the axis of the cervix; normally it faces posteriorly in the same plane as the anterior vaginal wall. Examine the *uterine corpus and fundus* bimanually by pushing the cervix anteriorly while the fingers of the left hand press into the abdomen posteriorly just above the mons pubis. Estimate the size of the uterus, its axis, tenderness, mobility, and characterize any nodules that may be present. To examine the *adnexa*, place the vaginal fingers on one side of the cervix and push their tips superiorly and posteriorly as far as possible. With the fingers of the left hand, locate a point on the same side of the abdomen 2 to 3 cm medially from the anterior superior iliac spine. Push the abdominal fingers deep so their tips approach the vaginal fingers. This should bring the approximated hands back to the uterine tubes and ovaries. If the structures are not felt at that point, move the fingertips of both hands inferiorly toward the pubis, so that the adnexa pass between the two hands. Exert abdominal pressure gently, but deeply, pressing the two hands a little closer each time the patient expires to avoid abdominal guarding. The role of the abdominal hand should be to displace the structures, while the vaginal hand feels them. The normal ovary and tube are usually not palpable. When the normal *Fallopian tube* is felt, it is approximately 4 mm in diameter, approximately half the size of a common pencil. It has the consistency of a piece of rubber tubing. The normal *ovary* is approximately 3 cm × 2 cm × 2 cm; the lateral face is, therefore, approximately the size of the distal phalanx of the examiner's thumb, but the thickness of the ovary is approximately half that of the digit. The ovary is soft and naturally tender to palpation. Look for enlargement or asymmetry of the adnexa, unusual tenderness, decreased mobility, and other masses or induration. Examine the pelvic floor, noting the size of the introitus, and, with the examining fingers facing posteriorly, press the pelvic floor inferiorly and posteriorly to determine the resistance or relaxation.

Rectovaginal examination.   Conclude the pelvic examination with a rectovaginal examination. Ordinarily, the female genitalia are felt much more satisfactorily through the vagina than the rectum. In the virgin, however, vaginal palpation may not be feasible, and enough may be learned by rectal examination to make or exclude diagnoses.

After changing gloves, insert the middle finger of the gloved right hand into the anal canal with the forefinger in the vagina palpating the rectovaginal wall between the two fingers. Thickening of the rectovaginal septum or parametrium occurs from spread of cervical carcinoma, puerperal infection, and pelvic inflammatory disease. Note any distortion or defects in the circular *anal sphincter muscle*, a common consequence of vaginal delivery. Next, palpate the *anal canal* for intrinsic lesions (see page 460). Palpate the anterior *rectal wall* (posterior vaginal wall) for tenderness and masses then systematically examine the lateral and posterior rectum and ampulla. While using the left hand to press on the lower abdomen as in the bimanual vaginal examination, palpate the pelvis. Through the anterior rectal wall, locate the cervix; attempt to feel the *body and fundus of the uterus*. This may be the only route by which a retroverted uterus is palpable. Insert your finger fully and palpate the anterior rectal wall in the region of the peritoneal *rectovaginal pouch* (cul-de-sac of Douglas; see Fig. 11–1).

Female Genital and Reproductive Symptoms

General Symptoms

> **KEY SYMPTOM** Pelvic Pain

Pain arises from inflammation, usually as the result of infection, distention of tubular structures or cysts, traction on serosal surfaces by masses or adhesions, hemorrhage, and invasion of sensitive structures by neoplasms or implantation of endometrial tissue. Visceral pain is poorly localized whereas serosal pain is usually well localized by the patient. Pain in the pelvis is common. It is essential to obtain a complete history of the patient's pain pattern, its relationship to menses, ovulation, bowel movements, urination, and physical and sexual activity. Describe the pain quality using the patient's words. The pelvic examination must be gentle and the patient relaxed for the examiner to localize the pain to a specific area or structure.

✔ *PELVIC PAIN—CLINICAL OCCURRENCE:* *Congenital* imperforate hymen, porphyria; *Endocrine* ectopic pregnancy, functional ovarian cysts; *Idiopathic* ovarian cysts, especially with hemorrhage or rupture, endometriosis, ovulation (mittelschmerz), diverticulosis; *Inflammatory/Immune* inflammatory bowel disease, appendicitis; *Infectious* cervicitis, endometritis, salpingitis, tuboovarian abscess, cystitis, diverticulitis and diverticular abscess, appendicitis; *Mechanical/Traumatic* ovarian torsion, tubal pregnancy; *Neoplastic* any locally invasive cancer (e.g., cervical, endometrial, rectal, bladder), metastases, degenerating leiomyoma; *Psychosocial* physical, emotional, and sexual abuse; *Vascular* ovarian infarction (torsion).

> **KEY SYMPTOM** Painful Menstruation (Dysmenorrhea)

Primary dysmenorrhea results from uterine ischemia caused by myometrial contraction under the influence of prostaglandins released during menstruation. Pain accompanying menses but arising from disease in the pelvis is secondary dysmenorrhea. The most prominent and most frequent complaint is severe abdominal cramps in the suprapubic region. Less severe are accompanying backache and headache. Dysmenorrhea may disappear after a pregnancy. Prostaglandin inhibitors can be quite helpful and may be used prophylactically. Secondary dysmenorrhea may result from endometriosis, pelvic neoplasms, and pelvic inflammations.

> **KEY SYMPTOM** Painful Intercourse—Dyspareunia

Physical stimulation of pelvic structures during vaginal intercourse can lead to pain preventing sexual enjoyment. Anxiety and fear increase perception of pain. Inquire whether the pain is felt superficially or deeply after penetration. Ask specifically whether the patient has sufficient stimulation to become sexually aroused, about the sufficiency of vaginal lubrication, whether the partner is so aggressive as to cause trauma, and any bleeding after intercourse. Inquire about sexual practices, including the use of foreign bodies as stimulants, rectal intercourse, and whether previous experiences have produced a fear of intercourse (for example, rape, incest, molestation, and physical and emotional abuse).   *CLINICAL OCCUR-RENCE:*   Insufficient foreplay, inadequate lubrication, postmenopausal estrogen deficiency with dryness of vaginal mucosa, vaginismus (reflex spasm of muscles around the lower vaginal opening), vulvar vestibulitis, lichen planus, perineal trauma and lacerations, pelvic and perineal infections, pelvic tumors.

> **KEY SYMPTOM**   Menstrual Disorders

See Female Reproductive Syndromes. Menstrual Disorders, page 559.

Vulvar and Vaginal Symptoms

> **KEY SYMPTOM**   Vulvar Pain

The vulva is somatically innervated and pain perception and localization are good. Infection, inflammation, and local trauma are the most common identifiable causes of pain. *Dysesthetic vulvodynia* may be neuropathic and *vulvar vestibulitis* may have an inflammatory basis.

Vaginal Pain—Vaginismus: Painful contraction of the pubococcygeus muscle around the lower third of the vagina results in severe pain that can be persistent or intermittent. The cause is unknown and treatment is difficult. Intercourse is painful or impossible.

> **KEY SYMPTOM**   Vulvar Pruritus

Itching of the vulva is usually the result of obvious disease or chemical irritation of the vulvar skin. *Candida* infection and lichen sclerosis are common etiologies.

> **KEY SYMPTOM**   Vaginal Bleeding

See Female Reproductive Tract Syndromes—Menstrual Disorders, page 559.

Female Genital and Reproductive Signs

Vulvar Signs

> **KEY SIGN**   Ambiguous Genitalia—Intersexuality

Refer to special works on this subject.

> **KEY SIGN**   Genital Ulcer

Trauma and sexually transmitted diseases are the most common causes. Painless ulcers are most typical of syphilis. Ulcers increase the risk of transmitting and acquiring sexually transmitted infections (STIs) including HIV. Ulcers may be both more painful and slower healing in women than in men because of persistent warmth and moisture. See also pages 562 and 581ff.   *CLINICAL OC-CURRENCE:*   lichen sclerosis, Behçet syndrome, vulvar vestibulitis, fixed drug reaction, lichen planus, herpes simplex types 1 and 2, chlamydia, syphilis, chancroid, lymphogranuloma venereum, HIV, cytomegalovirus, Epstein-Barr virus, granuloma inguinale, inadequate lubrication during intercourse, squamous cell cancer.

KEY SIGN Vulvar Rash

Determine if the rash is acute or chronic, pruritic, weeping or scaling, associated with bleeding or pain, or with the use of topical and systemic medications, creams, and lotions.

✔ VULVAR RASH—CLINICAL OCCURRENCE: See also Vulvar Inflammation—Vulvitis, below. *Endocrine* atrophic vulvovaginitis; *Idiopathic* lichen sclerosis; *Inflammatory/Immune* contact dermatitis; *Infectious* candidiasis, dermatophytes, cellulitis, abscess of skin and mucosal glands; *Metabolic/Toxic* diabetes mellitus; *Mechanical/Traumatic* abrasions and lacerations, tight-fitting clothing with poor ventilation; *Neoplastic* Bowen disease, vulvar carcinoma; *Psychosocial* pruritis vulvae, pruritis ani.

KEY SIGN Vulvar Inflammation—Vulvitis

The skin is often red, warm, and variably edematous and tender. The condition may be associated with vaginitis and discharge, or occur alone. Alternatively, the skin may appear thinned, atrophic or opaque, and white. The latter changes are more common in lichen sclerosis and lichen planus. *CLINICAL OCCURRENCE:* contact dermatitis, vulvar vestibulitis, lichen planus, lichen sclerosis, cellulitis, *candida*, dermatophyte, topical irritants, tight-fitting clothing, diffuse bowen disease.

Atrophic Vulvovaginitis: Withdrawal of estrogen leads to skin which is thinned, inelastic, and easily irritated and inflamed. A careful history focusing on menstrul pattern and symptoms of estrogen insufficiency, especially hot flushes, point to the diagnosis. Examination shows absent rugae and a thin dry mucosa (see page 552).

KEY SIGN Vulvar Swelling, Masses, and Growths

All the normal vulvar structures are susceptible to neoplastic change. Infection with human papilloma virus or syphilis can produce condylomas. Evaluation is identical to other skin growths with special respect for the sensitivity of the tissues and the need to maintain cosmesis. *CLINICAL OCCURRENCE:* *Inflammatory/Immune* granulomatous disease; *Infectious* condyloma latum (syphilis), condyloma acuminatum (human papilloma virus), histoplasmosis; *Mechanical/Traumatic* obstructed mucosal glands and Bartholin and Skene glands; *Neoplastic* Bowen disease, melanoma, invasive squamous cell cancer.

Diffuse Swelling of the Vulva: Obstruction of the lymphatic channels from any cause may produce lymphedema of the labia and surrounding tissues. Likewise, the labia will be edematous when systemic venous pressure is very high and dependent edema reaches above the inguinal ligaments, for example, advanced right ventricular failure or constrictive pericarditis. Irritation may produce hypertrophy of the labia. Look for local irritation and history and physical finding for systemic disease affecting the lymphatics or venous system.

Hematoma: A large, painful, bluish swelling of the labium may occur within a few hours after local trauma. Without a history of trauma, the condition may be confused with cellulitis of the vulva.

Labioinguinal Hernia: Failure of the peritoneal pouch to obliterate in the fetus may permit a hernia to descend from the abdomen into the labium majus. It is analogous to the scrotal hernia in the male and presents with visible swelling.

> **KEY SIGN**   **Abscess of the Greater Vestibular Gland (Bartholin Gland Abscess)**

Bartholin gland cysts are common and asymptomatic. Infection of the cyst leads to abcess formation, which may track to the skin or toward the ischiorectal fossa. The normal glands are not palpable and their ducts are not visible. Epidermal inclusion cysts are a common cause of swelling. Cysts and smaller abscesses are found only by vaginal examination (Fig. 11–4B). Inflammation causes a red spot in the mucosa at the site of the ductal orifice, and pus may be expressed from it. If the abscess is large, the posterior portion of the labium is swollen and fluctuant and the overlying skin is tender, hot, and red.

> **KEY SIGN**   **Urethral Meatus Abnormalities**

Urethritis.   See also *Urinary Syndromes, Urinary Tract Infections—Urethritis,* Chapter 10, page 539. A purulent discharge issues from the meatus. This is usually caused by the inflammation from *Neisseria gonorrhoea, Chlamydia trachomatis,* genital mycoplasmas or herpes simplex. Palpation of the anterior vaginal wall, beginning at the cervix and stroking toward the meatus, reveals tenderness and induration along the course of the urethra. Pus may be squeezed from the meatus in this manner. A urethral diverticulum may also produce pus.

Urethral Caruncle: This papilloma appears as a small red mass in the meatus or the visible portion of the urethra. It usually occurs as a complication of urethritis. It may be tender and painful on urination.

Inflammation of the Periurethral (Skene) Gland and Duct: The periurethral gland (the Skene gland) lies on either side of, and posterior to, the female urethra, just inside the meatus. Often it becomes the site of chronic infection. If inflamed, the mouth of the duct is visible and red, when reviewed on spreading of the meatus.

Prolapse of the Urethra: Slight gaping of the meatus is common in the multipara. When more severe, the urethral mucosa may protrude from the meatus and become tender and inflamed.

Vaginal Signs

> **KEY SIGN**   **Vaginal Ulcers**

The same types that occur on the vulva may involve the vaginal mucosa; see page 555.

> **KEY SIGN** Vaginal Discharge and Vaginitis

A clear to slightly white vaginal discharge containing mucous, epithelial cells, and commensal bacteria (particularly lactobacilli) at a pH of 4.0 is normal. Infection and/or inflammation lead to increased mucous production and exudation of white blood cells from the mucosa, producing vaginal discharges. Depending upon etiology, discharges vary from thick white to thin, frothy, and bloody with variable odor, pH, and accompanying pruritis. [Eckert LO. Acute vulvovaginitis. *N Engl J Med*. 2006;355:1244–1252] *CLINICAL OCCURRENCE:* atrophic vaginitis, contact dermatitis, bacterial vaginosis, *Candida, Trichomonas*, cytolytic vaginosis, retained tampons, pessary, foreign body, vaginal and cervical cancers (often bloody).

Vaginitis. Inflammation of the vaginal mucosa from infection, allergy, or irritants leads to erythema. History and examination of the vaginal secretions will usually yield a diagnosis. *CLINICAL OCCURRENCE:* contact dermatitis, Behçet disease, *Candida, Trichomonas*, bacterial vaginosis, viral enanthems, cytolytic vaginosis, retained foreign bodies, inadequate lubrication during intercourse, diffuse Bowen disease.

Vulvovaginal Candidiasis: Itching, pain, dyspareunia, with erythema and edema characterize infection with *Candida albicans*. The discharge has a normal vaginal pH (<4.6) and pseudohyphae and many neutrophils can be identified in a 10% KOH preparation. Culture may be needed to confirm the diagnosis and distinguish it from less-common noninfectious causes.

Trichomonas Vaginitis: *Trichomonas vaginalis* produces a tender, reddened mucosa, studded with small hemorrhagic spots. The resulting malodorous discharge is yellow-green to gray and is frequently frothy, with a pH of 5.0 to 6.0. In a more chronic stage, the vaginal mucosa contains scattered red papules, giving a granular appearance. Rapid diagnosis may be made by suspending a bit of discharge in isotonic saline solution and finding many neutrophils and mobile trichomonads by microscopic examination.

Atrophic Vaginitis: The vaginal mucosa is estrogen dependent and following menopause becomes thin, dry, and smooth without rugae. The thin and tender mucosa contains abraded patches and adhesions that bleed easily. Frequently, a serosanguinous discharge with a pH greater than 6.0 results.

Bacterial Vaginosis: This is one of the most common causes of vaginitis in women of childbearing age. They present with a thick, off-white, malodorous discharge with a "fishy smell" and a pH greater than 4.5. Diagnosis is confirmed by finding clue cells (exfoliated vaginal epithelial cells to which *Gardnerella vaginalis* adhere) in vaginal secretions. Cultures are of no value because *G. vaginalis* is present in 50% to 60% of healthy women.

Cytolytic Vaginosis: Overgrowth of Lactobacillus spp. produces a low vaginal pH leading to breakdown of epithelial cells and inflammation. The vaginal pH is between 3.5 and 4.5, and microscopic examination shows few polymorphonuclear cells, cytolytic changes in the epithelial cells, and no evidence of *Candida, Trichomonas*, or bacterial vaginosis.

Bluish vagina—cyanosis. The mucosa becomes cyanotic as a result of local venous engorgement in pregnancy or a pelvic tumor. The generalized cyanosis of congestive cardiac failure is also visible in the mucosal lining.

Vaginal mass—neoplasm.   Neoplasms in the vaginal mucosa may be primary or secondary to carcinoma of the uterus, rectum, bladder, or external genitalia.

Vaginal mass—vaginal Polyp.   Polyps can arise from the vaginal wall or extend from the cervix. Polypoid deformities of the vaginal apex following hysterectomy are common.

Masses in the rectovaginal pouch.   Because the rectovaginal pouch is the most dependent portion of the abdominal cavity, it collects fluid, exfoliated cells, and mobile masses from within the abdomen. Masses include prolapsed ovary, bowel loops, carcinoma of the colon, implants of endometriosis or ovarian carcinoma, a rectal shelf formed by other intraabdominal cancer, or an accumulation of pus, fluid, or blood from abdominal lesions.

Rectovaginal fistula.   Breakdown of the rectovaginal wall occurs after extensive radiation, obstetrical trauma, surgery, Crohn disease, and malignancy. A fistula from rectum to vagina is suggested by the history of fecal contamination of the vagina. The mouth of the fistula may be palpable as a small patch of induration in the posterior wall of the vagina and the orifice may be visible on speculum exam. The rectal wall may be indurated from scar tissue.

> **KEY SIGN   Pelvic Floor Relaxation**

The muscular pelvic floor is pierced by the rectum, vagina, and urethra. It is subject to extensive trauma during vaginal delivery, which stretches and may tear the muscles. Tearing of the urethral and anal sphincters may also occur. Inadequate support of the pelvic organs leads to loss of sphincter functions and prolapse of tissues. Patients complain of incontinence, feelings of pressure and fullness, and the occurrence of visible or palpable prolapsing tissues.

Enlarged entroitus: When the hymen is ruptured, the vaginal orifice normally admits the examiner's two fingers. When three fingers are accommodated, the introitus is definitely enlarged, usually indicating some degree of pelvic relaxation from childbirth.

Cystocele (bladder prolapse).   When the patient stands or strains, the anterior vaginal wall containing a portion of the bladder, bulges into the vagina and may emerge from the introitus as a soft, spheric tumor (Fig. 11–5B). This finding usually indicates pelvic floor laceration during childbirth.

Rectocele (rectal prolapse).   When the patient stands or strains, the posterior vaginal wall, containing a portion of the rectum, protrudes into the vagina and may emerge from the introitus (Fig. 11–5B). This is also evidence of pelvic floor laceration during childbirth. Examination in the left decubitus position may be better able to detect larger rectoceles than examination with the patient supine.

Uterine prolapse.   When the patient stands or strains, the cervix may protrude from the introitus. This results from loss of the normal ligamentous support for the uterus.

Cervical Signs

Cyanosis.   Bluish discoloration of the cervix is a sign of early pregnancy (Chadwick sign). It also occurs in tumors of the pelvis and in congestive cardiac failure.

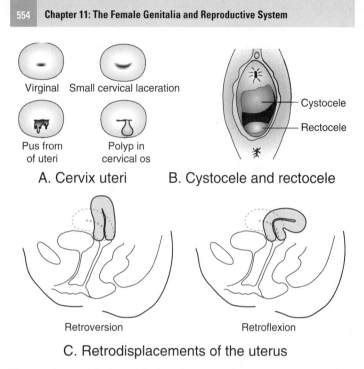

Virginal   Small cervical laceration

Pus from   Polyp in
of uteri   cervical os

Cystocele

Rectocele

A. Cervix uteri   B. Cystocele and rectocele

Retroversion   Retroflexion

C. Retrodisplacements of the uterus

Fig. 11–5 *Some Pelvic Signs. A. Lesions of the cervix:* *The lacerations of childbirth leave various scars. Pus or a polyp may be seen coming out from the os.* *B. Cystocele and rectocele:* *When the patient is asked to strain as if to defecate, the introitus widens and bulging may develop anteriorly (cystocele) or posteriorly (rectocele).* *C. Uterine displacements:* *If the axis of the uterus remains straight and the whole organ is tilted, it is called retroversion. If the axis of the uterus is bent, the condition is called retroflexion.*

Softening.   An early sign of pregnancy is softening of the cervix in the first trimester.

Lacerations.   During vaginal delivery, the cervix frequently sustains some laceration (Fig. 11–5A). Commonly, the tear is transverse and bilateral; occasionally, the laceration is unilateral, or multiple tears produce a stellate lesion. Recently torn edges appear raw. In a few weeks, healing leaves scarred fissures or notches. The cleft lips of the cervix may become everted; healing may be incomplete, causing an area of erosion. Healed lacerations of the cervix leave notches or fissures in the surface of the cervix that can be felt with the finger.

Eversion.   Velvety red mucosa, without ulceration, extending outward from the cervical os is usually the result of migration of the endocervical tissue onto the visible portions of the cervix.

> **KEY SIGN**   **Discharge—Endocervicitis**

While the vagina is quite resistant, the columnar epithelium of the endocervix is particularly susceptible to infection with gonorrhea, chlamydia, herpes, and genital mycoplasmas. A mucopurulent or purulent discharge emerges from the cervix os (Fig. 11–5A). The cervical lips are usually inflamed and eroded. The absence of tenderness on palpation of the uterine fundus suggests that the infection is limited to the cervical canal. Cervicitis is acute and is usually caused by gonorrhea or chlamydial infection. Extension into the uterine cavity and tubes produces endometritis and pelvic inflammatory disease, which can lead to tuboovarian abcess and sterility.

Endometritis: See Uterine Signs—Endometritis, page 556.

KEY SIGN Ulcer

There is a loss of epithelium and sloughing of underlying tissue. Specific causes are herpes simplex, chancroid, syphilis, tuberculosis, and carcinoma. Biopsy is indicated when tests for microbial diseases are negative. This may result from the abrasion of a pessary.

Hypertrophic cervix.   The lips of the cervix may enlarge and elongate. This most frequently occurs in parous women. In hypertrophy the fundus retains its normal position. In uterine prolapse the cervix is also more visible as fundus descends toward the vaginal orifice, but not enlarged. The cervix retains its normal contour in hypertrophy, whereas neoplasm distorts the proportions.

Cervical polyp.   A soft, bright-red, benign tumor, usually pedunculated, often emerges from the cervical os (Fig. 11–5A). It may cause discharge and bleeding.

Cervical cysts.   Occlusion of glands in the cervical mucosa causes 1 to 3 mm clear or white retention cysts, called *nabothian cysts*, that are visible on speculum examination.

Cervical carcinoma.   Frequently, a bloody discharge follows straining or coitus. Whereas a cervical polyp is small and soft, a hard mass in the cervix suggests a neoplasm, which should prompt Pap smear and cervical biopsy. A chronic ulcer of the cervix with induration is a late sign of carcinoma. In the later stages, extensive ulceration, induration, and nodularity make the diagnosis obvious.

Uterine Signs

Uterine positions.   (Fig. 11–5C.) The most common position of the uterine body is anteriorly in the same axis as the cervix.   *Retroversion*   is displacement of both fundus and cervix in a common axis and is present in 25% of normal women. The axis of the fundus and cervix is in the direction of the spine and the plane of the cervix faces the anterior wall of the vagina. The fundus encroaches upon the rectum. The uterine fundus may be felt through the anterior rectal wall when it cannot be palpated per vagina. When freely movable, it is symptomless; when fixed, it suggests endometriosis.   *Retroflexion*   is posterior displacement of the fundus. The plane of the cervix is in the normal position but the fundus is palpable through the posterior fornix and rectum (Fig. 11–5C).   *Lateral displacement*   of the uterus is frequently caused by adhesions or masses in the adnexa.

KEY SIGN Softening (Hegar Sign)

During the first trimester of pregnancy, junction of the cervix with the body of the uterus softens. This change in consistency is easily palpable; sometimes the contrast between fundus and isthmus is so pronounced that the cervix seems to separate from the fundus [Bastian LA, Piscitelli JT. The rational clinical examination. Is this patient pregnant? Can you reliably rule in or rule out early pregnancy by clinical examination? *JAMA.* 1997;278:586–591].

KEY SIGN   Tenderness—Endometritis

The appearance of the cervix is similar to that in endocervicitis, but tenderness of the uterine body or fundus indicates involvement of the endometrium. Endometritis is caused by sexually transmitted diseases (gonorrhea, chlamydia, and mycoplasmas) or by infection following childbirth or abortion.

KEY SIGN   Uterine Enlargement—Pregnancy

Generalized uterine enlargement in a woman of childbearing age should be considered a pregnancy until proven otherwise. Initially, the gravid uterus becomes globular or more rounded in shape. Other symptoms and signs of pregnancy are morning sickness, tenderness of the breasts, amenorrhea, cyanosis of the vaginal and cervical mucosa (Chadwick sign), softening of the cervix, and softening of the uterine isthmus (Hegar sign). Pregnancy testing is mandatory. The gravid uterus may be distinguished from large ovarian cysts by hearing the fetal heartbeat, remembering that concurrence of ovarian cysts with pregnancy is common. The height of the uterus reflects the stages of pregnancy: 3 months, at the pubis; 4.5 months, at the umbilicus; 9 months, at the xiphoid.

KEY SIGN   Uterine Enlargement—Leiomyoma (Fibroid)

Hard, often painless nodules, frequently multiple, are firmly attached to the uterus. The nodules and the fundus move freely together. An asymmetric gravid uterus is sometimes mistaken for a uterine fibroid in a woman of childbearing age. Fibroids are three to five times more common in blacks than in whites [Stewart EA. Uterine fibroids. *Lancet.* 2001;357:293–298].

KEY SIGN   Uterine Enlargement—Neoplasm of the Uterus

Carcinoma and sarcoma of the uterus produce more-generalized or less-generalized enlargement, which may be associated with bloody discharge. Evaluate with ultrasonography and seek gynecologic evaluation.

Adnexal Signs

Endometriosis.   See Female Genital and Reproductive Syndromes, Endometriosis, page 562.

KEY SIGN   Adnexal Tenderness

Pain arises from inflammation of structures, usually as the result of infection, and from distention of tubular structures or cysts, traction on serosal surfaces by masses or adhesions, hemorrhage, and invasion of sensitive structures by neoplasms or implantation of endometrial tissue. It is essential to obtain a complete history of the patient's pain pattern, its relationship to menses, ovulation, bowel movements, urination, and physical and sexual activity. The pelvic examination must be gentle and the patient relaxed for the examiner to localize the pain to a specific area or structure.

✔ *ADNEXAL TENDERNESS—CLINICAL OCCURRENCE:* *Congenital* imperforate hymen, porphyria; *Idiopathic* ovarian cysts, especially with hemorrhage or rupture, ovulation (mittelschmerz), endometriosis, diverticulosis; *Inflammatory/Immune* inflammatory bowel disease, appendicitis; *Infectious* cervicitis, endometritis, salpingitis, tuboovarian abscess, cystitis, diverticulitis and diverticular abscess, appendicitis; *Mechanical/Traumatic* ovarian torsion, tubal pregnancy; *Neoplastic* any locally invasive cancer, for example, ovarian, cervical, endometrial, rectal, bladder, metastatic, appendicitis; *Vascular* ovarian infarction (torsion).

KEY SIGN **Adnexal Mass—Pelvic Inflammatory Disease (Salpingitis, Hydrosalpinx, Pyosalpinx, Tuboovarian Abscess)**

Infection ascends from the cervix via the endometrium. Sexually transmitted organisms (gonorrhea, chlamydia, mycoplasmas) initiate infection, but aerobic and anaerobic enteric florae are frequent secondary complications in the advanced stages of infection. With acute infections, the Fallopian tubes are tender and swollen, which frequently obscures the separate structures in the adnexa. Movement of the uterus and cervix is extremely painful. In more chronic stages, the exudate and fibrosis around the tubes feel like an unyielding mass, termed *a frozen pelvis*. When adhesions or inflammation seal a tube at both ends it may become filled with fluid or pus, felt as a sausage-shaped mass, termed a hydrosalpinx and pyosalpinx, respectively. When the ovary and broad ligament become involved a tuboovarian abscess is formed. See also page 562, STIs.

KEY SIGN **Tubal Mass—Ectopic Pregnancy**

See page 558. Irregular vaginal bleeding and pelvic pain during childbearing years indicates ectopic pregnancy until proven otherwise. Thickening, or a mass, may or may not be appreciated in the adnexa. Softening of the cervix and fundus occurs with tubal pregnancy, as well as with intrauterine pregnancy. Movement of the uterus and cervix is painful. Occasionally, a bulging mass is felt in the rectovaginal pouch from a pelvic hematoma.

Ovarian Mass—Oophoritis: Although inflammation of an ovary causes it to enlarge, the change in size is usually not detected by palpation because the inflammatory process also involves the tubes making identification of the component structures difficult.

KEY SIGN **Ovarian Mass**

Neoplasm. Both benign and malignant neoplasms may involve the ovaries; diagnosis is made by pathology of a surgical specimen. The sensitivity of physical examination, even in experienced hands, is insuffficient to recommend it as screening for adnexal masses [Padilla LA, Radosevich DM, Milad MP. Accuracy of the pelvic examination in detecting adnexal masses. *Obstet Gynecol*. 2000;96:593–598].

Endometriosis. Enlargement of the ovaries is frequently encountered in endometriosis (page 562).

Cyst.   See Female Genital and Reproductive Syndromes—Ovarian Cysts, page 561. A firm or slightly fluctuant, nontender spheroidal mass is felt in the region of the ovary. Large cysts that emerge from the pelvis into the abdomen must be distinguished from other abdominal masses (see Chapter 9, page 520).

Rectal Signs

Healed Anal Laceration.   This is usually the result of childbirth, but it may be evidence of sexual abuse. Partial sphincter lacerations are common. If the laceration extended through the anal canal the edges of the anus are either not approximated or form an irregular line rather than a depression with puckered borders. Palpation reveals weakness and a defect in the sphincter. When the sphincter ani is severed, the condition is termed a third-degree laceration. See Fecal Incontinence in Chapter 9, page 468.

Female Genital and Reproductive Syndromes

➤ **KEY SYNDROME**   **Ectopic Pregnancy**

Implantation of the fertilized ovum normally occurs in the endometrium. Implantation can occur in the Fallopian tubes, ovary, or peritoneum. Presentation depends upon the site of implantation. Pain and bleeding are frequent. These pregnancies are not viable to term and must be aborted surgically or pharmacologically to protect the woman from life threatening hemorrhage [Dart RG, Kaplan B, Varaklis K. Predictive value of history and physical examination in patients with suspected ectopic pregnancy. *Ann Emerg Med.* 1999;33:283–290].

➤ **KEY SYNDROME**   **Abdominal Pain and Pallor—Rupture and Hemorrhage from Tubal Pregnancy**

Tubal pregnancy occurs most commonly as the result of previous pelvic inflammatory disease with tubal scarring or previous tubal surgery. Implantation of the fertilized ovum in the tube results in a tubal pregnancy, which stretches and finally ruptures the wall. Since the tube has become very vascular the result is a sudden, large-volume hemorrhage into the peritoneal cavity. Uterine bleeding or spotting is common. Because rupture of tubal pregnancy usually occurs in the first 8 weeks of gestation, menstrual irregularities may have been slight or unnoticed. Often, a previously healthy young woman presents with agonizing poorly localized abdominal and pelvic pain. Sometimes the pain begins in the suprapubic or pelvic region, probably from serosal inflammation and premonatory small volume bleeding prior to frank rupture. The abdomen is quiet, increasingly tender, and rigidity develops progressively. The abdomen becomes distended and evidence of free fluid may appear. Signs of hemorrhagic shock develop quickly. With subacute hemorrhage, the symptoms are not so severe. The patient may be seen after the first episode has subsided, when hemorrhage has ceased. Blood in the pelvis gives a sense of fullness when palpating the fornices. A definite mass of clot or liquid blood may be present in the rectouterine pouch. Urine pregnancy tests must be obtained in all women of childbearing age with abdominal pain. Transvaginal ultrasonography is diagnostic. One must suspect ectopic pregnancy in any fertile woman with acute abdominal pain. The severe attack must be distinguished from most other causes of acute abdominal pain. Ectopic pregnancy in other locations (ovary, broad ligament, abdomen) can also present with pain and abdominal bleeding.

> **KEY SYNDROME** Abdominal Pain and Pallor—Follicular and Corpus Luteum Hemorrhage

Rupture of the ovarian surface to release the ovum into the Fallopian tube can result in pain (*mittelschmerz*). Persistant bleeding, especially in women on anticoagulants, can occur. The corpus luteum matures over 7 to 10 days and rupture of a corpus luteum cyst usually occurs around the onset of menses. Minor bleeding may be symptomless, but, when heavy, the classic signs of intraabdominal hemorrhage result (see discussion of tubal pregnancy above). Sonography will show free fluid (blood) in the peritoneal cavity and may demonstrate the follicular or corpus luteum cyst.

> **KEY SYNDROME** Menstrual Disorders

Menstruation usually begins (*menarche*) between the ages of 12 and 15 years in temperate climates and at 9 or 10 years in the tropics. The anterior pituitary gland produces FSH and LH, in response to pulsitile hypothalamic secretion of gonadotropin-releasing hormone (GnRH). FSH causes the maturation of an ovarian graafian follicle by growth of its granulosa cells and the formation of follicular fluid. In combination with FSH, LH causes the theca interna to secrete estrogen. The mature follicle ruptures through the ovarian surface, releasing the ovum. It enters the fimbriated end of the Fallopian tube passing down the tube and, if fertilized, implants in the endometrium. The ruptured ovarian follicle becomes the corpus luteum, whose cells secrete both estrogen and progesterone under the influence of LH and FSH. If the ovum is not fertilized, the corpus luteum gradually degenerates and scarifies. Ovulation occurs approximately 2 weeks before menstruation. During the time when estrogen is the primary secretion (*follicular phase*), the uterine endometrium undergoes proliferation. Later, when the secretion of progesterone predominates (*luteal phase*), the endometrium differentiates into secretory endometrium. With involution of the corpus luteum and decline in estrogen and progesterone, the endometrium degenerates and sloughs as menstrual blood. The menstrual cycle usually recurs in periods of 27 to 32 days, although great variability exists. The menstrual flow lasts approximately 5 days. During the entire menses, the usual blood loss is from 60 to 250 mL, most during the first and second days. A menstrual pad is considered filled when it contains 30 to 50 mL of blood. The menopause may occur between the ages of 40 and 55 years. Menstrual disturbances may be caused by disorders of the anterior pituitary gland, the hypothalamus, the thyroid gland, the ovary, or the uterus.

It is first necessary to establish the woman's normal menstrual pattern starting at menarche, including the menstrual cycle length, the amount and duration of normal flow, and her history of conception, live births, abortions, stillbirths, and contraception. Determine the time of the last normal cycle and then seek specific information about the current problem. It is important to differentiate problems of cycle length (early or delayed menses), duration of flow (protracted or short), quantity of flow (too much or too little) and associated symptoms, for example, pain (dysmenorrhea). The terminology for these disorders can be confusing so use clear descriptions, avoiding Greek and Latin obscurations. Evaluation of menstrual abnormalities requires a thorough history, complete pelvic examination, and evaluation of the woman's hormonal status, frequently combined with imaging of the pelvis and/or endometrial sampling. Remember that pregnancy and menopause are the most common causes of menstrual disorder.

Profuse Menstruation—Menorrhagia: Menorrhagia is the condition in which menstruation persists longer or the daily volume of flow is greater than normal. Excessive blood loss with menorrhagia is a common cause of iron-deficiency with or without anemia. ***CLINICAL OCCURRENCE:*** persistence of the corpus luteum, anovulation, perimenopause, hypothyroidism, endocervical and endometrial polyps, endometriosis, SLE, endometritis, salpingitis, scurvy, uterine leiomyoma, endometrial hyperplasia or carcinoma, leukemia, coagulation defects (thrombocytopenia, von Willebrand disease, hemophilia).

Intermenstrual and Irregular Bleeding—Metrorrhagia: Irregular and intermenstrual bleeding suggests an abnormality of the endometrium. Although metrorrhagia is commonly synonymous with intermenstrual bleeding, it also refers to irregular bleeding. Some causes of heavy bleeding, in more severe form, produce irrregular bleeding as well. The most common causes are endometritis, uterine leiomyoma, endometrial polyp, cervical polyps, cervical and endometrial cancer, pregnancy, ectopic pregnancy, threatened abortion, and retained products of conception.

Primary Amenorrhea: Primary amenorrhea is failure to initiate regular menstrual cycles at a chronologically appropriate age. It results from genetic, endocrinologic, or anatomic abnormalities of sex chromatin, sexual differentiation, and/or sexual maturation. Severe psychologic stress can result in amenorrhea in otherwise normal individuals. The examination should focus upon the correlation of sexual and somatic maturation with chronological age and, if necessary, bone age. Obtain growth records from birth to identify long-standing growth problems. Estimate the stage of secondary sexual development by using the Tanner system of classification. In addition to confirming normal external genitalia by physical examination, imaging studies may be needed to confirm the presence of a normal vagina, uterus, and ovaries.

✔ *PRIMARY AMENORRHEA—CLINICAL OCCURRENCE:*   *Congenital* delayed puberty, uterine agenesis, imperforate hymen (cryptomenorrhea), ovarian agenesis or dysgenesis (Turner syndrome), and other disorders of sex chromosomes; *Endocrine* hypo- and hyperthyroidism, hypopituitarism, androgens; *Metabolic/Toxic* lead, mercury, morphine, alcohol, malnutrition, chemotherapy, excessive exercise, obesity, debilitating diseases; *Mechanical/Traumatic* hysterectomy, oophorectomy, pelvic irradiation; *Neoplastic* androgen-producing tumors, prolactinoma, craniopharyngioma; *Psychosocial* anorexia nervosa, depression.

Gonadal Dysgenesis—Turner Syndrome, Ovarian Agenesis: There is an inherited deficiency of one X chromosome. The karyotype is XO with no Y and a diploid number of 45 in 80% of cases. Congenitally fibrotic ovarian anlagen is associated with negative (male pattern) sex chromatin of buccal mucosal cells and neutrophils. There is short stature, webbed neck, a shield-like chest, cubitus valgus, short metacarpals, lymphedema, and infantile female genitalia and breasts. Sexual maturation is delayed with primary amenorrhea and delayed growth of axillary and pubic hair.

Secondary Amenorrhea: Secondary amenorrhea is the cessation of menstrual cycles after previous menstrual bleeding. It results from endocrinologic or anatomic abnormalities. Severe psychologic stress can result in amenorrhea in genetically, endocrinologically, and anatomically normal individuals. Evaluation of secondary amenorrhea requires a detailed personal medical, psychologic and menstrual history, a family history, and physical examination with attention to signs of endocrine disease. Secondary amenorrhea is expected in midlife, associated with ovarian aging (menopause). Pregnancy is the most common cause of secondary amenorrhea in women of childbearing age.

✔ SECONDARY AMENORRHEA—CLINICAL OCCURRENCE: *Congenital* polycystic ovary syndrome, adrenal hyperplasia; *Endocrine* pregnancy, menopause, hyper- and hypothyroidism, hypopituitarism, primary ovarian failure, hormonal contraceptives, elevated prolactin, diabetes; *Inflammatory/Immune* SLE, vasculitis; *Infectious* HIV, tuberculosis; *Metabolic/Toxic* lead, mercury, morphine, alcohol, malnutrition, chemotherapy, excessive exercise, obesity, debilitating diseases; *Mechanical/Traumatic* hysterectomy, oophorectomy, pelvic irradiation, after uterine curettage; *Neoplastic* androgen-producing tumors, prolactinoma; *Psychosocial* anorexia nervosa, depression.

Polycystic Ovary Syndrome: Increased production of androgenic steroids by the ovary, or, less commonly, the adrenal, is associated with insulin resistance and impaired fertility because of anovulation. Genetic factors are important, although the genes and mode of inheritance are unknown. Patients may present in adolescence or more commonly the third or fourth decade of life with oligomenorrhea, amenorrhea, infertility, obesity, and excessive hair growth. Approximately half the women with the metabolic abnormality have polycystic ovaries. There is an increased risk for diabetes [Ehrmann DA. Polycystic ovary syndrome. *N Engl J Med.* 2005;352:1223–1236].

KEY SYNDROME   Ovarian Cysts

See also Female Reproductive Tract Signs—Ovarian Cysts, page 558. Cystic change in the ovary can result from the follicles, the corpus luteum, the stroma, and the ovarian epithelium. Cysts can be degenerative or neoplastic (benign and malignant) or teratomas. Specific diagnosis can only be made pathologically.

KEY SYNDROME   Ovarian Cancer

Malignant tumors arise predominantly from the epithelium, although germ cell and stromal tumors are not rare. BRCA-1 and BRCA-2 genotypes increase the risk for ovarian cancer. Screening for ovarian cancer is not currently effective and the disease often presents as ascites after generalized peritoneal spread.

KEY SYNDROME   Endometrial Cancer

It is more common in women with increased levels of estrogen in the absence of progesterone-induced cycling. This is a disease predominately of postmenopausal women who present with vaginal spotting or bleeding. Diagnosis is by endometrial biopsy. Obesity, unopposed estrogen therapy, a positive family history, and atypical endometrial hyperplasia are risk factors.

Vaginal Cancer.   This is a rare disease. Clear-cell vaginal cancer was associated with the exposure of female fetuses to maternal diethylstilbestrol (DES), given in an attempt to prevent spontaneous abortion.

> **KEY SYNDROME**   Sexually Transmitted Infections (STIs)

STDs can present locally as ulcers or inflammation, systemically, or be asymptomatic. All sexually active women, especially those with new or multiple partners, should be screened for STDs. The presence of one STD increases the risk of acquiring or transmitting others. Barrier contraceptives (condoms) are somewhat effective at decreasing the risk of acquiring an STD. All persons with an STD must be screened for other treatable STDs, including HIV and syphilis, which are often acquired asymptomatically. Extension of infection to the tubes, ovaries and broad ligament results in pelvic inflammatory disease (see page 557), a frequent cause of female infertility. In addition, several infectious diseases, not usually defined as STDs, can be acquired sexually, for example, hepatitis B.

> **KEY SYNDROME**   Infertility

The capacity to become pregnant with a viable fetus requires the coordinated functioning of complex physiologic systems in an anatomically normal woman. Failure of any component of this system can result in infertility. Initial examination should focus on an assessment of general health and nutrition, the menstrual history, and a physical examination to confirm normal sexual development and anatomy. Evaluation of the sexual partner is also required. The etiology and evaluation of infertility is a complex subject. See specialized texts for further information.

> **KEY SYNDROME**   Endometriosis

Normal-appearing endometrial tissue forms implants in ectopic sites including the ovaries, posterior surface of uterus, sigmoid colon, uterosacral ligaments, and, less often, distant sites such as pleura. Cyclical bleeding is associated with pain and the development of adhesions. The cause is unknown. Patients present with dysmenorrhea and abdominal or pelvic pain that is often cyclical. Tender nodular masses surrounded with fibrosis may be felt. Frequently, the ovaries are enlarged. The uterus may be fixed or painful with movement. Infertility is common and diagnosis usually requires laparoscopy.

The Male Genitalia and Reproductive System

The identical embryologic anlage produce female or male external genetalia depending the level of testosterone. Lack of the SRY gene (typically found on the Y chromosome) leads to development of ovaries, with subsequent maturation of female sex organs. Conversely, the presence of this gene leads to testicular development, with masculinization of the reproductive tract. The scrotum and penis are cognates of the labia majora and clitoris, respectively. Ambiguous genitalia occur when development and maturation occurs with a mixed genetic substrate or hormonal environment.

The male reproductive organs are the testes, epididymis, vas deferens, seminal vesicles, prostate, and penis. The testes arise intraabdominally and descend through the inguinal canal into the scrotum, usually by birth. The scrotal location is more conducive to spermatogenesis being slightly cooler than body temperature. Leutenizing hormone causes testicular Leydig cells to produce testosterone. Spermatogenesis in the seminiferous tubules requires follicle-stimulating hormone and paracrine testosterone production. Sperm are collected in the epididymis and travel up the vas deferens to the level of the prostate and seminal vesicles in the spermatic cord. The spermatic cord also contains the testicular artery and vein and the lymphatics. Ejaculate contains sperm, prostatic, and seminal vesicle secretions.

Anatomy of the Male Reproductive System

At puberty, the mons pubes becomes covered with hair that extends onto the skin of the abdomen to form the *male escutcheon,* which describes an upright triangle with the apex near the umbilicus.

The Penis

The shaft of the penis is formed by three columns of erectile tissue, the two dorsolateral *corpora cavernosa* and the ventral smaller *corpus spongiosum* containing the urethra (Fig. 12–1). Fibrous tissue binds the three columns into a cylinder. The tip of the penis is an obtuse cone of erectile tissue, the *glans penis*, containing the urethral meatus. The glans has a corona at its junction with the shaft. A flap of skin, the *prepuce* or foreskin, covers the glans. The *frenulum* is a fold of the prepuce that extends ventrally into the ventral notch in the glans. Penile erection

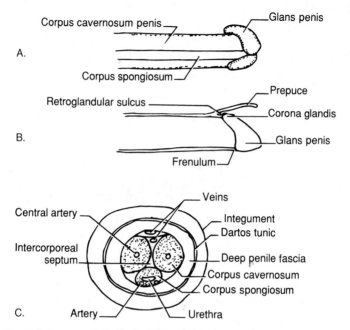

Fig. 12–1 *Structure of the Penis. A. The shaft in its ventrolateral aspect, with Integument removed. B. A sagittal section of the shaft with integument included. C. A cross-section of the shaft.*

and ejaculation are complex physiologic and hemodynamic processes that can be disrupted by vascular disease, drugs, injury to nerves, endocrine abnormalities, and anxiety. The male reproductive system is designed to produce and store sperm cells, which can be deposited at the entrance to the female cervix with forceful ejaculation of the sperm and spermatic fluids via the erect, penetrating penis. Successful reproduction is dependent upon the coordinated functioning of this system.

The Scrotum

This pouch is formed by a layer of thin, rugous skin overlying the tightly adherent dartos tunic consisting of muscle and fascia (Fig. 12–2C). The sac hangs from the root of the penis. The scrotal skin is bisected by a median raphe. Internally, the two halves of the pouch are separated by a septal fold of dartos tunic. Each half contains a testis with its epididymis and spermatic cord. The scrotal contents slide easily in a fascial cleft between the scrotal wall and the covering of the testis and cords. The skin of the scrotum is deeply pigmented and contains large, sebaceous follicles that have a tendency to form cysts. The *dartos muscle* tone determines scrotal size, with exposure to cold shrinking the sac and heat enlarging the pouch. In advanced age, the dartos muscle becomes relatively atonic. The action of the dartos muscles is independent of contractions of the *cremasteric muscles* that elevate the testes. The arterial, venous and lymphatic drainage of the scrotal

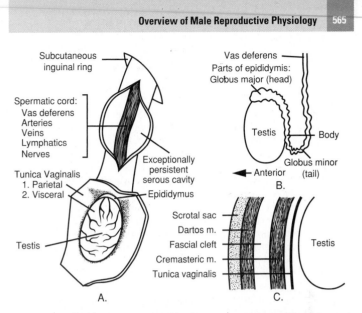

Fig. 12–2 *Anatomy of the scrotal wall and epididymis. A. Cavities of the tunica vaginalis are opened anteriorly to show testis and cord. B. Parts of the epididymis and cord. C. Layers of the scrotum.*

contents arises intraabdominally and reaches its scrotal location via the inguinal canal and spermatic cord. Lymphatics from the scrotal contents drain to the pelvic lymph nodes. The scrotal vascular and lymphatic supply is in continuity with the perineum and its lymphatics drain to the inguinal lymph nodes.

Testis, Epididymis, Vas Deferens, and Spermatic Cord

Toward the end of fetal development, the testis begins its descent from the abdomen to the scrotum. The peritoneum covering the testis becomes the *processus vaginalis*, and the *gubernaculum* leads the testis into its scrotal position. Normally, the spermatic cord portion of the peritoneal pouch is obliterated, leaving a cavity surrounding the testis and epididymis, except for their posterior aspect (Fig. 12–2A). This serous membrane is the *tunica vaginalis*. Abnormal persistence of this peritoneal connection leads to congenital hernias or funicular hydroceles. The *testis* is a smooth, solid ovoid, compressed laterally, and roughly 4 cm × 2 cm. The spermatic cord suspends the testis in the scrotum with the long axis nearly vertical. The head of the *epididymis* caps the upper pole of the testis. The body of the epididymis forms an elongated inverted cone attached vertically to the posterior surface of the testis. The apex of the cone, or tail of the epididymis, approaches the lower pole of the testis (Fig. 12–2B). The epididymis is continuous with the *vas deferens*, which joins other vessels to form the spermatic cord. The *spermatic cord* consists of the vas deferens, arteries, veins, nerves, and lymphatic vessels, all held together by the *spermatic fascia*. From the testis, the cord extends upward, entering the external inguinal ring and coursing through the inguinal canal to the internal inguinal ring, where its components diverge. In the abdominal cavity, the vas deferens continues backward and downward behind the peritoneum until it lies behind the bladder and anterior to the rectum, joining the duct of the seminal vesicle to become the *ejaculatory duct.*

The Prostate and Seminal Vesicles

The prostate contains glands dispersed in a stroma of smooth muscle and fibrous tissue. It is shaped roughly like a truncated cone the size of a walnut and is prone to hyperplasia with age. It lies in the pelvis approximately 2 cm posterior to the symphysis pubis; the cone is inverted so the base is superior and the apex inferior (Fig. 12–3B and C). The anterior and posterior surfaces are somewhat flattened. The basal surface is directed superiorly and is overlaid by the bladder; the apical surface faces inferiorly and rests on the *urogenital diaphragm.* The *prostatic urethra* pierces the basal or superior surface, slightly anterior to the center, and runs inferiorly in a vertical axis to emerge through the apical or inferior surface. The only palpable portion of the prostate is the slightly vertically convex posterior prostatic surface, which is in close contact with the rectal wall. A shallow *median furrow* divides all except the upper portion of the posterior surface into a right and left lobe. Near the superior edge of the posterior surface is a *transverse depression* made by the ejaculatory ducts which enter the prostate and converge to enter the urethra. The paired *ampullae* of the vas deferens and the seminal vesicles diverge superiorly from the prostate base. The ampulla of the vas is superior and medial to the seminal vesicles and both contact the posterior wall of the bladder. The *bulbourethral glands* of Cowper lie on each side of the midline just inferior to the caudal border of the prostate.

Physical Examination of the Male Genitalia and Reproductive System

Inspection and palpation reveal many disorders of the external and internal male reproductive organs and the lower urinary tract. Familiarity with the genital disorders demonstrated by inspection and palpation is necessary for any physician performing a physical examination.

Examination of the Penis

Wearing gloves, view the penis in its usual state, then have the patient retract the prepuce revealing the size of the foreskin orifice and the glans. Observe any superficial lesions of the corona or retroglandular sulcus. Palpate lesions for induration and tenderness. Palpate the length of the shaft, ventrally along the corpus spongiosum, and laterally over both corpora cavernosa, feeling for nodules and plaques. Compress the glans anteroposteriorly between the thumb and forefinger to open and inspect the meatus and terminal urethra. If urethral symptoms are present, strip the ventral penis from its base to the glans to collect a drop of urethral discharge for microscopic examination.

Examination of the Scrotum

The scrotum is examined by inspection and palpation. Because rugae are produced by contractions of dartos muscle, the walls should be inspected by spreading the layers between gloved fingers. Transillumination is readily performed; it is most informative for examining the scrotal contents.

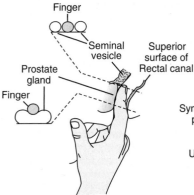

A. Digital examination of prostate

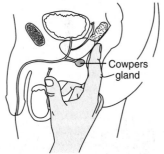

B. Sagittal section of male pelvis

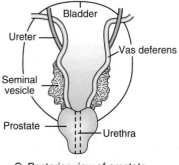

C. Posterior view of prostate

D. Cowper bulbourethral gland

Fig. 12–3 *Rectal Examination of the Male Genitalia. A. Relationship of the examining finger to the prostate and seminal vesicles: The lower section shows the finger at the prostate gland; the higher section shows the finger between the two seminal vesicles. B. A sagittal section of the male penis and pelvic organs. C. A posterior view of the prostate, seminal vesicles, and vasa deferentia. D. Palpation of the Cowper* **bulbourethral gland:** *There is one gland on each side of the urethra. The diagram shows a sagittal section of the male pelvis. The tip of the index finger is in the rectum with the pad facing the anterior rectal wall, between the inferior border of the prostate and the inner edge of the anal canal. The thumb is outside the rectum, pressing the perineum on the medial raphe toward the fingertip. A normal gland is not palpable, but an inflamed gland is tender. If it contains pus, it forms a palpable mass, from pea to hazelnut size (the round black spot).*

Examination of Scrotal Contents

Palpation and transillumination identify most structures within the scrotal sac. Examine the scrotum systematically in the following sequence: (1) testes, (2) tunica vaginalis, (3) epididymis (head, body, and tail), (4) spermatic cord, and (5) inguinal lymph nodes. The complete sequence should be followed in every routine physical examination. If the scrotum is swollen, first exclude an inguinal hernia descending into the scrotum, then examine for the structures normally in the scrotum.

Examination for Scrotal Hernia

Palpate the root of the scrotum to determine if the mass extends that high. If the fingers can get above the mass, a hernia is excluded. Insert a finger into the external inguinal ring and feel for a cough impulse from hernia. Inguinal hernias always descend in front of the spermatic cord and testes, so identify these structures and their anatomic relations to the mass. A swollen scrotum should be transilluminated by using a cool light source in a darkened room. With the thumb and forefinger, pull the scrotal wall tightly over the mass. Place the light in contact with the posterior wall of the scrotum, shining the light anteriorly through the mass to determine whether the structure is translucent or opaque. Most hernia contents are opaque, although occasionally a gas-filled loop of gut will transmit light. Listen with a stethoscope for peristaltic sounds.

Examination of the Testes

Examine the testes simultaneously by grasping one with each gloved hand, using thumb and forefinger. Determine their size, shape, consistency, and sensitivity to light pressure. Transilluminate each, even if they feel normal; one may be atrophied and the normal size attained by a hydrocele. Use scrotal ultrasonography to help distinguish between intratesticular and extratesticular masses or lesions [Junnila J, Lassen P. Testicular masses. *Am Fam Physician.* 1998;59:685–692].

Examination of the Epididymis

Locate each epididymis by palpating the smooth testis to find a vertical ridge of soft nodular tissue beginning at the upper pole and extending to the lower pole. Usually the epididymis is behind the testis, but in approximately 7% of males, the structure develops anterior to the testis, *anteversion of the epididymis.* Recognizing the anteversion, the examiner will expect the cavity of the tunica vaginalis to be posterior to the testis. Compare the findings from palpation in both epididymides, in their component segments of head, body, and tail.

Examination of the Spermatic Cord

Palpation of varicoceles is best done in the upright position, while it is easiest to examine the scrotal contents in the supine position. Compare the spermatic cords by simultaneously grasping each at the neck of the scrotum. With the thumb in front and the forefinger behind the scrotum, gently compress the cord (Fig. 12–4), then have the patient bear down to increase the intraabdominal pressure. The normal vas deferens is felt as a distinct hard cord, which can be separated from other cord structures. A varicocele looks and feels like a bag of worms. Other structures that may be palpable are spermatoceles that are separate from and rest superior to the testis and epididymal cysts. These can be confirmed by ultrasound examination. The other, less-definable strands are nerves, arteries, and fibers of cremasteric muscle. The vas may be congenitally absent. Trace the cords down to the testes.

Examination of the Inguinal Regions for Hernia

The tip of the index finger is placed at the most dependent part of the scrotum and directed into the subcutaneous inguinal ring by invaginating the slack scrotum

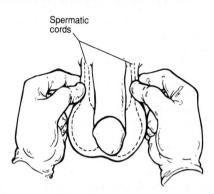

Spermatic cords

Fig. 12–4 *Palpation of the Spermatic Cords.* *Each gloved hand simultaneously grasps a cord between thumb and index finger, comparing the two structures. Normally, the vasa deferentia feel like distinct whipcords. The other components of the cord, arteries, veins, vessels, and nerves, feel like indefinite strands.*

with it (Fig. 12–5A). The patient coughs or strains so an impulse from the hernial sac may be felt on the fingertip.

Zieman inguinal examination. This procedure reveals direct and indirect inguinal hernias, and hernias of the femoral triangle. With the patient standing, stand at the patient's right side and place the palm of your right hand against the right lower abdomen. Spread your fingers slightly so your long finger lies along the inguinal ligament with its pulp in the external inguinal ring, your index finger is over the internal inguinal ring, and your ring finger palpates the region of the femoral canal and the opening of the saphenous vein (Fig. 12–5B). Have the patient take a deep breath, hold it, and bear down, as if to have a bowel movement. Then repeat the maneuver, standing at the patient's left side and palpating his left

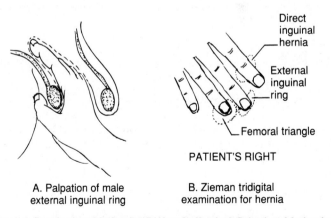

Direct inguinal hernia

External inguinal ring

Femoral triangle

PATIENT'S RIGHT

A. Palpation of male external inguinal ring

B. Zieman tridigital examination for hernia

Fig. 12–5 *Examination of the Inguinal Regions for Hernia. A. Palpation of the inguinal ring in the male. B. Zieman tridigital examination for hernia: The left side of the patient is examined from his left and with the examiner's left hand.*

groin with your left hand. A hernia in any of the three sites is perceived either as a gliding motion of the walls of the empty sac or as a protrusion of a viscus into the sac. When the internal ring is closed by the palpating finger, any herniating mass cannot be an indirect inguinal hernia.

Palpation of prostate and seminal vesicles. Place the patient in the lithotomy position, the knee-chest position, the left-lateral-prone position (Sims), or bent-over-the-table position. Three of these have been considered elsewhere (see Fig. 9–16, page 462). In the bent-over-the table position, the patient stands with legs apart, the trunk flexed on the thighs, and the elbows resting on the knees or the examining table. Whatever the position, the details of the procedure are the same. Cover the examining hand with a glove and generously lubricate the forefinger. Place the pad or pulp of the forefinger on the anal orifice with light pressure while the patient bears down gently until the sphincter relaxes, admitting the curve of the pad. Then incline the finger until the tip is also inserted. Gradually ease the tip past the anal canal and into the rectal ampulla. Keep the pad of the finger facing the anterior rectal wall.

As the finger moves cephalad from the anal canal, it encounters the elastic bulging surface of the *prostate* (Fig. 12–3A). Feel the median furrow that separates the lateral lobes. When the fingertip reaches the superior edge of the prostate, the median furrow thins out to the flat middle lobe. Superior to the prostate, the fingertip reaches the seminal vesicles on either side of the midline. Determine whether the prostatic surface is smooth or nodular; whether the consistency is elastic, hard, boggy, soft, or fluctuant; whether the shape is rounded or flat; whether the size is normal, enlarged, or atrophied; whether sensitivity to pressure is abnormal; whether there is normal mobility or fixation.

Normally, the *seminal vesicles* are not palpable because they are too soft; only diseased structures can be felt. The seminal vesicles are approximately 7.5 cm long, so only their lower portions can be reached. Examine each seminal vesicle for distention, sensitivity, size, consistency, induration, and nodules. Palpate in the region of the bulbourethral glands, they are normally not palpable. When enlarged, they are felt as rounded masses in the anterior rectal wall.

On completion of the examination, either clean the patient or provide tissue to the patient.

Male Genital and Reproductive Symptoms

KEY SYMPTOM Scrotal Pruritus

Scrotal skin is thin, rugated, and susceptible to irritation and infection because it is usually warm and often moist. Pruritus often indicates inflammatory or infectious dermatitis, but sometimes it persists without skin changes or evident cause.

Pelvic Pain. See Syndromes, Acute Prostatitis page 581 and Chronic Pelvic Pain Syndrome, page 583.

KEY SYMPTOM Pain in the Testis and Epididymis

Innervation of the testis and epididymis is somatic and sympathetic arising in the lower thoracic roots. Pain arising from these structures frequently radiates to the epigastrium and/or hypogastrium. If the scrotal wall or tunica vaginalis is involved, the pain is well localized. Pain arising in the testis may be mild or excruciating and is frequently accompanied by nausea. Look for a relationship to activities, sexual activities, and signs of systemic or sexually transmitted disease. A complete sexual history is essential.

✔ **TESTICULAR PAIN—CLINICAL OCCURRENCE:** *Congenital* very large hydrocele; *Idiopathic* inguinal hernia, large varicocele; *Infectious* acute orchitis (mumps, echovirus, lymphocytic choriomeningitis virus, arbovirus group B), chronic orchitis (leprosy, tuberculosis), acute epididymitis (gonorrhea, chlamydia, *Escherichia coli*, mycoplasma), and chronic epididymitis (leprosy, tuberculosis, syphilis, brucellosis); *Mechanical/Traumatic* blunt and penetrating trauma, testicular rupture, torsion, ureteral stone; *Neoplastic* testicular carcinoma, leukemia; *Neurologic* neuropathy; *Vascular* testicular infarction and hemorrhage.

> **KEY SYMPTOM** **Penile Curvature**

See Male Genitourinary Signs—Plastic Induration of the Penis, page 583.

> **KEY SYMPTOM** **Erectile Dysfunction and Impotence**

See Syndromes—Erectile Dysfunction and Impotence, page 591.

Male Genital and Reproductive Signs

Penis Signs

Ambiguous Genitalia—Intersexuality: See specify texts.

> **KEY SIGN** **Condyloma Acuminatum (Venereal Wart, Papilloma)**

Infection with human papillomavirus (HPV) produces the lesion. The condyloma is a villous projection (acuminata means pointed) that may be single or conglomerate (Fig. 12–6E). It can occur on the corona, in the retroglandular sulcus, on the shaft, and frequently about the anus, and occasionally it is found in the urethra. In the presence of moisture, secondary infection produces ulceration. In its uncomplicated form, the verrucous appearance is quite distinctive. An exuberant growth with much ulceration must be distinguished from carcinoma by biopsy.

> **KEY SIGN** **Condyloma Latum**

A flat and warty (Fig. 12–6D) growth (a *secondary syphilid*) occurs on the genitalia or anus. The flat appearance is diagnostic. When the lesion has an exuberant growth, it must be distinguished from the acuminate condyloma and carcinoma.

> **KEY SIGN** **Urethral Discharge**

See Urinary System Signs—Urethral Discharge, page 536, and Male Genital and Reproductive Syndromes—Urethritis, pages 546 and 590.

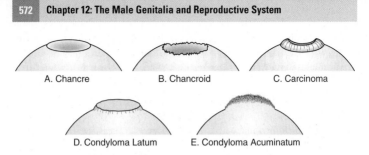

A. Chancre   B. Chancroid   C. Carcinoma

D. Condyloma Latum   E. Condyloma Acuminatum

Fig. 12–6 *Penile Lesions. A. Chancre:* *The border is smooth; there is no necrosis or suppuration. Induration surrounds the lesion so it can be picked up like a disk. **B. Chancroid:** The border is irregular without induration and the center is necrotic. There is profuse suppuration. **C. Ulcerating carcinoma:** The necrotic ulcer may resemble chancroid, but soon the process is surrounded by induration and nodulation. **D. Condyloma latum:** This is the flat, nonsuppurating nodule of secondary syphilis. **E. Condyloma acuminatum:** The lesions are moist, villous growths that protrude above the skin and undergo secondary ulceration.*

Penis—Hypoplasia and Hyperplasia.   Normal penis size varies widely, a range learned only from examination of many individuals. Striking discrepancies between penile size and the patient's age lead to the inference of hypoplasia or hyperplasia. Penile hypoplasia is either a feature of intersexuality or eunuchoidism occurring before puberty. In intersexuality, distinction between a hypoplastic penis with hypospadias and a hyperplastic clitoris may be difficult or impossible without histologic examination of the gonads. Hyperplasia is caused by tumors of the pineal gland, hypothalamus, Ledig cells or adrenal gland. An inaccurate impression of hypoplasia often occurs as men gain wieght and abdominal girth.

KEY SIGN   Generalized Penile Swelling

Edema.   Fluid accumulates in the loose tissue of the penis in generalized edematous states from any cause and with obstruction of the penile veins or lymphatics. The penis, and usually scrotum, are diffusely swollen without erythema, warmth, or tenderness. See also Scrotal Edema page 585.

Generalized Penile Swelling—Contusion: Especially during erection, trauma to the penis may cause extravasation of blood that is usually painless. In a few days, the skin of the penis and scrotum may be stained blue from degraded hemoglobin.

Fracture of the Shaft: Trauma during erection may rupture one or both corpora cavernosa penis. Severe pain occurs at the time of injury, with immediate subsidence of the erection and temporary relief of pain. Subsequent engorgement from extravasation of blood produces recurrence of pain. This is a urologic emergency. Rupture may not be distinguishable from contusion unless an operation is performed.

KEY SIGN   Genital Ulcer

Ulceration of the penile shaft, glans, or foreskin occurs at the site of trauma or inoculation of sexually transmitted infectious organisms. The character of the ulcer is diagnostically useful (Fig. 12–6). Inspect the base and edges; look for vesicles that ulcerate, noting especially the presence of pain. Palpate for induration of the surrounding tissue and base of the ulcer, and carefully feel for regional lymphadenopathy. Because these are usually sexually transmitted infections (STIs), serologic evaluation for syphilis and HIV are indicated, as are counseling on safe sexual practices and use of condoms. *CLINICAL OCCURRENCE:* Behçet syndrome, herpes simplex, syphilis, chancroid, lymphogranuloma venereum, molluscum contagiosum, traumatic sex, tight-fitting clothing, penile cancer.

Syphilitic Chancre (Hard Chancre): *Treponema pallidum* from sexual contact invades intact skin producing a silvery papule that erodes to form a superficial ulcer with serous discharge teeming with organisms. This is the primary lesion of syphilis (Fig. 12–6A). It commonly occurs on the glans or the inner leaves of the foreskin but is occasionally on the shaft or scrotum. Rarely, it is extragenital, usually on the lips. The chancre is painless, usually single, round or oval, with a smooth, slightly raised border. The underlying induration permits the superficial lesion to be lifted as a small disk between the thumb and forefinger. Regional inguinal lymph nodes undergo painless moderate enlargement. Neither the ulcer nor the lymph nodes suppurate. Physical signs are not conclusive and because the lesion appears before serologic tests for syphilis become positive, the diagnosis must be confirmed by demonstrating the *T. pallidum* in the serous exudate with the dark-field microscope.

Chancroid (Soft Chancre): Suppurative infection caused by the bacillus *Haemophilus ducreyi*, it usually involves the genitalia, although it may be extragenital. The lesion begins as a small red papule that quickly becomes pustular and enlarges to form a punched-out ulcer with undetermined edges (Fig. 12–6B). The base is covered with a gray slough, discharging pus profusely. Extensive necrosis ensues and multiple ulcers form. The lesions are quite painful. In one-third of the cases, the regional lymph nodes become swollen and tender (the bubo). These frequently suppurate. While the clinical appearance is quite typical, mixed infections must be excluded.

Lymphogranuloma Venereum (Lymphogranuloma Inguinale [LGV]): LGV is caused by *Chlamydia trachomatis*, a rickettsia-like organism, and primarily involves the lymphatic system. The painless and evanescent initial lesion, an erosion less than 1 mm in diameter, is frequently overlooked. Occasionally, the penile lesion becomes vesicular, papular, or nodular. One or 2 weeks after infection, the inguinal lymph nodes become swollen and tender, matting together with areas of softening and reddening of the overlying skin. Multiple small fistulas form, discharging creamy pus or serosanguineous exudate. Healing with much fibrosis occurs over many months. A cicatrizing proctitis may be a late complication. The late clinical appearance is fairly distinctive. In the early stages, syphilis, chancroid, and herpes simplex need to be excluded.

Herpes Simplex: Local discomfort on the glans, prepuce or shaft precedes a characteristic group of vesicles surrounded by erythema. The vesicles rupture, producing painful superficial ulcers that heal in 5 to 7 days. Recurrent relapsing painful vesiculation and ulceration is characteristic.

Behçet Syndrome: Painful aphthous ulcers with yellowish necrotic bases occur singly or in crops lasting 1 to 2 weeks, and resemble those seen in the oral mucosa.

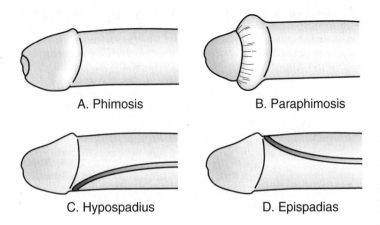

A. Phimosis

B. Paraphimosis

C. Hypospadius

D. Epispadias

Fig. 12–7 *Structural Abnormalities of the Prepuce (Foreskin). A. Phimosis:* The preputial orifice is too tight to permit retraction of the foreskin over the glans penis. *B. Paraphimosis:* A prepuce with small orifice has been retracted over the glans and the lips have impinged on the retroglandular sulcus, preventing return to the normal position. Edema occurs in the prepuce, the skin of the shaft, and the glans. *C. Hypospadias:* This is a developmental anomaly in which the urethral meatus opens on the underside of the shaft. *D. Epispadias:* A developmental anomaly in which the urethral meatus is on the dorsal side of the penis.

> **KEY SIGN** **Prepuce—Phimosis**

The orifice is too small for the foreskin to be retracted from the glans (Fig. 12–7A). The acquired type may be caused by adhesions to the glans as the result of infection. The lips of the prepuce are pallid, striated, and thickened. The narrow orifice may actually obstruct urination. Retained smegma leads to inflammation and even calculus formation. Circumcision is curative.

Paraphimosis: A tight foreskin once retracted becomes edematous and cannot be returned over the glans (Fig. 12–7B). The edema impedes the venous drainage of the glans causing swelling. Manual replacement of the prepuce may be attempted. Surgical incision or circumcision may be necessary.

> **KEY SIGN** **Glans—Balanitis**

Acute or chronic irritation, infection or inflammation of the glans resutls in epithelial erosions or thickening with papules or plaques. In erosive balanitis the skin of the glans desquamates with formation of erosions and small ulcers which may become confluent, involving the entire glans. *Zoon's balanitis* is due to plasma cell infiltration of unknown cause; it occurs mostly in uncircumsized middle-aged men. *Circinate balanitis* is characteristic of reactive arthritis (Reiter's syndrome). Primary cutaneous disease such as psoriasis, lichen planus and lichen sclerosis et atrophicus affect the glans. Infections include *Candida*, HPV (condylomata) and syphilis (primary, secondary and tertiary). Intraepithelial and invasive squamous cell cancers can mimic other causes of balanitis.

KEY SIGN — Carcinoma of the Penis

Squamous cell carcinoma occurs in areas of irritation or inflammation on the foreskin, glans or shaft; being uncircumcized increases risk. Commonly, the primary lesion involves the dorsal corona or the inner lip of the foreskin. A warty growth develops, ulcerates, and discharges watery pus. Parts of the tumor undergo necrosis and slough (see Fig. 12–6C). Metastasis occurs, most often to the inguinal lymph nodes. Often, the clinical appearance is not sufficiently typical to distinguish this from condyloma, so a biopsy is necessary.

Dorsal Shaft—Thrombosis of the Dorsal Vein: A thrombus in the dorsal vein of the penis causes a palpable cord, approximately 1 mm in diameter, in the midline dorsally. This condition is usually secondary to inflammation of the glans.

Dorsal Shaft—Varicose Veins: Varicosities of the dorsal veins of the penis may be visible and palpable. They may be sufficiently large to require surgical treatment.

Shaft—Cavernositis: An irregular hard mass may occur in the lateral or ventral cavernous corpora from inflammation. Priapism and edema usually accompany this condition. Suppuration may occur, with drainage through the skin or the urethra.

KEY SIGN — Priapism

Erection is sustained by reflex or central nerve stimulation, or by local mechanical causes, such as thrombosis, hemorrhage, neoplasm, injection of vasoactive agents, and inflammation in the penis. Prolonged, persistent, penile erection occurs without sexual desire. The condition is usually painful. It may complicate leukemia, sickle cell anemia and use of drugs for erectile dysfunction. Urgent treatment is required.

KEY SIGN — Plastic Induration of the Penis (Peyronie Disease)

This is a chronic disease of unknown cause, characterized by irregular fibrosis of the septum or sheath of the corpus cavernosum penis, extending into the tunica albuginea. It never affects the corpus spongiosom. It is considered a component of Dupuytren diathesis along with palmar and solar fibrosis. The patient may complain of curvature of the penis during erection. Firm, nontender plaques may be felt laterally in the corpora cavernosa penis or dorsally over the intercorporeal septum. The plaques may be single or multiple; they are not necessarily symmetrical.

Urethral Signs

KEY SIGN — Meatal Stricture

Narrowing of the urethral meatus is detected by anteroposterior pressure on the glans. Strictures in other portions of the urethra may be suggested by difficulty passing a urethral catheter.

Hypospadias: The urethral meatus appears on the ventral surface of the glans, the shaft, or at the penoscrotal junction (Fig. 12–7C).

Epispadias: Maldevelopment results in the meatus opening dorsally on the glans, shaft, or at the penoscrotal junction (Fig. 12–7D). This anomaly is often associated with exstrophy of the bladder.

Morgagni Folliculitis: The follicles of Morgagni open into the urethra laterally, immediately behind the meatal lips. When the urethral mucosa is inflamed, the mouths of these ducts become prominent, and pus can be seen exuding when the follicles are involved.

Papilloma: This benign tumor in the meatus may be visible when the orifice gapes from pressure on the glans.

KEY SIGN   Acute Urethritis

See also, Male Genital and Reproductive Syndromes—Urethritis, page 590. An acute indurating urethritis, especially as the result of infection from an indwelling catheter, may cause a palpable cord that extends the entire length of the ventral midline of the penis.

Periurethral Abscess: An accumulation of pus in the midportion of the penile urethra in the *Littre follicle* will produce visible swelling.

KEY SIGN   Urethral Stricture

A tunnel stricture of the urethra may cause a palpable, cord-like mass in the corpus cavernosum urethrae at the penoscrotal junction. Strictures in other parts of the penile urethra are usually not palpable.

Urethral Diverticulum: When located at the penoscrotal junction, a diverticulum frequently produces a visible swelling, felt as a soft midline mass.

Ventral Penile Shaft—Urethral Carcinoma: A urethral neoplam may occasionally be felt in an indurated mass in the corpus spongiosum.

Scrotum Signs

Blue papules—scrotal venous angioma (fordyce lesion).   Venous angiomas develop in the superficial scrotal veins in men older than 50. The papules are usually multiple, 3 to 4 mm in diameter, and filled with venous blood that colors them dark red, blue, or almost black. They are of no significance.

KEY SIGN   Scrotal Edema

Extracellular fluid collects in the dependent scrotum when venous or lymphatic outflow is obstructed and when urine extravasates from a ruptured urethra below the urogenital diaphragm. Acute obstruction of the lymphatics from any cause may produce lymphedema that pits on pressure; when long-standing, it will be nonpitting. Pitting edema occurs when systemic venous pressure is very high and dependent edema reaches above the inguinal ligaments (e.g., advanced right ventricular failure or constrictive pericarditis, thrombosis of the pelvic veins or inferior vena cava, nephrotic syndrome) and often in the setting of tense ascites.

> ### KEY SIGN Scrotal Gangrene

This necrotizing perineal infection (Fournier gangrene) is caused by polymicro-bial mixed aerobic and anaerobic, gram-positive and gram-negative organisms, often with gas production. The rapid progression results from subcutaneous vascular thrombosis leading to gangrene of the overlying dermis. It is most com-mon in diabetic patients beyond the sixth decade. Fever and signs of sepsis are accompanied by necrotic, foul-smelling, rapidly advancing lesions of scrotum; crepitation may be present. Prompt wide surgical debridement and antibiotics can be lifesaving.

Scrotal cysts—sebaceous cysts.   These common nodular lesions of the scrotal skin are benign. The white cyst content may be visible.

KEY SIGN Scrotal Carcinoma

The neoplasm is similar to those in other areas of skin. It is particularly common in workers with occupational exposure to tar or oil.

Testis, Epididymis, and Other Intrascrotal Signs

KEY SIGN Maldescended Testis—Cryptorchidism

During fetal development, the descent of the testis may be arrested in the ab-domen, inguinal canal, or at the puboscrotal junction; other locations are possi-ble. Either or both testes may be affected. An abdominal testis cannot be palpated. In the other locations, the testis is palpable, but smaller and softer due to atrophy. A maldescended testis is frequently associated with a congenital inguinal hernia on the same side resulting from persistence of the saccus vaginalis. Maldescended testis carries an increased risk of testicular cancer and decreased fertility.

KEY SIGN Small Testes—Atrophy

The testis may be smaller than normal from Klinefelter syndrome or Prader-Willi syndromes. Atrophy may occur after infarction, trauma, mumps orchitis, cir-rhosis, syphilis, filariasis, large varicocele or surgical repair of an inguinal hernia.

KEY SIGN Nontender Testicular Swelling—Neoplasm

A young man usually presents with regional or disseminated disease that is ag-gressive, yet curable. The testis is usually enlarged and harder than normal, and it frequently contains softer cystic regions (Fig. 12–8D and H). The testis with car-cinoma is denser than with orchitis or hydrocele. An orchiectomy by the transin-guinal (never transscrotal) approach is required for diagnosis; biopsy is never per-formed due to the high risk of disseminating a cancer. The presence of metastatic lesions elsewhere is presumptive evidence that a testicular nodule is neoplastic.

> ### KEY SIGN Tender Testicular Swelling—Testicular Torsion

The testicle is suspended within the scrotum on the spermatic cord. It is normally anchored at its distal pole. When the spermatic cord becomes twisted, venous and

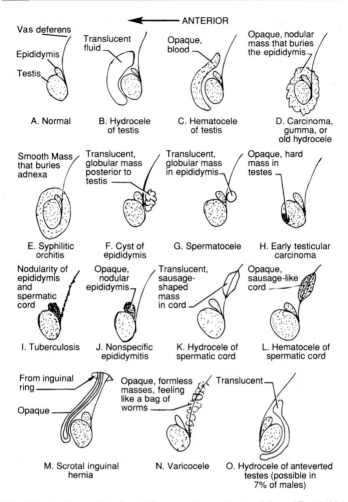

Fig. 12–8 *Swellings of the Scrotal Contents.* *(See text for descriptions of Fig. 12–8A to 12–8O).*

lymphatic obstruction occur first because of the thin vessel walls and lower pressures. This produces engorgement of the testicle, worsening circulation leading to arterial, as well as venous and lymphatic, occlusion. Pain is acute and severe, and may be referred to the abdomen. Palpation reveals a tender, irregular, edematous mass in the scrotum. The testicle lies in a horizontal position and the epididymis lies in an anterior location. The pain may be referred to the right lower quadrant of the abdomen, mimicking appendicitis. Occasionally, the twist in the cord can be felt. **DDX:** Torsion is frequently confused with acute epididymoorchitis and strangulated scrotal hernia. Five distinguishing features are: (1) The testis on the affected side lies higher than normal from the twisting of the cord and the spasm of the cremasteric muscles, (2) Palpation cannot distinguish between the testis and the epididymis. In acute epididymoorchitis, the epididymis can usually be felt separately from the testis, (3) Elevation and support of the scrotum for an hour usually relieves the pain of epididymoorchitis; it does not ameliorate the pain in torsion (*Prehn sign*), (4) In torsion, the leg of the involved side is often held in flexion, and (5) When a secondary hydrocele is present, the aspirated contents yield serosanguineous fluid from torsion, serous fluid in epididymoorchitis. Sometimes strangulated hernia cannot be distinguished from torsion without operation. Utrasound examination with Doppler flow analysis confirms the diagnosis. Temporary relief can be obtained by untwisting the cord: face the patient holding on to the testicular/cord mass and rotate it in an open book fashion. Urgent surgical intervention is required to prevent decreased function or atrophy of the testicle.

KEY SIGN   Tender Testicular Swelling—Acute Orchitis

Inflammation of one or both testes occurs frequently in mumps, and occasionally in other infectious diseases. The testis is swollen, tender, and usually extremely painful. Frequently, the inflammation causes acute hydrocele, but the inflammatory edema and the pain of palpation prevent accurate distinction. Often, primary or secondary epididymitis is associated. Orchitis is sometimes confused with torsion of the spermatic cord.

KEY SIGN   Non-tender Intra-scrotal Swelling

Normal and persistent fetal structures enlarge due to fluid accumulation or neoplasms. The differential diagnosis of painless intrascotal lesions requires a complete knowledge of the normal and developmental anatomy including arterial, venous and lymphatic circulations.

Hydrocele: Serous fluid accumulates in the cavity of the tunica vaginalis. Palpation reveals a smooth and resilient pear-shaped mass with the smaller pole upward terminating short of the root of the scrotum. The testis and epididymis are usually behind the mass (see Fig. 12–8B), except when anteversion is present and the structures are then anterior (see Fig. 12–8O). Transillumination can reveal the opaque shadow of the testis within the translucent mass. **DDX:** Hematoceles are opaque. Spermatoceles arise from the epididymis behind the testis. Hydrocele of the spermatic cord occurs above the testis.

Hydrocele of the Spermatic Cord: When the saccus vaginalis around the spermatic cord fails to obliterate a serous cavity persists; fluid accumulation forms a hydrocele. The hydrocele is smooth, resilient, and sausage-shaped; it is located above the testis and transilluminates (see Fig. 12–8K). Absent other abnormalities, these findings are diagnostic. When associated with a hernia, spermatocele, or testicular hydrocele, the distinction may be difficult or impossible without ultrasound or operation. Occasionally, there is a communication between the hydrocele and the peritoneal cavity, a communicating hydrocele, recognized by its variation in size.

Hematocele: The cavity of the tunica vaginalis is filled with blood. The swelling resembles that of a hydrocele, but blood is opaque to transillumination (Fig. 12–8C). A history of recent trauma suggests hematocele.

Hematoma of the Cord: When trauma causes bleeding around the spermatic cord, a boggy mass may be felt in the region. The mass is opaque to transillumination (Fig. 12–8L).

Chylocele: In filariasis, opalescent lymph may accumulate in the cavity of the tunica vaginalis. The mass is translucent and distinction from hydrocele can be made only by aspiration of the fluid.

Varicocele: Varicosities of the pampiniform plexus of veins form a soft, irregular mass in the scrotum. The condition occurs predominantly on the left side, occasionally it is bilateral and almost never is the right side involved exclusively. Palpation discloses a soft "bag of worms" sensation that is rarely mistaken for anything else (see Fig. 12–8N). **DDX:** To distinguish a varicocele from an indirect inguinal hernia containing omentum, have the patient lie down; the lesion should be gone. Place your gloved finger over the subcutaneous inguinal ring. When the patient stands, with your finger in place, the veins refill but the hernia will be held back.

Spermatocele: These are retention cysts of the epididymis. They are usually located behind the testis (see Hydrocele above). They are translucent and usually small, but can be up to 10 cm (Fig. 12–8G). **DDX:** Neoplams of the epididymis are rare; they are opaque on transillumination.

Syphilis: Nontender swelling and nodularity starts in the globus major extending then to the body of the epididymis (Fig. 12–8J). The cause is inferred from positive serologic tests for syphilis.

Tuberculosis: Hard, nontender nodularity begins in the body of the epididymis. The epididymis becomes adherent to the scrotum, and sinuses may form (Fig. 12–8I). The cause is usually inferred from the presence of tuberculosis elsewhere.

> **KEY SIGN**   Tender Epididymal Swelling—Acute Epididymitis

Infection of the epididymis occurs by extension from infections in the urethra, prostate, or seminal vesicles. Indwelling urethral catheters increase the risk of epididymitis. The painful, tender swelling of the epididymis may be accompanied by fever, leukocytosis, and pyuria. In young, sexually active men with multiple or new sexual partners, sexually transmitted organisms are expected; in men more than age 40 years of age and in those with catheters, enteric organisms are common.

Thickening of the Vas Deferens—Deferentitis: This is inflammation of the vas deferens. In acute diseases, the vas is tender and swollen. The inflammation is usually an extension from other structures. With chronic inflammation the vas may be thickened and indurated, with some nodularity (see Fig. 12–8I), suggesting either tuberculous or syphilis extending from other parts of the genitourinary tract.

Prostate and Seminal Vesicle Signs

> **KEY SIGN**   Non-tender Prostate Enlargement

The prostate may enlarge due to hyperplasia of normal prostatic tissues or by infiltration with chronic inflammation or neoplastic cells, or a combination of all of these. Diffuse enlargement with a normal consistency is expected as men age and most often represents benign hyperplasia (page 591). Asymmetrical enlargement, stoney hard nodules or diffuse hardness of the gland and obliteration of the normal sulcii suggest cancer (page 591). Chronic prostatitis, either infectious or primarily inflammatory, may present with a boggy or firm gland. Palpation is neither sensitive nor specific for the separation of these diagnoses.

> **KEY SIGN** Tender Prostatic Enlargement—Acute Prostatitis

In sexually active young men, chlamydia and gonorrhea are most likely, whereas in men over age 40 or those men with an indwelling urethral catheter, enteric organisms (*E. coli* or *Klebsiella*) are the cause. It may begin with dysuria, chills, and fever. Gentle palpation reveals an enlarged, tense or boggy and tender prostate, surrounded by edematous tissue. The urine specimen contains large mucous shreds. Vigorous massage of the prostate to obtain fluid for examination is contraindicated because it may induce bacteremia, and a urine specimen containing bacteria and white blood cells will be adequate for culture.

Palpable Seminal Vesicle—Vesiculitis. The normal seminal vesicle is not palpable. When the structure can be felt as a dilated or indurated mass, it is the site of acute or chronic infection or obstruction. The finger in the rectum may procure fluid for examination by massaging the vesicle toward the prostate, then milking the urethra to extrude the seminal fluid.

Palpable Cowper Gland—Inflammation of Bulbourethral Gland (Cowperitis). Normally the bulbourethral glands are not palpable. When they are inflamed, they are exquisitely tender. In chronic inflammation, they enlarge from the size of a pea to that of a hazelnut. When considered and examined appropriately, the findings are readily demonstrated. One gland lies on each side of the membranous urethra between the inferior edge of the prostate and the inner border of the anal canal. With the gloved forefinger in the rectum, explore the anterior rectal wall inferior to the prostate and superior to the edge of the anal canal (Fig. 12–3D). At the same time, the thumb is held outside on the median raphe of the scrotum just anterior to the anus. The tissue between the thumb and forefinger is compressed to detect tenderness or a mass.

Male Genital and Reproductive Syndromes

> **KEY SYNDROME** Inguinal Hernia

See Chapter 9, Hernias, page 529.

> **KEY SYNDROME** Sexually Transmitted Infections (STIs)

STIs can present locally as ulcers or inflammation, systemically, or be asymptomatic. All sexually active men, especially those with new or multiple partners, should be screened for a history of STIs. The presence of one STI increases the risk of acquiring and transmitting others. Barrier contraceptives (condoms) are somewhat effective at decreasing the risk of acquiring an STI. All persons with an STI must be screened for other treatable STIs, including HIV and syphilis, which are often acquired asymptomatically. In addition, several infectious diseases, not usually defined as STIs, can be acquired sexually, for example, hepatitis B and C.

KEY SYNDROME   Syphilis

T. pallidum acquired from sexual contact causes an acute ulcer (chancre) at the inoculation site followed by dissemination throughout the body. See page 581. *Primary syphilis* presents as a chancre (Fig. 12–6A), a single, firm, painless, punched-out ulcer on or near the genitalia or, uncommonly, on the lips, mouth, or woman's breast, with regional lymphadenopathy. *Secondary syphilis* presents 6 weeks after the chancre with headache, sort throat, myalgia, malaise, itching and a maculopapular rash on the soles, palms, and extremities. There may be lymphadenopathy, fever, and alopecia. *Tertiary syphilis* presents with various clinicopathologic pictures depending on tissues involved. Findings may include aortic insufficiency, tabes dorsalis, general paresis, or gumma formation.

KEY SYNDROME   Urethritis

Infection, usually by sexually transmitted organisms, results in inflammation and purulent discharge from the urethral orifice accompanied by burning pain with urination. The edges of the meatus may be reddened, edematous, and everted. A variable amount of pus or clear fluid discharges from the urethra. The lymphatic channels in the dorsum of the penis may be tender and palpable. Tender, swollen, palpable lymph nodes develop in the inguinal regions. Micturition and erection may be painful. The diagnosis is usually obvious by direct inspection and the presence of mucous shreds and pus in the first part of the urine specimen. In young, sexually active men, chlamydia, gonorrhea, and the genital mycoplasmas are the most common pathogens. In men over age 40, enteric bacteria predominate. Prostatitis may complicate urethritis by extension of infection into the prostatic ducts. Urethritis may constitute a member of the triad, along with conjunctivitis and arthritis, in reactive arthritis (Reiter disease); the urethritis frequently is the presenting sign.

KEY SYNDROME   Erectile Dysfunction: Impotence

Sexual arousal, rigid distention of the corpora cavernosum of the penis, orgasm, and effective ejaculation require intact endocrine, neurologic, and vascular function. Dysfunction anywhere in this complex and coordinated process can produce erectile dysfunction, the inability to sustain a penile erection of sufficient rigidity or duration to consummate satisfactory coitus. Many patients do not volunteer information about their inability to sustain an erection of sufficient rigidity or duration satisfactory for intercourse, although they may acknowledge the problem on a questionnaire. Commonly, however, this problem will not be identified unless you ask specifically about sexual performance. Awakening with early morning erections argues against an organic cause (neurologic, vascular, or endocrinologic), and suggests a functional problem. A thorough history focusing on the onset and progression of symptoms, libido, medications, surgery, and psychosocial issues is essential in the evaluation. Early morning erections militate against neurologic, vascular, or endocrinologic causes, and suggests a psychological problem. Screening for depression, hypothyroidism, hypogonadism and diabetes is useful. Full evaluation requires urologic referral [Morgentaler A. Male impotence. *Lancet.* 1999;354:1713–1718; Davis-Joseph B, Tiefer L, Melman A. Accuracy of the initial history and physical examination to establish the etiology of erectile dysfunction. *Urology.* 1995;45:498–502].

✔ *ERECTILE DYSFUNCTION—CLINICAL OCCURRENCE:* **Congenital** genetic disorders impairing sexual maturation (e.g., Prader Willi syndrome) or leading to hypogonadism (e.g., hemochromatosis); **Endocrine** primary hypogonadism, hypothyroidism, hypopituitarism, diabetes mellitus; **Idiopathic** hypertension, atherosclerosis; **Metabolic/Toxic** medications (antihypertensives, anxiolytics, antidepressants), alcohol, opiates, marijuana, chronic renal failure; **Mechanical/Traumatic** postradical prostatectomy, radiation, long-distance bicycling; **Neurologic** peripheral neuropathy, myelitis, spinal cord compression, multiple sclerosis, dementia; **Psychosocial** depression, anxiety; **Vascular** atherosclerosis, vasculitis.

> **KEY SYNDROME** Benign Prostatic Hyperplasia

Hyperplasia of the transitional zone places pressure on the bladder trigone and constricting the prostatic urethra. Benign prostatic hyperplasia affects men as they age, most often beginning after the fifth decade. Many experience urethral obstructive and/or irritative symptoms such as hesitancy, weak urinary stream, nocturia, and dribbling. When the prostate is enlarged, it is often elastic to rubbery or firm on palpation. Hyperplasia of the transitional zone may be difficult to detect when the gland protrudes anteriorly often producing urethral obstruction. Size cannot be used to judge propensity for obstruction.

> **KEY SYNDROME** Prostate Cancer

While local disease is usually asymptomatic, dysuria and symptoms of obstruction may occur in advanced disease. A discrete nodule may be palpated on the posterior surface of the prostate or the gland my feel diffusely enlarged. The entire gland may become stony hard, or there may be several hard nodules. The median furrow becomes obliterated. Early spread is often in the direction of the seminal vesicles. It is important to note the size of the mass, whether it involves one or both lobes, whether normal anatomic landmarks are preserved or obliterated, and whether there is extension beyond the prostate. Extension is palpable or inferred from fixation of the rectal mucosa to the posterior surface of the prostate. If the digital rectal examination is positive, ultrasound-guided needle biopsy is indicated.

> **KEY SYNDROME** Chronic Prostatitis

Palpation of the prostate may not reveal distinctive findings. Prostatic massage is accomplished by repeatedly and firmly stroking the posterior surface of the prostate from the lateral margins toward the midline, an often-painful procedure. The fluid is milked from the urethra and examined under the microscope. In prostatitis, the fluid contains many leukocytes. Chronic prostatitis may be either infective or noninfective, a distinction sometimes difficult to make.

Chronic Pelvic Pain Syndrome (Prostadynia): Chronic pain is not rare in otherwise healthy men. The onset may be acute or insidious. It is usually described as a deep boring persistent pain felt deep to the perineum. It may wax and wane, but rarely remits completely. It may be accompanied by mild urinary symptoms of decreased stream or hesitancy, but dysuria, uretheral discharge, hematuria and fever are absent. The cause is unknown, but usually attributed to chronic prostatic inflammation (chronic prostatitis), either infectious or idiopathic. The prostate may be normal, enlarged, diffusely softened (boggy) or firm; it is not tender. Routine urine cultures are negative; Meares-Stamey 4 glass test after prostatic massage may identify an infection or evidence of inflammation [Schaeffer AJ. Chronic prostatitis and the chronic pelvic pain syndrome. *N Engl J Med*. 2006;355:1690–1698]. Treatment is often unsatisfactory.

KEY SYNDROME   Reactive Arthritis (Reiter Syndrome)

This syndrome occurs following a STI or diarrheal illnesses. It involves chronic recurrent inflammation of the urethra, conjunctivae, skin, periarticular tissue, and large joints. Patients present with urethritis, conjunctivitis, arthritis, back pain, and/or characteristic skin disease on the feet and glans penis. Diagnosis rests on finding multisystem involvement in a patient with a compatible history and without other demonstrable disease. There is no diagnostic test.

KEY DISEASE   Behçet Syndrome

Patients frequently present with aphthous ulcers of the mouth or genital tract. See Chapter 8, page 418.

KEY SYNDROME   Klinefelter Syndrome

An abnormal complement of 47 chromosomes (XXY and variants) produces variable masculinization. Affected individuals are tall with long legs, atrophic testes and gynecomastia. They are subfertile [Lanfranco F, Kamischke A, Zitzmann M, et al. Klinefelter's syndrome. *Lancet*. 2004;364:273–283].

CHAPTER 13

The Spine, Pelvis and Extremities

The musculoskeletal system has four major functional components: the bones and ligaments, the synovial and fibrocartilaginous joints, the muscles and tendons, and the nerves innervating the muscles. Tendons anchor muscle to bone while ligaments anchor bone to bone. The overall shape and contour of the body is attributable to its bony structure and overlying muscles.

Major Systems and Their Physiology

Bones and Ligaments

Bones provide mechanical support for the body and protection for the viscera within the body cavities, vertebral column and skull. Mature bone forms by mineralization of osteoid laid down by osteoblasts on a cartilaginous matrix in the epiphyses of the long bones, endplates of the vertebrae and cartilaginous structures (endochondral bones of the skull and face). *Cortical bone* forms a thick cortex surrounding a central hollow, the marrow space. *Trabecular bone* forms an intricate lattice laid down along the lines of stress within the marrow cavity. Bone reabsorption by osteoclasts and new bone formation by osteoblasts is continuous. Bone must maintain strength sufficient to resist compression and tension applied by mechanical loading forces and muscle traction. Bone strength depends upon normal architecture, collagen, and mineralization; abnormality of any component results in susceptibility to fracture. The shape of mature bone is influenced by the pull of the muscles at their anatomic origins and insertions during skeletal maturation. Muscles that insert on a small portion of bone and exert large forces deform the bone into prominences. Adjacent bones are connected by *ligaments*, collagenous bands continuous with the collagen of the bone itself. Ligaments stabilize the bones relative to one another and the intervening joints.

Joints

Joints separate articulated bones. *Fibrocartilage* separates bones at joints where motion is minimal, for example, the intervertebral discs. *Synovial (diarthrodial) joints* separate bones where motion is extensive. The bone surfaces of diarthrodial joints are covered with *hyaline cartilage* architecturally designed to resist repeated axial loading with minimal deformation while providing a smooth, virtually friction-free surface for motion. The avascular cartilage derives its nutrition from the synovial fluid by diffusion. The diarthrodial joints are enclosed within a synovial envelope of collagen lined with a single synovial cell layer that secretes the proteoglycans necessary for joint lubrication. Joint integrity is maintained by ligaments anchoring bone to bone and the forces exerted by muscles whose tendons cross the joint.

Muscles, Tendons, and Bursae

See also Chapter 14, The Neurologic Examination. *Striated skeletal muscles* exert contractile force proximally on one bone at its origin and distally via a variably elongated *tendon* onto its insertion on another bone. Therefore, muscular contraction serves to change the relative position of the bones. Most muscles originate diffusely directly from the periosteum, while some attach by tendons at both their origin and insertion, for example, the long head of the biceps. Tendons are elongated, relatively avascular collagen structures that are continuous at their origin with the interstitial collagen of the muscle and at their insertion with that of the bone. Tendons may lie free in the tissue, but are often surrounded by synovial sheaths or bursae where they cross mobile joints or pass around bony prominences. *Bursae* are synovial-lined cavities serving to reduce friction between tendons or muscles and underlying bone. Muscles are highly vascular since they require maximal oxygen delivery to efficiently convert stored glycogen and fatty acids into effective mechanical power. Muscle is enclosed in an inelastic collagenous *fascia*. Muscle is susceptible to tearing from the force of its own contraction. Ischemic necrosis may occur when contracting with a compromised blood supply. Body contours result from muscles and subcutaneous fat overlying the skeleton. Asymmetry or abnormalities of body contour suggest changes in the underlying muscles, or less commonly, fat distribution.

Superficial Anatomy of the Spine and Extremities

See the descriptions of each anatomic location given under section on Physical Examination and texts on anatomy for artists. The bones of the spine are considered along with their ligamentous attachments, intervertebral disks, and musculature.

The Axial Skeleton: Spine and Pelvis

The Cervical Spine

There are seven cervical vertebrae (Fig. 13–1A); three of which are specialized: C1 is the atlas (bearing a globe, like the Greek god after whom it is named); C2 is the axis about which the atlas rotates; and C7 is the vertebra prominens. Nodding of the head occurs chiefly at the atlantooccipital joint. Flexion and extension involve the occiput—C1 and C3 to C7. All vertebrae permit lateral bending. Half of rotation occurs at the atlantoaxial joint, with the remainder distributed through the cervical spine. For measurements of cervical motion, see Fig. 13–1B.

Thoracolumbar Spine and Pelvis

Below the neck, there are 12 thoracic and 5 lumbar vertebrae, a fused mass of 5 sacral vertebrae articulated with the pelvic bones at the sacroiliac (SI) joint and 4 variously separated coccygeal vertebrae. Viewed laterally, the vertebral column presents four curves (Fig. 13–2A). Least pronounced is the cervical curve, which is concave backwards, beginning at C2 and ending at T2. The thoracic

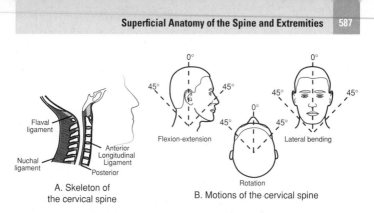

Fig. 13–1 *Anatomy and Motions of the Cervical Spine. A. The skeleton of the cervical spine. B. Motions of the cervical spine:* Normal range of motion exceeds the angles, which are shown as points of reference.

curve is convex backwards, beginning at T2 and ending at T12. The lumbar curve, more pronounced in the female, is concave backwards, from T12 to the lumbosacral joint. The pelvic curve, convex backwards and downward, extends from the lumbosacral joint to the tip of the coccyx. The spinal motions are flexion-extension, lateral bending, and rotation. For methods of measurement, see Fig. 13–2B.

Appendicular Skeleton Including Joints, Ligaments, Tendons, and Soft Tissues

The Hand

The hand includes the carpal, metacarpal, and phalangeal bones, their joints, and the covering soft tissues. Abnormalities in size and disproportions in a part are usually caused by bone abnormalities. The *posture of the hand* results from the relative tone of the finger and wrist flexors, extensors, and intrinsic hand muscles and the presence or absence of joint disorders.

The Wrist

The wrist includes the radiocarpal joint, the eight carpal bones in two parallel rows, and the overlying tendons and tendon sheaths (Fig. 13–3). The *radiocarpal joint* is the articulation of a concave with a convex surface. The proximal concave surface is formed by the distal end of the radius and the adjacent triangular *articular disk* that caps the distal end of the ulna. The distal convex surface consists of the curving sides of three carpal bones of the proximal row, the *navicular*, the *lunate*, and the *triquetrum* (from the radial to the ulnar side). The pisiform does not participate because it lies on the volar aspect of the triquetrum. The navicular is most commonly fractured, because the radius has wider contact with it than with the lunate, and the forces transmitted from the ulna to the triquetrum are cushioned by the articular disk. The major synovial cavity lies between radius and the navicular. A minor cavity separates the distal end of the ulna and the articular disk, extending proximally between the radius and ulna.

Knowledge of the topography is necessary to examination of the wrist (Fig. 13–4). **Volar Aspect of the Wrist:** The *pisiform* bone can be palpated as a bony prominence on the ulnar side, just distal to the palmar crease and proximal to the

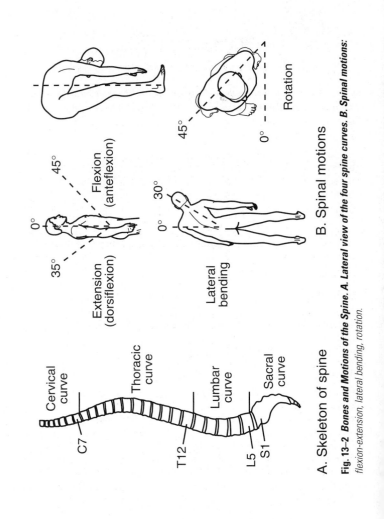

Extension
(dorsiflexion)

0°

35°

Flexion
(anteflexion)

45°

Lateral
bending

0°

30°

Rotation

45°

0°

B. Spinal motions

Cervical
curve

Thoracic
curve

Lumbar
curve

Sacral
curve

C7

T12

L5
S1

A. Skeleton of spine

Fig. 13–2 Bones and Motions of the Spine. A. Lateral view of the four spine curves. B. Spinal motions:
flexion-extension, lateral bending, rotation.

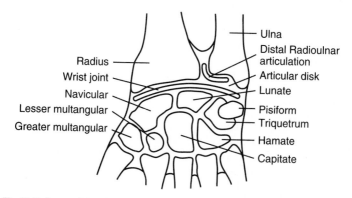

Fig. 13–3 *Bones of the Wrist.*

base of the hypothenar eminence. Four tendons can be palpated and often seen. With the digits slightly flexed and muscles tensed, three tendons are apparent in most persons. From the ulnar to the radial side, they are the *flexor carpi ulnaris, palmaris longus,* and *flexor carpi radialis.* The palmaris longus is absent in approximately 10% of persons. With the fist clenched hard, the tendon of the *flexor digitorum sublimis* also appears between the flexor carpi ulnaris and the palmaris longus. ***Dorsal Aspect of the Wrist:*** The most conspicuous prominence is the ulnar styloid process. Extension of the thumb accentuates the borders of the *anatomist's snuffbox,* a recess formed between the *extensor pollicis longus and brevis.*

The Forearm

The forearm extends from the elbow to the wrist. *Inspection* and *palpation* are used for examination. The radius and ulna articulate with the humerus proximally.

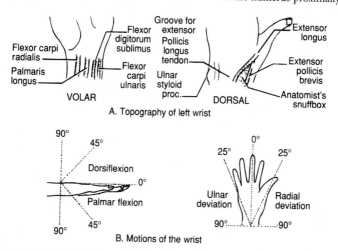

Fig. 13–4 *The Wrist. A. Topography of the wrist joint. B. Motions of the wrist joint.*

They are connected by an *interosseous membrane* throughout most of their length. The radius and ulna are practically subcutaneous, so their entire length can be palpated. The dorsal muscle mass is formed by the wrist and finger extensor muscles which insert on the lateral epicondyle of the humerus. The volar mass is the finger and wrist flexors inserting on the medial epicondyle.

The Elbow

There are two articulations in the elbow. The hinged *humeroulnar joint* is formed by the semilunar notch of the ulnar olecranon process embracing and moving around the transverse drum of the spool-shaped *trochlea* of the distal humerus (Fig. 13–5A). When the elbow is in full extension, the *olecranon process* fits into the *olecranon fossa* of the humerus just above the trochlea. The *trochlea* forms the medial two-thirds of the lower humeral articulation. The lateral third is the rounded *capitulum* on which a cup-shaped depression in the radial head pivots and glides to form the *humeroradial joint*. The radial head is a squat cylinder whose sides rotate in the *annular ligament* during pronation and supination of the forearm.

Viewed from the back (Fig. 13–6), the flexed elbow presents three bony prominences of an inverted equilateral triangle: the two basal points are the medial and lateral epicondyles of the humerus, the tip of the olecranon process forms the apex. During full extension, the three points form a straight transverse line.

The Shoulder

The shoulder girdle includes bones (humerus, scapula, clavicle, sternum), joints (glenohumeral, acromioclavicular, sternoclavicular, and scapulothoracic), their ligamentous connections, and the overlying muscles, tendons, and bursae. The shoulder joint is a ball-and-socket articulation with the hemispheric humeral head fitting into the shallow cavity formed by the scapular *glenoid* and its surrounding, fibrous *labrum* (Fig. 13–7). The articulating surfaces are enclosed by a short tube of joint capsule. The scapular *coracoid process* projects anterior and medial to the joint and the *acromion* forms a rigid fender above the joint. They are connected by the *coracoacromial ligament*. The clavicle is connected to the acromion by the superior *acromioclavicular ligament* and to the underlying coracoid process by the coracoclavicular ligament. From its origin within the joint capsule, the tendon of the long head of the biceps emerges anteriorly through a capsular opening between the greater and lesser tubercles of the humeral head. The joint capsule is lined by a synovial membrane with a prolongation forming a tubular sheath for the biceps tendon which follows the tendon distally to the surgical neck of the humerus.

The *joint capsule* is loose, exerting little tension except in extreme positions. Therefore, shoulder stability is maintained by muscle pull. The shoulder joint enjoys great freedom of motion from the shallowness of the glenoid cavity, the large articular surface of the humeral head and the lack of restraining ligaments, but this also makes it vulnerable to dislocation. The *scapula* is held to the thoracic wall entirely by its muscular attachments, its wing gliding freely over the thoracic muscles. Scapular movements add greatly to the mobility of the upper limb, so scapular motion must be distinguished from movements of the glenohumeral joint. The single ligament-bone connection of the shoulder girdle to the axial skeleton is via the *acromioclavicular joint*, the *clavicle*, and the *sternoclavicular joint*.

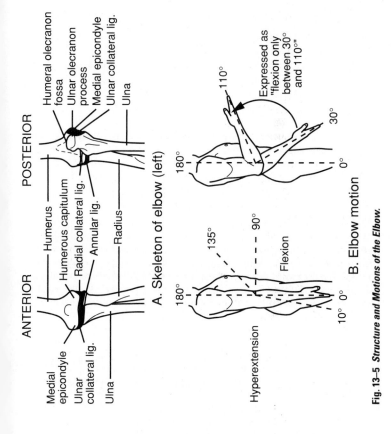

ANTERIOR

Medial epicondyle
Humerus
Humerous capitulum
Radial collateral lig.
Annular lig.
Radius

Medial epicondyle
Ulnar collateral lig.
Ulna

POSTERIOR

Humeral olecranon fossa
Ulnar olecranon process
Medial epicondyle
Ulnar collateral lig.
Ulna

A. Skeleton of elbow (left)

180°

135°

90°

10° 0°

Hyperextension

Flexion

180°

110°

Expressed as "flexion only between 30° and 110°"

30°

0°

B. Elbow motion

Fig. 13-5 *Structure and Motions of the Elbow.*

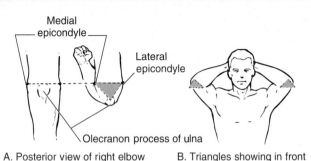

A. Posterior view of right elbow   B. Triangles showing in front

Fig. 13–6 *Topographic Relations of the Elbow.* *In extension, the ulnar olecranon process lies on a straight line between the medial and the lateral epicondyles of the elbow. In flexion, the olecranon process moves downward to produce an inverted equilateral triangle between the three bony prominences. Any distortion of this triangle after trauma points to a fracture involving one or more of its points.*

The principal bony landmarks of the shoulder form a right-angled triangle: the tip of the coracoid, the greater tubercle of the humeral head, and the acromion. The right angle is at the greater tubercle. The acromion is easily seen and felt beyond the end of the clavicle. The coracoid is palpated near the anterior border of the deltoid muscle on a horizontal line with the greater tubercle.

The Hip Joint and Thigh

In the diagnostic examination, the hip joint and thigh are considered together. The femoral axis slants medially toward the knee. The *greater trochanter* of the femur presents a lateral bony mass, palpable through the thigh muscles (Fig. 13–8A). On the medial side and a little distal is the *lesser trochanter*, smaller in size and inaccessible to palpation. Arising between the trochanters, the *femoral neck* slants proximally and medially, forming an angle with the femoral axis of

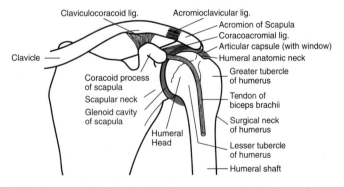

Fig. 13–7 *Anatomy of the Shoulder Joint.* *The anterior window in the joint capsule exposes the inner attachment of the biceps brachii muscle.*

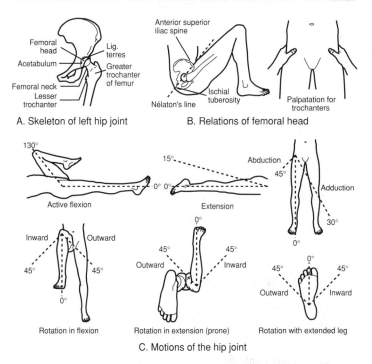

A. Skeleton of left hip joint

B. Relations of femoral head

C. Motions of the hip joint

Fig. 13–8 *Anatomy and Motions of the Hip Joint. A. Skeleton of the left hip joint.* ***B. Relations of the femoral head:*** *The femoral greater trochanter lies on the Nélaton line between the anterior superior iliac spine and the ischial tuberosity. The relative positions of the femoral heads with respect to the trochanters can be compared on the two sides as illustrated. The thumbs are placed on the anterior superior iliac spines, while the fingers rest on the greater trochanters of the femora. Small disparities in distance are readily detected.* ***C. Motions of the hip joint.***

120 to 160 degrees. An increase in the angle produces lateral deviation of the femoral shaft, *coxa valga*, a decrease in the angle deviates the shaft medially, *coxa vara*. The neck is surmounted by the globular *femoral head*, which fits into the cupped *acetabulum* of the pelvis, forming a ball-and-socket joint. This joint permits flexion-extension, abduction-adduction, and internal-external rotation (Fig. 13–8C). An important topographic relationship is defined by the *Nélaton line*, extending from the *anterosuperior iliac spine* to the *ischial tuberosity*. With the thigh flexed, the line passes through the tip of the greater trochanter; an upward deviation of 1 cm is considered normal (Fig. 13–8B).

The Knee

The knee region includes the *tibiofemoral and tibiofibular joints*, the *patella*, the adjacent segments of the femur, tibia, and fibula, their ligaments, menisci, and muscles. Viewed from below (Fig. 13–9), the articular surface of the femur is

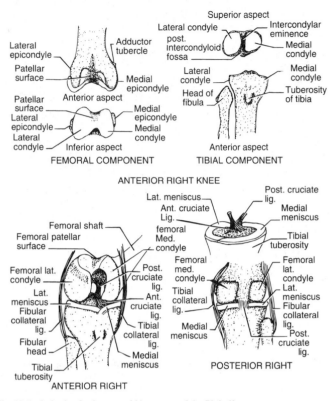

Fig. 13–9 *Articular Surfaces and Ligaments of the Right Knee.*

shaped like a horseshoe with its open end posterior. The two anteroposterior legs of the shoe are formed by nearly parallel *lateral and medial femoral condyles*, separated by the *intercondylar fossa*. The surface of the anterior bow is indented by a shallow median groove curving upward onto the anterior femur, the patellar articular surface. Superior to the articular surfaces of the condyles are the *medial and lateral epicondyles*. Viewed from above, the articular surface of the tibia presents two lateral almost flat, oval facets, the *medial and lateral tibial condyles*, separated by an *intercondylar fossa* with anterior and posterior segments. The lateral borders of the intercondylar fossa are the *intercondylar eminences*. On the central anterior tibia, slightly below the joint, is the *tibial tuberosity*.

The *knee joint has three articulations:* a medial and a lateral condylar articulation and an anterior joint where the patella glides over the femur (see Fig. 13–9). The femoral condyles may be likened to two thick disks with their edges resting on the almost flat tibial condyles. The small radius of curvature of the femoral condyles presents little apposing surface with the tibia in any position. The *lateral and medial menisci* are flattened crescents of fibrocartilage that rim the peripheral borders of the tibial condyles. Their radial cross-sections are wedge-shaped, with the thickest part outward. This arrangement deepens the articular surfaces of the

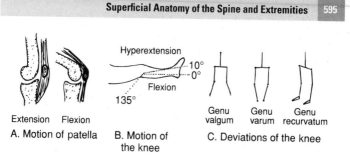

A. Motion of patella

B. Motion of the knee

C. Deviations of the knee

Fig. 13–10 *Motions and Deviations of the Knee.*

tibial condyles and fills the space between the curved femoral condyles and the flatter tibial surface. The ends of their crescents are attached to the intercondylar fossa.

The principal internal ligaments are the *anterior and posterior cruciate ligaments,* named for the positions of their tibial attachments and their crossing arrangement (see Fig. 13–9). The anterior cruciate ligament (ACL) begins in front of the anterior tibial intercondyloid eminence and passes upward, backward, and lateralward to the back of the lateral femoral condyle. The posterior cruciate ligament (PCL) attaches to the posterior intercondyloid fossa, passes upward, forward, and medially, to the front of the medial femoral condyle. The *lateral (fibular) collateral ligament* is a strong fibrous cord ascending vertically from the lateral aspect of the fibular head to the back of the lateral femoral condyle. Its opposite is the thinner and broader *medial (tibial) collateral ligament* ascending from the medial tibial condyle to the medial femoral condyle.

The flat triangular *patella,* a sesamoid bone, is embedded in the tendon of the quadriceps femoris. The distal extension of this tendon is the patellar ligament, attached distally to the tibial tuberosity. During extension of the knee, the patella rides loosely in front of the distal femur. In flexion, the patella opposes the lateral part of the medial femoral condyle (Fig. 13–10), while with active extension it is often pulled against the lateral femoral condyle.

The head of the *fibula* articulates with the lateral tibial condyle by an arthrodial joint. This joint is inferior to the knee joint and entirely separated from it. The fibula is held to the tibia by the joint capsule and anterior and posterior ligaments.

The *joint capsule of the knee* is a complex of fibrous sheets reinforced by bands from the muscle tendons crossing the joint. It is a single synovial sac that envelops the articular surfaces of both pairs of condyles forming the largest joint cavity in the body. A large *suprapatellar pouch* of the sac ascends anteriorly, first between the patella and the anterior aspect of the femur, then into a bursa between the quadriceps tendon and a fat pad in front of the femur. A precise understanding of the extent of this sac is diagnostically important.

The *principal bursae of the knee* are of diagnostic importance: (1) a bursa lying between the skin and the patella, the *prepatellar bursa,* (2) a smaller bursa between the skin and the patellar ligament, the *superficial infrapatellar bursa*; (4) a bursa between the skin and the tibial tuberosity, (3) the *anserine bursa* medial and inferior to the knee joint between the tibia and the tendons of the semitendinosus, gracilis, and sartorius muscles. The suprapatellar pouch of the knee joint extending superiorly between the quadriceps tendon and the femur is not a true bursa, although it functions as such. It may be erroneously called the suprapatellar bursa.

MEDIAL ASPECT OF RIGHT FOOT

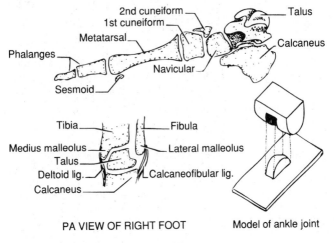

PA VIEW OF RIGHT FOOT   Model of ankle joint

Fig. 13–11 *Structure of the Ankle Joint and Foot.*

The Ankle

The ankle joint is a hinged articulation between the *tibia* proximally and the *talus* of the foot distally. The superior articular surface of the talus is rounded superiorly and tipped slightly medially and is continuous with the flattened, nearly vertical medial and lateral faces (Fig. 13–11). The upper curvature articulates with the flat surface of the lower tibia. The sides of the proximal portion of the joint are the *medial malleolus* of the tibia and the *lateral malleolus* of the fibula. These serve as the sides of a mortise, articulating with the flat lateral surfaces of the talus and stabilizing the joint laterally and medially. During ankle flexion and extension, the tibial surface glides over the curved surface of the talus changing the angle between leg and foot and rotating the leg medially on the foot with increasing dorsiflexion helping to transfer weight toward the medial foot and great toe during stance and push-off phases of gait. The lower ends of the tibia and fibula are bound together by the anterior and posterior *tibiofibular ligaments.* The medial malleolus is attached to the talus and calcaneus by a triangular band, the *deltoid ligament.* The lateral malleolus is attached below to the talus and the calcaneus by the *calcaneofibular ligament* and the anterior and posterior *talofibular ligaments.* The joint capsule surrounds the articulation and is lined with synovial membrane.

The motions of the ankle joint are dorsiflexion (extension) and plantar flexion (flexion) (Fig. 13–12). The only bony landmarks are the lateral and medial malleoli; the lateral is lower than the medial.

The Foot

The foot is a complex structure designed to withstand the enormous forces transmitted bidirectionally between the body and the ground during walking, running, and jumping. It is both flexible and strong, and able to adapt to virtually any

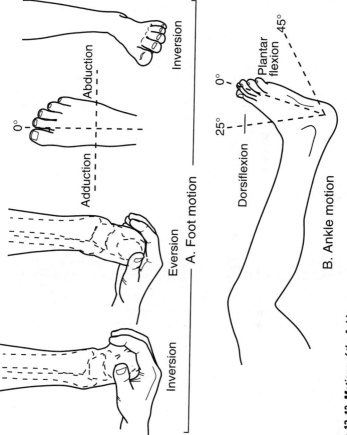

Inversion   Eversion

Adduction   0°   Abduction

Inversion

— A. Foot motion —

Dorsiflexion 25°   0°

Plantar flexion   45°

B. Ankle motion

Fig. 13–12 *Motions of the Ankle.*

ground surface. It is divided into the *hindfoot* (talus and calcaneus), *midfoot* (navicular, cuboid and medial, intermediate and lateral cuneiforms), and the *forefoot* (metatarsals, phalanges, and sesamoids). The hindfoot and midfoot are separated by the *transverse tarsal joint* separating the talus and calcaneus from the navicular and cuboid, respectively. The transverse tarsal joint is responsible for inversion and eversion. The midfoot is separated from the forefoot at the *tarsometatarsal joint*. The foot has two prominent arches: the *longitudinal arch* forms the instep medially from the tubercles of the calcaneus to the heads of the metatarsals; and the mediolateral *metatarsal arch* from the first to the fifth metatarsal heads. The calcaneus is palpable on all but its superior and distal surfaces. The bones of the midfoot and forefoot are best palpated dorsally where they are not covered by muscle. There is a bony prominence on the midlateral margin just above the sole formed by the tuberosity of the fifth metatarsal.

The foot can be visualized anatomically as a tripod constructed of a series of triangles, each with an apex and a base. The tripod has its apex at the tibio-talar joint and a triangular base made up of the calcaneus and the first and 5th metatarsal heads. This tripod allows stable weight bearing on uneven ground. One of the triangles is the longitudinal arch with its apex at the transverse tarsal joint and its base the calcaneus and first metatarsal head. Another is the metatarsal arch, with its base the first and fifth metatarsal heads and its apex the third metatarsal head. The tip of the great toe with the first and fifth metatarsal heads forms the stable triangular base for the pushoff phase of gait. Lastly, each toe forms a triangle with the apex at the proximal interphalangeal (PIP) joint and the base at the pad of the toe and the metatarsal head. These functionally interlocking structures give the foot extraordinary strength and dynamic stability. Any disruption of this complex architecture results in significant loss of function.

Physical Examination of the Spine and Extremities

Because the examination must integrate the observations of bones, joints, and muscles, most clinicians examine anatomic regions in a sequence dictated by convenience for the doctor and patient, rather than examining each component sequentially. This also requires constant cross-referencing to the nervous and peripheral vascular systems.

Examination of the Axial Skeleton: Spine and Pelvis

EXAMINATION OF THE CERVICAL SPINE

 Following trauma or suspected cervical injury, the cervical spine must ALWAYS be immediately IMMOBILIZED in a rigid collar PRIOR TO ANY MOVEMENT or examination of the patient.

In the absence of acute trauma, examine the patient in the seated position viewing the neck from the front, sides, and back for deformities and unusual posture. Have the patient point to the site of pain. Test active motions of the neck with the instructions: "chin to chest," "chin to right and left shoulder," "ear to right and left shoulder," and "head back." With the flat of the hand, palpate the paravertebral muscles for muscle spasm, tender points or trigger points. Palpate and percuss the spinous processes for tenderness.

GENERAL EXAMINATION OF THE THORACOLUMBAR SPINE AND PELVIS

Following trauma or suspected spinal injury, the spine must ALWAYS be immediately immobilized on a back board PRIOR TO ANY MOVEMENT or examination of the patient.

The patient should be gowned such that the spine can be easily observed while maintaining patient comfort. ***With the Patient Standing:*** Observe from the back and side for deformity, muscle wasting, local swelling, abnormal curvature or lateral deviations of the spine. If the spinal processes are not visible, palpate and mark each to disclose a scoliosis. When lateral curvature is present, have the patient bend forward observing the spine and the chest wall on either side of the spine. Note whether the spine straightens and any asymmetry of the chest wall. In structural scoliosis, one side will be higher than the other (Fig. 13–13); with muscle spasm or ligament and joint disease, the chest will be symmetrical. Have the patient tense the glutei to reveal wasting. Percuss each spinous process to elicit tenderness. Have the patient walk observing the gait. Have the patient hop on each foot to identify muscle weakness and pain. Direct the patient to flex, extend, and laterally bend the spine without assistance. Test rotation by grasping the hips while the patient turns first one shoulder, then the other. Palpate for tenderness, muscles spasm or tender, or trigger points. ***With the Patient Supine:*** Have the head pillowed and the knees slightly flexed for comfort. Do the *straight-leg-raising test*, (Fig. 13–14A) by grasping the ankle, with the knee held in extension, and lifting the lower limb to its limit. Note the location of pain elicited, especially contralateral radiation indicating nerve root compression (*Lasèque sign*). With the straight leg elevated at a little-less-than-complete flexion, dorsiflex the foot looking for aggravation of pain. An alternative test is to gradually extend the flexed knee, with the finger pressing on the tibial nerve in the popliteal fossa; this produces pain if there is irritation of the lower lumbar nerve roots. ***With the Patient Prone:*** Ask the patient to turn from the supine to the prone position and note the amount of guarding, an indication of pain severity. For comfort, place a pillow between the table and the patient's pelvis. See if the muscle spasm and spinal deformity observed while erect persists in the prone position. Reexamine for areas of tenderness and deformity. A step deformity between L5 and S1 indicates

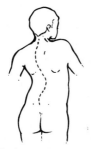

Scoliosis as demonstrated
by marking spinous processes

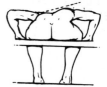

Scoliosis as viewed
with spine hyperflexed

Fig. 13–13 *Structural Scoliosis.* *Inspection of the flexed spine from behind shows the unequal elevation of the two erector spinae muscle masses.*

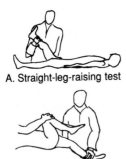

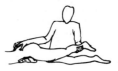

A. Straight-leg-raising test

Push upraised knee laterally

B. Patrick test

C. Passive hyperextension

D. Active hyperextension

Fig. 13–14 *Tests at the Hip and SI Joint. A. Straight-leg-raising test: The examiner lifts the supine patient's lower limb when the knee is held in extension. B. Patrick test: Lateral rotation of the hip is assessed by having the knee flexed and the foot of that leg placed on the opposite patella. The examiner then pushes the flexed knee down and out to rotate the head of the femur. C. Passive hyperextension of the thigh (Gaenslen test): While supine, the patient flexes the knee and femur on the affected side and holds the knee with the hands to eliminate lumbar lordosis. The examiner then hyperextends the unaffected thigh by letting it, sinks over the side of the table. In disease of the SI joint, this maneuver evokes pain. D. Active hyperextension: With the patient prone and the abdomen resting on a pillow, the patient lifts the spine against the resistance offered by the examiner's hand; SI disease causes pain.*

spondylolisthesis. With the heel of the hand, press along the spinous processes. Pain from light pressure suggests approximating spines with an intervening bursa; pain from deep pressure arises from intervertebral facets or disks. **With the Patient Sitting:** Examine for muscle wasting and check the knee and ankle reflexes.

Schober test for lumbar flexion. With patient standing erect, heels together, place a mark on the spine at the lumbosacral junction (the L5 spinous process or the point where a horizontal line between the posterior superior iliac spines intersects the spine). Have the patient bend forward maximally, trying to touch the fingers to the toes. Normally, the distance between the marks increases by ≥5 cm. If the distance increases <4 cm, mobility is restricted.

Additional exams for herniated disk. Test neurosensory function by assessing knee and ankle reflexes, flexion and extension strength at the knee and ankle, great toe extension strength, and sensation to touch. *Crossed-Straight-Leg-Raising Test:* Have the patient lie supine and lift the unaffected limb with the knee held straight. In the presence of herniated disk, this maneuver will exacerbate the pain in the affected limb, and may cause sciatic pain in the hitherto unaffected limb. This is considered by some writers to be pathognomonic of herniated disk. *Reverse Straight-Leg-Raising Test:* With the patient lying prone and the knee flexed maximally on the thigh, the normal person complains of quadriceps tightness in the anterior thigh. With true disk disease, as the root tightens over the involved disk and abdominal compression increases the subarachnoid pressure, the pain is felt in the back or in a sciatic distribution on the affected side.

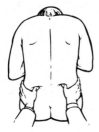

Fig. 13–15 *Palpation of the SI Joints.*

Testing the SI joint. Examine the patient while sitting facing away from you. Locate the posterior superior iliac spines by the dimples in the overlying skin or by placing your thumbs on the iliac crests with your hands around the patient's trunk (Fig. 13–15) and following the crests medially to the iliac spines. The portion of the SI joint most accessible to palpation is one fingerbreadth medial to the spines. As the patient bends forward slowly, press your thumbs deeply along the joint looking for tenderness. In the *Gaenslen test of the SI joint* (Fig. 13–14C), the supine patient holds the knee of the affected side with both hands, flexing the knee and the hip to fix the lumbar spine against the table; then hyperextend the other thigh by pushing it downward over the side of the table. An affected SI joint will be painful with this maneuver. Active prone hyperextension of the spine (Fig. 13–14D) may aggravate SI pain when the patient attempts to lift the spine against the resistance of the examiner's hand held in the lumbar region.

Low back pain—Magnuson pointing test for malingering. Low back pain is a favorite complaint of malingerers. Identify the painful spot by palpation and mark it with a skin pencil. After completing the rest of the examination, palpate once again for the painful spot. The patient with organic disease identifies the same point each time; the malingerer identifies a somewhat different spot.

Examination of the Appendicular Skeleton Including Joints, Ligaments, Tendons, and Soft Tissues

GENERAL EXAMINATION OF JOINTS

Examine all joints systematically from head to foot or in reverse sequence, comparing right and left. To minimize pain and guarding, place the patient so the joint to be examined is supported. *Inspect* the bony landmarks, the size and contour of the joint (visualizing the location of the joint capsule), the overlying skin color and any deformity (swelling, angulation, rotation, subluxation, contracture or ankylosis). *Palpate* gently, for skin temperature and for tenderness in the skin, muscles, bursae, ligaments, tendons, fat pads, and joint capsule. The normal synovium is not palpable, while a thickened synovium feels "doughy" or "boggy." *Test the joint for effusion* by placing the finger(s) of each hand on opposite sides of the joint, then compress with one hand; an effusion will displace the receiving fingers. *Test active range of motion* by directing the patient to move the joint through its full range. To *test passive range of motion*, anchor the joint proximally with one hand while the other moves the distal member gently to its full limits.

Observe how the motion terminates: muscle spasm, gelling that improves with repeated movement, effusion in the joint, locking from loose bodies in the joint or fibrosis cause "*soft arrests,*" while bony ankylosis causes a "*hard arrest.*" Palpate over the joint for crepitus with motion. *Test for ligament integrity* by anchoring the bone proximal to the joint while gently displacing the distal bone in the plane to be tested. The muscles must be relaxed when testing ligament stability. Always compare right and left since normal ligament tightness is quite variable, from tight to loose ("double jointed").

The Upper Limb

This anatomic region includes the structures of the neck, shoulder girdles, upper arms, forearms and hands. Its principle function is the placement and manipulation of the hands. The examination usually begins with the hands and works upward, the sequence used here.

Examination of the Hand

Hand structures are relatively superficial and easily examined. **Inspection:** The fingertips in extension form an arc with the apex at the middle finger. With flexion the finger tips align at the base of the thenar eminence with the nails in the same plane; if there is shortening or crossing of the fingertips then prior injury with shortening and/or rotation of the affected phalanges or metacarpal is present. Have the patient gently make a fist and observe the proximal knuckles, the distal metacarpal heads. There should be a smooth arc between the index and little fingers. Depression of a knuckle indicates shortening of the metacarpal. Observe the bulk of the intrinsic hand muscles on the dorsum of the hand and the web space between the thumb and index finger. Prominence of the tendons and bones occurs with loss of muscle mass, usually resulting from an ulnar nerve lesion. Inspect the palmar aspect of the hand for normal skin creases, the bulk of the thenar and hypothenar muscle masses, callosities or thickening of the palmar fascia. Inspect the nails and finger tips for deformities, ulcers, and signs of previous trauma. **Palpation:** Examine each joint for bony prominences, synovial thickening, or effusion. Palpate the thenar, hypothenar and first web space muscles both relaxed and with contraction. If bone injury is suspected, palpate the entire length of the bone. Squeeze the palm from front to back and laterally across the knuckles to detect tenderness.

Functional tests of fingers.   Complete functional examination of the hands is beyond the scope of this text, requiring an in-depth understanding of the anatomy of the bones, muscles, tendons, ligaments, and nerves of the hand and forearm. Here, we present a screening examination. The fingers are named thumb, index, long or middle, ring, and little, or they are numbered one through five. The phalangeal joints are termed *distal interphalangeal (DIP), proximal interphalangeal (PIP),* and *metacarpophalangeal (MCP).* The aspects of the fingers are dorsal (extensor surface) and volar (flexor or palmar surface). Figure 13–16 illustrates the functional assessment of the joints. Muscles testing is described on page 699. Test active flexion and extension against resistance at the DIP and PIP joints. The *superficial flexors* attach on the middle phalanx assisting flexion of the MCP and PIP. Flexion at the DIP is performed solely by the *deep flexors.* Next, test abduction and adduction of the fingers; these movements are powered by the *interosseus* and *lumbrical muscles* innervated by the *ulnar nerve.* Test the thumb flexion and

FINGER MOTIONS

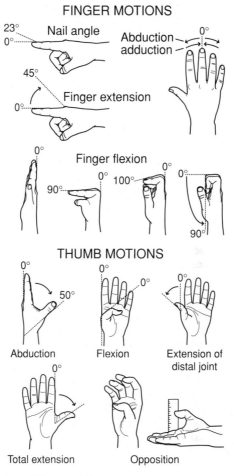

THUMB MOTIONS

Abduction   Flexion   Extension of distal joint

Total extension   Opposition

Fig. 13–16 *Motions of Fingers and Thumb.*

extension power at the MCP and IP, as well as abduction and adduction performed by the thenar muscles innervated by the median nerve.

EXAMINATION OF THE WRIST

Inspect and *palpate* the wrists for asymmetry, swelling, tenderness, deformities, and crepitus. **Testing Wrist Motion:** The primary motions of the wrist are extension-flexion (dorsiflexion and palmar flexion) and radial-ulnar deviation; Fig. 13–4 depict the methods of measurement.

EXAMINATION OF THE FOREARM

Inspect the muscle masses for symmetry; often the dominant arm is better muscled. Assess weakness and wasting in the muscles of the forearm that supply the

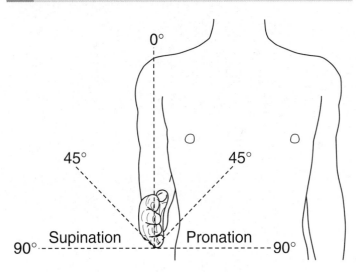

Fig. 13–17 *Forearm Motions.*

hand. Both the radial and ulnar arterial pulses are palpable proximal to the wrist. The motions of the forearm are *pronation* and *supination* (Fig. 13–17). Test for active and passive range of motion and power against resistance. Pain with resisted motion is especially important and the sites of pain should be palpated.

EXAMINATION OF THE ELBOW

Inspect and *palpate* the region for deformity, tenderness, and swelling. Swellings are more common on the extensor surface. Subcutaneous nodules are often found in the *olecranon bursa* and distally in the ulnar region. **Testing Elbow Motion:** The movements of the humeroulnar joint are extension-flexion. Pronation-supination principally involves the humeroradial and the distal radioulnar joints. Measurements of these motions are indicated in Fig. 13–5B. Test passive and active motion and strength by resisting active motion.

EXAMINATION OF THE SHOULDER

Inspection and palpation of the shoulder joint. Examine the disrobed patient from front and back while sitting with the arms relaxed (Fig. 13–18). *Inspect* the shoulder anteriorly and the scapula posteriorly for deformities and muscle wasting; nearly everyone carries one shoulder higher than the other. *Palpate* the scapular spine, following it forward to the acromion and the acromioclavicular joint. Palpate the sternoclavicular joint for deformity or tenderness. Next, palpate the subacromial space and the deltoid muscle and its subdeltoid bursa. Palpate the tendons of *the rotator cuff* for defects or tenderness and their insertions on the greater (*supraspinatus, infraspinatus*, and *teres minor* tendons) and lesser (*subscapularis tendon*) tuberosities of the humerus. Feel the *bicipital groove* between greater and lesser tuberosities for tenderness in the bicipital tendon sheath. Stand behind and to the side of the patient to palpate the *supraspinatus tendon* and the *subacromial bursa*. For the right shoulder, place your left hand over the shoulder

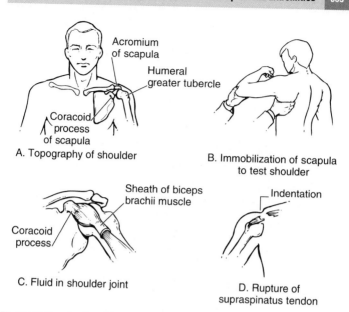

Acromium
of scapula

Humeral
greater tubercle

Coracoid
process
of scapula

A. Topography of shoulder

B. Immobilization of scapula
to test shoulder

Sheath of biceps
brachii muscle

Coracoid
process

Indentation

C. Fluid in shoulder joint

D. Rupture of
supraspinatus tendon

Fig. 13–18 *Examination of the Shoulder Joint. A. Topography of the shoulder:* The bony prominences of the humeral greater tubercle and the coracoid and acromial processes of the scapula form a right-angled triangle. *B. Immobilization of the scapula to test shoulder motion. C. Fluid in the shoulder joint:* The heavily stippled structures are the joint capsules distended with fluid. *D. Rupture of supraspinatus tendon.*

so your index finger palpates the tendon just behind its attachment on the greater tubercle of the humeral head, and your middle finger palpates the subacromial bursa. With your right hand on the patient's flexed elbow, move the arm backward and forward a few times to detect crepitus or tenderness at either point. Finally, place your fingers in the axilla with the pulps facing laterally and palpate the humeral head and the lateral aspect of the glenoid synovial sac.

Measurements of shoulder motion. Imagine the shoulder joint as the center of a sphere, marked as a globe with a north and south pole and meridians (Fig. 13–19). Then an anterior-posterior (parasagittal) plane through the shoulder joint describes an anterior meridian on the sphere's surface that is 0 *degrees of abduction-adduction.* Meridians lateral to it mark degrees of abduction and those medial to it are degrees of adduction. When the arm hangs at the patient's side, it is in 0 *degree of elevation and of abduction.* The arm can be lifted from the south pole to the north pole, or from 0 to 180 *degrees of elevation.* While elevating, the arm must follow in a meridian that designates abduction or adduction. If the arm is raised directly forward to the horizontal, the position is *90 degrees of elevation with 0 degrees of abduction;* this is the cardinal motion of FLEXION. When the arm is raised laterally to the horizontal, the position is *90 degrees of elevation with 90 degrees of abduction;* this is the cardinal motion of ABDUCTION. When the arm is raised directly posteriorly, the *position is elevation with 180 degrees of abduction;* this is the cardinal motion of EXTENSION. If, however, the arm is

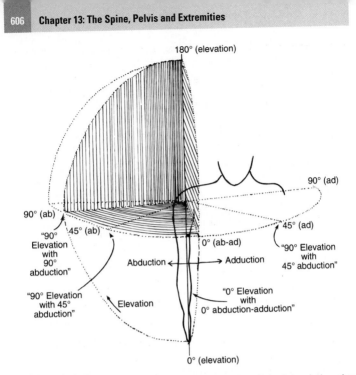

Fig. 13–19 *Motions at the Shoulder.* *There has been much confusion in terminology about shoulder motion. The system presented here leaves no room for misinterpretation. Elevation is a movement of the arm along any meridian, measured from position at the south pole. Elevation along the meridian in the parasagittal plane passing through the shoulder joint are flexion (forward) and extension (backwards). Movement medial to this is adduction; movement lateral to the plane is abduction. When the arm is elevated in any meridian other than the parasagittal one, the motion is expressed as "elevation in abduction" or "elevation in abduction." The amount of deviation from the parasagittal plane is noted in degrees, for example, "elevation in 70 degrees of abduction."*

raised to the horizontal in a meridian 20 degrees medial to 0 degrees, the position is *90 degrees of elevation with 20 degrees of adduction.*

Testing mobility of the shoulder. Shoulder mobility includes scapulothoracic and glenohumeral joint motions. Test the unaffected shoulder first and compare the affected side with it. The cardinal movements of the shoulder are **abduction** (*elevation at 90 degrees abduction*), **adduction** (*at 90 degrees elevation*), **flexion** (*elevation at 0 degrees abduction*), **extension** (*posterior elevation at 180 degrees abduction*) and **internal and external rotation**. Range of motion should be assessed both actively and passively. *Active motion* is accomplished by the patient and assesses joint mobility and muscle and tendon integrity and reveals limitations of motion as a result of pain. The examiner provides the power during *passive motion* while the patient relaxes, eliminating muscle and tendon limitations, to reveal the full range of motion available to each joint. *Elevation with abduction* involves both scapulothoracic and glenohumeral movement. Have the patient slowly raise the arm laterally from the side to straight overhead; the scapula should begin to move when elevation of the arm attains 60 degrees. *To test glenohumeral motion alone,* grasp the scapular wing and hold it fast to the thorax with one hand while the patient's arm is resting at his side (Fig. 13–18B). Alternatively, place one hand on top of the acromion to stabilize the scapula. Have the patient raise the arm laterally (90 degrees of abduction) and let the patient complete the motion as far as possible, with the scapula fixed. For *adduction (at 90 degrees elevation),* rest the fingers of one hand on the top of the patient's shoulder with your thumb behind, fixing the patient's scapula. Have the patient move the arm across the front of the chest as far as possible trying to place the wrist over the opposite shoulder. *Flexion (elevation at 0 degrees abduction)* is tested by having the patient elevate the arm forward from rest to straight overhead in the anterior-posterior plane. For *extension (posterior elevation at 180 degrees abduction),* have the patient push the arm straight backward in the same plane to the limit of motion. Test *internal and external rotation* with the arm at 90 degrees of abduction and 90 degrees of elevation, starting with the elbow flexed at 90 degrees and the palm facing the floor. For *internal rotation,* ask the patient to lower the hand, palm down, as far as possible without moving the elbow. For *external rotation,* start from the neutral position and have the patient raise the hand, palm forward, as far as possible without moving the elbow. When there is a deficit in active motion, test passive range of motion by repeating the maneuver with the patient relaxed and the examiner supporting the arm and gently putting it through the motion. Test for abduction strength and pain by resisting abduction at 30 degrees (supraspinatus) and 90 degrees (deltoid).

Auscultation of bony conduction through the shoulder. The olecranon-manubrium percussion sign is useful in evaluating patients with possible shoulder dislocations, clavicular fractures, or humeral fractures. Place the bell of the stethoscope over the manubrium with the patient's elbows flexed at 90 degrees and percuss the olecranons. Normally, with no disruption of bony conduction, percussion of right and left will produce equal crisp sounds. When dislocation or fracture disrupts bony conduction, the affected side will have decreased intensity and duller pitch.

The Lower Limb

This region includes the pelvis, buttocks, hip joints, thighs, knees, legs, ankles, feet, and toes. Its principal function is maintenance of an upright stance against gravity and locomotion.

EXAMINATION OF THE HIP AND THIGH

The patient should be disrobed from the waist down, covering the genitalia but not the buttocks.

Sites of pain. Have the patient point to the site of pain. An affected hip joint commonly causes pain in the inguinal region or in the buttocks posterior to the greater trochanter. *Pain from the hip joint may be felt only in the knee; this has led to many diagnostic errors.*

Begin the examination with the patient standing. Have the patient walk looking for abnormalities of gait: swinging the leg from the lumbar spine suggests ankylosis; a waddling gait is typical of bilateral hip dislocation; the gluteal gait

(*Trendelenburg gait*), with the trunk listing to the affected side with each step, suggests gluteus medias weakness, or, rarely, unilateral hip dislocation. With the patient standing still, look for a list to one side, asymmetry of the buttocks or other muscle masses, and scars or sinuses.

Lateral tilting of the pelvis. To determine if the pelvis is level, sit in front of the standing patient, with your thumbs on the anterior superior iliac spines; the interspinous line should be horizontal. Lateral tilting results either from adduction of one thigh or from shortening of the limb. Next, measure the distance between the greater trochanters and the anterior superior iliac spines: with your middle fingers, find the tips of the greater trochanters and palpate the distances to the spines. Small disparities can be detected in this manner (Fig. 13–8B). If the pelvis is not horizontal, place books or blocks under the foot of the shorter limb until the pelvis becomes horizontal; this provides an accurate measurement of shortening.

Next, *have the patient lie on the examining table. All the following tests except that for extension are made in the supine position.*

Test for rotation with extension. This motion should be tested first because it is gentlest; if it is painful, all other maneuvers should be carried out cautiously. With the patient supine, place a hand on each side of the lower thigh and rock it from side to side, watching the patella or the foot for the range of rotation (Fig. 13–20A). Alternatively, the foot may be rocked from side to side.

Test for rotation with flexion. Flex the knee and hip to 90 degrees, then move the foot maximally both medially (external rotation) and laterally (internal rotation) (Fig. 13–8C).

Test for abduction. Have the patient lie supine with the legs together. Place a hand on the iliac crest and grasp the ankle with your other hand; gradually abduct the patient's thigh until you feel the pelvis move, and note the angle attained (Fig. 13–8C).

Test for adduction. With each hand, grasp an ankle, holding one leg down in extension while you move the other thigh across it (see Fig. 13–8C). Note the angle attained from the neutral position. Normally, the thigh should cross the other at midthigh.

Test for hip flexion contracture. Flexion contracture of the hip is compensated for by a lumbar lordosis, allowing an upright stance that masks the contracture. Place your hand under the lumbar spine flexing the unaffected thigh until the spine presses your hand against the table to indicate that the lumbar lordosis has been straightened. Now, extend the other thigh. It should be able to lie flat on the examination table. Lack of full extension reveals a flexion contracture on the affected side, a positive *Hugh Owen Thomas sign* (Fig. 13–20C).

The anvil test. If other maneuvers have not been painful, raise the leg from the table with the knee in extension and strike the calcaneus with your fist, using a moderate blow in the direction of the hip joint (Fig. 13–20B). This may elicit pain in early disease of the joint.

Direction palpation of the hip joint. Facing the patient, examine the left hip with your right hand, and the right hip with your left hand. Hook your fingers about the greater trochanter with your thumb placed on the anterior superior iliac spine (Fig. 13–8B). With your thumb, follow the inguinal ligament medially until you feel the femoral artery, then move your thumb just below the inguinal ligament

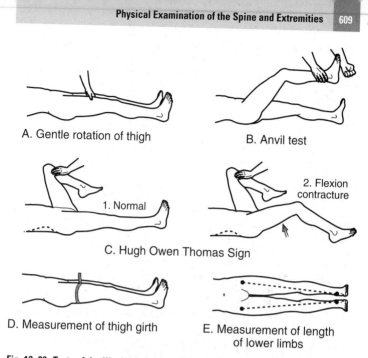

A. Gentle rotation of thigh

B. Anvil test

1. Normal

2. Flexion contracture

C. Hugh Owen Thomas Sign

D. Measurement of thigh girth

E. Measurement of length of lower limbs

Fig. 13–20 *Tests of the Hip Joint and Thigh. A. Gentle rotation of thigh. B. Anvil test. C. Hugh Owen Thomas sign for lumbar lordosis:* Flexion of the unaffected hip presses the lumbar spine against the table. If extension of the opposite hip is shown to be impaired when eliminating lumbar lordosis, it is a positive Hugh Owen Thomas sign. **D. Measurement of the girth of the thigh:** Mark similar levels on both limbs, measured down from the anterior superior iliac spines. Measure the girth at each level. **E. Measurement of length of limbs:** Have the two limbs approximated, or in the same relative positions from the midline. Measure from the anterior superior iliac spine to the medial malleolus, with the tape running medial to the patella.

and lateral to the artery; this should bring your thumb over the small portion of the femoral head that is extra acetabular. Exert, increasingly firm pressure to elicit pain from arthritis. Rock the femur gently, to feel crepitus. If the head does not move, fracture of the neck is probable. If the head cannot be felt, dislocation is suggested.

Patrick (FABER) test.   Passively flex the knee to a right angle and place the foot on the opposite patella. Push the flexed knee towards the table as far as the hip joint permits (Fig. 13–14B). This is also known by its acronym FABER (Flexion, Abduction, External Rotation). Painless and full external rotation (negative Patrick sign) excludes symptomatic disease of the hip joint and sacroiliac joints.

Test for extension.   *With the patient prone,* steady the pelvis with one hand while you raise the limb posteriorly (Fig. 13–8C). Normal extension is about 15 degrees.

Measurement of the lower limbs.   The girth of the thighs and legs is ascertained by measuring the circumferences with a tape measure at symmetrical levels, determined by measuring distances from the anterior superior iliac spines and marking them with a skin pencil (Fig. 13–20D). The length of the lower limbs is measured in straight lines from the anterior superior iliac spines to the medial malleoli of the tibiae (Fig. 13–20E). Care should be taken to have the tape in a straight line running medial to the patellae. Both extremities should lie exactly equidistant from the midline. If one limb cannot be placed in normal position, its opposite should be measured in a similar position. A difference of >1.5 cm suggests hip deformity in the shorter leg.

EXAMINATION OF THE KNEE

The normal movements of the knee are flexion and extension. For measurements, see Fig. 13–10B.

General examination of the knee. *Inspection:* Have the legs and thighs uncovered; observe the patient standing and supine. Inspect the knee region for deformities, swelling, redness, and muscle wasting. Note the position of the patella. *Palpation:* With the patient supine, test swellings for fluctuance, joint effusion, crepitation with motion, and points of localized tenderness in the ligaments, bones, and along the joint line. Palpate for doughy thickening of the synovium with obscuration of bony landmarks. Test the range of flexion and extension, test for abnormal anterior and posterior mobility of the tibia on the femur, and stress the medial and collateral ligaments for laxity or pain. Always compare right to left since considerable individual variation exists for joint stability. With a history of pain or locking, test for internal disorders as described on page 620ff.

Examination for knee effusion. *Inspection* may reveal bulging obliterating the natural hollows on both sides of the patellar tendon and in the suprapatellar pouch; it may assume a horseshoe shape around the patella (Fig. 13–21A). *Palpate* with the patient supine and the knees extended. Gently press the thumb and fingers of the right hand against the anterior femoral condyles at the medial and lateral sides of the distal patella slightly proximal to the joint line. Slide the left hand down the distal thigh with constant pressure until the patella rests in the space between the thumb and first finger; you will be compressing the suprapatellar pouch. If effusion is present, you will palpate and often see a bulge of fluid appear under the palpating thumb and/or fingers. Small amounts of fluid can be detected visually by compressing the swelling in one of the obliterated hollows beside the patella then watching for the hollow to slowly refill spontaneously or with compression of the suprapatellar pouch. Test for *patellar ballottement* (patellar tap or floating patella) by compressing the suprapatellar pouch, as described above, while the fingers of the other hand push the patella sharply against the femur (Fig. 13–21B). If fluid is present in sufficient quantity to elevate the patella from the femur, the brisk pressure on the patella will force it down against the femoral condyles with a palpable tap, the *patellar ballottement sign.*

Examination of the knee ligaments. This is part of the routine knee examination. Determine the degree of tightness or laxity of the anterior and posterior cruciates and both collateral ligaments.

Collateral Ligaments: With the patient supine, flex the knee to 10 degrees. Palpate the insertions proximally and distally and each ligament at the joint line. The rope-like lateral ligament is easily identified at the joint line posterolaterally.

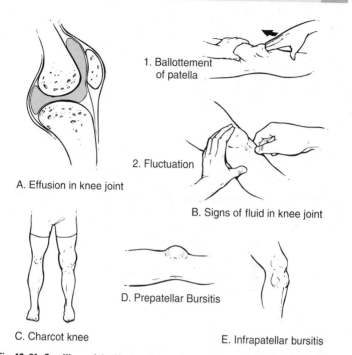

1. Ballottement of patella

2. Fluctuation

A. Effusion in knee joint

B. Signs of fluid in knee joint

C. Charcot knee

D. Prepatellar Bursitis

E. Infrapatellar bursitis

Fig. 13–21 *Swellings of the Knee and their Diagnosis. A. Knee effusion. B. Signs of knee effusions. C. Charcot knee. D. Prepatella bursitis. E. Infrapatellar bursitis.*

The broader medial ligament is more difficult to identify. Grasping the calf with one hand while the other hand supports and stabilizes the femur from behind with the thumb and fingertips on opposite joint margins overlying the collateral ligaments (Fig. 13–22). Stress first the lateral, then the medial collateral ligaments by exerting a varus then a valgus force on the calf while palpating over the ligaments at the joint margin. Feel for separation of the tibia from the femur while observing the amount of medial or lateral displacement of the tibia.

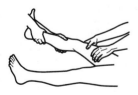

Assisted test for lateral stability of the knee

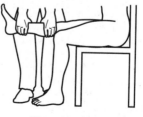

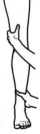

Unassisted tests for lateral stability of the knee

Fig. 13–22 *Tests for Lateral Stability of the Knee Joint.*

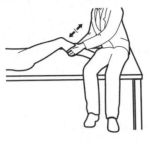 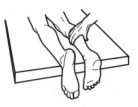

A. Lachman test for torn
cruciate ligament

B. Examination for ruptured
Achilles tendon

Fig. 13–23 *Testing the Cruciate Ligaments and Achilles Tendon. A. Lachman test for torn cruciate ligament: The patient is supine with the knee flexed at 30 degrees and the foot flat on the table. The examiner sits on the foot to anchor it, then pulls the head of the tibia toward himself to test the ACL. Forward motion of more than 1 cm is positive. Pushing the knee backward with the knee flexed at 90 degrees tests the PCL. B. Examination for ruptured Achilles tendon: The prone patient hangs the feet over the end of the table. Inspection shows less natural plantar flexion on the side of rupture. Simmonds Test: Squeeze the calf muscles transversely; a normal or partially ruptured tendon will produce plantar flexion; complete rupture will not respond.*

Cruciate Ligaments: Test the anterior cruciate with the *Lachman test* (Fig. 13–23A). Have the patient lie supine and flex the affected knee to an angle of 30 degrees. Sit on the patient's foot to fix it. Grasp the upper part of the leg with your fingers in the popliteal fossa and your thumbs on the anterior joint line. Pull the head of the tibia toward you so it glides on the femoral condyles. Forward movement of more than 1 cm is a positive Lachman test, indicating rupture of the ACL. To test the posterior cruciate, start as in the Lachman test and observe for sagging of the tibia posteriorly. Then push the head of the tibia posteriorly. Displacement should be less than 5 mm. Always compare the two knees because considerable individual variability in ligament tightness is normal; a discrepancy between the two sides is a sign of previous injury.

EXAMINATION OF THE INJURED KNEE

Obtain a detailed account of previous trauma, including the exact mechanism of injury. This is essential to understanding which structures might have been injured. Ask which motions cause discomfort or locking, and ascertain whether unlocking is sudden or gradual (as in muscle spasm). Have the patient point to sites of pain and demonstrate the position of fixation if locking has occurred. **Inspection:** Examine the patient supine on the table. Note evidence of joint effusion and muscle wasting. **Palpation:** Feel the knee carefully for point tenderness, especially over the quadriceps tendon, patellar tendon, collateral ligaments, anserine bursa, and along the joint line. Palpate the surface of the patella and under its edges, then push the patella aside and palpate the underlying femoral condyles. Feel for a click with pain while putting the knee through a full range of motion. A painless click is relatively unimportant as it may be caused normally by tendons moving over a bony prominence. Have the patient put the knee through a full range of active motion and compare with the range of passive motion by

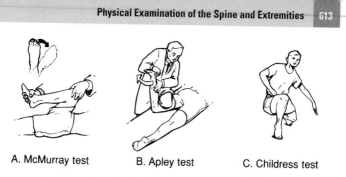

A. McMurray test   B. Apley test   C. Childress test

Fig. 13–24 *Tests for Tear of the Medial Meniscus. A. McMurray test. B. Apley test. C. Childress test.*

the examiner. Remember that joint effusion limits flexion and full extension. Immediately after injury, muscle spasm and swelling may make full examination impossible, in which case, immobilize the knee for a day or two and then reexamine it [Solomon DH, Simel DL, Bates DW, et al. The rational clinical examination. Does this patient have a torn meniscus or ligament of the knee? Value of the physical examination. *JAMA.* 2001;286:1610–1620].

Testing for meniscus injury. Several tests can be performed to identify meniscus injury.

McMurray Test (Fig. 13–24A): With the patient supine on the table, grasp the patient's knee with one hand so that your fingers press the medial and lateral aspects of the joint. Grasp the patient's heel with your other hand so that the plantar surface of the foot rests along your wrist and forearm. First, flex the knee until the heel nearly touches the buttock. To test the posterior half of the medial meniscus, rotate the foot laterally, and then slowly extend the knee fully. If a click is felt or heard during the extending motion, and the patient recognizes it as the sensation preceding pain or locking, the medial meniscus is torn. To test the lateral meniscus, repeat the maneuver with the foot rotated medially.

Apley Grinding Test (Fig. 13–24B): Have the patient lie prone on a low couch, approximately 2 feet (60 cm) high, with the patient's affected limb toward you. Grasp the foot with both your hands, flex the knee to 90 degrees, and rotate the foot laterally. This should cause little discomfort. Now, rest your knee on the patient's hamstrings to fix the femur, and pull the leg to further flexion while the foot is held in lateral rotation; pain indicates a lesion of the MCL. Next, compress the tibial condyles onto the femoral condyles by placing your body weight onto the plantar surface of the foot, still in lateral rotation. Pain from this maneuver indicates tear of the medial meniscus.

Childress Duck-Waddle Test (Fig. 13–24C): This test is strenuous and is reserved for athletes. Have the patient squat and waddle on the toes, swinging from side to side. With rupture of the posterior horn of the meniscus, complete flexion cannot be attained; the maneuver elicits pain or clicking in the posteromedial portion of the joint.

EXAMINATION OF THE ANKLE JOINT

Inspect and *palpate* the ankle for edema, effusion, or tenderness. Test, dorsiflexion and plantarflexion, by grasping the heel firmly with your left hand to immobilize the subtalar joints while your right hand grasps the midfoot and moves the ankle through the full range of flexion and extension. Test anterior stability (*drawer test*) by stabilizing the distal tibia with one hand while grasping the heel and pulling it directly forward with the other. Test *inversion* and *eversion* stability by stabilizing the tibia as above while alternately firmly inverting and everting the heel. Increased mobility with each test indicates injury to the ankle ligaments stabilizing that motion.

EXAMINATION OF THE FOOT

Inspect the shoes for uneven wear. Normal wear is on the lateral edge of heel and sole. Wear on the medial side of the heel and tilting of the vertical heel seam indicates abnormal foot mechanics. With the patient barefoot and standing inspect the heels from behind, the sides and the front. Always compare right to left. Look for the normal slight outward angulation of the heel which should rotate medially when standing on the toes. Note any deformities (e.g., hammertoes or bunion), the height of the pedal arches, and alignment (a plumb line hanging from the mid-patella should point between the first and second metatarsals). Have the patient point to the site of pain and palpate there for tenderness or crepitus. With the patient supine, inspect the sole for calluses and palpate the fat pads under the calcaneus and metatarsal heads. Test motion by supporting the heel with one hand while moving the foot in dorsiflexion, plantarflexion, eversion, and inversion with the other hand (see Fig. 13–12A).

Examination for flatfoot: Have the patient stand with the feet parallel and separated by approximately 10 cm. Note the height of the medial longitudinal arch. If it is flattened, see if it resumes a normal height when weight is removed. Test strength of the anterior leg muscles by having the patient stand on the heels. Test for shortening of the Achilles and peroneal tendons by dorsiflexion and inversion, respectively, in the supine position. Test eversion, which is limited in rigid flatfoot.

Muscle Examination

See Chapter 14, The Neurologic Examination, page 699.

BRIEF EXAMINATION FOR SKELETAL INJURIES

If pain or other symptoms or signs lead you to suspect injury to the spine, IMMEDIATELY IMMOBILIZE the patient and obtain radiographic confirmation of stability before moving the neck or spine or proceeding with the examination. Trauma of sufficient force to cause injury to major skeletal structures is frequently accompanied by internal visceral injuries, which ALWAYS take precedence over the skeletal injuries.

The following procedure is recommended for the rapid examination of injured but conscious persons to uncover skeletal lesions in the absence of specific complaints.

Head: Have the patient open and close his mouth and bite down when your fingertips are on the masseter muscles; if no pain is elicited, the facial bones are not affected. Palpate the zygomatic arch and nose for tenderness. Palpate the scalp for bruises and lumps. With your hands, press from opposite sides of the patient's head for the pain of a skull fracture.

Neck: Palpate the spines of the cervical vertebrae with your fingers before moving the neck. Have the patient roll his head gently from side to side while your fingers palpate the neck muscles for tenderness or spasm. Ask the patient to lift his head while you place your hand under it. Ask the patient to push down with his head to estimate his strength and discomfort.

 If PAIN is elicited with any of these maneuvers, IMMEDIATELY IMMOBILIZE the neck and cease further movement or examination until the neck is cleared by adequate radiologic examination.

Chest: Ask the patient to take a deep breath; if this is painful, place your hands on opposite sides of the patient's chest and squeeze to locate the point of tenderness of a rib fracture. Palpate the length of each clavicle.

Spine: With the patient supine, slip your hand under the patient's back, lift the patient's chest slightly, and run your fingers over the spinous processes for tenderness and angulation. Determine, if there is limitation of spinal motion.

 If PAIN is elicited with any of these maneuvers, IMMEDIATELY IMMOBILIZE the spine and cease further movement or examination until the spine is cleared by adequate radiologic examination.

Arms and Hands: Have the patient move his arms, hands, and fingers in succession and through a full range of motion. Palpate each finger for phalangeal and metacarpal injuries. Shake hands, both right and left, and ask the patient to twist his arm, with elbow both straight and flexed. Performance of these motions, with normal strength and painlessly, excludes injuries of hand, wrist, forearm, elbow, arm, shoulder, clavicle, and scapula.

Pelvis: Place downward pressure medially with a hand on each anterior ilium, then on the symphysis pubis. Place your clenched fist between the patient's knees and ask the patient to squeeze it; lack of pain excludes fractures of pelvis and femora.

Legs and Feet: Ask the patient to move first one leg, then the other, through a full range of motion. Palpate each toe. Have the patient stretch his legs flat on the table. Press his feet together and have him rotate them laterally against your resistance. If the patient employs normal strength without pain, you have excluded major injuries of legs and pelvis.

Musculoskeletal and Soft Tissue Symptoms

KEY SYMPTOM   Joint Pain—Arthralgia

Arthralgia means joint pain with or without objective signs of inflammation. Arthralgias may precede arthritis by weeks or months. The onset, location, severity, and temporal pattern of pain are important. Inquire for morning stiffness and whether activity makes the pain better or worse and how quickly it recurs with rest. Morning stiffness lasting more than 60 minutes suggests an inflammatory etiology, while a lesser duration of pain suggests noninflammatory conditions such as osteoarthritis.

> **KEY SYMPTOM** Bone Pain

Pain in bone is caused by mechanical injury, inflammation, infarction, increased intraosseous pressure, or stretching of the periosteum. Somatic afferent nerves carry the pain fibers and the pain is well localized, especially when the periosteum or endosteum is involved. Pain is often the only symptom of bone disease, although it may be accompanied by localized tenderness and swelling. Characteristically, bone pain is constant, well localized, worse at night and often intensified by movement or weight bearing. Bone pain may be referred to the nearest joint, but careful examination can usually distinguish between articular and bone pain. Squeezing the overlying muscles should exclude tender muscles as the source of pain. Bone pain should prompt imaging.

✔ **BONE PAIN—CLINICAL OCCURRENCE:** *Congenital* hemoglobin S and C (bone infarction), aseptic necrosis (Legg-Calvé-Perthes disease) of the femoral head; *Endocrine* hyperparathyroidism (osteitis fibrosa cystica); *Idiopathic* Paget disease, hypertrophic osteoarthropathy (HOA), osteoarthritis; *Inflammatory/Immune* eosinophilic granuloma; *Infectious* osteomyelitis, syphilis, tuberculosis; *Metabolic/Toxic* osteoporosis, osteomalacia, drugs (GCSF), erythropoietin; *Mechanical/Traumatic* fractures, tendon avulsions and ruptures, ligament avulsions, epiphyseal plate injuries; *Neoplastic* osteosarcoma, multiple myeloma, giant cell tumor, large cell lymphoma, Ewing tumor, metastases to bone, fibrosarcoma, chondrosarcoma; *Vascular* avascular necrosis (with glucocorticoids, hemoglobin S and C diseases).

> **KEY SYMPTOM** Muscle Pain—Myalgia

Muscle pain is carried on somatic sensory neurons and is generally well localized. Pain can result from external trauma, repetitive or sustained contraction, inflammation, ischemia, and metabolic disturbances. Chronic myofascial pain is of unknown etiology, but probably represents alterations in the peripheral or central pain circuits. Pain is frequently referred to and from muscles and regional structures. History is the key to diagnosis: note the onset, duration, and character of the pain, its relationship to activity, rest, and symptomatic therapy. Myalgias accompanying systemic inflammatory illnesses are often more severe at night or with prolonged inactivity. Neuromuscular examination is performed looking for wasting, hypertrophy, spasm, tenderness, trigger points, tender points, weakness, or fasciculations.

✔ **MYALGIA—CLINICAL OCCURRENCE:** *These are examples, only.* *Congenital* McArdle disease (paroxysmal myoglobinuria); *Endocrine* hyper-/hypoparathyroidism, hypothyroidism; *Idiopathic* osteoarthritis; *Inflammatory/Immune* rheumatic fever (RF), Rheumatoid Arthritis (RA), dermatomyositis, polymyositis, systemic lupus erythematosus (SLE), vasculitis, polymyalgia rheumatica (PMR); *Infectious* Any acute infection, e.g. influenza, (less common but important: malaria, rubella, dengue, rat-bite fever, trichinosis, leptospirosis, typhus, rickettsiosis, Bartonella), epidemic pleurodynia, pyomyositis; *Metabolic/Toxic* fever, acute hyponatremia, hypocalcemia, hypophosphatemia, hypomagnesemia, dehydration, diuresis, osteomalacia, drugs (statins and others); *Mechanical/Traumatic* trauma, strain, hematoma, march myoglobinuria, hypertonia, spinal stenosis; *Neoplastic* paraneoplastic myopathy and dermatomyositis; *Neurologic* fibromyalgia, neurogenic claudication;

Psychosocial abuse; *Vascular* compartment syndromes, ischemia, athero-emboli, vasculitis.

Trichinosis: Heavy infection with Trichinella spiralis after ingestion of incompletely cooked infected meat (pork, bear meat) may cause severe disease and, infrequently, death. The organisms localize in muscle. One to four days after ingestion, the patient complains of nausea and vomiting, diarrhea, and abdominal pain. Within 10 days, there are fever, dyspnea, anorexia, myalgia, and asthenia. Physical findings include periorbital edema, scarlatiniform rash, splinter hemorrhages under nails, tremors, and involuntary movements.

KEY SYMPTOM   Back Pain

Discomfort in the back may be acute and/or chronic; the quality may be sharp or aching. It is useful to think of back pain in terms of the anatomic structures that cause pain in or radiating to the back. It is essential to remember that pain from internal organs can be referred to the back. Acute pain is usually sharp and severe and results from mechanical forces applied to the back. Chronic pain, usually of an aching quality, can be the consequence of any acute injury or a repetitive use disorder. [Deyo RA, Weinstein JN. Low back pain. *N Engl J Med.* 2001;344:363–370; Deyo RA, Rainville J, Dent DL. The rational clinical examination. What can the history and physical examination tell us about low back pain? *JAMA.* 1992;268:760–765]. *CLINICAL OCCURRENCE: Acute Bones and Ligaments:* fractures, dislocations, torn or avulsed ligaments; *Cartilages:* herniated intervertebral disk, diskitis; *Joints:* reactive arthritis; *Muscles:* strain, myositis, hematoma; **Nerves:** radiculopathy (disk compression, diabetes), epidural mass or abscess, subarachnoid hemorrhage, polio, tetanus; *Referred Pain:* dissecting aortic aneurysm, angina, retrocecal appendicitis, pancreatitis, cholecystitis, biliary colic, pneumothorax, pleurisy, nephrolithiasis, pyelonephritis. *Chronic Bones and Ligaments:* osteoporosis, osteomalacia, osteomyelitis, diffuse idiopathic skeletal hyperostosis (DISH), spondylolysis and spondylolysthesis spondyloarthritides, tuberculosis, syphilis, Paget disease, primary or secondary bone neoplasm, spina bifida; *Cartilage:* herniated intervertebral disk; *Joints:* osteoarthritis; *Muscles:* chronic muscle strain, fibromyalgia, myositis; *Nerves:* syringomyelia, Chiari malformation, arachnoiditis; *Referred Pain:* esophageal carcinoma, peptic ulcer, chronic pancreatitis, pancreatic carcinoma, renal cell carcinoma, retroperitoneal lymphoma, hepatomegaly from any cause, spinal cord tumor, aortic aneurysm.

KEY SYMPTOM   Pain in the Upper Arm, Forearm, and Hand

When pain is well localized to one part of an extremity, the diagnosis is relatively simple. However, often the pain is more or less diffuse throughout the upper limb, so an anatomic classification of causes is useful. Limb pain does not always arise in musculoskeletal sources, for example, pain may be referred to the upper arm from myocardial ischemia. *CLINICAL OCCURRENCE: Well-Localized Pain* arthritis, bursitis, bone fracture, tendon rupture, tenosynovitis, cellulitis, muscle strain, neoplasm, ischemia and claudication. *Diffuse Pain* herniated cervical intervertebral disk, PMR, spondylitis, spinal tuberculosis, neoplasm of bone, Pancoast tumor, syringomyelia, radiculitis, carpal tunnel syndrome, ulnar tunnel syndrome, complex regional pain syndrome (reflex sympathetic dystrophy).

KEY SYMPTOM   Pain in the Shoulder

Shoulder pain is common but may be poorly localized. Diagnosis requires identifying the provocative and palliative movements, the quality of the pain; the anatomic region of the pain; its severity; and timing. It is helpful to consider the common conditions arranged by anatomic location [Steinfeld R, Valente RM, Stuart MJ. A common sense approach to shoulder problems. *Mayo Clin Proc.* 1999;74:785–794]. Attention should focus on identifying the structures involved and shoulder stability. Several physical examination maneuvers are helpful in shoulder examination but none are definitive for identifying instability [Luime JJ, Verhagen AP, Miedema HS, et al. Does this patient have an instability of the shoulder or a labrum sesion? *JAMA.* 2004;292:1989–1999].

✔ *SHOULDER PAIN—CLINICAL OCCURRENCE:*   *Shoulder Joints* arthritis of sternoclavicular, acromioclavicular, and glenohumeral joints; subluxations of humeral head, acromioclavicular joint, sternoclavicular joint; *Bursae* subacromial and subdeltoid bursitis. *Tendons* supraspinatus tendonitis, tear of supraspinatus tendon (partial or complete), other rotator cuff tears, rupture of long tendon of the biceps, bicipital tenosynovitis; *Muscles* strain, fibromyalgia (tender points), myositis, hematoma, muscle rupture (complete or incomplete), PMR; *Bones* fractures of humeral neck, scapular neck, clavicle; *Nerves* nerve compression by the scalenus anticus muscle (*scalenus anticus syndrome*), first rib and clavicle (*costoclavicular syndrome*); complex regional pain syndrome (*shoulder-hand syndrome*); *Vascular* aneurysm or thrombosis of the subclavian artery.

Pain referred to the shoulder.   Pain is referred to the shoulder from many sites in the chest, especially those innervated by the phrenic or vagus nerves or cervical sympathetic chain. When the diaphragm is involved (phrenic nerve) patients present with aching or sharp pain usually felt over the top of the shoulder or in the trapezius at the base of the neck (See Pleuritis, and Fig. 8.43, page 391). Angina is most often referred to the inner arms, jaw, and shoulder. Pain from nerve injury is often burning in quality and follows the appropriate dermatome. The following anatomic sites and conditions must be considered.

✔ *REFERRED SHOULDER PAIN—CLINICAL OCCURRENCE:*   *Cardiovascular* angina pectoris (to either or both shoulders), aortic aneurysm or dissection; *Pleura* pleuritis of the central part of diaphragm, pneumonia, tuberculosis, pneumothorax, or carcinoma of the superior sulcus (*Pancoast syndrome*); *Spleen* (left shoulder only) infarction, rupture; *Diaphragm* subphrenic abscess, leaking peptic ulcer; *Stomach and Duodenum* gastritis, peptic ulcer, gastric carcinoma; *Liver and Gallbladder* cholelithiasis, cholecystitis, hepatitis, hepatic cirrhosis or carcinoma, hepatic abscess; *Pancreas* chronic pancreatitis, carcinoma, calculus, or pseudocyst; *Nerves* herpes zoster, brachial plexitis, neoplasm of cervicothoracic vertebrae, myelitis, spinal cord tumor.

KEY SYMPTOM   Pain in the Hip, Thigh, Knee or Leg

Pain in the lower extremity requires distinguishing between the primary lesion and pain resulting from redistribution of weight bearing to favor the original disorder. For example, limping on a chronically painful foot causes muscle strain in the back, pelvic girdle, and both lower limbs. Painful structures are identified by localization of palpable tenderness and accentuation of the pain with specific movements. Pain arising in somatic tissues (muscle, bone, tendon, ligament) is usually well localized by the patient. Pain also is frequently referred to regional structures innervated by the same spinal segment. As an example, lesions involving the femoral neck frequently produce pain in the medial aspect of the knee. An anatomic organization for diagnostic purposes is useful. Patients will often describe pain in the general region of a joint as arising from the joint so a broad approach should be maintained to "hip", "knee", and "ankle" pain.

✔ *HIP, THIGH, AND LEG PAIN—CLINICAL OCCURRENCE: Muscle* strains and tears, hematoma, PMR, fibromyalgia, ischemia and infarction, infection, tumors; *Soft Tissues* herniation of fat through muscle fascia, bursitis; *Tendons* tenosynovitis, strain and rupture; *Joints* arthritis (inflammatory, septic, crystal-induced, osteoarthritis), dislocations, sprains; *Bones* fractures, neoplasms, osteomyelitis, osteoporosis, osteomalacia, aseptic necrosis, spondylolisthesis; *Arteries* thrombosis, embolism (thrombus, atheroma, fat, septic vegetations), vasculitis, aneurysm; *Veins* thrombosis, thrombophlebitis, venulitis, venous insufficiency; *Nerves* herniated intervertebral disk, epidural mass, contusion, vasculitis (mononeuritis multiplex), tabes dorsalis, neoplasms (especially neurofibromas), postherpetic neuralgia, peripheral neuropathies (e.g., diabetes and others).

Musculoskeletal and Soft Tissue Signs

(STOP) *Fractures are discussed in this section only for the purpose of illustrating relatively common physical findings. This text should not be used as a guide for the definitive diagnosis of traumatic musculoskeletal injuries. Orthopedic texts should be consulted for details, differential diagnosis, and as a guide to diagnosis and management.*

General Signs

KEY SIGN   Painless Nodules Near Joints or Tendons

Several diseases produce painless nodules in joint capsules, tendons, ligaments, or the surrounding connective tissue. *Subcutaneous nodules* of **rheumatoid arthritis** are usually over bony prominences in the periosteum or the deeper layers of the skin. *Gouty tophi*, although usually in bursae, are also formed in the Achilles tendon and the pinna of the ear. Subcutaneous nodules of *rheumatic* fever are freely movable and occur especially over bony prominences or tendons. The diagnostic *xanthomas* of **hypercholesterolemia** occur in tendons of the hands and in the Achilles tendon and patellar tendon. *Juxtaarticular nodes* (*Jeanselme nodules*) occur near joints in syphilis, yaws, and other *treponemal diseases*. Periarticular *calcium deposits* occur in the **CREST syndrome** and **tumoral calcinosis**.

Synovial cyst, mucoid cyst. These are either bursae or tendon sheaths distended by fluid or protrusion cysts herniated by hydrostatic pressure from joint capsules.

They are usually nontender and fluctuant. The protrusion cysts may collapse under pressure. Synovial cysts occur in the course of *RA*, usually on the dorsal aspects of the PIP joints. In osteoarthritis, they commonly occur over the DIP joints of the hands and feet. When cysts arise from the extensor sheaths of the wrists, they cause oval swellings on the dorsa of the hands often called *ganglions*. The protrusion cyst of the knee is known as a *Baker* or *popliteal cyst*.

Bursitis.　Some periarticular bursae communicate with the joint space. Effusions occur as a result of repetitive use trauma, direct blunt or penetrating trauma, crystal deposition, or infection. The history and examination combined with knowledge of the local anatomy is essential for diagnosis.

KEY SIGN　Noisy Joints

Normal joint surfaces produce a smooth, gliding motion without palpable or audible friction or noise. Inflammation, cartilage injury, and loose bodies are often associated with demonstrable friction, clicks or crepitation on movement. Moving joints may emit several types of sounds. The knees or hips especially may produce creaking. Crepitus is a grating sound whose vibrations may also be palpated. It is produced by the roughened surfaces of cartilage rubbing together and indicates significant damage to the surface of the joint. Some persons have apparently normal joints that crackle or pop under certain conditions.

KEY SIGN　Muscle Tenderness

Pain reproduced by gently squeezing the muscles identifies pain arising in muscles and distinguishes it from referred pain. Tonic muscle contraction is identified as palpable persistent muscle firmness. Both muscle and joint pain are intensified by movement. Neuritic pain is associated with tenderness over the nerve trunk with radiation in the distribution of its branches. Chronic neuritic pain may stimulate secondary tonic muscle contractions.

KEY SIGN　Increased Joint Mobility

Passive joint motion is restrained by the ligaments attaching the bones on either side of the joint. Active motion is also restrained by muscular contraction. Excessive motion implies disorders of the ligaments. Abnormalities can be congenital or acquired. Acquired laxity results from acute or chronic injury to the ligament(s) leading to loss of support. It is limited to the affected joint and involves only the motion usually restrained by the affected ligament. There is asymmetry between the affected and the unaffected side. Diffuse joint laxity results from congenital disorders of connective tissue in the *Ehlers-Danlos syndromes*. Increased laxity of the skin, easy bruising, and poor scar formation are among the more common manifestations of these syndromes. *Benign hypermobility syndrome* is more common and can be associated with loose joints, daytime pain and nighttime awakening with discomfort, especially after exercise. It is more common in females and is an important cause of musculoskeletal pain in children and young adults.

Axial Musculoskeletal Signs
Neck Signs

> **KEY SIGN**   **Neck Pain**

Nuchal Headache: Onset of dull pain is unilateral in the occipital region, progressing in a few hours to the back of the eye, where it may persist for hours to days and become throbbing. Palpation of the posterior cervical muscles may disclose one or more trigger points that reproduce the pain, although the muscle itself is not tender. The pain may be reproduced or accentuated by pressing on the vertex of the skull when the neck is bent laterally. Passive extension of the neck may relieve the pain. The physical signs in the neck distinguish the condition from migraine, occipital neuritis, trigeminal neuralgia, and brain tumor.

Pain in the Neck and Shoulder—Pancoast Syndrome (Superior Sulcus Syndrome): Lung cancer at the thoracic apex invades locally to involve the pleura, thoracic muscles, and neurovascular bundles, including the brachial plexus and cervical sympathetic chain. Pain is felt in local structures and is referred in the distribution of the involved nerves. Severe pain is present in the posterior part of the shoulder and axilla, often shooting down the arm, with paresthesia of the arm and hand. Paresis or wasting of arm muscles may occur. In addition to neck and shoulder pain, the complete syndrome includes *Horner syndrome* (unilateral miosis, ptosis, and absence of sweating on the ipsilateral face and neck). It may be confused with rupture of the supraspinatus tendon, cervical spondylosis, and peripheral neuritis.

Pain in the Neck and Shoulder—Cervical Spondylosis (Cervical Osteoarthritis): Spondylosis results from degeneration of the intervertebral disks. Osteophytes may encroach on the intervertebral neural foramina or protrude into the spinal canal. Pain is usually present in the neck or scapula and frequently extends to the shoulder, occiput, or down the arm (see Nuchal Rigidity with Arm Pain—Cervical Radiculopathy below). Numbness and tingling of the hands are frequent, but muscle wasting is rare. Active and passive motions of the neck are restricted and may be painless, but often produce subjective and objective crepitus. Coughing with the head held in extension may reproduce the pain.

Nuchal Rigidity with Arm Pain—Cervical Radiculopathy: Contusion of a cervical root in the neural foramen produces severe pain in the nerve distribution. Commonly, the cause is narrowing of intervertebral foramina or compression of nerve roots by osteophytes. Uncommonly, the lesion is caused by protrusion of an intervertebral disk or by C1–C2 instability from RA. Usually, minor trauma precedes the onset of pain. Painful spasm of the neck muscles causes temporary torticollis, with the head tilted away from the painful side. Sharp, shooting pains spread slowly down the shoulder, the lateral aspect of the upper arm, and the radial aspect of the forearm, to the wrist. The neck muscles are rigid on the affected side. The biceps tendon reflex is frequently diminished or absent with a radiculopathy of C5 or C6. The triceps reflex is decreased with a radiculopathy of C7. There may be tingling and numbness in the thumb, index and middle fingers. Extend and laterally rotate the neck; when pain is elicited, *Spurling's sign* is present. Other causes, such as incomplete rupture of the supraspinatus, Pancoast tumor, and peripheral neuropathy must be excluded. Symptoms remit gradually over days to weeks [Carette S, Fehlings MG. Cervical radiculopathy. *N Engl J Med.* 2005;353:392–399].

Stiff Neck, with or without Pain—Tuberculous Spondylitis (Cervical Pott Diseases): Tuberculosis of the spine is an indolent osteomyelitis of the anterior vertebral endplates with extension to the paravertebral soft tissues. The neck is held stiffly and spontaneous rotation of the head is absent. There may be pain in the neck, but often the neck is painless. When seated, the patient may support the head with the hands (*Rust sign*). An abscess of the cervical vertebra may track to the retropharyngeal space.

 KEY SIGN   Posttraumatic Neck Pain

(STOP) *Following trauma or suspected cervical injury, the cervical spine must ALWAYS be immediately IMMOBILIZED in a rigid collar PRIOR TO ANY MOVEMENT or examination of the patient.*

Whiplash Cervical Injury: Sudden, forceful hyperextension of the neck with flexion recoil commonly occurs to a passenger in an automobile that is struck from behind (Fig. 13–25). Posterior neck pain develops slowly over hours or days. Nerve-root irritation produces spasm of the neck muscles and torticollis. Occipital headache develops, sometimes with blurring of vision. The chin is turned toward the painful side of the neck. Palpation over the lower cervical spinous processes elicits tenderness. An effusion with soft crepitus can sometimes be felt over the lowest part of the ligamentum nuchae. The biceps reflex may be diminished or absent on one or both sides. Occasionally, the pupil is dilated on the affected side.

Fracture of a Spinous Process: The long, thin, spinous process of vertebrae near the cervicothoracic junction break readily from a direct blow or from violent muscular contraction, such as raising a heavy load with a shovel. Sudden, severe pain extends from the neck to the shoulder, accentuated by flexion and rotation of the neck. Tenderness is exquisite over the fracture site. Sometimes the fractured process is mobile laterally and crepitus can be felt.

➤ **Flexion Fracture of the Neck:** The C5 vertebral body is most frequently fractured when there is forceful hyperflexion of the neck, for example, when a diver strikes his head on the bottom. The patient who escapes immediate death

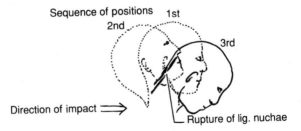

Fig. 13–25 *Extension Injury (Whiplash) of the Cervical Spine.* *Violent impact from behind produces rapid translation between three sequential positions, causing rupture of the ligamentum nuchae.*

or quadriplegia may be unable to walk without supporting his head with his hands. Pain restricts all motions of the neck. The spinous process of the affected vertebra is tender and may be somewhat prominent.

➤ **Partial Dislocation from Hyperextension:** A fall or blow on the forehead may hyperextend the neck and rupture the anterior longitudinal ligament. There is intense pain in the neck. One spinous process may seem more prominent. Paraplegia frequently occurs.

➤ **Fracture of the Atlas (C1) or the Odontoid Process (C2):** Disruption of the ring of bone and ligament restraining the odontoid process or fracture at the base of the odontoid produces instability of C1 on C2 leading to compression of the cervical spinal cord. If immediate death does not result, the patient supports his head with his hands; he is unwilling to nod his head. There is severe occipital headache. The patient cannot rotate the head. If the clinical diagnosis is not made immediately and the neck completely immobilized, sudden death may ensue. In RA, pannus may erode the transverse ligament of C1 that supports the posterior odontoid leading to C1-C2 instability with trivial trauma. A high index of suspicion is required to make the diagnosis.

Thoracolumbar Spine and Pelvis Signs

Dorsal protrusion from the spine—spina bifida cystica. Failure in fusion of the neural arch of a vertebra is spina bifida. When the meninges form a sac protruding through the defective arch, it is a *meningocele* (Fig. 13–26A). When the sac contains spinal cord or cauda equina, it is termed a *myelomeningocele*. In spina bifida occulta, there is no protrusion of the meninges; the only external manifestation may be a dimple in the skin, a patch of hair, or a lipomatous nevus. The sac is covered by healthy skin; the local swelling is filled with spinal

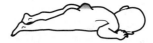

A. Meningocele in an infant

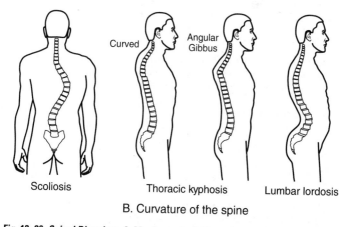

Scoliosis   Thoracic kyphosis   Lumbar lordosis

B. Curvature of the spine

Fig. 13–26 *Spinal Disorders. A. Meningocele. B. Curvatures of the spine.*

fluid, so it is fluctuant and translucent. With *myelomeningocele*, the overlying skin is frequently defective and transillumination may show cord or nerve fibers. Transmission of pressure from the open fontanelle to the meningocele shows the communication to be wide. Sometimes, a sinus leads from a spina bifida occulta to the skin of the sacral region, a congenital *sacrococcygeal sinus*, often mistaken for a pilonidal sinus.

Scoliosis. Lateral curvature of the thoracic spine is usually accompanied by some rotation of the vertebral bodies, but only the lateral deviations of the spinous processes are visible. Minor *functional scoliosis* forms a single lateral curve, usually with convexity to the right. With structural changes, the lateral curve in the thorax produces an opposite compensatory curve inferiorly, so the line of spinous processes forms an S-shaped curve. The spinous processes always rotate toward the concave side. On the convex side, rotation of the vertebral bodies causes flattening of the ribs anteriorly and bulging of the chest posteriorly, elevation of the shoulder, and lowering of the hip. Scoliosis is most often idiopathic, occurring most commonly in adolescent girls. Viewed from the patient's back, the posterior bulge is augmented with anteflexion of the spine (see Fig. 13–2). Lateral deviation with a single curve is usually postural, as proved by its disappearance in extreme spinal flexion. An S-shaped or other complex curve may be compensatory or structural (Fig. 13–26B). *Compensatory scoliosis* occurs with torticollis, thoracoplasty, congenital dislocation of the hip, and shortened lower limb. *Structural scoliosis* occurs in congenital deformities and paralysis of back or abdominal muscles.

Kyphosis. The forward concavity of the thoracic curve is accentuated, producing a hunchback (see Fig. 13–26B). A smooth curve results from faulty posture, rigid kyphosis of adolescence (*Scheuermann disease*), ankylosing spondylitis, Paget disease, osteoporosis (*dowager's hump*), acromegaly, and senile kyphosis. Of these, only the curve of faulty posture disappears with spinal extension. An abrupt angular curve caused by the collapse of one or more contiguous vertebrae (*Gibbus deformity*, see Fig. 13–26B), results from osteoporosis, osteomyelitis, tuberculosis, neoplasm (e.g., multiple myeloma), or trauma. In either *curved or angular kyphosis*, the spinal flexion may force the thorax to permanently assume the inspiratory position, with increased anteroposterior diameter and horizontal ribs. The thoracic distortion is identical with the barrel chest of pulmonary emphysema, but the auscultatory signs of emphysema are absent.

Kyphoscoliosis: The thoracic deformity of scoliosis is accentuated and compounded when kyphosis is also present. The thoracic cavity may be so reduced as to compromise cardiopulmonary function.

Backward spinal curvature—lordosis. The normal posterior concavity of the lumbar curve is accentuated (see Fig. 13–26B). Weakness of the anterior abdominal muscles is a common cause. This may occur to counterbalance a protuberant abdomen in pregnancy and obesity. It compensates for other spinal deformities in spondylolisthesis, thoracic kyphosis, flexion contracture of the hip joint, congenital hip dislocation, coxa vara, and shortening of the Achilles tendons. Muscular weakness from copper deficiency myopathy is associated with swayback. Accentuation of the lumbar curve throws the thoracic spine backward and the thoracic cage becomes flattened from the pull of the abdomen, causing an expiratory position to be assumed.

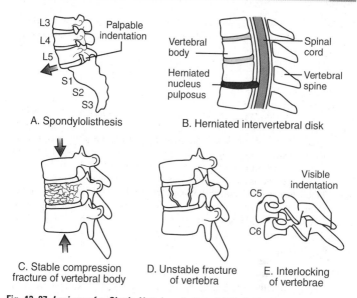

Fig. 13–27 *Lesions of a Single Vertebra. A. Spondylolisthesis. B. Herniated intervertebral disk. C. Stable compression vertebral fracture. D. Unstable compression vertebral fracture. E. Interlocking or subluxation of vertebra.*

KEY SIGN   Low Back Pain with Spinal Indentation—Spondylolisthesis

Usually L5 slips forward on S1 (Fig. 13–27A) because of an inherited defect of the lamina or fracture or degeneration of the articular processes of the neural arch. If symptoms occur, there is low back pain, often referred to the coccyx or the lateral aspect of the leg (L5 dermatome). Inspection frequently discloses a transverse loin crease. Palpation of the lumbar spine reveals a deep recession of the spinous process of L5. There is restricted flexion of the lower spine.

KEY SIGN   Posttraumatic Mid-Back Pain

Stable Compression Fracture of Vertebral Body (with Intact Spinal Ligaments): The thoracic or lumbar vertebrae are fractured by trauma that crushes their bodies, such as forceful hyperflexion of the spine, falling and landing on the feet or buttocks, or a downward blow on the shoulders (Fig. 13–27C). Pain and tenderness at the fracture site may be mild or even absent for weeks, so fracture may not be suspected until a radiograph is obtained. Occasionally, slight kyphosis is present.

▶ **Unstable Compression Fracture of Vertebral Body (with Torn Spinal Ligaments):** Rupture of the interspinal and supraspinal ligaments, accompanying the compression fracture, permits the articular facets of two adjacent vertebrae to slide apart; on recoil, they may interlock (Fig. 13–27E). This dangerous condition may be suggested clinically by palpating a gap between two spinous processes (Fig. 13–27D).

➤ **Fracture-Dislocation of Vertebrae:** Violent hyperflexion of the spine, in addition to fracturing the vertebrae, may tear the supporting ligaments, permitting vertebral dislocation and consequent damage to the spinal cord. This is a potentially unstable condition requiring immediate immobilization and evaluation. This should be suspected when the palpating finger finds a gap between two spinous processes.

Fracture of a Transverse Process: Usually, the transverse process of a lumbar vertebra is fractured from violent contraction of the attached muscles. There is severe pain in the lumbar region, with intense muscle spasm. The spinous processes are not tender. If caused by a direct blow, look for blood in the urine to identify a concomitant kidney injury.

KEY SYNDROME **Chronic Back Pain—Ankylosing Spondylitis**

See page 686.

Appendicular Skeleton, Joint, Ligament, Tendon, and Soft-Tissue Signs

Finger Signs

Some abnormalities of the fingers have been included in consideration of the entire hand; the more localized disorders are discussed here.

Thumb pain following a fall—ulnar collateral ligament sprain. There is a history of a fall onto the palm, often while grasping an object with the thumb. The patient complains of pain in the MCP joint of the thumb and an inability to exert significant pressure on the pad of the thumb tip without pain or giving way. Examination shows tenderness and laxity of the ulnar collateral ligament.

KEY SIGN **Painless Nodules on the Interphalangeal Joints—Heberden and Bouchard Nodes**

These findings are a result of marginal osteophytes on the DIP and PIP joints. Heberden nodes of the DIP joints are hard nodules, 2 to 3 mm in diameter, one on either side of the dorsal midline (see Fig. 13–34K). They are usually painless, motion is slightly limited, and deformity is progressive, but function is preserved. They are more pronounced on the dominant hand. Involvement begins in several joints most commonly in peri- or postmenopausal women. The condition in women is usually hereditary and the process is a result of osteoarthritis. A single Heberden node may result from trauma. Nodules on the PIP joints are called Bouchard nodes. They occur together with Heberden nodes, but somewhat less frequently than the latter.

KEY SIGN **Clubbing of the Fingers**

The mechanism is proven but recent evidence suggests that vascular endothelial growth factor (VEGF) reaching the systemic circulation either from the lung or via extra pulmonary shunts may play a role (Martinez-Lavin M. Exploring the cause of the most ancient clinical sign of medicine: finger clubbing. Semin Arthritis Rheum 2007;36:380–5). Clubbing has intrigued physicians since Hippocrates because of its association with serious systemic disorders. Clubbing is reversible when the cause is removed. The three key observations are floating of the nail base, loss of the unguophalangeal angle, and increased longitudinal convexity of the nail plate. Clubbing is painless and usually bilateral. With long-standing clubbing, the soft tissue and terminal phalanx become thickened, the convexity of the nail plate is extreme, and the fingers are bulbous. In the literal sense, the term clubbing should be reserved for this late stage, but it is now applied to the general process in all stages, from the first sign of floating nail. The floating nails and alteration of the unguophalangeal angle distinguish clubbing from all other conditions. Convexity alone is seen in other conditions or as a normal variant.

Demonstrating clubbing. *Obliteration of the Unguophalangeal Angle (Lovibond Angle):* Inspect the profile of the terminal digit. Normally, the nail makes an angle of 20 degrees or more with the projected line of the digit. With clubbing, this angle is diminished or may be obliterated or extend below the projected line of the digit (Fig. 13–28). *Floating Nail:* Palpate the proximal nail with the tip of your finger. You can feel and see the springy softness as the root of the nail is depressed (see Fig. 13–28). This may be simulated as follows: with your right index finger press the mantle of your left middle finger; the plate rests snugly against the bone without movement. Now depress the free edge of the nail with your left thumb and test the mantle again with your right index finger; the plate root now sinks with pressure and springs back when released. *Convexity of the Nail:* A month or so after the floating nail and nail angle changes occur, a transverse ridge appears in the plate from beneath the mantle. The ridge marks the change from the normal distal curve to a new curve of smaller radius in the proximal nail.

The floating nail and flattened angle occur rapidly, for example, within 10 days after a tonsillectomy complicated by lung abscess. With chronic illness of more than 6 months, the entire nail has abnormal convexity. The sequence of changes can occasionally be observed in a patient with subacute bacterial endocarditis. When first seen with a 3-month history of illness, a transition ridge is visible (see Fig. 13–28). After treatment of the infection a second ridge appears, this one marking the transition between distal abnormal curvature and proximal normal profile.

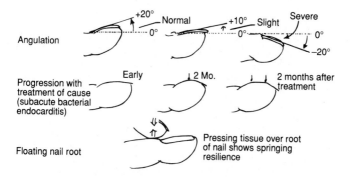

Fig. 13–28 *Characteristics of Clubbed Fingers.* There are three principal signs of clubbing of the fingers: 1. Angulation; 2. Curvature of the nail; and 3. Floating nail root.

✔ *CLUBBING—CLINICAL OCCURRENCE:* *Congenital* cyanotic congenital heart disease, familial, cystic fibrosis; *Endocrine* hypothyroidism; *Idiopathic* COPD, bronchiectasis; *Inflammatory/Immune* inflammatory bowel disease, biliary cirrhosis, alcoholic cirrhosis; *Infectious* infective endocarditis, lung abscess, pulmonary tuberculosis; *Neoplastic* lung cancer, metastatic cancer to lung, mesothelioma; *Vascular* HOA, pulmonary arteriovenous malformations (including dialysis shunts).

Hypertrophic Osteoarthropathy: See page 689.

KEY SIGN   Finger Swelling

Dactylitis, sausage digits.   Enthesitis of one or more fingers produces diffuse "sausage-like" swelling with or without joint effusion. Dactylitis is seen in reactive and psoriatic arthritis and hand-foot syndrome of sickle cell or sickle-thalassemia disease.

Fusiform monarticular swelling—sprain of an interphalangeal joint.   A painful fusiform joint swelling may persist for several months. In most cases, there is a history of trauma.

Localized swelling over a joint—synovial or mucous cyst.   A synovial cyst results from myxomatous degeneration of a joint capsule. A small, tense nodule appears over an interphalangeal joint; frequently it is mistaken for a sesamoid bone. It may be so tense that it feels bony hard; usually, it is not fluctuant. Pressure may elicit slight tenderness. Often there is slight transverse mobility.

KEY SIGN   Finger Deformity

Flexion Deformity of Distal Finger Joint—Mallet Finger: This is caused by rupture or avulsion of the extensor tendon that inserts on the distal phalanx. The DIP is flexed and cannot be voluntarily extended (Fig. 13–30A).

Extension Deformity of the PIP Joint—Swan Neck Deformity: Fixed extension of the PIP joint occurs when the flexor tendons are injured or sublux to the dorsum of the joint, holding the joint in extension. This deformity is common in RA and SLE. In the latter, it is usually reducible, *a Jaccoud deformity.*

Flexion Deformity of the PIP Joint—Boutonnière Deformity: This results from rupture of the central band of the extensor tendon that inserts on the middle phalanx. Volar subluxation of the intact lateral band to the distal phalanx holds the PIP in flexion. The finger is flexed at the PIP and lacks voluntary extension (Fig. 13–29B). Extension followed by flexion of the PIP joint may produce a palpable or audible diagnostic click, as the lateral slips of the distal extensor tendons diverge and slip laterally over the head of the proximal phalanx, hence, buttonhole rupture.

Flexion Deformity of the Thumb—Saluting Hand: Extension at the thumb MCP and interphalangeal joint is performed by the extensor pollicis longus tendon; rupture leads to loss of function. This is approximately the position of the hand in an American military salute (Fig. 13–29C). The thumb is limply flexed in the palm and cannot be voluntarily extended. The tendon is often worn through by moving over the fragments of a Colles fracture.

Snapping or Locking of Finger—Trigger Finger: A nodular thickening forms in the long flexor tendon just proximal to the metacarpal head as a result of inflammation or repetitive trauma. In extension, the nodule lies within

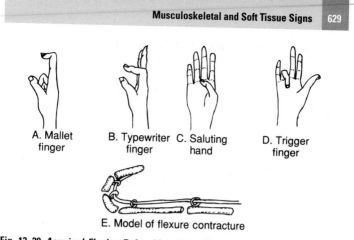

A. Mallet finger
B. Typewriter finger
C. Saluting hand
D. Trigger finger
E. Model of flexure contracture

Fig. 13–29 *Acquired Flexion Deformities of the Fingers.* **A. Mallet finger.** **B. Boutonnière deformity:** *There is permanent flexion of the PIP joint from rupture of the extensor tendon inserting on the middle phalanx, giving a position similar to that employed when using a typewriter or computer keyboard.* **C. Saluting hand:** *The thumb is limply flexed in the palm and cannot be voluntarily extended.* **D. Trigger finger:** *The fourth or ring finger moves into flexion painlessly, but attempted extension is temporarily impeded. Extension is accomplished with a palpable snap.* **E. Flexure contractures of the fingers:** *With sheath adhesions, passive motion of the tendon is nil, even with wrist flexion.*

the flexor tendon sheath; during flexion, it is easily pulled from the proximal end of the sheath. The constricted mouth of the sheath resists reentry of the nodule during extension until it is suddenly achieved with a noticeable click. The middle or ring finger is usually involved (Fig. 13–29D). Flexion of the finger feels normal, but extension is accompanied by a snap that the patient sometimes refers to the region of the PIP joint. The nodule can be palpated moving with the tendon on active or passive flexion-extension. Triggering may or may not be painful.

Contracture of a Flexor Tendon—Tendon Adhesions or Tendon Shortening: Adhesions between a tendon and its sheath are caused by tenosynovitis. Fibrotic shortening of the tendon without synovial adhesions occurs in Volkmann ischemic contracture (page 647). Distinction between the two mechanisms can be made with the wrist flexed. Grasp the tip of the flexed finger and pull it into extension. With the slack provided by wrist flexion, the shortened tendon permits partial extension; adhesions to the sheath or palmar fascia entirely prevent extension (Fig. 13–29E).

> **KEY SIGN** **Tight Skin—Sclerodactyly**

See *Scleroderma,* page 170. All digits are usually involved, Raynaud phenomenon is nearly always present, and calcinosis of the skin may occur. In constrast, the skin is normal with muscle contracture or tendon adhesions.

> **KEY SIGN** **Digital Infection**

It is essential to distinguish superficial from deep tissue infections in the fingers. The latter are initially limited to specific tissue compartments giving characteristic signs.

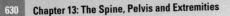

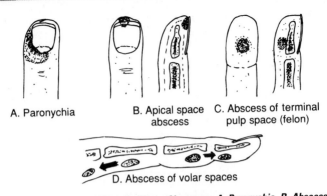

A. Paronychia

B. Apical space abscess

C. Abscess of terminal pulp space (felon)

D. Abscess of volar spaces

Fig. 13–30 *Common Locations for Finger Abscesses. A. Paronychia. B. Abscess of the apical spaces:* The apical space is located in the nail bed near the free margin of the nail plate. *C. Abscess of the terminal pulp space (felon):* The stippled region on the volar surface represents the site of rupture through the skin. *D. Abscess of the volar spaces:* The stippled regions are the sites of abscesses; the arrows point in the direction of burrowing to reach the flexor creases of the finger.

Paronychia: The skin over the matrix of the nail and the lateral nail folds is swollen, reddened, painful, and tender (Fig. 13–30A). When infection is over the nail root, light palpation of the inflamed area provokes exquisite pain. Pain from pressure on the nail plate indicates *subungual abscess*, which occurs between the nail plate and periosteum.

Chronic Paronychia: *Candida* paronychia is minimally tender and does not drain. Chronic ulceration of the nail mantle and lateral folds occurs in occupations requiring frequent immersion of the hands in water or contaminated oil. The ulcers are indolent; abscess formation is rare.

Abscess of the Apical Space: Symptoms follow a puncture wound beneath the nail. The distal nail bed becomes red and extremely painful without much swelling (Fig. 13–30B). Maximum tenderness is proximal to the free edge of the plate, unlike a felon, which produces tenderness at the fingertip. When the abscess ruptures, drainage is at the free edge of the nail plate.

Abscess of the Terminal Pulp Space (Felon): Infection of the finger pad is confined within small fascial compartments attached to the periosteum (Fig. 13–30C). There is swelling of the fingertip and dull pain that becomes intense and throbbing with exquisite tenderness. Induration of the pulp indicates the presence of pus. The abscess may drain through the volar surface of the finger pad; osteomyelitis may occur.

Abscess of the Middle Volar Pulp Space: The finger is held in partial flexion to reduce the pain. A tender swelling occurs on the volar aspect of the finger between the PIP and DIP joints (Fig. 13–30D). The symptoms resemble those of a felon. Osteomyelitis may occur or the abscess may drain after burrowing to the distal flexor crease.

Abscess of the Proximal Volar Pulp Space: An abscess forms on the volar aspect between the MCP and PIP joints (Fig. 13–30D). The symptoms and signs are similar to those in the middle space, except the infection burrows proximally to involve the web space.

Barber's Pilonidal Sinus: Short hair shafts may penetrate the soft skin in the finger webs producing inflammation. One or more nodules are felt which are drained by sinuses; seen as black dots between the fingers.

> **KEY SIGN** Nodules in Finger Pads

Osler's Nodes: Septic emboli from infective endocarditis lodge in the cutaneous vessels producing microscopic abscesses. These pea-sized, tender bluish or pink nodules, sometimes with a blanched center, occur on the pads of the fingers, palms of the hands, and soles of the feet in some patients with infective endocarditis.

Janeway Spots: Janeway spots are only a few millimeters in diameter. They appear over a few hours or days as crops of erythematous or hemorrhagic, macular or nodular lesions. They occur in the palms, soles, or distal finger pads. Although painless and nontender, they may ulcerate. Most writers consider them hallmarks of bacterial endocarditis or mycotic aneurysm. The causative organisms have been isolated from the lesions.

Circulatory disorders of the fingers: See Chapter 8, pages 387 and 430ff.

> **KEY SIGN** Fingernail Signs

See Chapter 6, pages 138ff.

Palm Signs

Yellow palms—carotenemia: See page 136.

Granular palms—hyperkeratoses. Palpation with the fingertips discloses rough granular excrescences in the horny layer. The most common cause is chronic arsenic poisoning. A rare cause is *hyperkeratosis (tylosis) palmaris et plantaris*, an autosomal dominant disease.

> **KEY SIGN** Thenar Wasting

The thenar eminence is formed by the bellies of *opponens pollicis, abductor pollicis brevis and flexor pollicis brevis* innervated by the median nerve. Wasting suggests a lesion of the median nerve, most commonly carpal tunnel syndrome or severe osteoarthritis at the base of the thumb, or it may accompany wasting of all intrinsic hand muscles with axonal neuropathies (Fig. 13–31B).

> **KEY SIGN** Hypothenar Wasting

The hypothenar eminence is formed by the bellies of *palmaris brevis, abductor digiti quinti, flexor digiti quinti,* and *opponens digiti quinti* innervated by the ulnar nerve. Wasting suggests damage to the ulnar nerve (Fig. 13–31C). If both thenar and hypothenar wasting are present, consider cervical myelopathy.

> **KEY SIGN** Localized Thickening of Palmar Fascia—Dupuytren's Contracture

See page 645. Nontender, nodular thickening in the palmar fascia precedes actual contracture (Fig. 13–34I).

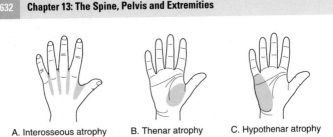

A. Interosseous atrophy   B. Thenar atrophy   C. Hypothenar atrophy

Fig. 13–31 *Wasting of the Intrinsic Muscles of the Hand*: *Regions of atrophy are indicated by stippling.*

KEY SIGN   Hand Infections

Painful Palmar Swelling—Web Space Infection: Fever, malaise, and diffuse pain in the hand and dorsal edema occur early. The two involved fingers are separated at their bases by a tender erythematous swelling; tenderness is maximal on the palmar surface (Fig. 13–32A).

Painful Palmar Swelling—Infection of the Thenar Space: The thenar eminence is swollen, tender, and may have erythema and warmth. **DDX:** Deep hematoma gives similar symptoms and signs but with a history of blunt trauma. Extension of the IP joint is not painful as it is in tenosynovitis of the flexor pollicis longus.

➤ **Painful Palmar Swelling—Deep Abscess of the Palm:** There is usually a history of penetrating trauma, often minor. There is pain, swelling and limited motion. In addition to severe dorsal edema, the concavity of the palm is obliterated, or even elevated; the raised area is tender and erythematous; the erythema may extend to the volar wrist extending *under* the flexor retinaculum. This is a surgical emergency.

➤ **Painful palmar and digital swelling—acute suppurative flexor tenosynovitis.** Throbbing pain begins in a finger, progressing toward the palm. The finger and

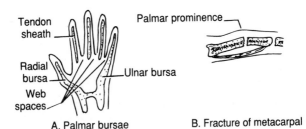

Tendon sheath   Palmar prominence

Radial bursa   Ulnar bursa

Web spaces

A. Palmar bursae   B. Fracture of metacarpal

Fig. 13–32 *Swellings of the Hand. A. Palmar bursae:* *The locations of the bursae are indicated by stippling. Note the tendon sheaths ending proximally near the palmar crease; there is a connection between the radial and ulnar bursae. The radial bursa is continuous from the thumb to the region of the thenar eminence. The web spaces are indicated as sites of abscesses. **B. Fracture of a metacarpal bone:** Diagram shows displacement of the fragments into the palm, where an abnormal prominence may be noted.*

dorsum of the hand are swollen. The finger is held slightly flexed; the patient resists moving it. Passive extension of adjacent fingers is painful, of the affected finger, exquisitely so. Test for the point of maximum tenderness by gently palpating the palm and flexor surface of the finger with the blunt end of an applicator or tongue depressor. If it is located at the proximal end of the tendon sheath of the index, middle, or ring finger, involvement of the sheath is certain. If there is no localization, the sheath may have ruptured.

Painful Palmar Swelling—Infection of the Ulnar Bursa: There is dorsal edema and fullness on the ulnar side of the palm (Fig. 13–32A). The point of maximum tenderness is halfway between the lunate and the fifth MCP joint.

Painful Palmar Swelling—Infection of the Radial Bursa: The interphalangeal joint of the thumb is flexed and passive extension produces pain. There is tenderness and swelling over the sheath of the flexor pollicis longus.

> **KEY SIGN** Painful Palmar Swelling—Fracture of a Metacarpal Bone

In a transverse fracture, the fragments of the metacarpal bone are bowed into the palm to produce a painful prominence (Fig. 13–32B). The prominence may be obscured by soft-tissue swelling, but dorsal palpation will localize tenderness at the fracture site. In a spiral fracture, proximal slippage of the distal fragment produces shortening revealed by loss of prominence in the corresponding knuckle when the fist is closed. Rotation of the distal fragment is present if the affected finger is not aligned with the unaffected fingers when the tips are flexed onto the base of the thenar eminence. *Bennett fracture* is an oblique break through the base of the first metacarpal, frequently with subluxation of the carpal-metacarpal joint. The thumb is semiflexed, and it cannot be opposed to the ring or little finger and the fist cannot be clenched.

Hand and Wrist Signs

> **KEY SIGN** Swelling of the Wrist

Physical examination can identify which structure(s) is swollen. Periarticular edema in the subcutaneous tissues around the joint, but outside the synovium, pits with pressure. With thickening of the joint capsule and synovium the tissues feel boggy. When the synovial envelope is bulging and fluctuant, fluid is present. Effusion, pus, or blood are identified by aspiration.

Painful Swelling or Limited Motion of the Wrist—Arthritis: With active inflammation, there is swelling accompanied by variable degrees of pain and tenderness. The overlying skin may be warm and reddened. In RA, there is limited motion. The joint is swollen, red, hot, and tender with gout, pseudogout, and septic arthritis. Primary osteoarthritis does not affect the wrist.

Painful Swelling in the Anatomic Snuffbox: Inflammation in the tendon sheaths of the *extensor pollicis longus and brevis* as they pass under a fibrous band near the radial styloid causes pain and tenderness. Pain is felt in the region of the snuffbox. The patient has pain with pinching, thumb extension and ulnar deviation of the wrist. When the fist is clenched over the flexed thumb, gentle but firm ulnar deviation of the hand by the examiner elicits pain at the

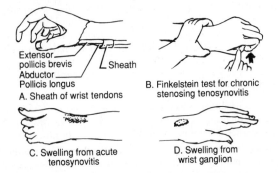

Fig. 13–33 *Some Disorders of the Wrist. A. Sheaths of the wrist tendons: This shows the sheath, which swells to obstruct the motion of the tendons of extensor pollicis brevis and abductor pollicis longus in chronic stenosing tenosynovitis. B. Finkelstein test for tenosynovitis: The patient clenches his fist on his thumb while the examiner pushes the fist toward the ulna. A positive test elicits pain at the radial styloid process. C. Swelling from acute nonsuppurative tenosynovitis. D. Frequent site of ganglion of the wrist: The swelling is painless and sometimes translucent.*

radial styloid process (*Finkelstein test*, see Fig. 13–33B). This pain may be transmitted down the thumb or toward the elbow. Passive extension of the thumb is painless. Crepitus may be felt or auscultated over the tendon sheath during thumb flexion-extension.

Acute Tenosynovitis: A sausage-like swelling; approximately 4 cm long (Fig. 13–33C), involves the tendon sheaths at the radial border of the snuffbox. The cause is usually trauma, although inflammation can be produced by gout, pseudogout or gonococcal infection.

Chronic Stenosing Tenosynovitis (De Quervain Tenosynovitis): The symptoms are similar to the acute process and are frequently chronic and recurrent, exacerbated by repetitive movements of the wrist and thumb. Chronic inflammation involves all layers of the tendon sheath.

Localized Painless Swelling on the Dorsum—Ganglion: This is a protrusion cyst of the joint capsule usually seen on the dorsum of the naviculolunate joint (see Fig. 13–33D). It is painless, round, sessile, tense, translucent and more prominent in flexion.

Numbness, tingling, and pain in the hand—carpal tunnel syndrome (compression neuropathy of the median nerve in the carpal tunnel): See page 767.

> **KEY SIGN** **Normal and Abnormal Hand Posture**

Position of anatomic rest. The relaxed posture of the hand is with the wrist slightly extended and the fingers and thumb flexed, the index finger less bent than the others (Fig. 13–34C). Injury or inflammation with the hand or the muscles and tendons powering it produces this posture to reduce painful tension on the involved structures.

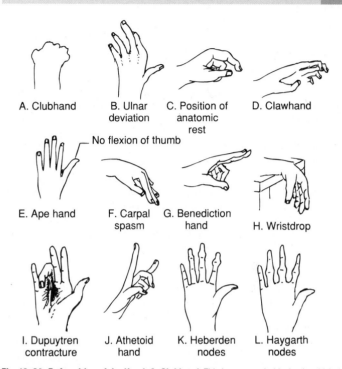

Fig. 13–34 *Deformities of the Hand. A. Clubhand:* This is a congenital lesion in which the hand development is rudimentary; the stub may be surmounted by rudimentary or normal digits. *B. Ulnar deviation:* Also called ulnar drift. *C. Position of anatomic rest. D. Clawhand. E. Ape hand. F. Carpal spasm. G. Benediction hand. H. Wrist-drop. I. Dupuytren contracture. J. Athetoid hand. K. Heberden nodes. L. Haygarth nodes:* The spindle-shaped enlargements of the middle interphalangeal joints occur in RA.

Ulnar Deviation or Drift of Fingers: The fingers deviate at the MCP joints toward the ulna. There may also be subluxations of the MCP joint (Fig. 13–34B). It results from erosion of the joint capsules and ligaments with subluxation of the extensor tendons to the ulnar sides of the joints.

Diabetic Hand, Diabetic Cheiropathy: In long-standing diabetes, the soft tissues of the hand become thick and contracted, bending the fingers into a slightly flexed position. Have the patient attempt to place the palms together; a space will remain between the palms and fingers in a "prayer sign."

> **KEY SIGN** **Dupuytren Contracture (Palmar Fibrosis)**

There is a painless nodular thickening of the palmar aponeurosis from hyalinization of collagen fibers beginning near the base of the digit. It extends to form a plaque or band adhering to the palmar fascia and producing retraction and dimpling of the palmar skin and flexion contracture of the fingers. It usually begins after age 40 years as an inconspicuous hard nodule fixed to the skin in the distal palm. Both hands may be involved. The ring finger is more often affected than the little, long, index or thumb. Fascial retraction pulls the finger(s) into partial flexion (Fig. 13–34I). Palpation reveals a hard cord over the tendon that is raised in extension making it readily seen. With progression, a painless contracture of the digit(s) results requiring surgical correction. Other fibrosing conditions that may be part of the same diathesis, occurring singly or in combination, are plantar fibrosis (*Lederhosen syndrome*) and fibrosis of the corpus cavernosum (*Peyronie disease*). The condition occurs exclusively in Caucasians, predominately men and 40% have a positive family history. It is more common in patients with alcoholism, epilepsy, or diabetes mellitus; the cause for these associations is unknown.

Carpal Spasm: The thumb is flexed on the palm, the wrist and MCP joints are flexed, while the interphalangeal joints are hyperextended and the fingers are adducted in the shape of a cone. All the hand muscles are rigid. The spasm is involuntary and usually painless. This posture occurs in tetany; when present, it is involuntary and cannot be altered by the patient (Fig. 13–34F). It is also seen in *hand dystonia* associated with repetitive hand activities.

Clawhand: This occurs from the predominant pull of the extensor communis digitorum and the flexor digitorum against weak or paralyzed interosseus and lumbrical muscles. The claw is caused by hyperextension of the MCP joints and flexion of the interphalangeal articulations (Fig. 13–34D). Paralysis may result from brachial plexus, ulnar and median nerve injuries, syringomyelia, the muscular atrophies, or acute poliomyelitis.

Ape Hand: The thumb is held in extension by its inability to flex (Fig. 13–34E). This may occur in syringomyelia, progressive muscular atrophy, or amyotrophic lateral sclerosis.

Benediction Hand (Preacher's Hand): The ring and little fingers cannot be extended while the other digits move normally and may be extended to produce the posture (Fig. 13–34G). This occurs in ulnar nerve palsy, syringomyelia, and extensor tendon rupture in RA. It is named from the ecclesiastical gesture of pronouncing benediction. Do not confuse with Dupuytren contracture of the palmar fascia.

Wrist-Drop: When the pronated hand is held horizontally, it drops from the wrist because of weak wrist extensors (Fig. 13–34H) which are unable to overcome gravity. The cause is radial nerve injury of any etiology.

Athetoid Hand: A grotesque pattern is seen in athetosis in which involuntary muscle contractions produce simultaneous flexion of some digits and hyperextension of others, resembling the writhing of a snake (Fig. 13–34J).

KEY SIGN   Large Hands

Acromegaly and Gigantism: See page 673. Soft-tissue overgrowth increases the finger girth and thickens the palm, called a paw or spade hand. Arthritis is frequently present.

Large hands—HOA.   See page 689. All dimensions of the hands are increased, as in acromegaly, but the condition is invariably accompanied by finger clubbing.

Enlargement of one hand—hemihypertrophy and local gigantism.   An entire side of the body may be enlarged in a congenital deformity known as hemihypertrophy. Local gigantism is often the result of a congenital arteriovenous fistula of the upper limb. In either case, the hand is normally proportioned.

KEY SIGN — Long, Slender Hands—Spider Fingers (Arachnodactyly, Marfan Syndrome)

All the long bones of the hands are slender and elongated, often with hyperextensible joints (Plate 29). The *wrist sign* is useful to distinguish elongated fingers from long, normal fingers. The patient encircles his own wrist, with his thumb and little finger proximal to the styloid process of the ulna. In normal persons, the encircling digits scarcely touch, but in arachnodactyly they may overlap by 1 to 2 cm due to the combination of long digits and narrow wrist. The thumb sign (*Steinberg sign*) may also be positive: when the fingers are clenched over the thumb, the end of the thumb protrudes beyond the ulnar margin of the hand (Plate 29) [Falk RH. The "thumb sign" in Marfan's syndrome. *N Engl J Med.* 1995;333:430]. Neither sign is specific for Marfan syndrome.

KEY SIGN — Interosseous Wasting

The hands show prominence of the extensor tendons and metacarpals on the dorsum. There is loss of muscle mass, most easily detected in the first dorsal interosseous between the thumb and index finger. Adduction-abduction of the fingers is weak. Wasting suggests injury to the ulnar nerve (ulnar nerve entrapment at the elbow, diabetic neuropathy) or severe disuse (RA).

KEY SIGN — Swelling of the Dorsum

Painless Swelling: Edema arising from the deep spaces of the hand accumulates in the loose subcutaneous tissue dorsally, rather than the palmar surface, because of the restricting palmar fascia. Causes include infection, obstruction of the superior vena cava, anasarca, and *relapsing symmetrical seronegative synovitis with pitting edema* (RS3PE). Unilateral edema may also occur from occlusion of the venous or lymphatic drainage of the upper arm.

Painful Dorsal Swelling: Infection and extensor tenosynovitis cause edema, erythema, and localized tenderness. Fluctuation may not be present with an abscess. A rare cause is thyroid arcopathy associated with Graves disease and treatment of hyperthyroidism.

KEY SIGN — Pain in Ulnar Side of Hand—Ulnar Tunnel Syndrome

The ulnar nerve passes posterior to the medial humeral epicondyle in the ulnar groove, and then deep to the superficial flexors and above the deep flexors of the forearm, where it is stretched and compressed during vigorous muscular activity. Injury to the ulnar nerve at the elbow causes pain or numbness in the little finger, the ulnar half of the ring finger, and the ulnar side of the palm. Wasting of the hypothenar eminence and interosseus muscles may result from prolonged compression. The ulnar nerve may be stretched or injured by a cubitus valgus deformity or an old elbow fracture. Other risk factors for ulnar entrapment include alcoholism and diabetes. Press on the ulnar nerve in its groove behind the median epicondyle; tingling in the ulnar distribution of the hand suggests ulnar tunnel syndrome.

Forearm and Elbow Signs

> **KEY SIGN** **Forearm Pain and Weakness—Flexor Compartment Syndrome and Volkmann Ischemic Contracture**

Ischemic necrosis of muscle results from either primary arterial events (compression, vascular spasm, arterial injury or embolism) or secondary to hemorrhage or swelling within the confining fascia of the flexor muscle compartment (compartment syndrome, page 692). Volkmann contracture, the fibrosis and shortening of the muscles, is a late finding. Early recognition of the initial ischemic phase may prevent damage leading to contracture. The onset of ischemia is indicated by *the five P's: Pain, Puffiness, Pallor, Pulselessness, and Paralysis.* Passive extension of the fingers produces pain in the forearm. The fingers may be cyanotic and are often edematous. The radial pulse is absent, the skin over the hands is cool and median nerve sensation is diminished. Emergent surgical consultation is required. In Volkmann contracture, the fingers are fixed in flexion by shortening of the fibrotic bellies of the digital flexors in the forearm. Because the flexor tendons are free to move in their sheaths, slight extension of the fingers is permitted when the wrist is held in flexion. This distinguishes it from adhesions of flexor tendons to their sheaths. Precipitating events are forearm and supracondylar fractures and circumferential bandages or casts applied shortly after trauma.

> **KEY SIGN** **Forearm Deformity**

Traumatic forearm deformities are common; Their gross appearance and mechanism of injury are accurate guides to the radiographic findings.

Silver-Fork Deformity—Colles Fracture: The most common cause is a fall on the outstretched hand. The radius is fractured within 2.5 cm of its distal end (Fig. 13–35A). Fracture of the ulnar styloid process occurs in half the cases. When the pronated arm is laid on the table, its profile resembles a dinner fork lying horizontally with the tines pointing downward, so the base of the tines forms an upward curve. The corresponding hump in the fractured arm occurs from dorsal displacement of the distal radial fragment.

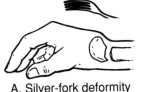

A. Silver-fork deformity of colles fracture

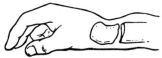

B. Deformity of Smith fracture (reversed silver-fork)

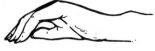

C. Madelung deformity of the wrist

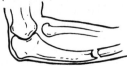

D. Fracture of the ulnar shaft

Fig. 13–35 *Traumatic Deformities of the Forearm.*

Reversed Silver-Fork Deformity—Smith Fracture (Reversed Colles Fracture): Like the Colles fracture, this is a break of the distal end of the radius, but the distal fragment is displaced volarward, making a deformity somewhat resembling the silver fork with its tines pointing upward (Fig. 13–35B). The fracture usually results from a blow or fall on the hyperflexed hand.

Pain and Tenderness in the Bony Shafts—Radial and Ulnar Fractures: In fractures of the ulnar shaft, the bone is well splinted by the radius, so displacement and deformity are rare (Fig. 13–35D). The only physical signs are localized tenderness and swelling. Ulnar fractures accompanied by volar dislocation of the radial head (*Monteggia fracture/dislocation*), especially common in children, permit considerable bowing of the fractured ulna. A fractured radial shaft presents variable degrees of bowing, especially with concomitant dislocation of the lower radioulnar joint.

Painful Angular Deformity—Fractures of Both Forearm Bones: Greenstick fractures produce little deformity, but complete fractures of the radius and ulna present easily recognizable deformity.

Dorsal Angulation of the Wrist—Madelung Deformity: The pronated hand presents a profile in which the wrist is deformed by a sharp protrusion upward (dorsally) of the lower ulna (Fig. 13–35C). This is caused by a nontraumatic dorsal subluxation of the distal end of the ulna, usually in young women.

Smooth Forearm Curvature—Diseases of Osseous Growth. Smooth curves of the radius and ulna are usually attributable to syphilis, rickets, osteomalacia, or Paget disease.

> **KEY SIGN** Posttraumatic Elbow Pain

Fracture of the Coronoid Process of the Ulna: Fracture of the ulnar coronoid process, which forms the distal elbow joint, is easily missed if not considered and searched for.

Posttraumatic Elbow Pain—Fracture of the Olecranon Process: Pronounced swelling results, particularly around the dorsum of the elbow. The olecranon process is tender. When the fracture is complete, the patient cannot extend the flexed forearm (Fig. 13–36A). The bony equilateral triangle may be flattened.

Deformity of the Elbow—Cubitus Valgus and Varus. The normal elbow carrying angle is approximately 170 degrees as measured on the lateral side of the arm and forearm, an angle less than 165 degrees is a valgus deformity, and one greater than 175 degrees is a varus deformity (Fig. 13–37A). A difference of >10 degrees between right and left is also abnormal.

> **KEY SIGN** Swelling of the Elbow

Effusion in the Elbow Joint: The synovial sac of the elbow joint is very loose and easily distended with fluid, giving a characteristic outline. There is fluctuant bulging posteriorly, on both sides of the olecranon process and triceps tendon (see Fig. 13–37B). It is most easily palpable laterally between the lateral epicondyle, radial head, and olecranon. The elbow is held in semiflexion to accommodate maximal fluid volume. The joint may be distended by synovial fluid, pus, or blood.

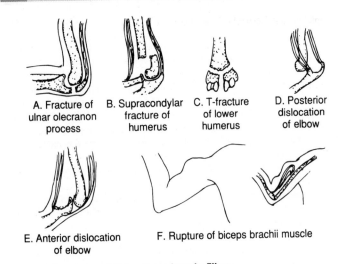

A. Fracture of ulnar olecranon process

B. Supracondylar fracture of humerus

C. T-fracture of lower humerus

D. Posterior dislocation of elbow

E. Anterior dislocation of elbow

F. Rupture of biceps brachii muscle

Fig. 13–36 *Fractures and Dislocations about the Elbow.*

Arthritis of the Elbow: Any type of arthritis may involve the elbow joint. *Suppurative arthritis* produces painful swelling, with pus in the joint. *Rheumatic fever* and *rheumatoid arthritis* cause painful swelling; the chronic stage of RA often results in limited extension. *A loose body* in the joint is suggested by a history of locking. An enlarged, painless joint, suggesting *osteoarthritis* but unilateral, may be *neurogenic arthropathy* (Charcot joint); when encountered in the elbow, syringomyelia is the most likely cause.

Olecranon Bursitis (Miner's Elbow, Student's Elbow): Trauma, inflammation, infection or gout produces an accumulation of fluid in the olecranon bursa, a subcutaneous space overlying the olecranon process (Fig. 13–37C). The swelling is fluctuant. The location of the bulge readily distinguishes it from fluid in the joint.

> **KEY SIGN** **Elbow Pain**

Lateral and Medial Epicondylitis (Tennis Elbow): Repetitive forceful wrist and/or finger flexion and extension focus tension on the common proximal tendon insertions at the lateral (extensors) and medial (flexors) humeral

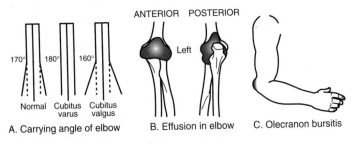

ANTERIOR   POSTERIOR

170°   180°   160°

Normal   Cubitus varus   Cubitus valgus

A. Carrying angle of elbow

Left

B. Effusion in elbow

C. Olecranon bursitis

Fig. 13–37 *Disorders of the Intact Elbow.*

epicondyles. *Lateral Epicondylitis* causes pain in the lateral aspect of the elbow, accentuated by use of the hand during a power grip (when the wrist extensors are also contracting), as in lifting objects. Palpation discloses tenderness over the lateral epicondyle and 1 cm distally. Having the patient hold the long finger in full extension against resistance reliably reproduces the pain. In the *Cozen test* (resisted wrist extension), the patient is asked to keep the fist clenched while extending the wrist against resistance reproducing the patient's lateral epicondylar pain. In the *Mill maneuver*, have the elbow held in extension with the wrist flexed; when you pronate the forearm against the patient's resistance, epicondylar pain is elicited. *Medial Epicondylitis* is less common. The pain is located just distal to the medial epicondyle in the flexor tendons and is reproduced by maneuvers requiring wrist and finger flexion or arm pronation against resistance.

Posttraumatic Elbow Pain—Subluxation of the Radial Head: This usually occurs in childhood (the "pulled elbow"). There is no deformity of the elbow and tenderness is maximum near the radial head. Flexion-extension elicits pain, but pronation and supination are painless.

Posttraumatic Elbow Pain—Fracture of the Radial Head: Usually this results from a fall on the outstretched hand. Swelling is minimal and there is no deformity; the bony equilateral triangle is normal. Flexion and extension are painless, but there is severe restriction of pronation-supination and the radial head is tender.

Upper Arm Signs

This region includes the shaft of the humerus and its covering muscles, principally the biceps brachii and the triceps brachii.

> **KEY SIGN** Pain in the Upper Arm

Bicipital Tenosynovitis: Inflammation in the tendon sheath of the biceps where it emerges anteriorly from the capsule of the shoulder joint is usually the result of overuse. Pain is located near the insertion of the pectoralis major on the humerus and may shoot down the arm. Shoulder motions are somewhat limited, especially flexion of the arm. Palpation of the bicipital groove reproduces the pain. *Yergason Sign:* With the elbow flexed to 90 degrees and the forearm pronated, ask the patient to supinate against resistance; pain in the anteromedial aspect of the shoulder is a positive test.

Pain in the Shoulder—Coracoiditis: Repeated acute or chronic arm work produces inflammation at the origin of the short head of the biceps and the coracobrachialis muscles on the tip of the coracoid process. There is a history of trauma with pain and tenderness at the tip of the coracoid process. The pain is reproduced by adduction and external rotation of the humerus, or having the patient perform against resistance either supination of the forearm with the elbow flexed, forward flexion of the shoulder, or adduction of the flexed shoulder.

Bicipital Humps—Rupture of the Biceps Brachii: The smooth profile of the biceps is interrupted by one or two humps. One hump results with rupture of the tendon or muscle sheath. Rupture of the belly causes two humps. Rupture occurs during lifting and is usually painful. Absence of this history suggests degeneration of the bicipital long-head tendon in the shoulder joint, often associated with chronic impingement or shoulder synovitis. Rupture of the long-head tendon is most common, resulting in mild weakness. Rupture of the muscle may not greatly impair strength.

Painful Immobility of the Upper Arm—Fracture of the Humeral Shaft: These are painful injuries, and the arm is useless, being held in the opposite hand. Transverse fracture is usually caused by a direct blow and there is unmistakable deformity. Spiral fracture, commonly from a fall on the hand, may not cause deformity. Lacking deformity, gently palpate the lateral and medial aspects of the humerus for local tenderness and swelling. Shaft fractures can lacerate the radial nerve and distal brachial artery as they lie in contact with the posterior upper third of the humerus. In all cases of fractured humerus, feel the radial arterial pulse and test for radial nerve injury. Test the motor function of the nerve by having the patient flex the elbow with the forearm pronated and look for wrist-drop. Anesthesia on the radial dorsum of the hand is evidence of sensory loss of the radial nerve.

Shoulder Signs

> **KEY SIGN** **Deficits of Arm Abduction**

See Fig. 13–38. Full painless abduction effectively excludes serious injury to the shoulder. Pain with elevation or limited active range of motion suggest pathology in the shoulder. Pain between 60 degrees and 120 degrees of elevation, with the remainder of the arc painless, suggests partial rupture of the supraspinatus tendon, supraspinatus tendinitis, or subacromial bursitis. Minimal elevation and support of the arm with the opposite hand point to fracture, dislocation, or complete rupture of the supraspinatus; in the latter case, passive motions of the joint are normal. Pain throughout the range of elevation indicates arthritis. Descriptions of these conditions follow.

Partial rupture of the supraspinatus tendon, supraspinatus tendinitis, and subacromial bursitis—pain between 60 degrees and 120 degrees of abduction (painful arc, impingement sign). During arm abduction the supraspinatus

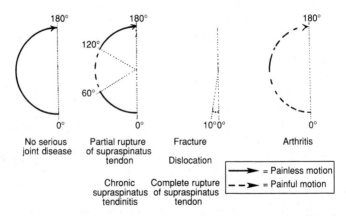

Fig. 13–38 *Causes of Pain and Limited Motion with Elevation of the Arm in Abduction.*

tendon and its insertion on the proximal greater humeral tuberosity must pass beneath the acromion. The subacromial bursa is positioned to decrease the friction, or impingement, which occurs with this motion. Repetitive forceful motion causes mechanical irritation to the tissues eliciting inflammation of the tendon and bursa. Sudden or severe loading of the shoulder may result in incomplete or complete tears of the tendon. These three conditions present with similar signs and symptoms. A history of sudden onset favors partial tear of the tendon, whereas repetitive shoulder motion and subacute or chronic symptoms favor tendonitis or bursitis. All have painful abduction between 60 degrees and 120 degrees, often prohibiting full active range of motion. Less painful passive range of motion is preserved. Precise distinction between the three is not possible with physical examination.   ***Partial Rupture of the Supraspinatus Tendon:***   When the tendon is only incompletely torn, the rotator cuff is intact. Pain is referred to the humeral insertion of the deltoid muscle, but there is no tenderness at that point. Sometimes the pain extends down the arm to the elbow or beyond. Tenderness is elicited just beneath the acromial tip or in the notch between greater and lesser humeral tubercles. DDX: If weakness of the supraspinatus, weak external rotation and impingement signs are all present, a rotator cuff tear is likely [Murrell GA, Walton JR. Diagnosis of rotator cuff tears. *Lancet.* 2001;357:769–770].   ***Acute Supraspinatus Tendinitis:***   This usually occurs in a person 25 to 45 years of age, with a dull ache developing in the shoulder without antecedent trauma. The pain steadily worsens and may be excruciating. The diagnostic test is abduction to 90 degrees and then full internal rotation, which reproduces pain. Tenderness is pronounced beneath the acromial tip.   ***Chronic Supraspinatus Tendinitis:***   Dull shoulder pain develops in a patient who is usually between 45 and 60 years old and without preceding trauma. Abduction is painless to 60 degrees, where the patient feels a jerk with pain in the region of the deltoid muscle. Pronounced tenderness can be elicited in the notch between the greater and lesser tubercles of the humeral head or beneath the acromial tip. Crepitus may also be present. Lying on the shoulder produces pain that prevents sleeping on the affected side for months.   ***Subacromial Bursitis:***   This can be acute or chronic and often accompanies supraspinatus tendonitis. The pain is constant and aggravated by elevation in abduction. There is often a history of heavy arm use.

Complete Rupture of the Supraspinatus Tendon, Torn Rotator Cuff—Minimal Arm Elevation and Support with the Opposite Hand: The supraspinatus muscle initiates arm abduction from 0 to 45 degrees, where the deltoid engages. Inability to initiate elevation in 90° abduction indicates rupture of the supraspinatus tendon. This usually occurs after age 40. The patient cannot elevate the arm against minimal resistance at 30 degrees elevation and 90 degrees abduction, but passive motion is free and painless. Initial shoulder motion is mostly with the scapula. There is resistance to external rotation when the arm is held at the side with elbow flexed. As the arm is moved forward, one may palpate a jerk, fine crepitus, or an indentation in the subacromial region between the greater and lesser humeral tubercles (Fig. 13–18D, page 613). Wasting of the supraspinatus and infraspinatus occurs after 3 weeks.

Shoulder Dislocation—Minimal Arm Elevation with Support of Opposite Hand: When the hand or arm are forcefully abducted and externally rotated, the humeral head dislocates out of the glenoid tearing through the anterior rotator cuff. The humeral head is usually displaced anteriorly and medially from its normal location to under the coracoid process (Fig. 13–39A). The

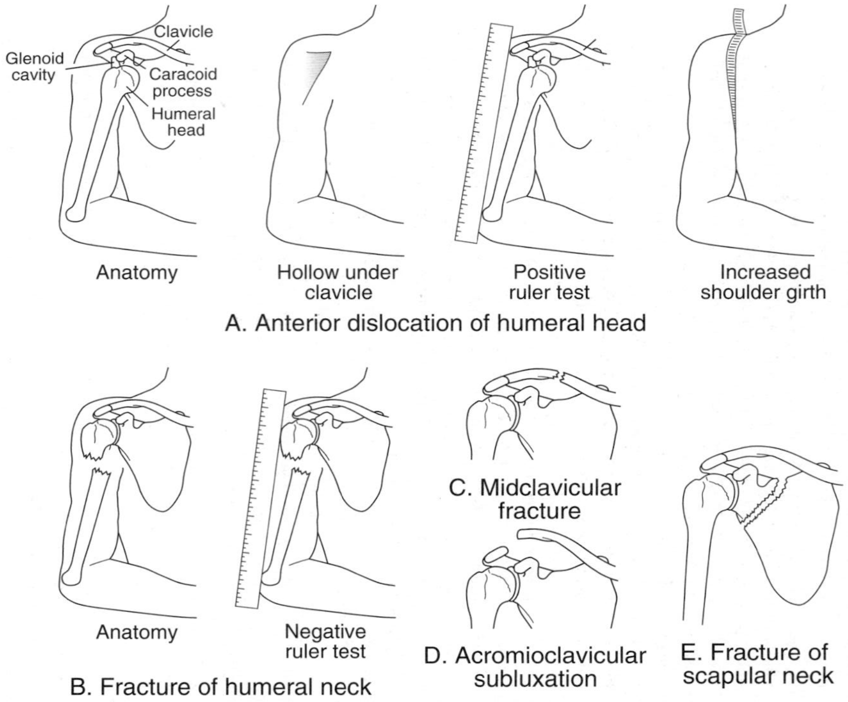

Fig. 13–39 *Traumatic Disorders of the Shoulder. A. Anterior dislocation of the humeral head. B. Fracture of the humeral neck. C. Midclavicular fracture. D. Acromioclavicular subluxation. E. Fracture*

A. Anterior dislocation of humeral head

Anatomy

Hollow under clavicle

Positive ruler test

Increased shoulder girth

Clavicle
Glenoid cavity
Caracoid process
Humeral head

B. Fracture of humeral neck

Anatomy

Negative ruler test

C. Midclavicular fracture

D. Acromioclavicular subluxation

E. Fracture of scapular neck

shoulder profile in anterior dislocations is flattened and the bony triangle is disrupted. The humeral head can be palpated medially in the normally soft belly of the upper third of the deltoid. With the *ruler test of Hamilton*, a straight edge can rest simultaneously on the acromial tip and the lateral epicondyle of the elbow; normally, the humeral head intervenes. The test is also positive in fracture of the humeral neck. The *Calloway test*, useful in obese patients, consists of measuring the girth of the two shoulder joints. A tape measure is looped through the axilla and the girth measured at the acromial tip; the girth of the affected joint is increased. In the *Dugas test*, the patient cannot adduct the arm sufficiently to place the hand on the opposite shoulder. Posterior dislocations are rare. The humeral head is felt posteriorly under the spine of the scapula near the base of the acromial process. A common cause of this uncommon dislocation is a major motor seizure. Shoulder dislocation can be identified by a scapular Y-view X-ray without manipulation of the shoulder. Dislocation of the humeral head can damage adjacent structures including the labrum of the glenoid and the axillary nerve (causing paralysis and later wasting of the deltoid). Palpate the pulses of the arm to detect compression of the axillary vessels.

Humeral Neck Fracture—Minimal Arm Elevation And Support with Opposite Hand: Usually, this results from a fall on the outstretched hand. There is pain in the shoulder and the arm is supported by the opposite hand. Viewed from the side there may be an anterior angular deformity (Fig. 13–39B). The axillary aspect of the arm and the chest wall may be ecchymotic. Rotate the arm gently, while palpating the humeral head; if the fracture is not impacted, the head will not move with the shaft, confirming the diagnosis. When displacement is present, the ruler test of Hamilton (see *Shoulder Dislocation* above) may be positive. If a break is not obvious, consider impacted fracture and measure the distance from acromial tip to epicondyle on the two sides; the impacted side should be shorter.

Clavicular Fracture—Minimal Arm Elevation and Support with Opposite Hand: Fractures at the center of the shaft are most common. Because the fragments are usually displaced, diagnosis can be made by inspection and palpation (Fig. 13–39C). Greenstick or impacted fractures may be detected by tenderness and swelling.

Acromioclavicular Subluxation—Minimal Arm Elevation and Support with Opposite Hand: There is pain and tenderness over the acromioclavicular joint with reluctance to elevate the arm; the distal clavicular tip is often elevated. Have the patient place the hand of the affected side on the opposite shoulder and press firmly on the distal end of the clavicle. The end of the clavicle moves downward and the maneuver is painful (Fig. 13–39D). When the patient holds weights in both hands, the end of the clavicle on the affected side becomes more prominent.

Sternoclavicular Subluxation—Minimal Arm Elevation and Support with Opposite Hand: The more common injury is forward dislocation and subluxation, causing painful clicking in the joint with elevation of the arm in abduction. The deformity is usually obvious to inspection. The rarer backward dislocation is seen as a hollow where the normal clavicular head protrudes. If the mediastinum is invaded, dyspnea and cyanosis may occur.

Scapular Fracture—Minimal Arm Elevation and Support with Opposite Hand: There is pain in the shoulder preventing elevation of the arm (Fig. 13–39E).

Sit at the patient's affected side supporting the forearm while palpating the shoulder. Abduct the forearm to 90 degrees; crepitus in the joint strongly suggests fracture of the scapular neck when the clavicle is intact.

KEY SIGN　Restriction of All Shoulder Motions—Trauma and Arthritis

All types of arthritis may involve the shoulder. In the early stages of inflammatory processes, motions are inhibited by pain; later, adhesions restrict motion. Osteoarthritis may be associated with crepitus in the joint, but effusions are relatively rare. Over time, there is progressive loss of glenohumeral motion. With chronically limited motion, generalized muscle wasting occurs. Joint effusion suggests RA, crystal arthritis (calcium pyrophosphate dihydrate deposition) or less-common disorders such as villonodular synovitis.

Adhesive Capsulitis (Frozen Shoulder): Chronic inflammation of the rotator cuff and joint capsule leads to shortening of the usually loose tendinous cuff and to progressive loss of motion. This often follows unresolved subacromial bursitis or supraspinatus tendinitis. At onset, pain is that of the original injury. Progressive limitation of motion ensues until capsular contraction and fibrosis abate the pain with associated muscle wasting.

KEY SIGN　Painful Nodules in Shoulder Muscles—Trigger Points

Pain is usually present on arising or after inactivity, while exercise diminishes or abolishes the pain. Small nodules may be palpated on the surface of the trapezius or other muscle. Pressure on the nodule reproduces the pain, often with radiation to the neck and upper arm.

Shoulder-pad Sign—Amyloidosis. Bilateral anterolateral swelling of the shoulder joints is a conspicuous, although uncommon, sign of amyloid disease. The periarticular swellings feel hard and rubbery.

Winged Scapula—Paralysis of the Long Thoracic Nerve. Paralysis of the serratus anterior permits the scapula to be separated posteriorly from the thoracic wall, a winged scapula. Have the patient stand and push the hands against a wall while you observe the scapulae (Fig. 13–40A). Injury to the long thoracic nerve is caused, by stretching, during heavy lifting or surgical trauma.

Conditions of the Entire Upper Limb

Flail arm. Lower motor neuron or peripheral nerve injuries produce muscular denervation with flaccid paralysis and muscular wasting. After injuries to the brachial plexus or poliomyelitis, the arm may hang limply at the side with the flexed palm facing backward (Fig. 13–40B).

Spastic arm. Injury to upper motor neurons leads to uninhibited muscular contraction with the antigravity flexors overpowering the weaker extensors. With hemiplegia, the arm is carried with flexion of the elbow, wrist, and fingers (Fig. 13–40C).

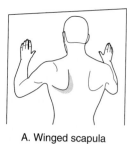
A. Winged scapula

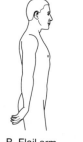
B. Flail arm

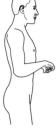
C. Spastic arm

Fig. 13–40 *Disorders of the Intact Shoulder. A. Winged scapula:* When the patient pushes the hands against a wall the involved scapula protrude posteriorly, forming a winged scapula. *B. Flail arm:* The arm hangs limply at the side with palm posterior and fingers partially flexed. *C. Spastic arm:* The arm assumes flexion at the elbow with the upper arm at elevation, flexion at the wrist and fingers, with slight adduction of the humerus; the forearm is in pronation.

Hip, Buttock, and Thigh Signs

> **KEY SIGN** Sacral Pain

Lesions of the Cauda Equina: Compression of the cauda equina ("horse's tail": the spinal roots below the level of the spinal cord termination, or conus), results in compromise of nerve function in one or more lumbar or spinal nerves, often accompanied by pain. Pain is localized to the sacrum and inner thigh and the skin may be anesthetic. Bladder symptoms (including decreased urinary stream, hesitancy, and urinary retention), anal sphincter laxity, absent anal wink, and impotence are common. Compression occurs from a herniated intervertebral disk with posterior protrusion, epidural hematoma or abscess, and neoplasms.

Sacroiliac Pain—SI Arthritis: On arising, there is painful stiffness in the upper medial buttocks, which improves with exercise. Pain may be referred to the upper outer quadrant of the buttock, or the posterolateral aspect of the thigh. Sometimes there is a limp. Spinal rotation accentuates pain. The joint is tender to palpation or percussion. SI arthritis is characteristic of the spondyloarthropathies (page 686).

Sacroiliac Pain—SI Strain: Mechanical strain or postpartum relaxation of the ligaments about the joint is followed by inflammation. The patient complains of pain in the joint or in the upper inner quadrant of the buttock or the posterolateral aspect of the thigh (dermatomes L4, L5, S1). The joint is tender. The pain is accentuated by compressing the anterior iliac crests while the patient lies supine. The tendon reflexes in the lower limbs are normal.

> **KEY SIGN** Ischial Tuberosity Pain and Ischiogluteal Bursitis

The gluteal muscles cover the ischial tuberosities when standing. With thigh flexion, such as sitting, the muscles slide upward exposing the tuberosities and their tendon insertions to pressure, protected only by intervening skin, subcutaneous tissue and the ischiogluteal bursa. Irritation of the bursa and/or tendon insertions can lead to secondary sciatic nerve irritation. This is more common with occupations characterized by sitting on a poorly cushioned seat. The pain is aggravated by sitting, coughing, walking, and standing on tiptoe. The patient stands and walks with a list toward the affected side and the stride is shortened with circumduction of the affected foot. The patient sits with the affected buttock elevated and on lying supports the pelvis on that side. There is point tenderness on the ischial tuberosity. The straight-leg-raising test causes pain. The *FABER sign* is present. On rectal examination a region of tender, bulging, doughy tissue may be palpated in the lateral rectal wall. **DDX:** Patients with herniated disk and lumbosacral disease lie quietly and lack the Fabere sign. This bursa may also be affected by gout. Pain is referred to the tuberosity from intramedullary lesions of the femoral head.

> **KEY SIGN** **Painless Limping—Osteonecrosis, Aseptic Hip Necrosis**

Ischemia of the femoral head leads to necrosis of bone and to the collapse and mushrooming of the femoral head. It may be unilateral or bilateral. Although the cause may be unknown, use of corticosteroids, diabetes, obesity, and alcohol are each associated with an increased risk. Osteonecrosis of the epiphysis in childhood (*Legg-Calvé-Perthes disease*) is relatively painless, whereas osteonecrosis in adults may be painful. Usually it begins with a painless limp and all motions of the hip are slightly impaired. Later, there is severe limitation of abduction and rotation. Muscle wasting and shortening of the limb are common. The *Trendelenburg gait* (page 615) suggests hip dislocation.

> **KEY SIGN** **Pain in the Hip**

Septic Arthritis of the Hip: Usually, there is groin pain, fever, leukocytosis, and prostration. The thigh may be held in slight abduction and lateral rotation to best accommodate the joint effusion. All motion of the hip is painful. Rarely, fluctuation can be felt in the joint. Because pain may be referred only to the knee, knee pain should always prompt examination of the hip. Early diagnosis is urgent because the joint cartilage may be irreparably damaged in a few hours without proper drainage and antibiotics. Tuberculous arthritis is more insidious, often presenting with a limp and pain only after exertion.

Slipped Capital Femoral Epiphysis: The femoral head dislocates on the femoral neck at the relatively weak growth plate during rapid growth in adolescence. A limp with hip pain, usually in boys who are either obese or unusually tall and thin. The distinguishing feature is painful limitation of internal rotation when thigh and knee are both flexed. This may be succeeded by shortening and outward rotation from anterosuperior displacement of the femoral neck.

Torn Labrum: A tear in the acetabular labrum occurs due to trauma. Patients are usually young men with persistent hip pain without limitation of motion. There may be no history of specific injury, or only of injury thought to be minor at the time. Instability of the hip is increased.

Osteoarthritis: See page 679. Boring pain in the groin and buttocks, sometimes with referral to the knee is frequent. Initially, stiffness on arising disappears with exercise, but later walking is limited by pain. The thigh is held in

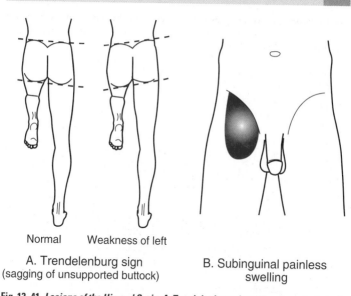

Normal   Weakness of left

A. Trendelenburg sign
(sagging of unsupported buttock)

B. Subinguinal painless swelling

Fig. 13–41 *Lesions of the Hip and Groin. A. Trendelenburg sign:* When the patient stands on one foot, the buttock falls. *B. Subinguinal painless swelling:* Swelling below the inguinal ligament may be either a psoas abscess or an effusion in the psoas bursa.

adduction. Passive motion is restricted in internal rotation and abduction and may be painful. Palpable and audible crepitus may be present with motion.

KEY SIGN   Pain and Limping—Chronic Hip Dislocation

Dislocation of the hip may be congenital or acquired. Weakness of the supporting muscles (from nerve or muscle injury), joint infections, and trauma lead to dislocation in adults. Prosthetic hips are especially susceptible to dislocation with flexion and external rotation. For congenital hip dislocation, consult pediatric texts. In adults, *Trendelenburg gait* (page 615) is present. With the patient supine and the hips and knees flexed, the knee of the affected leg will be lower when observed from the foot of the bed. Inspect the buttocks with the patient standing on one leg; normally, the free buttock is raised when the pelvis tilts (Fig. 13–41A). In the *Trendelenburg sign*, the free buttock falls because the muscles are not strong enough to sustain the position when the femur is not engaged in the acetabulum. The sign is also positive with disease of the glutei, fracture of the femoral head, and in severe degrees of coxa vara. In adults, there is hip pain and premature osteoarthritis of the affected joint.

KEY SIGN   Posttraumatic Hip Pain

Dislocation of the Hip: A blow on the knee while a person is sitting drives the femoral head posteriorly out of its socket, frequently fracturing the rim of the acetabulum (Fig. 13–42A). The rare anterior traumatic dislocation occurs

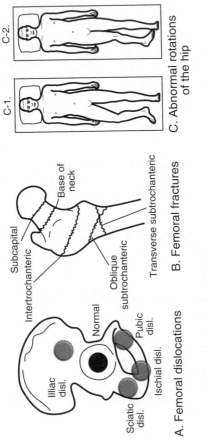

Subcapital

Base of neck

Intertrochanteric

Oblique subtrochanteric

Transverse subtrochanteric

B. Femoral fractures

Illiac disl.

Normal

Pubic disl.

Ischial disl.

Sciatic disl.

A. Femoral dislocations

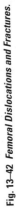

C-1.

C-2.

C. Abnormal rotations of the hip

Fig. 13–42 *Femoral Dislocations and Fractures.*

from landing on the feet in a fall. Dislocation of prosthetic hips is particularly common with abduction and external rotation with minimal forces applied. **Posterior Dislocation:** Inguinal and thigh pain is severe and constant. The thigh lies in extreme internal rotation, adduction, and slight flexion (Fig. 13–42C-2) and only the foot can be actively moved without pain. The greater trochanter is abnormally prominent, while palpation for the femoral head beneath the inguinal ligament yields an indentation. The limb is shortened and passive rotation of the femur is absent. **Anterior Dislocation:** The joint is fixed in abduction, outward rotation, and slight flexion (Fig. 13–42C-1). There is no shortening of the limb, because the head is impaled anteriorly in the iliofemoral ligament.

Fracture of the Femoral Neck: The femoral neck may be fractured below the capsule, a *low fracture*, or within the capsule, a *high fracture* (Fig. 13–42A). In the *extracapsular fracture*, the femur is shortened and externally rotated in the supine position (Fig. 13–42C-1). With an *intracapsular fracture*, the tense joint capsule restrains rotation and swelling of the upper thigh is considerable. If the patient can lift the foot off the bed, the fracture is impacted. In *impacted fractures*, the patient can sometimes walk with little pain, so a fracture may not be suspected. However, passive rotation of the thigh will usually yield some pain.

➤ **Fracture of the Femoral Shaft:** This may lead to shock because of blood loss, so careful observation is required. The thigh is rotated externally, often with obvious deformity and shortening as a consequence of muscle spasm and overlap of the proximal and distal femur.

KEY SIGN   Mass in the Femoral Triangle

Psoas Abscess: A painless abscess is usually an extension of spinal tuberculosis. Painful abscess suggests purulent infection from an intraabdominal source. A conical mass appears beneath the inguinal ligament (see Fig. 13–41B). **DDX:** There is a similar swelling in the iliac fossa distinguishing it from effusion in the psoas bursa. Abscess must be distinguished from fluctuant lymphadenopathy.

Psoas Bursitis: A painless effusion in the psoas bursa, occasionally associated with osteoarthritis of the hip, produces tense, nonfluctuant, immobile conical swelling beneath the inguinal ligament (see Fig. 13–41B). The absence of a mass in the iliac fossa excludes psoas abscess.

Lymphadenopathy: See page 101.

Femoral Hernia: See pages 532 and 590 and Fig. 9–36, page 530.

Knee Signs

KEY SIGN   Painless Unilateral Knee Deformity

Neurogenic Arthropathy (Charcot Joint): See Fig. 13–21C and *Charcot Joint* on page 678.

Genu Varum (Bowleg): The legs deviate toward the midline so that the knees are farther apart than normal when the medial malleoli are together (see Fig. 13–10C). The feet are turned inward when walking. The most common cause is medial knee compartment osteoarthritis. Other causes are rickets affecting the upper tibial and lower femoral epiphyses, Paget disease and occupational stress.

Genu Valgum (Knock-Knee): The legs deviate away from the midline, often bilaterally (see Fig. 13–10C). The most common cause is osteoarthritic narrowing of the lateral knee compartment.

KEY SIGN   Knee Swelling

Fluid Within the Joint: An excess of synovial fluid in the knee joint is an *effusion*. Blood in the joint space is *hemarthrosis*. The presence of pus indicates suppurative arthritis. Fluid signs are independent of fluid type, so specific diagnosis can only be made by aspiration. Effusion is commonly caused by trauma, RA, osteoarthritis, gout, other crystalline arthritides (calcium pyrophosphate, basic calcium phosphate) or intermittent hydrarthrosis. Traumatic hemarthrosis suggests intracapsular fracture or ligament disruption. Nontraumatic hemarthrosis occurs with hemophilia and neoplasms.

Anterior Knee Swelling—Prepatellar Bursitis: A fluctuant subcutaneous swelling occurs anterior to the lower patella and patellar ligament, the distribution of the prepatellar bursa (Fig. 13–21D). It is often found associated with occupational trauma to the tissue overlying the patella. This differs from fluid in the joint cavity that produces swelling beside the patella.

Anterior Knee Swelling—Infrapatellar Bursitis: Swelling occurs in a bursa on both sides of the patellar ligament near the tibial tuberosity (Fig. 13–21E). Fluctuation can be demonstrated from one side of the ligament to the other. This often results from occupations requiring kneeling, such as roofing and laying floors.

Anterior Knee Swelling—Infrapatellar Fat Pad: The infrapatellar fat pad becomes inflamed, causing tenderness and swelling on both sides of the patellar ligament. The tenderness and lack of fluctuance distinguish it from bursitis and synovitis.

Popliteal Swelling—Semimembranosus Bursitis: Fluid accumulates in the bursa between the head of the gastrocnemius and the tendon of the semimembranosus, forming the upper medial border of the diamond-shaped popliteal fossa (Fig. 13–43). Extension of the knee causes painful tensing of the bursa, while flexion relaxes it. Fluctuation is difficult to demonstrate.

Popliteal Swelling—Baker Cyst: The cyst is a pressure diverticulum of the synovial sac protruding through the posterior joint capsule of the knee. Sometimes, dull pain is present. The cyst is best seen by inspection of the fossa when the patient is standing. In contrast to the semimembranosus bursitis, the swelling is in the midline at or below the tibiofemoral junction (see Fig. 13–43). The cyst protrudes when the knee is extended and, unless it is very large, is not visible with flexion. When the cyst freely communicates with the joint, gradual, steady pressure on the sac forces some fluid back into the joint cavity, temporarily reducing the swelling. The swelling may be translucent. Baker cysts often complicate RA and osteoarthritis. Large cysts can compress the popliteal vessels. If the artery is compressed, forced extension of the knee or strong dorsiflexion of the foot may obliterate the pedal pulse.

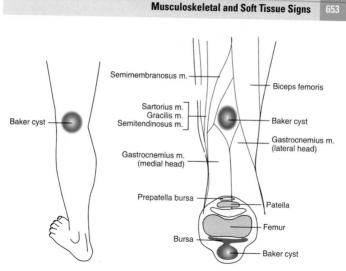

Fig. 13–43 _The Popliteal Fossa._

➤ **Popliteal Mass—Popliteal Aneurysm:** This feels like a cyst and only a conscious effort to detect pulsation will identify it.

Medial Knee Swelling—Cyst of the Medial Meniscus: This is a developmental anomaly of the medial meniscus felt as a fluctuant joint line swelling. Dull pain may be present on standing. The oval, transversely elongated cyst may protrude either anterior or posterior to the MCL. Knee flexion makes it more prominent.

Lateral Knee Swelling—Cyst of the Lateral Meniscus: This congenital cyst occurs at the tibiofemoral junction, posterior to the fibular collateral ligament. Flexion accentuates the transverse fluctuant swelling. It may be painful and, occasionally, protrudes into the popliteal fossa.

KEY SIGN Medial Knee Pain—Anserine Bursitis

The anserine bursa lies superficial to the tibial collateral ligament and deep to the _pes anserina_ (goose foot) formed by the tendons of the sartorius, gracilis, and semitendinosus (see Fig. 13–43). The patient complains of pain in the anterior medial aspect of the knee 2 to 3 cm distal to the joint line. Pain is aggravated by walking; especially while climbing up the stairs. Tenderness, usually without swelling, is palpated on the medial aspect of the knee.

KEY SIGN Anterior Knee Pain

Chondromalacia Patellae: Degeneration of the articular surface of the patella occurs from unknown cause. It is more common in women than men. Pain is felt anteriorly and is aggravated by prolonged sitting and walking down stairs. A small effusion may be present. Passive joint motion is painless. Rocking the patella in the femoral groove frequently elicits pain, often with palpable crepitation.

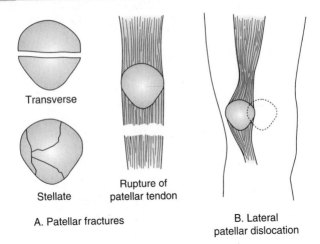

Transverse

Stellate

A. Patellar fractures

Rupture of patellar tendon

B. Lateral patellar dislocation

Fig. 13–44 *Some Traumatic Injuries to the Anterior Knee.*

Quadraceps and Patellar Tendonitis: Pain is felt in the anterior knee either above (quadraceps) or below (patellar) the patella. It usually occurs following an unusual level of activity (running, lifting, climbing, up and down sqatting); it may occur as a result of chronic overuse. Pain is well localized to the involved tendon and reproduced by direct pressure and resisted knee extension.

> **KEY SIGN** Posttraumatic Patellar Pain

Patellar Fracture: This results from a direct blow to the patella, usually from falling onto the flexed knee. Stellate fractures are often not displaced and are easily missed without proper radiologic examination. With nondisplaced fractures, active extension is preserved but painful. Transverse fractures are most likely to be displaced. If there is separation of the bone fragments, the joint is semiflexed and active extension is impossible (Fig. 13–44A). To identify a separation, palpate down the surface of the patella feeling for a crevice. Hemarthrosis always occurs with displaced fractures.

Rupture of the Patellar Tendon: The pathognomonic sign is an upward shift of the patella. After the swelling subsides, the ruptured tendon may be palpated (Fig. 13–44A). Tenderness at the tibial tuberosity suggests concomitant avulsion of the tuberosity.

Sudden Collapse with Locking Knee—Patellar Dislocation: This frequently recurrent problem may be diagnosed from the history. The knee abruptly gives way with pain and subsequent swelling. Acutely, the patella is displaced laterally (Fig. 13–44B). Between episodes, there is increased lateral mobility of the patella and quadriceps wasting may be seen.

> **KEY SIGN** Knee Pain and Recurrent Locking—Loose Body in the Joint

A history of intermittent joint pain with recurrent effusions or locking suggests a loose body in the joint or a torn meniscus. Crepitus may be present; rarely, the examiner may be able to palpate a mass. Loose bodies are usually a chip of bone; resulting from previous injury.

Subacute and Chronic Knee Pain—Osteonecrosis and Stress Fractures: In the absence of direct trauma or signs of disease within the joint, tibial plateau stress fractures and osteonecrosis of the femoral condyles or tibial plateau should be considered.

> **KEY SIGN** **Posttraumatic Knee Pain**

Once femoral and tibial fractures have been excluded, other etiologies need to be explored. The evaluation of patients with knee injuries starts with a detailed history emphasizing the mechanism of injury. A complete knee examination should be attempted, but may be limited by pain. See page 620 and the following reference for further discussion. [Stiell IG, Greenberg GH, Wells GA, et al. Prospective validation of a decision rule for the use of radiography in acute knee injuries. *JAMA*. 1996;275:611–615].

Posttraumatic Pain Proximal to the Patella—Rupture of the Rectus Femoris Muscle: The muscle fibers of the rectus femoris attach to the tendon well above the patella. Traumatic muscular tears often occur at the musculotendinous junction. The injury is painful and the knee is held in semiflexion. Shortening of the torn fibers may form a lump that enlarges when the thigh muscles are contracted; the normal muscle mass is not felt distal to the lump in the suprapatellar region.

MCL Injury: Injuries of the MCL occur from valgus stress to the knee, such as a blow to the lateral side of the knee during weight bearing. Usually the femoral attachment is torn. The ligament is tender and somewhat swollen. Because the medial meniscus attaches to the midportion of the ligament, MCL injury often accompanies medial meniscus injury. With incomplete rupture, pain in the region is severe, medial stability is present, but valgus stress elicits pain; function is not completely lost and movement may be resumed in a few hours. When complete rupture occurs there is medial instability seen as palpable separation of the tibia from the medial femoral condyle with valgus stress. Always compare the injured to the uninjured side, as there is considerable individual variation in the baseline degree of joint stability.

Medial Meniscus Injury: The meniscus is usually injured when the femur is rotated medially while the knee is flexed and the foot and tibia are fixed by bearing weight. The cartilage may be split longitudinally, or either the anterior or posterior horn may be torn. Most commonly, there is a bucket-handle tear in which the horns remain attached while the curved portion is torn. Locking may occur. The most constant sign is joint line tenderness over the MCL when the knee is flexed. Tearing of the posterior horn causes tenderness posterior to the MCL. *McMurray* and *Apley tests* may be positive. MCL injuries are often coexistent.

Lateral Collateral Ligament Injury: A varus force on the knee with external rotation of the femur on the fixed tibia tears the fibular attachment and the head of the fibula may be avulsed. Tenderness is found on the lateral aspect of the knee between the lateral femoral epicondyle and the fibular head. With a complete tear the defect in the ligament may be palpable. Crepitus indicates avulsion of the fibular head. Stability is tested by placing a varus stress on the knee while palpating for opening of the lateral joint line. The common peroneal nerve may be injured simultaneously, so test the strength of the anterior and lateral muscles of the leg and the short extensors of the toes.

Lateral Meniscus Injury: The trauma may be so slight as to escape attention. Pain may be felt either laterally or medially. Tenderness is found in the lateral joint line. *McMurray* and *Apley tests* may be positive. Locking is uncommon.

ACL Injury: Partial tear or complete rupture of the ACL occurs as the result of high-impact injury where the tibia is driven anterior relative to the femur. There is severe pain and the joint is held in slight flexion. Testing of the ligament is difficult or impossible acutely because of pain and limited mobility secondary to tense hemarthrosis. After aspiration or resolution of the hemarthrosis, examination shows a positive *Lachman test* for anterior instability (see page 620) with complete tears.

PCL Injury: Posterior cruciate injury results from a direct blow on the head of the tibia while the knee is flexed. The tibia may sag posteriorly with both knees are flexed at 90 degrees. The acute and late signs are similar to injury of the ACL except that there is a positive *posterior* drawer sign. This is elicited by pushing the tibial head backward on the femoral condyles with the knee flexed at 90 degrees. Also, with the knee in 90 degrees of flexion, a sharp blow to the proximal anterior tibia will elicit pain.

Leg Signs

> **KEY SIGN** Posttraumatic Calf Pain

Injury to the Gastrocnemius and Soleus: Both muscles insert into the Achilles tendon, powering ankle plantar flexion. Forceful dorsiflexion of the foot rapidly loads both muscles and knee extension additionally loads the gastrocs, since this muscle originates on the femoral condyles. The most common injury is a strain of one or both felt as pain in the distal belly of the calf at the musculotendinous junction.

Gastrocnemius Tear: A forceful combination of knee extension and ankle dorsiflexion is felt like a blow to the posterior calf, sometimes with an audible snap. Immediately, walking is intensely painful in the posteromedial midcalf and there is tenderness and a palpable defect in the medial belly of the gastrocnemius. After a few hours, swelling obscures the defect for a few days. The power of plantar flexion is diminished and ecchymoses develops over days extending from the calf to the heel, ankle, and foot.

Soleus Tear: Trauma causing extreme dorsiflexion of the foot may tear the soleus muscle. This produces severe pain and tenderness in the mid-calf.

> **KEY SIGN** Posttraumatic Leg and Calf Pain

Rupture of the Achilles Tendon: The most common scenario is a man, more than 45 years of age, attempting unusual and vigorous activities requiring sudden accelerations or jumping. Complete rupture usually occurs approximately 5 cm above the calcaneal insertion. There is sudden excruciating pain and walking is not possible. Examine the patient in the prone position, with the feet hanging over the end of the table (see Fig. 13–23B, page 620). The affected foot is less plantar flexed and passive dorsiflexion is excessive. With incomplete rupture, squeezing the calf muscles transversely produces plantar flexion of the foot (*Simmonds test*); when the tendon is severed completely no motion occurs, a gap can be felt in the tendon, the distal portion of the tendon is thicker and less taut, and the calf muscles are shortened into a visible lump.

Posttraumatic Anterior Leg Pain—Fracture of the Fibular Shaft: A direct blow on the anterolateral aspect of the leg is the most common cause. Fracture proximal to the ankle may also accompany severe inversion ankle injuries. There is pain at the site of injury, but, usually, the patient can walk. Compressing the tibia and fibula together causes pain at the fracture site.

Postexercise Tibial Pain—Stress Fracture of the Tibia: An incomplete cortical fracture of the tibia results from repeated strenuous use of the leg. Dull aching pain begins gradually with progressively shortening intervals after exercise and persists for hours. There is localized tenderness over the tibia, frequently along the medial border. Pain at the fracture site may be elicited by springing the tibia: with the patient supine, place one hand on the knee and the other on the heel; pull the tibia laterally against your knee as a fulcrum.

Exertional Calf Pain—Intermittent Claudication: See Chapter 8, page 430.

➤ **Postexercise Anterior Leg Pain—Anterior Tibial Compartment Syndrome:** See page 692. Several hours after unusually strenuous leg exercise, stiffness followed by severe pain occurs in the anterior tibial muscular compartment. The region becomes swollen, tense, tender, and warm. Ischemic necrosis of the muscles may occur if the pressure is not relieved by fasciotomy.

Postexercise Subpatellar Pain—Osteochondritis of Tibial Tubercle (Osgood-Schlatter Disease): Before closure of the epiphysis of the tibial tubercle during adolescence, vigorous exercise produces chronic traction injury with partial avulsion of the tubercle. Pain occurs after exercise and a tender, hard swelling is seen and felt at the attachment of the patellar tendon.

Thickened achilles tendon. Thickening is most easily detected by inspection and palpation when the foot is dorsiflexed. Several diseases may produce inflammation (e.g., seronegative spondyloarthropathies, RA) or deposits in the tendon (e.g., xanthomas).

Ankle Signs

KEY SIGN   Swelling of the Ankle Joint—Joint Effusion

The foot is held in slight dorsiflexion and inversion. The distended joint produces bulging beneath the extensor tendons, near the talotibial junction and in front of the lateral and medial malleolar ligaments.

KEY SIGN   Posttraumatic Ankle Pain

Ankle trauma is common and the examiner needs a practical approach to the evaluation. The most common mechanism of injury is inversion of the flexed ankle. Ligament injuries are expected, but fractures may occur; this is the diagnostic dilemma. Careful prospective studies indicate that radiographs of the ankle are necessary, only if there is pain near the malleoli and the patient is older than

55 years of age, is unable to bear weight immediately after the injury or take four steps when examined, or has bone tenderness at the posterior edge or tip of either malleolus. If these conditions are not met, fracture is very unlikely [Stiell IG, Greenberg GH, McKnight RD, et al. Decisions rules for the use of radiography in acute ankle injuries. *JAMA*. 1993;269:1127–1132; Bachmann LM, Kolb E, Koller MT, et al. Accuracy of Ottawa ankle rules to exclude fractures of the ankle and mid-foot: Systematic review. *BMJ*. 2003;326:417].

Rupture of the Joint Capsule: Forceful plantarflexion with eversion of the foot may disrupt the anterolateral portion of the articular capsule. Pain and tenderness occur just anterior to the lateral malleolar ligaments (calcaneofibular and talofibular). A hematoma in the site rapidly appears, accompanied by some edema.

Rupture of the Calcaneofibular Ligament, Common Ankle Sprain: This results from forced inversion of the foot. The tenderness is anterior and inferior to the lateral malleolus. With complete rupture, careful passive inversion of the foot demonstrates tilting of the talus. When the lateral malleolus is fractured, the posterior-lateral malleolus itself is tender.

Rupture of the Deltoid Ligament: This ligament is rarely injured in isolation. It may occur as part of severe fracture dislocation of the ankle.

Pain or Click During Dorsiflexion with Eversion—Recurrent Slipping of Peroneal Tendons: The *tendons of the peroneus longus and brevis* curve behind and under the lateral malleolus, held in a groove by the ligamentous band; the *superior peroneal retinaculum*. Relaxation of the retinaculum may permit slipping of the tendons during dorsiflexion with eversion. Pain or click occurs with the slipping. Physical examination at rest is normal but active motion may produce palpable tendon subluxation.

Pain on Inversion of the Foot—Chronic Stenosing Tenosynovitis of the Peroneal Tendon Sheath: This causes pain only on inversion of the foot. Tenderness and swelling occur in the sheath behind and below the lateral malleolus.

Foot Signs

Nodules in the Foot—Fibroma. Fibromas are benign growths of fibrous tissue that can occur anywhere on the foot (or elsewhere), usually following minor soft tissue trauma. They frequently are painful, especialy on the sole or where they are impinged upon by footwear. They are felt as firm, discrete, rubbery and ocassionally tender nodules usually fixed to the underlying soft tissues, not to bone.

> **KEY SIGN** **Deformed Foot**

Talipes: The five principal varieties are *talipes varus* (inversion), *talipes valgus* (eversion), *talipes equinus* (plantar flexion), *talipes calcaneus* (dorsiflexion), and *talipes or pes cavus* (hollowing the instep) (Fig. 13–45). Combined deformities are *talipes equinovarus* (clubfoot), *talipes equinovalgus*, *talipes calcaneovarus*, and *talipes calcaneovalgus.* The diagnosis is usually made by inspection.

Pes Planus (Flatfoot): One or more of the pedal arches are lowered (Fig. 13–45). A functional classification includes *relaxed flatfoot*, in which the arch is lowered only while bearing weight; *rigid flatfoot*, caused by bony or fibrous

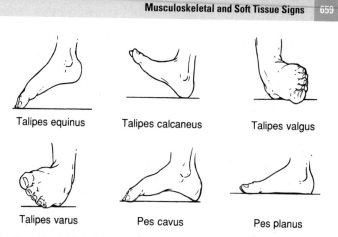

Talipes equinus   Talipes calcaneus   Talipes valgus

Talipes varus   Pes cavus   Pes planus

Fig. 13–45 *Deformities of the Foot.*

ankylosis; *spasmodic flatfoot*, from contraction of the peronei; and *transverse flatfoot*, from flattening of the transverse arch.

> **KEY SIGN** **Posttraumatic Heel Pain—Calcaneal Fracture**

Landing on the heel during a fall may cause fracture of the calcaneus (os calcis) (Fig. 13–46A). The heel appears broader than normal from the back and the hollows beneath the malleoli are obliterated. Tenderness is maximal in the calcaneus near the insertion of the Achilles tendon. Palpation below the malleolus discloses the sides of the calcaneus to be flush with the malleolus, rather than indented. All motions of the ankle are restricted by pain. A hematoma forms in the sole of the heel. Signs of fracture may be subtle, so a high index of suspicion is required.

> **KEY SIGN** **Pain in the Heel**

Retrocalcaneal Bursitis: The bursa between the Achilles tendon and the calcaneus may be inflamed, causing pain, swelling, and tenderness near the tendon insertion (Fig. 13–46B). The lesion is caused by pressure from footwear, especially high-heeled shoes or stiff-backed boots.

Plantar Fasciitis: The plantar fascia is a thick band of fibrous tissue arising from the medial tuberosity of the calcaneus and spreading like a fan across the sole to insert on the proximal phalanges of the toes. Unusual or prolonged weight-bearing activity leads to microtrauma, which is concentrated at the calcaneal insertion. Pain is present in the plantar aspect of the heel and is usually worst with the first steps in the morning. Pain improves with activity, only to recur after rest. Tenderness is elicited at the insertion of the plantar fascia on the distal calcaneus somewhat medially [Buchbinder R. Plantar fasciitis. *N Engl J Med.* 2004;350:2159–2166].

Inflammation of the Calcaneal Fat Pad: Fibrous bands extend from the calcaneal periosteum to the skin; their interstices are filled with fat. Infection or inflammation is compartmentalized by the fibrous bands leading to increased tissue pressure and intense pain. The region is too tender to permit weight

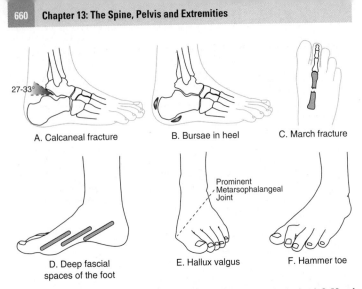

Fig. 13–46 *Lesions of the Foot. A. Calcaneal fracture. B. Bursae in the heel. C. March fracture of a metatarsal bone. D. Deep fascial spaces of the foot. E. Hallux valgus:* This deformity shows lateral deviation of the great toe, with prominence of the 1st MTP joint. *F. Hammertoe:* The second toe is always affected. There is permanent flexion of the PIP joint.

bearing. Usually edema accumulates around the ankle; fluctuation occasionally is present.

Tarsal Tunnel Syndrome: The tarsal tunnel is behind and inferior to the medial malleolus of the tibia. Its bony floor is roofed by the *flexor retinaculum* extending from the medial malleolus to the calcaneus. Through the tunnel pass several tendons and the *posterior tibial nerve*, which divides into the *calcaneal nerve* to the skin of the heel, the *medial plantar nerve* to the skin and muscles of the medial aspect of the sole, and the *lateral plantar nerve* to the lateral portion of the sole. Compression of the nerves in the tunnel causes numbness, burning pain, or paresthesias in portions of the sole. Paresis or paralysis of some small muscles of the foot may occur. Occasionally, a tender area is palpated at the posterior margin of the medial malleolus. The diagnosis is confirmed by nerve conduction studies. Precipitating conditions include fracture or dislocation of the bones near the tunnel, traumatic edema, tenosynovitis, chronic stasis of the posterior tibial vein and foot strain.

> **KEY SIGN** **Metatarsal Pain**

Metatarsalgia: Loss of the normal transverse metatarsal arch from the first to the fifth metatarsal heads leads to abnormal weight bearing on the second to fourth metatarsal heads, which are insufficiently padded. Ask the patient to point to the site of the pain. Pain occurs in the region of the distal metatarsal heads. Examination may show callus under the second to fourth metatarsals and decreased callus under the first and fifth. Pressure on the callus reproduces the pain. Symmetrical bilateral metatarsalgia may be an early symptom of

RA. Fibroneuroma may also be the cause, so squeeze the foot transversely to see if the pain is reproduced.

Metatarsal Stress Fracture: Excessive walking or standing may cause a fracture of the metatarsal shaft (Fig. 13–46C). Pain develops gradually. Muscle cramps and slight swelling may occur. Motion of the corresponding toe is painful. Pain is usually localized several centimeters proximal to the metatarsal head.

Infection in the Interdigital Space: Puncture of the sole may cause infection in one of the four interdigital subcutaneous spaces. The abscess may point between two metatarsals causing swelling on the dorsum of the foot. Walking produces pain between the metatarsals. Tenderness is localized to the interdigital space.

Localized Swelling on the Dorsum—Ganglion. This is a cyst arising from a tarsal joint capsule or an extensor tendon.

Pain in the Instep—Infection in the Deep Fascial Spaces. The central plantar space has four compartments between the sole and the pedal arch (Fig. 13–46D). Infection of the spaces occurs from direct puncture or backward extension from an interdigital space. There is tenderness in the instep (midfoot), dorsal edema, and the curve of the instep becomes obliterated.

Contracture of plantar fascia. Unilateral or bilateral asymptomatic thickening of the plantar fascia is associated with Dupuytren contracture of the palms and Peyronie syndrome.

> **KEY SIGN**   **Lateral Deviation of the Great Toe—Hallux Valgus**

Lateral deviation and rotation of the great toe produces abnormal prominence of the first metatarsophalangeal (MTP) joint (Fig. 13–46E). The second toe may overlap the first, or it may be a hammertoe. The great toe retains good motion. Pain is caused by accompanying hammertoe, an inflamed bursa over the prominent metatarsophalangeal joint (*bunion*), or metatarsalgia from transverse flatfoot (*splay foot*). The most common causes are improper shoes and primary osteoarthritis.

> **KEY SIGN**   **Stiffened Great Toe—Hallux Rigidus**

A prominent osteophyte is usually present on the dorsal aspect of the joint. Pain may occur with walking and climbing. Extension of the MTP is severely limited and flexion is present mainly in the interphalangeal joint.

> **KEY SIGN**   **Deformity of the Second to Fifth Toes—Hammertoes**

The MTP is fixed in dorsiflexion and the PIP is fixed in plantarflexion, while the DIP is freely movable (Fig. 13–46F). A corn or inflamed bursa frequently occurs over the PIP joint. Hammertoes are usually bilateral with several toes on each foot involved. It often accompanies hallux valgus.

Painful Swelling of a Toe—Fractured Phalanx. No matter how trivial the trauma seems, consider the possibility that the bone has been fractured.

> **KEY SIGN**   **Painful Swelling of the Metatarsal Phalangeal Joint—Gout**

This is the classic lesion (*podagra*) of early gout, described on page 675.

Toenail Signs

See Chapter 6, *The Skin and Nails*, page 142.

Muscle Signs

See also Chapter 14, *The Neurologic Examination*.

> **KEY SIGN** **Muscular Wasting**

Loss of muscle substance occurs from disuse or damage to muscle tissue or motor nerves. Fasciculation of the muscles indicates denervation; the history will disclose injury and disuse.

> **KEY SIGN** **Muscle Contracture**

Prolonged disuse, immobilization, ischemia leading to muscle necrosis, or inflammatory processes result in fibrosis of muscle with inelastic shortening. The shortened muscle does not permit full range of joint movement. The joints, however, are normal as distinct from joint contracture. The muscle is firm to hard and atrophic.

> **KEY SIGN** **Muscle Hypertrophy**

Increased muscle volume results from enlargement of normal muscles or infiltration of the muscle by cellular or extracellular material. Resistance exercise increases muscle bulk and power. Hypertrophy may also occur with anabolic steroid use, hypothyroidism, congenital myotonia, Duchenne muscular dystrophy, and focal myositis.

> **KEY SIGN** **Muscle Masses**

To prove that a mass is intramuscular the mass must be freely movable transversely to the long axis with the muscle relaxed. Tensing the muscle must limit the transverse mobility. A mass may result from rupture of a muscle, herniation of a muscle through its sheath, intramuscular hemorrhage, neoplasm, abscess or localized myositis ossificans.

> **KEY SIGN** **Trigger Points—Myofascial Pain**

Painful firm nodules or bands occur in muscles under frequent tonic contraction. The patient complains of pain, often with projection of pain in a nondermatomal pattern around the area and distally into the arm from trigger points in the upper back and neck, or into the leg from trigger points in the pelvic girdle. The pain often has a burning quality. Motor strength and sensation are normal. Trigger points are characteristic of myofascial pain syndromes. They occur most commonly in large muscles of the back and in proximal extremities. Injection of local anesthetic, heat, massage, and stretching, combined with avoidance or changes in precipitating postural activities, is effective therapy. Left untreated, changes may occur in central and peripheral pain pathways leading to chronic persistent pain syndromes.

> ### KEY SIGN   Tender Points—Fibromyalgia

Persistent reproducible pain is elicited by palpation of specific muscles. The patient does not complain specifically of pain in these sites, unlike trigger points. Eighteen symmetrically located sites in the neck, back, and extremities have been standardized for the diagnosis of fibromyalgia (page 690).

Musculoskeletal and Soft Tissue Syndromes

General Syndromes

> ### KEY SYNDROME   Complex Regional Pain Syndrome—Reflex Sympathetic Dystrophy

See Chapter 4, page 87.

➤ ### KEY SYNDROME   Necrotizing Soft-Tissue Infection

Rapid expansion of infection in subcutaneous tissue planes produces local vascular thrombosis leading to ischemia of fat, connective tissue, skin and underlying muscle. Infection and necrosis spread proximally and distally along tissue planes and invade deeper structures along neurovascular bundles that penetrate these planes. When the muscular fascia is involved the term *necrotizing fasciitis* is applied. Pain and fever accompanied by signs of inflammation (erythema, warmth, tenderness) result from infection with group A streptococci or polymicrobial (mixed aerobic/anaerobic) soft-tissue infections. Systemic hypotension, tachycardia, and delirium develop rapidly, and outcome is fatal without complete surgical debridement. Predisposing factors include diabetes mellitus, immunosuppression, and minor puncture wounds. Urgent surgical debridement is mandatory to save limb and life. [Hoadley DJ, Mark EJ. Weekly clincopathological exercises: Case 28-2002: A 35-year-old long-term traveler to the Caribbean with a rapidly progressive soft-tissue infection. *N Engl J Med.* 2002;347: 831–837].

> ### KEY SYNDROME   Acromegaly and Gigantism

The hands enlarge from overgrowth of bone and soft tissues, stimulated by an excess of growth hormone, usually from an adenoma of the anterior pituitary gland. When the condition occurs before the epiphyses close, the enlarged skeleton is well proportioned and the condition is termed gigantism. When growth occurs after epiphyseal closure, the skeletal pattern is called acromegaly, in which the hands, feet, face, head, and soft tissues are thickened. Patients often have diffuse muscular or joint stiffness and may complain of headaches and back pain. Examination shows thickening of the soft tissues, particularly apparent in the face, hands, and feet. Widening without lengthening of the bones leads to prominence of the jaw, wide spacing of the teeth, prominent supraorbital ridge, and enlarged hands and feet. Osteoarthritis is common. In advanced disease with suprasellar extension of the tumor, signs of hypopituitarism and bitemporal hemianopsia may be present.

> **KEY SYNDROME** **Marfan Syndrome**

This is a congenital disease, frequently inherited as an autosomal dominant, but sporadic cases occur. It affects the development of bone, ligaments, tendons, arterial walls, and supporting structures in the heart and eyes. Many persons show only a few stigmas, while the complete syndrome is striking. The long, slender phalanges, spider fingers, have given the name *arachnodactyly* to the disease (Plate 29); some patients lack this sign. The skull is long and narrow, and the palate is high and arched. The long bones are thin and elongated, so the finger-to-finger span with the outspread arms exceeds the body height. Thoracic deformities may be either *pectus excavatum* (funnel breast) or *pectus carinatum* (pigeon breast). The spine may exhibit fused vertebrae or spina bifida. Joint laxity permits hyperextension (double-jointedness), dislocations, kyphoscoliosis, pes planus, or pes cavus. The ears may be long and pointed, satyr ear. Weakness of the supporting structures of the eye produces elongation of the globe (myopia), retinal detachment, lenticular dislocation, and blue sclerae. Degeneration of the vascular elastic media leads to aneurysmal dilatation of the aorta or pulmonary artery. Subsequent dissection or rupture are common causes of early death. Deformities of the cardiac valve cusps are sites for bacterial endocarditis. The foramen ovale may remain patent.

Conditions Primarily Affecting Joints

> **KEY SYNDROME** **Arthritis—Inflammatory and Noninflammatory Joint Disease**

The diagnosis of *arthritis* requires the examiner to confirm signs of acute or chronic joint inflammation: redness, warmth, tenderness, synovial thickening, effusion, bony enlargement, or erosive changes on X-ray. The most diagnostically useful descriptive classification of joint diseases is based upon the history and physical findings. First, the number of joints actively involved is assessed as *monarticular* (1 joint), *oligoarticular* (2–4 joints) or *polyarticular* (>4 joints). For patients with oligo- or polyarthritis, note the pattern of joint involvement: (1) *large more proximal joints or distal small joints*, (2) *axial joints and/or peripheral joints*, and (3) whether involvement is *symmetric* or *asymmetric*. Widespread and symmetrical joint involvement increases the likelihood of a systemic inflammatory disease primarily involving the joints (e.g., RA, SLE).

Careful attention during the physical examination is necessary to distinguish involvement of the joint (synovium and articular cartilage: *arthritis*) from inflammation of the periarticular tendon and ligament insertions into bone (the enthesis: *enthesitis*), the tendons and their sheaths (*tendonitis* and *tenosynovitis*) or the underlying bone (*osteitis*). When tendon inflammation is suspected, listen with the stethoscope for a rub over the painful site.

No classification system is perfect and the examiner must always be alert to evolution of the pattern over days to weeks or years. Remember that polyarthritic diseases may initially present with single joint involvement. Correct rheumatologic diagnosis requires patience and an open mind.

> **KEY SYNDROME** **Monarticular Arthritis**

Arthritis involving a single joint is likely caused by local mechanical, inflammatory, or infectious factors. Less commonly, it is the initial manifestation of a systemic process that will involve other joints. Sequential involvement of single joints with intervening remissions suggest an underlying systemic disorder (congenital or acquired) with superimposed local precipitating events, for example, trauma in hemophilia.

✓ MONOARTHRITIS—CLINICAL OCCURRENCE: *Congenital* hemophilia; *Endocrine* hyperparathyroidism, hypothyroidism; *Idiopathic* osteoarthritis; *Inflammatory/Immune* postinfectious reactive arthritis (e.g., Reiter syndrome, viral exanthems), psoriasis, RA (initial presentation), SLE, amyloidosis; *Infectious* acute septic arthritis (*Staphylococcus aureus*, gonococcemia, others), Lyme disease, syphilis, mycobacteria, osteomyelitis, viral (e.g., HIV, parvovirus, others); *Metabolic/Toxic* crystal-induced diseases (e.g., gout, calcium pyrophosphate deposition, calcium hydroxyapatite, calcium oxalate), scurvy; *Mechanical/Traumatic* blunt trauma, hemarthrosis, fracture, repetitive use/overuse; *Neoplastic* sarcoma (bone, synovium, or cartilage), metastases to bone, benign tumors (e.g., osteochondroma, osteoid osteoma, pigmented villonodular synovitis), leukemia; *Neurologic* neuropathy producing a Charcot joint; *Vascular* osteonecrosis.

➤ **Septic Arthritis:** Direct extension of bacterial infection (most commonly with *S. aureus*) from skin, soft tissue, or periarticular bone or hematogenous spread (e.g., bacterial endocarditis, gonorrhea bacteremia) produces infection within the joint. Release of lysosomal enzymes can rapidly destroy the joint. Usually one joint is involved, often the knee, but in gonococcal arthritis, three-fourths of the patients have an initial transient (2–4 days) migratory oligoarthritis and/or tenosynovitis. Symptoms often begin suddenly with chills and fever. The joint swells rapidly, the overlying skin is red and warm, and the joint is painful and tender to touch. The swelling becomes fluctuant, indicating fluid in the synovial cavity. In immunosuppressed patients signs of infection are frequently absent. Joint aspiration discloses purulent fluid that must be cultured to identify the causative organism. [Margaretten ME, Kohlwes J, et al. Does this adult patient have septic arthritis? *JAMA.* 2007;297:1478–1488] **CLINICAL OCCURRENCE:** In addition to *S. aureus* and gonorrhea, less-common organisms to consider are streptococci, meningococci, *Haemophilus influenzae* (especially in unimmunized infants and children), and, rarely, brucellosis, typhoid fever, glanders, blastomycosis, granuloma inguinale, tuberculosis, fungi, and others.

Gout: Uric acid accumulates in tissue and extracellular fluid as a result of genetic (primary gout) or acquired (secondary gout) causes of uric acid overproduction or underexcretion. When the fluid becomes supersaturated, crystals form in the tissue. When crystals are shed into the joint fluid and phagocytosed by polymorphonuclear neutrophils, acute inflammation results [Choi HK, Mount DB, Reginato AM. Pathogenesis of gout. *Ann Intern Med.* 2005;143:499–516]. The initial attack presents the chief diagnostic problem because a history of recurrent stereotypic episodes is very suggestive of gout. Frequently, the patient is awakened from sleep by severe burning pain, tingling, numbness, or warmth in a joint. The joint rapidly swells and becomes excruciatingly tender, intolerant to the pressure of the bedclothes. Typically, the overlying skin becomes red or violaceous. There may be malaise, headache, fever, and tachycardia. Untreated, the attack lasts for 1 to 2 weeks. In more than half the cases, the MTP joint of the great toe is affected initially (*podagra*) (Plate 30). Other sites are the midfoot (instep), ankle, knee, elbow, or wrist. Acute gout in the midfoot resembles cellulitis. The attacks may be triggered by trauma, surgery, acidosis, infection, exposure to cold, changes in atmospheric pressure, overindulgence in alcoholic beverages, or any acute illness. Large tissue deposits of uric acid (*tophi*) occurring around joints over bony prominences are not usually inflamed.

Calcium Pyrophosphate Dihydrate Deposition Disease (Pseudogout, Chondrocalcinosis): Calcium pyrophosphate dihydrate, shed from articular cartilage, crystalizes within the joint into small, rhomboidal, weakly positive birefringent crystals that trigger the inflammation. Articular fibrocartilage may calcify and be detected by X-ray (*chondrocalcinosis*) in the knee or wrist. This disorder is quite similar to true gout in both its acute and chronic forms. The attack begins abruptly with painful swelling and heat, usually in a single joint, occasionally in two or more joints. The knee, ankle, and wrist are most commonly affected. Untreated, the pain and tenderness are intense for 2 to 4 days, then they gradually subside during the next 1 to 2 weeks. It is commonly associated with increasing age and osteoarthritis and may be a clue to hyperparathyroidism or hemochromatosis (approximately 5% of calcium pyrophosphate dihydrate deposition disease).

Tuberculosis: There is chronic swelling of a single joint with only moderate pain. Joint effusion may be present with thickening of the synovium. Most commonly affected are the hips, knees, and spine. Previous intraarticular or oral corticosteroids and immunosuppressive drugs are major risk factors. Cultures of aspirated joint fluid or synovial biopsy yield *Mycobacterium tuberculosis*.

Painless Effusions of the Knees: The patient experiences episodes of painless swelling and joint effusion in one or both knees, with no constitutional symptoms over a number of years, with an average duration of 3 to 5 days. The cause is unknown, though, occasionally, the condition presages the onset of RA.

Trauma: Mechanical trauma as a result of falls, sports, or other activities causes bleeding (*hemarthrosis*) or effusion with pain as a consequence of damage to the joint capsule, intra- or periarticular ligaments, cartilage, or bone. The knee and ankle are commonly affected, but any joint can be injured. The exact mechanism of injury, time course of pain (immediate versus delayed), and physical examination will assist in suggesting the type and degree of injury. Guidelines for the proper use of radiologic examination for injuries to the ankle and knee have been developed.

Charcot Joint: See page 680.

> **KEY SYNDROME** Oligoarthritis and Polyarthritis

Arthritis involving several joints, either simultaneously or sequentially, is termed oligoarthritis (2–4 joints) and polyarthritis (>4 joints). The pattern of involvement can be useful in helping to identify the exact diagnosis. Generally, oligoarthritis involves larger joints and is *asymmetric* while the classic polyarthritis syndromes (RA, SLE) involve *symmetric* joints, including the small joints of the hands and feet. These are only guidelines and must not be interpreted as hard-and-fast rules.

✔ **OLIGO- AND POLYARTHRITIS—CLINICAL OCCURRENCE:** Congenital hemophilia, familial Mediterranean fever, hemochromatosis, sickle cell disease, alkaptonuria/ochronosis;   *Endocrine*   hyperparathyroidism, hypothyroidism, acromegaly;   *Idiopathic*   inflammatory and noninflammatory osteoarthritis; *Inflammatory/Immune*   postinfectious reactive arthritis (e.g., Reiter syndrome, viral exanthems, inflammatory bowel disease), psoriasis, RA, SLE, RF, ankylosing spondylitis, systemic sclerosis (scleroderma), polymyositis/dermatomyositis, Still disease, Behçet syndrome, relapsing polychondritis, amyloidosis, sarcoidosis, erythema multiforme, erythema nodosum, drug reactions, serum sickness; *Infectious*   septic arthritis, Lyme disease, viral (e.g., HIV, parvovirus, rubella, mumps, others), Whipple disease, mycoses (coccidioidomycosis, histoplasmosis, blastomycosis, cryptococcosis), actinomycosis, secondary syphilis, brucellosis, typhoid fever;   *Metabolic/Toxic*   crystal-induced diseases (e.g., gout, calcium pyrophosphate deposition, calcium hydroxyapatite, calcium oxalate), ochronosis, scurvy;   *Neoplastic*   sarcoma (bone, synovium, or cartilage), metastases to bone, benign tumors (e.g., osteochondroma, osteoid osteoma, pigmented villonodular synovitis);   *Vascular*   osteonecrosis, systemic vasculitis, HOA.

Gonococcal Arthritis—Migratory Oligoarthritis: *Neisseria gonorrhoeae* infects the urethra or uterine cervix and then disseminates hematogenously to synovial membranes and skin, causing local inflammation. Infectious arthritis, tenosynovitis, and skin lesions are the most common extragenital complications of gonorrhea. One to 4 weeks after the onset of urethritis, inflammation may suddenly occur in the knees, wrists, and ankles, although other joints may be affected. The most common pattern is a migratory oligoarthritis and tenosynovitis. Small amounts of thin fluid may accumulate in joint cavities. In other cases, suppurative arthritis develops, with inflammation of a single joint and production of purulent exudate. Tenosynovitis in the hands, wrists, or ankle is more common in gonorrhea than in arthritis from any other cause. The diagnosis may not be easy because the gonococcus is difficult to culture from the joints. Pustular skin lesions on an erythematous base are seen with gonococcal bacteremia and help to distinguish gonococcal arthritis from other conditions. Genital, rectal and throat specimens for culture or polymerase chain reaction testing of urine for gonococcus and chlamydia should be obtained. *Reiter syndrome* (nonspecific urethritis, arthritis, and conjunctivitis) following nongonococcal urethritis may cause confusion, because conjunctival infection is present in up to 10% of patients with gonorrhea.

Spondyloarthritides and Ankylosing Spondylitis: See page 686.

Tophaceous Gout: See page 675. Tophi are masses of sodium urate crystals deposited in the tissues often over bony prominences and around joints where they erode bone. Acting as foreign bodies, they stimulate low-grade inflammation that may extrude the tophi through the skin. The asymmetrical nodular swellings and cartilage degeneration may impair joint function. Clinical signs of inflammation are variable, from mild to moderately severe. The olecranon, bunion and prepatellar bursae, and hands are most frequently affected.

Rheumatoid Arthritis—Deforming Symmetrical Distal Polyarthritis: RA is characterized by proliferation of inflamed synovial tissue (*pannus*) that enters the joint cavity in tongue-like projections. The pannus erodes cartilage, periarticular bone, and soft tissues, including tendons and ligaments. Untreated, the result is destruction of the joint surfaces and supporting structures producing subluxation, deformity, and loss of joint function. The onset may be insidious with morning stiffness and pain followed by swelling and tenderness of the joints, proceeding over weeks to months into a small and large joint polyarthritis. Less commonly, the onset is sudden with pain and swelling occurring simultaneously in several joints accompanied by fever and prostration. Smaller joints of the hands (MCP, PIP), feet (MTP), wrists, and ankles are typically involved early and symmetrically; onset in a single larger joint, usually a knee, is not rare. Interphalangeal joints become fusiform from joint effusion (fluctuant) or thickening of the joint capsule (nonfluctuant). DIP joints are invariably spared. Tenderness is confined to the region of the capsule. Joint motion is initially limited by pain or effusion, later by fibrosis or muscle shortening. Muscle weakness and wasting may be rapid and disproportionate to the degree of disuse. Although remissions may occur, the disease is usually progressive over a period of years. Joint contracture and subluxations are frequent, with subluxation of the MCP joints producing characteristic ulnar deviation of the fingers. Tenosynovitis is manifest as swelling of the tendon sheaths. In 20% to 35% of cases, subcutaneous rheumatoid nodules develop over bony prominences and tendon sheaths. They are painless, firm, and freely movable over bones, similar to those in RF. A serious late complication is instability of the cervical spine as from subluxation of C1 on C2, that may present as neck pain or upper motor neuron signs. Diagnosis is based upon clinical and laboratory criteria. Frequently, the patient must be observed for many months before the diagnosis is secure. **DDX:** RA frequently involves the temporomandibular joint unlike RF. In RF, arthritis is migratory, while it is persistent in RA. Reactive arthritis (Reiter syndrome, postdysentery, or urethritis) is usually oligoarticular and mainly affects large joints, especially ankles and knees. An initial monarthritis may suggest an infectious or crystalline arthritis; however, aspiration of joint fluid excludes these possibilities.

Variants of RA. *Felty's syndrome* is the triad of RA, splenomegaly, and leukopenia. *Palindromic rheumatism* presents as multiple afebrile attacks of mono- or oligoarthritis lasting for only 2 or 3 days, leaving no residua. *Secondary Sjögren's syndrome* is diagnosed when keratoconjunctivitis sicca and xerostomia accompany RA. *Vasculitis* may accompany RA and involve the skin (necrosis and nodules) and lung. *Juvenile idiopathic arthritis* is a group of disorders which may overlap with the adult disease [Hashkes PJ, Laxer RM. Medical treatment of juvenile idiopathic arthritis. *JAMA.* 2005:294:1671–1684]. See pediatric texts for descriptions and details.

Systemic Lupus Erythematosus—Nondeforming Symmetrical Distal Polyarthritis: The cause is unknown, but the disease involves inflammation of multiple tissues and organs accompanied by antibodies to specific nuclear antigens usually degraded in the nucleosome. The role of these antibodies in the pathogenesis of the syndrome is unclear. SLE is a chronic inflammatory multisystem disease, more common in women than men. No one symptom or sign is pathognomonic of SLE; rather, the diagnosis is established by clinical criteria. The most common symptoms and signs are fatigue, malaise, or fever (90% of cases), arthritis or arthralgias (90%), and skin rashes (50–60%). The arthralgias, myalgias, and joint inflammation resemble mild RA, but deformities usually do not develop. The malar ("butterfly") rash is a macular to maculopapular, sometimes scaly, erythematous process forming the "wings" of the butterfly on each malar prominence, with the "trunk" on the bridge of the nose. It may be more intense after exposure to sunlight. In addition, there may be skin atrophy, telangiectasia, and mucosal ulcers. Serositis is common, presenting as pleurisy (with effusion and/or pleural rubs), abdominal pain, or pericarditis. Nonbacterial endocarditis with valvular insufficiency (usually mitral), central nervous system disease (with personality change, psychosis, or seizures) and glomerulonephritis can occur at any time, and may be the presenting syndrome. Other signs are recurrent urticaria, mononeuritis multiplex and lymphadenopathy. Fetal wastage and thromboembolic disease are associated with antiphospholipid antibodies [D'Cruz DP, Khamashta MA, Hughes GRV. Systemic lupus erythematosus. *Lancet.* 2007;369:587–596; Caro I, Zembowicz A. Case 5-2003: A 16-year-old girl with a rash and chest pain. *N Engl J Med.* 2003;348:630–637].

Osteoarthritis (Degenerative Joint Disease)—Noninflammatory Polyarthritis of Large Joints: This is a disease of articular cartilage with degradation of the proteoglycan matrix leading to fissuring, thinning, and loss of articular cartilage, and secondary thickening of subchondral bone. In late stages, the bone ends rub directly on each other so their surfaces become worn and polished. The joint capsules are little affected, so adhesions are not formed, and although joint motion is restricted, ankylosis does not result. The bony margins proliferate to form spurs, lipping, and exostoses. Genetic and acquired factors (trauma, surgery, obesity, excessive use) contribute to the pathogenesis. Symptoms are usually first noticed in the weight-bearing joints after age 40 and signs of inflammation are relatively slight. Symptoms correlate poorly with the objective extent of joint disease. The most common symptom is pain with use that disappears with rest. The patient may note grating during motion. Initially, the range of motion is normal, with a gradual decrease occurring as the disease progresses. Enlargement of the distal and PIP joints of the fingers (Heberden and Bouchard nodes, respectively), is frequently encountered. Painless knee effusion is frequent as is asymmetric loss of knee cartilage leading to valgus or varus deformity.

Hemochromatosis: The second and third MCP joints and the radiocarpal joint of the wrist are most commonly affected. *Chondrocalcinosis* is present. Symmetric noninflammatory arthritis of the MCP joints should initiate a search for an iron-storage disorder.

Rheumatic Fever—Migratory Polyarthritis: This disease is a delayed inflammatory reaction following infection with specific Lancefield groups of group A beta-hemolytic streptococci. Tissues affected include the heart, joints, skin and central nervous system. The disease is protean in its clinical manifestations. The classic presentation begins from 1 to 4 weeks after streptococcal pharyngitis, with gradual onset of malaise, fatigue, anorexia, and fever. A single large joint becomes painful, tender, and swollen, and the overlying skin is red and hot. An effusion forms that is turbid and sterile. While the fever and other signs of illness persist, the joint inflammation spontaneously subsides in a few days, only to reappear in another joint, and later in another joint—a *migratory polyarthritis*. Joint involvement may be so mild that pain is unaccompanied by physical signs of inflammation. Months of observation may be required to distinguish it from RA; involvement of the temporomandibular joint often occurs in RA, practically never in RF. RF leaves no residual joint deformity. At onset, the inflammation of a single joint with effusion requires distinction from suppurative arthritis. *Carditis* is manifest as tachycardia, muffled heart sounds, heart enlargement, valvular insufficiency murmurs, pericardial friction rub, or gallop rhythm on examination. The electrocardiogram may show PR prolongation. Two distinct types of *skin lesions* may be associated with RF, although neither is pathognomonic. *Erythema marginatum or circinatum* is characterized by coalescing circular erythematous areas over the trunk and extremities, migratory and transitory, changing within the hour. With chronic disease, subcutaneous *rheumatic nodules* may appear as firm, nontender masses over the joint prominences and tendon sheaths of the limbs, scalp, and spine. They are loosely attached to the underlying tissue; when numerous, their distribution tends to be symmetrical. *Sydenham chorea* may appear several months after onset. There are no diagnostic laboratory tests, but the full clinical picture is fairly distinctive. Diagnosis is based upon the Jones criteria of major and minor manifestations.

Relapsing Symmetrical Seronegative Synovitis with Pitting Edema (RS3PE): This condition of unknown cause presents with recurrent episodes of symmetrical synovitis of the hands and wrists with pitting edema and erythema of the dorsum of the hands. Pain is relatively mild and the condition usually remits after several days to a couple of weeks. When RS3PE occurs as a paraneoplastic condition, it may be more chronic.

Charcot Joints: Absence of pain or proprioceptive sensation in a joint leads to loss of joint integrity. Repeated injuries cause successively three stages of articular damage: swelling, joint degeneration, and formation of new bone. In the initial stage, erythema and swelling are the only findings. The course is progressive with hypermobility, traumatic osteophyte formation, and subluxation leading to painless deformities and crepitus on movement. In any stage, the diagnostic clue is the absence of the expected pain with movement and loss of pain sensation and proprioception in the involved limb. A single joint may be affected, or, commonly, all the joints in an anatomic region (e.g., the midfoot joints) are involved. Physical examination should try to determine if the neuropathy is part of a local or systemic neuropathic process. Classic clinical conditions, causing Charcot joints, include tabes dorsalis (knee most commonly involved (Fig 13–21C); hip, ankle, lower spine, less frequently involved), diabetes mellitus (tarsal and metatarsal joints most commonly, ankle occasionally, knee rarely), syringomyelia (usually joints of the upper limbs), and leprosy [Hartemann-Heurtier A, Van GH, Grimaldi A. The Charcot foot. *Lancet.* 2002;360:1776–1779].

Conditions Primarily Affecting Bone

> **KEY SYNDROME** Osteoporosis

Bone resorption exceeds bone formation, leading to decreased bone mass and decreased mechanical strength. Trabecular bone is affected more than cortical bone. Increased resorption of bone results from immobilization, inflammation, multiple myeloma, and hyperparathyroidism. Decreased bone formation results from gonadal hormone deficiency and glucocorticoid steroid excess, and with advanced age. Trabecular bone deficiency is especially important in the vertebrae and pelvic bones, while cortical bone loss is predominant in long bones. Osteoporosis is asymptomatic until insufficiency fractures occur, usually in the thoracic or lumbar spine and pelvis. Thoracic kyphosis results from anterior wedging of thoracic vertebrae. Bone mineral density is assessed by dual X-ray absorptiometry scan. The bones are much more susceptible to fracture with minor trauma; hip and wrist fractures from falls should initiate evaluation for osteoporosis in both men and women [Green AD, Colón-Emeric CS, et al. Does this woman have osteoporosis? *JAMA.* 2004;292:2890–2900].

OSTEOPOROSIS—CLINICAL OCCURRENCE: *Congenital* vitamin D-resistant rickets, Marfan syndrome, hemochromatosis, Ehlers-Danlos syndrome, hemophilia, thalassemia, positive family history; *Endocrine* postmenopausal estrogen deficiency, premature menopause, hypogonadism, hyperthyroidism, hyperparathyroidism, Cushing syndrome, glucocorticoid use, diabetes mellitus, pregnancy, adrenal insufficiency, acromegaly, hyperprolactinemia; *Idiopathic* advanced age; *Inflammatory/Immune* sarcoidosis, amyloidosis, RA, ankylosing spondylitis; *Metabolic/Toxic* vitamin D deficiency, malnutrition, chronic renal insufficiency, heparin, cirrhosis, postgastrectomy, parenteral nutrition, cigarette smoking, low body weight; *Mechanical/Traumatic* immobilization, disuse, and nonweight bearing; *Neoplastic* multiple myeloma, paraneoplastic (parathyroid hormone-related protein secretion), lymphoma, prolactinoma; *Neurologic* paralysis, stroke, multiple sclerosis; *Psychosocial* anorexia nervosa; *Vascular* hyperemia of bone.

KEY SYNDROME   Osteomalacia

Vitamin D deficiency, hypocalcemia, or hypophosphatemia after the epiphyses are closed prevents calcification of newly formed bony matrix. Early there are no symptoms or signs, while later, bone pain and tenderness occur. Low back pain and striking muscle weakness are common. Low serum calcium levels may produce spontaneous carpopedal spasm with the Chvostek and Trousseau signs. Insufficiency (stress) fractures are common and pseudofractures may be seen by X-ray.

OSTEOMALACIA—CLINICAL OCCURRENCE: *Congenital* vitamin D-resistant rickets; *Endocrine* hyperparathyroidism, rapid deposition of calcium and phosphorus in the tissues after ablation of the parathyroid glands in osteitis fibrosa cystica, hypoparathyroidism; *Inflammatory/Immune* celiac disease; *Metabolic/Toxic* vitamin D deficiency, hypocalcemia, hypophosphatemia, malabsorption, pancreatic insufficiency, malnutrition, chronic renal insufficiency, renal tubular acidosis, Fanconi syndrome, ureterosigmoidostomy, essential hypercalciuria, drugs (anticonvulsants, e.g., phenytoin, glucocorticoids, etidronate), fluoride and aluminum intoxication.

Rickets: Vitamin D deficiency in childhood before epiphyseal closure results in inadequate calcification of cartilage and new bone. See Chapter 8, Fig. 8–30, page 346. Softening of bone produces widening of the cranial sutures and fontanelles (craniotabes), Parrot bosses, rachitic rosary, Harrison grooves, thoracic kyphosis or lordosis, genu valgum or varum, and a contracted pelvis. With the sole exception of the rosary, all deformities are permanent stigmas of childhood disease.

KEY SYNDROME   Paget Disease

Increased resorption of bone combines with rapid growth of new bone with disordered architecture and decreased mechanical strength. The cause is unknown.

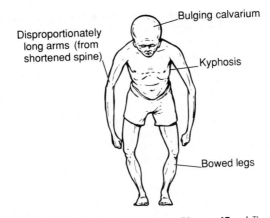

Fig. 13–47 *Bony Signs of Osteitis Deformans (Paget Disease of Bone). The chief features of Paget disease are the enlarged calvarium (contrasting with the normal-sized face underneath), kyphosis and shortening of the spine, shortening of the spine so the arms look proportionately longer than the trunk, and bowed legs. The figure represents a collection of features, which are unlikely to occur together in the same person.*

Bone pain may occur but is seldom severe. With the exception of the hands and feet, any bones may be involved. The skin over affected bones may be warm. The classic osseous deformities are increased girth of the calvarium, thoracic kyphosis, genu varum, and shortening of the spine by flattening of the vertebrae, giving the appearance of disproportionately long arms (Fig. 13–47). Spontaneous or stress fractures can occur and rarely osteogenic sarcoma develops. Increased blood flow through the spongy bone may produce an arteriovenous fistula leading to high-output cardiac failure.

KEY SYNDROME   Hyperparathyroidism, Primary (Osteitis Fibrosa Cystica)

Increased production of parathyroid hormone (PTH) causes bone resorption to exceed new bone formation, leading to hypercalcemia, hypercalciuria, hyperphosphaturia, and hypophosphatemia. The disease may be asymptomatic, although diffuse musculoskeletal aching and fatigue is seen in many patients. Late findings are bone tenderness, muscle weakness, and waddling gait. Subperiosteal cysts in the skull and long bones can cause visible and palpable swellings. Peptic ulcer and urolithiasis should prompt a search for hyperparathyroidism.

Hyperparathyroidism, Secondary and Tertiary: Hyperphosphatemia and hypocalcemia combined with disordered vitamin D metabolism in chronic renal failure (renal osteodystrophy), or osteomalacia from other causes, leads to increased production of PTH, hyperplasia of the parathyroid glands, and progressive bone disease. Combinations of dietary, hormonal, and renal replacement therapies can help control the disorder. When PTH production is not suppressible with appropriate treatment, it is termed tertiary hyperparathyroidism.

KEY DISEASE   Multiple Myeloma

This malignant clonal proliferation of immunoglobulin-producing plasma cells (terminally differentiated B cells) in the bone marrow causes destruction of bone by activation of osteoclasts leading to hypercalcemia. Normal immunoglobulin production is suppressed, there is production of monoclonal plasma proteins (heavy chains, light chains, and intact immunoglobulin), and anemia and thrombocytopenia develop. Renal insufficiency results from tubular toxicity of light chains (Bence-Jones proteins), hyperuricemia, and hypercalcemia. This is the most common malignant tumor primarily affecting bone. Fatigue or generalized aching discomfort may be the only early symptoms. The most common specific symptom is bone pain. With spinal compression fractures, localized pain in the back with radicular distribution occurs. The presenting complaints may be referable to anemia, renal failure, or a pathologic fracture. Multiple myeloma should be considered in patients, more than 45 years of age, with back pain and anemia.

KEY SYNDROME   Metastasis to Bone

Metastatic disease presents as a localized swelling or pain in a bone, a pathologic fracture, or is found incidentally on radiographs taken for another reason. The most frequent primary lesions are carcinomas of the breast, lung, and prostate.

KEY SYNDROME   Fractures

Fractures are mechanical disruptions of the mineralized bone and its collagenous matrix. Forceful localized trauma fractures the entire bone. Fracture of the mineralized bone leaving the collagenous matrix intact results from trauma in children (*greenstick fracture*) and repetitive activities in adults (*stress fracture*). If the bone is inherently weak because of local destructive disease, it may fracture at usual loads (*pathologic fracture*). When fracture fragments penetrate the skin, it is an *open fracture*. When fracture is suspected, immobilize the part and assess neurovascular function distal to the injury. Inspection often reveals deformity. Unavoidable movement reveals abnormal mobility, and bone crepitus, distinctive signs of fracture one should not deliberately try to elicit. Muscle contraction attempting to splint the fracture often aggravates pain. Localized bone tenderness indicates the site of the fracture. Shortening of a long bone may be the crucial sign of an impacted fracture.

Spontaneous or Pathologic Fracture: This is a fracture that occurs with trauma insufficient to break a normal bone. Judging the amount of trauma is difficult, hence spontaneous fractures are easily mistaken for traumatic fractures; a high index of suspicion is warranted. X-ray signs of generalized or local bone disease should be sought if pathologic fracture is suspected. Sometimes spontaneous fractures are less painful than those of healthy bone. Osteomalacia, osteoporosis, Paget disease, hyperparathyroidism, multiple myeloma, osteogenesis imperfecta, and primary and metastatic neoplasms in bone are common underlying conditions.

Fat Embolism: After trauma to large bones, and especially after fractures, fat globules embolize via the veins to the lungs, brain, and other tissues. The pathogenesis remains controversial. The onset of fat embolism is sudden, with restlessness and vague pain in the chest. Symptoms reach a maximum in approximately 48 hours. Dyspnea and cyanosis are common and purulent sputum occasionally containing diagnostic fat droplets may be produced. Fever occurs with a disproportionately high pulse rate. Cerebral symptoms and signs are extremely variable; delirium and coma indicate a grave prognosis. Fat droplets may be seen in retinal or conjunctival vessels. On the second or third day, petechiae may appear over the shoulders and chest as well as in the conjunctivae and retinae. Fat embolism should be considered in acutely ill patients with trauma to long bones or skull, insertion of prostheses, chronic alcoholism, diabetes mellitus, and sickle cell disease.

KEY SYNDROME   Osteomyelitis

Acute: Bloodborne bacteria from superficial infections are carried to the terminal capillary loops of the metaphyseal cortex, causing a necrosing infection that erodes to the periosteum. The initial infection is in the metaphysis, near but not involving the epiphysis. *S. aureus* is the most common organism. Osteomyelitis is most common in children. The onset is usually sudden, with fever and pain. Older children may be able to point to the painful site, although the pain may be referred to the nearest joint where sympathetic effusion may be noted. Localized swelling and redness of the overlying skin with increased warmth may be seen. Light bone percussion frequently discloses tenderness; localize the site with finger pressure on the bone moving toward the suspected site until the point of maximum tenderness is located. The proximal femoral metaphysis is within the hip joint in children, so they present with a septic hip. Sometimes deep cellulitis cannot be distinguished clinically from osteomyelitis.

Chronic Osteomyelitis: After the acute phase, the purulent discharge from the necrosing bone breaks through the periosteum and drains through sinuses in the skin. The circulation of the cortex becomes impaired, producing islands of dead bone, *sequestra*. A sequestrum may be absorbed or discharged through the sinus or surrounded by new bone, the *involucrum*. Continuing necrosis of bone and retention of sequestra cause persistence of the infection.

KEY SYNDROME   Osteogenesis Imperfecta

An inherited disorder of type I collagen results in decreased mechanical strength of all bones and pathologic fractures during the first decade of life. Autosomal dominant inheritance occurs in 60% of cases, but four different types have been recognized. The bones are harder and more brittle than normal, so spontaneous or pathologic fractures are common. The fractures are sometimes painless. Blue sclerae may be observed. Short stature is usual and skull deformity is often present. Hypermobility of joints is common.

KEY SYNDROME   Bony Swellings

Swelling is detected by inspection and palpation, but the signs are rarely diagnostic. The location of the swelling in a long bone may be distinctive. Hamilton Bailey formulated the following diagnostic aids: (1) Swelling in all diameters of the bulbous end of a long bone is most likely caused by *giant cell tumor*; (2) Swelling on one aspect of a bone, near the epiphyseal line, is most likely an *epiphyseal exostosis*; (3) Swelling in all diameters, beginning at the metaphysis and extending toward the center of gravity, may be *Brodie abscess, osteoid osteoma,* or *osteosarcoma*; (4) Swelling in all diameters, at the center of gravity, may be *Ewing tumor, eosinophilic granuloma,* or *bone cyst*; and (5) Consider that any localized bone tumor may be *metastatic from a distant primary,* so complete examination is indicated. X-ray findings may be distinctive, but biopsy is often indicated.

KEY SYNDROME   Bony Nodules (Occupational)

Repeated trauma to a limited region of soft tissue and underlying bone during work or sport may cause bosses of the bones with overlying calluses. Examples are *surfer's nodules* on the dorsa of the feet (from pressure on the surfboard as the surfer sits cross-legged) and *painter's bosses* on the subcutaneous surface of the tibia at the junction of the upper and middle thirds (from standing on a ladder and resting the tibias against the next higher rung).

Fibrous Dysplasia of Bone: The cause of this disease is unknown. The architecture of one or more bones is distorted by fibrosis; the cranium and long bones are especially involved. There is asymptomatic bowing of the affected long bones. The skin often contains melanotic spots with jagged borders. In young girls, precocious puberty may occur.

Hereditary Multiple Exostoses—Osteochondromatosis: The autosomal dominant disease is characterized by exostoses arising from the bony cortex, deforming the metaphyseal region of some long bones. Involvement is usually bilateral but not symmetrical. The ulna may be shortened, producing ulnar deviation of the hand. Valgus deformities of the ankle are common. The only symptom may be mechanical interference with normal joint function.

Axial Skeleton: Spine and Pelvis Syndromes

KEY SIGN   Spondyloarthritis

Inflammation at the insertion of ligaments and tendons into bone (*the enthesis, enthesitis*) leads to joint and tendon sheath effusions and calcification of periarticular structures. Genes (HLA-B27) and acquired illness (inflammatory bowel disease, infectious colitis, nongonococcal urethritis, psoriasis) predispose to these disorders. Asymmetric oligoarthritides of the large joints with prominent involvement of the spine and SI joints and negative tests for rheumatoid factor are described as the *seronegative spondyloarthritides.* Patients present with back pain and stiffness, and occasionally with fever, malaise, and weight loss. Look for extraarticular disease, such as genitourinary or gut symptoms, eye involvement (*uveitis*), and skin disease. [Khan MA. Update on spondyloarthropathies. *Ann Intern Med.* 2002;136:896–907]. ***CLINICAL OCCURRENCE:*** ochronosis, disk disease, DISH, ankylosing spondylitis, reactive arthritis (e.g., Reiter), enteropathic arthritis (inflammatory bowel disease), psoriasis, after diarrheal and genitourinary infections (see reactive arthritis, Reiter syndrome).

Ankylosing Spondylitis: Inflammation of the ligamentous attachments to the vertebrae (*enthesitis*), the SI joints and the junction of the annulus fibrosis and the vertebral end plates leads to new bone formation and bridging resulting in ankylosis. This chronic, progressive arthritis begins with SI involvement and progresses proximally often leading to severe ankylosis. Nonspecific symptoms often begin in adolescence and occur intermittently for

5 or 10 years. Pain and morning stiffness are felt in the lumbar region, but-tocks, and SI region. Fatigue, fever, and weight loss may occur. Decreased lum-bar spinal motion is an early sign with the normal lumbar lordosis straight-ened, diminished anterior flexion, and spinal rotation and lateral bending impaired. Slowly, the process ascends the lumbar and thoracic spine, the cervical region may be involved late. Episodes of acute or subacute arthritis may involve hip, knee, shoulder, sternoclavicular, or manubriosternal joints. Tenderness is found over the involved joints. *Iridocyclitis* occurs in one-fifth of the cases. *Aortic regurgitation* is a late complication in 3% of patients. Idiopathic ankylosing spondylitis needs to be distinguished from psoriatic arthritis and reactive spondyloarthritis (Crohn disease, ulcerative colitis, Reiter disease), Whipple disease, and diffuse idiopathic spinal hyperostosis (DISH).

Reactive Arthritis (Reiter Syndrome): Following infection of the urethra (chlamydia) or gut (Shigella, Salmonella, Yersinia, Campylobacter) an oligoarthritis, predominately of the lower extremities, develops. It may be accompanied by enthesitis of the hands, ankles, and feet, conjunctivitis, ure-thritis, and rash on the glans penis (*circinate balanitis*) and feet (*keratoderma blenorrhagica*). Sacroiliitis and spine involvement may occur. 85% of patients are HLA-B27-positive.

Enteropathic Arthritis: Inflammatory asymmetric arthritis predominately of the ankles and knees may occur in association with inflammatory bowel disease (ulcerative colitis and Crohn disease). Enthesitis is common, especially at the Achilles tendon insertion, and symmetrical SI and spinal involvement occurs. The arthritis may precede clinical manifestations of the inflammatory bowel disease.

Psoriatic Arthritis: The joint disease is usually an asymmetrical oligo- or pol-yarthritis of small and large joints. It is occasionally a symmetrical polyarthri-tis resembling RA. Destructive arthritis of the DIP joints is seen in psoriatic arthritis but not in RA. Spondylitis and sacroiliitis occur in up to 25% of patients with psoriatic arthritis, especially those with HLA-B27. Enthesitis may predominate in some patients. The arthritis may precede, accompany, or follow onset of the skin rash. Physical examination should include a careful skin examination, especially of the scalp (the rash may be hidden by hair or dismissed as seborrhea) and fingernails (looking for pits and onycholysis).

Diffuse Idiopathic Skeletal Hyperostosis (DISH): Asymmetric osteophytes de-velop at multiple levels of the spine leading to bridging of multiple interver-tebral spaces and irregular ankylosis with decreased spinal motion, especially in the cervical and lumbar regions. The disk spaces are preserved. Women are affected more often than men.

Rigid Spine Syndrome: The clinical syndrome of rigid spine, proximal muscle weakness, scoliosis and joint contractures can have several different etiologies. The combination of restrictive chest disease and muscle weakness can lead to respiratory failure [Janssen WJ, Collard HR, et al. A perfect storm. *N Engl J Med.* 2005;353:1956–1961].

> **KEY SIGN** Infectious Spondylitis

Spinal infection most commonly starts in the disks (*diskitis*) and anterior end-plates of the vertebrae leading to vertebral erosion and collapse. Infection may extend anteriorly into the psoas or posteriorly into the epidural space leading to spinal cord compression. Pain and tenderness of the spinous vertebral processes are usually present over the site of infection, often with spasm of the sacrospinalis. The pain may be referred along a spinal nerve to be mistaken for appendicitis, pleurisy, or sciatica, if the back is not examined. Collapse of the vertebral body causes a gibbus and paraplegia may result. Psoas abscess, classic in tuberculosis, may form along the sheath of the psoas and point beneath the inguinal ligament. Pain in the spine may be localized by the heel-drop test: have the patient rise onto tiptoes, and then drop onto the heels; pain will be elicited at the site of infection. Infections with pyogenic organisms (*S. aureus*) are most common. Tuberculosis, Salmonella, brucellosis, fungi, and actinomycosis are less common.

Tuberculosis of the Spine (Pott Disease): Patients present with fever, night sweats, and back pain, and may develop signs of spinal cord compression with epidural extension. Rarely, cold abscess present as an inguinal mass from prevertebral extension.

➤ **KEY SYNDROME** Epidural Spinal Cord Compression

Masses in the closed epidural space may erode bone, compress spinal nerves, and compress the spinal cord. Most epidural masses extend from the adjacent vertebrae or from retroperitoneal malignancy to press on the anterior or anterolateral cord. Progressive axial, radicular, or referred back pain, unrelieved by recumbency, should prompt an immediate search for spinal cord compression. Pain is the most common presenting symptom followed by leg weakness, constipation, incontinence, and sensory disturbances. The latter indicate advancing cord compression, from which there is less chance for complete recovery. Paraplegia may occur in a matter of hours after the onset of neurologic signs. The pain may occur at any level and is increased by straight-leg raising, Valsalva maneuver, neck flexion, and movement. MRI of the entire vertebral column and cord is the most sensitive and specific test. ***CLINICAL OCCURRENCE:*** Breast, prostate, or lung cancer are the most frequent causes. Other cancers in adults include multiple myeloma, malignant lymphoma, renal carcinoma, sarcoma, and melanoma. In children, consider lymphoma, sarcoma, and neuroblastoma. Epidural abcess complicates infectious spondylitis.

KEY SYNDROME Lumbosacral Strain

Mechanical injury commonly occurs to the soft tissues (muscles, tendons, and ligaments) of the low back where the mobile lumbar spine meets the fixed sacrum, concentrating mechanical forces at the transition zone. Injury can be the result of a single, large loading force or of a repetitive loading with lesser forces. Usually the patient complains of aching pain near L5 and S1. The pain may radiate laterally or to the lateral aspect of the thigh. There is an increased lumbar lordosis and attempted spinal motion is accompanied by muscle spasm. Spinal flexion is limited and painful. The patient cannot lie flat without flexing the knees and hips to relieve pain. The straight-leg-raising test is negative except that lumbosacral pain occurs at extreme flexion. Have the patient lie prone with the pelvis resting on four pillows to separate the spinous processes. In this position, palpation of the spines and supraspinous ligament may reveal tenderness above or below the spine of L5; sometimes a depression is found indicating spondylolisthesis.

KEY SYNDROME   Sciatica

Compression or direct injury to the sciatic nerve produces pain, altered sensation (dermatomes L4-S3), loss of muscle reflexes (ankle jerk), and, if severe, muscle power and in the distribution of the nerve (e.g., ankle flexion, extension, inversion and eversion, great toe extension). Sciatica is pain in the distribution of the sciatic nerve. Pain is initially felt in the buttock and posterior thigh, and may extend to involve the posterolateral aspect of the leg to the lateral malleolus, the lateral dorsum of the foot and the entire sole. When nerve function is compromised, paresthesias are felt in the same distribution. Pain and paresthesias are intensified by coughing or straining. The nerve trunk is tender when palpated at the sciatic notch or stretched when the leg is extended while the thigh is flexed (*Lasègue sign* or straight-leg raising). Rectal examination should always be done to look for pelvic masses. A pulsating rectal mass associated with sciatica suggests aneurysm of the internal iliac or common iliac artery. Most cases are caused by herniated intervertebral disk.

KEY SYNDROME   Herniated Intervertebral Disk

Herniation of a desiccated nucleus pulposus through tears in the annulus fibrosa produces pressure on nerve roots in the neural foramina laterally or directly on the cauda equina, conus or spinal cord if the extrusion is directly posterior (see Fig. 13–27B, page 633). The onset of pain may be gradual or sudden and is partially relieved in recumbency. Sciatica may be the presenting symptom with pain in the buttock radiating to the thigh. In severe cases, the pain involves the leg, usually the lateral aspect, and some or all of the toes (dermatomes L4 to S3). Coughing, sneezing, or the Valsalva maneuver accentuates the pain. Chronic herniated disk is attended by symptom-free periods; continuous back pain is usually caused by some other lesion. On examination, the spine may be flexed, frequently with a lateral deviation toward the affected side. Active flexion and extension of the spine are limited, more so than lateral bending and rotation. Muscle spasm is most severe over the ipsilateral sacrospinalis with rigidity and tenderness, most pronounced on the affected side 5 cm lateral to the midline. Palpate for muscle rigidity, and other areas of tenderness including fibrositis tender points and trigger points. Have the patient heel-and-toe walk and extend the great toe against resistance. Pain with the straight leg test often occurs at less than 40 degrees with a prolapsed disk; when pain occurs only at much greater angles, there may be another cause. If the straight-leg-raising test is positive, repeat it and as the painful angle is approached, dorsiflex the foot sharply stretching the sciatic nerve to test its irritability. Check sensation noting the dermatome involved [Vroomen PC, de Krom MC, Knottnerus JA. Diagnostic value of history and physical examination in patients suspected of sciatica due to disc herniation. *J Neurol.* 1999;246:899–906; Vroomen PC, de Krom MC, Knottnerus JA. Consistency of history taking and physical examination in patients with suspected lumbar nerve root involvement. *Spine.* 2000;25:91–96].

KEY SYNDROME   Spinal Stenosis

Compression of the lower lumbar and sacral roots occurs from overgrowth of bony tissue from congenital narrowing or degenerative disk disease that narrows the spinal canal. *Pseudoclaudication* is pain in the buttocks, bilateral posterior thighs, and calves while standing or walking upright, that is relieved by sitting or bending forward (reversing the lumbar lordosis and decreasing the degree of stenosis). **DDX:** Unlike intermittent claudication from vascular insufficiency, pain occurs while standing without walking. Sitting gives relief, in contrast to lumbar disk disease. Osteoporosis, spondylolisthesis, trauma, laminectomy, spinal fusion, spondylosis, scoliosis, acromegaly, and Paget disease are all potential contributors. Congenital narrowing of the canal also occurs.

Appendicular Skeletal Syndromes (Including Joints, Tendons, Ligaments, and Soft Tissues)

KEY SYNDROME   Hypertrophic Osteoarthropathy (HOA)

This is a periostitis of unknown cause with: (1) clubbing of the fingers, (2) new subperiosteal bone in the long bones, (3) swelling and pains in the joints, and (4) autonomic disturbances of the hands and feet, such as flushing, sweating, and blanching. The earliest sign is finger clubbing (see page 636). With progression, bone pain occurs while swelling and pain in the joints may become severe and tenderness is elicited by palpation over the distal forearms and legs. In advanced cases, sweating and flushing of the hands and feet may alternate with the Raynaud phenomenon. The condition may be congenital, with signs appearing in childhood, or acquired. Primary hereditary HOA (*Marie-Bamberger syndrome*) is an autosomal dominant syndrome, which is expressed much more commonly in males. It has clubbing, greasy thickening of the skin, especially noticeable on the face, and hyperhidrosis of the hands and feet. Acquired HOA results from systemic disease.

HOA—CLINICAL OCCURRENCE: *Congenital* familial, cyanotic congenital heart disease, cystic fibrosis; *Endocrine* Grave disease, pregnancy; *Idiopathic* emphysema, cirrhosis; *Inflammatory/Immune* ulcerative colitis, Crohn disease, chronic interstitial pneumonitis, sarcoidosis, dysproteinemia; *Infectious* lung or liver abscess, bronchiectasis, tuberculosis, bacterial endocarditis, dysentery; *Metabolic/Toxic* malabsorption, chronic hypoxemia; *Neoplastic* lung, pleural, and gastrointestinal cancer, metastatic disease to lung; *Vascular* aortic aneurysm.

KEY SYNDROME   Chronic Painless Enlargement of the Legs

Several causes must be distinguished. **Adiposity.** Although some evidence of obesity is present elsewhere in the body, the fat about the ankles may be disproportionately great, while the feet are spared. The tissue has the consistency of fat, and pitting edema is absent. **Chronic deep venous obstruction** usually is preceded by a history suggesting thrombophlebitis. The venous deficit may produce pain in the legs. Some pitting edema is usually present, although it may be obscured by thickening of the skin from chronic inflammation (*dermatoliposclerosis*). The skin is stained with hemosiderin and may be cyanotic. Superficial veins may be dilated. **Postphlebitic syndrome** results from previous occlusion of the deep veins either without recanalization or resulting in destruction of the valves with persistent venous incompetence. One-third of patients with acute deep vein thrombosis will develop postphlebitic syndrome (page 434). The leg is persistently enlarged, usually with pitting edema. Sensations of fullness and pain occur with prolonged sitting or standing and chronic stasis changes are common. Early treatment decreases long-term disability. **Varicose veins** are readily recognized when they are associated with edema. Chronic edema from any cause leads to subcutaneous and cutaneous fibrosis with woody induration that does not pit. **Lymphedema** causes a firm, nonpitting swelling with no venous engorgement or cyanosis.

Muscle Syndromes

See also Chapter 14, *The Neurologic Examination*.

> **KEY SYNDROME**   **Fibromyalgia**

See *Tender Points*, page 673. Fibromyalgia is more common in women than men. It is characterized by widespread, diffuse, aching musculoskeletal pain, stiffness, nonrestorative sleep, and fatigue. Although the cause and pathogenesis are unknown, it has been associated with antecedent trauma, surgery, medical illness, and emotional stress. The diagnosis is based upon clinical criteria; laboratory studies are normal. The American College of Rheumatology criteria for diagnosis include a history of pain in all four body quadrants for at least 3 months with at least 11 of 18 paired, bilateral tender points elicited on physical examination: suboccipital muscle insertion, low cervical, trapezius, supraspinatus, second rib, lateral epicondyle, gluteal, greater trochanter, and knee (Fig. 13–48).

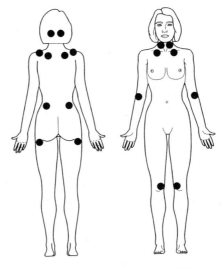

Tender points of fibromyalgia
in at least 11 of 18 sites

Fig. 13–48 *The Tender Points of Fibromyalgia.* There should be tenderness in at least 11 of the 18 points to diagnose fibromyalgia.

KEY SYNDROME   Myofascial Pain Syndrome

Afferent signals from the trigger areas are believed to remodel spinal and possibly thalamic pain pathways to cause reflex muscle spasm and diminished blood flow, which, in turn, increase the sensitivity of the trigger area. See *Trigger Points*, page 672. Chronic recurrent pain occurs roughly in the distribution of one or more muscles and their distribution of referred pain. The pain may be lancinating, aching, boring, or a feeling of muscular stiffness. Often, the patient relates the onset to some specific trauma or activity. The distinguishing feature is the presence of one or more trigger points, with or without palpable muscle spasm. The examiner should palpate the entire region carefully with firm pressure of the fingertips. Often, the trigger point is discovered some distance from the referred pain area. The diagnosis is confirmed when the pain is relieved by injection of the primary trigger point with a local anesthetic.

KEY SYNDROME   Polymyalgia Rheumatica

This inflammatory disease of unknown origin is characterized by pain in proximal muscle groups, with inflammation demonstrable by MRI in the shoulder girdle tendon sheaths and bursae, and less commonly the shoulder joint itself. It usually occurs after the sixth decade and is most common in women. Pronounced morning stiffness of the neck, shoulder, and upper back muscles usually begins gradually. Some patients have sudden onset and can note the day and time of their first symptoms. Muscles of the low back, pelvic girdle and thighs are less prominently involved and/or may develop later. It is common in patients with temporal arteritis, but only 15% of patients presenting with PMR develop temporal arteritis. Although spontaneously painful, the muscles are seldom very tender, trigger points are not characteristic, and the stiffness is improved by activity. The erythrocyte sedimentation rate is usually >80 and symptoms are promptly relieved by low-dose corticosteroids.

► KEY SYNDROME   Compartment Syndrome

Edema, hemorrhage and inflammation from injury to muscle enclosed within a constricting fascial compartment leads to increasing pressure within the compartment, ischemia and further injury. A high index of suspicion is required to recognize this serious disorder before irreversible muscle injury occurs. The patient complains of severe pain often disproportionate to apparent injury. Palpation of the affected compartment reveals tense distention of the fascia with severe pain. If major arteries or nerves pass through the compartment, distal pulses may be diminished and sensation impaired. Without relief of pressure, muscle necrosis leads to fibrosis, shortening, and loss of function. Diagnosis is made by measuring compartment pressure; treatment is surgical fasciotomy.

ADDITIONAL READING

1. Mense S, Simons DG. *Muscle Pain.* Philadelphia, PA: Lippincott Williams & Wilkins; 2001.

2. Sheon RP, Moskowitz RW, Goldberg VM. *Soft Tissue Rheumatic Pain. Recognition, Management and Prevention.* 3rd ed. Baltimore, MD: William & Wilkins; 1996.

3. Letha Yurko Griffin. *Essentials of Musculoskeletal Care*, 3rd ed. Rosemont, IL: American Academy of Orthopedic Surgeons; 2005.

4. Klippel JH, Stone JH, Crofford LeJ, White PH, eds. *Primer of the Rheumatic Diseases*. 13th edition corrected. Atlanta, GA: The Arthritis Foundation; 2001.

5. Travell JG, Simons DG. *Myofascial Pain and Dysfunction. The Trigger Point Manual*, 2nd edition, Baltimore, MD: Williams & Wilkins; 1999.

CHAPTER 14

The Neurologic Examination

The diagnostic examination of the nervous system requires testing of its specific functional components, in addition to the traditional physical examination modalities of inspection and palpation.

Many nervous system components are evaluated while taking the history and examining the body by regions. The patient's speech and behavior reflect cerebral function. When examining the head, some, if not all, of the cranial nerves (CN) are tested. Muscle mass and strength are assessed by inspection and observation of gait and movement. Tendon reflexes are elicited during examination of the extremities. When evidence of nervous system malfunction is encountered, a complete, systematic neurologic examination is required.

The first objective of the systematic neurologic examination is to identify all cognitive, sensory, motor, and coordination deficits. From this inventory, the site(s) and mechanism(s) of injury can by hypothesized using the following general principles:

1. *Deficits of intellect, memory, or higher brain function* imply lesions of the cerebral hemispheres.

2. *Deficits of consciousness* indicate lesions of the brainstem reticular activating system or bilateral cerebral damage.

3. *Paralysis with loss of deep tendon reflexes* indicates a lower motor neuron (LMN) lesion interrupting the reflex arc. This can be at the spinal cord, spinal root, plexus or peripheral nerve level. Acute upper motor neuron (UMN) lesions can be associated with decreased reflexes initially, but produce increased reflexes after hours to days.

4. *Paralysis with an accentuated deep tendon reflexes* (spasticity) indicates an UMN lesion. This may reflect disease of the hemisphere, brainstem, or spinal cord.

5. *Unilateral loss of touch and position sensation and contralateral loss of temperature and pain sensation* indicate a unilateral lesion of the spinal cord ipsilateral to the loss of touch and position. This happens because the ascending tracts for touch and position sensation decussate in the medulla, while the ascending tracts for pain and temperature sensation cross near where they enter the spinal cord.

6. *Paralysis is contralateral to lesions above the medulla and ipsilateral below.* This is because the descending motor tracts, like the tracts for discriminative sense, decussate in the medulla.

7. *An LMN paralysis accompanied by anesthesia in an appropriate distribution usually indicates a peripheral nerve lesion,* because many nerves carry both

motor and sensory fibers. Sometimes spinal root or segmental cord lesions cause similar signs.

8. *Muscle wasting with fasciculation results from an LMN lesion;* without fasciculation, wasting is often attributable to intrinsic muscle disease.

Overview of the Nervous System

Interpretation of the neurologic examination requires a comprehensive understanding of the anatomy and functional organization of the nervous system. A complete description of the anatomy and the functional components of the nervous system is beyond the scope of this book. The reader should consult anatomy and neurology texts for detailed discussions of neuroanatomy and functional physiology.

Anatomic Organization

For diagnostic purposes, the nervous system is divided anatomically into the brain, the spinal cord and the peripheral nerves.

The central nervous system (CNS).   The **brain** consists of the cerebrum, the brainstem, and the cerebellum. The *cerebrum* performs cognitive functions, is the site of emotion and mood formation and determines personality and behavior. The deep cerebral structures modulate motor and sensory function and control endocrine and appetitive functions. The *brainstem* consists of the midbrain, the pons and the medulla and contains nuclei of CN III to CN XII. The *cerebellum* is involved in many motor and sensory pathways and controls the coordination of complex motor activities.

   The **spinal cord** contains the ascending sensory tracts, the descending motor and autonomic tracts and the LMN which activate skeletal muscles. The dorsal and ventral *spinal roots* contain the sensory and motor tracts, respectively. The *dorsal root ganglia* contain the cell bodies of afferent sensory nerves.

The peripheral nervous system.   The **peripheral nervous system** is equally complex. Cranial and spinal nerves come together to form *ganglia* and *plexuses* (brachial, lumbar, sacral) where the sensory and motor components of the cranial and spinal segments are redistributed into peripheral nerves directed to specific anatomic areas of the periphery.

Functional Organization of the Nervous System

It is also necessary to have an understanding of the functional organization of the nervous system. Function can be systematically described as follows: *cognition* (intellect, language, registration, memory, attention, orientation, spatial discrimination); *mood and affect; special sensory* (sight, hearing, balance, taste, smell); *somatic and visceral sensation* (touch, position, pain, temperature, vibration, pressure, two-point discrimination); *motor function* (pyramidal tracts and extrapyramidal system); *posture, balance, and coordination* (cerebellar, vestibular, and basal ganglia function); and *autonomic function*. The autonomic nervous system is divided into the *parasympathetic* and *sympathetic* systems. The parasympathetic outflow is from the cranial, cervical, and sacral roots, with ganglia close to the organs they innervate. The sympathetic outflow is from the thoracic and lumbar roots via the sympathetic spinal ganglia.

Superficial Anatomy of the Nervous System

The brain is encased within the rigid skull and the spinal cord within the spinal canal of the vertebral column. The segmental organization of the nervous system is most evident in the chest and abdomen, much less so in the head and extremities. The ganglia, plexuses, and nerve trunks are inaccessible to physical examination lying deep to the muscles and bones of the spine, chest, abdomen, and pelvis. The peripheral nerves, however, are distributed in the neurovascular bundles, along with their corresponding arteries and veins, and may be accessible to palpation where they exit the trunk and in the extremities.

The Neurologic Examination

MENTAL STATUS SCREENING EXAMINATION: See chapter 15, page 767 for a *complete discussion.*

During the history and physical examination, the clinician is evaluating the patient's mental status. In addition, screening tests like the Mini-Mental State Examination (MMSE) and the Mini-Cog can be used. These are described in Chapter 15, page 777ff. The components of the mental status examination of most interest for neurologic disease are the level of consciousness, memory and language.

Cranial Nerve Examination

The 12 pairs of CN emerge from the brain and pass through foramina in the base of the skull. They are designated by Roman numerals I to XII in relation to their position from forebrain to brainstem. The physical examination of several of the CN is contained in the discussion of the head and neck in Chapter 7.

Olfactory Nerve (CN I)

The olfactory mucosa lining the upper third of the nasal septum and the superior nasal concha contains the receptors and ganglion cells. Their fibers converge into approximately 20 branches that pierce the cribriform plate of the ethmoid bone and consolidate to form the olfactory tract.

Testing smell. Evaluate the nasal passages for patency. With the eyes closed, test each nostril while the other is occluded, with familiar odors, such as coffee, cloves, or peppermint. Noxious chemicals such as ammonia or alcohol should not be used since they stimulate nociceptors from the trigeminal nerve giving a false positive response.

Optic Nerve (CN II)

The examinations of the retina, vision and function of the optic nerve, chiasm, and tract are discussed in Chapter 7, pages 198ff.

Oculomotor Nerve (CN III)

This is the motor nerve to five extrinsic eye muscles: the levator palpebrae superioris, medial rectus, superior rectus, inferior rectus, and inferior oblique. Its nucleus lies in the posterior midbrain, subdivided into a part for each muscle.

Testing for oculomotor paralysis. See Chapter 7, page 198.

Trochlear Nerve (CN IV)

CN IV innervates the superior oblique muscle.

Testing for trochlear paralysis. See Chapter 7, page 198.

Trigeminal Nerve (CN V)

CN V is the largest CN; it has three divisions. Its sensory root supplies the superficial and deep structures of the face and the deep structures of the head; its motor root innervates the muscles of mastication. The *first division, or ophthalmic branch (CN V1)*, contains sensory fibers from the cornea, ciliary body, conjunctiva, nasal cavity and sinuses, and skin of the eyebrows, forehead, and nose. The *second division, or maxillary branch (CN V2)*, contains sensory fibers from the skin on the side of the nose, the upper and lower eyelids, the palate, and maxillary gums. The *third division, or mandibular branch (CN V3)* is a mixed nerve with sensory and motor nerves: its sensory fibers are from the temporal region, the external ears, lower lip, lower face, mucosa of anterior two-thirds of the tongue, mandibular gums, and teeth; the motor root supplies the muscles of mastication: masseter, temporalis, and internal and external pterygoid.

Testing the trigeminal nerve. *Motor Division:* Inspect for muscle wasting in the temporal region, jaw tremor and trismus (spasm of the masticatory muscles). Palpate the temporal and masseter muscles comparing the muscle bulk and tension on the two sides while the patient clenches the teeth (Fig. 14–1A). If there is malalignment of the incisors when the mouth is opened, paralysis of the pterygoid muscle on the weak side is indicated. *Sensory Division:* With the eyes closed, test light touch, pain and temperature in each division comparing the two sides (Fig. 14–1B). The *jaw jerk* tests both the motor and sensory components of the trigeminal nerve. Test the *corneal reflex* by having the patient look upward while you gently touch the cornea (not the sclera) with a small shred of sterile gauze; this normally induces blinking. The corneal reflex is a bilateral reflex testing the fifth and seventh CN on the side stimulated and the seventh consensually.

Abducens Nerve (Cranial VI)

The abducens is the motor nerve to the lateral rectus.

Testing for abducens paralysis. See Chapter 7, page 198.

Facial Nerve (CN VII)

The facial nerve contains motor, autonomic, and sensory fibers. It supplies motor fibers to the muscles of the scalp, face, and auricula as well as to the buccinator, platysma, stapedius, stylohyoideus, and the posterior belly of the digastricus. Autonomic motor fibers in the *chorda tympani* nerve, a branch of CN VII, supply the submandibular and sublingual salivary glands. CN VII carries sensation from

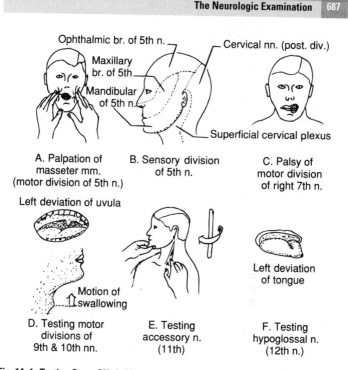

A. Palpation of masseter mm. (motor division of 5th n.)

B. Sensory division of 5th n.

C. Palsy of motor division of right 7th n.

D. Testing motor divisions of 9th & 10th nn.

E. Testing accessory n. (11th)

F. Testing hypoglossal n. (12th n.)

Fig. 14–1 *Testing Some CN. **A. Motor division of the fifth (trigeminal) nerve:** See text.* ***B. Sensory division of the fifth (trigeminal):*** *The three branches of the sensory trigeminal are ophthalmic, maxillary, and mandibular, as indicated by the areas.* ***C. Motor division of the seventh (facial):*** *When the patient opens the mouth to show clenched teeth, only the unparalyzed side of the face retracts; the cheek muscles form creases on the normal side; the eyelid fissures are increased. The paralyzed side remains smooth with eyelid open.* ***D. Motor division of the ninth (glossopharyngeal) and tenth (vagus) nerves:*** *When the patient opens the mouth and says "ah," the uvula deviates toward the strong side. Upon swallowing, the larynx normally elevates, as indicated by the motion of the thyroid cartilage in the neck (Adam's apple); it does not rise in bilateral paralysis.* ***E. The accessory (eleventh nerve):*** *The patient is asked to rotate the head toward the midline against the resistance of the examiner's hand while the other hand palpates the tension in the sternocleidomastoid muscle. The trapezius can likewise be tested for paralysis.* ***F. The twelfth (hypoglossal) nerve:*** *The protruding tongue deviates to the paralyzed side; muscle atrophy may also be present.*

the ear canal and behind the ear as well as from the taste organs on the anterior two-thirds of the tongue.

Testing the facial nerve. *Motor:* Inspect the face in repose for paralysis or spasm. Have the patient perform the tasks below to demonstrate asymmetry indicating unilateral paralysis and to determine whether the cause is an LMN or an UMN lesion: (1) inspect the face in repose noting the palpebral fissures, nasolabial folds and corners of the mouth; (2) elevate the eyebrows and wrinkle the forehead or have them look up and inspect the forehead wrinkles; (3) frown; (4) tightly close the eyes; (5) show the teeth; (6) whistle and puff the cheeks; and (7) smile. *Sensory:* Test taste on the anterior two-thirds of the tongue with sugar, vinegar (dilute acetic acid), quinine, and table salt. Write the words sweet, sour, bitter, and salty on a piece of paper and have the patient identify the sensation. Holding the tongue in gauze, touch the anterior two-thirds successively on one side then the other with an applicator saturated with the test substance. Remember, sweet receptors are located on the tip of the tongue. Get the patient's response before testing the other side. Have the patient rinse the mouth with water between tests.

Acoustic Nerve (CN VIII)

The eighth nerve is a relatively short trunk consisting of the *cochlear* and *vestibular sensory nerves.* They are morphologically and functionally distinct. The cochlear nerve supplies the *organ of Corti,* while the vestibular nerve furnishes sensory endings for the semicircular ducts.

Testing the acoustic nerve. *Cochlear Portion:* The tests for hearing are described in Chapter 7 on pages 196. *Vestibular Portion:* Note spontaneous nystagmus; use the labyrinthine tests described in Chapter 7 on pages 197.

Glossopharyngeal Nerve (CN IX)

CN IX contains sensory, motor, and autonomic fibers. It contains sensory nerves for pain, touch, and temperature from the mucosa of the pharynx, fauces, and palatine tonsil; in addition, it is the nerve of taste for the posterior third of the tongue. Somatic motor fibers travel through both the glossopharyngeal and vagus to innervate the muscles of the pharynx.

Testing the glossopharyngeal nerve. This is tested with the vagus nerve.

Vagus Nerve (CN X)

Most extensive of the CN, the vagus carries motor, sensory, and autonomic fibers to and from the neck, thorax, and abdomen. It exits the skull in the jugular fossa. Its cervical branches are the pharyngeal, superior laryngeal, recurrent laryngeal, and superior cardiac nerves. The thoracic branches are the inferior cardiac, anterior and posterior bronchials, and esophageal nerves. In the abdomen, its major branches are the gastric and hepatic nerves and the celiac and superior mesenteric ganglia.

Testing of the glossopharyngeal and vagus nerves. Listen for voice quality and normal variation of tones. *Pharynx:* While inspecting the pharynx, have the patient say "ah," noting elevation of the uvula. Note whether the faucial pillars converge equally. Test the gag reflex by touching the back of the tongue with a tongue blade. Test the pharyngeal mucosa for areas of anesthesia by touching with an applicator. *Larynx:* Watch the laryngeal contours in the neck to ascertain if they rise with swallowing (Fig. 14–1D). Have the patient swallow water observing for coughing or reflux into the posterior nose. Examination of the vocal cords is described in Chapter 7 on page 209.

Accessory Nerve (CN XI)

The accessory nerve is the motor nerve to the trapezius and sternocleidomastoid.

Testing of the accessory nerve. Palpate the upper borders of the trapezii while the patient raises his shoulders against the resistance of your hands. Look for scapular "winging" as the patient leans against a wall with palms and arms extended. Test the sternocleidomastoid by having the patient turn his head to one side and attempt to bring his chin back to the midline against the resistance of your hand (Fig. 14–1E). Note the strength of rotation and the prominence of the tensed muscles in the neck.

Hypoglossal Nerve (CN XII)

The hypoglossal is the motor nerve to the tongue.

Testing of the hypoglossal nerve. First, inspect the tongue while it is at rest in the floor of the mouth for wasting and fasciculations; the contracting muscles of the protruded tongue may normally fasciculate. When one side is paralyzed, the protruded tongue deviates toward the weak side (Fig. 14–1F). Occasionally, deviation of the tongue results from an UMN lesion. Test muscle strength by having the patient push the tongue against the cheek while your hand resists from the outside. Test lingual speech by having the patient repeat "La, La, La" (linguals; see Chapter 7, page 209 for K, L, M test).

Motor Examination

Normal motor function requires that the skeleton, muscles and motor nerves (pyramidal and extrapyramidal) are intact. Assessment of muscle movements requires motion at the joints; hence, orthopedic, rheumatologic, and neurologic examinations are interdependent.

Inspect for Muscle Wasting

Compare the muscle masses side to side and the relative masses in different regions.

Evaluate Muscle Tone

Ask the patient to relax, then assess muscle tone by resistance to passive range of motion. When the patient has difficulty relaxing, test tone when their attention is diverted. Gently rocking or lifting a limb and letting it fall reveals the tone. When the patient sits on the end of the examination table, the freedom with which the dangling legs swing indicates their tone.

Test Muscle Strength

Have the patient actively move the joint through its range of motion. Then, have the patient attempt to move against your resistance while you palpate the contracting muscle (Fig. 14–2). If the patient cannot move the limb against gravity, position the limb so the patient can move it unaffected by gravity. An arbitrary scale is used for grading muscle strength.

Grading of Muscle Strength (Oxford Scale)

Grade 0   No muscle movement
Grade 1   Muscle movement without joint motion
Grade 2   Moves with gravity eliminated

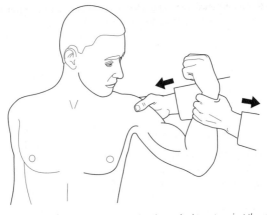

Fig. 14–2 *Testing Muscle Strength.* The patient is required to act against the resistance of the examiner.

Grade 3   Moves against gravity but not resistance

Grade 4   Moves against gravity and light resistance

Grade 5   Normal strength

Lower extremity muscle strength will usually exceed arm strength in the examiner, so mild degrees of leg weakness are easily missed with resisted motion. Therefore, the following tests are useful. (1) Watch the patient get up after sitting on the floor. Use of both arms or raising the buttocks first by working the hands on the floor toward the feet and then up the legs, indicates proximal muscle weakness (*Gowers sign*). (2) Ask the sitting patient to stand without using their arms for assistance; if they do this easily, see if it can be done one leg at a time using the hands for balance only. (3) Have the patient hop on the balls of the feet, then on each foot individually. Normally, the heel will not strike the ground. Having the patient hop on a piece of paper will accentuate the sound of the heel strike (creating a "gallop" rhythm), indicating gastrocnemius and soleus muscle weakness.

Examination of Reflexes

In the screening examination, the clinician usually tests a few reflex arcs, representative of various levels in the cord and brainstem. A normal reflex confirms the integrity of each element in the reflex arc and proper function of the descending motor tracts. When an abnormality is encountered, lesions can be localized by mapping the normal and abnormal reflexes to their known spinal cord and brainstem levels.

Brainstem Reflexes

These are tested during CN examination. The CN innervation of the afferent and efferent limbs are shown in parentheses.

Direct pupillary reaction to light.   The iris constricts when bright light is shone upon the retina (afferent CN II; efferent ipsilateral CN III).

Consensual pupillary reaction to light. Light stimulation of one retina produces constriction of the contralateral pupil (afferent CN II; efferent contralateral CN III).

Ciliospinal reflex. Pinching the skin on the back of the neck causes pupillary dilatation (afferent cervical somatic nerves; efferent-cervical sympathetic chain).

Corneal reflex. Touching the cornea causes blinking of the eyelids (afferent CN V; efferent CN VII).

Jaw reflex. When the mouth is partially opened and the muscles relaxed, tapping the chin causes the jaw to close. The reflex center is in the mid-pons (afferent CN V; efferent CN V).

Gag reflex. Gagging occurs when the pharynx is stroked. The reflex center is in the medulla (afferent CN IX, -X; efferent CN IX, -X).

The Muscle Stretch Reflexes

Muscle stretch reflexes are often misnamed "tendon" reflexes. The muscle is stretched by a brisk tap on its taut tendon of insertion. The muscle stretch reflex is a simple reflex arc containing a muscle cell, a sensory, and a motor neuron (Fig. 14–3). The muscle spindle is innervated by the dendrite of a sensory neuron whose cell body is in the dorsal root ganglion and whose axon enters the spinal cord where it synapses with the axon and the dendrite of the LMN in the anterior horn. The efferent limb of the arc consists of the LMN, the muscle synapse, and the muscle fibers of the motor unit. The reflex arc is broken if any one of its elements malfunctions. The physical sign of an interrupted reflex arc is a diminished or absent reflex. When the descending motor pathway (the pyramidal tract) in the spinal cord is injured above the level of the reflex arc, normal cortical inhibition is lost, producing a hyperactive or spastic reflex.

General principles for eliciting muscle stretch reflexes. The limb should be relaxed. Identify the tendon of the muscle to be tested. Position the limb so that the muscle is slightly stretched. Strike a brisk blow on the tendon with the finger or reflex hammer; if the tendon cannot be struck directly, place your thumb on the tendon and strike your thumb. If no reflex is present, a heavier hammer can be tried. If there is still no reflex, reinforcement can be used: have the patient concentrate on a voluntary act such as pulling on interlocked fingers or clenching the fists while you test the reflex.

There is considerable variability in normal reflexes, from absent to brisk. Significant asymmetry between right and left at the same level is abnormal. Clonus,

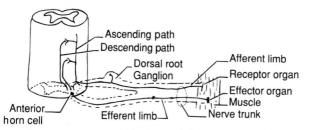

Fig. 14–3 *Components of a Spinal Reflex Arc.*

the sustained repetitive maintenance of the reflex arc with tonic stretch of the muscle is always abnormal. A four-point scale, denoted by numbers or pluses, is commonly used to grade the reflex response.

0, 0	No response
1, +	Detectable only with reenforcement
2, + +	Easily detectable
3, + + +	Brisk with at most a few beats of clonus
4, + + + +	Sustained clonus

The reflexes below are listed by descending level of the reflex center in the spinal cord. The peripheral nerves carrying the afferent and efferent signal are listed in parentheses.

Reflex center at C5 to T1—pectoralis reflex (medial and lateral anterior thoracic nerves). Support the arm in 10 degrees of elevation at 90 degrees of abduction (Fig. 14–4A). Place the fingers of your left hand on the patient's shoulder with your thumb extended downward pressing firmly on the tendon of the pectoralis major. Strike a blow directed upward toward the axilla. The muscle contraction can be seen or felt.

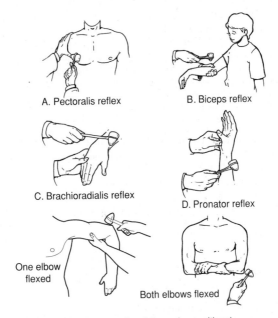

A. Pectoralis reflex

B. Biceps reflex

C. Brachioradialis reflex

D. Pronator reflex

One elbow flexed

Both elbows flexed

E. Triceps reflex (alternative positions)

Fig. 14–4 Deep Reflexes I. A. Pectoralis reflex. B. Biceps brachii reflex. C. Brachioradialis reflex. D. Pronator reflex. E. Triceps brachii reflex: There are two alternative positions: Hold the patient's arm at 90 degrees abduction, allowing the relaxed forearm to dangle with the elbow at flexion, or have the patient fold the arms and grasp the forearms with the hands (reinforcement can be obtained by having the patient tighten the grasp on the arms).

Reflex center at C5 to C6: biceps reflex (musculocutaneous nerve). Place the elbow at 90 degrees of flexion with the arm slightly pronated. Grasp the elbow with your left hand so that the fingers are behind and your thumb presses the biceps tendon (Fig. 14–4B). Strike a series of blows on your thumb varying your thumb pressure with each blow until the most satisfactory response is obtained. The normal reflex is elbow flexion.

Reflex center at C5 to C6: brachioradialis reflex (radial nerve). Hold the patient's wrist with your left hand with the forearm relaxed in pronation (Fig. 14–4C). With a vertical stroke, tap the forearm directly, just above the radial styloid process. The normal response is elbow flexion and forearm supination.

Reflex center at C6 to C7: pronator reflex (median nerve). Hold the patient's hand vertically so the wrist is suspended (Fig. 14–4D). From the medial side, strike the distal end of the radius directly with a horizontal blow. The normal response is pronation of the forearm. An alternate method is to strike the distal end of the ulna directly with a blow mediad.

Reflex center at C7 to C8: triceps reflex (radial nerve). Hold the patient's arm at 90 degrees abduction and elevation, allowing the relaxed forearm to dangle with the elbow at 90 degrees flexion (Fig. 14–4E). Tap the triceps tendon just above the olecranon process. The normal response is elbow extension. Alternatively, have the patient flex both elbows, bringing the arms parallel across the chest (Fig. 14–4E). Have each hand grasp the other forearm. Reinforcement can be obtained by having the patient grasp harder and extending the elbow slightly.

Reflex center at T8 to T9: upper abdominal muscle reflex. Tap the muscles directly near their insertions on the costal margins and xiphoid process (Fig. 14–5A).

Reflex center at T9 to T10: middle abdominal muscle reflex. Stimulate the muscles of the mid-abdomen by tapping an overlaid finger or doubled-tongue blades (Fig. 14–5B).

Reflex center at T11 to T12: lower abdominal muscles. Tap the muscle insertions directly, near the symphysis pubis (Fig. 14–5C).

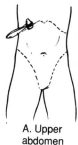
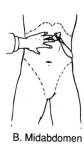
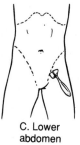

A. Upper abdomen   B. Midabdomen   C. Lower abdomen

Fig. 14–5 *Abdominal Muscle Reflexes. A. Upper abdomen:* *Tap the abdominal muscles directly with the reflex hammer, near their attachments to the costal margin.* ***B. Mid-abdomen:*** *Place your finger or a double-tongue blade on the muscles and tap the pleximeter.* ***C. Lower abdomen:*** *Tap the lower abdominal muscles directly at their attachments near the symphysis pubis.*

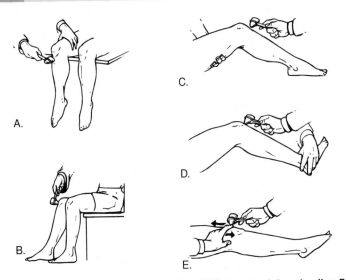

Fig. 14–6 *Knee Jerk (Alternative Positions). A. With the patient's legs dangling. B. Sitting. C. With the patient Supine, Method 1. D. With the patient supine, Method 2. E. With the patient supine and knee extended, Method 3.*

Reflex center at L2 to L4: quadriceps reflex (femoral nerve). Several methods are available. In each, a normal response is extension of the knee and contraction of the quadriceps can be palpated. *Legs Dangling (Fig. 14–6A):* Grasp the lower thigh with your left hand while your right hand delivers a hammer tap on the patellar tendon. *Sitting, Feet on the Floor (Fig. 14–6B):* The patient sits on a chair or low bed. Have the patient's toes curled in plantarflexion and knee slightly extended from a right angle. Tap the patellar tendon directly. **Lying Supine (Three Methods):** *Method 1* With your hand under the popliteal fossa, lift the patient's knee from the table. Tap the patellar tendon directly (Fig. 14–6C). *Method 2* Grasp the patient's foot, flexing the hip and knee, and rotate the knee outward and dorsiflex the foot. Tap the patellar tendon directly (Fig. 14–6D). *Method 3* With the knee extended and the limb lying on the table, push the patellar tendon distad with your index finger on the insertion of the quadriceps tendon. Tap downward on the index finger (Fig. 14–6E). The muscle contraction pulls the patella proximally.

Reflex center at L2 to L4: adductor reflex (obturator nerve). With the patient supine, place the limb in slight abduction (Fig. 14–7A). Directly tap the adductor magnus tendon just proximal to its insertion on the medial epicondyle of the femur. Normally, the thigh adducts. If the quadriceps reflex is absent and the adductor reflex is present, this indicates a lesion of the femoral nerve.

Reflex center at L4 to S2: hamstring reflex (sciatic nerve). Have the patient supine with hips and knees flexed at about 90 degrees and the thighs rotated slightly outward. Place your left hand under the popliteal fossa so the index finger compresses the medial hamstring tendon (a bundle of tendons from semitendinosus, semimembranosus, gracilis, sartorius) (Fig. 14–7B). Tap your finger. The normal response is flexion of the knee and contraction of the medial mass

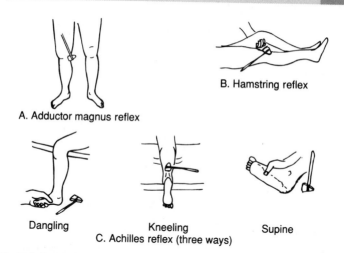

Fig. 14–7 *Deep Reflexes II. A. Adductor magnus reflex. B. Hamstring reflex. C. Achilles reflex (three ways):* Leg dangling, kneeling, and supine.

of hamstring muscles. Test the lateral hamstrings in a similar manner: with your finger compress the lateral hamstring tendon just proximal to the fibular head and tap your finger. The normal response is contraction of the lateral hamstring mass (biceps femoris) and flexion of the knee.

Reflex center at L5 to S2: Achilles reflex (tibial nerve). The normal response is contraction of the gastrocnemius and plantarflexion of the foot. *Legs Dangling (Fig. 14–7C):* With your left hand, grasp the patient's foot and pull it into dorsiflexion to find the degree of Achilles stretch that produces the optimal response. Tap the tendon directly. *Kneeling (Fig. 14–7C):* Have the patient kneel with the feet hanging over the edge of a chair, table, or bed. With your left hand dorsiflexing the foot, tap the tendon directly. Assess both the contraction and relaxation of the muscle; delayed relaxation (hung-up reflex) is characteristic of hypothyroidism. *Supine (Fig. 14–7C):* Partially flex the patient's hip and knee while rotating the knee outward as far as comfort permits. With your left hand, grasp the foot and pull it into dorsiflexion, then tap the Achilles tendon directly.

The Superficial (Skin) Reflexes

These reflex arcs have receptor organs in the skin rather than in muscle fibers. Their adequate stimulus is stroking, scratching, or touching. If there is no response, a painful stimulus should be tried. The superficial reflexes are lost in disease of the pyramidal tract.

Reflex center at T5 to T8: upper abdominal skin reflex. Have the patient supine and relaxed, with the arms at the sides and knees slightly flexed. Use a fresh (previously unused) pin to stroke the skin over the lower thoracic cage from the midaxillary line toward the midline (Fig. 14–8A). Watch for ipsilateral contraction of the muscles in the epigastric abdominal wall. When the muscle contractions cannot be seen, observe for umbilical deviation toward the stimulated side. In

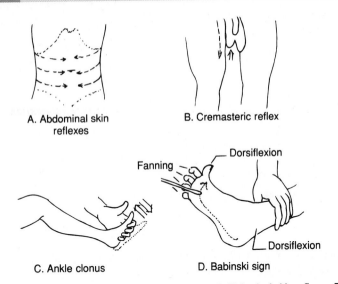

A. Abdominal skin
reflexes

B. Cremasteric reflex

C. Ankle clonus

D. Babinski sign

Fig. 14–8 *Skin Reflexes and Pyramidal Tract Signs. A. Abdominal skin reflexes. B. Cremasteric reflex. C. Ankle clonus: With the patient supine, lift the knee in slight flexion with the muscles relaxed. Grasp the foot and jerk it into dorsiflexion, then hold it under slight tension in that direction. In a positive response, the foot reacts with a number of cycles of alternating dorsiflexion and plantarflexion. The motion may die in a few cycles (unsustained clonus), or it may persist as long as the tension is held (sustained clonus).* **D. Babinski sign.**

very obese persons, retract the umbilicus toward the opposite side to feel it pull toward the side of stimulation.

Reflex center at T9 to T11: mid-abdominal skin reflex.   Make similar strokes from the flank toward the midline at the umbilical level.

Reflex center at T11 to T12: lower abdominal skin reflex.   Make similar strokes from the iliac crests toward the midline of the hypogastrium.

Reflex center at L1 to L2: cremasteric reflex.   In males, stroke the inner aspect of the thigh from the inguinal crease down (Fig. 14–8B). Normally, this causes contraction of the cremaster with prompt elevation of the testis on the ipsilateral side. A slow and irregular rise of the testis results from muscular contraction in the dartos tunic and is not the reflex response.

Reflex center at L4 to S2: plantar reflex.   Grasp the patient's ankle with your left hand. With a blunt point and moderate pressure, stroke the sole near its *lateral* border, from the heel toward the metatarsal heads, where the course should curve medially following the bases of the toes (Fig. 14–8D). For the blunt point, use a wooden-tip applicator, the end of a split wooden tongue blade, or the dull handle end on a reflex hammer. If no response is observed, a pin should be used as this is a nociceptive reflex. Normally, this produces plantarflexion of the toes and, often, the entire foot responds with plantarflexion. The presence of an extensor plantar response is called *Babinski sign;* it should be noted as present or absent. In disease of the pyramidal tract, this reflex results, with some or all of four components: dorsiflexion of the great toe, fanning of all toes, dorsiflexion of the ankle, and flexion of the knee and thigh.

Reflex center at S1 to S2: superficial anal reflex (*anal wink*). Stroke the skin or mucosa of the perianal region. Normally, the anal sphincters contract.

Posture, Balance, and Coordination: The Cerebellar Examination

Precise voluntary movement requires graded contraction of the agonist, or prime mover, with a corresponding graded relaxation of the antagonist about each joint. Other muscles act to fix the joint with proper tension. The total integration of these movements, called *coordination*, is partially mediated through efferent and afferent tracts of the cerebellum. The vestibular apparatus and the cerebral cortex also participate. Maintenance of posture and balance requires sensory input from the joints, muscles, tendons, and vestibular system, and coordinated motor outputs mediated by the cerebral cortex and basal ganglia.

Test Station (Equilibratory Coordination)

Ask the patient to stand comfortably with the hands at the sides. Observe the position of the feet. Normally, the feet will be just a few centimeters apart and the knees opposed. A wide stance suggests an accommodation to instability of stance. Next, have the patient put the feet together and observe for stability. Note swaying of the trunk or elevation of the arms to maintain balance. Now, have the patient close her eyes while again observing for loss of balance. Be ready to support her should she lose her balance and reassure her you will protect her. Falling during the test is the ***Romberg sign.*** If she remains stable, tell her you are going to tap her gently to assess her stability. Gently push her laterally on each upper arm, forward on the upper back and, last, backward on the chest. With normal proprioception, vestibular function, cerebellar and motor pathways she will remain stable throughout. Have her open her eyes, and, after fair warning, push more firmly on her chest to check for maximal stability.

Test for Diadochokinesia

Normal coordination includes the ability to arrest one motor motion and substitute its opposite. Loss of this ability (*dysdiadochokinesia*) is characteristic of cerebellar disease. Many simple tests may be employed to test for dysdiadochokinesis. *Alternating Movements (Fig. 14–9A):* (1) Have the patient hold his forearms vertically and alternate pronation and supination in rapid succession. In cerebellar disease, the movements overshoot, undershoot, or are irregular and inaccurate; the motions may be slowed or incomplete in disease of the pyramidal tract; (2) Have the patient rapidly tap his fingers on the table, or close and open the fists; (3) Holding the arms at 90 degrees elevation and 0 degrees abduction may show the affected arm deviating in abduction; and (4) *Stewart-Holmes Rebound Sign* (Fig. 14–9A): While the patient clenches his fist, with elbow flexed and forearm pronated, grasp his fist from above and pull strongly attempting to extend his elbow against his resistance; suddenly release your grip and observe for rapid control of rebound. The examiner must guard against injury to the patient. With cerebellar disease, the forearm may rebound in several cycles of extension-flexion, or the patient may strike himself if not guarded.

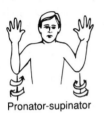

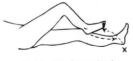

Pronator-supinator
Stewart-Holmes
rebound sign

A. Tests for diadochokinesia

B. Finger-to-nose test

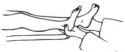

C. Heel-to-knee test

D. Hoover sign of hysteria

Fig. 14–9 *Test for Cerebellar Disease. See text for full descriptions. **A. Tests for diado-chokinesia:** The ability to perform alternating movements may be tested by having the patient hold the forearms vertically; then ask the patient to quickly alternate pronation and supination in the vertical position. Another method is the Stewart-Holmes rebound test, in which the patient is requested to flex the biceps brachii muscle by pulling against the wrist held by the examiner. While at full strength, the examiner suddenly releases the wrist and observes for control of the rebound. **B. Finger-to-nose test. C. Heel-to-knee tests. D. Hoover sign of hysteria:** This distinguishes hysterical paralysis of the lower limb from paralysis with an organic cause. Take a position at the foot of the supine patient. Cradle each of the patient's heels in one of your palms and rest your hands on the table. Have the patient attempt to raise the affected limb. In organic disease, the associated movement causes the unaffected heel to press downward; in hysteria, the associated movement is absent.*

Test for Dyssynergia and Dysmetria

Finger-to-Nose Test: With the eyes open, have the patient fully extend his elbow and, in a wide arc, rapidly bring the tip of the index finger to the tip of his nose (Fig. 14–9B). In cerebellar disease, this action is attended by an action tremor. When the maneuver is performed with the eyes closed, the sense of position in the shoulder and elbow is tested. In a variant of this maneuver, have the patient make wide arcs with both arms to approximate the tips of his index fingers in front of him. *Heel-to-Shin Test:* With the patient supine and the lower limbs resting in extension, ask the patient to raise one heel and place it on the opposite knee, then slide the heel down the shin (Fig. 14–9C). The moving foot should be dorsiflexed, and the motion should be performed slowly and accurately. In cerebellar disease, the arc of the heel to the knee is jerky and wavering, the knee is frequently overshot, and the slide down the shin is accompanied by an action tremor. With the eyes closed, the motions are inaccurate in posterior spinal column disease. Frequently, the heel slides off the shin, but action tremor is absent.

Testing Skilled Acts

Ask the patient to write a sentence to inspect handwriting. Test the patient's facility at buttoning and unbuttoning a coat or shirt. Have the patient pick up pins or thread a needle. Test the patient's skill at cutting figures out of paper with scissors.

Testing the Vestibular Apparatus

Past pointing and other tests are described in Chapter 7 on page 197.

The Gait

The gait is influenced by the rate, rhythm, and the character of the movements employed in walking. In assessing the neurologic contribution to gait, painful and restrictive conditions of the joints, muscles, and other structures must be excluded. Observe the patient's usual gait in a well-lighted hallway. Note the posture of the head, neck and trunk, swing of each arm, leg swing, width of stance, size of steps and clearance of the toe from the floor. Be sure to observe all three phases of gait: touch down, which should occur with the lateral heel; stance, which should be centered; and push-off which should come off the great toe. Foot strikes are normally in a nearly straight line. Also, observe the turn for loss of balance or multiple small steps to get turned around. Next, have the patient walk away from you on the toes, observing from behind, turn and walk toward you on the heels observing from the front; note how far the heels and toes, respectively, are held off the ground. Examine the wear on the patient's shoes; abnormal wear pattern is a good clue to disorders of the foot and gait.

SENSORY EXAMINATION

A complete assessment of sensory functions is not made in the routine physical examination. But a history of diabetes, localized pain, numbness, or tingling, or the finding of motor deficits, calls for a detailed sensory examination.

The patient must be lucid and have adequate attention to cooperate with the examination. The clinician must have a detailed knowledge of segmental and peripheral nerve distribution in the skin (refer to Figs. 14–10 and 14–11) and make a drawing of the distribution of sensory deficits. The diagram may be used for immediate comparison on retesting; abnormal sensory examinations should be repeated for consistency, progression or resolution. Disparities in examinations may indicate factitious findings.

The detailed examination of the CN includes testing of the special senses and the cutaneous sensibility of the head. For the remainder of the body, the distribution of sensibility for cutaneous pain, touch, pressure, position, and vibration should be evaluated. If a deficit in pain sensation is detected, temperature sensation must be tested. When an area of altered cutaneous sensibility is found, the borders should be marked with a skin pencil, and a diagram should be made in the patient's record.

Basic Sensory Modalities

Testing pain and touch sense. *Superficial Pain (Sharp-Dull):* Have the patient close his eyes. Use the point and the dull guard end of a sterile open safety pin as a stimulus (Fig. 14–12A). Hold it lightly between your thumb and index finger so that the pin slides slightly with each application and ask, "What do you feel?". If there is doubt about the response, mix sharp and dull stimuli from the point and head of the pin. Compare side-to-side with the same degree of pressure and ask, "Is it the same"; it is better if the patient reports differences than if you suggest them. In mapping deficit borders, slowly stimulate the skin from nonsensitive to

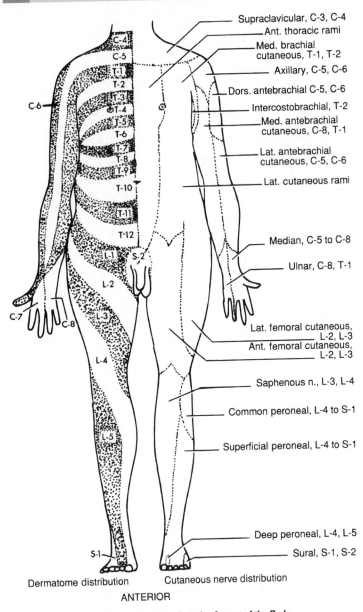

Dermatome distribution | Cutaneous nerve distribution

ANTERIOR

Fig. 14–10 *Cutaneous Sensation in the Anterior Aspect of the Body.*

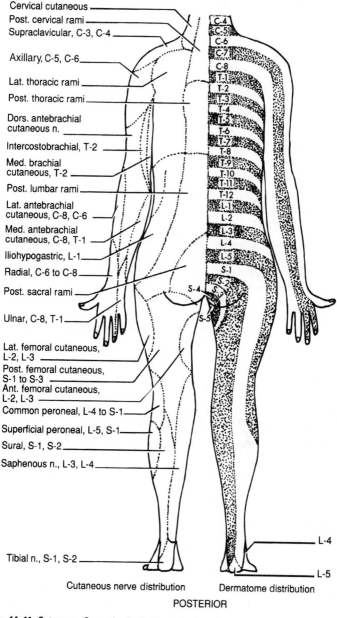

Cervical cutaneous

Post. cervical rami

Supraclavicular, C-3, C-4

Axillary, C-5, C-6

Lat. thoracic rami

Post. thoracic rami

Dors. antebrachial cutaneous n.

Intercostobrachial, T-2

Med. brachial cutaneous, T-2

Post. lumbar rami

Lat. antebrachial cutaneous, C-8, C-6

Med. antebrachial cutaneous, C-8, T-1

Iliohypogastric, L-1

Radial, C-6 to C-8

Post. sacral rami

Ulnar, C-8, T-1

Lat. femoral cutaneous, L-2, L-3

Post. femoral cutaneous, S-1 to S-3

Ant. femoral cutaneous, L-2, L-3

Common peroneal, L-4 to S-1

Superficial peroneal, L-5, S-1

Sural, S-1, S-2

Saphenous n., L-3, L-4

Tibial n., S-1, S-2

C-4, C-5, C-6, C-7, C-8, T-1, T-2, T-3, T-4, T-5, T-6, T-7, T-8, T-9, T-10, T-11, T-12, L-1, L-2, L-3, L-4, L-5, S-1, S-2, S-3, S-4, S-5

L-4

L-5

Cutaneous nerve distribution   Dermatome distribution

POSTERIOR

Fig. 14–11 *Cutaneous Sensation in the Posterior Aspect of the Body.*

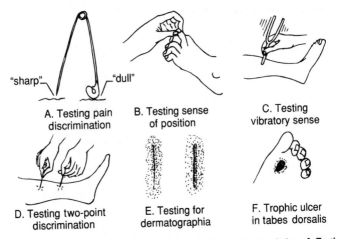

"sharp" — "dull"

A. Testing pain discrimination

B. Testing sense of position

C. Testing vibratory sense

D. Testing two-point discrimination

E. Testing for dermatographia

F. Trophic ulcer in tabes dorsalis

Fig. 14–12 *Sensory Testing and Other Phenomena. See text for descriptions.* **A. *Testing "sharp-dull" with a safety pin.* B. *Testing position sense in the toes.* C. *Testing vibratory sense.* D. *Testing two-point discrimination.* E. *Testing for dermatographism:* Stroke the skin with a blunt object; the normal response is a pale line along the path of stimulation, the "white line." The abnormal responses are a "red line" in which the area becomes bright red and then extends with red mottling, and, with more exaggerated response, the line develops a wheal that becomes raised, edematous, and pale. F. *Trophic plantar ulcer in tabes dorsalis.***

sensitive skin, having the patient indicate where the sensation changes. Sensibility to pain may be increased (*hyperalgesia*), normal, reduced (*hypalgesia*) or absent (*analgesia*). **Deep Pain:** Test for deep or protopathic pain by pressure on the nerve trunks, and tendons. For example, in the *Abadie sign* for tabes dorsalis, the normal pressure tenderness of the Achilles tendon is lost.

Testing temperature sense. When pain sense is impaired, test for temperature sensibility; the pathways are closely associated. Ask the patient to distinguish between warm and cold. With the eyes closed, touch the skin with glass tubes of hot and cold water. Alternatively, test cold perception with a cold tuning fork and warm perception by exhaling on the skin through your widespread lips.

Testing tactile sense. With the patient's eyes closed, compare sensation right to left by stroking the skin with a shred of sterile gauze and having the patient indicate when and where you touch him. If you suspect that he is using his eyes, make sham tests near but without touching the skin. Grade the results as *hyperesthetic, normal, anesthetic,* or *hypesthetic.*

Testing proprioception: position sense. With the patient's eyes closed, grasp a finger on the sides (avoid grasping on the top and bottom or touching adjacent fingers because that provides touch cues). Extend or flex the finger at one joint and ask the patient to state its position (Fig. 14–12B). Similarly, test the position sensation in the metatarsalphalangeal joint of the great toe. Normal young patients discriminate 1 to 2 degrees of movement in their distal finger joints and 3 to 5 degrees of the great toe. Test position sense in the leg or arm with the eyes closed. Place one limb in a position and ask the patient to place its counterpart in a symmetrical position.

Vibratory sense: pallesthesia. Place the handle of a vibrating 128-Hz tuning fork over bony prominences, such as the styloid processes of the radii, the subcutaneous aspects of the tibiae, the malleoli of the ankles, or the interphalangeal joint of the great toe (Fig. 14–12C). Compare symmetrical points. When the patient indicates that the vibration of the fork has ceased, place the handle on your own wrist to detect any persistence of vibration. Young patients feel vibration for approximately 15 seconds in the great toe and 25 seconds in the distal joint of the finger, whereas 70-year-olds feel it for 10 and 15 seconds, respectively. Make sham tests by setting the fork in vibration and unobtrusively stopping it with your finger before applying the handle to the patient.

Pressure sense. Standardized monofilaments are available to precisely check for protective pressure sensation. Anesthesia to a 10-g monofilament is a sensitive test for loss of protective sensation to pressure injury. All diabetics should be tested at least once a year with this technique [Caputo GM, Cavanagh PR, Ulbrecht JS, et al. Assessment and management of foot disease in patients with diabetes. *N Engl J Med.* 1994;331:854–860]. Test the patient's ability to discriminate objects of different weight in their palms. Test the ability to distinguish between pressures from the head of a pin and the tip of your finger. Press over the joints and subcutaneous aspects of bones for perception of pressure.

Testing Higher Integrative Functions

Stereognosis. Simple sensory perception should be normal. With their eyes closed, test the patient's ability to identify objects placed in their hands. Use coins, pencils, glass, wood, metal, cloth, and other familiar articles.

Two-Point discrimination. Test the ability to distinguish the separation of two simultaneous pinpricks (Fig. 14–12D). Find the distance at which the patient perceives two points rather than one as the stimuli are moved farther apart. Test and compare symmetric regions. The normal distance varies in different parts of the body, from 1 mm on the tongue, to 2 to 8 mm on the fingertips, 40 mm on the chest and forearm, and 75 mm on the upper thigh and upper arm.

Perception of figures on the skin (graphesthesia). Tell the patient you will write numerals or letters "right-side up." Then, while their eyes are closed, ask the patient to identify figures 1 cm high traced with a blunt point on the distal pad of the index finger. The figures should be at least 2 cm high on other body parts.

Testing Specific Peripheral Nerves

Exclusion test for major nerve injury in the upper limb. Normal sensibility to pinprick in the tips of the index and little fingers excludes major injury to the median and ulnar nerves. Normal ability to extend the thumb and fingers excludes injury of the radial nerve (Fig. 14–13).

Testing the median nerve. *Motor Function:* *Ochsner Test* (Fig. 14–14A). Have the patient clasp the hands firmly together; the index finger cannot flex when the innervation of the *flexor digitorum sublimis* has been injured anywhere below the antecubital fossa. *Flexion of the Thumb* (Fig. 14–14B). Hold the patient's

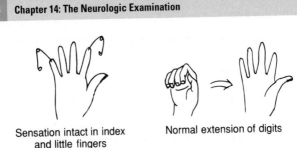

Sensation intact in index
and little fingers

Normal extension of digits

Fig. 14–13 *Exclusion Test for Major Nerve Injury in the Upper Limb.* Sensation is intact in the palmar tips of the index and little fingers; extension of the digits of the hand is unimpaired.

first metacarpophalangeal joint with your thumb and index fingers so that the metacarpal bone is extended and ask the patient to bend the interphalangeal joint; failure indicates paralysis of the *flexor pollicis longus,* innervated by the volar interosseus that branches from the median nerve in the middle third of the forearm. **Abduction of Thumb.** Test the *abductor pollicis brevis,* innervated exclusively by the median nerve, to distinguish it from low-level paralysis of the ulnar nerve by two methods: (1) *Wartenberg Oriental Prayer Position* (Fig. 14–14C). Have the patient extend and adduct the four fingers of each hand, with thumbs extended, then raise the two hands in front of the face so they are side by side in the same plane, with thumbs and index fingers touching tip to tip.

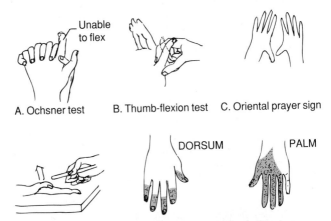

A. Ochsner test   B. Thumb-flexion test   C. Oriental prayer sign

D. Pen-touching test   E. Areas of anesthesia (blue)

Fig. 14–14 *Median Nerve Paralysis.* See text for descriptions. **A. Ochsner test:** The patient cannot flex the index finger on the paralyzed side. **B. Thumb flexion test:** The patient cannot flex the distal joint of the thumb. **C. Wartenberg oriental prayer sign:** Paralysis prevents extension of the thumb so its tip cannot reach its mate. **D. Pen-touching test:** The thumb cannot abduct to touch the object when the median nerve is paralyzed. **E. The area of anesthesia:** This includes the radial three digits of the palmar aspect and folds over the tips to the dorsal aspect where it covers the distal phalanges of the same digits (blue).

Paralysis of the abductor pollicis brevis prevents full range of thumb abduction, so thumbs do not come together when index fingers touch. (2) *Pen-Touching Test* (Fig. 14–14D). Have the patient rest the supinated hand on a table holding the fingers flat. Ask the patient to raise his thumb in straight up off the table to touch a pen or pencil held horizontally above the thumb. *Sensory Function: Phalen test* is performed by having the patient flex the wrists at 90 degrees and press the backs of their hands together for one minute. Numbness and tingling in the thumb and fingers indicates compression of the median nerve, as in the carpal tunnel syndrome (Fig. 14–14E). The *Tinel sign* (page 758) is often useful.

Testing the ulnar nerve. *Motor Function:* Weakness of finger adduction results from paralysis of the *interosseus palmaris.* This is demonstrated by pulling a sheet of paper from between the patient's extended and adducted fingers to assess the pressure exerted by the sides of the fingers (Fig. 14–15A). Paralysis of the *adductor pollicis* can be tested by asking the patient to grip each end of a folded paper between thumbs on top and index fingers underneath. Have the patient pull the hands apart while gripping the paper. The thumb with an inadequate adductor becomes flexed at its interphalangeal joint from involuntary use of the flexor pollicis longus, innervated by the median nerve (Fig. 14–15B). In lesions at or below the elbow, test for paralysis of the *flexor carpi ulnaris* by having the patient's supinated hand lie on the table. Hold all digits but the little finger flat against the table. Have the patient abduct the little finger maximally; if there is no paralysis, the tensed tendon may be seen or palpated at the wrist (Fig. 14–15C). *Sensory Function:* An area of anesthesia covers the ulnar digits and the corresponding region of the palm. A similar distribution occurs on the dorsal

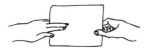

A. Paper-pulling test

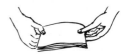

B. Test of adductor pollicis

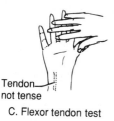

Tendon not tense
C. Flexor tendon test

PALM

DORSUM
D. Areas of anesthesia (stippled)

Fig. 14–15 *Ulnar Nerve Paralysis. See text for descriptions. **A. Paper-pulling test:** This tests the adductors of the fingers by having the patient hold a piece of paper between two adducted fingers; the examiner pulls the paper to test the strength of compression exerted by the adductors. **B. Adductor pollicis test:** In ulnar paralysis, the thumb cannot exert enough pressure in adduction, so it flexes involuntarily from action of the flexor pollicis longus. **C. Test of flexor carpi ulnaris:** The patient attempts to flex the free finger, but the paralyzed tendon in the wrist does not tense. **D. Area of anesthesia:** The ulnar 1.5 digits on both aspects of the hand (blue).*

aspect, except when the nerve lesion is at the wrist so the area is constricted to the distal half of the little finger (Fig. 14–15D).

Movements of Specific Muscles and Nerves

It is frequently desirable to identify the muscles and nerves involved in a deficit of bodily movement. The following is a compilation of the principal muscle movements, their causative muscles, and their innervation (in parentheses). This survey starts with CN and precedes distally identifying movements served by cervical, thoracic, lumbar, and sacral roots sequentially. The reader can use the list in several ways: an abnormal movement can be traced to the peripheral nerve and spinal roots; abnormal movements can be predicted for each peripheral nerve or spinal segment.

Eyebrow, elevation. Frontalis (CN VII from inferior pons).

Eyebrow, depression downward and inward, wrinkling of the forehead. Corrugator (CN VII from inferior pons).

Upper eyelid, elevations. Levator palpebrae superioris (CN III from upper midbrain).

Eyelids, closing, wrinkling of forehead, compression of lacrimal sac. Orbicularis oculi (CN VII from inferior pons).

*Eyeball, elevation and adduction.** Superior rectus (CN III from upper midbrain).*

*Eyeball, elevation and outward rotation.** Inferior oblique (CN III from upper midbrain).

*Eyeball, depression and rotation downward and inward.** Inferior rectus (CN III from upper midbrain).

*Eyeball, depression and rotation downward and outward.** Superior oblique (CN IV from midbrain) or primary downward rotation, secondary inward (intorsion) rotation, and tertiary weak outward rotation.

*Eyeball, adduction.** Medial rectus (CN III from upper midbrain).

*Eyeball, abduction.** Lateral rectus (CN VI from inferior pons).

Pupil, constriction. Ciliary (CN III and parasympathetic from upper midbrain).

Lips, retraction. Zygomatic (CN VII from inferior pons).

Lips, protrusion. Orbicularis oris (CN VII from inferior pons).

Mouth, opening. Mylohyoid (CN V from pons), digastricus (CN VII from pons).

Mandible, elevation and retraction. Masseter and temporalis (CN V from midpons).

Mandible, elevation and protrusion. Pterygoid (CN V from mid-pons).

Pharynx, palatine elevation and pharyngeal constriction. Levator veli palatini and pharyngeal constrictor (CN IX and X from medulla).

---

*Ophthalmologic Interpretation of Muscle Action.** The items marked with asterisks constitue the actions of the oculorotatory muscles, as assigned by the anatomists and some neurologists. Sharply divergent interpretations are furnished by the opthalmologists on the basis of clinical findings. The direction of movement of the eyes is a result of the actions of synergists and antagonists producing six cardinal positions of gaze, corresponding to the six extraocular muscles. Paralysis of a single muscle results in the inability of the eye to attain its cardinal position, which, in four of the six muscles, does not correspond to the prediction of the anatomists.

Tongue, depression and protrusion. Genioglossus (CN XII from medulla).

Neck, rotation of the head. Sternocleidomastoid and trapezius (CN XI from medulla and upper cervical cord).

Neck, flexion. Rectus capitis anterior (C1 to C3).

Neck, extension, and rotation of the head. Splenius capitis et cervicis (C1 to C4).

Neck, lateral bending. Rectus capitis lateralis (C1 to C4 and suboccipital nerve).

Spine, flexion. Rectus abdominis (T8 to T12).

Spine, extension. Thoracic and lumbar intercostals (thoracic nerves from T2 to L1).

Spine, extension and rotation. Semispinalis (thoracic nerves from T2 to T12).

Spine, extension and lateral bending. Quadratus lumborum (lumbar plexus from T10 to L2).

Ribs, elevation and depression. Scaleni and intercostal (cervical and thoracic nerves from C4 to T12).

Ribs, elevation. Serratus posterior superior (from T1 to T4).

Diaphragm, elevation and depression. The diaphragmatic muscles (phrenic nerve from C3 to C5). Remember diaphragmatic innervation by the phrenic nerve with the rhyme, "C3, 4, and 5 to keep the man alive."

Scapula, rotation and extension of neck. Upper trapezius (CN XI from C3 to C4).

Scapula, retraction with shoulder elevation. Middle and lower trapezius (CN XI from C3 to C4).

Scapula, elevation and retraction. Rhomboids (dorsal scapular nerve from C5).

Arm, elevation. Supraspinatus (suprascapular nerve from C5 to C6), upper trapezius (CN XI from C3 to C4).

Arm, elevation and rotation. Deltoid (axillary nerve from C5 to C6).

Arm, depression and adduction. Middle pectoralis major (anterior thoracic nerve from C5 to T1).

Arm, depression and medial rotation. Subscapularis (subscapular nerve from C5 to C7), teres major (thoracodorsal nerves from C5 to C7).

Arm, depression and lateral rotation. Infraspinatus (suprascapular nerve from C5 to C6).

Elbow, flexion. Biceps brachii, brachialis (musculocutaneous nerve from C5 to C6).

Elbow, extension. Triceps brachii (radial nerve from C7 to T1).

Elbow, supination. Biceps brachii (musculocutaneous nerve from C5 to C6), brachioradialis (radial nerve from C5 to C6).

Elbow, supination and elbow flexion. Brachioradialis (radial nerve from C5 to C6).

Elbow, pronation. Pronator teres (median nerve from C6 to C7).

Wrist, extension and adduction. Extensor carpi ulnaris (radial nerve from C7 to C8).

Wrist, extension and abduction of hand. Extensor carpi radialis longus (radial nerve from C6 to C7).

Wrist, extension of the hand. Extensor digitorum communis (radial nerve from C7 to C8).

Wrist, flexion and abduction. Flexor carpi radialis (median nerve from C7 to C8).

Wrist, flexion and adduction. Flexor carpi ulnaris (ulnar nerve from C7 to C8).

Thumb, adduction and opposition. Adductor pollicis longus (ulnar nerve C8 to T1).

Thumb, abduction and extension. Abductor pollicis longus and brevis (median and radial [and posterior interosseous nerves] from C7 to C8).

Thumb, extension of distal phalanx. Extensor pollicis longus (radial nerve from C7 to C8).

Thumb, extension of proximal phalanx. Extensor pollicis brevis (radial nerve from C7 to C8).

Thumb, flexion of distal phalanx. Flexor pollicis longus (median nerve from C7 to T1).

Thumb, flexion of proximal phalanx. Flexor pollicis longus and brevis (median nerve from C7 to T1).

Thumb, flexion and opposition. Opponens pollicis (median nerve from C8 to T1).

Fingers, flexion and adduction of little finger. Opponens digiti minimi (ulnar nerve from C8 to T1).

Fingers, adduction of four fingers. Palmar interossei (ulnar nerve from C8 to T1).

Fingers, abduction of four fingers. Dorsal interossei (ulnar nerve from C8 to T1).

Fingers, extension of hand. Extensor digitorum communis (radial nerve from C7 to C8).

Fingers, flexion of hand. Palmar interossei (interosseous nerves from C7 to T1), lumbricales (ulnar and median nerves from C7 to T1).

Fingers, extension of interphalangeal joints. Interossei palmaris and lumbricales (interosseous nerve; median and ulnar nerves from C7 to T1).

Fingers, flexion of the distal phalanges. Flexor digitorum profundus (median and ulnar nerves from C7 to T1).

Fingers, flexion of middle phalanges. Flexor digitorum sublimis (median nerve from C7 to T1).

Abdomen, compression with flexion of trunk. Rectus abdominis (lower thoracic nerves from T6 to L1).

Abdomen, flexion of abdominal wall obliquely. Obliquus abdominis externus (lower thoracic nerves from T6 to L1).

Hip, flexion. Iliacus (femoral nerve), psoas (L2 to L3), sartorius (femoral nerve from L2 to L3).

Hip, extension. Gluteus maximus (inferior gluteal nerve from L4 or S2), adductor magnus (sciatic nerve and obturator nerve from L5 to S2).

Hip, abduction. Gluteus medius (superior gluteal nerve from L4 to S1), gluteus maximus (inferior gluteal nerve from L4 to S2).

Hip, adduction. Adductor magnus (sciatic and obturator nerves from L5 to S2).

Hip, outward rotation. Gluteus maximus (inferior gluteal nerve from L4 to S2), obturator internus (branches from S1 to S3).

Hip, inward rotation. Psoas (branches from L2 to L3).

Knee, flexion. Biceps femoris, semitendinosus, semimembranosus, gastrocnemius (all through sciatic nerve from L5 to S2).

Knee, extension. Quadriceps femoris (femoral nerve from L2 to L4).

Ankle, plantar flexion. Gastrocnemius and soleus (tibial nerve from L5 to S2).

Ankle, dorsiflexion. Anterior tibial (deep peroneal nerve from L4 to S1).

Ankle, inversion. Posterior tibial (tibial nerve from L5 to S1).

Ankle, eversion. Peroneus longus (superficial peroneal nerve from L4 to S1).

Great toe, dorsiflexion. Extensor hallucis longus and brevis (superficial peroneal nerve from L4 to S1).

Neurologic Symptoms

General Symptoms

KEY SYMPTOM Headache

See page 731ff.

KEY SYMPTOM Memory Loss

There are four components of memory that can be distinguished by function and location in the brain. *Episodic memory* records episodic events in the medial temporal and frontal cortex (cingulate gyrus). *Semantic memory* records names, general knowledge and information in the lateral temporal lobes. *Procedural memory* retains the ability to perform complex behaviors and tasks in the frontal lobes, basal ganglia and cerebellum. *Working memory* stores immediately useful information at which attention is directed in the frontal lobes, amygdala and parietal cortex. Information from working memory is either stored or deleted if not recalled or used. Patients often complain of forgetfulness, especially of people's names. Paradoxically, it is rarely the patient who is concerned about memory loss who has a serious problem. Changes in behavior, failure to complete expected tasks, difficulty with instrumental activities of daily living, especially managing finances, are more likely to be clues to significant impairments in memory and cognition. Always formally screen for cognitive impairment if there is any concern. [Budson AE, Price BH. Memory Dysfunction. N Eng J Med 2005;352:692–9.]

KEY SYMPTOM Spells

The patient experiences one or more episodes of altered perception or behavior, usually of a duration measured in seconds or minutes. When multiple, they are usually described as stereotypic. The spell may have only subjective symptoms, or be associated with behavioral changes observed by others. The patient may be aware throughout the spell or be amnestic for the episode. When accompanied by changes in consciousness, behaviors or motor events, the reports of observers are often key to making the diagnosis. Inquire about triggering events or sensations, associated symptoms and signs (such as loss of muscle tone with falling, injury or incontinence), the duration of the spells and the patient's responsiveness during and after the spell. Spells generally indicate a primary or secondary brain event. **CLINICAL OCCURRENCE:**   Seizures, especially complex partial and absence seizures; transient ischemic events; stroke; nonconvulsive seizures; tics; conversion disorder; panic attacks; hyperventilation; narcolepsy; delirium; drug toxicity or intoxication.

> ### KEY SYMPTOM   Insomnia

Disorders of sleep are common, especially in shift workers and following long distance air travel. A careful history of the onset and pattern of disrupted sleep with close attention to sleep hygiene will often disclose the sources of sleep disruption. Several different patterns are recognized and should be distinguished: *initial insomnia* is the inability to get to sleep at the usual time; *terminal insomnia* results from early awakening and specifically produces deficits in rapid eye movement sleep. **CLINICAL OCCURRENCE:**   poor sleep hygiene, medications, illicit drug and alcohol use, depression, anxiety disorder, panic disorder, obstructive sleep apnea and hypomania or mania.

Cranial Nerve Symptoms

> ### KEY SYMPTOM   Visual Loss

See Chapter 7, page 216.

Absent or Abnormal Taste and Smell—Ageusia, Dysgeusia, Anosmia

See Chapter 7, page 216.

> ### KEY SYMPTOM   Ringing in the Ears—Tinnitus

See Chapter 7, page 214.

> ### KEY SYMPTOM   Hearing Loss

See Chapter 7, page 286.

> ### KEY SYMPTOM   Vertigo

See Chapter 7, page 287.

> ### KEY SYMPTOM   Double Vision—Diplopia

See Chapter 7, page 214.

> ### KEY SYMPTOM   Difficulty Swallowing—Dysphagia

See Chapter 7, pages 216 and 291.

> ### KEY SYMPTOM   Difficulty Speaking—Dysarthria

See Chapter 7, pages 209 and 760.

KEY SYMPTOM   Difficulty Speaking—Aphasia

See page 760.

KEY SYMPTOM   Pain in the Face

Trigeminal neuralgia (tic douloureux), see Chapter 7, page 213.

KEY SYMPTOM   Asymmetrical Face or Smile

See page 714, Facial Nerve Signs.

KEY SYMPTOM   Hoarseness

See Chapter 7, page 272.

KEY SYMPTOM   Neck and Shoulder Weakness

See Chapter 13, pages 618 and 642, and page 727.

Motor Symptoms

KEY SYMPTOM   Weakness

See page 689. Weakness may arise from lesions in the brain, spinal cord, peripheral nerves, motor endplate, or muscle. Either primary disease of the tissue or generalized metabolic abnormalities can be the cause. Weakness is a common complaint that requires a complete evaluation. A careful history is required to identify the specific activities that are impaired. Difficulty with rising from a chair or climbing stairs suggests proximal muscle weakness, whereas difficulty writing, opening jars and doors, and catching the toes while walking suggest distal weakness. Global weakness can be seen with generalized muscle diseases, myasthenia gravis, and polyneuropathies (e.g., Guillain-Barré syndrome). During the physical examination, observe for fasciculations, assess muscle mass, tone, and strength, and evaluate the reflexes. Hysterical weakness is not rare and malingering is perhaps more common; these diagnoses can only be made after organic disease is excluded by a thorough evaluation.

KEY SYMPTOM   Acute Episodic Weakness—Cataplexy

Episodic loss of motor and postural control is precipitated by laughter or strong emotions. There is momentary loss of voluntary motor power including speech, without loss of consciousness or postural tone. Cataplexy is seen in patients with narcolepsy.

KEY SYMPTOM   Muscle Pain—Myalgia

See also Chapter 13, page 616 and 680. This is a common, but nonspecific finding. Generalized myalgias, especially in the back and proximal limb muscles frequently accompany febrile illness of any cause. Severe myalgias are common in several infectious diseases (e.g., Lyme disease, trichinosis, and dengue); other elements of the history are of more use than the presence of myalgia in making the specific diagnosis. Drugs (e.g., statins) also cause myalgias so a complete medication and herbal therapy history is mandatory. In persons older than 50 years of age, abrupt onset of myalgias in the proximal muscles (shoulders > pelvic girdle) suggests polymyalgia rheumatica.

> **KEY SYMPTOM** **Muscle Stiffness**

Overuse of skeletal muscle induces a damage-repair cycle that is felt by the patient as pain and stiffness. Underuse leads to muscle wasting, which may be accompanied by stiffness. The unconditioned patient often complains of sore, stiff muscles 1 to 2 days following unaccustomed exercise (weekend athlete syndrome). Examination shows no abnormalities other than tenderness and occasionally mild spasm in the affected muscles. Patients with inherited disorders of muscle metabolism or electrolyte disorders can develop severe myonecrosis with exercise. **DDX:** Abrupt onset of proximal muscles stiffness in a person older than 50 years of age without a clear-cut precipitating event suggests polymyalgia rheumatica. Generalized cramps with tetany are seen with hypocalcemia. Bradykinesia and increased muscle tone seen in Parkinson syndromes is often describe by the patient as stiffness. Rare causes are stiff person syndrome, myotonia and hypocalcemia.

> **KEY SYMPTOM** **Twitches and Tics**

See pages 716 and 724.

> **KEY SYMPTOM** **Irresistible Leg Movements—Restless Legs Syndrome**

See page 763.

> **KEY SYMPTOM** **Muscle Spasm—Cramps, Dystonias**

See page 755.

Posture, Balance, and Coordination Symptoms

> **KEY SYMPTOM** **Loss of Balance—Falling**

See page 730.

> **KEY SYMPTOM** **Difficulty Walking**

See page 722.

> **KEY SYMPTOM** **Vertigo**

See Chapter 7, page 287.

> **KEY SYMPTOM** **Tremors**

See page 723.

Sensory Symptoms

> **KEY SYMPTOM** **Altered Sensation—Tingling and Numbness, Paresthesias**

Tingling and numbness of a body part indicate impairment of the normal sensory modalities of pressure, pain, and/or touch. Numbness implies neural damage and tingling stimulation of the nervous system. The pattern of the symptoms gives a good indication of the anatomic level of the nerve injury: symptoms on one side of the entire body indicate a problem in the thalamus or cortex; loss on one side of the body below a specific level suggests spinal cord injury; symptoms in a peripheral nerve distribution implies injury to that nerve; and symmetrical distal paresthesia (stocking-glove distribution) suggests a generalized sensory (with or without motor) axonal neuropathy. Test for the specific modalities of sensation are required. Unilateral loss of touch and position sensation and contralateral loss of temperature and pain sensation indicate a unilateral lesion of the spinal cord ipsilateral to the loss of touch and position.

> **KEY SYMPTOM** **Pain with Non-painful Stimuli—Allodynia**

See page 725.

> **KEY SYMPTOM** **Altered Sensation—Pain**

See page 725.

Neurologic Signs

Cranial Nerve Signs

The signs of CN dysfunction are the deficits of normal function demonstrated by the physical examination. The signs of CN dysfunction can be mimicked by nonneurologic end-organ diseases that must be searched for as part of *the head and neck examination* discussed in Chapter 7. Therefore, these signs are discussed fully in Chapter 7. Once end-organ disease is excluded, the challenge is to decide whether the neurologic lesion is central (brain) or peripheral (nerve). The following is a brief list of some specific CN signs.

> **KEY SIGN** **Anosmia—Olfactory Nerve (CN I)**

see Chapter 7, page 254.

> **KEY SIGN** **Visual Field Loss—Optic Nerve (CN II)**

see Chapter 7, page 234.

> **KEY SIGN** **Abnormalities of Gaze. Oculomotor (CN III), Trochlear (CN IV) and/or Abducens (CN VI) Nerve**

see Chapter 7, page 230ff and Figure 14–16. Unilateral complete paralysis is usually caused by direct pressure from tumor, aneurysm, or herniating brain. Less

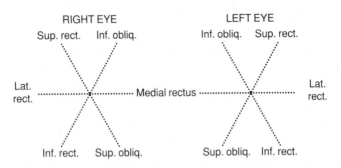

Fig. 14–16 The Cardinal Positions of Gaze. *Each of the six positions is the result of synergists and antagonists acting with a specific muscle. Paralysis of the specific muscle prevents the eye from attaining the cardinal position for the muscle.*

common are cavernous sinus thrombosis and granulomatous process at the base of the brain, for example, tuberculous meningitis and Tolosa-Hunt syndrome. Transient pupillary-sparing oculomotor and abducens nerve palsies may complicate diabetes mellitus.

KEY SIGN   Abnormal Pupils

Oculomotor nerve (CN III), Optic nerve (CN II), or cervical sympathetic chain, see Chapter 7, page 241ff.

KEY SIGN   Abnormal Corneal Reflex

Trigeminal (CN V) and/or Facial (CN VII) nerves. The corneal reflex is a bilateral reflex testing the fifth and seventh CN on the side stimulated and the seventh consensually. With an afferent (CN V) lesion, the response from both sides will be depressed. With an ipsilateral efferent (CN VII) lesion, the direct reflex is lost, but the consensual is preserved.

KEY SIGN   Jaw Weakness and Spasm

Trigeminal nerve (CN V). Jaw closure may be weak and/or asymmetric. The jaw jerk may be absent or hyperreflexic. Irritative lesions of the motor root may cause spasm or trismus.

KEY SIGN   Facial Weakness and Paralysis

Facial nerve (CN VII). Because the LMNs of the lids and forehead are innervated bilaterally by the UMNs, UMN lesions do not affect the upper lid or forehead. The following are key observations to help localize the lesion and resulting functional impairments: (1) Face in repose: shallow nasolabial folds in both UMN and LMN; palpebral fissure widened in LMN; (2) Eyebrow elevation and forehead wrinkling is absent in LMN, but present in UMN; (3) Frowning: lowering of the eyebrow is absent in LMN, present in UMN; (4) Tight closing of an eye is absent in LMN, with an associated upturning of the unclosed eye (*Bell phenomenon*).

The lids close normally in UMN. When the eyes are tightly closed, weakness of one upper lid can be detected by forcing the lids open with the thumb. Irritation of the cornea (*keratitis*) and conjunctivae (*keratoconjunctivitis sicca*) may occur as a result of inadequate lid closing; (5) Showing teeth: the lips do not retract fully in either UMN or LMN (see Fig. 14–1C); (6) Whistling and puffing cheeks are absent or diminished in both UMN and LMN. Weakness may be manifest by pocketing of food in the cheeks and difficulty with efficient mastication; and (7) A natural smile: the lips and corners of the mouth do not fully elevate with LMN lesions. The paralysis of the mouth is overcome by motions responding to emotion, so a symmetrical smile may occur in UMN disease. Abnormalities of taste will accompany LMN lesions. Facial spasm, clonic contractions of the facial muscles, may occur following partial denervation of the facial muscles.

CLINICAL OCCURRENCE: The cause of peripheral palsies of the facial nerve is usually unproven. They occasionally occur in sarcoidosis, tumors of the temporal bone and cerebellopontine angle, poliomyelitis and post-polio syndrome, neoplasms, infectious polyneuritis (Guillain-Barré syndrome), Lyme disease, herpes simplex, AIDS, and syphilis. In the *Ramsay-Hunt syndrome*, varicella-zoster virus infects the geniculate ganglion of the sensory branch of the facial nerve to produce a facial palsy, loss of taste on the anterior two-thirds of the tongue, and pain and vesicles in the external auditory canal on the same side. Herpetic lesions in the ear canal is the clue to diagnosis. Idiopathic facial nerve paralysis is *Bell palsy.*

KEY SIGN **Abnormal Hearing—Auditory Nerve (CN VIII)**

see page 223.

KEY SIGN **Abnormal Balance. Auditory Nerve (CN VIII)**

see page 223.

KEY SIGN **Dysarthria**

Glossopharyngeal (CN IX) and/or Vagus (CN X) Nerve: Patients will have difficulty with articulation and the pharyngeal phase of swallowing. Examination shows poor and/or asymmetric elevation of the soft palate and uvula. Absence of elevation indicates bilateral paralysis while unilateral elevation deviates the uvula toward the strong side (see Fig. 14–1D).

KEY SIGN **Dysphagia—Glossopharyngeal (CN IX) and/or Vagus (CN X) Nerve**

See Chapter 7, page 291. Laryngeal paralysis (CN X, recurrent laryngeal nerve) may cause coughing or reflux into the posterior nose when swallowing liquids.

KEY SIGN **Hoarseness—Vagus Nerve (CN X)**

See Chapter 7, pages 272 and 294. Hoarseness may indicate unilateral vocal cord paralysis, while dyspnea and inspiratory stridor are associated with bilateral involvement.

> **KEY SIGN** **Sternocleidomastoid and Trapezius Weakness**

Accessory Nerve (CN XI). Patients will have weakness of head rotation and shoulder shrug.

> **KEY SIGN** **Tongue Deviation and Wasting**

Hypoglossal Nerve (CN XII), see page 266.

Motor Signs

Most abnormal movements are responses of normal muscle to abnormal neural control signals.

> **KEY SIGN** **Weakness—Muscle Paralysis, Paresis, and Palsy**

Paralysis is defined as complete loss and *paresis* as diminution of muscle power from abnormalities of the UMN, LMN, peripheral nerve or muscle fibers. *Palsy* is a nonspecific descriptive term that indicates varying degrees of paralysis and/or paresis. Increased tone and uninhibited reflexes (*spasticity*) occur with UMN lesions, whereas LMN and peripheral nerve lesions result in *flaccid paralysis* and *muscle wasting*. Primary disease of muscle is associated with flaccid paralysis and variable changes in muscle bulk. It is essential to take a careful history to assess the onset of paralysis: acute, subacute, or chronic.

✒ *MUSCLE PARALYSIS—CLINICAL OCCURRENCE:* *Congenital* porphyria, muscular dystrophy, familial periodic paralysis, paramyotonia congenita, cerebral palsy; *Endocrine* hyperthyroidism; *Idiopathic* noninflammatory myopathies; *Inflammatory/Immune* Guillain-Barré syndrome, chronic idiopathic demyelinating polyneuropathy, myasthenia gravis, polymyositis, dermatomyositis, multiple sclerosis (MS), vasculitis; *Infectious* poliomyelitis, post-polio syndrome, West Nile virus; *Metabolic/Toxic* electrolyte disturbances (high or low potassium, magnesium, calcium, low copper), drugs (muscle relaxants, anesthetics, aminoglycosides-rarely), heavy metal poisoning, beriberi, anemia, pernicious anemia, amyloidosis; *Mechanical/Trauma* brain and spinal cord trauma, peripheral nerve trauma; *Neoplastic* epidural metastases; *Neurologic* polyneuropathy, transverse myelitis; *Psychosocial* hysteria, malingering; *Vascular* stroke, spinal cord infarction, subdural and epidural bleeding, vasculitis.

Muscle Wasting: Loss of the trophic effect of motor nerves on muscle fibers results in the severe muscle wasting typical of LMN lesions. A lesser degree of wasting results from peripheral nerve injury and much less with UMN lesions. Wasting becomes apparent weeks to months following the nerve injury. *Fasciculations* (see below) are seen with LMN lesions, but are absent with UMN lesions. Generalized weakness and wasting accompanied by fasciculations, often most evident in the tongue and small muscles of the hands, along with UMN signs, suggest primary motor neuron disease, for example, amyotrophic lateral sclerosis. Segmental disease is characteristic of poliomyelitis, West Nile virus and diseases of the spinal cord and nerve plexuses.

KEY SIGN   Hypotonia

Decreased resting muscle tone occurs with LMN injury, such as poliomyelitis, a root syndrome, and peripheral neuropathy. It is also encountered in cerebellar and other central lesions.

KEY SIGN   Hypertonia

Extrapyramidal lesions, such as parkinsonism, produce increased resting muscle tone.

Cogwheel Rigidity: On passive motion of a limb, the examiner feels muscular resistance as a series of stepwise relaxation-arrest cycles, rather than a smooth giving way. This is an expression of the increased muscle tone in Parkinson disease. It disappears during sleep.

KEY SIGN   Spasticity

In UMN paralysis, uninhibited stretch reflexes produce continuous clonic contraction (spasticity) when the muscle is stretched. When the limb is moved against its spastic muscles, the resistance may suddenly cease, giving a *clasp-knife* effect. Long, continued spasticity results in muscle fibrosis and shortening, known as *contracture.*

KEY SIGN   Myoclonus

A single, sudden jerk, or a short series, occurring succession, may be so powerful as to throw the patient to the floor. Unlike tremor, myoclonus may not disappear with sleep and is frequent at sleep onset. It is a common complication of chronic meperidine use and other metabolic encephalopathies.

KEY SIGN   Myotonia

The muscles continue in contraction after a voluntary or reflex action has ceased. Similarly, relaxation of a contraction induced by tapping the muscle belly with a reflex hammer is prolonged. After shaking hands, the fingers are slow to relax. When the fingers are flexed on the supinated palm, attempted extension is slow and difficult. The movement is typical of myotonia congenita and myotonic dystrophy [Nanayakkara PW, Hartdorff CM, Steovwer CD, et al. A man with fever and a persistent handgrip. *Lancet.* 2003;362:1038].

KEY SIGN   Tetany

The threshold for muscular excitability is lowered such that involuntary sustained contractions occur, either painless or painful. Any cause of a low ionized serum calcium can result in tetany, including hypoparathyroidism, acute hyperventilation, and hypomagnesemia. The contracting muscles feel rigid and unyielding. Spasm may be preceded by numbness and tingling in the lips and limbs. Contractions of the hands and feet are collectively termed *carpopedal spasm.* In carpal spasm, the wrist is flexed and flexion at the metacarpophalangeal joints is combined with extension of the interphalangeal joints. The hyperextended fingers are also adducted to form a cone and the thumb is flexed on the palm. In latent tetany, carpal spasm may be induced by occluding the brachial artery for 3 minutes with an inflated sphygmomanometer cuff; tetany induced by this maneuver is called the *Trousseau sign*. Tapping the facial nerve against the bone just anterior to the ear produces ipsilateral contraction of facial muscles; this is *Chvostek sign*. It is uniformly present in latent tetany, but contraction occurs in some normal persons.

> **KEY SIGN   Fasciculations**

Damage to the nerve supplying a muscle results in spontaneous motor unit firing that is visible as a twitching of muscle fibers. Coarse twitches are often caused by exposure to cold, fatigue, or other conditions, and are not serious. Fasciculations must be carefully sought when the muscle is relaxed because they are not powerful enough to move a joint or a part. In the presence of muscle wasting or weakness, their presence is attributable to progressive denervation of the muscle. *Fibrillations* are twitches of individual muscle fibers; they are invisible, but can be demonstrated by electromyography.

Reflex Signs
Abnormal Reflexes in Pyramidal Tract Disease

> **KEY SIGN   Altered Normal Reflexes**

A lesion of the pyramidal tract almost invariably causes complete suppression of the normal superficial reflexes caudal to the level of the lesion. On the contrary, the muscle stretch reflexes are hyperactive except during the acute stage of damage, as in spinal shock, when they are absent.

Clonus and Spasticity: Normally central inhibition of the spinal cord limits the stretch reflex to a single beat. Loss of inhibition allows the reflex to become self-perpetuating. Spasticity occurs with complete loss of cortical inhibition, leading to sustained contractions of opposing muscle groups, the flexors dominating in the arms, and the extensors in the back and legs. A hyperactive reflex may produce clonus, a rhythmic contraction of muscles initiated by stretching. Clonus may be unsustained, lasting for only a few jerks despite continued stretching, or it may be sustained (more than seven beats), persisting as long as stretching is applied.

   Ankle Clonus: With the patient's knee flexed, grasp the foot and briskly dorsiflex it. Rhythmic contractions of the gastrocnemius and soleus cause the foot to alternate between dorsiflexion and plantar flexion (see Fig. 14–8C).

   Patellar Clonus: With the patient supine and the relaxed lower limb extended, grasp the patella and push it quickly distal. The patella will jerk up and down from the rhythmic contractions of the quadriceps femoris.

   Wrist Clonus: Grasp the patient's fingers and forcibly hyperextend the wrist. The wrist will alternate rhythmically between flexion and extension due to contraction of the wrist flexors.

   Hoffmann Sign—Finger Flexor Reflex: This is also called the finger flexor reflex and has the same significance as other muscle stretch reflexes. Hold the patient's pronated hand in your hand, with fingers extended and

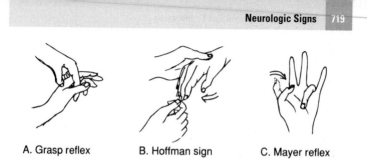

A. Grasp reflex   B. Hoffman sign   C. Mayer reflex

Fig. 14–17 *Some Pathologic Reflexes. See text for descriptions.* **A. Grasp reflex:** *In lesions of the premotor cortex, the patient may be unable to release her grasp.* **B. Hoffmann sign:** *In pyramidal tract disease, the patient's thumb may flex and adduct asymmetrically.* **C. Mayer reflex:** *Have the patient present her relaxed supinated hand to you. Firmly flex the ring finger at the metacarpophalangeal joint. The normal response is adduction and flexion of the thumb. Absence of this occurs in pyramidal tract disease.*

relaxed. Support the patient's extended middle finger by your right index finger held transversely under the distal interphalangeal joint crease (Fig. 14–17B). With your thumb, press the patient's fingernail to flex the terminal digit. The abnormal reflex is flexion and adduction of the thumb. The other fingers may also flex. When the reflex is present bilaterally, it may be a normal variant.

Babinski Sign: Perform the test for the plantar reflex, page 706. Alternate methods of eliciting Babinski reflex have been described as eponymic signs. In the *Oppenheim sign*, great toe dorsiflexion is elicited with pressure applied by the thumb and index finger or knuckles to the anterior tibia. The pressure stroke should begin at the upper two-thirds of the bone and be continued to the ankle. In *Chaddock sign*, the stimulus is a scratch with a dull point. The path of stimulation should curve around the lateral malleolus of the ankle, then along the lateral aspect of the dorsum of the foot. If a dull stimulus does not elicit the sign, a painful stimulus should be used such as the scratch of a pin. The normal response is plantar flexion of the toes and foot. The complete Babinski sign is: (1) dorsiflexion of the great toe, (2) fanning of all toes, (3) dorsiflexion of the ankle, and (4) flexion and withdrawal of the knee and hip. All of these signs are pathologic responses to noxious stimuli in or spreading to the S1 dermatome. Partial responses include only dorsiflexion of the great toe, failure of the small toes to abduct or fan, and fanning of small toes without great toe dorsiflexion. Complete and partial responses are all indicative of different degrees of pyramidal disease, so the details of response should be accurately recorded.

Primitive Reflexes (Release Signs)

All of these signs may indicate diffuse cerebral disease, but are sometimes present in normal individuals.

Grasp Reflex: Place your index and middle fingers between the patient's thumb and index finger, laying them across the patient's palm. Gently pull them across the palm with a stroking motion. Grasping with the thumb and index finger is a positive response (Fig. 14–17A). When the grasp reflex is present, the patient cannot release the fingers at will. Though normal in infants, in adults it indicates a lesion of the premotor cortex.

Palmomental Reflex: Scratching or pricking of the thenar eminence causes ipsilateral contraction of the muscles of the chin. This occurs in diffuse cerebral disease.

Snout/Suck Reflexes: Scratching or gentle percussion of the upper lip may induce a puckering or sucking movement.

Spinal Automatisms

Spinal automatisms occur when the central inhibitions of reflexes are lost in severe disease of the spinal cord or brain.

Spinal Reflex Reactions: In extensive lesions of the cord or midbrain, painful stimulation of a limb may produce ipsilateral flexion of both upper and lower extremities, called *ipsilateral mass flexion reflex*, spinal withdrawal, or shortening reflex.

Mass Reflex: A transverse lesion of the cord may produce flexion followed by extension of the limbs below the level of lesion. In complete transection, only flexion occurs, accompanied by contractions of the abdominal wall, incontinence of urine and feces, and autonomic responses, such as sweating, flushing, and pilomotor activity. This complex is termed *mass reflex*. Involuntary urination may be stimulated by stroking the skin of the thighs and abdomen, an *automatic bladder*. Priapism and seminal ejaculation may be induced by similar mechanisms. In the *crossed extensor reflex*, flexion of one limb may be associated with extension of its counterpart. In some cases, the *extensor thrust reaction* is encountered: pressure on the sole causes extension of the leg. When the leg is placed in flexion, scratching on the skin of the thigh induces extension of the leg. Painful stimulation of the arm or chest may result in abduction and outward rotation of the shoulder.

► **KEY SIGN**   **Signs of Meningeal Irritation**

Irritation of the meninges by meningitis, subarachnoid hemorrhage, drugs, and increased intracranial pressure cause abnormal contraction of various muscle groups, which are identified on physical examination.

Nuchal Rigidity: The patient cannot place the chin on the chest. Passive flexion of the neck is limited by involuntary muscle spasm, while passive extension and rotation are normal.

Kernig Sign: With the patient supine, passively flex the hip to 90 degrees while the knee is flexed at about 90 degrees (Fig. 14–18A). With the hip kept in flexion, attempts to extend the knee produce pain in the hamstrings and resistance to further extension. This is a reliable sign of meningeal irritation, which may occur with meningitis, herniated disk, or tumors of the cauda equina.

Brudzinski Sign: With the patient supine and the limbs extended, passively flex the neck. Flexion of the hips, a sign of meningeal irritation, is a positive Brudzinski sign (Fig. 14–18B).

Spinal Rigidity: Movements of the spine are limited by spasms of the erector spinae. In extreme cases, the spinal muscles are in tetanic contraction,

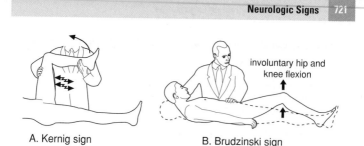

A. Kernig sign   B. Brudzinski sign

Fig. 14–18 *Two Signs of Meningeal Irritation. A. Kernig sign:* With the patient supine, flex the hip and knee, each to about 90 degrees. With the hip immobile, attempt to extend the knee. In meningeal irritation, this attempt is resisted and causes pain in the hamstring muscles. *B. Brudzinski sign:* Place the patient supine and hold the thorax down on the bed. Attempt to flex the neck. With meningeal irritation this causes involuntary flexion of the hips.

producing rigid hyperextension of the entire spine with the head forced backward and the trunk thrust forward. The condition is termed *opisthotonos*.

Posture, Balance, and Coordination Signs: Cerebellar Signs

Perfect execution of skilled acts is *eupraxia*. *Apraxia*, the loss of previous skills, is the inability to convert an idea into a skilled act. Maintenance of postural equilibrium at rest and with movement requires the proper function of proprioceptive mechanisms, the vestibular apparatus, and the cerebellum. Loss of coordination in maintaining proper posture is *ataxia*. The patient who is incoordinate lying down has *static ataxia;* if the condition is only evident on standing or moving, it is *kinetic ataxia*.

KEY SIGN Dysdiadochokinesis

Loss of the ability to arrest one motor impulse and substitute its opposite, dysdiadochokinesis, is characteristic of cerebellar disease (see page 697).

KEY SIGN Dyssynergia and Dysmetria

Failure to coordinate the contraction of synergistic muscle during a movement is *dyssynergia*. Inability to control the distance, power and speed of a movement is *dysmetria*. **Finger-to-Nose Test:** In cerebellar disease, this action is attended by an action tremor. When the maneuver is performed with the eyes closed, the sense of position in the shoulder and elbow is tested. **Heel-to-Shin Test:** In cerebellar disease, the arc of the heel to the knee is jerky and wavering, the knee is frequently overshot, and the slide down the shin is accompanied by an action tremor. In posterior column disease, the heel may have difficulty finding the knee, and the ride down the shin weaves from side to side, or the heel may fall off altogether.

KEY SIGN Wide Stance

Ataxia from proprioceptive, vestibular, or cerebellar disease is less when the patient stands on a broad base, the feet widely apart.

> **KEY SIGN** **Instability of Station**

Visual Compensation: Cerebellar ataxia is not ameliorated by visual orientation, while the ataxia from posterior column disease involves disordered proprioception and only appears or is worsened when the eyes are closed (*Romberg sign*). *Direction of Falling:* In disease of the lateral cerebellar lobes, falling is toward the affected side. Lesions of the cerebellar midline or vermis may cause falling indiscriminately, depending entirely on the initial stance of the patient.

> **KEY SIGN** **Gait Ataxia**

Gait is a complex activity requiring normal sensory input from the feet, spinal cord, and vestibular system, and normal motor and cerebellar function. Impairments in any of these systems leads to characteristic changes in the gait. Careful inspection of gait can greatly aid identification of the site of the lesion.

Cerebellar Ataxia: The gait is staggering, wavering, and lurching walk and not visually compensated. With a lesion in the mid-cerebellum, instability is in all directions; when one lobe is involved, staggering is toward the affected side. The ataxia is partially compensated by a wide base. Ataxia secondary to vestibular disease may appear similar.

Impaired Proprioception: The gait and stance are facilitated by a wide stance. In walking, the feet are lifted too high, and frequently are set down with excessive force. The eyes are used to compensate for loss of proprioception, so the ataxia is much greater with the eyes closed. The lesion may be in peripheral sensory nerves (e.g., diabetes) or posterior column of the spinal cord (e.g., vitamin B_{12} or copper deficiency, tabes dorsalis); in either case, proprioceptive impulses to the brain are defective.

Dementia: Ataxia of gait in patients without dementia predicts a significantly increased risk for the development of non-Alzheimer dementia during a follow-up of over 6 years [Verghese J, Lipton RB, Hall CB, et al. Abnormality of gait as a predictor of non-Alzheimer's dementia. *N Engl J Med.* 2002;347:1761–1768].

Foot Drop (Steppage Gait): Paralysis of the ankle dorsiflexors causes the foot to slap down onto the floor. To compensate for the toe drop, the patient must raise the thigh higher, as if walking upstairs. Unilateral toe drop usually results from injury of the peroneal nerve. Bilateral paralysis may occur from polyneuropathies, poliomyelitis, lesions of the cauda equina, or peroneal atrophy in Charcot-Marie-Tooth disease.

Peroneal Muscular Atrophy—Charcot-Marie-Tooth Disease: This is a hereditary disease of unknown cause. Presenting symptoms are foot drop, pain, weakness, numbness and paresthesias of the lower legs. The syndrome is slowly progressive with clawfoot and foot drop, from weak peronei, tibialis anterior, and extensor longus digitorum. Muscle stretch reflexes are absent and there is cutaneous hypesthesia and the steppage gait. The forearm may be affected.

Hemiplegic Gait: The patient walks with the affected lower limb extended at the hip, knee, and ankle, and the foot inverted. The thigh may swing in a lateral arc (*circumduction*) or the patient may push the inverted foot along the floor.

Spastic Gait, Scissors Gait: In paraparesis with adductor spasm, the knees are pulled together so the body must sway laterally away from the stepping limb to allow it to clear the floor. The feet may overstep each other laterally, alternately crossing across the line of travel with each step.

Parkinsonian Gait (*Festinating Gait*): The trunk and neck are rigid and flexed. The arm swing is diminished or lost unilaterally or bilaterally. The steps are short and shuffling and become faster in an attempt to avoid falling forward (chasing the center of gravity: *festination*). Turns are slow and in-block, without evident turning of the head on the trunk or the trunk on the pelvis.

Magnetic Gait: The stance is wide and the steps are short and shuffling. The feet are not lifted from the floor, as if held down by magnets. This indicates diffuse cerebral disease or multisystem damage.

Huntington Chorea: Walking is attended by grotesque movements caused by the interposition of purposeless involuntary chorea on gait movements.

Waddling Gait—Muscular Dystrophy: The patient walks with a broad base. The thighs are thrown forward by twisting the pelvis to compensate for the weak quadriceps muscles. A similar gait is employed by those with bilateral dislocations of the hips.

> **KEY SIGN** Tremors

Coarse, poorly coordinated, contractions of opposing muscle groups are unable to maintain stable posture and/or smooth movement resulting in oscillating movements at one or more joints. The amplitude may be either fine or coarse, and the rate either rapid or slow. Movements may be rhythmic or irregular. All tremors disappear during sleep. Examine the affected part at rest with the muscles relaxed (repose), with maintenance of posture against gravity and with movement.

Essential Tremor: This is an accentuation of the normal fine motor movements made to maintain posture. It is accentuated with increased adrenergic stimulation of muscle and may be a familial trait. All persons have this tremor, but it is usually at an amplitude below the limit of visible detection. It is accentuated with anxiety and is characteristic of hyperthyroidism and alcohol withdrawal. The tremor is rapid and fine. It is absent is repose and accentuated by trying to maintain a posture [Pahwa R, Lyons KE. Essential tremor: Differential diagnosis and current therapy. *Am J Med*. 2003;115:134–142; Louis ED. Essential tremor. *N Engl J Med*. 2001;345:887–891].

Parkinson Tremor: This is a result of damage to the extrapyramidal motor system of the substantia nigra in Parkinson disease. The tremor is present at rest and diminished or absent with movement. It is slow and coarse, and often described as "pill-rolling" from the characteristic movements of the fingers and wrist. Parkinson tremor is usually asymmetric at onset [Utti RJ. Tremor: How to determine if the patient has Parkinson's disease. *Geriatrics*. 1998;53:30–36].

Cerebellar Tremor: Poor cerebellar coordination of muscle contraction associated with movement leads to limb oscillation, often accentuated with attempts at fine control. Action or intention tremor occurs in MS and cerebellar disease in which voluntary movements initiate and sustain a slow oscillation of wide amplitude.

> **KEY SIGN** Tics

Normal movements of muscle groups, such as grimacing, winking, or shoulder shrugging, are repeated at inappropriate times. The reaction is stereotyped for the individual. Tics may be acquired behavioral habits or a sign of organic disease, for example, Tourette syndrome. They may be abolished by diverting the patient's attention and they disappear during sleep.

> **KEY SIGN** Dyskinesia

Dyskinesias are complex abnormalities of muscle movement. They are centrally mediated. Several characteristic patterns are recognized:

Chorea: Rapid, purposeless, jerky, asynchronous movements involve various parts of the body. Although some are spontaneous, many are initiated and all are accentuated by voluntary acts, as in extending the arms or walking. They commonly occur in both Sydenham and Huntington chorea; in the latter, the movements are coarser and more bizarre. They disappear with sleep.

Athetosis: In contrast to choreiform movements, these are slower and writhing, resembling the actions of a worm or snake. The distal parts of the limb are more active than the proximal. Grimaces are more deliberate than in chorea. The grotesque athetoid hand is produced by flexion of some digits with others extended. They disappear with sleep. The mechanism is not understood, but the movements are frequently associated with diseases of the basal ganglia and levodopa therapy for Parkinson disease.

Hemiballismus: One side of the body is affected by sustained, violent, involuntary flinging movements of the limbs. These result from a lesion in the contralateral *subthalamic nucleus of Luys*, usually secondary to stroke. They disappear with sleep.

> **KEY SIGN** Asterixis

When the arms are held straight forward from the shoulders with the fingers and wrists extended and fingers spread, there is sudden loss of wrist and interphalangeal extensor tone. This loss and regaining of tone results in a flapping motion. The fingers deviate laterally and exhibit a fine tremor. A similar flap occurs at the ankle when the leg is elevated and the foot dorsiflexed. Ask the obtunded patient to squeeze two of the examiner's fingers; asterixis is felt as an alternately clenching and unclenching grip. Asterixis occurs in any form of metabolic encephalopathy including liver failure, uremia, and hypercapnia as a consequence of respiratory failure.

> **KEY SIGN** Muscle Cramps—Dystonias

See page 755.

> **KEY SIGN** Lost Associated Movements (Synkinesia)

Associated movements, or *synkinesias*, are involuntary motor patterns, more complex than reflexes, that normally accompany voluntary acts: examples include swinging the arms while walking, facial movements of expression, and motions accompanying coughing and yawning. Frequently, these are lost in disease of the pyramidal tract or the basal ganglia; for example, the patient with parkinsonism walks without swinging the arms. An early sign of corticospinal tract damage may be loss of synkinetic movements. Knowledge of normal and abnormal patterns of synkinesis can assist in the identification of the patient with factitious neurologic illness. The detailed testing of synkinesis is beyond the scope of this text. The reader should consult textbooks of neurologic diagnosis.

Sensory Signs

Loss of normal sensation can result from injury to either the peripheral or CNS. The distribution of the sensory loss, the modalities involved and the presence or absence of motor involvement are useful in distinguishing peripheral nerve from plexus, root, and central injury.

> **KEY SIGN** Abnormal Pain Sensation

Changes in pain sensation can result from injury to any portion of the pain pathway (peripheral nerve, spinal cord, or brain). Sensibility to pain may be normal, reduced (*hypalgesia*), absent (*analgesia*), or increased (*hyperalgesia*).

Allodynia: Allodynia indicates damage to the sensory pathways, usually in the dorsal root or spinal cord; it is not a sign of peripheral nerve injury. *Allodynia* (*allo* = differing from normal; *dynia* = pain) is the perception of pain with stimuli that are normally not painful such as light touch or vibration. Patients complain of pain with the touch of clothing or bedding and with weight bearing on the feet. Lightly touch and stroke the skin over the suspected area and apply a tuning fork to look for allodynia. Use a mildly uncomfortable stimulus like the sharp end of a broken tongue depressor to elicit hyperesthesia. DDX: Allodynia (pain with normally nonpainful stimuli) indicates damage to sensory nerves and is commonly seen with post-herpetic neuralgia, diabetic radiculopathy, and complex regional pain syndrome.

Hyperalgesia: The skin is stroked lightly with the point of a sterile pin and asked if the sensation is painful. Observe the patient's facial expression for signs of discomfort. Alternatively, a fold of skin is plucked lightly between thumb and index finger, pulling the fold of skin away from the underlying tissue; care should be taken not to pinch the skin. The sensation is more intense, but not painful in areas of cutaneous hyperesthesia.

Analgesia and Hypalgesia: Decreased or absent pain sensation indicates damage to the peripheral or central pain pathways. The distribution of the lost sensation (peripheral nerve, deratome) will indicate the level of the lesion. Look for loss of other modalities, especially temperature and touch.

Hysterical Anesthesia: Hysteria may be revealed by outlining the borders of an area of "anesthesia" stimulating from the center to the border in a zigzagging line and then in the opposite direction; also repeat the test after examining other areas. Disparities between successive tests supports this diagnosis.

Loss of Pain and Temperature Sensation: Pain and temperature fibers cross near their entry into the cord. Disruption of the crossing fibers leads to loss of these modalities with preservation of other regional sensation. Ask the patient to distinguish between hot and cold. Temperature and pain discrimination is lost in syringomyelia while tactile sense is retained.

> **KEY SIGN** **Tactile Extinction Test**

In parietal lobe disease, the patient may perceive touch accurately when the stimulation is applied to the right and left consecutively; if the points are stimulated simultaneously, the patient no longer perceives, or *extinguishes*, the affected side.

> **KEY SIGN** **Loss of Position and Vibration Sense**

Position and vibration sense are carried in the posterior columns of the spinal cord. Damage to the posterior columns results in impaired proprioception leading to abnormalities in stance and gait. Posterior column diseases include vitamin B_{12} or copper deficiency and tabes dorsalis.

> **KEY SIGN** **Loss of Integrative Function—Astereognosis**

Inability to recognize familiar objects by touch is astereognosis. Assuming the primary sensory modalities are intact, it is a sign of cortical disease, an inability to integrate the multiple inputs.

Autonomic Nervous System Signs

Temperature Regulation: See Chapter 4, page 51ff. Some instances of hyperthermia occur from hypothalamus or high cervical cord lesions. Hypothermia is encountered in insulin shock and myxedema, although the role of the autonomics in the latter condition is doubtful.

Perspiration: Localized areas of sweating may occur in syringomyelia, peripheral nerve injury, or neuropathy. *Anhidrosis* is a component of Horner syndrome, autonomic insufficiency (severe combined degeneration), and anticholinergic medications or poisoning. Increased perspiration can be seen with use of β-blockers.

> **KEY SIGN** **Trophic Disturbances**

Loss of innervation leads to functional deficiencies of the sweat and oil glands of the skin. Combined with decreased sensation, the skin is more vulnerable to injury and infection. The skin becomes shiny, smooth, thin, and dry. Painless ulcers may develop over bony prominences of the feet in peripheral neuropathy from diabetes or tabes dorsalis, and syringomyelia (see Fig. 14–12F). Charcot joints (Chapter 13, page 670) are a neuropathic arthropathy caused by loss of proprioception and protective sensation required to maintain joint alignment.

Pilomotor Reactions: Scratching the midaxillary skin produces pilomotor erection (gooseflesh). The normal response is abolished below the level of a transverse cord lesion. An exaggerated reaction may occur on the affected side in hemiplegia.

> **KEY SIGN** **Blood Pressure Regulation**

See Chapter 4, page 72ff. Orthostatic hypotension without tachycardia is common with autonomic nervous system diseases.

> **KEY SIGN** **Bladder/Bowel Function**

Patients with autonomic nervous system diseases often lose control of bladder and bowel function producing incontinence and/or urinary and fecal retention.

Some Peripheral Nerve Signs

> **KEY SIGN** **Sciatic Nerve Signs**

Sciatica: See Chapter 13, page 678.

Weak Ankle Plantar Flexion—Tibial Nerve Palsy (Sciatic Component): The tibial nerve is the motor nerve to the *gastrocnemius* group and *intrinsic muscles in the sole of the foot*. Paralysis causes a calcaneovalgus deformity from the unopposed action of the dorsiflexors and evertors (Fig. 14–19A); plantar flexion and inversion of the foot are weak and the ankle jerk is absent. Since the nerve is sensory to the skin of the sole, damage results in an anesthetic sole vulnerable to pressure ulcers.

Weak Ankle Dorsiflexion—Common Peroneal Nerve Palsy (Sciatic Component): The common peroneal nerve is the motor nerve to the muscles of the anterior and lateral compartments of the leg and the short extensors of the toes; it is sensory to the dorsum of the foot and ankle. Peroneal paralysis causes an equinovarus deformity with inability to dorsiflex the foot and toes—a foot drop (Fig. 14–19B). An area of anesthesia covers the dorsum of the foot and sometimes extends up the lateral side of the leg. The nerve is susceptible to pressure injury where it winds around the fibular head.

> **KEY SIGN** **Femoral Nerve Sign**

Lack of Knee Extension: Femoral Nerve Palsy: The femoral nerve is the motor nerve for the *quadriceps femoris*. When the nerve is injured, patients cannot walk and standing is unstable. Extension of the knee is impossible (Fig. 14–19C). Anesthesia is widespread over the anteromedial aspect of the thigh, knee, leg, and the medial aspect of the foot.

> **KEY SIGN** **Shoulder Weakness**

Dorsal Scapular Nerve Paralysis: The nerve supplies the *rhomboids* that elevate and retract the scapula. These muscles ascend obliquely from the medial border of the scapula to the spinous processes of the upper thoracic vertebrae. Although covered by the trapezius, they may be palpated when the shoulders are drawn backward.

Suprascapular Nerve Paralysis: The nerve supplies the *supraspinatus* and the *infraspinatus*. Paralysis results in weakness in the first 30 degrees of shoulder abduction and of external rotation. Wasting of these muscles is seen as depressions above and below the scapular spine.

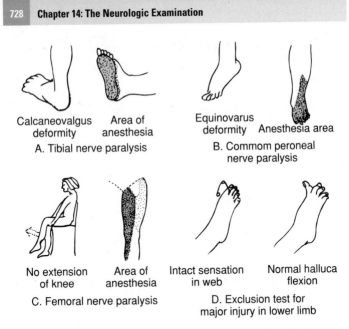

Calcaneovalgus   Area of
deformity   anesthesia
A. Tibial nerve paralysis

Equinovarus
deformity   Anesthesia area
B. Commom peroneal
nerve paralysis

No extension   Area of
of knee   anesthesia
C. Femoral nerve paralysis

Intact sensation   Normal halluca
in web   flexion
D. Exclusion test for
major injury in lower limb

Fig. 14–19 *Nerve Lesions of the Lower Limb. A. Tibial nerve paralysis:* The foot assumes the posture of calcaneovalgus from paralysis of the plantar flexors. The sole of the foot is anesthetic (blue). ***B. Common peroneal nerve Paralysis:*** The foot assumes the position of equinovarus; it cannot be dorsiflexed—a foot drop. The dorsum of the foot and frequently the lateral aspect of the leg, are anesthetic (blue). ***C. Femoral nerve paralysis:*** The knee cannot be extended when sitting. The region of anesthesia covers the major portion of the anterior thigh and medial aspect of the leg. ***D. Exclusion test for major nerve injury in lower limb:*** Sensation is intact in the web between the great toe and second toe; extension (dorsiflexion) of the great toe is normally performed.

Long Thoracic Nerve Paralysis: The nerve supplies the *serratus anterior* that holds the scapula to the thorax. Paralysis produces a winged scapula (see Fig. 13–40A, page 646) when the patient pushes forward against a wall.

Weak Abduction of the Arm—Axillary Nerve Paralysis: The *deltoid* is paralyzed and atrophied. Elevation of the arm above 30 degrees in 90 degrees of abduction is impossible. A patch of sensory loss on the lateral aspect of the shoulder is often found. This can result from humeral neck fracture, shoulder dislocation or scapular fracture.

Weak Adduction and Depression of the Arm—Anterior Thoracic Nerve Paralysis: This nerve supplies the *pectoralis major and minor*. Paralysis is demonstrated when the patient presses the hands down on the hips (Fig. 14–20B).

Weak Adduction and Depression of the Arm—Thoracodorsal Nerve Paralysis: This nerve innervates the *latissimus dorsi*. Paralysis is demonstrated by grasping the posterior axillary muscle fold just below the scapular angle when the patient coughs. Normally the muscle tenses (Fig. 14–20C), a *synkinesis*; failure to tense or asymmetry suggests nerve damage.

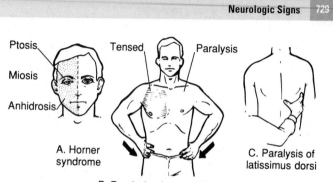

Fig. 14–20 *Nerve Lesions of the Upper Trunk. A. Horner syndrome:* Injury to the superior cervical sympathetic ganglion on one side causes ipsilateral ptosis of the eyelid, miosis, and anhidrosis of the face. *B. Paralysis of the pectoralis major muscle:* Injury to the anterior thoracic nerve causes paralysis of the pectoralis major and minor muscles. When the patient is asked to press the hands down on the hips, the normal pectoralis muscle is tensed but the paralyzed one is not. *C. Paralysis of the latissimus dorsi muscle:* The examiner grasps the latissimus muscles in his hands and asks the patient to cough. A paralyzed muscle does not tense with coughing.

Flail Arm (Erb-Duchenne Paralysis)—Brachial Plexus Injury: LMN paralysis of the brachial plexus may occur from forceful depression of the shoulder during birth or a blow on the shoulder later in life. The arm hangs limply with the fingers flexed and turned posteriorly, a *flail arm* (see Fig. 13–40, page 656). The biceps reflex is lost and there is muscle wasting. With partial recovery, motions of the elbow and hand may be regained.

> **KEY SIGN** Weak Elbow Flexion

Musculocutaneous Nerve Paralysis: The *biceps brachii* and *brachialis* are supplied by this nerve. Paralysis can usually be demonstrated by inspection of the arm when the elbow is flexed against resistance. A small area of anesthesia occurs on the volar surface of the forearm.

> **KEY SIGN** Radial Nerve Paralysis—Incomplete Extension of Wrist and Fingers

Motor deficits depend upon the level of injury. Injury in the axilla causes paralysis of the *triceps brachii, anconeus, brachioradialis*, and *extensor carpi radialis longus*. A lesion at the level of the upper third of the humerus spares the triceps while damage between the humeral upper third and 5 cm above the elbow also spares the brachioradialis. Innervation of the wrist extensors may be injured at a lower level. Any lesion involving the *extensor carpi radialis longus* prevents fixation at the wrist in grasping, producing a wrist-drop (Fig. 14–21A). Paralysis of the *extensor digitorum communis* prevents extension of the wrist and fingers with thumb and finger drop. When the deep branch of the radial nerve is injured, radial deviation of the wrist may occur without wrist-drop. Sensory loss on the dorsum of the hand extends from the radial border to the dorsum of the fifth metacarpal; the dorsum of the thumb is involved (Fig. 14–21B). The distribution of anesthesia

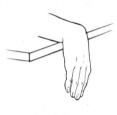

Wrist drop

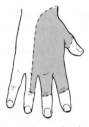

Area of anesthesia

Fig. 14–21 *Radial Nerve Paralysis.* *The extensors of the wrist are paralyzed, so the hand droops when it is placed at the end of the table with no support; this sign is called wrist-drop. The region of anesthesia includes the dorsal aspect of the radial three digits (blue shading).*

is quite irregular, but it usually includes dorsum of thumb to first phalanx and web. Injury commonly results from external pressure on the nerve in the spiral groove of the humerus (*Saturday night palsy*) or from fracture of the humerus.

> **KEY SIGN   Median Nerve Paralysis—Incomplete Flexion of Thumb and Fingers**

The nerve is exposed to trauma in the antecubital fossa. It supplies the flexors of the wrists, digits, and pronators of the forearm: pronator teres, pronator quadratus, flexor carpi radialis, flexor digitorum sublimis, flexor digitorum profundus (except the fourth and fifth digits), flexor pollicis brevis, flexor pollicis longus, opponens pollicis, lumbrical, abductor pollicis longus, and brevis. All these muscles are innervated below the elbow. The most common site of median nerve entrapment is at the carpal tunnel (see *Carpal Tunnel Syndrome* page 757).

> **KEY SIGN   Ulnar Nerve Paralysis—Adductor Weakness of Fingers**

The ulnar nerve is most vulnerable near the elbow where it curves posteriorly around the medial epicondyle. The chief motor disability from palsy is loss of the finer intrinsic motions of the hand. Inspection will show an abduction deformity of the little finger from paralysis of the interossei, interosseous muscle wasting, and partial clawhand from interphalangeal flexion deformities of the ring and little fingers.

Clawhand—Klumpke Paralysis: An LMN lesion at the brachial plexus or ulnar nerve produces paralysis of the intrinsic hand muscles results in the clawhand. Sensation on the ulnar aspect of the arm, forearm, and hand may be lost.

Neurologic Syndromes

Falling

> **KEY SYNDROME   Loss of Balance and Falls**

Falls are a common problem, especially at more than 75 years of age. Many patients will not volunteer information about falls; they must be asked. Maintaining balance requires normal proprioceptive sensory nerves and tracts, vestibular system, motor tracts and nerves, muscles, cerebellum, and basal ganglia. Major abnormalities in any one of these pathways can produce falls; more commonly, there are less severe impairments in several systems. When proprioceptive function is impaired, patients compensate with their eyes to locate themselves in space; visual impairment (including use of bi- and trifocal lenses) is a frequent contributor to falls. Skeletal abnormalities, especially of the joints, are a common precipitant. Decreased mentation and reaction times because of drugs (e.g., benzodiazepines, anticholinergics) or aging frequently contribute to a risk of falling. A complete neurologic examination is required to identify all the contributing abnormalities. Prevention of falls is a major focus of the geriatric assessment. The major risk for falls in the future is a history of previous falls [Ganz DA, Bao Y, Shekelle PS, et al. Will my patient fall? *JAMA*. 2007;297:77–86].

Headache

> **KEY SYNDROME** Headache

The head contains many pain-sensitive structures, most innervated by the trigeminal nerve (CN V). Mechanisms of headache include inflammation, infection, arterial dilation, hemorrhage, changes of pressure within closed spaces, expanding mass lesions producing traction or compression of structures, trauma, tissue ischemia, and tissue destruction. The common extracranial cause of headache is sustained contraction of the muscles of the head, neck, and shoulders. Headache refers to more than momentarily pain in the cranial vault, orbits or nape of the neck; pain elsewhere in the face is not included. An urgent search for serious pathology is required if a severe headache is unlike any experienced in the past [Steiner TJ, Fontebasso M. Headache. *BMJ*. 2002;325:881–886].

HEADACHE—CLINICAL OCCURRENCE: **Congenital** arteriovenous malformations, hydrocephalus; **Endocrine** pheochromocytoma; **Idiopathic** idiopathic intracranial hypertension; **Inflammatory/Immune** giant cell arteritis, sarcoidosis; **Infectious** meningitis, encephalitis, rickettsial infections, sinusitis, otitis, mastoiditis, non-CNS viral infections (e.g., influenza, cytomegalovirus, varicella), parasites (e.g., malaria, neurocysticercosis), protozoa (e.g., toxoplasmosis); **Metabolic/Toxic** analgesic rebound headache, hypoxia, hypercapnia, hypoglycemia, alcohol and illicit drug withdrawal, carbon monoxide poisoning, caffeine abstinence; **Mechanical/Trauma** accelerated and malignant hypertension, trauma (concussion), muscule tension, temporomandibular joint disease, increased intracranial pressure, glaucoma, decreased intracranial pressure (cerebrospinal fluid [CSF] leak); **Neoplastic** primary and metastatic brain tumors; **Neurologic** migraine, cluster headache, paroxysmal hemicrania, trigeminal neuralgia, occipital neuralgia; **Psychosocial** stress; **Vascular** migraine, intracranial aneurysm, hemorrhage (intracerebral, subdural, epidural, and subarachnoid), venous sinus thrombosis, stoke, cerebral vasculitis.

Clinical Examination for Headache

History: Inquire carefully for the attributes of pain (PQRST): **Provocative and Palliative Factors** trauma, medications, substance abuse, position of the head and body, coughing, straining, emotional state, relief with massage, and resolution with sleep; **Quality** whether burning, aching, deep or superficial, lancinating, throbbing, or continuous; *Region Involved and Radiation* cranial, facial, orbital, unilateral, bilateral; *Severity* use the 1 to 10 scale; and *Timing* when headaches began, frequency, time of day, duration, pattern of intensity. Inquire about family members with a headache history. Identify associated symptoms, for example, fever, stiff neck, nausea and vomiting, constipation or diarrhea, diuresis, rhinorrhea, visual disturbances (e.g., photophobia, scotomata, tearing, diplopia), cerebral symptoms (e.g., confusion, slurred speech, aura, paresthesias, anesthesias, motor paralysis, vertigo, mood, and sleep disturbances). *Physical Examination:* Inspect the skin and scalp for bulges and areas of erythema. With deep pressure palpate and percuss the bones of the cranium and face for tenderness and irregularities of contour. Palpate the neck muscles and the upper borders of the trapezii for tenderness. Palpate the carotid and temporal arteries for pulsations and tenderness. Examine the eyes for pupil contour and response to light and near point, conjunctival injection or abnormal extraocular motion; use the confrontation test (page 200) to detect gross defects in the visual fields. Examine the fundus for choked disks and retinal hemorrhages. Auscultate the cranium for bruits. Perform a thorough neurologic examination with special attention to the CN and the deep tendon reflexes.

► **KEY SYNDROME**   Thunderclap Headache

The sudden onset of a severe excruiating headache that at maximal intensity within seconds of onset is often termed a thunderclap headache. A first severe headache meeting this description must be evaluated urgently. If accompanied by a change in the level of consciousness, nausea, visual changes, vertigo, paralysis or paresthesias, the likelihood of a serious intracranial problem is increased. [Linn FH, Wijdicks EF. Causes and management of thunderclap headache: A comprehensive review. *Neurologist* (United States). 2002;8:279–289] *CLINICAL OCCURRENCE:* Classically, this is attributed to subarachnoid hemorrhage, but it may occur with intracerebral hemorrhage, migraine, cluster headache, stroke, with intercourse (*coital headache*), cerebral venous thrombosis or cerebral vasoconstriction [Calabrese LH, Docick DW, Schwedt TJ, et al. Narravtive review: Reversible cerebral vasoconstriction syndromes. *Ann Intern Med.* 2007;146: 34–44].

KEY SYNDROME   Traction, Displacement, Inflammation Causing Intracranial Headaches

The pain-sensitive intracranial structures are the dura and the arteries at the base of the brain, the cerebral arteries in the same region, the great venous sinuses, and certain nerves (CN V, -IX, -X, and C1–3). The greater portion of the dura and cranium is insensitive. Mechanisms producing headaches from intracranial disorders include: (1) traction on the superficial cerebral veins and venous sinuses, (2) traction on the middle meningeal arteries, (3) traction on the basilar arteries and their branches, (4) distention and dilatation of the intracranial arteries, (5) inflammation near any pain-sensitive region, and (6) direct pressure or traction by tumors on cranial and cervical nerves. The resulting headaches may be throbbing when arteries are involved; otherwise the pain is steady. Headaches are often intensified by movements of the head, certain postures, and rapid changes in CSF pressure.

Brain Tumor: Benign and malignant intracranial neoplasms compress and place traction on surrounding structures. Headache may be the first symptom. It can be intermittent or constant. The pain may be mild or excruciating and occur anywhere in the cranium. The headaches are not characteristic of any defined headache syndrome. *Pulse synchronous tinnitus* identifies the headache as caused by raised intracranial pressure. **DDX:** Brain tumor should be suspected whenever the onset is recent, pain is persistent and worsening rather than episodic, a recent change in the customary headache pattern has occurred, or an apparent migraine aura persists after the headache subsides.

➤ **Brain Abscess:** A localized region in the brain parenchyma becomes infected and encapsulated, enclosing liquefied brain and pus. Infection is either hematogenous or from local extension. Symptoms and signs of brain mass appear coincident with or after infection in the ears, paranasal sinuses, lungs or, rarely, osteomyelitis or other source. When the primary infection has not been recognized, the distinction from brain tumor may not be evident until imaging is obtained. Less than half the patients with brain abscess exhibit the classic triad of fever, headache, and focal deficit. *CLINICAL OCCURRENCE:* *Direct Extension* from otitis or sinusitis; *Hematogenous* pneumonia, endocarditis (especially *Staphylococcus aureus*), osteomyelitis, other bacteremias (patients with cyanotic congenital heart disease and right-to-left shunts are particularly susceptible), systemic arteriovenous malformations; *Penetrating Trauma* after neurosurgery, gunshot wounds, open skull fractures.

➤ **KEY SYNDROME** Epidural Hematoma

Trauma in a young person, before the dura is firmly attached to the skull, results in laceration of the middle meningeal artery and expansion of a hematoma between the skull and the dura. The lenticular hematoma compresses the brain. This is always the result of trauma. Pain is uniform and attributable to the skull fracture in the temporal parietal area. Loss of consciousness, progressive mental clouding or focal motor or sensory defects suggest epidural hemorrhage; urgent head CT is mandatory.

➤ **KEY SYNDROME** Subdural Hematoma

This is most common in older adults due to a decrease in brain volume producing increased traction on the veins spanning the space between the mobile arachnoid and brain substance and the dural sinuses which at this age are fixed to the skull. Trauma leads to tearing of these small veins, producing low-pressure bleeding and slowly accumulating hematoma. Symptoms and signs of expanding intracranial mass occur some time following head trauma. After a severe head injury, the immediate accumulation of blood in the subdural space is not unexpected and offers no diagnostic difficulty. However, minor head trauma may be followed by a latent period of days, weeks, or months before the onset of headaches or other neurologic symptoms. The progression, timing, and attributes of the pain are similar to those of a brain tumor with relatively rapid expansion. Often no physical signs are present initially; later, localizing signs of an expanding intracranial mass become evident. Drowsiness, mental confusion, or coma may appear without headache or other signs, especially with bilateral frontal subdurals. The diagnosis is confirmed by CT or MRI imaging.

► **KEY SYNDROME** Intracerebral Hemorrhage

Hypertensive bleeding is usually from deep striatal vessels. The site is usually intracerebral; rarely is it subarachnoid. Cerebral amyloid angiopathy weakens vessel walls; it is associated with intracerebral hemorrhage without preceding hypertension. In approximately half the patients, the onset is marked by a sudden, severe, generalized headache, followed by rapidly evolving neurologic signs. Frequently, the patient vomits; often, there is nuchal rigidity. Seizures and/or coma may supervene. The sequence of events and the neurologic manifestations vary with the site and volume of hemorrhage. *Putamen:* A sensation of intracranial discomfort is followed in 30 minutes by dysphagia, hemiplegia, and sometimes anesthesias. *Thalamus:* Hemiplegia and hemianesthesias with dysphasia, homonymous hemianopsia, and extraocular paralyses are common. *Cerebellum:* Slowly developing, with repeated vomiting, occipital headaches, vertigo, paralysis of conjugate lateral gaze, and other ocular disorders. *Pons:* Prompt unconsciousness and death within a few hours. [Qureshi AI, Tuhrim S, Broderick JP, et al. Spontaneous Intracerebral hemorrhage. *N Engl J Med.* 2001;344;1450–1460] *CLINICAL OCCURRENCE:* Hypertension, aneurysm (traumatic, inflammatory, saccular or mycotic), angiomas, cerebral amyloid angiopathy, erosion from neoplasm, complicating cerebral infarction (embolism, thrombosis), hemorrhagic disorders, primary CNS lymphoma and coagulation defects.

► **KEY SYNDROME** Subarachnoid Hemorrhage

Subarachnoid hemorrhage usually results from rupture of a saccular (berry) aneurysm of the circle of Willis. Often, rupture is preceded by leakage, in contrast to the rupture of an artery from hypertension. New onset of severe headache between age 14 and 50 should suggest a ruptured aneurysm; prompt diagnosis and therapy may be lifesaving. CN III signs may be seen and should always suggest a ruptured aneurysm; stiff neck may be present, but its absence does not exclude a ruptured aneurysm. The patient usually reports having the worst headache of his life. Excruciating generalized headache may be succeeded by nuchal rigidity, coma, and often death. Small hemorrhages may be missed, especially in patients with normal mental status, leading to adverse clinical outcomes [Kowalski RG, Claassen J, Kreiter KT, et al. Initial misdiagnosis and outcome after subarachnoid hemorrhage. *JAMA.* 2004;291:866–869; Edlow JA, Caplan LR. Avoiding pitfalls in the diagnosis of subarachnoid hemorrhage. *N Eng J Med.* 2000;342:29–36].

Lumbar Puncture Headache: CSF is lost through the puncture hole in the dura, decreasing the CSF volume. A few hours or days after a lumbar puncture, the patient develops a constant or throbbing, usually bifrontal or suboccipital, deep headache. Moderate neck stiffness may occur. The pain is intensified when standing, shaking the head, or with bilateral jugular vein compression. It is lessened by the horizontal posture and flexion or extension of the neck.

Idiopathic Intracranial Hypertension: Symptoms resemble those of a brain tumor. Elevated CSF pressure is found, with no structural abnormality. The typical patient is a young obese woman with recent rapid weight gain. Funduscopic examination reveals papilledema; if longstanding, the disks may be pale. Transient *visual obscurations* are common. Prevention of visual loss requires prompt diagnosis and therapy. The headache is much like common migraine except that it is often daily. *Pulse synchronous tinnitus* is commonly present and identifies increased intracranial pressure.

➤ | **KEY SYNDROME** Bacterial Meningitis

Headache is a prominent early symptom of meningitis. It is generalized, throbbing or constant, and accompanied by fever and stiff neck. Because the meninges are inflamed, the headache is intensified by sudden movements of the head. The headache may be accompanied or followed by drowsiness or coma. Signs of meningeal irritation are nuchal rigidity and Kernig and Brudzinski signs. Although many febrile illnesses are accompanied by some degree of head pain, the headache of meningitis is especially severe. When headache is associated with stiff neck, a lumbar puncture is indicated [Attia J, Hatala R, Cook DJ, Wong JG. Does this adult patient have acute meningitis? *JAMA.* 1999;282:175–181].

| **KEY SYNDROME** Tension-Type Headache

Pain is attributed to sustained contraction of the neck, head, and shoulder muscles. Chronic intermittent headaches occur in the occiput and temporal regions, often with tenderness in the neck and trapezii. Usually the pain has recurred irregularly for many years, without periodicity. The sensation is described as mild or moderate discomfort, vise-like, a heavy feeling, a sense of pressure, a tight band, cramping, aching, or soreness; it is steady rather than throbbing. The pain is not augmented by coughing, straining at stool, or shaking the head. It usually begins in the occiput and extends upward to the temporal regions and down the nape of the neck to the shoulders. It may last for a few hours, with intensification near the day's end; or it may persist for many days, waxing and waning throughout. The onset of an episode is often related to emotional strain or to occupational activity. The pain is relieved by external support of the head, the application of hot packs or massage to the neck and mild analgesics. *Physical Signs.* Tenderness may be found in the upper border of the trapezii or the intrinsic neck muscles. DDX: The symptoms and signs are characteristic. Tension-type headaches are the only type not intensified by coughing or straining at stool; they are also the only type ameliorated by shaking the head. It common to have features of both tension type and migraine headache.

| **KEY SYNDROME** Migraine

Migraine occurs in approximately one quarter of the population. Its exact pathogenesis is uncertain, but genetic factors are important. Some patterns have a defined genetic basis, for example, 50% of patients with familial hemiplegic migraine have an identified genetic abnormality. Spreading cortical depression is characteristic, perhaps initiated in the trigeminal projection system of the brainstem. Vascular constriction and dilation occur in many, but not all patients; constriction can rarely lead to ischemic cerebral events. Release of substance P and neurogenic inflammation may play a role. Serotonin, dopamine, and noradrenaline are all important in the migrainous process and their receptor blockers are used in treatment. This is heritable disorder with periodic unilateral headache frequently preceded by an aura (*classic migraine*). Generalized throbbing headache is associated with nausea, light and sound sensitivity and frequently allodynia ipsilateral to the headache. The prevalence of migraine is estimated to be up to 25% (more common in women than in men) in the United States. Patients with migraine have an increased incidence of Raynaud phenomenon. Onset is usually in adolescence, but may occur at any age; many have experienced motion sickness in childhood. The attacks occur from a few times a year to several times per week. Periods of frequent attacks may be separated by periods of none or few attacks. Often, migraine is coincident with some phase of the menstrual cycle. The clinical pattern varies so much among individuals that each individual must be considered separately. Persons with recurrent "sick" or "sinus" headaches, without definite documentation of infection, most likely have migraine [Goadsby PJ, Lipton RB, Ferrari MD. Migraine—Current understanding and treatment. *N Engl J Med*. 2002;346:257–270; Cady R, Dodick DW. Diagnosis and treatment of migraine. *Mayo Clin Proc*. 2002;77:255–261].

Migraine with Aura (Classic Migraine): Migraine with aura has four phases. *The Prodrome:* An attack is often triggered or preceded by a period of anxiety, tension, or sluggishness. Triggers include bright lights, loud noise, strong odors, skipped meals, various foods and beverages, and changes in sleep patterns. A day or so before the attack, the patient may feel depressed or feel a sense of unusual well-being; occasionally, hunger is noted. *The Aura:* Migrainous phenomena are typically unilateral, but are occasionally bilateral; the side may vary in different attacks. Patients tend to repeat their distinctive aura in successive attacks. *Visual Disturbances:* A *scintillating scotoma*, usually involving both eyes, presents as flashing lights; sometimes there are black and white wavy lines, like the shimmering made by heat waves rising from pavement. *Fortification spectra* may be exhibited, with zigzag colored patterns with dark centers moving slowly across the visual field. Distinct patterns of the aura are associated with migraine variant syndromes (see *Migraine Variants,* below). *Other Neurologic Events:* Neurologic symptoms occurring during the aura define special migraine syndromes discussed below. *The Headache:* The attack may begin any time of the day or night; it is frequently present on awakening. Some patients have a typical aura without succeeding headache. Usually, as the aura diminishes, unilateral headache appears on the side opposite to unilateral visual or somatosensory symptoms during the aura. The pain may start above one orbit and spread over the entire side of the head to the occiput and neck, or it may begin in the back of the head and move forward. Rarely, the site of pain is below the eye, in front of the ear, behind the mandibular angle, in the nape of the neck, or in the shoulders. Over an hour, the pain spreads and intensifies to a severe throbbing, boring, aching headache. Constant nonthrobbing pain occurs in 50% of patients. The pain is often augmented by reclining and lessened by sitting or standing. Shaking the head, coughing, or straining at stool intensifies the pain. Although the pain may be severe, it usually does not disrupt sleep. The pain is usually lessened by lying in a dark, quiet room. Nausea and, less commonly, vomiting often accompany the headache. *Photophobia, phonophobia*, and annoyance from odors (*hyperosmia*) are common during the headache. *Physical Signs During Headache:* The patient may appear normal or be incapacitated with cold limbs and pale skin. Lacrimation, conjunctival injection, nasal congestion and rhinorrhea are not rare, leading to the misattribution of "sinus headache." The duration of the paroxysm is usually from 2 to 6 hours; it is relieved by sleep. *The Recovery:* When an attack terminates with sleep, the patient awakens without headache and experiences a sense of buoyancy and well-being. DDX: The diagnosis is easy in a long-established case with relatively typical symptoms. When the onset is recent and the symptoms unusual, other intracranial disorders must be excluded. *Ophthalmoplegic migraine* can simulate an aneurysm in the circle of Willis. Although hemiplegia can be a migrainous phenomenon, more serious causes should be sought.

Migraine Variants: These variant forms of migraine with aura are distinguished by the particular pattern of the aura.

Migraine without Aura (Common Migraine): The onset is slower than classic migraine and the duration is often longer, 4 to 72 hours. It may persist through sleep. The headache is unilateral or bilateral. In other respects, common and classic migraine are similar. There is considerable overlap of common migraine and tension type headache.

Ophthalmic Migraine: This rare disorder may have scotomata that are succeeded by momentary blindness, anopsia, in the entire field, or in the lower or upper quadrants; or the pattern may be bitemporal or homonymous hemianopsia.

Ophthalmoplegic Migraine: Transient unilateral paralysis of CN III (oculomotor) produces lateral deviation and ptosis. This occurs in young girls.

Basilar Artery Migraine: The scotomata and anesthesias of the face and limbs are bilateral, and vertigo or CN palsies may be present from brainstem nuclear ischemia. The transition from aura to headache may be accompanied by momentary loss of consciousness or light sleep.

Hemiplegic Migraine: This is spectacular but rare. The paralysis is most likely to occur in migrainous patients experiencing paresthesias. The right side is more often involved. The patient complains of numbness or "woodenness" of the affected limbs. Although weakness may be the complaint, it may only be manifest by exaggeration of the deep tendon reflexes and Babinski sign. The paralysis lasts for 10 to 40 minutes, but may persist for 2 to 3 days; usually there are no permanent sequelae. Many neurologists are reluctant to make this diagnosis without excluding more serious and irreversible disorders. The diagnosis is strongly supported by a family history of hemiplegic migraine.

KEY SYNDROME   Cluster Headache

The headache is produced by dilatation of branches of the internal carotid artery, especially those supplying the meninges innervated by the trigeminal nerve. Although the syndrome can be simulated by the injection of histamine into the internal carotid artery, there is no conclusive evidence that histamine plays a role in the natural disorder. Cluster headache is five to six times more common in men than women with onset typically in the third or fourth decade of life. A family history of migraine or cluster headaches is not uncommon. Cluster headache is most commonly episodic occurring several times a day or week for several weeks, with long intermissions between episodes. However, it may be chronic with headaches persisting for more than a year without intermission. The headache begins without aura and lasts 15 to 120 minutes (average 40 minutes). It is unilateral, severe, boring, and throbbing. It recurs consistently on the same side. It is usually maximal just inferior to the medial canthus of the orbit, but may occur in the temple or in the side of the face, and it may spread to the neck and shoulder. Flushing, edema and sweating of the skin, lacrimation, conjunctival injection, nasal congestion, rhinorrhea, partial Horner syndrome, and temporal artery dilatation may occur on the affected side [May A. Cluster headache: Pathogenesis, diagnosis, and management. *Lancet*. 2005;366:843–855]. DDX: Paroxysmal hemicrania is briefer and more common in women; in Raeder syndrome, the pain is identical in quality but is persistent without discreet attacks; trigeminal neuralgia is much briefer lancinating pain, though overlap syndromes exist.

Paroxysmal Hemicrania: The cause is unknown; women are more commonly affected than men. It is more often chronic than episodic. The headache is indistinguishable from cluster headache, but the pattern is distinct. Headaches are short, lasting on average 15 minutes, more frequent, up to 40 times per day, and uniformly abolished by indomethacin.

> **KEY SYNDROME** **Chronic Daily Headache—Transformed Migraine, Rebound Headache**

Long term use of analgesics leads to rebound headaches when medication use is interrupted for a few hours. This common cause of chronic daily headache occurs in patients with a history of tension-type or migraine headache who have developed daily persistent headache relieved only temporarily by medication. A history of regular daily use of prescription or over-the-counter analgesics and the absence of aura, neurologic findings, or other causes of headache are the keys to diagnosis. Overuse of caffeine in migraineurs will also precipitate chronic daily, rebound headaches. The treatment is complete abstinence from analgesics for 2 weeks. Migraineurs should not use analgesics more than 2 days a week. If this proves inadequate, prophylactic therapy should be instituted.

Ice Cream Headache: See Chapter 7, page 281.

Hypertensive Headache: The evidence points to segmental dilatation of branches of the external carotid artery. In patients with mild to moderate hypertension, the incidence and types of headache are no different than in normotensive persons. The diastolic pressure must exceed 120 mm Hg to cause headache. In accelerated hypertension without encephalopathy, half of the patients experience headache. The headaches are often occipital and there is no aura.

> **KEY SYNDROME** **Headache Present on Awakening**

Headaches present on awakening should suggest migraine, carbon monoxide poisoning, sleep apnea, and analgesic rebound headache. Tension headaches are not present on first awakening.

Carbon Monoxide Poisoning: Excessive amounts of carboxyhemoglobin are formed from inhalation of carbon monoxide gas leading to decreased oxygenation. This results from inhalation of products of combustion in poorly ventilated spaces, for example, cars with malfunctioning exhaust systems, homes with malfunctioning gas furnaces or wood stoves, and burning charcoal in an enclosed space. Symptoms consist of headache, dizziness, nausea and vomiting, mental confusion, and visual disturbances progressing to obtundation, coma and death. The key sign is cherry-red skin and mucosa accompanied by a bounding pulse, hypertension, muscular twitching, stertorous breathing, and dilated pupils.

Fever: See Chapter 4, page 52ff.

> **KEY SYNDROME** Giant Cell Arteritis

See Chapter 8, page 414.

Occipital Neuritis: See page .

> **KEY SYNDROME** Paranasal Sinusitis

See page 289. There is considerable debate as to the incidence of headache related to pathology of the nasal sinuses. Many experts, based upon an extensive literature, believe that many, if not most of the conditions labeled "sinus headache," are migraine [Schreiber CP, Hutchinson S, Webster CJ, et al. Prevalendce of migraine in patients with a history of self-reported or physician-diagnosed "sinus" headache. *Arch Intern Med.* 2004;164:1769–1772]. Sinus and nasal symptoms are common in association with both migraine and cluster headache. No consensus has been reached [Cady RK, Dodick DW, Levine HL, et al. Sinus headache; A neurology, otolaryngology, allergy, and primary care consensus on diagnosis and treatment. *Mayo Clin Proc.* 2005;80:908–916].

Seizures

> **KEY SYNDROME** Seizures

Seizures are caused by paroxysmal disordered electrical activity in the brain that may be focal, focal in onset with generalization, or generalized at the onset. Seizures are classified as generalized or partial. Partial seizures are defined as those with a focal onset, regardless of whether they generalize later in their course [Chabolla DR. Characteristics of the epilepsies. *Mayo Clin Proc.* 2002;77:981–990].

✔ **SEIZURES—CLINICAL OCCURRENCE:** *Congenital* congenital brain injury; *Endocrine* hypoglycemia; *Idiopathic* idiopathic epilepsy; *Inflammatory/Immune* vasculitis; *Infectious* meningitis, encephalitis, brain abscess, neurocysticercosis; *Metabolic/Toxic* fever, drug withdrawal (alcohol, barbiturates, benzodiazepines, anticonvulsant medications), amphetamines, cocaine, phencyclidine, theophylline, hypoglycemia, hypocalcemia, uremia, liver failure, hypoxia, penicillins and other β-lactams; *Mechanical/Trauma* head trauma; *Neoplastic* primary or metastatic cancer, insulinoma; *Neurologic* epilepsy, degenerative diseases of the CNS; *Psychosocial* drug abuse, physical abuse; *Vascular* stroke, vasculitis, hemorrhage.

Evaluation of a Patient with Seizure

When the patient has a seizure the immediate approach is to prevent injury and support cardiorespiratory function if necessary. However, the physician rarely observes the event, so a thorough history and examination are essential to identify the cause and to exclude other causes of impaired consciousness. In a patient treated for seizures, look for causes of relapse and evaluate adequacy of therapy. For patients with new onset of seizures, seek the cause, supplementing your neurologic examination with appropriate imaging and laboratory studies.

KEY SYNDROME   Partial Seizures

Partial seizures begin within a specific region of the brain identified by the initial symptoms. They may remain localized, spread to a larger but limited area of the cortex, or progress to a generalized seizure involving both hemispheres. Partial seizures are classified as *simple* if the event is limited to a small portion of one cortex and consciousness is not altered. *Complex* partial seizures involve larger areas of the cortex and consciousness is impaired, although not lost.

Partial Motor Seizure: The seizures are caused by a focal lesion in the motor cortex. The seizure begins in a single body region with muscle twitching that becomes more violent with increasing amplitude. It may spread to contiguous muscle groups until the entire ipsilateral side is involved in clonic contractions. The seizure may stop at any stage of spread, or the contralateral side may be affected producing a generalized motor seizure. Consciousness is retained unless the attack is generalized.

Partial-Complex (Psychomotor) Seizure: These are often accompanied by an aura of an abnormal psychic event that can be olfactory, visual, or gustatory disturbances, or déjà vu. The attack may last from a few minutes to a few hours. Sudden but subtle loss of higher levels of consciousness occurs in which the patient is unaware of what transpires but retains motor functions and ability to react in an automatic fashion. The patient may respond to questions, but the answers disclose lack of understanding. This may be the only objective clue. Repetitive movements, which are often stereotyped, may be reported. Patients generally do not become violent or assaultive during an attack. Only occasionally are there tonic muscle spasms of the limbs. Amnesia for the attack is partial or complete. This condition should prompt a search for a focal lesion in the temporal lobe.

KEY SYNDROME   *Secondary Generalized Seizure*

Most major motor seizures begin from a unilateral small focus in one hemisphere then progress to involve the ipsilateral hemisphere and cross the corpus callosum to involve the contralateral hemisphere, producing a secondary generalized seizure. There may or may not be a warning or aura. Several hours or days before the attack, prodromata may be noted, with feelings of strangeness, dreamy states, increased irritability, lethargy or euphoria, ravenous appetite, feeling of impending disaster, headaches, or other symptoms. The aura is a partial seizure, and the patient learns its significance. The patient may experience vague epigastric sensations such as nausea or hunger and palpitation, vertigo, or sensations in the head. Any aura or focal seizure reflects focal brain disease. Consciousness is lost suddenly and simultaneously with the epileptic cry from sudden expulsion of air through the glottis. The patient is helpless and falls, often incurring injuries. Tonic spasm of all muscles occurs which may be so violent as to fracture bones. Breathing ceases from spasm of the thoracic muscles and cyanosis may be deep. Suddenly, the tonic state subsides, followed by clonic movements that increase in strength with repetition then cease. Foaming at the mouth results from forced expulsion of air and saliva. Clonic movements of the jaws cause biting of the tongue, cheeks and lips. Frequently, there is involuntary defecation and urination. Unconsciousness usually lasts a few minutes, but may last hours. On return of consciousness, patients are often confused and amnestic for the seizure and preceding events and complain of headache, stiffness, and sore muscles. Seizures are frequently followed by a deep sleep.

KEY SYNDROME   Generalized Seizure

Generalized seizures involve the entire cerebral cortex at onset so they do not have an aura. History obtained from bystanders is critical in determining whether a seizure was generalized or focal at onset.

Absence Seizure (Petit Mal): There is a sudden decrease in or loss of consciousness lasting up to 90 seconds, with no abnormal muscle movements; the patient's eyes are wide open and staring. Full consciousness is rapidly and completely restored. Injuries may result from the momentary lapse, but not from falls since there is no loss of postural tone. The patient is vaguely aware of having "missed something."

Major Motor Seizure (Grand Mal): This seizure is identical to the secondary generalized seizure except for the absence of an aura or any evidence of focal onset of the event. Consciousness is lost without warning and the patient is amnestic for the event.

KEY SYNDROME   Sudden Unexplained Death in Epilepsy (SUDEP)

There is an increased risk of sudden death in patients with epilepsy. The causes are not certain, but may be linked to centrally-triggered cardiac arrhythmias. Risk of traumatic deaths including drowning are also increased.

Impaired Consciousness

Disturbances of consciousness may be classified according to severity. *Lethargy* is drowsiness caused by a condition other than normal sleep. *Stupor* is a somnolent state from which the patient may be momentarily aroused by questions or painful stimuli. *Coma* is the deepest state of unconsciousness in which the patient is motionless and unresponsive to stimuli. *Syncope* is a brief loss of consciousness that presents a different diagnostic problem from that of coma. *Confusion* denotes decreased attentiveness and may be present with any level of consciousness. The hallmark of confusional states is impaired perception, memory and awareness of surrounding; *delirium* is confusion accompanied by hallucinations. Although delirium is sometimes accompanied by agitation and violent emotional responses, the patient may be quiet and withdrawn.

Episodic Impaired Consciousness

KEY SYNDROME   Narcolepsy

Narcolepsy is idiopathic or occurs secondary to brain injury. There is impaired ability to voluntarily maintain wakefulness associated with immediate onset of rapid eye movement sleep. The idiopathic form usually occurs in young adults and may be associated with sudden loss of motor tone without loss of consciousness (*cataplexy*), inability to move upon awakening (*sleep paralysis*), and visual or auditory hallucinations at sleep onset (*hypnagogic hallucinations*) or on awakening (*hypnopompic hallucinations*). The patient experiences unexpected, inappropriate, and irresistible short spells of sleep. There may be several attacks per day of brief somnolent periods with no deterioration of mentation.

➤ **KEY SYNDROME   Syncope**

Syncope results from transient arrest of cerebral or brainstem function. This usually results from momentary arrest of effective cerebral or brainstem perfusion. Impaired brain perfusion may occur from ineffective cardiac contraction (myocardial insufficiency or dysrhythmias), peripheral vasodilation producing hypotension, or from vascular reflexes. In the erect position, consciousness is lost when the mean arterial pressure declines to 20 to 30 mm Hg or when the heart stops for 4 to 5 seconds. In the horizontal position, more extreme conditions can be tolerated. The patient may complain of "weak spells," "light-headedness," or "blackouts." A careful history must be obtained from both the patient and witnesses. The history and initial physical examination are of the greatest usefulness in establishing a specific etiology. Extensive investigations are unlikely to be useful, unless the history or examination direct you to a specific diagnosis [Kapoor WN. Syncope. *N Engl J Med*. 2000;343:1856–1862]. The most common cause of syncope is the vasovagal or vasodepressor faint. Other considerations are cardiac dysrhythmias (Adams-Stokes attacks—either tachy- or bradycardia), seizure, or autonomic dysfunction with orthostatic hypotension, pulmonary embolism, aortic stenosis, and cerebrovascular disease. Neurogenic causes can nearly always be differentiated with a good history or eyewitness report.

Neurocardiogenic Syncope (Vasovagal Syncope, Fainting): Sudden vasodilation leads to decreased cardiac filling and forceful myocardial contraction on an underfilled ventricle. This triggers myocardial receptors that reflexively cause strong vagal outflow, leading to bradycardia, further hypotension, and syncope. With recumbency, the venous return improves and recovery ensues. The attack is induced in healthy persons by fear, anxiety, or pain. A hot environment, fatigue, illness, alcohol consumption, and hunger increase susceptibility. The patient usually has a prodrome that is brief and often begins in the erect position with feeling light-headed and unsteady. Yawning, dimming of vision (as a consequence of the intraocular pressure collapsing arterioles), nausea and vomiting, and sweating are common. The face becomes pale or ashen. If the patient reclines promptly, the attack may be aborted. The syncopal stage consists of loss of postural tone and impaired consciousness. The patient falls to the floor either slowly or abruptly, usually avoiding injury. The patient may be mentally confused but still hear voices and dimly see the surroundings. Unconsciousness may be complete and last for a few seconds to at most a few minutes. Usually the muscles are utterly flaccid and motionless, although sometimes there are a few clonic jerks of arms and legs (convulsive syncope) but seldom a full tonic-clonic convulsion. Urinary or fecal incontinence is rare. The skin appears strikingly pale or cyanotic and the pulse is weak or absent. Bradycardia is accompanied by arterial hypotension and extremely shallow, quiet breathing. Recovery follows assumption of the horizontal position. During recovery the patient remains weak, but is awake and lucid, the face gradually suffuses with pink, the blood pressure rises, the pulse becomes palpable and accelerated, the breathing deepens and quickens, the eyelids may flutter. The patient awakens with immediate awareness of the surroundings and memory for the prodrome. The muscle weakness persists for some time, so attempts to rise prematurely may induce another attack [Fenton AM, Hammill SC, Rea FR, et al. Vasovagal syncope. *Ann Intern Med.* 2000;133;714–725].

Orthostatic Syncope: See Chapter 4, page 77. In the erect position pooling of blood in the lower limbs is prevented by vasoconstriction mediated through the autonomic nervous system. When there is decreased intravascular volume or the compensatory mechanism is blocked, blood pools in the legs and arterial hypotension results. Distinctive features of autonomic insufficiency are normal heart rate, and absence of pallor and sweating. Recovery occurs in the horizontal position.

Adams-Stokes Syndrome: The attacks of unconsciousness occur when effective cardiac contractions are absent for more than 5 seconds in the vertical position or 10 seconds in the horizontal. Usually, asystole results during the transition from a partial to a complete heart block or from the onset of paroxysmal tachycardia or ventricular fibrillation. When the heart rhythm is regular and the rate less than 40 per minute, heart block can be distinguished from sinus bradycardia by the variation in intensity of the first heart sounds. An ECG is required for confirmation. This form of syncope occurs in any position without a prodrome.

Valvular Heart Disease: Muscular vasodilation with exercise in patients with a fixed cardiac output leads to cerebral hypoperfusion and syncope. Exertion may induce typical syncope in a patient with aortic stenosis or, less commonly, aortic regurgitation or pulmonary hypertension.

Carotid Sinus Syncope: This occurs most commonly in patients older than 60 years with hypertension or occlusion of one carotid artery. Rotation of the head or a tight collar puts pressure on the carotid bulb, inducing vagal stimulation that results in one of three responses: (1) sinoatrial block, (2) hypotension without bradycardia, or (3) syncope with normal pulse rate and blood pressure. Syncope related to specific motions of the neck suggest carotid sinus syncope. Carotid sinus massage is dangerous and should not be used to support the diagnosis as cerebral infarction and death have resulted from this maneuver. Never palpate both carotids simultaneously. **DDX:** Rotation of the neck may precipitate syncope in patients with severely impaired vertebrobasilar circulation.

Hyperventilation: Hyperventilation results in hypocapnea that induces diminished cerebral blood flow. Before the attack, the patient is usually anxious or emotionally upset. The patient feels tightness in the chest or suffocation accompanied by numbness and tingling of arms and face, sometimes with carpopedal spasm. Loss of consciousness may be prolonged compared with most other types of syncope. The symptoms are reproduced by having the patient overventilate. Rebreathing into a paper bag will arrest the attack and demonstrate a method of self-treatment.

Cough Syncope (Tussive Syncope): Severe paroxysms of coughing, laughing or vomiting may induce syncope; this is rare in women. The history is usually diagnostic. The mechanism is disputed.

Micturition Syncope: Voiding a large volume, particularly after arising from a warm bed, may precipitate syncope. Similarly, the rapid decompression of an overfilled bladder by catheterization or the removal of large volumes of ascitic fluid may also cause syncope.

Akinetic Epilepsy: Common features in akinetic epilepsy, but rare in syncope, are lack of pallor, sudden onset without prodrome, injury from falling, tonic convulsions with upturned eyes, urinary or fecal incontinence, and postictal mental confusion with headache and drowsiness. Most of these features occur occasionally with syncope.

Hysterical Syncope: This is the swoon of Victorian novels. It usually occurs in the presence of witnesses. The fall is graceful and harmless. The skin color, heart rate, and blood pressure are all normal. Either the patient lies motionless or makes resisting movements.

Coma

➤ **KEY SYNDROME** **Coma**

Coma results from serious disruption of brain function that impairs the reticular activating system such that consciousness is lost. Coma is a state of prolonged unconsciousness. Since the patient cannot give a history or cooperate, the examination requires a special approach. The correct diagnosis can be rapidly established in most cases by a structured complete physical and neurologic examination and use of radiologic and laboratory testing. Two axioms must always be kept in mind: (1) Finding one cause for coma is not sufficient. For instance, a comatose patient with alcohol on the breath may have sustained a head injury while intoxicated; a person injured in an automobile accident may have had an antecedent stroke leading to the accident; or an unconscious patient with a few sedative tablets at the bedside may have taken the drug for symptoms of meningitis or brain tumor and (2) A complete neurologic examination is necessary but not sufficient. All other systems must also be assessed: finding atrial fibrillation raises the possibility of cerebral embolism; the retinae may contain signs of diabetes; demonstration of a consolidated lung suggests lobar pneumonia or pneumococcal meningitis; examination of the abdomen has discovered a distended bladder, leading to a diagnosis of uremia from bladder outlet obstruction. The differential diagnosis and management of coma is beyond the scope of this text. The reader should consult textbooks of medicine, neurology, and emergency medicine.

History of the Comatose Patient: Interview the relatives, acquaintances, attendants, or police officers who discovered the patient. *Circumstances of Discovery:* How was the patient found? Were there any drugs or poisons nearby? Do the surroundings suggest poisoning from carbon monoxide or other fumes? Was there evidence of trauma? What was known about the patient's antecedent intake of food and fluids? Who prepared the food? What were the symptoms and actions before the onset of coma? Did the patient have pain, diarrhea, or vomiting? *Past History:* Was the patient known to have epilepsy, diabetes, hypertension, or alcohol or drug addiction? Did the patient have suicidal thoughts? Was the patient ever hospitalized in a mental institution? Was the patient known to be taking medicines? Had there ever been operations for malignancy? Has this happened before?

Physical Examination of the Comatose Patient: Assess patency of the airway and the presence of adequate respirations and pulse. *Vital Signs:* Note any abnormalities. *General Inspection:* Note posture; look for tremors or muscle jerks; inspect the respiratory movements for bradypnea, tachypnea, Kussmaul breathing, Cheyne-Stokes breathing. *Color:* Look for pallor, icterus, the cyanosis of methemoglobinemia, the cherry-red color of carbon monoxide hemoglobin. *Scalp and Skull:* Look for contusions, lacerations, gunshot wounds; palpate for depressed skull fractures and inspect the mastoid for hematoma of basilar skull fracture (*Battle sign*). *Eyes:* Inspect for periorbital bruising (*raccoon sign*) of basilar skull fracture. Lift the eyelids and let them close; lagging of one lid suggests hemiplegia. The patient with hysteria resists opening by closing the lids tighter. In coma, the eyes remain fixed or oscillate slowly from side to side; oscillation is lacking in hysteria in which the eyes may wander but fix momentarily. Conjugate deviation of the eyeballs is toward the affected side in destructive lesions of the frontal lobe, away from the affected side in irritative lesions. The presence of extraocular muscle palsies assists in localizing an intracranial lesion. After confirming the absence of neck injury, open the eyelids and quickly turn the head from side to side. The eyes of the comatose patient with cerebral damage turn in the opposite direction in a conjugate movement if the brainstem is intact (*doll's eyes*). This *oculocephalic reflex* is lost with lesions of the pons or midbrain. Caloric studies, in which you test an *oculovestibular reflex*, provide information of similar significance. These are performed by irrigating the ear canal with 30 to 50 mL of ice water and noting that, with cerebral dysfunction and an intact brainstem, a tonic conjugate deviation of the eyes toward the cold ear lasts for 30 to 120 seconds. Bilateral, widely dilated pupils occur in profound posttraumatic shock, massive cerebral hemorrhage, encephalitis, poisoning with atropine-like drugs, and the end stages of brain tumor. Bilateral pinpoint pupils suggest opiate poisoning or a pontine hemorrhage. A unilateral unreactive pupil indicates a rapidly expanding lesion on the ipsilateral side, as in subdural or middle meningeal epidural hemorrhage or brain tumor. Examine the ocular fundi for the exudates and hemorrhages of diabetes and nephritis, and the choked disks of increased intracranial pressure. *Facial Muscles:* Asymmetry of the face may indicate hemiplegia. The mouth droops on the affected side; the cheek puffs out with each expiration. Painful pressure on the supraorbital notch causes the mouth to grimace in an asymmetric pattern to reveal the weak side. *Oral Cavity:* Examine the tongue for lacerations from biting during a seizure. Look for a diphtheritic membrane, other signs of pharyngitis, or ulceration or discoloration from poisons. *Breath:* Smell the breath for acetone, ammonia, alcohol or its successor aldehydes, paraldehyde, and other odors. *Ears:* Look for pus, spinal fluid, or blood emerging from the external acoustic meatus or blood behind the drum from basilar skull fracture. *Neck:* Test for nuchal rigidity, Kernig sign, and Brudzinski sign, looking for evidence of meningeal irritation. *Chest:* Percuss and auscultate the chest for pneumothorax, consolidation, wheezing, or crepitation. *Heart:* Auscultate for rhythm, rate, and strength of the heart sounds and any abnormal sounds. *Abdomen:* Auscultate for bruits and palpate for masses or rigidity suggesting peritonitis or fluid. *Limbs:* Test each limb successively for flaccidity by lifting it and letting it fall to the bed. If any muscle tone is retained, a difference in the two sides indicates a hemiplegia. The reflexes on the paralyzed side are absent during the stage of spinal shock, but in deep coma, all reflexes are lost. In deep coma, the Babinski reflex is present bilaterally, so it cannot be employed to localize a lesion. If some reflexes are retained, a difference in the two sides is significant. *Sensory Examination:* In semicoma, only the responses to painful stimuli can be evaluated. The patient will show defensive reactions when pricked in sensitive areas, but no response is forthcoming

Table 14–1 Glasgow Coma Scale

Response		Score
Eyes Open		
_____	Spontaneous	4
_____	To speech	3
_____	To pain	2
_____	Absent	1
Verbal		
_____	Converses/oriented	5
_____	Converses/disoriented	4
_____	Inappropriate	3
_____	Incomprehensible	2
_____	Absent	1
Motor		
_____	Obeys	6
_____	Localizes pain	5
_____	Withdraws (flexion)	4
_____	Decorticate (flexion) rigidity	3
_____	Decerebrate (extension) rigidity	2
_____	Absent	1

when analgesic regions are stimulated. If the stimulated region is sensitive but paralyzed, a defense or withdrawal movement may occur on the opposite side; the facial expression will indicate pain. Deep pressure sense should be tested by compression of the Achilles tendon, the testis, and the supraorbital notch.

Classify the seriousness of cerebral dysfunction by using the Glasgow Coma Scale (Table 14–1) in which mild is 13 through 15, moderate is 9 through 12, and severe is 3 through 8 points. Patients with scores less than 8 are in coma [Booth CM, Boone RH, Tomlinson G, et al. Is this patient dead, vegetative, or severely neurologically impaired? Assessing outcome for comatose survivors of cardiac arrest. *JAMA.* 2004;291:870–879]. Recently an alternative scoring system for coma has been proposed and validated by one group, the FOUR (Full Outline of UnResponsiveness) Score (Table 14–2) [Wolf CA, Wijdicks EFM, Bamlet WR, et al. Futher validation of the FOUR score scale by intensive care nurses. *Mayo Clin Proc.* 2007;82:435–438]. It is able to be used in patients on ventilators and has high interobserver reliability. Scores are from 0 to 16.

Differential Diagnosis of Coma: The multiple etiologies of coma can be conveniently divided into three categories, which may be suggested by findings from the history and physical examination.

Metabolic Encephalopathy: Metabolic derangements or toxin exposure impairs brain function and leads to coma. Coma occurs with normal pupillary responses, normal brainstem reflexes and no focal neurologic deficits. Asterixis, myoclonus, and Cheyne-Stokes respiration occur. Treatment is correction of the metabolic disturbance. *CLINICAL OCCURRENCE:* Hypoglycemia, hypoxia, hypercarbia, hyponatremia,

Table 14-2 FOUR Score Coma Scale

Response	Points				
	0	1	2	3	4
Eyes	Eyelids open, tracking and blinking on command	Eyelids open, but not tracking	Eyelids closed but open to loud voice	Eyelids closed but open to pain	Eyelids remain closed to pain
Motor	Thumbs up, fist or peace sign to command	Localizing to pain	Flexion response to pain	Extensor posturing to pain	No response to pain or generalized myoclonus; status epilepticus
Brainstem Reflexes	Pupillary and corneal reflexes present	One puli wide and fixed	Pupillary or corneal reflexes absent	Pupillary and corneal reflexes absent	Absent pupillary, corneal and cough reflexes
Respirations	Not intubated, regular breathing	Not intubated, Cheyne-Stokes pattern	Not intubated, irregular breathing pattern	Breathing above ventilator rate	Breathing at ventilator rate or apnea

Adapted from Demaerschalk BM, Meschia JF, et al: Advantages of the Mayo Clinic FOUR Coma Score over the Glasgow Coma Scale in the intensive care unit. Mayo Clinic Neurosciences Update.

intoxications (e.g., alcohol, benzodiazepines, barbiturates, opiates), hepatic insufficiency, advanced kidney failure, severe hypothyroidism, and many others.

Hypoglycemic Coma: The prodrome may resemble a vasovagal spell but confusion is prominent. The syncopal stage is frequently prolonged and loss of consciousness is usually incomplete. Instead, there is muscle weakness with mental confusion. The blood sugar is usually below 30 mg/100 mL; the symptoms are relieved by the intravenous administration of glucose or injection of glucagon.

Transtentorial Herniation: An expanding supratentorial mass forces the uncus to herniate. Typically, the uncus of the temporal lobe compresses the third nerve and then the midbrain initially producing focal deficits. Progression from the focal deficits to coma and death can be rapid. *CLINICAL OCCURRENCE:* Brain tumor (primary or metastatic), bleeding (intracerebral, subdural, epidural), cerebral edema associated with infarction (arterial or venous), abscess, encephalitis, or massive liver necrosis.

Brainstem Injury: The brainstem reticular activating system that runs from the upper pons to the lower diencephalon is responsible for maintaining consciousness; damage results in coma. The onset is usually abrupt, either following trauma or acute severe headache. Emergent neuroimaging is required. *CLINICAL OCCURRENCE:* Trauma and spontaneous hemorrhage are the most common etiologies.

Chronic Vegetative and Minimally Conscious States

> **KEY SYNDROME** **Chronic Vegetative State**

This condition results from severe injury to the cortex, thalamus and/or white matter of the brain. The clinical syndrome is one of wakefulness and sleep without awareness or responsiveness to the environment. The cycling of wakefulness and sleep is distinct from coma [Bernat JL. Chronic disorders of consciousness. *Lancet.* 2006;367:1181–1192].

> **KEY SYNDROME** **Minimally Conscious State**

These patient show some awareness behaviors and imaging suggests that some may have considerable awareness without the ability to respond akin to the locked in state. Clinicians should always assume that even apparently comatose patients are able to perceive what is done to them and hear and comprehend what is said at the bedside. The prognosis is very difficult to predict.

Cerebrovascular Syndromes

➤ > **KEY SYNDROME** **Transient Ischemic Attack (TIA)**

TIA results from a failure of perfusion due to hemodynamic causes or microembolism. Less common causes are in situ arterial thrombosis, arterial dissection and venous sinus thrombosis. The symptoms reflect the area of ischemia. TIA is, by definition, the acute onset of a focal neurologic deficit in a specific vascular distribution with full recovery within 24 hours of onset. Events usually last 5 to 20 minutes. Neurologic signs are usually absent between attacks. The correct diagnosis and prompt evaluation of TIA are important because it is an indication of possible impending cerebral infarction; up to 25% of patients with a new TIA will have a stroke within 24 hours [Johnston SC. Transient ischemic attack. *N Engl J Med.* 2002;347:1687–1692]. The risk for stroke within 7 days of a TIA is predicted by a simple clinical score (ABCD) based upon Age, Blood pressue, Clinical features and Duration [Rothwell PM, Giles MF, Flossman E, et al. A simple score (ABCD) to identify individuals at high early risk of stroke after transient ischaemic attack. *Lancet.* 2005;366:29–36]. **DDX:** Diplopia, syncope, transient confusion, and paraparesis are uncommon symptoms of TIA. The differential diagnosis of TIA includes convulsions, syncope, migraine, focal cerebral masses, such as subdural hematomas, cardiac diseases, and labyrinthine disorders.

Carotid Artery TIA: Symptoms and signs are related to the ipsilateral cerebral hemisphere and/or retina. Findings include contralateral weakness, clumsiness, numbness of the hand, hand and face, or entire half of the body, dysarthria, aphasia, and ipsilateral *amaurosis fugax* with monocular visual loss, usually described as a shade coming down. Visual loss may be complete blindness or sector visual loss. Carotid bruits or retinal emboli may be found.

Amaurosis Fugax: Cholesterol (from ruptured atherosclerotic plaques in the common or internal carotid artery) or other types of emboli transiently occlude flow to the retinal artery. There is sudden onset of monocular blindness, often described as a shade being pulled down, which lasts a few minutes and resolves spontaneously.

Vertebrobasilar Artery TIA: Symptoms and signs are related to the posterior circulation and may affect vision and CN function. Frequent complaints are combinations of binocular visual disturbance or loss, vertigo, dysarthria, ataxia, unilateral or bilateral weakness or numbness and drop attacks (sudden loss of postural tone and collapse without loss of consciousness).

➤ **KEY SYNDROME** Ischemic Stroke

Arterial obstruction by thrombosis, embolism or dissection produces tissue ischemia resulting in neuronal infarction. The area of infarction is surrounded by a penumbra of ischemic tissue which is salvagable with prompt resoration of perfusion. Ischemic stroke is painless and the patient remain conscious. Symptom onset may be abrupt or stuttering (see TIA, above). The specific symptoms reflect the functional loci within the distribution of the affected vessel [Goldstein LB, Simel DL. Is this patient having a stoke? *JAMA.* 2005;293:2391–2402]. The *middle cerebral artery* is most commonly affected with the arm more severely affected than the leg. With *anterior cerebral artery* stroke, the leg is more affected than the arm. *Posterior cerebral* strokes result in homomynous hemianopsia. *Basilar artery* strokes are frequently associated with vertigo, diplopia, dysarthria or Horner syndrome; hemiparesis is not a feature. *Cerebral venous sinus* thrombosis presents with symptoms and signs of cerebral vascular disease with less discrete evidence of focal lesions [Stam J. Thrombosis of the cerebral veins and sinuses. *N Engl J Med.* 005;352:1791–1798; Thaler DE, Frosch MP. Case 16-2002. Case Records of the Massachusetts General Hospital. *N Engl J Med.* 2002;346:1651–1658].

The National Institutes of Health Stroke Scale: (Table 14–3) This is the preferred tool for evaluating the severity of initial stroke symptoms and signs and the response to therapy.

Table 14-3 National Institutes of Health Stroke Scale

Domain	Score					
	0	1	2	3	4	5
Level of Consciousness (LOC)	Alert	Drowsy	Stuporous	Coma		
LOC Questions: ask month and age	Both correct	One correct	None correct			
LOC Commands: close eyes, make fist	Both correct	One correct	None correct			
Best Gaze	Normal	Partial gaze palsy	Forced deviation			
Visual Fields	No loss	Partial hemianopsia	Complete hemianopsia	Bilateral hemianopsia		
Facial Palsy	Normal	Minor	Partial	Complete		
Right Arm	No drift	Drift but does not hit the bed	Drifts down to the bed	No effort against gravity	No movement	Amputation or joint fusion
Left Arm	No drift	Drift but does not hit the bed	Drifts down to the bed	No effort against gravity	No movement	Amputation or joint fusion
Right Leg	No drift	Drift but does not hit the bed	Drifts down to the bed	No effort against gravity	No movement	Amputation or joint fusion
Left Leg	No drift	Drift but does not hit the bed	Drifts down to the bed	No effort against gravity	No movement	Amputation or joint fusion
Limb Ataxia	Absent	Present in one limb	Present in two limbs			
Sensation to Pin	Normal	Partial loss	Severe loss			
Best Language	No aphasia	Mild-moderate aphasia	Severe aphasia	Mute		
Dysarthria	None	Mild-moderate	Near to unintelligible or worse	Intubated or other barrier		
Extinction and Inattention	No neglect	Partial neglect	Complete Neglect			

Adapted from Lewis SL, Ende J, et al. MKSAP 14: Neurology. 2006. American College of Physicians. Also available at www.ninds.nih.gov/doctors/NIH_Stroke_Scale_Booklet.pdf

Middle Cerebral Artery—Hemiparesis: Paresis of either the right or left side of the body indicates contralateral disease of the brain or ipsilateral high spinal disease. The most common cause is vascular occlusion of the middle cerebral artery. Paralysis Is partial or complete. Sensory loss occurs In the same distribution. Consciousness is not impaired. The patient may not be aware of the deficit with right-sided infarcts. Lesions in the left hemisphere often affect Broca's area disrupting speech while comprehension remains intact. If the visual pathways are affected, a homonymous hemianopsia will be found.

Hemiparesis—Conversion Reaction: In patients with complaints of unilateral weakness or paralysis of the legs but confusing findings, try to elicit the *Hoover sign*, which depends on the absence of a normal associated movement (synkinesia). Place the patient supine, stand at the foot of the table, and place a palm under each heel. Ask the patient to raise the affected limb (Fig. 14–9D). In organic disease, the unaffected limb will press downward in the effort to raise the affected limb, it is absent in conversion reaction. The sign is helpful only when the patient has, or claims to have, paralysis of one leg. Paraplegia must be excluded. Hysterical arm paralysis may be identified by dropping the flaccid arm onto the face. With organic paralysis, the arm will strike the face; in hysteria, it always misses.

> **KEY SYNDROME   Cavernous Sinus Thrombosis**

Thrombosis with occlusion of the cavernous sinus results from bacterial infection of the upper lip, tooth socket, eyes, or face. Patients present with pain in the eye and forehead, chills, fever, and impaired vision. Physical findings include chemosis, edema of the eyelids, exophthalmos, hyperemia, papilledema, orbital tenderness, and CN palsies of CN III, -IV, and -VI. Progression leads to leptomeningitis, blindness, intracerebral abscess, septicemia, and death.

Hemorrhagic Stroke: See *Headache*, page 734.

Other CNS Syndromes

> **KEY SYNDROME   Trigeminal Neuralgia—Tic Douloureux**

See Chapter 7, page 213.

> **KEY SYNDROME   Parkinson's Disease and Parkinsonism**

Parkinson's disease is caused by depletion of the dopaminergic neurons of the substantia nigra leading to decreased dopamine delivery to the striatum. Parkinson's disease is one of a family of conditions affecting the extrapyramidal motor system and presenting with abnormalities of posture and movement. The onset of Parkinson's disease is asymmetric and gradual; familial forms exist. Tremor is present in two-third of patients, usually beginning in one hand. It is a slow (~6 Hz) repose tremor absent with movement and sleep. Other classic features are slowed voluntary movements (*bradykinesia* leading to *masked face*), *rigidity*, *postural instability*, and a gait marked by small steps (*march au petit pas*) with difficulty lifting the feet, absent arm swing and difficulty turning smoothly. Features that may be found early in the disease, if sought, include *micrographia*, decreased blink rate and *anosmia*. Cognitive and emotional disturbances are late findings [Rao G, Fisch L, Srinivasan S, et al. Does this patient have Parkinson disease? *JAMA*. 2003;289:347–353] **DDX:** Absence of tremor, though not rare, should raise the suspicion for one of the other Parkinsonian syndromes. Early cognitive or emotional instability, fluctuating mental status and hallucinations suggest *Lewy body disease*. Symmetrical onset without tremor but with eye findings, particularly paralysis of upward gaze, and falls suggests *Progressive Supranuclear Palsy*. Orthostatic hypotension, urinary incontinence and dysarthria, also without tremor, should suggest *Multisystem Atrophy* (Shy-Drager Syndrome). Drug induced Parkinsonism is common with metoclopramide and the antipsychotics most commonly described.

> **KEY SYNDROME** **Multiple Sclerosis**

Multifocal demyelinization occurs in the nervous system presumed to be mediated by autoimmune mechanisms. The onset is usually abrupt over hours to a few days, with remissions occurring over weeks, if at all. Optic neuritis with transient visual loss lasting weeks to months is a common presenting symptom. Other symptoms include incoordination, paresthesias, weakness, and loss of sphincter control. The signs depend upon the location of the demyelinating lesion(s): ataxia, dysarthria, intention tremor, ocular palsies, visual loss, hyperactive deep reflexes, diminished abdominal reflexes, and trophic changes in skin. The *Charcot triad* of signs is intention tremor, nystagmus, and scanning speech. The disease may be progressive from onset with inexorable loss of function, or relapsing-remitting with complete resolution of the symptoms and signs between relapses. Many patients with initially relapsing-remitting disease will progress to chronic progressive disease with incomplete remissions of each relapse [Compston A, Coles A. Multiple sclerosis. *Lancet*. 2002;1221–1231].

Neuromyelitis Optica (Devic Syndrome): IgG antibodies to a unique class of CNS membrane channel proteins has been identified in this syndrome. This is thought to be a form of MS that results in repeated attacks of optic neuritis and lesions involving long segments of the cervical spinal cord. Symptoms are visual loss and paresthesias, painful spasticity and weakness in the arms and legs.

> **KEY SYNDROME** **Neurosyphilis**

Chronic infection with *Treponema pallidum* produces degeneration of the spinal cord posterior columns, dorsal roots, and dorsal root ganglia. Brain infection produces a tertiary syphilis syndrome of degenerative brain disease. The patient is often unaware of having been infected and with many years intervening the history of a chancre may be lost. Other signs of tertiary syphilis may be present, such as aortitis with aortic insufficiency and gumma formation. Two CNS syndromes are recognized.

Tabes Dorsalis: Spinal cord involvement produces lightning-like pains in the trunk and lower limbs, paresthesias, urinary incontinence, and impotence. There is loss of position sense, ataxic wide-based gait, footdrop, and loss of reflexes. Loss of position sense leads to joint destruction with Charcot deformities. *Tabetic crisis* is abdominal pain and vomiting with a relaxed abdominal wall.

General Paresis: The brain findings can be recalled using the pneumonic *PARE-SIS:* Personality, Affect, loss of Reflexes, Eye findings (Argyll-Robinson pupil), Sensory changes, Intellectual deterioration (*dementia precox*), and Speech changes.

➤ **KEY DISEASE   Rabies**

Infection by this neurotropic virus is transmitted by the bite of infected mammals. Onset is marked by local dysesthesia radiating from the site of entry, malaise, nausea, and sore throat. Later, restlessness and hallucinations occur. There is hyperesthesia of the wound and later, dysarthria, dysphagia for fluids, convulsions, delirium, and opisthotonos stimulated by lights or noises. Breathing becomes shallow and irregular with hoarseness or aphonia. The stretch reflexes are hyperactive and there is nuchal rigidity, Babinski sign followed by flaccid paralysis, and death. A high index of suspicion is required to make the diagnosis and to protect contacts to body fluids. Many patients diagnosed in the United States do not have an identified source of infection; bats are the most common identified source.

KEY SYNDROME   Syringomyelia and Chiari Malformations

There is cavitary expansion within the cervical spinal cord that damages the centrally crossing sensory tracts and the pyramidal tracts. The cause is unknown. Syringomyelia is frequently associated with herniation of the cerebellar tonsils through the foramen magnum (Chiari type 1). Patients present with decreased pain and temperature sensation in the arms and shoulders, LMN weakness in the arms and UMN weakness with spasticity in the legs. Chiari type 2 malformation (incomplete closure of the spinal canal) is always accompanied by myelomeningocele.

KEY SYNDROME   Paraparesis

Loss of motor power to both legs indicates a transverse lesion of the spinal cord. The level is determined by the sensory findings. Frequent causes of paraparesis are trauma and transverse myelitis, which may follow several different types of viral infection. Extrinsic cord compression by herniated disk or epidural abcess or neoplasm are less common but potentially treatable. Dural arteriovenous malformations cause venous congestion and spinal cord ischemia without infarction; the deficits are fully reversible if the diagnosis is made and treatment closes the malformation [Atkinson JLD, Miller GM, Kraus WE, et al. Clinical and radiographic features of dural arteriovenous fistula, a treatable cause of myelopathy. *Mayo Clin Proc.* 2001;76:1120–1130].

KEY SYNDROME   Quadriparesis

Paresis or paralysis of all limbs without changes in consciousness indicates impairment of the descending corticospinal (pyramidal) tracts. The most common cause is traumatic injury to the cervical spine; in this case the bulbar muscles are spared. Less common, but not rare, causes, usually with some bulbar involvement, are multiple sclerosis, primary motor system disease (e.g., amyotrophic lateral sclerosis), and botulism. Onset of nontraumatic generalized weakness or paralysis over a few hours or days suggests an electrolyte disturbance (most commonly severe hypokalemia). In the hospital, other causes to be considered are inadvertently high spinal anesthesia, paralytic drugs, and the polyneuropathy of severe illness.

> **KEY SYNDROME** **Hemisection of the Spinal Cord—Brown Sequard Syndrome**

Hemisection of the cord damages the ipsilateral descending motor pathways and ascending proprioceptive pathways (cross in the brainstem), and the contralateral sensory pathways for pain and temperature (cross at their spinal root levels). Patients have motor paralysis with spasticity and loss of proprioception on the side of the lesion and absent pain and temperature sensation on the opposite side, below the level of the injury.

> **KEY SYNDROME** **Amyotrophic Lateral Sclerosis**

Degeneration of upper and LMNs leads to progressive weakness and muscle wasting. The disease begins gradually, proceeds progressively, and ends fatally in 2 to 3 years. Muscle aches and cramps are accompanied by weakness of distal upper limbs, spreading to the lower extremities; dysarthria, dysphagia, and drooling indicate bulbar involvement. Muscle fasciculation and severe wasting are seen, especially in upper limbs. Fasciculations may be evident in the tongue. Hyperreflexia and spasticity of lower limbs indicate upper motor neuron involvement [Rowland LP, Shneider NA. Amyotrophic lateral sclerosis. *N Engl J Med.* 2001;344:1688–1700; O'Neill GN, Gonzalez RG, Cros DP, et al. Case 22-2006: A 77-year-old man with rapidly progressive gait disorder. *N Engl J Med.* 2006;355:296–304].

> **KEY SYNDROME** **Poliomyelitis and West Nile Virus**

Infection of the spinal cord by West Nile or polio virus leads to destruction of LMNs with muscle weakness and atrophy. Polio still occurs outside the Western Hemisphere, despite efforts to eradicate it through vaccination. Fever, headache, sore throat, stiff neck, and pain in the back and limbs is followed by inability to move one or more muscle groups. Signs are varying deep reflexes, weakness, fasciculations, hyperesthesia, paresthesias, and lymphadenopathy. Kernig and Brudzinski signs may be present. Healing may lead to complete return of function or be followed by muscular atrophy. Bulbar involvement leads to weakness of the pharyngeal muscles and diaphragm. Many years after recovery, insidious weakness may recur in the affected muscles, *postpolio syndrome.* A very similar syndrome is being reported with West Nile Virus infection.

Post-Polio Syndrome: Recovery from poliomyelitis involves reinervation of denervated muscle fibers by branches from remaining motor axons. After many years, axonal degeneration with elimination of these axonal twigs results, once again, in denervation, weakness and atrophy. Patients present with weakness in the muscle groups most severely affected at the time of initial infection. The course is slowly progressive with increasing weakness and functional decline.

> **KEY SYNDROME** Dystonias

Dystonias are abnormally prolonged tonic contractions of a muscle or muscle group. Dystonias are often associated with certain activities and can become disabling. The patient will refer to them as a cramp. Examples are writer's cramp, torticollis, and dystonias associated with playing musical instruments [Tarsy D, Simon DK. Dystonia. *N Engl J Med.* 2006;355;818–829].

> **KEY SYNDROME** Posterior Column Disease

Deficiencies of vitamin B_{12} and copper and neurosyphilis (tabes dorsalis) lead to degeneration of the posterior columns with loss of proprioception in the lower extremities leading to abnormalities of gait and balance. Nitrous oxide anesthesia may precipitate severe B12 deficiency in patients with minimal stores. **DDX:** Glossitis, macrocytic anemia and dementia accompany severe B12 deficiency; a spastic gait disorder may accompany copper deficiency [Kumar M. Copper deficiency myelopathy (human swayback). *Mayo Clin Proc.* 2006;81:1371–1384].

Other Motor and Sensory Syndromes

> **KEY SYNDROME** Peripheral Neuropathy

Lesions are classified as axonal if the nerve cell axon is primarily involved, or demyelinating if the lesion is in the myelin coating of the nerve. Single nerve trunk lesions may be traumatic, ischemic, or inflammatory. Peripheral nerve dysfunction in the absence of CNS disease is common. Patients present with complaints of numbness, burning, unsteadiness (often described as dizziness), falling, or weakness. Physical examination may show sensory impairment (pressure, vibration, position, pain and temperature or simple touch depending on the size of nerves involved), muscle weakness and wasting with fasciculations, and/or diminished reflexes. Release signs are not present and plantar response is flexor. *Demyelinating neuropathies* present acutely or more slowly with involvement of both motor and sensory nerves; often the motor component dominates with weakness and areflexia. They may involve any nerve at any level from root distally so the pattern is usually asymmetrical and involves proximal as well as distal muscles. *Axonal neuropathies* are diffuse, symmetrical, slowly progressive and usually sensory at onset with later involvement of motor nerves; they are primarily distal and progress proximally affecting the feet before the hands. Isolated nontraumatic involvement of all components of a single nerve is called *mononeuritis multiplex*, usually resulting from an inflammatory lesion causing ischemia; recovery is common and complete [Hughes RAC. Peripheral neuropathy. *BMJ.* 2002;324:466–469; Poncelet AN. An algorithm for the evaluation of peripheral neuropathy. *Am Fam Physician.* 1998;57:755–764].

✔ PERIPHERAL NEUROPATHY—CLINICAL OCCURRENCE: **Congenital** Charcot-Marie-Tooth disease, porphyria, Fabry disease, familial neuropathy; **Endocrine** diabetes; **Idiopathic** ICU polyneuropathy, idiopathic polyneuropathy; **Infectious** leprosy, rabies (early at inoculation site), postherpetic neuralgia; **Inflammatory/Immune** acute and chronic inflammatory demyelinating polyneuropathy, vasculitis, SLE, amyloidosis, celiac disease, monoclonal gammopathy; **Mechanical/Trauma** contusion and laceration, repetitive use, vibration (e.g., jackhammers, pneumatic drills), cold injury (chilblains and frostbite), electrical injury; **Metabolic/Toxic** amyloidosis, porphyria, diabetes, Fabry disease, poisoning (arsenic, other heavy metals, pyridoxine), drugs (e.g., vincristine), nutritional deficiency (vitamins B_{12}, copper and B_6); **Neoplastic** paraneoplastic syndromes, metastatic invasion of nerves; **Psychosocial** substance abuse producing unconsciousness with pressure-induced ischemia; **Vascular** vasculitis.

Diabetic Neuropathies: Diabetes types 1 and 2 are associated with peripheral nerve injury with a latency of approximately 15 years from onset for type 1. Damage is thought to be metabolic in most forms, and ischemic in the acute reversible forms. Several forms of diabetic neuropathy are recognized. **Distal sensorimotor axonal neuropathy** is most common, presenting as numbness or burning pain in the feet and progressing proximally with loss of protective sensation, trophic skin changes, pressure-induced ischemic ulceration, and infection leading to amputation, if preventive measures are not taken. Limbs at risk are insensitive to a 10-g monofilament test [Smieja M, Hunt DL, Edelman D, et al. Clinical examination for the detection of protective sensation in the feet of diabetic patients. International Cooperative Group for Clinical Examination Research. *J Gen Intern Med.* 1999;14:418–424]. In severe forms, muscle wasting and Charcot joints occur. **Autonomic neuropathy** frequently involves the stomach with gastroparesis and delayed gastric emptying which may make control of blood sugars very difficult. Sudomotor injury contributes to skin fragility and ulceration. Impotence is common and colon and bladder dysfunction not rare. The sensorimotor and autonomic neuropathies are delayed or prevented by tight control of blood glucose. **Diabetic amyotrophy or polyradiculopathy** is an acute, painful, inflammatory or ischemic injury to one or more spinal roots. Patients present with severe back, chest, abdominal or proximal leg pain, and progressive weakness, and may have bowel and bladder dysfunction. It is usually acute in onset and asymmetric. Recovery is expected over months in most people. Isolated **CN palsies,** especially CN III, -IV, and -VI are not uncommon and often mistaken for much more serious intracranial pathology. The pupil is spared in CN III lesions. Diabetic amyotrophy and CN lesions are not clearly related to the duration of diabetes or degree of blood sugar control.

➤ **KEY SYNDROME** **Acute Inflammatory Demyelinating Polyneuropathy (AIDP, Guillain-Barré Syndrome)**

This is an immune-mediated demyelinating disorder occurring 1 to 3 weeks after viral infection, *Campylobacter jejuni* gastroenteritis, or, rarely, after surgery or with malignant lymphoma. There is usually rapidly progressive ascending motor weakness with pain in back and limbs, and distal numbness and tingling. Nausea and vomiting can occur. There is ascending flaccid paralysis with diminished deep and superficial reflexes. CN involvement causes dysphasia, dysphagia and dysarthria. With chest wall involvement, respiratory failure supervenes.

KEY SYNDROME **Chronic Inflammatory Demyelinating Polyneuropathy (CIDP)**

Chronic immune mediated demylination of nerve roots, plexuses and peripheral nerves. There is sudden or gradual onset of motor and sensory symptoms and signs referrable to a spinal root, plexus or peripheral nerve. Multiple nerves may be involved often in an asymmetric pattern. Symptoms may progress gradually or remit and relapse. Weakness and areflexia accompany sensory findings indicating involvement of mixed nerves [Koller H, Kieseier BC, Jander S, et al. Chronic inflammatory demyelinating polyneuropathy. *N Engl J Med.* 2005;352: 1343–1356].

KEY SYNDROME Numb Chin Syndrome

Infiltration of mental or inferior alveolar nerve(s) branches of CN IX by malignant cells, most commonly an aggressive lymphoma. The patient is ususaly a young adult presenting with a numb lower lip and chin, no other complaints and a normal physical examination other than decreased sensation on the chin. The patient should not be reassured; further evaluation is indicated.

KEY SYNDROME Autonomic Neuropathy

Damage to the subcortical autonomic control systems in the hypothalamus and brainstem and/or damage to the peripheral nerves results in loss of normal autonomic regulation. Patients present with abnormalities of cardiovascular, gastrointestinal, urogenital and sudomotor function; loss of activity is more common than overactivity. *Orthostatic hypotension*, not accompanied by a rise in pulse, and not infrequently combined with hypertension when supine is the most frequent presenting sign. They have abnormal heart rate and blood pressure responses to the Valsalva maneuver and carotid massage and absent heart rate variation with deep breathing. Other frequent symptoms are constipation or diarrhea, absent or excessive sweating, problems with bladder function (difficulty voiding or incontinence) and erectile and ejaculatory dysfunction. Patients with anhydrosis are susceptibel to overheating in warm, especially humid, environments. **CLINICAL OCCURRENCE:** Long standing diabetes is the most common encountered association, but multisystem atrophy, subacute combined degeneration, Parkinson disease, Fabry disease, syringomyelia, porhyrias, paraneoplastic neuropathies and amyloidosis, among others, must be considered.

KEY SYNDROME Compression Neuropathies

Nerves are vulnerable to compression injury at sites of frequent motion, trauma, external pressure or excessive traction. Symptoms are usually pain and dysethesia initially but may progress to weakness if the nerve is a mixed motor and sensory nerve. Knowledge of the distribution and exact anatomic locations of vulnerable portions of the peripheral nerves will greatly assist in diagnosis. Reproduction of the symptoms by *gently* tapping the nerve at the sight of compression (Tinnel's sign) supports the diagnosis; however, not that all sensory nerves are positive if struck hard enough (e.g., the ulnar nerve "funny bone"). Some common examples are listed below.

Carpal Tunnel Syndrome: The median nerve is compressed beneath the volar transverse carpal ligament of the wrist (Fig. 14–22) producing dysesthesia and pain, then loss of fine (two-point) sensation, and, finally, thenar muscle atrophy and weakness. The patient complains of numbness and tingling in the hand, particularly at night. There may be associated pain, limited to the hand or running up the forearm. Ultimately, there is progressive weakness and awkwardness in the finer movements of the fingers. It may be unilateral

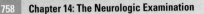
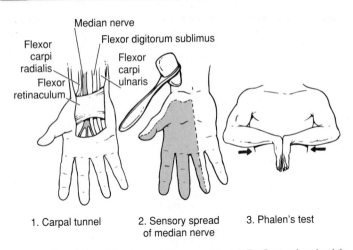

1. Carpal tunnel   2. Sensory spread   3. Phalen's test
of median nerve

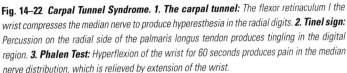

Fig. 14–22 Carpal Tunnel Syndrome. 1. The carpal tunnel: *The flexor retinaculum I the wrist compresses the median nerve to produce hyperesthesia in the radial digits.* **2. Tinel sign:** *Percussion on the radial side of the palmaris longus tendon produces tingling in the digital region.* **3. Phalen Test:** *Hyperflexion of the wrist for 60 seconds produces pain in the median nerve distribution, which is relieved by extension of the wrist.*

or bilateral. Although patients frequently describe tingling of the entire hand, hypoesthesia is distributed on the palmar aspects of the 3.5 radial digits and the distal two-thirds of the dorsal aspects of the same fingers. Light percussion on the radial side of the palmaris longus tendon may produce a tingling sensation (*Tinel sign*, Fig. 14–22). Flexion of the wrists at 90 degrees with the dorsal surfaces of the hands in apposition for 60 seconds (*Phalen test*) may reproduce the pain (Fig. 14–22). Neither maneuver is particularly sensitive or specific for the finding of nerve injury by nerve conduction studies. The condition is most common with repetitive use injury, for example, meat-packing workers, grocery clerks, and keyboard operators [Katz JN, Simmons BP. Carpal tunnel syndrome. *N Engl J Med.* 2002;346:1807–1812; D'Arcy CA, McGee S. The rational clinical examination. Does this patient have carpal tunnel syndrome? *JAMA.* 2000;283:3110–3117]. **CLINICAL OCCURRENCE:** congenitally small carpal tunnel, hypothyroidism, diabetes, acromegaly, pregnancy, osteoarthritis, rheumatoid arthritis, amyloidosis, sarcoidosis, gout, Paget disease, repetitive wrist flexion and extension, posttraumatic arthritis, multiple myeloma, MGUS.

Lateral Femoral Cutaneous Nerve (Meralgia Paresthetica): The lateral femoral cutaneous nerve is entrapped under the anterior superior iliac spine and inguinal ligament or directly compressed by tight fitting restraints or work belts. It results in numbness of the lateral thigh. Since it is a pure sensory nerve, there are no motor signs. It frequently occurs in the setting of obesity or pregnancy.

Tarsal Tunnel Syndrome: There is entrapment of the posterior tibial nerve in the tarsal tunnel under the medial malleolus giving pain and tingling on the sole of the foot and toes. It may be aggravated by standing.

Cubital Tunnel Syndrome: The ulnar nerve is entrapped at the elbow behind the medial humeral condyle. It is aggravated by flexion of the elbow putting the nerve on stretch. Symptoms are numbness of the fourth and fifth fingers progressing to weakness of the intrinsic hand muscles.

Radial Nerve: The radial nerve is compressed where it wraps around the upper third of the humerus. This is often associated with prolonged unconsciousness due to injury or overdose with the arm weight resting on a hard object. Numbness of the dorsum of the arm and hand is associated with weakness of finger and wrist extensors.

Common Peroneal Nerve: The common peroneal nerve wraps around the head of the fibula laterally where it is vulnerable to compression from tight casts, crossed legs or unconsciousness with compression against a hard surface. Symptoms are a foot drop on that side. There may be numbness on the lateral calf and dorsum of the foot.

KEY SYNDROME   Myasthenia Gravis

An autoantibody binds to the acetylcholine receptor at the neuromuscular junction blocking neuromuscular transmission, especially with repetitive excitation. There is an association with thymoma. Affected individuals complain of increased fatigability, transient muscle weakness, diplopia, ptosis, easy fatigue with chewing and talking, regurgitation, and dysphagia. During an exacerbation there may be lack of facial expression, abnormal speech or aphonia and disconjugate gaze. In extreme cases, the patient cannot lift his head from the pillow. Muscle function is normal and diplopia absent on awaking, when the most acetylcholine is stored. The levator and, to a lesser extent, the other ocular muscles recover after rest. Ptosis is quickly relieved by neostigmine, but the other paralyses do not respond as dramatically. [Scherer K, Bedlack RS, Simel DL. Does this patient have myasthenia gravis? *JAMA.* 2005;293:1906–1914]

➤ KEY SYNDROME   Botulism

Neurotoxins produced by *Clostridium botulinum* may be ingested or absorbed from contaminated wounds. Symptom onset is over hours with variable combinations of weakness, headache, dizziness, dysphagia, abdominal pain, nausea and vomiting, diarrhea, and diplopia. Physical findings include fixed and dilated pupils, nystagmus, ptosis, irregular respiration, swollen tongue, hyporeflexia, and incoordination [Sheridan EA, Cepeda J, De Palma R, et al. A drug user with a sore throat. *Lancet.* 2004;364:1286]. Improperly canned foods prepared in the home and wound and skin infections are the most common causes.

➤ KEY SYNDROME   Tetanus

Tetanus is caused by the toxin of *Clostridium tetani* acting on myoneural junctions. A single muscle or many groups become rigid with sustained tonic spasm. The masseter is frequently involved early, hence the term lockjaw (*trismus*). Loud noises, bright lights, or pain induce superimposed violent generalized spasms. The condition should not be confused with tetany, which it resembles only in name.

Disorders of Language and Speech

> **KEY SYNDROME** **Disorders of Language—Aphasia**

Language is instantiated in the dominant hemisphere, which is the left hemisphere in >99% of right- and left-handed people. Damage to specific language-processing areas produces distinct aphasias. Language is the symbolic representation and interpretation of meaning in voice sounds and written symbols (*symbolization*). It is a far more complex activity than speech, requiring extensive central interconnectivity. An acquired inability to use language correctly is termed *aphasia* and indicates acquired disease of the brain. Congenital or developmental disorders of language are called *dysphasias*. Language is evaluated during history taking and with the MMSE. Six domains are assessed: (1) speech expression, both spontaneous and automatic sequences (e.g., singing, nursery rhymes, and cursing); (2) naming; (3) speech comprehension; (4) repetition; (5) reading; and (6) writing [Damasio AR. Aphasia. *N Engl J Med*. 1992;326:531–539].

Broca Aphasia: There is damage to the Broca area of the left frontal lobe. The speech is nonfluent, often leaving out pronouns, prepositions, and the like; reading and writing are also affected. Patients are aware of their difficulty and become frustrated. They appear to know what they want to say. Speech comprehension is relatively spared for simple communication.

Wernicke Aphasia: Speech is fluent but words are jumbled and substituted, obscuring all meaning (*paraphasia*). Writing is similarly affected. Reading and verbal comprehension are poor. The patient is unaware of their deficit and may become angry when not understood.

Global Aphasia: This is a combination of Broca and Wernicke aphasia.

Other Aphasias: See neurology texts for discussion of conduction, anomic, transcortical, and subcortical aphasias.

> **KEY SYNDROME** **Alexia and Agraphia**

Alexia is the inability to read. *Dyslexia* is an impairment of reading ability. *Agraphia* is the inability to write.

> **KEY SIGN** **Disorders of Speech. Dysarthria, Dysphonia, Ataxia, and Apraxia**

Normal speech has many qualities, each of which may be specific to an individual allowing precise recognition of individual voices. Specific qualities to be noted are articulation, phonation, fluency, and repetition.

Articulation—Dysarthria and Dyslalia: Articulation is the production of sounds and their combinations into syllables. Disorders of the brain produce *dysarthria*; specific dysarthrias are identified by the types of sounds which are improperly formed (see Chapter 7, page 209). *Dyslalia* is impaired articulation from non-neurologic structural defects or hearing loss.

Voice—Dysphonia: This concerns coordination and control of the larynx and resonating qualities of the pharynx. *Dysphonia* is the disturbance in pitch, quality, and volume. *Hypernasality* and *hyponasality* refer to nasal resonance.

Rhythm—Ataxia: This deals with the timing and sequence of syllables. Irregular, slow speech with pauses and bursts of sounds is called *scanning speech* and indicates a cerebellar disorder, for example, MS. Faltering or interruptions in speech are termed *stuttering;* this is frequently inherited or may be a developmental disorder.

Sound Selection—Apraxia: This is the inability to properly and consistently program a correct sequence of sounds, especially consonants. Have the patient repeat the word "artillery" five times; each sound is formed correctly, but they are misplaced and no two attempts may be alike. The problem is evident with writing as well as speech.

Syndromes of Impaired Mentation

> **KEY SYNDROME** Delirium

See Chapter 15, page 776 for the full discussion of delirium.

➤ **Hepatic Encephalopathy:** Severe hepatocellular dysfunction and/or portal hypertension with portal-systemic shunting allows accumulation of toxic metabolites leading to cerebral dysfunction. This presents four features—only the last two are distinctive: (1) altered mental state varying from slight loss of memory to confusion, slurred speech, sedation, and coma; (2) asterixis, also present in cerebrovascular disease, uremia, and severe pulmonary insufficiency; (3) signs of abnormal liver function such as jaundice, palmar erythema, spider angiomata, hepatomegaly, and ascites; and (4) fetor hepaticus, smelling something like old wine, acetone, or new-mown hay; if present, it is distinctive of hepatic coma.

➤ **Wernicke-Korsakoff Syndrome:** Thiamine deficiency is common in alcoholism and symptoms may occur when administration of glucose causes acute thiamine deficiency (*Wernicke encephalopathy*) leading to chronic brain injury (*Korsakoff syndrome*). Wernicke syndrome presents with confusion, nystagmus, ataxia, ophthalmoplegia, impaired memory, and decreased attention. It is essential to recognize and treat the patient immediately with parenteral thiamine. Korsakoff syndrome is an irreversible chronic encephalopathy with antegrade and retrograde amnesia and confabulation. Thiamine deficiency may be a late complication of surgical treatments for obesity.

> **KEY SYNDROME** Mild Cognitive Impairment

This represents a decline in cognitive function exceeding that expected for age but not resulting in significant impairment of daily life. Memory is the most frequently observed abnormality. More than half of patients with mild cognitive impairment progress to dementia within five years; others remain stable for variable lengths of time [Gauthier S, Reisberg B, Zaudig M, et al. Mild cognitive impairment. *Lancet.* 2006;367:1262–1270].

> **KEY SYNDROME** Dementia

Dementia is a decline in cognitive function sufficient to impair function. It includes memory loss (recent more than remote; i.e., loss of orientation) and at least one of the following: aphasia, apraxia, agnosia, or abnormal executive function. It is chronic and usually progressive, although the rate of progression is quite variable. Personality changes and loss of normal social inhibitions are late findings in most cases. Dementia is easily missed early in its course if not specifically sought. There are no early physical findings, the release signs being late manifestations of advanced disease. Screening with the MMSE, clock drawing task or Mini-Cog are useful. Medical illness can present as dementia so it is essential to exclude the many potentially reversible medical conditions such as hypothyroidism, other endocrinopathies, medication side effects, and vitamin B_{12} deficiency. There are many causes of dementia, but Alzheimer disease is most common [Karlawish JHT, Clark CM. Diagnostic evaluation of elderly patients with mild memory problems. *Ann Intern Med.* 2003;138:411–419]. Most reversible causes are accompanied by some blunting of consciousness.

✔ **DEMENTIA—CLINICAL OCCURRENCE:** *Congenital* Familial Alzheimer disease, adrenoleukodystrophy, Huntington disease, lipopolysaccharidoses, Wilson disease, mitochondrial disease, porphyria, Down syndrome (trisomy 21); *Endocrine* hypothyroidism, Addison disease, Cushing syndrome, hyper- and hypoparathyroidism; *Idiopathic* Alzheimer disease, Pick disease, Lewy body disease, progressive supranuclear palsy, frontotemporal dementias; *Inflammatory/Immune* vasculitis, subacute sclerosing panencephalitis, sarcoidosis; *Infectious* HIV infection, syphilis, prion disease (Creutzfeldt-Jacob disease [CJD], bovine spongiform encephalopathy [variant CJD (vCJD)], and others), progressive multifocal leukoencephalopathy (papovavirus), Whipple disease, postencephalitis; *Metabolic/Toxic* chronic alcoholism, vitamin B_{12}, thiamine, and nicotinic acid deficiency, uremia, liver failure, aluminum toxicity (dialysis dementia), postanoxia, drug intoxication; *Mechanical/Trauma* acute and chronic head trauma, normal pressure hydrocephalus, chronic subdural hematoma; *Neoplastic* paraneoplastic limbic encephalitis, brain tumors, and metastatic cancer; *Neurologic* nonconvulsive seizures, Parkinson disease; *Psychosocial* depression (pseudodementia), schizophrenia; *Vascular* vascular dementias (multi-infarct, Binswanger disease).

Alzheimer Disease: Neurofibrillatory tangles and plaques with extracellular deposition of amyloid precursor protein accumulate in the brain. The cause is partly genetic and possibly partly environmental. Slowly progressive dementia usually begins in the seventh or eighth decade of life; it may occur at younger ages, especially in the hereditary syndromes. The identical syndrome occurs uniformly in patients with trisomy 21 (Down syndrome) at an earlier age, usually in the fourth decade of life. The mental deterioration begins insidiously with memory loss, depression, anxiety, suspicion, and later amnesia, agnosia, aphasia, shuffling gait, and rigidity. The diagnosis is clinical, after excluding treatable forms of dementia. Imaging reveals diffuse atrophy of the cerebral cortex with symmetrical enlargement of the lateral and third ventricles. **DDX:** If severe psychiatric symptoms are present (e.g., hallucinations, psychosis), consider Lewy body disease. If the dementia is rapidly progressive, consider CJD or vCJD, bovine spongiform encephalopathy).

Dementia with Lewy Bodies: This accounts for approximately 20% of diagnosed dementias. It is accompanied by fluctuating mental status with periods of delirium separated by more clear times, visual hallucinations and parkinsonism. Fluctation is defined as any three of the following: sleeping for more than 2 hours during the day; daytime sleepiness not related to inadequate nighttime sleep; prolonged staring episodes; and garbled speech with clear words but unorganized content. Patients have more visual spatial problems than Alzheimer patients. Syncope, frequent falls, difficulty sleeping and depression are common as well. When you feel the need for both a neurologist and a psychiatrist you may be dealing with Lewy body disease [Neef D, Walling AD. Dementia with Lewy bodies: An emerging disease. *Am Fam Physician.* 2006;73:1223–1229].

Normal Pressure Hydrocephalus: Enlargement of the ventricular system at normal CSF pressure is accompanied by dementia, gait apraxia and urinary incontinence. The symptoms and signs are reversible with appropriate treatment so a high index of suspicion should be maintained.

> **KEY SYNDROME**   Psychosis

See Chapter 15, page 783.

Other Syndromes

> **KEY SYNDROME**   Tourette Syndrome

This is a neurodevelopmental disorder presenting in childhood. Patients have a complex array of vocal and facial tics, echolalia and coprolalia that often impair social function. The tics may be suppressed by the patient with great effort. Obsessive-compulsive disorder and attention-deficit disorder hyperactivity disorder occur in association with Tourette syndrome [Jankovic J. Tourette's syndrome. *N Engl J Med.* 2001;345:1184–1192].

> **KEY SYNDROME**   Restless Legs Syndrome

The patient complains of leg discomfort at rest, often prior to sleep. The sensation may be aching, drawing, pulling, prickling, restlessness, formication, or completely nondescript. Always bilateral, the sensations are relieved by walking or massage. There are no pertinent physical findings. The cause is unknown, but has been reported with iron and folate deficiency and uremia. Familial forms occur. Many patients also have periodic limb movements of sleep. Diagnosis is based upon four criteria: onset of symptoms at rest, urge to move, symptoms relieved by movement and symptoms worse in the evening. Most patients obtain some relief with dopamine agonists [Earley CJ. Restless legs syndrome. *N Engl J Med.* 2003;348:2103–2109].

> **KEY SYNDROME**   Horner Syndrome

A lesion of the cervical sympathetic chain produces the following signs on the ipsilateral side: (1) partial ptosis of the upper eyelid (weakness of Mueller muscle) and some elevation of the lower lid ("inverse ptosis"), (2) constriction of the pupil, miosis, accompanied by pupil dilation or delay after a light reflex (dilation lag), and (3) absence of sweating on the forehead and face of the affected side (Fig. 14–20A, page 729). If damage to the sympathetics occurs early in life, pigmentation of the iris may be affected; for example, the affected iris may remain blue when the other changes to brown if the patient is brown-eyed. Horner syndrome occurs with ipsilateral mediastinal tumor and has been reported with spontaneous pneumothorax and brainstem stroke.

> **KEY SYNDROME** **Complex Regional Pain Syndrome—Reflex Sympathetic Dystrophy, Causalgia**

See Chapter 4, page 87.

Repeated Bell Palsy—Melkersson Syndrome: This is a triad of scrotal tongue (lingua plicata) with repeated attacks of Bell palsy and painless, nonpitting, facial edema. The cause is unknown.

> **KEY SYNDROME** **Death**

Death is an obvious fact of life. Most adults can make a reasonably accurate diagnosis of death, but occasional cases prove complicated. One of the horror stories in medical history is a probably apocryphal episode in the life of Vesalius. In 1564, during the height of his European fame as an anatomist, he was appointed physician to Philip II of Spain. He is said to have conducted an autopsy in Madrid on a young nobleman who had been his patient. According to the custom of the time, this was carried out before a large crowd of citizens. When the thorax of the body was opened, the heart was seen to be beating, and the anatomist was compelled to leave Spain hastily. Such experiences have made it necessary to have a physician or other trained person pronounce the death of a patient.

Biological death is the cessation of function of all bodily tissues. In the process of dying, tissues and organ functions deteriorate at varying rates, so a precise end point is difficult to define. For ordinary purposes, it is conclusive to recognize the irreversible cessation of circulatory, respiratory, brain, or brainstem functions. This is partially assessed by unconsciousness and absence of the "vital signs" (cardiac activity, respirations, and maintained body temperature), but these indicators have proved inadequate in victims of cold water drowning, for example, when unconsciousness, apnea, and imperceptible heartbeat are still compatible with resuscitation and full recovery. Different criteria are also required for patients receiving mechanical respiration and cardiac pacing.

Death Examination for Most Patients: Examine for evidence of heart contraction by palpating for pulsations in the carotid arteries and auscultating the precordium for heart sounds. An ECG will determine if cardiac electrical activity is present in the absence of mechanical contraction. Search for respiratory activity by placing the diaphragm of your stethoscope over the patient's mouth while listening for breath sounds. Also, hold a cold mirror at the nostrils and mouth to detect a deposit of water vapor. Neurologic function is assessed by several tests: call to the patient to test responsiveness; retract the eyelids to observe the pupillary reaction to light (fixed dilated pupils are seen with death and some drug intoxications); rotate the head from side to side with the lids retracted to observe whether the eyes remain fixed in their orbits or move in conjugate (doll's eyes), indicating an intact brainstem; perform ice water caloric stimulation, if there are no eye movements; press the sternum and squeeze the Achilles tendons to look for a response to deep pain; lift and let fall the limbs to test for muscle tone; check for gag and corneal reflexes [Wijdicks EFM. The diagnosis of brain death. *N Engl J Med.* 2001;344:1215–1221].

Supplementary Death Examination, Especially for Near-Drowning and Patients with Mechanical Ventilators and Pacemakers: Victims of cold water immersion drowning experience rapid total body cooling (severe hypothermia) and may meet all the preceding criteria of death yet still be capable of resuscitation with excellent neurologic function after immersion of up to 1 hour. A reasonable practical guideline is that such patients are not dead until they are warm (core temperature $> 35°C$) and dead. Other patients needing special consideration are those sustained by mechanical ventilation and pacemakers who fail to meet the cardiac and respiratory criteria for death, but who may be dead by irreversible loss of brain function. The clinician should always seek consultation from a neurologist in these complicated clinical situations.

CHAPTER 15

The Mental Status, Psychiatric, and Social Evaluations

Psychiatric and social disorders are common in medical settings. They are associated with an increased risk for nonpsychiatric illness and frequently confound the evaluation of patients presenting with nonspecific complaints. The student of medicine at all levels should read more specialized texts that deal with psychiatric illness and seek formal psychiatric consultation whenever doubt exists concerning psychiatric diagnosis. It is imperative to recognize that the presence of a psychiatric diagnosis in no way decreases the probability of serious organic disease in a patient with appropriate signs or symptoms. The challenge is to render appropriate diagnosis and therapy for all coexistent psychiatric and nonpsychiatric illnesses simultaneously, not sequentially. Delay in the diagnosis of organic disease in patients with psychiatric illness is all too common and should caution the clinician to take extra care in the evaluation of patients with psychiatric symptoms.

The distinction between what we classify as neurologic or psychiatric illness is a function of our understanding of brain physiology and pathophysiology. The distinction often rests on the presence of identifiable structural, genetic, physiological, or biochemical disorders in the neurologic category and their absence in psychiatric disease. Many psychiatric syndromes show genetic predispositions and respond to medications that alter brain function. Functional imaging studies are increasingly identifying localized abnormalities of brain function in some psychiatric disorders. For the practitioner, it is sufficient to recognize that the disorders we classify as psychiatric, although representing disorders of brain function, will be recognized by their clinical signs with abnormalities of thought, mood, affect, and behavior rather than specific tests of brain structure and clinical laboratory testing.

Social behavioral disorders and violence are also common problems in our society. To properly evaluate and care for patients, clinicians must be knowledgeable about the social situation of their patient. Social factors lead to patients presenting with a wide variety of complaints both physical and psychiatric. A complete social and psychiatric history with attention to current safety, a history of abuse (such as physical, sexual, emotional, financial, etc.), and the resources available to the patients for their care is essential in the evaluation of all patients.

This chapter does not provide a complete diagnostic approach to psychiatric illness. Rather, our purpose is to alert the clinician to the common psychiatric syndromes likely to be encountered in clinical practice and to provide some guidance to their recognition. The *Diagnostic and Statistical Manual of Mental Disorders, Fourth Edition* (*DSM-IV*), published by the American Psychiatric Association, is a particularly valuable resource with which all practitioners should become familiar [American Psychiatric Association. *Diagnostic and Statistical Manual of*

Mental Disorders. 4th ed. Washington, DC: American Psychiatric Association; 1994]. In addition to diagnostic criteria, the manual provides an overview of the epidemiology and presentation of mental disorders.

SECTION 1

The Mental Status and Psychiatric Evaluation

The Mental Status Evaluation

Psychiatric diagnosis is based upon the patient interview and the exclusion of medical illness by appropriate history, physical examination, and, if needed, a selection of laboratory tests. The psychiatric interview requires time, patience, and experience. A wide variety of screening questionnaires are available to assist the clinician in the evaluation of psychological symptoms. Useful screening tools include the Mini-Cog, the Mini-Mental State Examination, clock drawing test, Beck Depression Inventory, Hamilton Depression Scale, and the Prime MD instruments [Spitzer RL, Williams JBW, Kroenke K, et al. Utility of a new procedure for diagnosing mental disorders in primary care: The Prime-MD 1000 study. *JAMA*. 1994;272:1749–1756]. Overreliance upon these tools is not encouraged, but they can assist in the evaluation and selection of patients for referral.

The clinician is assessing the mental status during the history and physical examination. When problems are suspected, formal testing is indicated. The MMSE (Table 15–1), an efficient inventory of cognitive function.

The Mini-Cog is a validated screening test that uses the registration and recall questions from the MMSE and the clock drawing exercise. The latter is performed by drawing a circle and placing the numeral "12" in its proper clock position. Then ask the patient to fill in the remaining numerals followed by indicating a particular time such as "4:35" [Scanlan J, Borson S. The Mini-Cog: Receiver operating characteristics with expert and naive raters. *Int J Geriatr Psychiatry*. 2001;16:216–222]. Errors in either task indicate the need for detailed evaluation of cognitive function.

The psychiatric evaluation addresses several dimensions of mental processes that are briefly discussed below.

- **Level of Consciousness.** See page 741. Patients are described as alert, lethargic, stuporous, or in coma. These are arbitrary categories and the patient's mental status may fluctuate. Although patients with mental illness may be lethargic from medications or intoxications, all patients who are less than fully alert should be assumed to have an organic neurologic disorder until such has been excluded.

- **Orientation.** This has four dimensions: person, place, time, and situation. Does the patient know who he and others in the room are? Does he know their names and roles? Does he know where he is—the place, city, state, country? Does he know the year, season, day, and date?

Table 15-1   Mini-Mental State Examination

Orientation	Points
_____What is the time (date/day/month/year)?	5
_____Where are we (state/county/city/hospital/ward)?	5
Registration _____Name three objects and ask the patient to repeat them until all three are learned. Record the number of trials.	3
Attention and Calculation _____Ask the patient to subtract serial 7s for five times.	5
Recall _____Ask the patient to recall the three objects named above.	3
Language	
_____Naming: Pencil and watch.	2
_____Repetition: "No ifs, ands, or buts."	1
_____Three-stage command: "Take paper in your right hand, fold it in half, and put it on the floor."	3
_____Reading: Obey instruction given in writing: "Close your eyes."	1
_____Writing: "Write a sentence." _____"Copying: Construct a pair of intersecting pentagons and ask the patient to copy them.	1

Source: Crum RM, Anthony JC, Bassett SS, Folstein MF. Population-based norms for the Mini-Mental State Examination by age and educational level. *JAMA.* 1993;269:2386–2391.

- **Attention.** This is the ability to stay on task and follow the course of a conversation and interview avoiding distractions. Attention deficits are the hallmark of confusional states and delirium and should alert the clinician to the possibility of a metabolic disorder. Decreased attention is too frequently attributed to a lack of cooperativeness when, in fact, the patient is unable to cooperate. Tests of serial 7s, serial 3s (subtract 3 sequentially, starting at 20), and attempting to spell "world" backwards are tests of attention. Always consider the patient's level of education in interpreting these tasks. A nonverbal task is the tap-no-tap test. Have the patient tap his or her hand twice when you tap once; if you tap twice they are not to tap.
- **Memory.** This is the ability to register and retain material from previous experience. Memory is a complex phenomenon. It is usefully classified as immediate recall (registration), short- and long-term memory. Immediate recall is the ability to register items presented. Short-term memory is the ability to recall the registered items within 5 to 10 minutes. Long-term memory is the ability to recall events from the more distant past from days to years. Specific tests of immediate recall and short-term memory are included in the MMSE. Short- and long-term memory are evaluated while taking the history. Find out what the patient is really interested in (such as politics, sports, cooking, etc.) and ask them, specific detailed questions about it, questions that demand specific quantitative, rather than vague qualitative answers.

- **Thought.** This is how the brain communicates consciously with itself. Thought has several dimensions. The ***content*** of thought is what the patient is thinking about. Is it appropriate to his or her situation and a reasonable perception of the world? The ***sequence*** of thoughts is also important. How are they linked one to the next? Can the patient digress and get back to the original point? The logic a person uses to connect events and explanations should be evaluated. What is the nature of cause and effect in his or her life? What are the reasons he gives for seeking care? ***Insight*** is the ability to look at one's self and situation with comprehension and understanding. Lack of insight into the nature or consequences of behaviors or thoughts is an important clue to mental illness. ***Judgment*** is the ability to make reasonable assessments of the external world and choices between alternative actions. How are decisions made? How does the patient evaluate alternatives? How are potential benefits and risks considered?

- **Perception.** This is a global term for the way in which a person experiences the world through the senses. Distortions of perception can be symptoms of either neurologic or psychiatric disease. ***Hallucinations*** are sensory experiences perceived only by the patient, not by an observer. They may be auditory, visual, tactile, gustatory, or olfactory. Auditory hallucinations are particularly common in psychosis, whereas visual hallucinations are more common in delirium. Gustatory and olfactory hallucinations are common in partial seizure disorders (temporal lobe epilepsy). ***Illusions*** are the incorrect perception of objects seen by both the patient and the observer. These are particularly common with sensory impairment such as visual loss. ***Structural perception*** is the ability to place objects and shapes in relation to one another. It can be tested by having the patient copy interlocked pentagons (MMSE) or perform clock drawing.

- **Intellect.** Intellect is generally held to be an innate brain faculty, though it is difficult to separate deficits of intellect from deficits of education. The clinician must know the patient's ***educational and literacy level*** in order to properly evaluate his or her intellect. Culture greatly influences tests of intellect and it is hazardous to make assessments across cultures. There are several dimensions of intellect. What is his or her ***information level***? Does he know about important local, national, or international events? What are his or her sources of information? ***Calculations***, the ability to manipulate numbers are tested by simple and gradually more complex arithmetic tasks. ***Abstraction*** is the ability to see general principles in concrete statements. Abstractions are tested by asking the patient to interpret proverbs, for example, "people in glass houses shouldn't throw stones" = "don't criticize others for things you have probably done yourself." Interpretation at the simplest level, for example, "they would break the windows," is indicative of a concrete thinking and a deficit in abstract thinking. Remember that proverbs are culturally bound and may not be recognizable to people from different cultural backgrounds. ***Reasoning*** is the ability to solve problems involving simple logical sequences. ***Language*** is what one brain uses to communicate with another brain. It is tested in the interview and by having the patient follow both written, verbal instructions and write a sentence (MMSE). Assess the patient's vocabulary and the complexity of the patient's spoken language. Other dimensions of language are fluency of speech, body language, facial expression, and other nonverbal forms of communication; all should be thought of as language.

- **Mood.** Mood is the sustained affective state of the patient: how they feel. It is more like the tidal flow of emotion than the waves of affect. Mood is classified as normal, depressed, or elevated. Mood should be assessed, by asking the patient, how his or her mood has been over the last 2 weeks. Other questions used to evaluate mood include questions regarding how the patient feels about his or her life, the patient's thoughts of the future, the patient's confidence in his or her abilities, and the patient's hopes, and the intensity of these feelings. If depression is suspected, it is mandatory to inquire about suicidal thoughts or plans. Depressed patients may show blunted affect with little range.

- **Affect.** This is the more transient state of emotion, which varies from minute to minute and day to day, depending upon the setting and types of social and personal interactions in which a person is engaged. Affect is the clinician's assessment of emotion and is assessed by facial expression, tone, and modulation of voice and specific questions about how the patient feels. Affect is also measured by considering intensity and range of expression. Affective states include happy, sad, angry, fearful, worried, and wary.

- **Appearance and Behavior.** Close observation of the patient during the interview will provide important information. How is the patient dressed and groomed? How is the patient's personal hygiene? Does the patient make and sustain eye contact? Does the patient answer questions promptly and fully? Are there areas of questioning that the patient avoids or tries to deflect? What is the patient's body language? Is the patient fidgeting or unusually still? What is the patient's tone of voice, volume, and speech rhythm?

Psychiatric Symptoms and Signs

This chapter discusses symptoms and signs together because in psychiatric illness the symptoms and signs manifest together as the patient's behaviors and the patient's perception and description of those behaviors.

Abnormal Perception

We perceive the world through our senses, which we take as reliable and valid measures of the external environment. Sensory perceptions are distorted as a result of injury to the sensory organs or pathways, from abnormal processing of the sensory perceptions or from false perceptions arising within the brain. Abnormal perceptions arising from primary injury to the sensory organs and their pathways are often negative (loss of perception) or represent an exaggeration or distortion of the normal sensory signal (e.g., tinnitus, paresthesia, hyperalgesia, allodynia). Abnormal perceptions arising in the processing centers and cortex are more often complex.

KEY SYMPTOM   Hallucinations

Hallucinations are abnormal sensory perceptions (such as auditory, visual, olfactory, tactile/somatic, or gustatory) that the patient may or may not recognize as unreal. They arise without external cues. Auditory hallucinations are common in schizophrenia, whereas visual hallucinations are more typical of delirium. Olfactory and gustatory hallucinations are common with partial seizures.

Illusions: Illusions are a misinterpretation of real sensory events. Illusions are commonly associated with delirium during which poor attentiveness leads to false attribution of sensory phenomena such as misidentification of people and behaviors.

> **KEY SYMPTOM**   Confusion—Delirium

See page 776.

> **KEY SYMPTOM**   Abnormal Sleep Perceptions—Parasomnias

These are disorders of perception or behavior associated with the sleeping state. The most common parasomnias are *nightmares* and *sleep terrors*. Auditory hallucinations occurring upon falling asleep (hypnogogic) and awakening (hypnopompic) are common, and do not indicate pathology in the absence of other hypnagogic symptoms.

Sleepwalking: This is classified as a parasomnia, like sleep terrors and nightmares. The patient may perform complex activities while asleep and awakens with no recollection. Hypnotic drugs are associated with an increased risk of sleepwalking behaviors related to the induction of antegrade amnesia.

Periodic Leg Movements of Sleep: Frequent leg movements during sleep are associated with arousals in obstructive and central sleep apneas. They can be quite disturbing to the bed partner, but the patient is unaware of the activity, other than finding the partner absent or the bedding disrupted. When the patient complains of an inability to hold the legs still on going to bed, consider restless legs syndrome.

Abnormal Affect and Mood

Feelings are the way we react emotionally to the perceptions and events of our lives. Normally, we have a range of feelings throughout the day and the intensity of our feelings may vary over time, from periods or relative intensity to periods of less intensity. Abnormal extremes of feelings, either in degree or in duration, may indicate psychiatric disorders.

> **KEY SYMPTOM**   Change in Behavior or Mood

Any significant change in a person's behavior should raise the possibility of underlying medical or psychiatric illness. Changes in school or job performance and withdrawal from social activities should raise concerns about disorders of mood, thought, or substance abuse.

Elevated Affect and Mood: Elevation of mood is a normal transient response to positive events. The diagnosis of *mania* requires an abnormally elevated, expansive, or irritable mood lasting at least 1 week plus three or more of the following: inflated self-esteem or grandiosity, decreased need for sleep, more talkative, flight of ideas, distractibility, increase in goal-directed activity, or excessive involvement in pleasurable activities with a high potential for painful consequences (such as physical, sexual, financial). *Hypomania* is similar, although the duration is at least briefer and the symptoms are milder and less florid.

Depressed Affect and Mood: *Depressed affect* is a transient normal response to negative events and feelings. *Depression of mood* can be accompanied by a loss of interest in activities or pleasure, anorexia, weight loss, insomnia or somnolence, psychomotor agitation or retardation, fatigue, inappropriate guilt and/or a sense of worthlessness, loss of the ability to concentrate, thoughts of death, and suicidal ideation. When persistent for more than 2 weeks and accompanied by changes in sleep, eating, and behavior, it may indicate an episode of *major depression. Dysthymia* is a persistent, usually lifelong form of mildly depressed affect, not meeting criteria for a major depression.

Anxiety: This is a state of apprehension or fear accompanied by increased sympathetic nervous system activity. It is a normal response to threats, either physical or psychological, which resolves with resolution of the threat. It is abnormal when the feeling occurs or persists in the absence of real danger.

Phobias: These are irrational fears of situations, events or objects that produce uncontrollable fear, and anxiety in the patient. They are pathological, when they lead to alterations in social or psychological function.

Anhedonia: This is an absence of pleasure from normally emotionally rewarding activities, including eating, sexual stimulation, social activities, and personal or business success. It is characteristic of depression.

Depersonalization: This is a feeling of being outside the body, an observer of yourself and surroundings. It is accompanied by a loss of affective connection with the people and events in one's environment. It is normal during highly stressful, traumatic events, but abnormal in other situations, especially, if persistent or recurrent. Depersonalization may occur with anxiety disorders.

Abnormal Thinking

Thinking is the process by which we connect and explain events to ourselves and others. It is a relational activity of great complexity. Thought disorders may be manifested by verbal symptoms expressed by the patient or by abnormal behaviors resulting from the disordered thoughts.

KEY SYMPTOM Paranoia

This is a feeling of being systematically threatened or persecuted by a person, persons, or organizations. It is pathological when the paranoia results from a fixed delusion and leads to alterations in activities. Paranoia may be a relatively mild personality trait or a manifestation of psychosis.

KEY SYMPTOM Disordered Thinking

Thinking is usually logical and linked to an explicit rational system of cause and effect. The train of thought connecting each sequential idea is either apparent to an observer or readily explained by the patient and comprehensible to the observer. Disordered thinking is unconnected from thought to thought or connected by irrational or incomprehensible explanations. It is a sign of schizophrenia.

KEY SYMPTOM   Delusions

Delusions are unreal perceptions of the causal relations between perceptions, events, and people. They have their basis in real sensory perceptions and occurrences, but the linkage between the real people or events is illusory. Delusions are often described as fixed, false beliefs and are pathological when they continue to be believed despite strong, otherwise persuasive, evidence to the contrary. Delusions are characteristic of schizophrenia, manic psychosis, and delirium.

KEY SYMPTOM   Obsessions

Obsessions are recurrent, intrusive thoughts or fears that the person is unable to suppress or control despite recognizing that they are unreasonable. When disruptive of function, they indicate obsessive-compulsive disorder.

KEY SYMPTOM   Compulsions

Compulsive activities are repetitive stereotypic behaviors that the patient feels compelled to perform in order to reduce distress or fear of an unavoidable outcome should they not be done. When disruptive of function, they indicate obsessive-compulsive disorder.

Abnormal Memory

The hippocampus and temporal lobes are essential to memory formation and storage. Abnormal memory can result from failure to register, retain or recall information. Memory for names is frequently impaired with normal aging and is not a cause for concern. Short-term memory loss and inability to make new memories lead to disorientation, behavioral changes, and severe functional impairment. Memory loss is the most common characteristic of the dementias and may be the only finding is mild cognitive dysfunction.

KEY SIGN   Amnesia

Amnesia is a loss of memory. It can be retrograde for events of the past, or antegrade, the inability to form new memories. It can be either global or selective for particular events or domains of memory. It is indicative of brain injury or psychological disorder.

Confabulation: Confabulation occurs in the setting of severe memory loss. The patient constructs fabulous explanations for events and behaviors for which the memory of the correct explanation is lost. This is typical of Korsakoff's syndrome.

Abnormal Behaviors

How we behave, our actions in private and public, are the result of how we feel, how we think, and how we perceive the constraints and rewards of the social environment. Behavior is culturally bound such that behaviors appropriate in one culture or setting may be quite inappropriate in another. Normative evaluations of thought, feelings, and private behavior are problematic at best; however, public behaviors are reasonably and readily subject to normative evaluation. Behaviors which are consistently abnormal or unacceptable are indicative of personality or psychiatric disorders.

➤ **KEY SYMPTOM** **Suicidal Behavior**

Expressed suicidal ideation, threats, gestures, and attempts are progressively more serious signs of a potentially life-threatening situation. All such behaviors should be taken seriously. The patient's safety is the first concern; identification and treatment of the underlying problems should be undertaken either primarily or with referral.

KEY SIGN **Stereotypic Behaviors**

Activities, movements, or vocalizations that are stereotypically repeated without appropriate precipitants or explanation suggest either tics or compulsions or possibly complex partial seizures.

➤ **KEY SIGN** **Catatonia**

Catatonic patients often exhibit a profound retardation in motor activity, retaining postures, expressing negativism, and repeating the phrases or motions of other persons (*echolalia, echopraxia*). However, patients can have excessive motor activity, which is apparently purposeless and not influenced by external stimuli. Catatonia is most common in affective disorders, but is also seen in psychosis.

KEY SYMPTOM **Abnormal Sexual Feelings and Behaviors—Paraphilias**

Paraphilias are abnormal and/or unusually intense feelings of sexual arousal toward inappropriate sexual objects such as children, animals, or nonhuman objects, or the need for inappropriate behaviors such as sadism or masochism during sexual activity. Paraphilic thoughts are not necessarily abnormal, but when acted upon, especially with nonconsenting partners or children, they are indicative of psychiatric illness.

KEY SIGN **Bulimia**

Bulimia is alternating binge eating and purging with either induced vomiting or other cathartic activity. When the pattern is sustained and secretive, it is indicative of a major eating disorder.

KEY SYMPTOM **Anorexia Nervosa**

See Psychiatric Syndromes—Anorexia Nervosa and Bulimia Nervosa, page 781.

KEY SYMPTOM **Dyssomnias**

These include difficulty getting to or maintaining sleep (*insomnia*), abnormal daytime sleepiness or sudden sleep onset (*narcolepsy*), sleep-disorder breathing (obstructive or central sleep apnea, and other disorders of the circadian sleep cycle (e.g., jet lag). The system review should always include questions about sleep quality and disruption. Abnormal sleep patterns may result from or lead to psychiatric disorders. Terminal insomnia is associated with major depression, while initial insomnia characterizes atypical depressive disorder [Schenek CH, Mahowald MW, Sack RL. Assessment and management of insomnia. *JAMA.* 2003;289:2475–2479].

Psychiatric Syndromes

The disorders in this section are presented to help the clinician recognize them for the purposes of treatment or referral to a psychiatrist. Indications for psychiatric consultation or referral include suicidal or homicidal ideation, psychotic symptoms, severe anxiety or depression, mania, dissociative symptoms, and failure to respond to therapy.

To facilitate research, the American Psychiatric Association developed criteria for the diagnosis and classification of mental disorders. These have proved reliable and have improved the diagnosis and therapy of these problems. Practitioners should have a copy of its manual, the *Diagnostic and Statistical Manual of Mental Disorders*, Fourth Edition, Text Revision (*DSM-IV-TR*) published by the American Psychiatric Association [American Psychiatric Association. *Diagnostic and Statistical Manual of Mental Disorders.* 4th ed. Text Revision. Washington, DC: American Psychiatric Association; 2004] for assistance in your practice.

Multiaxial Assessment

The *DSM-IV* uses a multiaxial assessment method that provides a systematic approach to the description of each patient's disorders. Every clinician should be familiar with this system.

Axis I: Clinical Disorders; Other Conditions That May be a Focus of Clinical Attention

These are the major psychiatric and behavior syndromes addressed in the *DSM-IV*. If more than one disorder is present, the principle disorder or reason for the current visit is listed first.

Axis II: Personality Disorders; Mental Retardation

These are listed separately from Axis I disorders because they may coexist and complicate the diagnosis and management of Axis I problems.

Axis III: General Medical Conditions

Here are listed medical conditions, by system, which may be important in the understanding and management of the Axis I and II disorders.

Axis IV: Psychosocial and Environmental Problems

Problems in the psychosocial and physical environment of the patient, which influence the diagnosis, management, or prognosis of the Axis I, II, and III problems are enumerated here.

Axis V: Global Assessment of Functioning

The practitioner's assessment of the patient's global level of function is recorded using the Global Assessment of Functioning Scale, a 0 to 100 scale descriptive of the degree of function and impairment as a consequence of the psychiatric (Axis I and II) disorders. The full scale is available in the *DSM-IV-TR*.

There are few, if any specific signs or laboratory findings of psychiatric disease, so diagnosis depends principally upon an experienced observer obtaining a complete history from the patient and a collateral informant. The reader is encouraged to review specialized publications in the field.

Acute and Subacute Confusion

> **KEY SYNDROME** Delirium

Metabolic abnormalities (including prescription and nonprescription drugs), pain, restraints, or sleep deprivation impair cognitive function, particularly attention, judgment, and perception. This is usually a metabolic encephalopathy; failure to recognize and treat delirium is associated with a high incidence of long-term morbidity and increased mortality. Delirium is frequently confused with a primary psychiatric disorder, especially by examiners who have not known the patient in his or her premorbid state. The symptom complex is characterized by loss of attentiveness, fluctuations of mental status, progressive loss of orientation, and confusion. Persons at highest risk are the older adults, especially those on multiple medications at the time of hospitalization. The chief features are *decreased attentiveness* (distractibility, loss of train of thought), *alteration of consciousness* (from hypervigilance and agitation to lethargy or coma), *disorientation* (for time and place), *illusions* (misinterpreted sensory impressions), *hallucinations* (mostly visual), *wandering and fragmented thoughts, delusions, recent memory loss*, and *affective changes*. The patient may be restless, or picking at the bedclothes. A hypoactive delirium may occur as well. Myoclonus may be present. Some forms of delirium, for example, alcohol withdrawal, produce prominent autonomic dysfunction with fever, tachycardia, and hypertension (*delirium tremens*).   *CLINICAL OCCURRENCE:*   Common causes of delirium include drug intoxication or withdrawal (e.g., narcotics, sedatives, tranquilizers, alcohol, steroids, salicylates, digitalis, alkaloids), liver disease, uremia, hypoxia, hypoventilation, congestive heart failure, electrolyte abnormalities, urinary retention, fever, and infection. In hospitalized patients, sensory deficits, restraints, Foley catheters, and invasive procedures are associated with an increased incidence of delirium.

Anxiety Disorders

> **KEY SYNDROME** Generalized Anxiety Disorder

Anxiety is an experienced emotional state caused by activity in the deep cortical structures of the limbic system. In addition to the subjective feelings, anxiety triggers stress responses via the autonomic nervous system, which are felt by the patient and may heighten the sense of anxiety. Most persons experience some anxiety in response to stress, but excessive or continuous unfocused anxiety may be so debilitating as to require therapy. The causes of anxiety may be real, potential, or imagined. Autonomically-mediated symptoms and signs include palpitations, tachycardia, tremor, chest pain, hyperventilation with paresthesias and dizziness, faintness, fatigue, diaphoresis, nausea, vomiting, diarrhea, and abdominal distress. The Hamilton Anxiety Rating Scale can be used to assess the severity of the symptoms. Significant impairment of social, occupational, or other important functioning is required for diagnosis.

Panic Attack: Sudden intense fear or discomfort occurs often without an evident external cue. Symptoms include palpitations, sweating, tremor, shortness of breath, choking, chest pain, nausea, faintness or dizziness, paresthesias, and/or flushing accompanied by overwhelming cognitive turmoil, as in fear of dying, losing control, or "going crazy." Symptoms peak within 10 minutes and rarely last more than 30 minutes, leaving the patient feeling exhausted.

Panic Disorder: This is the condition of recurrent panic attacks accompanied by an ongoing apprehension of recurrent attacks, worry about the prognostic implications of the attacks (their physical and psychologic meaning), or significant changes in behaviors as a result of the attacks.

Agoraphobia: This is a persistent fear of situations which might cause embarrassment or discomfort without escape, or which might precipitate a panic attack. These are often social situations involving groups of people, particularly within confined surroundings such as classrooms, churches, and stores. Agoraphobia commonly accompanies panic disorder.

Social Phobia: These patients have a compelling desire to avoid social contact, fearing embarrassment or humiliation.

Specific Phobias: Phobia may develop for almost any specific type of event or interaction. To qualify as a phobia, the anxiety must be consistently produced by the exposure, the fear must be excessive and unreasonable and recognized as such by the patient who then alters her usual patterns of behavior in order to avoid the situation, leading to social disruption or extreme distress.

Acute and Posttraumatic Stress Disorders: Persons experiencing an event involving threatened or actual injury or death to themselves or others may develop significant anxiety either soon afterward in an acute stress disorder or later with recurrences in a posttraumatic stress disorder. Flashbacks, depersonalization, denial, avoidance of stimuli that induce the memories, and enhanced arousal are manifestations of stress disorders [Yehuda R. Posttraumatic stress disorder. *N Engl J Med.* 2002;346:108–114].

> **KEY SYNDROME** Obsessive-Compulsive Disorder

Obsessive thoughts and compulsive behaviors occur in any combination. The patient recognizes the unreasonableness of a connection between the behavior and the feared event or outcome. The obsessive and compulsive behaviors, such as handwashing, door locking, or checking, cleaning or arranging of possessions, consume more than 1 hour a day and interfere with social functioning.

Disorders of Mood

Mood is the sustained affective state of the patient. Mood can be depressed or elevated, or can cycle between depression and elevation. It is important to ascertain both the *amplitude* of the swings (the severity of the depression or elevation) and the *rate of cycling* between the states. Depressed and elevated moods are part of normal life. Grieving for a lost spouse or loved one may last for several months, but does not globally impair function.

> **KEY SYNDROME** Dysthymia

This is a chronic state of mildly depressed mood that is persistent, but not sufficiently severe to meet the criteria for major depression. Unlike depression, which is episodic, dysthymia is more chronic, a trait rather than a state.

KEY SYNDROME Depression

Depression is a sustained lowering of mood every day, or loss of interest or pleasure, for at least 2 weeks accompanied by change in weight, sleep, psychomotor activity, fatigue, feelings of worthlessness, difficulties with concentration and recurrent thoughts of death. Depression accompanies many serious medical illnesses or the medications prescribed for their treatment; this must be considered before a diagnosis of major depression is made. Depression can occur at any age, but first episodes are most common in the fourth and fifth decades. Depression has psychological, behavioral, and somatic manifestations: loss of appetite and change in weight (up or down); sleep disturbances, most frequently terminal insomnia, although increased sleep can be seen; decreased energy for activities; decreased interest in usual activities and decreased pleasure from usually pleasurable activities; restlessness or listlessness; feelings of guilt and worthlessness; inability to concentrate, initate activities or make decisions; and thoughts of death or suicide, either passive or active. If depressed mood is accompanied by four or more of these symptoms sustained more than 2 weeks, depression is present [William JW, Noel PH, Cordes JA, et al. The rational clinical examination. Is this patient clinically depressed? *JAMA*. 2002;287:1160–1170].

KEY SYNDROME Hypomania, Mania, Bipolar Disorder, and Mixed Episodes

Mania is characterized by episodes of abnormally elevated mood lasting for at least 1 week. Hypomania is less extreme and functionally successful, as opposed to the destructive consequences of mania. Mania or depression may occur alone (*unipolar*), or the patient may cycle between mania and depression sequentially over weeks, months, or years (*bipolar*), or within a single day (*mixed episode*).

➤ ## KEY SYNDROME Suicide

A suicide attempt is a common and frequently fatal manifestation of psychiatric illness. Persons at highest risk include older men and adolescents, those with a specific plan, those with the intent to use firearms in their possession, those who use substances, especially alcohol, and those with previous aborted attempts. All threats of suicide and expressions of suicidal ideation or intent should be taken seriously and immediate psychiatric consultation should be obtained. The practitioner's first obligation is to ensure the safety of the patient pending psychiatric evaluation.

Personality Disorders

Abnormal behaviors and personality disorders. Personality is a global description of how we think, feel, and interact with the world around us. Acceptable feelings and behaviors are culturally determined. Personality disorders are defined as persistent (rather than episodic) lifelong patterns of maladaptive feelings, thoughts, and behaviors. Patients have two or more of the following: *abnormal cognition*, that is, how they perceive other people, actions, and themselves; *abnormal feelings* about themselves, people, and events, either in type, intensity, or duration; *difficulty functioning* with other people socially, educationally, or occupationally; *difficulty with impulse control*, leading to inappropriate behaviors. The personality traits are consistent over time, regardless of changes in the social surroundings, and produce significant stress and disruption of their lives. These disorders are pervasive and inflexible; they do not change over time with or without therapy. Treatment is aimed at helping people function within the bounds of their disorder. Underlying medical disorders and substance abuse must be excluded before the diagnosis can be made. Examples include narcissism, borderline, antisocial, histrionic, dependent, avoidant, and obsessive-compulsive personality disorders.

Personality Disorder Clusters

Personality disorders are divided into three clusters that assist us in identifying patients and the patterns of their perceptions and behaviors. Understanding these clusters and the specific personality types within each is helpful in learning to manage these individuals and their medical problems effectively. Remember that everyone has some of these traits; *it is the disruption of global function that identifies a disorder.*

Many clinicians would rather avoid dealing with people with personality disorders; we can use the normal emotional responses to these interactions to assist us in both recognizing the specific disorders and dealing effectively with them. Remember that the patients have not chosen these personalities and the personality disorder stands between you and effective management of the medical problems.

Cluster A: The Odd and Eccentric: Generally, people with these disorders avoid the medical profession. When they do present, they frequently have somatic complaints such as chronic fatigue and pain.

Paranoid. These individuals have a pervasive suspiciousness of others. They are always questioning the motivations of those around them and suspect that they are not being dealt with honestly.

Schizoid. These individuals are detached and do not form personal or social relationships. They only come to physicians for specific indications or services and otherwise prefer to be socially and personally isolated. The range of their emotional responses is restricted.

Schizotypal. These people are recognized by their eccentric behaviors and often eccentric dress. They have social deficits and unusual cognitive and perceptual experiences. Think of the people who have been abducted by aliens or see UFOs, but otherwise function appropriately in their relationships.

Cluster B: The Dramatic, Emotional, and Erratic: This is the group we often think about when we discuss personality disorders. These are the patients who consume an inordinate amount of physician time and emotion without ever getting better; the folks you fear to see on your clinic schedule. Learning to deal with them effectively will help both you and your staff practice more effectively. Characteristically, these patients bring more pain and suffering to others than to themselves. Cluster B patients present with somatic complaints and may be seeking disability or drugs. They often have a history of reactions to many medications, "I don't react like other people, my metabolism is different."

Antisocial. There is a disregard for the rights of others and a lifelong pattern of difficulty with social and legal limits on behavior. They do not seem to have a conscience nor display regret or guilt for violating the rights of others.

Borderline. Borderline patients are emotionally labile and never happy or satisfied. Life is a constantly dysphoric experience. Their relationships are unstable and they are given to impulsive actions, not infrequently with self-harm. The emotional lability and intensity of their experiences often makes their caregivers uncomfortable [Lieb K, Zanarini MC, Schmahl C, et al. Borderline personality disorder. *Lancet.* 2004;364:453–461].

Histrionic. These patients have excessive emotionality, acting out their feelings in the office. They are often sexually provocative and attention seeking. They may be inappropriately dressed (e.g., revealing clothing, excessive make up and jewelry, overly formal or casual, etc.) and have provocative attention-seeking behaviors when alone with the clinician.

Narcissistic. The need to be admired and recognized as exceptional in some, if not all their activities distinguishes these individuals. They are often grandiose and disclose their close relationships with the rich and famous. They are self-centered and lack empathy or insight into the feelings of others.

Cluster C: The Anxious and Fearful: These people are never satisfied. They have constant fears that produce avoidant, dependent, or obsessive behaviors that disrupt their lives; they bring more suffering on themselves than those around them. These patients present to clinicians with anxiety manifest as seeking second opinions or needing reassurance. They often have somatic complaints and/or many sensitivities to medications or environmental exposures.

Avoidant. The patient feels inadequate in personal and social interactions, so tends to avoid social situations. They are overly sensitive to negative evaluations of every type; such evaluations are taken a statement of personal weakness not as an opportunity for improvement. No amount of reassurance is adequate to overcome this pervasive feeling.

Dependent. These patients need to be cared for. They are submissive and clinging and are fearful of separation from others. They often become very dependent upon their providers if given the opportunity. They do not take responsibility for their care but shift that to others.

Obsessive-Compulsive. These are the perfectionists who must have control at all times of their environment and their relationships. They are orderly in the extreme.

Other Personality Disorders

> **KEY SYNDROME   Somatoform and Related Disorders—Hysteria, Hypochondriasis, Briquet Syndrome**

Patients with these disorders have many physical complaints which occur in the absence of a medical explanation to account for them. They have usually visited several physicians, who "can't seem to find out what's wrong with me." The diagnosis should not be made until organic causes for the complaints are excluded by thorough examination. Patients have often had many extensive evaluations so, absent serious abnormalities on the screening physical and laboratory examinations, the clinician should always obtain complete records of all previous workups before initiating expensive or invasive evaluations [McCahill ME. Somatoform and related disorders: Delivery of diagnosis as the first step. *Am Fam Physician.* 1995;52:193–203].

Somatization Disorder: This is more common in women, begins before age 30 and leads to frequent medical visits for evaluation and treatment. Symptoms are of a degree that social, school, and job performances are impaired. Diagnostic criteria include pain in at least four different sites, two or more nonpainful gastrointestinal symptoms, at least one sexual or reproductive symptom without pain, and one pseudoneurologic symptom. The symptoms cannot be explained by a known general medical condition or result from medications or abuse of alcohol or illicit drugs. Unlike factitious disorder, the patient is not fabricating the symptoms or causing self injury [Barsky AJ, Borus JF. Functional somatic syndromes. *Ann Intern Med.* 1999;130(11):910–921].

Hypochondriasis: Hypochondriac patients persist in expressing the fear of a serious illness despite the reassurance of concerned physicians who have searched thoroughly for clinical evidence of organic disease and found none [Barsky AJ. Clinical practice. The patient with hypochondriasis. *N Engl J Med.* 2001;345:1395–1399].

> **KEY SYNDROME** **Factitious Disorders**

In these disorders, patients consciously and intentionally produce symptoms and/or signs of disease to gratify psychological needs.

Munchausen Syndrome: Munchausen syndrome is dramatic or dangerous behavior resulting in frequent hospitalizations for presumed severe illness. The most common symptoms and signs simulated by persons engaged in factitious behavior are bleeding from the urinary or gastrointestinal tract, diarrhea, fever, seizures, and hypoglycemia.

Malingering: This represents intentionally deceptive behavior in which persons claim to have symptoms or signs of disease that will benefit them in some way, for example, obtaining narcotics for pain relief or financial support for disability.

> **KEY SYNDROME** **Eating Disorders**

Marked changes in food selection and abnormal eating behaviors can indicate either organic disease or psychiatric disease.

Anorexia Nervosa. Anorexia nervosa is most common in adolescent and young women with an overwhelming concern about body image and weight. It is accompanied by a distortion of the perceived body image—the patient seeing an overweight person where observers see normal body form or even emaciation. The patients may be obsessed with food, preparing meals for others but not eating themselves. Excessive exercise may accompany the anorexia as a means of achieving the desired body image. Appetite is severely suppressed or absent. Patients become severely malnourished with retardation of secondary sexual maturation, absent menses, and osteoporosis. Patients are at high risk for death from complications of malnutrition. Early recognition and intensive treatment is essential.

Bulimia Nervosa. Bulimia is recurrent, secretive, binge eating. The patient feels unable to control the compulsive eating and resorts to induced vomiting, purging with laxatives, and/or abuse of diuretics to avoid weight gain. Clues include erosion of tooth enamel from acid emesis, abrasions on the roof of the mouth and callus on the backs of the fingers from induced vomiting, and electrolyte disorders from use of laxatives and diuretics. Nutritional deficiencies and malnutrition are uncommon [Mehler PS. Bulimia nervosa. *N Eng J Med*. 2003;349:875–881].

Binge Eating Syndrome. Large meals are eaten rapidly and accompanied by guilt and discomfort when eating. In addition to eating rapidly, patients eat alone and/or secretively despite feeling full and not being hungry. They often express self-disgust at their eating habits; depression may be increased. These patients do not vomit or increase exercise to compensate for their increased intake. If the above symptoms are present for more than two days per week for >6 months, the diagnosis of binge eating syndrome can be made.

Night Eating Syndrome. Patients with this disorder consume >50% of their total daily energy intake *after* the evening meal. They may snack continuously after the meal as well as awaken frequently to eat. They feel tension and anxiety that is relieved by eating. They are not hungry on awakening and tend to eat refined sugars and high carbohydrate snacks at other times.

> **KEY SYNDROME** **Alcohol-Related Illness**

Alcoholic beverages are ubiquitous in our society and commonly used social lubricants. Problems related to alcohol use have biological, social, and psychological roots. Each person lies somewhere on the continuum from abstinence to alcoholism; the clinician's task is to identify each person's use of alcohol, now and in the past, and the risk for addiction and social disruption. All patients should be asked about the frequency, amount, and type of beverages consumed; whether their use is in a social context or if they drink alone; whether they drink to become intoxicated; and whether they have memory losses, driving, or other infractions of the law related to alcohol. Alcohol intake should not exceed two drinks per day for males and one for females. There is great variability in individual tolerance to the effects of alcohol; increased tolerance develops with increased use. CAGE is an acronym helping the physician to recall questions that focus on *cutting* down, *annoyance* by criticism, *guilty* feeling, and *eye openers* (early morning drinks). Positive responses to the CAGE questions should raise the index of suspicion for chronic alcohol abuse. Alcohol abuse is commonly associated with other forms of substance abuse, including tobacco [Saitz R. Unhealthy alcohol use. *N Engl J Med*. 2005;352:596–607; Kitchens JM. The rational clinical examination. Does this patient have an alcohol problem? *JAMA*. 1994;272:1782–1787].

Problem Drinking. This alcohol consumption in excess of the recommended amounts but without dependence or serious social, legal, or occupational issues. Binge drinking in young adults is a common form of problem drinking.

Alcohol Abuse. Regular use of alcohol in excess of the recommended limits, without dependence, but associated with impairments in social functioning, interpersonal and relationship conflicts, legal issues, occupational difficulty, or repeated risky behaviors, such as driving while intoxicated indicates alcohol abuse.

Alcohol Dependence. This common condition is a compulsive behavioral disorder of drinking ethyl alcohol in biologically damaging quantities and repeatedly creating circumstances that are physically and socially damaging. Two key elements are increasing *tolerance* so that escalating amounts are consumed and *withdrawal symptoms* with attempts to discontinue or moderate drinking. The diagnosis is assured when behaviors that do damage to the drinker's health and reputation occur repeatedly. Such behavior is socially stigmatized; the patient is often reluctant to reveal it to the physician and may use subterfuges and untruths to conceal the truth. To circumvent this and uncover the facts, the clinician must be persistent and gain the patient's confidence. Often, the questioning must be oblique instead of blunt. Details are sought that are pertinent to the diagnosis but not recognizable to the patient as being associated with alcoholism. A history of previous treatment for alcoholism, injury without explanation, unexplained seizures ("rum fits"), job loss, and arrests for driving under the influence are important. Physical signs consistent with chronic alcoholism include vascular spiders on the skin, hepatomegaly, wristdrop, peripheral sensorimotor neuropathy, cerebellar ataxia, and alcohol or aldehyde on the breath.

KEY SYNDROME   Impulse Control Disorders

This group of disorders includes repetitive behaviors that range from the relatively minor (hair twisting and pulling: trichotillomania), to the socially disruptive (compulsive gambling, explosive disorder), to the criminal (kleptomania, pyromania). Repetitive impulsive socially disruptive behaviors may be the result of psychiatric disorders, epilepsy, or tics (Tourette syndrome).

KEY SYNDROME   Adjustment Disorders

Sudden, especially unwanted, disruptions of the social environment can produce profound changes in mood and behavior. Failure to adjust in a reasonable period of time with restoration of normal mood or persistent maladaptive or self-destructive behaviors is indicative of an adjustment disorder with or without accompanying anxiety or depression. Common events requiring adjustment are termination of an intimate relationship, divorce, changing schools or communities, loss of employment, getting married, and becoming a parent.

KEY SYNDROME   Prolonged Grieving

Grieving the loss of a loved one is a normal event, an adjustment to a new type of life. The form and pattern of appropriate grieving is both individually and culturally determined [Maciejewski PK, Zhang B, Block SD, et al. An empirical examination of the stage theory of grief. *JAMA.* 2007;297:716–723]. Normal grieving is a gradual process resolving the acute loss with a developing new appreciation for the lost person. With this resolution comes a restoration of a sense of purpose and the ability to find joy in life. Grieving associated with social withdrawal and depression disrupting normal activities and relationships and persisting for more than 2 months may indicate transition from the normal grief process to a psychiatric disorder.

Thought Disorders

KEY SYNDROME   Psychosis: Schizophrenia

Schizophrenia is now considered to comprise a group of diseases that are probably etiologically distinct. Primary psychotic disorders occur in adolescence or young adult life. Onset of psychotic symptoms at older ages should raise concern about organic brain disease, drug intoxication or withdrawal, or psychosis complicating major depressive or bipolar disease. Schizophrenia involves problems in thinking, affect, socializing, action, language, and perception. *Positive symptoms* represent an exaggeration or distortion of normal functions, including delusions and hallucinations, especially auditory. *Negative symptoms* reveal loss of normal functions such as affective flattening, alogia, anhedonia, and avolition. *Disorganizational symptoms* include disorganized speech or behavior and short or absent attention span. Several subtypes are recognized. *Catatonic* patients exhibit a profound change in motor activity, retaining postures, expressing negativism, and repeating the phrases or motions of other persons (echolalia, echopraxia). *Paranoid* patients are preoccupied with at least one systematized delusion or auditory hallucination related to a single subject. *Disorganized* schizophrenic patients are disorganized in their speech and behavior and display a superficial or inappropriate affect.

Other Disorders

Other major categories of psychiatric syndromes which we do not have space to present inclusively include substance-related disorders; disorders usually first diagnosed in infancy, childhood, or adolescence (including mental retardation, learning disorders, autism, attention-deficit and disruptive behavioral disorders, and tic disorders); dissociative disorders; sexual and gender identity disorders; sleep disorders; impulse-control disorders; adjustment disorders; relational problems (e.g., parent to child, siblings); and problems related to abuse or neglect. The reader should consult the *DSM-IV-TR* for detailed discussion of these diagnoses.

SECTION 2

THE SOCIAL EVALUATION

Evaluation of Social Function and Risk

Health status is strongly correlated with socioeconomic standing. Among the factors known to correlate with health status are family income, community of residence, education, social connectedness (the number and strength of interpersonal relationships), marital status, and employment status. In addition to any role the social environment plays in the incidence of ill health, it often places significant limitations on the ability of an individual and family to cope with the financial and social demands of illness. The result is a vicious spiral of unmet needs.

Evaluation of the patient's social environment should be part of a global patient assessment. The clinician should inquire about marital status, living arrangements, financial limitations and concerns, health insurance, education, literacy (do not assume that several years of elementary and secondary education equates to being able to read or write), interpersonal relationships and personal support system, use of community social support systems, and sense of personal safety and security. For the older adults and chronically ill, it is important to inquire about the availability of heat in the winter and air conditioning in the summer.

When questions arise; or problems are identified, consultation with your local social service agencies is strongly advised. They are often able to assist patients with medications, transportation, and a wide variety of other services. ***Identification of abuse or neglect is especially important and the caregiver is required to report to the appropriate social agency children (younger than age 18 years), elders (older than age 64 years), or dependent adults of any age who may be victims of abuse or neglect.*** The first priority in this situation is securing the safety of the patient, which may require hospitalization.

A description of a complete social evaluation is beyond the scope of this text. Axis IV of the *DSM-IV* lists the following specific areas of psychosocial and environmental problems. This list is an excellent organizational scheme for identification and classification of these problems:

1.   Problems with primary support group.
2.   Problems related to the social environment.
3.   Educational problems.
4.   Occupational problems.
5.   Housing problems.
6.   Economic problems.
7.   Problems with access to health care services.
8.   Problems related to interaction with the legal system/crime.
9.   Other psychosocial and environmental problems.

Common Social Syndromes and Problems

KEY SYNDROME   Abuse and Neglect

Abuse is common and can affect persons of any age and either sex. Child and elder abuse affects both males and females, while women are much more commonly affected in midlife. Abuse can be physical, sexual, emotional, or financial. The examiner should first inquire whether the patients have ever felt unsafe in a relationship, then whether they have concerns about their current safety, and last whether they wish help in dealing with the current problems. The safety of the patient, not the identification of a perpetrator, is the first and most important goal of the interview. Remember that reporting of child, elder, and dependent adult abuse and neglect are mandatory.

Domestic Violence. Violence in the home or between intimate sexual partners is common and often difficult to assess. In surveys of ambulatory practice, more than 20% of women have been abused at one time and 5% of women have been abused within the last year [McCauley J, Kern DE. The "battering syndrome": prevalence and clinical characteristics of domestic violence in primary care internal medicine practices. *Ann Intern Med.* 1995;123:737–746]. Sensitive questioning and a willingness to to provide assistance are the basis for diagnosing these problems [Eisenstat SA, Bancroft L. Domestic violence. *N Engl J Med.* 1999;341:886–892].

Elder Abuse. This is an increasingly recognized problem. It can take many forms, and because many elders are dependent upon others for many of their personal needs, they may be unwilling to volunteer a complaint. This is further complicated when family members are the offending individuals. Abuse may take place in the home or in institutional settings. An empathetic nonjudgmental approach to patient evaluation and including questions designed to elicit the patient's feelings ("Do you feel safe?") may help identify problematic situations [Lachs MS, Pillemer K. Elder abuse. *Lancet.* 2004;363:1263–1272].

KEY SYNDROME   Illiteracy

Inability to read and/or write is not uncommon. The patient is often embarrassed by the problem and will not volunteer this information. Learn to inquire tactfully and nonjudgmentally about the patient's educational and literacy skills. Illiteracy should be suspected when poor adherence to therapy plans and follow-up is identified [Bass PF, Wilson JF, Griffith CH. A shortened instrument for literacy screening. *J Gen Intern Med.* 2003;18:1036–1038].

KEY SYNDROME   Homelessness

Homeless persons are at high risk for medical illness and abuse and have high rates of serious psychiatric illness.

KEY SYNDROME   Isolation

Social isolation is common, especially in the older adults, in those with impaired motor or communication skills, and in those with financial limitations. Isolation makes dealing with chronic illness more difficult and may increase the rate of cognitive decline in the older adults.

KEY SYNDROME   Institutionalization

A significant proportion of our society spends time living in various institutional settings from the relatively benign, such as boarding schools, to the punitive, such as prisons. Other institutional settings that may impact on health status are nursing homes and homes for the developmentally disabled. It is important to know the stresses and limitations each of these environments places on our patients.

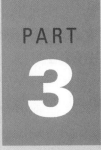

PART

3

Preoperative Evaluation

The Preoperative Evaluation

Introduction to Preoperative Screening

Preoperative medical screening strives to estimate the patient's risk for, and minimize the occurrence of, perioperative medical complications, without unnecessarily delaying surgery or causing undue morbidity or expense. To appropriately counsel the surgeon and patient, your history, physical examination, and other studies should assess the risks for myocardial infarction (MI), arrhythmias, heart failure, endocarditis, stroke, pulmonary insufficiency, venous thrombosis and pulmonary embolism (PE), hemorrhage, diabetic acidosis, renal or hepatic failure, and, in the immunocompromised host, infection. When needed, you must make recommendations to minimize these risks by specific preoperative evaluations or treatments or with specific perioperative management strategies. The consultant, surgeon and patient must balance the risks of proceeding directly to surgery against the risks of delaying a necessary procedure.

The History

First, determine the type and urgency of the proposed surgery and the patient's age and functional capacity. Ask, if your patient can climb a flight of stairs comfortably. Patients who have symptoms with activities of less than four metabolic equivalents (METs) have poor functional capacity and an increased for perioperative risk for cardiovascular events. One MET is defined as the energy expenditure for sitting quietly. This is equivalent to an oxygen consumption of 3.5 mL/kg body weight per minute, for the average adult. Activities that correlate with 4 to 5 METs of activity include mopping floors, cleaning windows, painting walls, pushing a power lawnmower, raking leaves, weeding a garden, or walking up 1 flight of stairs. Walking 4 miles (6.4 km) per hour or cycling 10 miles (16 km) per hour on level ground constitutes 5 to 6 METs of activity. The ability to accomplish these activities without symptoms correlates with moderate or greater functional capacity and a lower perioperative risk. If the patient cannot perform these activities, what are the symptoms that limit them?

Find out, if complications have occurred with previous operations. Then focus the history and physical examination upon the specific areas of concern as outlined below.

Assessment of Cardiovascular and Pulmonary Risk from History

The most frequent cause of nonsurgical perioperative morbidity and mortality is acute MI. The patient's current history is the best method of risk assessment. The American College of Cardiology and the American Hospital Association have published guidelines for perioperative cardiovascular evaluation [Eagle KA, Berger PB, Calkins H, et al. ACC/AHA guideline update for perioperative cardiovasculoar evaluation for noncardiac surgery—executive summary. *J Am Coll Cardiol.* 2002;39:542–553]. The recommendations are based upon three factors: clinical predictors, functional capacity, and surgery specific risks.

Pneumonia is a not infrequent postoperative complication. A multifactorial risk assessment tool has been published which predicts the risk for pneumonia. The derivation and validation cohorts were a large veterans population so applicability to other populations is not known [Arozullah AM, Khuri SF, Henderson WE, et al. Development and validation of a muiltifactorial risk index for predicting postoperative pneumonia after major noncardiac surgery. *Ann Intern Med.* 2001;135:847–857]. The traditional test of stair climbing ability also stratifies patients' risk for postoperative complications [Girish M, Trayner E, Dammann O, et al. Symptom-limited stair climbing as a predictor of postoperative cardiopulmonary complications after high-risk surgery. *Chest.* 2001;120:1147–1151]. The subject of pulmonary risk assessment and perioperative pulmonary risk reduction has recently been extensively reviewed by the American College of Physicians and a guideline has been published [Qaseem A, Snow V, Filterman N, et al. Risk assessment for and strategies to reduce perioperative pulmonary complications for patients undergoing noncardiothoracic surgery: A guideline from the American College of Physicians. *Ann Intern Med.* 2006;144:575–580].

Ischemic Heart Disease: Determine whether your patient has angina and if so, find the frequency, precipitating factors, and response to rest and nitroglycerin. Especially, worrisome are increasing frequency at lower levels of provocation and less prompt response to nitroglycerin. Examine the electrocardiogram (ECG) for evidence of prior MI or ongoing ischemia. If prior cardiac catheterizations or coronary revascularizations have been performed, obtain the reports. Successful revascularization within 3 years confers a low risk; the presence of drug eluting stents presents unique challenges since clopridogrel must be continued for at least one year post procedure.

Heart Failure: Inquire for symptoms of congestive heart failure now or in the past, such as exertional dyspnea, orthopnea, paroxysmal nocturnal dyspnea, cough, or peripheral edema. If prior estimates of cardiopulmonary function, such as cardiac catheterization or echocardiography have been performed, obtain the results.

Dysrhythmias and Pacemakers: Ask about palpitations, syncope, or other symptoms of arrhythmias, or whether arrhythmias been documented on prior ECGs or ambulatory monitoring. Examine current and old ECGs for high-grade atrioventricular block, symptomatic ventricular arrhythmias (especially in association with structural heart disease) or supraventricular tachycardias at uncontrolled rates. If the patient has a pacemaker, determine the type and model, date of implantation and when the battery life and performance were last interrogated.

Valvular and Congenital Heart Disease: The presence of intracardiac shunts or valvular abnormalities may require endocarditis prophylaxis. If present, determine when the last echocardiographic evaluation done and the results. Look especially for evidence of severe valvular heart disease (e.g., aortic stenosis) that might require cardiac surgical intervention before proceeding with elective noncardiac surgery.

Cerebrovascular Disease: The presence of symptomatic cerebrovascular disease (transient ischemic attack or stroke) is associated with an increased risk for perioperative cardiovascular morbidity including stroke. Ask if there have been prior evaluations or interventions performed on the carotid or peripheral arteries and obtain the results if these tests have been performed.

Venous Thromboembolism: A history of deep venous thrombosis or PE perioperatively or without provocation is associated with an increased risk for perioperative deep vein thrombosis/PE. Inquire whether studies for thrombophilia (e.g., factor V Leiden mutation, lupus anticoagulant, antithrombin III, protein C or S) were performed and obtain the results if possible.

Pulmonary Disease: Record any symptoms of current pulmonary disease and ask if there have been pulmonary complications after previous surgeries. Ask if patients with known lung disease have had pulmonary function testing and if so, obtain the results.

Assessment of Bleeding Risk from History

A negative history assures you that the patient is not at increased risk for bleeding in the absence antiplatelet and/or antithrombotic medications. If concerns arise from the history, a laboratory evaluation may be indicated. Screening tests in a patient with a negative history are not helpful.

Personal and Familial Coagulation Disorders: Ask about excessive bleeding with dental extractions, surgery, or childbirth or if there is a family history of excessive bleeding in those circumstances. Ask specifically, if the patient been recently hospitalized or received heparin for any reason; heparin induced thrombocytopenia and thrombosis may occur on reexposure.

Platelet and Vessel Disorders: Determine whether the patient experiences gingival bleeding, epistaxis, menorrhagia, hematuria, melena, or excessive bleeding or bruising at venipuncture sites or from minor cuts and whether they have noticed petechiae, spontaneous bruising, or bruises larger than a silver dollar with minor trauma.

Transfusion History: Has the patient ever had a blood transfusion or received procoagulant factor replacement at surgery? If so, determine when, which type of blood product, and the approximate volume of transfusion. Remember that patients will confuse reinfusion of autologous blood for a "transfusion."

Assessment of Metabolic Risk: Diabetes, Renal, and Hepatic Insufficiency

Metabolic abnormalities are assessed so that they can be controlled preoperatively and managed through the perioperative period.

Glucose Intolerance, Hyperglycemia, and Diabetes: Screen for symptoms of diabetes by asking about polyuria, polydipsia, or weight loss. Ask about a personal or family history of diabetes mellitus; ask women about gestational diabetes. If the patient is known to have diabetes, assess the use of use of oral hypoglycemic agents and control. If the patient uses insulin, record the types, schedule, and doses. Determine, the frequency and severity of hypoglycemia and whether hypoglycemia unawareness is likely.

Kidney Disease: Ask about any history of kidney disease and if present determine the stage and whether the patient has ever required dialysis.

Liver Disease: Inquire about a history of liver disease and the etiology and severity. Determine the current state of the liver disease, especially, the albumin and prothrombin/international normalized ratio.

Family History

Ask about a family history of adverse reaction to anesthesia (e.g., malignant hyperthermia), deep venous thrombosis or PE, bleeding problems, diabetes mellitus, elevated cholesterol, hypertension, or heart disease.

Medications

Most chronic medications can be continued through the perioperative period. The exceptions are aspirin; thienopyridines (clopidogreal or ticlopidine); warfarin; and nonsteroidal anti-inflammatory drugs for certain procedures and hypoglycemic agents whose dose should be reduced or held on the morning of surgery. All unnecessary medications should be discontinued. Avoid altering a chronic medication program just prior to surgery. The goal is to manage the medications and the medical problems through the perioperative period.

β-Blockers have been shown to reduce cardiovascular complications in patients undergoing high-risk surgery. If the patient is taking a β-blocker, it should always be continued throughout the perioperative period.

Cardiovascular Drugs: Review the patient's medications, to see, if they are taking cardiac, antiarrhythmic, or antihypertensive medications. Digitalis preparations are especially problematic.

Drugs Affecting Hemostasis: Ask specifically about any drugs that would affect hemostasis or increase the risk for thromboembolism, for example, nonsteroidal anti-inflammatory drugs, antiplatelet agents (including aspirin, clopidogrel or ticlopidine), warfarin, oral contraceptives, estrogens.

Because of recent concerns about coronary artery stent thrombosis following discontinuation of antiplatelet therapy (aspirin plus one of the thenopyridines), a joint advisory was issued electronically on January 16, 2007, that included the following recommendation: "Elective procedures that carry a risk of bleeding should be delayed until a month after the patient has completed a course of thienopyridine therapy, which is ideally 12 months after receiving a drug-eluting stent in patients who are not at high risk of bleeding, and at least 1 month after a bare metal stent. For patients who receive a drug-eluting stent and who must have procedures that mandate stopping thienopyridine therapy, aspirin should be continued if at all possible, and the thienopyridine restarted as soon as possible after the procedure."

Pulmonary Mediations: Record the use of bronchodilators for asthma or obstructive lung disease including the strength, frequency of use and response to rescue inhalers.

Corticosteroids: Steroid-induced adrenal suppression may persist for up to a year after even relatively short courses of corticosteroids in doses above 10 mg/d. If this has occurred, coverage with stress doses of steroids starting just before surgery and continuing for 48 to 72 hours is advised. Determine when, how much, for what reason, and for how long the patient took a steroid.

Insulin and Hypoglycemics: See diabetes, above.

Allergies and Drug Intolerances: Has the patient had an adverse reaction to any substance, including medications and radiology contrast materials? If so, describe the adverse reaction and response to treatment.

Personal Habits

Knowledge of a patient's habits will help you be alert for problems in the perioperative period such as drug or alcohol withdrawal.

Substance Use and Abuse: Has the patient been using alcohol or illicit or addicting drugs? If so, which drugs and when was the last time they were used? Drug withdrawal should be anticipated in the postoperative period if addicting drugs, including alcohol, were used recently.

Tobacco: Does the patient smoke? If so, how many cigarettes daily? Quitting smoking for at least 8 weeks prior to surgery is optimal. A shorter duration of abstinence may increase pulmonary complications while decreasing cardiovascular complications.

Mechanical and Positioning Risks

Musculoskeletal Conditions: Patients with rheumatoid arthritis may have cervical spine instability that can result in serious or fatal injury at the time of endotracheal intubation. Also, determine if the patient requires particular care in positioning to avoid excessive pressure on deformed limbs.

The Physical Examination

The physical examination is directed to identifying active medical problems in key organ systems that could increase the surgical risk or change perioperative management.

Vital Signs: Obtain vital signs including blood pressure, heart rate and regularity of rhythm, rate and ease of respiration, and temperature. Systolic blood pressure >180 mm Hg, diastolic pressure >110 mm Hg, or hypotension with clinical evidence of hypoperfusion or shock should be stabilized before proceeding to nonurgent surgery.

Heart Examination: Look for significant heart murmurs, extra sounds (S3, S4), ventricular systolic or diastolic dysfunction, elevated central venous pressure and peripheral edema.

Vascular Examination: Examine for carotid, abdominal, and femoral bruits.

Lung Examination: Examine the lungs for crackles, wheezes, decreased breath sounds, prolonged expiratory phase, effusions, and estimate pulmonary reserve. Limited inspiratory reserve with flattened diaphragms is suggested by failure of the thyroid cartilage to depress by 2 cm with deep inspiration or finding the top of this cartilage <4 cm above the suprasternal notch [McAlister FA, Khan NA, Straus SE, et al. Accuracy of the preoperative assessment in predicting pulmonary risk after nonthoracic surgery. *Am J Respir Crit Care Med.* 2003;167: 741–744].

Skin Signs of Hemostatic Disorder: Examine for integrity of the skin, evidence of venous stasis in the lower extremities, petechiae, and unusual bruises.

Mental Status

Assess the patient's mental status. This is especially important in the elderly patient because cognitive dysfunction, which is easily missed without specific testing, greatly increases the risk for postoperative delirium [Inouye SK, Charpentier PA. Precipitating factors for delirium in hospitalized elderly persons. *JAMA.* 1996;275:852–857].

Laboratory Tests

Based on the results of the history and physical examination, select the appropriate laboratory studies for confirmation and quantification of abnormalities. Routine laboratory tests are not useful unless there is a specific medical indication.

Electrocardiogram: Current evidence indicates that an ECG is not indicated for asymptomatic subjects undergoing low-risk procedures including endoscopic procedures, superficial procedures, transurethral prostate resection, cataract surgery, and breast surgery.

Obtain a 12-lead resting ECG for all patients with a recent episode of chest pain or ischemic equivalent (e.g., shortness of breath), patients with diabetes, and for intermediate or high-risk patients scheduled for intermediate or high-risk procedures.

Many, but not all, agree that an ECG should be obtained on all patients with prior coronary revascularization procedures, patients with prior hospitalization for heart disease, and on asymptomatic male patients older than 45 years of age or females patients older than 55 years of age with two or more risk factors for atherosclerosis.

Myocardial Perfusion Imaging: If the patient has known or suspected active coronary artery disease and an intermediate risk of perioperative cardiac complications, an intermediate-risk surgery, and poor functional capacity, or is to undergo a high-risk surgical procedure (aortic and other major vascular procedures or surgery with anticipated prolonged operative times associated with large fluid shifts and/or blood loss), consider further risk stratification using pharmacologic stress echocardiography or radioisotope myocardial perfusion imaging.

Intermediate-risk patients have two or more of the following: mild stable angina pectoris (Canadian class I or II), insulin-treated diabetes mellitus, pathological Q waves on the ECG, a history of MI or congestive heart failure, and/or renal insufficiency (creatinine ≥ 2.0). Some clinicians also include advanced age in this list. The need for surgery is not an independent indication for invasive coronary diagnostic or therapeutic procedures.

Revascularization of coronary arteries prior to surgery in asymptomatic patients by either coronary artery bypass grafting or coronary angioplasty with or without stenting does not reduce the perioperative cardiac morbidity or mortality risk [McFalls EO, Ward HB, Moritz TE, et al. Coronary-atery revascularization before elective major surgery. *N Engl J Med.* 2004;351:2795–2804].

Chest X-Ray: A chest X-ray is indicated for all patients with new respiratory symptoms, suspected congestive heart failure, valvular heart disease, or cardiac shunts.

Pulmonary Function Tests: If you identify severe pulmonary disease and the patient is undergoing a thoracic or upper abdominal procedure (higher risk for pulmonary complications), obtain pulmonary function tests with measurement of arterial blood gas.

Serum Chemistries: Serum chemistries are not required for low-risk procedures. For intermediate- and high-risk procedures, in the presence of diabetes mellitus, cardiac or renal disease, or when surgery is anticipated, to be prolonged or associated with significant blood loss, obtain blood urea nitrogen, serum creatinine, blood glucose, and a complete blood cell count. Serum electrolytes, or at least a creatinine and potassium, should be included for patients with hypertension, those taking medications likely to alter renal function or electrolyte balance and patients more than 40 years of age undergoing intermediate or high risk surgery. A low serum albumin has been associated with an increased risk of pulmonary complications.

Coagulation Studies: Obtain coagulation studies only for patients with a personal or family history suggesting a bleeding diathesis or thrombophilia.

All the above studies should be obtained for patients with poor or unstable general medical conditions.

Summative Risk Assessment

The purpose of the preoperative assessment is to estimate the risk for serious medical morbidity and death so that the surgeon and patient can make reasonable choices regarding the timing and risks of the planned surgical procedure. It is not the task of the medical consultant to either stop a planned surgical procedure or "clear" a patient for surgery. The consultant's task is to provide a sound risk assessment to the patient and surgeon. Avoid the common medical vernacular of "surgical clearance." The final decision of whether to operate, and when, is to be made by the patient and surgeon after reflection on the medical risk attendant to the surgery.

Biologic capacity declines with age, but it has been difficult to identify age as an independent risk factor for surgery. Perioperative morbidity and mortality are positively correlated with age [Polanczyk CA, Marcantonio E, Goldman L, et al. Impact of age on perioperative complications and length of stay in patients undergoing noncardiac surgery. *Ann Intern Med.* 2001;134:637–643], but, absent other risks, mortality is low in patients even greater than age 80 years.

The major nonsurgical cause of perioperative mortality is MI. Beginning with Goldman in 1977, a series of articles and guidelines have been published to assist the clinician in estimating the risk for cardiovascular complications in patients undergoing major surgery. These risk indices have been tested and refined over the years. A review of this literature is beyond the scope of this text; readers are encouraged to review the January 2003 issue of Medical Clinics of North America for a complete discussion of these topics, which is a collection of 15 essays on preoperative and perioperative care [Cohn SL, ed. Preoperative medical consultation. *Med Clin North Am.* 2003;1:1–28].

One of the most recent and well-validated indices is that of Lee et al., the Revised Cardiac Risk Index [Lee TH, Marcantonio ER, Mangione CM, et al. Derivation and prospective validation of a simple index for prediction of cardiac risk of major noncardiac surgery. *Circulation.* 1999;100:1043–1049]. They identify six independent risk factors for cardiac complications: high-risk surgery, a known history of ischemic heart disease, congestive heart failure (current or by history), cerebrovascular disease, insulin-treated diabetes, and a creatinine ≥ 2.0. The risk for complications, if 0 or 1 risk factor was present was $<1.0\%$; for 2 risk factors, 1.3%; for 3 risk factors, 4%; and for >3 risk factors, 9%. In 2005, a retrospective validation study was published that suggested that specification of age and type of surgery might add predictive accuracy [Boersma E, Kertai MD, Schouten O, et al. Perioperative cardiovascular mortality in noncardiac surgery: Validation of the Lee cardiac risk index. *Am J Med.* 2005:118:1134–1141]. This is a simple and easy to use index, but the clinician still must combine this with an assessment of the significant noncardiac risks.

As per the recommendations of the AHA/ACC 2006 Guideline, "Beta blockers should be continued in patients undergoing surgery who are receiving beta-blockers to treat angina, symptomatic arhythmias, hypertension or other ACC/AHA guideline indications. Beta blockers should be given to patients undergoing vascular surgery at high cardiac risk owing to the finding of ischemia on preoperative testing. Beta blockers are probably recommended for patients undergoing vascular surgery in whom preoperative assessment identifies coronary heart disease, for patients in whom preoperative assessment for vascular surgery identifies high cardiac risk as defined by the presence of multiple clinical risk factors, and for patients in whom preoperative assessment identifies coronary heart disease or high cardiac risk as defined by the presence of multiple clinical risk factors and who are undergoing intermediate- (intraperitoneal and intrathoracic surgery, carotid endarterectomy, head and neck surgery, orthopedic surgery, prostate surgery) or high-risk (emergent major operations particularly in the elderly, aortic and other major vascular surgery, peripheral vascular surgery, and anticipated prolonged surgical procedures associated with large fluid shifts and/or blood loss) procedures."

Revascularization of coronary arteries prior to surgery in asymptomatic patients by either coronary artery bypass grafting or coronary angioplasty with or without stenting does not reduce the perioperative cardiac morbidity or mortality risk [McFalls EO, Ward HB, Moritz TE, et al. Coronary-atery revascularization before elective major surgery. *N Engl J Med.* 2004;351:2795–2804].

ADDITIONAL READING

1. ACC/AHA Task Force Report. Guideline update for perioperative cardiovascular evaluation for noncardiac surgery. *Circulation.* 2002;105:1257–1268; *J Am Coll Cardiol.* 2002;39:542–553.

2. ACC/AHA 2006 Guideline updatae on perioperative cardiovascular evaluation for noncardiac surgey: Focused update on perioperative beta-blocker therapy.

3. Kajani AS, Taubert KA, Wilson W, et al. Prevention of bacterial endocarditis: Recommendations by the American Heart Association. *JAMA.* 1997;277:1794–1801.

4. Palda VA, Desky AS (Clinical Efficacy Assessment Subcommittee of the American College of Physicians). Guidelines for assessing and managing the perioperative risk from coronary artery disease associated with major noncardiac surgery. *Ann Intern Med.* 1997;127:309–328.

5. Smetana GW. Preoperative pulmonary evaluation. *N Engl J Med.* 1999;340:937–944.

6. Velanovich V. Preoperative laboratory evaluation. *J Am Coll Surg.* 1996;183:79–87.

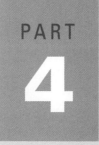

PART 4

Use of the Laboratory and Diagnostic Imaging

Where is the wisdom we have lost in knowledge?

Where is the knowledge we have lost in information?

T.S. Eliot
Choruses from "The Rock"

Principles of Diagnostic Testing

Diagnostic accuracy has been greatly enhanced by the sensitive and specific tests available in modern clinical laboratories and the rapid advances in clinical imaging. However, it is essential to recognize that proper use of the laboratory and imaging modalities is dependent upon accurate clinical hypotheses generated by the clinician at the bedside. Laboratory tests and diagnostic imaging can provide reliable and valid answers to well-conceived clinical questions, but they are also liable to overinterpretation and can be quite misleading if not interpreted in the clinical context as answers to particular questions. Beyond a few screening tests, these studies should be used to test the physiologic and diagnostic hypotheses generated during the history and physical examination. The laboratory and the radiology suite are not the places to go looking for ideas; they are the place to test your ideas. If you are unable to generate testable hypotheses after the history, physical examination, and screening tests, it will be more useful to seek consultation than to begin an undirected series of laboratory and radiologic studies.

A full discussion of the proper use of diagnostic tests is beyond the scope of this text. The reader is referred to the reading list at the end of this chapter. *Clinical Epidemiology: The Essentials* is especially valuable. The reader is advised to read this text and incorporate the principles of clinical epidemiology into your everyday practice.

Principles of Laboratory Testing

Laboratory testing is principally done for two reasons: (1) to obtain information that cannot be determined clinically, but which is often important in forming hypotheses and (2) to test hypotheses.

Tests in the first category are those commonly described as "routine" testing and include serum electrolytes, blood urea nitrogen, creatinine, complete blood counts, urinalysis, and, less commonly, transaminases and erythrocyte sedimentation rate or C-reactive protein. Some, or all, of these tests are performed in patients with significant illness in order to help the clinician identify significant abnormalities in major organ function or laboratory signs of inflammation or infection.

Tests in the second category are innumerable, and more are being developed as you read. They are used to identify specific abnormalities and diseases. The diagnostic performance of these tests is highly dependent upon the patient population tested. Tests in this category are most useful when the diagnosis in question is in the mid-range of probability on the basis of your clinical assessment—that is, the probability for the disease being present is roughly between 20% and 80%.

To understand why this is so, it is necessary to understand the measures of test performance and how interpretation is dependent on both the diagnostic criteria for a disease or condition and the pretest probability that the disease is present.

Principles of Testing for Disease

Disease Present or Absent

The first question is, how do we determine who has the disease and who does not? This is done with an independent test or set of criteria accepted as establishing "the diagnosis." The assumption is that a disease is either present or absent. Although this may seem obvious for diseases such as cancer or an infection where a tissue biopsy or culture are the diagnostic standards, most biologic measurements are continuous variables, not either/or determinations; it is often difficult to say whether rheumatoid arthritis is present or not, or which level of creatinine determines renal failure.

Most diseases have variable clinical severity; hence the diagnostic standard used to establish the disease can be either very inclusive (sensitive) or more exclusive (specific). A good example is, the American Rheumatologic Association criteria for the diagnosis of rheumatic syndromes. These criteria were developed because no laboratory tests of sufficient accuracy are available to identify these patients. The goal was to identify persons eligible for inclusion in research studies of the specific diseases. Hence, the criteria for diagnosis of these syndromes is set to be quite specific; that is to say, patients meeting the criteria are very likely to have the syndrome. However, it cannot be concluded that patients not meeting the criteria, who have many of the features and no other explanation, do not have the syndrome.

Test Positive or Negative

The definition of normal for continuous variables is a statistical determination (see the discussion of cholesterol in Chapter 18 for an exception). At what point "abnormal" becomes an illness or disease is a judgment based upon the desire to identify those with disease (*true positives*), but not include a significant portion of patients without the disease (*false positives*). Furthermore, most tests are not positive in all the patients with a given disease, so there will be patients with the disease who are missed by the test (*false negatives*). Finally, we want to be sure that a very high proportion of patients who do not have the disease, have a negative test (*true negatives*).

The decision of what cut point constitutes an abnormal test is determined by comparing the distribution of the test results in patients with the disease (determined as above) and in those without the disease (Fig. 17–1). When the two populations overlap in part of their range, a cut point is chosen to minimize the misallocation of patients (false positives and false negatives).

Note, however, that much of the information is lost in looking at tests of continuous variables as positive or negative: very abnormal tests are more likely to be associated with disease than mildly abnormal tests. As we discuss below, likelihood ratios (LR) are a good way to capture this information for making diagnostic decisions.

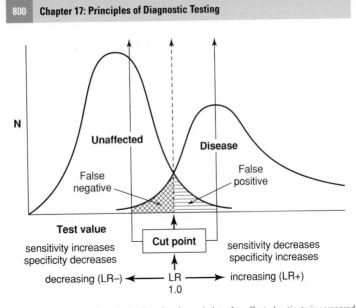

Fig. 17–1 *Interpretation of Test Results. A population of unaffected patients is compared with a population of diseased patients. The cut point for determining normal-abnormal is the value with the best compromise between sensitivity and specificity. LR can be calculated for test values above and below the usual cut point.*

Probability and Odds

Probability is a ratio or proportion of one part of a population to the population as a whole. A racehorse that wins 1 race in 20 has a 5% probability of winning (1/20 = 0.05).

Odds are the ratio of two probabilities. Because most events are uncommon (otherwise we would not need to make all these calculations), odds are customarily expressed as the odds against an event. For our horse, the probability of losing is 0.95; while the probability of winning is 0.05, that is, the odds are 19:1; that it will lose.

Odds and probabilities can be derived from one another:

$$\text{Odds} = \text{Probability}/(1 - \text{Probability})$$

$$\text{Probability} = \text{Odds}/1 + \text{Odds}$$

Pretest Probability and Prior Odds

We have generated a set of hypotheses at the bedside and have formulated a differential diagnosis (see Chapter 1). An essential part of the differential diagnosis process is to make a conscious estimate of the probability for the patient to have each disease in the differential diagnosis. If, we were to see 100 patients exactly like the patient before us—same age, sex, comorbidities, presenting symptoms and physical signs—how many would have each condition? This estimate is the *pretest probability*. Expressed as odds (the probability of having the disease over the probability of not having the disease); this known as the *prior odds*.

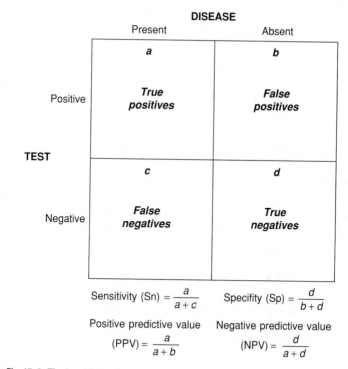

Fig. 17–2 *The 2 × 2 Table: Sensitivity, Specificity, and PPVs and NPVs.*

2 × 2 Tables

Tests can be systematically evaluated in a 2-cell × 2-cell table whose parameters are whether the disease is present or absent and whether the test is positive or negative (Fig. 17–2) by predetermined criteria. The four cells, conventionally labeled as a, b, c, and d, represent the true positive tests (disease present and test positive), the false-positives tests (disease absent, but test positive), the false-negative tests (disease present, but test negative), and the true negative tests (disease absent and test negative), respectively.

Prevalence of Disease

What additional information is in the table? We can see in the first column all the patients who have the disease ($a + c$) and in the second column all the patients who are free of disease ($b + d$). The ratio of the first column to the sum of the two columns is the prevalence of disease in the group of patients who generated the data in the table:

$$prevalence = (a + c)/(a + b + c + d).$$

To know how to interpret this prevalence, we need to know how the patients were selected for inclusion in each column. If this was a randomly selected, population-based sample, then the prevalence is that of the disease in the population, often a useful number. On the other hand, the investigators may have selected a group of patients with the disease and another group known not to have the disease in a predetermined ratio or by some nonrandom method. If this is the case, the "prevalence" is essentially meaningless for understanding disease prevalence in any useful clinical sense.

Aids in the Selection and Interpretation of Tests

Sensitivity (Sn)

Sensitivity is the number of patients with the disease who have a positive test, divided by the total number with the disease: *sensitivity = a / (a + c)*, a probability. *With highly sensitive tests, the vast majority of patients with the disease have a positive test (very few false negatives).* Tests with high sensitivity (>0.95) are most useful when negative, thereby making the diagnosis less likely. Note that the sensitivity of a test, because it is calculated only in those with the disease, is independent of the prevalence of the disease. Sensitivity can be increased by changing the cutoff for defining a positive test to a less abnormal value (see Fig. 17–1).

Because sensitivity is independent of prevalence, it is susceptible to overinterpretation when disease prevalence is very low (see Example 1 below). In this case, the false-positive tests (*b*) may significantly out number the true positives (*a*).

Sensitive tests are used when you do not wish to miss a serious disease because of the consequences of a delayed diagnosis. A negative result makes the disease unlikely and helps to reassure the patient and clinician, and serves to narrow the diagnostic possibilities. A positive test needs to be confirmed with more specific tests before a diagnosis can be established.

Specificity (Sp)

Specificity is the proportion of patients without the disease who have a negative test: *specificity = d / (b + d)*, a probability. *With highly specific tests, the vast majority of patients without the disease have negative tests (very few false positives).* However, the test may also be negative in those with the disease. Note that patients with the disease do not enter into the determination of specificity; it, like sensitivity, is independent of disease prevalence. Specificity can also be improved by changing the cut point for defining abnormal to a more abnormal value (see Fig. 17–1).

Because specificity is independent of prevalence, it is susceptible to overinterpretation when disease prevalence (pretest probability) is high (see Example 4 below). In this case, the false-negative tests (*c*) may significantly out number the true negatives (*d*).

Highly specific tests are used to confirm a diagnosis. This is especially important when the consequences of the diagnosis are serious for the patient, either for prognosis or therapy.

Setting Your Positive/Negative Cut Point

For most diagnostic tests, the clinical laboratory supplies a reference range (see Chapter 18). This range is determined by testing hundreds of samples of unselected patients, patients with the disease, and patients known to not have the disease. From this data, graphs such as Fig. 17–1 can be generated. The data are analyzed to determine the statistical best fit for distinguishing the diseased from the nondiseased populations.

For many clinical tests, such as treadmill exercise tests, interpretation of imaging studies, and application of diagnostic tests, the clinician must decide, based upon the clinical scenario and the type of diagnostic question being asked (screening, case finding, hypothesis testing) what cut point will best serve to answer the question. Consultation with specialists in laboratory medicine and with experts in the diseases in your differential diagnosis can assist you in determining what should be regarded as a positive or negative test in each specific clinical situation.

Predictive Values

When we do a test, we are not really interested in the test (sensitivity and specificity), but in how it can help us in understanding our patient's problem: does the presence of a positive test predict that the patient has the disease (*positive predictive value [PPV]*) and does a negative test predict the absence of the disease (*negative predictive value [NPV]*). Predictive values are calculated from 2 × 2 tables (see Fig. 17–2). As we shall see, the predictive values for a test are dependent upon the population which was used to generate the data in the 2 × 2 table; different populations have different disease prevalences. To generate meaningful predictive values, the patients generating the data must be chosen randomly from a clinical population that is relevant to your question and patient.

Positive predictive value. The PPV is calculated from our 2 × 2 table. It is the proportion of patients with a positive test who have the disease: $PPV = a/(a + b)$, a probability. Tests with a high PPV have few false-positive tests, therefore a positive test supports the diagnosis. Note, however, that if the disease is rare in the population (therefore $(b + d) >> (a + c)$, the test will have to be extremely specific (low false positives, b) for the true positives to be greater than the false positives (see examples). Therefore, when the pretest probability of disease is low (low prevalence), even seemingly good tests (sensitivity, specificity) may perform badly for predicting the presence of disease.

Negative Predictive Value. The NPV is the proportion of patients with a negative test who do not have the disease: $NPV = d/(c + d)$, a probability. Tests with a high NPV have few false negatives, therefore a negative test argues against the disease. When the condition is prevalent in the population to begin with, a negative test may not be very helpful; that is, the NPV may be low and the disease may be present despite a negative test.

Consequently, to use the PPV and NPV, the clinician must know, or have a good estimate of, the prevalence of the condition being tested for, in the population which the patient represents. Most clinicians do not have this data readily available. What we do have is our clinical estimate of the probability of disease that we have generated from our history and physical examination in generating our differential diagnosis.

Likelihood Ratios

Another way of expressing the usefulness of a test is in LR. *A positive likelihood ratio (LR +)* is the ratio of the probability of a positive test in people with the disease (the sensitivity) to the probability of a positive test in people without the disease: $LR + = [a/(a + c)] \div [b/(b + d)]$. *A negative likelihood ratio*

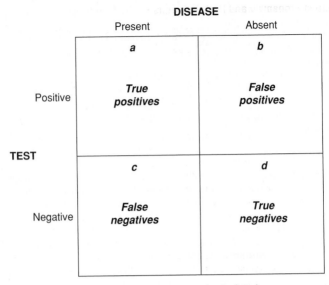

Positive likelihood ratio (LR+)
LR+ = [c/(a + c)] ÷ [b/(b + d)]

Negative likelihood ratio (LR−)
LR− = [c/(a + c)] ÷ [d/(b + d)]

Fig. 17–3 *Positive and Negative LR.*

(LR-) is the probability of a negative test in patients with the disease divided by the probability of a negative test in people without the disease (the specificity): $LR- = [c/(a + c)] ÷ [d/(b + d)]$ (Fig. 17–3). LR, the ratio of two probabilities, *are odds.*

LR show how well a result more abnormal (LR+) or less abnormal (LR-) than a given value for the test (the cut point for "test positive" in the 2 × 2 table) discriminates between those with and without the disease. They are a function of the defined parameters of the test and are independent of the prevalence of the disease (see the examples). LR contain all the sensitivity and specificity information and express the relationship between sensitivity and specificity for positive and negative results.

A big advantage of LR is that they can be calculated for a range of test values, rather than the single normal/abnormal cut point used for sensitivity and specificity. Thus, *LR allow us to use all the information, rather than the limited information in a single normal/abnormal cut point.*

As the LR+ becomes larger, the likelihood of the disease increases; as the LR- approaches zero, the disease becomes much less likely. Generally speaking, LR between 0.5 and 2.0 are not useful and those <0.5 but >0.2 or >2.0 but <5.0 are suggestive but not conclusive. Values of LR >5 argue for the disease whereas LR <0.2 argue against the disease.

Posttest Probability and Posterior Odds

LR include information from each cell of the 2 × 2 table; they are not susceptible to the errors that occur in the application of predictive values to conditions of low and high prevalence, respectively, as discussed above. This makes them much more useful diagnostically.

Because LR are a ratio of probabilities, they are an expression of odds. We can use them to derive a new probability for the disease based upon the test result. Because this new probability is determined after the test is done, it is the *posttest probability* (PP). To calculate the posttest probability, convert the pretest probability to pretest odds and then multiply by the LR to get the posttest odds (*posterior odds*). Then, convert the posttest odds back to the posttest probability (see example 1). The posttest probability can be calculated for both a positive test and a negative test.

Clinicians should learn to think in terms of the LR for the parameter ranges of the tests they use. This is the implicit reasoning that experienced and efficient clinicians use in selecting and interpreting their laboratory tests. It is useful to make this process explicit. This allows us to actually do the calculations in the occasional situation where it will be useful, but also helps us to understand and dissect our decision-making processes and to avoid misinterpretation of the significance of either normal or abnormal laboratory results [Barry HC, Ebell MH. Test characteristics and decision rules. *Endocrinol Metab Clin North Am* 1997;26:45–65].

Examples

Four examples of clinical testing scenarios are given, each with different estimated disease prevalence. For each example, the test is assumed to have 95% sensitivity and 95% specificity. These examples should help you to understand the concepts discussed above.

Example 1: Disease Prevalence 1% (Fig. 17–4)

Of 10 000 patients, only 100 have the disease (99:1 odds against). False positives are five times more likely to be found than true positives. The calculations will only be shown for this example.

Calculation of Positive and NPVs:

$$\text{PPV} = \frac{a}{(a+b)} = \frac{95}{(95+500)} = 0.16$$

$$\text{NPV} = \frac{c}{(c+d)} = \frac{5}{(5+9400)} = 0.999$$

Calculation of Positive and Negative LR:

$$\text{LR}+ = [a/(a+c)] \div [b/(b+d)]$$

$$= [95/(95+5)] \div [500/(500+9400)] = 19$$

$$\text{LR}- = [c/(a+c)] \div [d/(b+d)]$$

$$= [5/(95+5)] \div [9400/(500+9400)] = 0.05$$

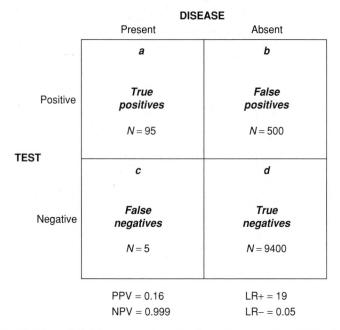

DISEASE

Fig. 17–4 *Example 1: Disease Prevalence 1%.* The test has a sensitivity of 0.95 and a specificity of 0.95.

The PPV (0.16) is better than the baseline risk (0.01), but is still quite low; so a positive test does not even make the diagnosis very probable. The NPV is 0.999 (1 in 10 000), which sounds good, but is actually not much better than the already low baseline risk of 0.01 (1 in 100).

Has this highly sensitive and specific test helped you in this situation? Not much. Although the likelihood of disease is much higher with a positive test (from 99:1 to 16:1), still most positive tests are false positives and further evaluation is necessary.

This example is typical of a screening situation for an uncommon disease in an asymptomatic population. The test has to be very sensitive and very specific to be useful. An example of such a test is HIV testing in pregnant women, but most clinical tests have neither the sensitivity nor specificity required to be effective when disease prevalence is low.

Example 2: Disease Prevalence 10% (Fig. 17–5)

Of 1000 patients, 100 have the disease (9:1 odds against).

$$PPV = 0.65 \quad LR+ = 19$$
$$NPV = 0.999 \quad LR- = 0.05$$

In this scenario, 65% of the patients with a positive test have the disease; a definite improvement over the 10% at baseline. A positive test is twice as likely

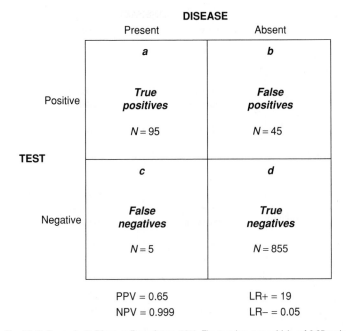

DISEASE

	Present	Absent
Positive	**a** *True positives* N = 95	**b** *False positives* N = 45
Negative	**c** *False negatives* N = 5	**d** *True negatives* N = 855

PPV = 0.65   LR+ = 19
NPV = 0.999   LR− = 0.05

Fig. 17–5 *Example 2: Disease Prevalence 10%.* *The test has a sensitivity of 0.95 and a specificity of 0.95.*

to be a true positive as a false positive. The NPV is quite low, so a negative test is helpful in reducing the likelihood of disease.

Are either the positive or negative results likely to be diagnostically sufficient? A negative test is useful to reduce the posttest probability of disease below any reasonable clinical threshold. A positive test will need to be followed with more specific testing to confirm the diagnosis (raise the probability of disease above the level needed for clinical certainty). This is especially true for any disease with an adverse prognosis or for which therapies are potentially toxic.

This scenario is representative of a case finding strategy in an at risk population. A test with 95% sensitivity and specificity could be used to separate the population into a low-risk pool and a high-risk pool, the latter to undergo further testing.

Example 3: Disease Prevalence 50% (Fig. 17–6)

You have worked up a patient and your clinical impression is that the patient has a 50% chance (1:1 odds) of having the disease (disease prevalence of 0.5). You construct a 2 × 2 table with what you know.

PPV = 0.95   LR+ = 19
NPV = 0.95   LR− = 0.05

The PPV and NPV are both significant improvements more than the baseline risk of 0.5. There are relatively few false positives or false negatives.

DISEASE

		Present	Absent
		a	**b**
TEST	Positive	True positives N = 95	False positives N = 5
		c	**d**
	Negative	False negatives N = 5	True negatives N = 95

PPV = 0.95   LR+ = 19
NPV = 0.95   LR− = 0.05

Fig. 17–6 Example 3: Disease Prevalence 50%. For these examples, the test has a sensitivity of 0.95 and a specificity of 0.95.

Does the test help you in this clinical situation? The test is clinically useful regardless of the result. Both a positive and a negative test make substantial changes in the disease probability, and both probably exceed the level of certainty required in most clinical situations.

This example is representative of the situation in which laboratory testing is most useful, i.e., true uncertainty, with even odds for and against the disease. Selecting tests with good LR in this setting will have a profound impact on your diagnostic process.

Example 4: Disease Prevalence 90% (Fig. 17–7)

You have worked up a patient and your clinical impression is that the patient has a 90% chance (9:1 odds in favor) of having the disease (disease prevalence of 0.9). You construct a 2×2 table with what you know.

PPV = 0.95   LR+ = 19
NPV = 0.73   LR− = 0.05

It is quite likely the patient has the disease based upon your clinical assessment. A positive test (PPV) only minimally improves your accuracy. A negative test (NPV) reduces the probability, but it is still the most likely diagnosis, and one-third of those with a negative test will be misclassified (false negatives).

Has the test helped you in reaching your predetermined levels of certainty required to either diagnose the disease or exclude it from further consideration? No, a positive result adds nothing and a negative result is likely to be an error.

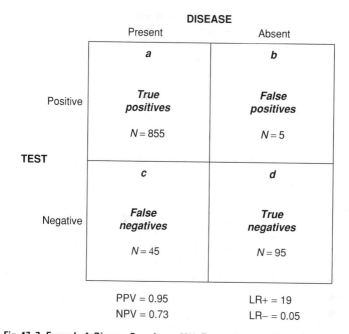

Fig. 17–7 *Example 4: Disease Prevalence 90%. The test has a sensitivity of 0.95 and a specificity of 0.95.*

This scenario is representative of a situation when too high a level of certainty is expected for the clinical situation. Neither a positive or negative test is helpful.

Comment.   Note that our test has excellent LR, and the LR are the same regardless of the prevalence of disease. Like sensitivity and specificity, LR are a function of the value of the test chosen as the cut point. This confirms that the LR tells how well a positive and negative test discriminate the population into higher and lower risk groups. However, the interpretation and usefulness of the test still depends upon the baseline probability of disease (pretest probability): a 20 times improvement in very long odds is still long odds (999:1 to 49:1), and a 20 times decrease in very short odds is still an almost even proposition (1:24 to 20:24).

The reader is encouraged to construct their own examples and vary the prevalence of disease and the sensitivity and specificity of the test in order to familiarize themselves with these concepts. The formal calculations are rarely done in clinical practice, but the principles and concepts are used every day by skilled clinicians in deciding how to evaluate their differential diagnoses.

As demonstrated in Example 3, diagnostic testing is most useful when true uncertainty exists with nearly even odds for and against the condition. The purpose of forming a probabilistic differential diagnosis is to identify the conditions which are truly uncertain (approximately even odds) where testing can improve your probability assessment. Most physical findings do not have positive LR of sufficient magnitude to be used as a clinical test of the hypotheses; they do not establish a diagnosis [McGee S. *Evidence-Based Physical Diagnosis*. Second Edition,

Philadelphia, PA: WB Saunders; 2007]. The history and physical examination are for hypothesis generation and estimation of pretest probabilities (prior odds). Many laboratory tests have LR that allow accurate diagnostic discrimination: the laboratory is the best place to test your specific hypotheses. When clinical probability estimates are either very high or very low, further testing is not useful, and is often misleading.

2 × 2 Tables Revisited: Caveat Emptor

If you plan to use the sensitivity, specificity or LR generated from a 2 × 2 table, it is necessary to understand the methods used for selection of the test sample that produced the data. Each of these parameters is dependent upon the inclusion criteria for the categories disease-present and disease-absent, and the method for identifying the population(s) that were tested.

Severity of Disease

Most diseases have a broad spectrum of severity that is generally reflected in the amount of aberration in the tests characteristic of the disease: more-severe disease, more abnormal tests; less-severe disease, less abnormal or even normal test results. As can be seen from Fig. 17–1 and the preceding discussion, if the investigators choose to define the presence of disease as those with more-severe disease (cut point moved to the right), the test will appear more specific and less sensitive, and the positive LR will improve, while the negative LR becomes less useful. If they choose an inclusive definition to reflect the broad range of those with the disease (cut point moved to the left), the test will be more sensitive and less specific, and the negative LR will improve, while the positive LR becomes less useful. In addition, if the 2 × 2 table was constructed using patients with unusually severe disease (as may be seen in an academic referral practice), the sensitivity and specificity calculated may be inappropriately high if applied to a more representative population of patients.

Sampling

Broadly speaking there are three methods of identifying patients to generate data for a 2 × 2 table.

By far the easiest method is to take patients from a known diseased group (e.g., patients with known systemic lupus erythematosus, attending a rheumatology clinic) and another group of patients from a nondiseased population (e.g., blood donors) and apply the test (e.g., an antinuclear antibody test) to both groups. This will generate a 2 × 2 table weighted to more severe disease because the patients are already diagnosed and attending a clinic (see Severity of Disease above). The apparent prevalence is not a real population prevalence; it is an a priori choice of the investigators as to how many people they want in each group. Tests evaluated by this method often appear very good when you calculate the sensitivity, specificity, and LR. Because the population of the table is really two independent populations, the PPV and NPV have no meaning. The clinical usefulness of information generated by this sampling method is marginal at best when the clinician attempts to apply the test parameters to an unselected population.

The second, far more difficult, method is to select a population of patients that represent the community at large (e.g., a random sample of adults), perform the test on all of them, and also evaluate all of them by the gold-standard criteria for the disease. When diseases have a low prevalence in the population (e.g., systemic lupus erythematosus), huge numbers of patients would need very thorough evaluations at tremendous expense to identify enough cases to produce any meaningful data. Hence, this method is only applied to the evaluation of screening tests proposed for large populations (e.g., fecal occult blood testing for colon cancer). This method also does not generate clinically useful data for the clinician outside of the screening paradigm.

The most clinically useful information is generated by selecting patients from a population that presents with the challenge faced by the physician: patients who might have the disease based upon history and physical examination (an intermediate pretest probability, near even odds). A consecutive series of such patients is identified and the test and diagnostic gold standard are applied to all. The data generated in this way is far more useful to the clinician when faced with a diagnostic challenge. The test parameters (LR, sensitivity, and specificity), the prevalence of disease, and the PPV and NPV are much more likely to be applicable to clinical decision making. The clinician still must assess whether the gender, ethnic mix, ages, and comorbidities of the test population are representative of their patient population.

Rule In; Rule Out

The phrases "rule in" and "rule out" are commonplace in the clinical vernacular, but are discouraged.

Some diagnoses can be *confirmed* by specific pathologic tests (e.g., neoplasms, vasculitis), by laboratory tests (e.g., HIV infection, myocardial injury, sickle cell disease), and by microbiologic tests (e.g., cultures and polymerase chain reaction [PCR] identification of specific organisms).

It is impossible, short of necropsy, to "rule out" a diagnosis. When tests with highly negative LR are negative in patients with intermediate or low pretest probability for the disease, the *probability* of the disease becomes very small, but never zero. In each clinical case, we empirically set a clinical level of certainty required to confirm a diagnosis, as we discussed in Chapter 1. We also determine a level of clinical certainty needed to effectively exclude a diagnosis from further consideration. This will depend upon the patient, the clinical scenario, and the risk associated with drawing a false-negative conclusion. When we have assured ourselves that the diagnosis is less probable than our threshold, we can say it is excluded clinically, but it is never "ruled out."

Furthermore, many clinical conditions, especially syndromes (e.g., rheumatoid arthritis), have no gold-standard diagnostic test or exclusion criteria.

Summary

The skilled clinician uses a patient's history and physical examination to generate pathophysiologic and diagnostic hypotheses. A differential diagnosis includes those diseases with the highest estimated probability of being present *in this patient*, and less likely diseases associated with severe morbidity if not promptly diagnosed. An explicit estimation of the probability for each is made. Tests are selected for which the result (positive, negative, or a specific value or finding) will generate a posttest probability (applying the LR) of a clinically significant high or low level. On the basis of the first round of test results and repeat examination of the patient, a refined differential diagnosis is generated and a second round of tests may be ordered. This process is repeated until the posttest probability for the diagnosis exceeds the threshold required by the clinical situation. At that point, a working diagnosis is established.

Principles of Diagnostic Imaging

Imaging techniques include standard radiography and computed axial tomography using X-rays with or without contrast, magnetic resonance imaging, ultrasonography (including Doppler flow measurements), and radioisotope imaging (standard nuclear medicine and positron emission tomography [PET]). The amount of information contained in an imaging study is enormous, especially with computed axial tomography and magnetic resonance imaging technologies. This increase in information may be essential for the care of patients, or it may be a distraction in the diagnostic process. Imaging techniques are rapidly evolving, so it is essential to work closely with your radiologist to select the appropriate imaging studies to answer your questions.

Static images reveal the structure of the body; the questions they are able to answer are anatomic, not physiologic questions. Images tell us where anatomy is altered and suggest how it is altered. Images cannot make pathologic, microbiologic or physiologic diagnoses. Be sure, your radiologist describes the images and the anatomic abnormalities using descriptive language, rather than conclusions. Radiologists cannot diagnose granulomas, tuberculosis, cancer or infection. They can describe lesions with characteristics suggestive of these diagnoses.

Dynamic imaging allows accurate evaluation of the mechanical properties of certain organs, such as blood flow in arteries and veins and heart muscle and valve function. They also allow reasonably good estimates of intravascular pressure gradients from the Bernoulli equation, which relates flow to the pressure gradient across areas of restricted flow.

As with all tests you order, beyond the most standard laboratory evaluation discussed above, each imaging study must be ordered to answer a specific clinical question. Ordering imaging studies without a hypothesis or specific question is a bad practice and often leads to the identification of incidental findings (anatomic variants, degenerative conditions, benign neoplasms, cysts, and hemangiomas) that distract the attention of the clinician, even when they have no plausible bearing on the patient's presenting complaints. It is easy to begin evaluating the imaging studies (and the laboratory abnormalities) rather than the patient.

The conclusions drawn from an imaging study need to be drawn by the clinicians who are familiar with the patient. You want the diagnostic and physiologic hypotheses of the radiologists, but only after you have their descriptions. Again, an easily made mistake is to let the imaging specialist begin to direct the evaluation, often of incidental findings or clinically irrelevant questions. Clinically important questions relevant to the presenting problem should be the drivers of the imaging evaluation. Incidental findings can be followed up, if needed, at a later time. It is extremely uncommon for incidental findings to have major significance for the patient.

ADDITIONAL READING

1. Fletcher RH, Fletcher SW, Wagner EH. *Clinical Epidemiology: The Essentials.* 3rd ed. Baltimore, MD: Williams & Wilkins; 1996.

2. McGee S. *Evidence-Based Physical Diagnosis.* Second edition, Philadelphia, PA: WB Saunders; 2007.

CHAPTER 18

Common Laboratory Tests

This chapter discusses normal and pathologic values for commonly ordered tests of the blood (cells and chemistries), urine, cerebrospinal fluid (CSF), and serous fluids. The tests discussed are commonly used to formulate physiologic and diagnostic hypotheses. The much more numerous, specific tests used for confirming the diagnosis of a specific disease should not be used until a narrow differential diagnosis has been established. These more specific tests are not discussed here.

Laboratory tests are ordered for one of four reasons:

1. **Screening:** A small number of tests have been demonstrated to find "silent" disease in the patient who has no symptoms or signs or specific risk factors for the disease. Common examples include testing for hemochromatosis with iron studies and for hypercholesterolemia.
2. **Case finding:** Some tests are used to identify affected symptomatic individuals within specific at risk populations. This differs from screening because a specific high-risk population, rather than the general population, has been selected for testing. An example is, testing the children of patients with breast cancer related to the BRCA genes for this genetic abnormality.
3. **Diagnosis:** This is the use of tests to assist in making (or excluding) a diagnosis suggested by the patient's symptoms and signs. See the discussion in Chapter 17, for a summary of the proper approach to diagnostic testing.
4. **Monitoring:** Tests are often used to monitor the progress of disease, response to therapy, or concentration of medication.

Many laboratory tests are used for more than one, or even for all, of these reasons, depending on the clinical situation. For example, blood glucose is used to screen for diabetes mellitus, to identify cases amongst obese patients with a family history of diabetes who are at high risk for diabetes, to confirm the diagnosis, and to monitor treatment in patients found to have the disease.

The decision as to which tests, if any, should be obtained routinely can be debated interminably. Certainly, the prevalence of the disease in the population of which your patient is a member should affect the selection [Sox HC. Probability theory in the use of diagnostic tests. *Ann Intern Med.* 1986;104:60–66]. In addition to assisting in the diagnosis, quantitative test results help to grade the severity of the physiologic abnormalities and provide objective verification for the purposes of documentation. Tests and their usefulness continually change, so the clinician must keep abreast of current indications for and uses of tests available in his clinical laboratory. Consultation with the pathologist in charge of the clinical laboratory is often useful when questions arise.

The reference ranges are presented for purposes of illustration only. Because each clinical laboratory determines its own reference ranges, those we have listed are not intended to be definitive.

Many organizations, including the American Medical Association, have supported the proposal of the American National Metric Council to convert units of measurement to Système International d'Unités (SI) units. Citing what they perceive to be good reasons, the US physicians and staffs of laboratories and hospitals have been reluctant to convert to SI units introduced in the mid-1980s. Indeed, excellent medical journals have chosen to use conventional (or both) units rather than to insist on conformity. For the non-American reader's convenience, we have included values with SI units in parentheses following the conventional units. Most of the laboratory reference values were adopted from *Harrison's Principles of Internal Medicine*, 16th ed., Appendix A [Kasper DL, Braunwald E, Fauci AS, et al. *Harrison's Principles of Internal Medicine*. 16th ed. New York, NY: McGraw-Hill; 2004].

Each test is followed by lists of diseases and disorders in which abnormal values occur. The lists of associated diseases, syndromes, and conditions highlight the more prevalent causes of the abnormalities and some important rarer diseases. The lists are not inclusive of all possibilities, but should be used as a guide for your thinking.

Consult textbooks of laboratory medicine for more complete discussions.

Blood Chemistries

ALBUMIN   See Proteins, page 826.

ALKALINE PHOSPHATASE, SERUM   This includes a number of cellular enzymes that hydrolyze phosphate esters. They are named from their optimum activity in alkaline media. High concentrations of the enzymes occur in the blood during periods of rapid growth, either physiologic or pathologic, and from cellular injury. The enzymes are normally plentiful in hepatic parenchyma, osteoblasts, intestinal mucosa, placental cells, and renal epithelium. Abnormally rapid growth or cell destruction will raise the concentration of these enzymes.

Normal Alkaline Phosphatase: 30 to 120 U/L (SI Units: 0.5–2.0 nkat/L).   It is high in newborns, declining until puberty and then rising every decade after 60 years of age.

Increased Alkaline Phosphatase.   This is usually associated with disorders of bone, liver or the biliary tract. *CLINICAL OCCURRENCE: Technical Error* dehydration of blood specimen; *Endocrine* hyperparathyroidism (osteitis fibrosa cystica), acromegaly, hyperthyroidism (effect on bone), subacute thyroiditis, last half of pregnancy; *Idiopathic* Paget disease, benign transient hyperphosphatasemia; *Infectious* liver infections (hepatitis, abscesses, parasitic infestations and infectious mononucleosis), chronic osteomyelitis; *Inflammatory/Immune* primary biliary cirrhosis, sarcoidosis; *Mechanical/Trauma* healing fractures, common bile duct obstruction from stone or carcinoma, intrahepatic cholestasis, passive congestion of the liver; *Metabolic/Toxic* osteomalacia, rickets, drug reactions (intrahepatic cholestasis), chlorpropamide, ergosterol, sometimes intravenous injection of albumin, pernicious anemia, hyperphosphatasia, dehydration, rapid loss of weight; *Neoplastic* osteoblastic bone tumors, metastatic carcinoma in bone, myeloma, liver metastases, cholangiocarcinoma; *Neurologic* cerebral damage; *Psychosocial* abuse with skeletal trauma; *Vascular* myocardial, renal, and sometimes pulmonary infarction.

Decreased Alkaline Phosphatase. *CLINICAL OCCURRENCE:* *Technical Errors* use of oxalate in blood collection; *Endocrine* hypothyroidism; *Idiopathic* osteoporosis; *Inflammatory/Immune* celiac disease; *Metabolic/Toxic* vitamin D toxicity, scurvy (vitamin C deficiency), milk-alkali syndrome, pernicious anemia/B_{12} deficiency.

ANION GAP, SERUM The anion gap is the difference between the concentrations of measured cations and the measured anions in the blood, measured in milliequivalents per liter, mEq/L: AG = $[Na^+] - ([Cl^-] + [HCO_3^-])$. The anion gap accounts for phosphates, sulfates, amino acids, and albumin.

Normal Anion Gap: 12 ± 2.

Increased Anion Gap. An increased anion gap indicates the accumulation of organic acids and the presence of an *anion gap metabolic acidosis.* *CLINICAL OCCURRENCE:* Ketoacidosis (diabetes, alcoholism, starvation), intoxication with salicylates, methanol or ethylene glycol, lactic acidosis, or renal failure.

Decreased Anion Gap. This occurs uncommonly and suggests the accumulation of positively charged proteins in the blood. *CLINICAL OCCURRENCE:* Multiple myeloma.

ALANINE AMINOTRANSFERASE (ALT), SERUM This enzyme occurs mostly in hepatocytes with smaller quantities in skeletal and heart muscle. It is released into the circulation when cells are damaged or necrotic.

Normal Concentration—0 to 35 U/L (SI units: 0–0.58 mkat/L).

Increased ALT. Increased ALT usually indicates damage to the liver, although severe damage to skeletal muscle can produce significant elevations. *CLINICAL OCCURRENCE:* *Infectious* viral hepatitis, infectious mononucleosis, liver abscess; *Mechanical/Trauma* passive liver congestion, extrahepatic biliary obstruction; *Metabolic/Toxic* drug-induced liver disease, alcohol; *Neoplastic* hepatocellular carcinoma, liver metastases.

ASPARTATE AMINOTRANSFERASE (AST), SERUM This enzyme is concentrated mostly in the cells of the heart, liver, muscle, and kidney; lesser amounts are in pancreas, spleen, lung, brain, and erythrocytes. Tissue injury releases the enzyme into the extracellular fluids, but not necessarily in amounts proportionate to the injury.

Normal AST: 9 to 40 U/L.

Increased AST. This usually reflects damage to the liver, the muscles, including the heart, and, less commonly, to other organs. It usually rises in concert with the ALT. When the AST is ≥2.0 times the ALT, alcohol abuse with cirrhosis or alcoholic hepatitis should be suspected. *CLINICAL OCCURRENCE:* *Technical Error* false-positive from opiates and erythromycin, dehydration of blood specimen; *Congenital* muscular dystrophy; *Endocrine* diabetes mellitus; *Idiopathic* Paget disease, cholecystitis; *Infectious* viral hepatitis, pulmonary infections; *Inflammatory/Immune* hemolytic diseases, polymyositis, pancreatitis, regional ileitis, ulcerative colitis; *Mechanical/Trauma* severe exercise, clonic and tonic seizures, crushing or burning or necrosis of muscle, inflammation from intramuscular injections, rhabdomyolysis, peptic ulcer, extrahepatic biliary obstruction; *Metabolic/Toxic* hepatic necrosis and drug-induced hepatitis, uremia, myoglobinemia, pernicious anemia, drugs (salicylates, alcohol), dehydration; **Neoplastic** bone metastasis, myeloma; **Vascular** myocardial, renal and cerebral infarction.

Decreased AST. CLINICAL OCCURRENCE: Endocrine pregnancy; **Metabolic/Toxic** chronic dialysis, uremia, pyridoxine deficiency, ketoacidosis, beriberi, severe liver disease.

BICARBONATE, TOTAL SERUM (HCO$_3$-, CO$_2$ CONTENT)
Bicarbonate (HCO$_3$-) is formed in the kidney by carbonic anhydrase and diffused through the body fluids as ionized bicarbonate in association with sodium. Bicarbonate is the major buffer consumed when protons (H$^+$) are produced by the metabolism of amino acids or the increased production or ingestion of organic acids. Renal production of bicarbonate buffers the acidosis of hypoventilation (increased PaCO$_2$). In respiratory alkalosis with a low PaCO$_2$, the kidney excretes bicarbonate to maintain the blood pH and the bicarbonate concentration falls.

Normal Serum Bicarbonate: 22 to 26 mEq/L (SI: 22–26 mmol/L).

Increased Bicarbonate. This indicates a metabolic alkalosis, either primary or secondary to a respiratory acidosis. **CLINICAL OCCURRENCE: Endocrine** hyperaldosteronism, Cushing disease, severe hypothyroidism; **Metabolic/Toxic** primary metabolic alkalosis (diarrhea, gastric suction, nausea, and vomiting), diuretics (especially loop diuretics), hypercapnia; **Psychosocial** bulimia, purging.

Decreased Bicarbonate. A decreased bicarbonate concentration indicates the presence of a metabolic acidosis. These are further classified by the anion gap, see page 815. **CLINICAL OCCURRENCE: Endocrine** Addison disease; **Metabolic/Toxic** hypocapnia from hyperventilation, metabolic acidosis, for example, renal failure, ketoacidosis (diabetic, alcoholic, starvation), lactic acidosis, salicylate intoxication, methanol or ethylene glycol intoxication, renal tubular acidosis.

BILIRUBIN, TOTAL SERUM
See Jaundice, page 470. Four-fifths or more is derived from the catabolism of the heme from aging erythrocytes. Bilirubin is insoluble in water and is bound to plasma proteins until conjugated with glucuronic acid in the liver. The water-soluble conjugated bilirubin is normally excreted in the bile. If the serum level exceeds 0.4 mg/dL, the water-soluble form appears in the urine.

Normal Serum Bilirubin: 0.3 to 1.0 mg/dL (SI Units: 5.1–17 mmol/L).

Increased Bilirubin: Hyperbilirubinemia. Increased bilirubin indicates an increased breakdown of red blood cells (RBCs) or failure of hepatic excretion. **CLINICAL OCCURRENCE:** See Jaundice, Chapter 9, page 470.

Unconjugated Hyperbilirubinemia. This is caused by hemolysis, ineffective erythropoiesis, decreased hepatic uptake of unconjugated bilirubin (Gilbert syndrome), or impaired hepatic conjugation (neonatal jaundice, drugs or Crigler-Najjar syndrome).

Conjugated Hyperbilirubinemia. Because the liver is able to conjugate bilirubin, the problem is either hepatocyte excretion (Dubin-Johnson syndrome, Rotor syndrome), intrahepatic cholestasis (hepatitis, drugs, granulomatous disease), or bile duct obstruction.

Decreased Bilirubin: Hypobilirubinemia. Nonhemolytic anemias and hypoalbuminemia.

BLOOD UREA NITROGEN, SERUM—BUN
Molecular weight 60. Urea is synthesized in the liver from ammonia derived from the metabolism of protein in the body and gut. It is filtered and reabsorbed by the kidney; reabsorption is inversely related to the rate of urine flow.

Normal Serum Blood Urea Nitrogen (BUN): 10 to 20 mg/dL (SI Units: 3.6–7.1 mmol/L).

Increased BUN. An increase indicates decreased glomerular filtration and/or increased tubular reabsorption, or increased production in the gut from ingested protein or blood. *CLINICAL OCCURRENCE:* *Prerenal* hypotension, hemorrhage, dehydration (vomiting, diarrhea, excessive sweating), Addison disease, hyperthyroidism, heart failure, sepsis, upper gastrointestinal hemorrhage, increased protein ingestion; *Renal* any cause of acute or chronic renal insufficiency; *Postrenal* obstruction of the ureters, bladder, or urethra.

Decreased BUN. *CLINICAL OCCURRENCE:* Low-protein diets, muscle wasting, starvation, cirrhosis, cachexia, high urine flow.

BUN: Creatinine Ratio >10:1. This indicates relatively preserved glomerular filtration with either increased urea production or decreased urine flow. *CLINICAL OCCURRENCE:* Excessive protein intake, blood in the gut, excessive tissue destruction (cachexia, burns, fever, corticosteroid therapy); postrenal obstruction, inadequate renal circulation (heart failure, dehydration, shock).

BUN: Creatinine Ratio <10:1. This indicates decreased urea production. *CLINICAL OCCURRENCE:* Low protein intake, multiple dialyses, severe diarrhea or vomiting, hepatic insufficiency.

B-TYPE NATRIURETIC PEPTIDE
Both systolic and diastolic heart failure are accompanied by increased ventricular and atrial wall tension leading to release of natriuretic peptides types A and B. This test is used to identify patients with dyspnea and pulmonary infiltrates who have heart failure from those with primary pulmonary disorders.

Normal Concentration: <50 pg/mL.

Increased B-type Natriuretic Peptide. Systolic and diastolic right and left ventricular failure.

CALCIUM, SERUM (Ca^{2+})
Ninety-nine percent of total body calcium is bound to phosphate and carbonate as insoluble salts within the bone matrix, in equilibrium with a small amount in the extracellular fluid. The plasma level varies with the rate of Ca^{2+} absorption from the small intestine and the proximal renal tubular reabsorption rate, under the control of parathyroid hormone (PTH). Calcium is present in the three forms: *ionized or free Ca^{2+}* that is physiologically active; *protein-bound or nondiffusible* Ca^{2+}, most of which is loosely bound to plasma albumin; and *complexed or complex-bound* Ca^{2+}, which forms relatively soluble fractions complexed with carbonates, citrates, or phosphates. *Parathormone (PTH)* accelerates release of Ca^{2+} and PO$_4^{3-}$ from bone and promotes renal excretion of PO$_4^{3-}$ and reabsorption of Ca^{2+}. PTH stimulates renal conversion of vitamin D$_3$ to the active 1,25-(OH)$_2$ form. *Calcitonin* inhibits bone resorption and decreases serum and extracellular Ca^{2+}.

Normal Serum Calcium: 9.0 to 10.5 mg/dL (SI Units: 2.2–2.6 mmol/L).

➤ **Increased Calcium: Hypercalcemia.** Hypercalcemia indicates increased bone breakdown, decreased renal excretion and/or vitamin D intoxication. *CLINICAL OCCURRENCE:* *Endocrine* primary hyperparathyroidism, hyperthyroidism, hypothyroidism, Cushing disease, Addison disease; *Idiopathic* osteoporosis, Paget disease; *Inflammatory/Immune* sarcoidosis; *Mechanical/Trauma* immobilization; *Metabolic/Toxic* vitamin D intoxication, milk-alkali syndrome, hyperproteinemia (sarcoidosis, multiple myeloma), drugs (thiazide diuretics), poisons (berylliosis); *Neoplastic* tumor metastatic to bone, lymphoma, multiple myeloma, leukemia, release of PTH-like peptide.

Decreased Calcium: Hypocalcemia. A low serum calcium can be caused by decreased binding proteins, vitamin D deficiency or resistance, precipitation of calcium phosphate salts or calcium soaps, or PTH deficiency. *CLINICAL OCCURRENCE:* *Endocrine* hypoparathyroidism (postthyroidectomy, idiopathic or pseudohypoparathyroidism), hypothyroidism, late pregnancy; *Inflammatory/Immune* acute pancreatitis with fat necrosis; *Metabolic/Toxic* renal insufficiency, excessive fluid intake, malabsorption of calcium and vitamin D or dietary vitamin D deficiency (osteomalacia and rickets), hypoproteinemia (cachexia, nephrosis, celiac disease, cystic fibrosis of the pancreas), drugs (antacids), corticosteroids.

CHLORIDE, SERUM (Cl^-) Chloride is the principal anion in the extracellular fluid. By contrast, in the intracellular fluid the chief anions are phosphate and sulfate. The serum Cl^- is usually proportionate to Na^+ (see discussion of anion gap, page 815).

Normal Serum Chloride: 98 to 106 mEq/L (SI Units: 98–106 mmol/L).

Increased Chloride: Hyperchloremia. *CLINICAL OCCURRENCE:* *Technical Error* bromide in blood gives false test for Cl; *Endocrine* hyperparathyroidism, diabetes mellitus, diabetes insipidus; *Metabolic/Toxic* renal tubular acidosis, acute renal failure, respiratory alkalosis, nonanion gap metabolic acidosis, drugs (acetazolamide, ammonium salts, salicylates), dehydration.

Decreased Chloride: Hypochloremia. The chloride concentration is low when organic acids accumulate in anion gap metabolic acidosis or bicarbonate replaces chloride in metabolic alkalosis. *CLINICAL OCCURRENCE:* *Endocrine* diabetic ketoacidosis, Addison disease, primary aldosteronism; *Mechanical/Trauma* congestive cardiac failure, pyloric obstruction; *Metabolic/Toxic* anion gap metabolic acidosis, metabolic alkalosis, pulmonary emphysema, excessive sweating, diarrhea, malabsorption, drugs (diuretics).

CHOLESTEROL, SERUM Cholesterol is insoluble in water. It is carried in the circulation in association with lipoproteins. The low-density lipoproteins (LDLs) have the highest concentration of cholesterol. Cholesterol is ingested and also synthesized by the liver. Cholesterol is essential to every cell; it is a precursor to adrenal steroids, gonadal steroids, and bile salts. Elevated cholesterol, particularly LDL cholesterol, is associated with accelerated atherogenesis. In contrast, elevated high-density lipoprotein (HDL) cholesterol is protective.

Normal Concentrations: See Tables 18–1 to 18–3. *It is of particular note, that cholesterol and triglycerides are the only serum chemistries reported as socially*

Table 18–1 ATP III Classification of Total Cholesterol and Triglycerides

	Total Cholesterol		Triglycerides	
	In mg/dL	In SI, mmol/L	mg/dL	In SI, mmol/L
Desirable	<200	<5.2	<150	<1.69
Borderline	200–239	5.20–6.18	150–199	1.69–2.25
High High	≥240	≥6.21	≥200	≥2.26

determined "desirable" and "undesirable" levels, rather than biologically determined population-based normal ranges.

Increased Cholesterol: Hypercholesterolemia. *CLINICAL OCCURRENCE:* *Congenital* familial hypercholesterolemia and combined hyperlipidemia; *Endocrine* hypothyroidism, diabetes mellitus; *Inflammatory/Immune* chronic nephritis, amyloidosis, SLE, polyarteritis; *Mechanical/Trauma* biliary obstruction (gallstone, carcinoma, cholangiolitic cirrhosis); *Metabolic/Toxic* obesity, metabolic syndrome, nephrotic syndrome, maldigestion and malabsorption, cirrhosis, lipodystrophy, alcohol; *Vascular* renal vein thrombosis.

Decreased Cholesterol: Hypocholesterolemia. *CLINICAL OCCURRENCE:* *Congenital* Tangier disease; *Infectious* chronic infections; *Inflammatory/Immune* cirrhosis, severe hepatitis; *Metabolic/Toxic* malnutrition, alcohol, starvation, uremia, steatorrhea, pernicious anemia, drugs (lipid-lowering agents, cortisone, adrenocorticotropic hormone [ACTH]).

C-REACTIVE PROTEIN (CRP) This is an acute-phase reactant with a short half-life, so it rises rapidly within 4 to 6 hours of the onset of inflammation or tissue injury, and declines relatively rapidly (T 1/2 5–7 h) with resolution.

Normal CRP: Consult local labs.

Elevated CRP. CRP rises with any acute or chronic inflammation, infection or tissue damage. Levels tend to correlate with the erythrocyte sedimentation rate (ESR), see page 847, but respond more rapidly to changes in the patient's status

Highly Sensitive CRP (hs-CRP). hs-CRP levels correlate positively in prospective studies with the likelihood for developing an acute coronary event. The

Table 18–2 ATP III Classification of LDL Cholesterol

	LDL Cholesterol	
	In mg/dL	In SI, mmol/L
Optimal	<100	<2.59
Desirable	<130	<3.36
Borderline High	130–159	3.36–4.11
High	160–189	4.14–4.89
Very High	≥190	>4.91

Table 18–3   ATP III Classification of HDL Cholesterol

	HDL Cholesterol	
	In mg/dL	In SI, mmol/L
High	$\geq$60	$\geq$1.55
Low	$\leq$39	$\leq$1.01

strength of the association is equivalent to and additive with LDL-cholesterol elevations [Labarrere CA, Zaloga GP. C-reactive protein: from innocent bystander to pivotal mediator of atherosclerosis. *Am J Med.* 2004;117;499–507]. The mechanism is unknown, but implicates an IL-6 driven inflammatory process.

CREATINE KINASE (CK), SERUM   CK catalyzes the transfer of high-energy phosphate between creatine and phosphocreatine, and between adenosine diphosphate and adenosine triphosphate. Major concentrations are found in cardiac and skeletal muscle and in the brain. Erythrocytes lack this enzyme, so autolyzed serum specimens are acceptable for testing.

Normal CK: Males—25 to 90 mU/mL (SI Units: 0.42–1.50 μkat/L); females— 10 to 70 mU/mL (SI Units: 0.17–1.17 μkat/L). African Americans may have significantly higher normal levels.

Increased Creatine Kinase. Increased CK suggests muscle or brain damage. The isoenzyme pattern (CK-MB from cardiac muscle, CK-BB from brain) can indicate the likely source. *CLINICAL OCCURRENCE:* *Congenital:* progressive muscular dystrophy; *Endocrine:* hypothyroidism, last few weeks of pregnancy; *Infectious:* pyomyositis; *Inflammatory/Immune:* polymyositis, dermatomyositis, inclusion-body myositis, pancreatitis; *Mechanical/Trauma:* severe exercise, muscle spasms, clonic and tonic seizures, muscle trauma (crush syndrome, postoperatively for about 5 days), electroshock for defibrillation, muscle necrosis and atrophy, intramuscular injections for 48 hours, dissecting aneurysm; *Metabolic/Toxic* megaloblastic anemia, drugs (statins, salicylates, alcohol) *Vascular* myocardial and cerebral infarction.

Decreased Creatine Kinase. *CLINICAL OCCURRENCE:* *Technical Error* drug interference; *Endocrine* early pregnancy; *Inflammatory/Immune* pancreatitis; *Metabolic/Toxic* decreased muscle mass.

CREATININE, SERUM   Creatinine is an organic acid product of creatine metabolism in muscle. It is distributed throughout the body water. Creatine is synthesized by the liver and pancreas from arginine and glycine and taken up by muscle where it is converted to creatine phosphate, catalyzed by the CK enzyme. Creatine decomposes to creatinine at a rate of 1% or 2% per day. The amount of creatinine produced increases with muscle mass and decreases with muscle wasting. Creatinine is cleared by the glomerular filtration (75%) and tubular secretion (25%), without reabsorption. The rate of urinary creatinine excretion is an indicator of glomerular filtration.

Normal Serum Creatinine: <1.5 mg/dL (SI Units: 133 μmol/L).

Increased Creatinine. Elevated creatinine indicates decreased renal function, particularly glomerular filtration, from prerenal, renal, or postrenal causes. Because creatinine is dependent upon muscle mass, decreased renal function may be masked in patients with decreasing muscle mass, especially in women and the elderly. See Table 10–1, page 537, for staging of clinical kidney disease. *CLINICAL OCCURRENCE:* *Technical Error* drug interference with the assay (cephalosporins, ketones); *Endocrine* acromegaly; *Idiopathic* renal insufficiency of any cause; *Mechanical/Trauma* burns, crush injury; *Metabolic/Toxic* increased muscle mass, ingestion of red meat, excessive intake of protein, dehydration, ureterocolostomy with urinary resorption, medications (cimetidine, probenecid, trimethoprim); *Vascular* inadequate blood flow to the kidneys, renal failure, heart failure.

Decreased Creatinine. *CLINICAL OCCURRENCE:* Cachexia, decreased muscle mass, and increased glomerular filtration (e.g., the osmotic diuresis of early diabetes).

CREATININE CLEARANCE Creatinine is filtered by the glomerulus and secreted by the proximal tubule. The clearance of creatinine from the blood, measured in mL/min, is a commonly used estimate of glomerular filtration rate. Creatinine clearance is measured directly with 24-hour urine collections. This is cumbersome and often urine collections are incomplete. An estimate of creatinine clearance is obtained with the Cockcroft-Gault formula:

Creatinine Clearnace (mL/min) = [(140-age) × (lean body weight in kg)] ÷ [plasma creatinine (mg/dL) × 72]

Multiply by 0.85, for estimating creatinine clearance in women.

Normal Creatinine Clearance: Females—100–110 mL/min · per 1.73 m^2; males—120–130 mL/min · per 1.73 m^2.

Increased Creatinine Clearance. See Increased GFR, below.

Decreased Creatinine Clearance. See Decreased GFR below and Acute and Chronic Kidney Failure, Chapter 10, page 537ff.

FERRITIN, SERUM. Ferritin is the major iron-storage protein in the body. Ferritin is an acute-phase reactant and is, therefore, best interpreted with a test of the acute-phase reaction such as the CRP or ESR.

Normal Ferritin: Females—10 to 200 ng/mL (SI 10–200 μg/L); males—15 to 400 ng/mL (SI Units: 15–400 μg/L).

Increased Serum Ferritin. *CLINICAL OCCURRENCE:* Increased body iron stores (from transfusion hemosiderosis, anemias of chronic disease, leukemias, Hodgkin disease), excess dietary iron, hemochromatosis (usually >400 ng/dL, often >1000 ng/dL), inflammation, infection, or cancer. Ferritin >10 000 occurs only with Still's disease and hemophagocytic syndromes.

Decreased Serum Ferritin. *CLINICAL OCCURRENCE:* Iron deficiency.

GLOMERULAR FILTRATION RATE (GFR). The glomerular filtration rate is determined by the filtration pressure gradient between the glomerular capillary and Bowman's space, the glomerular capillary filtration area and the state of the glomerular endothelium, basement membrane and epithelial cells. GFR is the most reliable measure of functioning nephron mass as it is independent of tubular absorption and secretion. Direct measurement of GFR is difficult, so various clinical formulae are utilized to estimate GFR. The creatinine clearance is an estimate of GFR, but since creatinine is both reabsorbed and secreted and these mechanisms are enhanced or impaired by drugs, it is not an accurate measure of GFR, especially as kidney disease advances. The formula developed by the investigators in the Modification of Diet in Renal Disease (MDRD) study is more accurate in chronic renal disease. Both the Cockcroft-Gault and MDRD formulas require knowledge of the patient's age and weight. Newer methods are being developed which may not have these limitations [Stevens LA, Coresh J, Greene T, Levey AS. Assessing kidney function—measured and estimated glomerular filtration rate. *N Engl J Med.* 2006;354:2473–83].

Normal GFR: Females—100–110 mL/min · per 1.73 m²; males—120–130 mL/min · per 1.73 m².

Increased GFR. Osmotic diuresis and constriction of the efferent arteriole will both increase the GFR. Clinically, increased GFR is seen with hyperglycemia in early diabetic nephropathy.

Decreased GFR. Loss of nephron mass, damage to the glomuerular capillary loops with vasculitis and glomerulopathies and damage to the glomerular basement membrane and obstruction to urine flow all result in decreases in GFR and renal insufficiency. *CLINICAL OCCURRENCE:* See Acute and Chronic Kidney Failure, Chapter 10, page 537.

GLUCOSE, SERUM This six-carbon monosaccharide is a primary energy source for metabolism. The serum level remains fairly constant during fasting; there is a moderate rise after the ingestion of food. Hepatocytes convert other carbohydrates to glucose. Surpluses of glucose are converted to glycogen in the liver and muscle, or fat that is deposited throughout the body, predominately in adipocytes. Glucose uptake by the liver, muscle, and adipocytes is insulin dependent. After an average meal, the blood sugar normally rises to approximately 180 mg/dL serum, returning to fasting levels within 2 hours. Higher blood glucose levels result from excessively rapid absorption or impaired peripheral disposition, usually related to insulin insufficiency or resistance. High blood glucose concentrations exceed the renal tubular reabsorption threshold and glucose is excreted in the urine (*glycosuria*). The normal renal threshold occurs at a serum glucose of 160 to 190 mg/dL. This may be higher in a damaged kidney.

Normal Serum Glucose: 75 to 110 mg/dL (SI Units: 4.2–6.4 mmol/L).

Diagnostic Criteria for Diabetes.

1. A fasting glucose of ≥126 mg/dL (SI Units: ≥7.0 mmol/L); or
2. Symptoms of diabetes plus a random glucose of ≥200 mg/dL (SI Units: ≥11.1 mmol/dL); or
3. A plasma glucose ≥200 mg/dL (SI Units: ≥11.1 mmol/L) 2 hours following a 75-g oral glucose load.

The abnormal test must be confirmed on another day.

Diagnosis of Impaired Fasting Glucose (IFG). A fasting glucose of 110 to 125 mg/dL (SI Units: 6.1–7.0 mmol/L).

Diagnosis of Impaired Glucose Tolerance (GT). A blood glucose of 140 to 199 mg/dL (SI Units: 7.8–11.0 mmol/L) 2 hours after a 75-g oral glucose load.

Increased Glucose: Hyperglycemia. Hyperglycemia indicates insulin resistance, diabetes or release of stress-associated hormones (epinephrine, cortisol, growth hormone). *CLINICAL OCCURRENCE:* *Endocrine* diabetes mellitus, impaired glucose tolerance, acromegaly, hyperthyroidism, Cushing disease, increased adrenalin, ACTH, pheochromocytoma, pregnancy, toxemia of pregnancy; *Infectious* any acute severe infection, for example, pneumonia; *Inflammatory/Immune* systemic inflammatory response syndrome, regional enteritis, ulcerative colitis; *Metabolic/Toxic* drugs (corticosteroids, diazoxide, epinephrine), poisoning (streptozotocin); *Neurologic* Wernicke syndrome, subarachnoid hemorrhage, hypothalamic lesions, convulsions; *Vascular* myocardial infarction, pulmonary embolism, hemorrhage.

Decreased Glucose—Hypoglycemia. Inability to maintain a normal blood glucose indicates excessive insulin secretion or administration, or severely impaired hepatic gluconeogenesis. *CLINICAL OCCURRENCE:* *Congenital* galactosuria, maple syrup urine disease, hepatic glycogenoses; *Endocrine* hypopituitarism, hypothalamic lesions, hypothyroidism, Addison disease; *Infectious* sepsis; *Inflammatory/Immune* pancreatitis; *Mechanical/Trauma* postgastrectomy dumping syndrome, gastroenterostomy; *Metabolic/Toxic* insulin administration, oral hypoglycemics, glycogen deficiency, hepatitis, cirrhosis, malnutrition; *Neoplastic* insulinoma, some sarcomas.

HEMOGLOBIN A$_{1C}$: GLYCOHEMOGLOBIN
Glycosylation of cellular and extracellular proteins occurs at a rate dependent upon the ambient plasma glucose concentration. Hemoglobin is glycosylated in this manner and the amount of glycosylated hemoglobin is an accurate measure of the average blood sugar over the average life of the circulating erythrocytes, approximately 6 weeks. Measurement of one glycosylated form of hemoglobin, hemoglobin A$_{1C}$, is used to estimate the average blood sugar as a determinate of diabetes control.

Normal Hemoglobin A$_{1C}$: 3.8% to 6.4% (SI Units: 0.038–0.064).

IRON, SERUM (FE^{2+})
The body contains about 3 to 4 g of iron. It is a component of hemoglobin, the cytochromes, and other cellular metalloproteins. Approximately 1 mg of iron is absorbed and excreted each day. Most of the iron circulates in erythrocyte hemoglobin (1.0 mg/1.0 mL packed erythrocytes), with the rest stored bound to ferritin, in myoglobin, and with a small fraction incorporated into respiratory enzymes and other sites. Iron is absorbed in the duodenum by a complex pathway regulated at the level of the enterocyte; most ingested iron is either not absorbed or is sloughed with the enterocytes, never entering the plasma. Absorbed iron is bound to transferrin. Iron is cleared from the plasma with a half-time of 60 to 120 minutes, and 80% to 90% is incorporated into new circulating erythrocytes over the subsequent 2 weeks. The serum concentration of iron decreases by 50 to 100 mg/dL with the diurnal acceleration of erythropoiesis in the afternoon, so the time of day the specimen is drawn and its relationship to meals should be known. Iron deficiency is a very common disorder.

Normal Serum Iron: 50 to 100 μg/dL (SI Units: 9–27 μmol/L).

Increased Serum Iron: Hyperferremia. An increase in serum iron may be seen following a high-iron meal, or with hemochromatosis and liver disease. *CLINICAL OCCURRENCE:* *Congenital* hemochromatosis, thalassemia; *Inflammatory/Immune* acute hepatic necrosis, aplastic anemia, hemolytic anemia; *Metabolic/Toxic* excessive absorption (iron therapy, dietary excess), cirrhosis, pernicious anemia.

Decreased Serum Iron: Hypoferremia. Low serum iron results from inadequate dietary intake, excessive blood loss (both with increased iron-binding capacity), or chronic inflammation (decreased iron-binding capacity). *CLINICAL OCCURRENCE:* *Endocrine* iron loss to the fetus during gestation; Infectious tuberculosis, osteomyelitis, hookworm; *Inflammatory/Immune* celiac disease, rheumatoid arthritis (RA), SLE; *Mechanical/Trauma* intravascular hemolysis with hemoglobinuria (paroxysmal nocturnal hemoglobinuria, march hemoglobinuria, prosthetic heart valves); *Metabolic/Toxic* iron deficiency, repeated phlebotomy, diminished absorption (decreased ingestion, celiac disease, pica, postgastrectomy); *Neoplastic* gastrointestinal cancers, loss of transferrin in nephrotic syndrome; *Psychosocial* poverty; *Vascular* intrapulmonary hemorrhage (e.g., idiopathic pulmonary hemosiderosis), chronic bleeding (e.g., menorrhagia, hematuria, peptic ulcer disease, gastritis, polyps, ulcerative colitis, colon carcinoma).

IRON-BINDING CAPACITY, SERUM TOTAL The total iron-binding capacity mainly reflects transferrin and, with the serum iron, helps to distinguish iron deficiency anemias from the anemia of chronic inflammation.

Normal Iron-Binding Capacity: 250 to 370 μg/dL (SI Units: 45–66 μmol/L).

Increased Iron-Binding Capacity. This generally reflects a response to iron deficiency. *CLINICAL OCCURRENCE:* Iron deficiency, acute or chronic blood loss, hepatitis, late pregnancy.

Decreased Iron-Binding Capacity. Transferrin falls with chronic inflammation. *CLINICAL OCCURRENCE:* Anemias of chronic disorders (infections, inflammations, and cancer), thalassemia, cirrhosis, nephrotic syndrome.

LACTIC DEHYDROGENASE (LDH), SERUM LDH catalyzes the reversible oxidation of lactate to pyruvate. It is found in all tissues, so an elevation of the blood level is a nonspecific indicator of tissue damage.

Normal LDH: 100 to 190 U/L (SI Units: 1.7–3.2 mkat/L).

Increased LDH. Elevations of LDH suggest injury to the muscles, liver, hemolysis, or rapid cell division as in lymphomas. *CLINICAL OCCURRENCE:* *Congenital* muscular dystrophy in 10% of cases, progressive muscular dystrophy, myotonic dystrophy (CK is more specific for muscle than LDH); *Endocrine* hypothyroidism; *Infectious* hepatitis with jaundice, infectious mononucleosis; *Inflammatory/Immune* polymyositis in 25% of cases, dermatomyositis, hemolytic anemias; *Mechanical/Trauma* cardiovascular surgery, common bile duct obstruction, intestinal obstruction; *Metabolic/Toxic* muscle necrosis, celiac disease, untreated pernicious anemia, alcohol; *Neoplastic* 50% of cases of lymphoma and leukemia; *Vascular* acute myocardial infarction, pulmonary embolism or infarction.

Decreased LDH. *CLINICAL OCCURRENCE:* Irradiation, ingestion of clofibrate.

PHOSPHATE, SERUM INORGANIC Serum phosphate measures the inorganic phosphorus of ionized HPO_4^{2-} and H_2PO_4 which are in equilibrium in the serum; only 10% to 20% is protein bound. Phosphorus is necessary for synthesizing nucleotides, phospholipids, and the high-energy adenosine triphosphate. Phosphates are excreted by the kidney; parathormone (PTH) increases phosphate excretion. When glycolytic energy demands are increased, the serum inorganic P decreases.

Normal Phosphate: 3.0 to 4.5 mg/dL (SI Units: 1.0–1.4 mmol/L).

Increased Phosphate: Hyperphosphatemia. Increased phosphate results from defects of vitamin D metabolism, breakdown of bone, release of intracellular stores by tissue damage and/or failure of renal excretion. *CLINICAL OCCURRENCE:* *Congenital* Fanconi disease; *Endocrine* acromegaly, hyperparathyroidism; *Idiopathic* Paget disease; *Infectious* sepsis; *Inflammatory/Immune* sarcoidosis; *Mechanical/Trauma* healing fractures, crush injury, high intestinal obstruction; *Metabolic/Toxic* acute and chronic renal failure, vitamin D deficiency (rickets, osteomalacia), muscle necrosis, milk-alkali syndrome, respiratory alkalosis, excess of vitamin D; *Neoplastic* multiple myelomas, osteolytic metastases, myelocytic leukemia.

Decreased Phosphate: Hypophosphatemia. Low serum phosphate results from dietary insufficiency, failure to absorb dietary phosphate, excessive uptake in bone or renal phosphate wasting. *CLINICAL OCCURRENCE:* *Congenital* primary hypophosphatemia; *Endocrine* hyperparathyroidism, diabetes mellitus; *Metabolic/Toxic* renal tubular defects (Fanconi syndrome), anorexia, vomiting, diarrhea, lack of vitamin D, in refeeding after starvation, malnutrition, gout, ketoacidosis, respiratory alkalosis, hypokalemia, hypomagnesemia, primary hypophosphatemia, drugs (intravenous glucose, anabolic steroids, androgens, epinephrine, glucagon, insulin, salicylates, phosphorus-binding antacids, diuretic drugs, alcohol).

POTASSIUM, SERUM (K$^+$) Potassium is the predominant intracellular cation, while sodium predominates in the extracellular fluids. Approximately 90% of the exchangeable K$^+$ is within the cells; less than 1% is in the serum. Small shifts of K$^+$ out of cells causes relatively large changes in serum [K$^+$]. Intracellular acidosis causes an extracellular shift of K$^+$ buffering H$^+$ shifting to the intracellular compartment. Plasma [K$^+$] is tightly regulated by the kidney: hyperkalemia leads to aldosterone secretion and potassium excretion; hypokalemia leads to excretion of urine nearly devoid of potassium. Changes in serum concentration of K$^+$ produce profound effects on nerve excitation, muscle contraction, and in cardiac conduction. Because the concentration of K$^+$ in the erythrocytes is about 18 times as great as that in the serum, hemolysis occurring during sample collection falsely elevates the reported serum K$^+$.

Normal Potassium: 3.5 to 5.0 mEq/L (SI Units: 3.5–5.0 mmol/L).

➤ **Increased Potassium: Hyperkalemia.** (Note: high levels of serum K$^+$ pose great danger of producing cardiac arrest.) *CLINICAL OCCURRENCE:* *Technical Error* hemolysis in performing venipuncture or intentional clotting in collecting blood specimens, especially with thrombocytosis; *Congenital* hyperkalemic periodic paralysis; *Endocrine* primary and secondary hypoaldosteronism, adrenal insufficiency (Addison disease, adrenal hemorrhage); *Mechanical/Trauma* rhabdomyolysis, crush injury, hemolyzed transfused blood, urinary obstruction; *Metabolic/Toxic* acute and chronic renal failure, acidosis (metabolic or respiratory), muscle necrosis, drugs (amiloride, spironolactone, triamterene, angiotensin-converting enzyme inhibitors), foods (fruit juices, soft drinks, oranges, peaches, bananas, tomatoes, high-protein diet), dehydration; *Neurologic* status epilepticus; *Vascular* gastrointestinal hemorrhage, hemorrhage into tissues.

Decreased Potassium: Hypokalemia. This is almost always associated with depletion of in total body K$^+$. *CLINICAL OCCURRENCE:* *Endocrine* diabetes mellitus, Cushing syndrome, hyperaldosteronism; ***Mechanical/Trauma*** ureterosigmoidostomy with urinary reabsorption, adynamic ileus; ***Metabolic/Toxic*** vomiting, gastric suction, postgastrectomy dumping syndrome, gastric atony, laxative abuse, polyuria, renal injury, salt-losing nephritis, metabolic alkalosis (from diuresis, primary aldosteronism, pseudoaldosteronism), metabolic acidosis (from renal tubular acidosis, diuresis phase of tubular necrosis, chronic pyelonephritis, diuresis after release of urinary obstruction), malabsorption and malnutrition, drugs (diuretics, estrogens, salicylates, corticosteroids) ***Neoplastic*** aldosteronoma, villous adenoma, colonic cancer, Zollinger-Ellison syndrome.

PROTEIN, TOTAL SERUM

Most serum proteins are synthesized in the liver (albumin and many others) or by mature plasma cells (immunoglobulins). Increases or decreases in serum proteins represent a balance between synthesis and protein catabolism or loss into third spaces or in the urine. Total protein is the sum of serum albumin and globulins; the fibrinogen was discarded in the clot that separated from the plasma to form the serum specimen. The quantity of the total serum protein, minus the albumin fraction, gives an estimate of the serum globulins.

Normal Total Protein: 5.5 to 8.0 g/dL (SI Units: 55–80 g/L).

Increased Total Protein: Hyperproteinemia. This represents increased concentration of normal proteins, or excessive production of immunoglobulins. ***CLINICAL OCCURRENCE:*** Water depletion, multiple myeloma, macroglobulinemia, and sarcoidosis.

Decreased Total Protein: Hypoproteinemia. This is caused by decreased synthesis, increased catabolism because of malnutrition, or loss into third spaces or into the urine in nephrotic syndrome. ***CLINICAL OCCURRENCE:*** Congestive cardiac failure, ulcerative colitis, nephrotic syndrome, chronic glomerulonephritis, cirrhosis, viral hepatitis, burns, malnutrition.

PROTEIN: ALBUMIN, SERUM

Molecular weight about 65 000. Normally, albumin comprises more than half the total serum protein. Because its molecular weight is low compared to that of the globulins (between 44 000 and 435 000), its smaller molecules exert 80% of osmotic pressure of the plasma. Albumin is a protein store that can be metabolized during starvation, so low levels may indicate protein malnutrition. It also serves as a solvent for fatty acids and bile salts and as a transport vehicle by loosely binding calcium, hormones, amino acids, drugs, and metals; low albumin levels must be taken into account when interpreting the serum concentrations of these substances.

Normal Albumin: 3.5 to 5.5 g/dL (SI Units: 35–55 g/L).

Increased Albumin: Hyperalbuminemia. No significant correlation with diseases.

Decreased Albumin: Hypoalbuminemia. This can only be due to decreased production (liver), increased metabolism or loss into third spaces or urine. ***CLINICAL OCCURRENCE:*** ***Congenital*** analbuminemia; ***Endocrine*** diabetes mellitus; ***Infectious*** viral hepatitis; ***Inflammatory/Immune*** ulcerative colitis, protein-losing enteropathies, chronic glomerulonephritis, lupus erythematosus, polyarteritis, RA, rheumatic fever; ***Mechanical/Trauma*** peptic ulcer; ***Metabolic/Toxic*** congestive cardiac failure, cirrhosis, nephrotic syndrome, malnutrition, drugs (estrogens); *Neoplastic* multiple myeloma, Hodgkin disease, lymphocytic leukemia, macroglobulinemia.

PROTEIN: GLOBULINS, SERUM The difference between the values for total serum protein and for serum albumin is referred to as the serum globulin fraction of the total serum protein. When the globulin level is increased, fractionation of the globulins is indicated to identify each component. This is accomplished by serum protein electrophoresis (SPEP).

SPEP. The proteins are separated by electrophoresis; the proteins migrate, each at its own rate, dependent on its charge and molecular weight. A serum specimen contains proteins that separate into several zones according to their mobility. The proteins are named for the zone in which they are found (named with Greek lowercase letters): alpha 0 (for albumin), alpha 1 (α_1), alpha 2 (α_2), beta (β), gamma (γ), and phi (ϕ) (for fibrinogen).

PROTEIN: α_1-GLOBULINS α_1-Globulins include α_1-antitrypsin, oromucil, and some cortisol-binding globulin.

Increased α_1-Globulins. Hodgkin disease, peptic ulcer, ulcerative colitis, cirrhosis, metastatic carcinoma, protein-losing enteropathy.

Decreased α_1-Globulins. Viral hepatitis.

PROTEIN: α_2-GLOBULINS α_2-globulins include macroglobulins, haptoglobin, HS glycoprotein, ceruloplasmin, and some immunoglobulins.

Increased α_2-Globulins. Hodgkin disease, peptic ulcer, ulcerative colitis, cirrhosis, nephrotic syndrome, chronic glomerulonephritis, systemic lupus erythematosus (SLE), polyarteritis nodosa, RA, metastatic carcinoma, protein-losing enteropathies.

Decreased α_2-Globulins. Cirrhosis, viral hepatitis.

PROTEIN: β-GLOBULINS β-Globulins include transferrin, hemopexin, and some immunoglobulins.

Increased β-Globulins. RA, rheumatic fever, analbuminemia.

Decreased β-Globulins. Nephrotic syndrome, lymphocytic leukemia, metastatic carcinoma.

PROTEIN: γ-GLOBULINS γ-Globulins are predominately immunoglobulins of the IgG class. Increases in γ-globulins can be *monoclonal*, arising from a clonal proliferation of plasma cells or lymphocytes, or *polyclonal* reflecting an inflammatory response. Polyclonal γ-globulins produce a *broad-based pattern* in the gamma zone, indicating the presence of proteins from many cell lines. Plasma immunoglobulins are increased either from acute and chronic inflammatory conditions (polyclonal) or neoplastic (benign or malignant) expansion of a single clone of cells (monoclonal).

Increased Polyclonal γ-Globulins. Cirrhosis, myelocytic leukemia, lupus erythematosus, RA, analbuminemia.

Decreased Polyclonal γ-Globulins. Nephrotic syndrome, lymphocytic leukemia, common variable immunodeficiency, hypogammaglobulinemia, protein-losing enteropathies.

PROTEIN: IMMUNOGLOBULIN IgG   Molecular weight 160 000. This is the smallest immunoglobulin and the only one that can cross the placenta. Consequently, it protects the fetus and newborn until the child's own immunoglobulins can be generated. IgG is synthesized after IgM in response to a new antigen. IgG producing plasma cells are the major humoral effector of chronic inflammation.

Normal IgG: 800 to 1500 mg/dL (SI Units: 8.0–15.00 g/L).

Increased IgG.   *CLINICAL OCCURRENCE:*   *Infectious*   pulmonary tuberculosis, hepatitis, osteomyelitis; *Inflammatory/Immune*   SLE, RA, vasculitis; *Metabolic/Toxic*   cirrhosis; *Neoplastic*   myeloma, monoclonal gammopathy of undetermined significance.

Decreased IgG.   *CLINICAL OCCURRENCE:*   *Congenital*   lymphoid aplasia, agammaglobulinemia; *Inflammatory/Immune*   common variable immunodeficiency, nephrotic syndrome; *Neoplastic*   heavy-chain disease, IgA myeloma, macroglobulinemia, CLL.

PROTEIN: IMMUNOGLOBULIN IgA   Molecular weight 170 000. IgA is especially involved in the protection against viral infections. It has an *excretory form* with a molecular weight of 400 000, found in colostrum, saliva, tears, bronchial secretions, gastrointestinal secretions, and nasal discharges. It has a special action against viruses of influenza, poliomyelitis, adenoviral diseases, and rhinoviruses.

Normal IgA: 90 to 325 mg/dL (SI Units: 0.90–3.2 g/L).

Increased IgA.   *CLINICAL OCCURRENCE:*   *Congenital*   Wiskott-Aldrich syndrome; *Inflammatory/Immune*   SLE, RA, sarcoidosis; *Metabolic/Toxic*   cirrhosis; *Neoplastic*   IgA myeloma.

Decreased IgA.   *CLINICAL OCCURRENCE:*   *Congenital*   absent in some people, hereditary telangiectasia, lymphoid aplasia; *Inflammatory/Immune*   nephrotic syndrome, Still disease, SLE, common variable immunodeficiency, agammaglobulinemia; *Metabolic/Toxic*   cirrhosis; *Neoplastic*   heavy-chain disease, ALL, CLL, CML.

PROTEIN: IMMUNOGLOBULIN IgM   Molecular weight 900 000. This is the largest of the immunoglobulins. It is formed during a primary antibody response. The rheumatoid factor and the isoantibodies anti-A and anti-B belong mostly to this class.

Normal IgM: 45 to 150 mg/dL (SI Units: 0.45–1.5 g/L).

Increased IgM.   *CLINICAL OCCURRENCE:*   *Infectious*   hepatitis, trypanosomiasis; *Inflammatory/Immune*   biliary cirrhosis, RA, SLE; *Neoplastic*   macroglobulinemia.

PROTEIN: IMMUNOGLOBULIN IgD   Molecular weight 185 000. There is no known specific activity for this protein.

Normal IgD: 0 to 8 mg/dL (SI Units: 0–0.08 g/L).

Increased IgD. Chronic infections, IgD myeloma.

PROTEIN: IMMUNOGLOBULIN IgE   Molecular weight 200 000. IgE is bound to mast cell membranes. Specific antigen (allergen) binding to the bound IgE causes mast cell degranulation and an allergic or anaphylactic response. IgE is essential for allergic and atopic reactions.

Normal IgE:,0.025 mg/dL (SI Units: 0.00025 g/L).

Increased IgE. Allergic asthma (60%), hay fever (30%), atopic eczema, parasitic infestations, IgE myeloma, hyper IgE syndromes.

PROTEIN: MONOCLONAL γ-GLOBULINS

The SPEP has a sharp and *narrow spike* (M-spike) in the gamma region indicating a monoclonal protein. The exact nature of the immunoglobulin is determined by immunoelectrophoresis. Monoclonal gammopathies are characterized by a marked elevation one or, rarely, more of the five human immunoglobulins normally present in human serum: IgG, IgA, IgM, IgD, and IgE. Each contains a specific heavy chain (H chain) coupled to one of two types of light chains (L chains). The heavy chains are named with lowercase Greek letters, corresponding to the capital letters designating immunoglobulin type: IgA (α), IgG (γ), IgM (μ), IgD (δ), IgE (ε). The light chains are called kappa (κ) and lambda (λ). The five immunoglobulins can be identified by immunofixation electrophoresis. In this procedure, after electrophoresis, specific antibodies are used to identify the H and L chains.

Monoclonal Immunoglobulin *CLINICAL OCCURRENCE:* Multiple myeloma, macroglobulinemia, malignant lymphoma, amyloidosis, monoclonal gammopathy of undetermined significance.

SODIUM, SERUM (Na⁺)

Molecular weight 23. This is the predominant cation in the extracellular fluid. Together with Cl^-, it makes the major contribution to the plasma osmotic pressure of the plasma. Loss of Na^+ is frequently accompanied by an equivalent amount of water (as an isotonic solution), so normal levels of serum Na^+ do not exclude total body loss of Na^+. Assessment of total body Na^+ status is done by assessing extracellular volume. To maintain extracellular volume, the kidney retains sodium, and with it, enough water to maintain normal osmolarity. Because water moves between the intracellular and extracellular compartments to maintain iso-osmolarity between the two, an increase or decrease in the $[Na^+]$ represents an inverse change in the total body water, that is, an increased serum Na^+ indicates a water deficit and a decreased serum Na^+ indicates water excess.

Normal Sodium: 136 to 145 mEq/L (136–145 mmol/L).

Increased Serum Sodium: Hypernatremia. This always indicates a relative total body water deficit, regardless of the extracellular volume status [Adrogué HJ, Madias NE. Hypernatremia. *N Engl J Med.* 2000;342:1493–1499]. *CLINICAL OCCURRENCE:* *Endocrine* diabetes insipidus, diabetes mellitus, hyperparathyroidism, hyperaldosteronism; *Metabolic/Toxic* water loss greater than Na loss (vomiting, sweating, hyperpnea, diarrhea), drugs (corticosteroids, diuretics), diuretic phase of acute tubular necrosis, diuresis after relief of urinary obstruction, excessive sodium intake, hypercalcemia, hypokalemic nephropathy; *Neurologic* thalamic lesions.

Decreased Serum Sodium: Hyponatremia. This always indicates a relative total body water excess, from excess water ingestion or inability of the kidney to excrete a sufficiently dilute urine, regardless of the extracellular volume status [Adrogué HJ, Madia NE. Hyponatremia. *N Engl J Med.* 2000;342:1581–1589]. *CLINICAL OCCURRENCE:* *Technical Error* spuriously normal serum osmolality (hyperlipidemia, hyperglycemia); *Endocrine* Addison disease; *Infectious* pneumonia, meningitis, brain abscess (all cause syndrome of inappropriate antidiuretic hormone secretion); *Metabolic/Toxic* congestive heart failure (CHF), salt-losing nephropathy, cirrhosis with ascites, fluid and electrolyte loss with replacement by hypotonic fluids, for example, water (vomiting, sweating, diarrhea, diuresis), malnutrition, syndrome of inappropriate antidiuretic hormone secretion; *Neoplastic* antidiuretic hormone-secreting tumors, especially lung cancers; *Psychosocial* anorexia nervosa, psychogenic polydipsia.

TRIGLYCERIDES Triglycerides are absorbed from the gut following ingestion of a fatty meal. They are transported in chylomicrons to the adipose tissue where they are cleaved by lipoprotein lipase, leading to the formation of less triglyceride enriched very low density (VLDL) and intermediate density (IDL) lipoproteins. Triglycerides are the major form of energy storage, mostly in adipose tissue. They are broken down to free fatty acids which are a highly efficient cellular energy source.

Normal Triglycerides: See Table 18–1, page 819.

Increased Triglycerides: Hypertriglyceridemia: *CLINICAL OCCURRENCE:* *Congenital* lipoprotein lipase deficiency, familial combined hyperlipidemia; familial hypertriglyceridemia, dysbetalipomotanemia; *Endocrine* diabetes, hypothyroidism; *Metabolic/Toxic* alcohol ingestion, high fat diets, metabolic syndrome, drugs (oral contraceptives).

UREA NITROGEN: See *Blood Urea Nitrogen*, page 817.

URIC ACID, SERUM Molecular weight 169. Uric acid is the end product of purine metabolism. Normally uric acid is produced at the rate of 10 mg/kg per day in a healthy adult. The body pool is about 1200 mg, distributed in the body water. Increased nucleic acid breakdown results in increased uric acid production. Uric acid leaves the body through renal excretion and by bacterial catabolism of uric acid in the gut. Renal excretion of uric acid is increased by expansion of body fluids (salt or osmotic diuresis). Excretion of uric acid is decreased by dehydration and diuretics.

Normal Uric Acid: Males—2.5 to 8.0 mg/dL (SI Units: 150–480 mmol/L); Females—1.5 to 6.0 mg/dL (SI Units: 90–360 mmol/L).

Increased Uric Acid: Hyperuricemia. *Note: High values for uric acid are among the most common abnormalities encountered in routine testing. This probably accounts for the much-too-frequent diagnosis of gout. The serum uric acid is elevated in only two-thirds of the cases of gouty arthritis, but the same elevation is noted in 25% of the cases of acute nongouty arthritis, and in 25% of relatives of gouty patients.* *CLINICAL OCCURRENCE:* *Congenital* polycystic kidneys, sickle cell anemia, Wilson disease, Fanconi disease, von Gierke disease, Down syndrome, certain normal populations (Blackfoot and Pima Indians, Filipinos, New Zealand Maoris); *Endocrine* hypothyroidism, hypoparathyroidism, primary hyperparathyroidism, toxemia of pregnancy; *Infectious* resolving pneumonia; *Inflammatory/Immune* psoriasis, hemolytic anemias, sarcoidosis; *Metabolic/Toxic* renal failure, drugs (diuretics, small doses of salicylates), high-protein low-calorie diet, high-purine diet (sweetbreads, liver), starvation, gout, relatives of gouty patients, poisons (acute alcoholism, lead poisoning, berylliosis), hypertension, metaboblic syndrome; *Neoplastic* leukemia, multiple myeloma, polycythemia vera, lymphoma, other disseminated cancers.

Decreased Uric Acid: Hypouricemia. *CLINICAL OCCURRENCE:* *Congenital* xanthinuria, Fanconi syndrome, Wilson disease, healthy adults with

Dalmatian-dog mutation (isolated defect in tubular transport of uric acid); *Endocrine* acromegaly; *Inflammatory/Immune* celiac disease; *Metabolic/Toxic* drugs (uricosuric medication, allopurinol, ACTH, glyceryl guaiacolate, X-ray contrast media); *Neoplastic* carcinomas, Hodgkin disease.

Hematologic Data

Blood Cells

BLOOD FILM EXAMINATION Examination of the stained blood film provides an opportunity to directly examine the circulating cellular elements of the blood (RBC, white blood cell [WBC], platelets) and to confirm results of automated blood analyzers. Here we give examples of information that can be obtained; the reader is encouraged to consult standard textbooks of hematology for comprehensive treatment of these subjects. Appreciate that cellular morphology may vary depending on the preparation technique, stain, and part of the smear you examine. Select an area where the erythrocytes are close but do not touch each other.

Erythrocyte Morphology. Evaluate color, size, shape, and contents. *Macrocytes* reticulocytosis, liver disease, megaloblastic anemia. *Hypochromic Microcytes* defects in hemoglobin synthesis (iron deficiency, thalassemias, sickle cell disease, and other hemoglobinopathies). *Spherocytes* hereditary spherocytosis, immune hemolysis. *Schistocytes* microangiopathic hemolytic anemias (disseminated intravascular coagulation [DIC], thrombotic thrombocytopenic purpura, hemolytic uremic syndrome, vasculitis, thrombotic microangiopathy, prosthetic heart valves, malignant hypertension, scleroderma renal crisis). *Teardrops (Dacryocytes)* marrow damage, for example, extramedullary hemopoiesis, myelophthisic anemia. *Erythroblasts* extramedullary hemopoiesis, myelophthisic anemia, severe hemolytic anemia, erythroleukemia. *Howell-Jolly Bodies* postsplenectomy, megaloblastic anemia. *Basophilic Stippling* lead poisoning, hemolytic disease. *Malaria, Babesia, Borrellia and Bartonella infection.*

Leukocyte Morphology. Confirm the automated differential leukocyte count. *Toxic Granulation of Neutrophils and Metamyelocytes* bacterial infections. *Giant Cytoplasmic Granules* Chediak-Higashi syndrome. *Bilobed Neutrophils* hereditary Pelger-Huet anomaly or pseudo-Pelger-Huet anomaly in acute leukemia. *Hypersegmented Neutrophils* nuclear maturation defect, for example, pernicious anemia, vitamin deficiency, folate deficiency, myeloproliferative diseases. *Neutrophil Inclusions* granulocytic ehrlichiosis and anaplasmosis. *Myeloblasts, Promyelocytes, Myelocytes* depending on the number and appearance of immature cells, consider AML, acute promyelocytic leukemia, CML, myelofibrosis, polycythemia vera. *Atypical Lymphocytes* viral infections, especially Ebstein-Barr virus (acute infectious mononucleosis) and cytomegalovirus (CMV). *Large Granular Lymphocytes* natural killer cells of T-gamma lymphoproliferative disease. *Lymphoblasts* acute lymphoblastic leukemia, prolymphocytic leukemia, malignant lymphoma, chronic lymphocytic leukemia, infectious mononucleosis. *Monocyte Inclusions* monocytic ehrlichiosis. *Plasma Cells* multiple myeloma.

Platelet Morphology. Confirm the automated platelet count. In oil immersion fields at 1000 magnification, where the erythrocytes are close but not touching, the number of platelets in an average field multiplied by 15×10^3 is approximately equal to the platelet count per mm^3. Scan the sides of the smear for clumps of platelets that may have been counted inaccurately by instrument. *Megathrombocytes* platelets greater than 2 μm in diameter may be increased in conditions of accelerated platelet production compensating for increased destruction (e.g., idiopathic thrombocytopenic purpura), B_{12} deficiency, folate deficiency, myeloproliferative diseases, Bernard-Soulier syndrome.

ERYTHROCYTE MEASUREMENTS: COUNTS, HEMOGLOBIN CONTENT, AND HEMATOCRIT
The volume of erythrocytes in the blood is determined by the hematocrit expressed as a percent of the blood volume occupied by erythrocytes in a centrifuged specimen. The hemoglobin measures the grams of hemoglobin per deciliter of whole blood. The total number of erythrocytes per mm^3 is counted by machine or a hemocytometer.

Normal Values: Hematocrit—Males, 42% to 52%; females—37% to 48%; hemoglobin: males—13 to 18 g/dL; females—12 to 16 g/dL; erythrocyte count: 4.15–4.903 $\times 10^6$ per mm^3.

ERYTHROCYTIC INDICES These values are all calculated from the RBC counts, hemoglobin content, and hematocrit.

Normal Values: Mean corpuscular hemoglobin: 28 to 33 pg/cell; mean corpuscular volume: 86 to 98 fL; mean corpuscular hemoglobin concentration: 32 to 36 g/dL.

High RBC Count: Erythrocytosis. This usually represents intravascular and extracellular fluid volume loss, chronic hypoxia, iatrogenic or endogenous erythropoietin excess, or polycythemia vera. *CLINICAL OCCURRENCE:* ***Endocrine*** diabetic acidosis, third to ninth month of pregnancy and to third week postpartum; ***Inflammatory/Immune*** chronic obstructive and restrictive lung disease with hypoxia; ***Mechanical/Trauma*** burns (contracted plasma volume), high-altitude hypoxia; ***Metabolic/Toxic*** contracted plasma volume (dehydration, diarrhea, burns, shock), carboxyhemoglobinemia, sulfhemoglobinemia, secondary polycythemia, drugs (erythropoietin, androgens, diuretics); ***Neoplastic*** polycythemia vera, renal cyst or carcinoma; ***Vascular*** venous-arterial shunt (right-to-left shunt), endothelial damage with diffuse capillary leak.

Low RBC Count: Anemia. See also Chapter 5, page 103. Anemia results from decreased RBC production, hemorrhage, increased RBC destruction (hemolysis), dilution or sequestration in hypersplenism. *CLINICAL OCCURRENCE:* ***Congenital*** thalassemia; ***Idiopathic*** bone marrow failure; ***Inflammatory/Immune*** hemolysis; ***Mechanical/Trauma*** hemolysis or bleeding; ***Metabolic/Toxic*** renal failure, oliguria, macrocytic anemia (pernicious anemia/vitamin B_{12} deficiency), folate deficiency, myelodysplasia, normocytic normochromic anemias (hemolysis, chronic disease, infections, renal failure, liver disease), microcytic hypochromic anemias (Fe deficiency, pyridoxine responsive anemia, hemoglobinopathies); ***Neoplastic*** refractory anemia; ***Vascular*** CHF, acute hemorrhage.

RETICULOCYTE COUNT Reticulocytes are immature erythrocytes just released from the bone marrow. The retained ribosomal RNA is revealed as basophilic stippling with supravital stain. At normal rates of erythrocyte production, this staining disappears within 24 to 48 hours. When erythropoeisis is accelerated RBCs may be released a day or two earlier than usual and hence the cells may stain as reticulocytes for 2 to 2.5 days. Values are expressed as a percent of erythrocytes or as an absolute number. Increased absolute numbers of reticulocytes reflect accelerated erythropoiesis.

Normal Reticulocytes: 0.5% to 1.8%; 29 to 87 × 10⁹/L.

Increased Reticulocytes: Accelerated Erythropoiesis. *Note:* There must be adequate iron, folate, and protein. *CLINICAL OCCURRENCE:* hemorrhage or hemolysis, response to erythropoietin from tissue hypoxia or from its therapeutic administration, and response to therapy of nutrient deprivation (iron, folate, protein).

Decreased Reticulocytes: Decreased Effective Erythropoiesis. *CLINICAL OCCURRENCE:* *Nutrient deprivation* (iron deficiency, pernicious anemia/B₁₂ deficiency, folate deficiency, starvation), *anemia of chronic disease* (inflammation, infection, cancer) and *bone marrow failure* (alcohol abuse, idiosyncratic drug reactions, cancer chemotherapy, total body irradiation, aplastic anemia, leukemia, lymphoma, multiple myeloma, and other cancers invading bone marrow).

ERYTHROCYTE SEDIMENTATION RATE (ESR)
Erythrocytes sediment as a result of gravity. Increased plasma proteins (especially fibrinogen, other acute-phase reactants, and immunoglobulins) decrease the repulsive force between erythrocytes allowing aggregation of larger clumps of cells (seen on the smear as rouleaux formation), which accelerates the rate of sedimentation.

Normal ESR: Males—1 to 17 mm/h; females—0 to 25 mm/h.

Increased ESR. This is a nonspecific finding indicating increased inflammation associated with infection, inflammatory diseases, and some cancers. *CLINICAL OCCURRENCE:* *Endocrine* hyperthyroidism, hypothyroidism, normal pregnancy from third month to termination plus 3 weeks postpartum, menstruation; *Infectious* many, but especially tuberculosis, endocarditis, osteomyelitis, and pelvic inflammation; *Inflammatory/Immune* RA, SLE, PMR, giant cell arteritis, vasculitis; *Metabolic/Toxic* hyperglobulinemia, hypoalbuminemia, dextran or polyvinyl plasma substitutes; *Neoplastic* many cancers; *Vascular* vasculitis.

LEUKOCYTES, TOTAL COUNT: WBC COUNT
This cellular compartment of the blood contains the neutrophils, eosinophils, basophils, lymphocytes, and monocytes.

Normal WBC: 4.3 to 10.83 × 10³/mm³.

Normal Neutrophil Count: 45% to 74% of total.

Increase in All Cellular Elements of the Blood (Erythrocytes, Leukocytes, Platelets): Pancytosis. *CLINICAL OCCURRENCE:* *Metabolic/Toxic* dehydration; *Neoplastic* polycythemia vera, the myeloproliferative syndromes.

Decrease in All Cellular Elements of the Blood (Erythrocytes, Leukocytes, Platelets): Pancytopenia. *CLINICAL OCCURRENCE:* *Idiopathic* marrow failure (aplastic anemia), paroxysmal nocturnal hemoglobinuria; *Infectious* bacterial (tuberculosis); viral (hepatitis); *Inflammatory/Immune* SLE; *Mechanical/Trauma* irradiation; *Metabolic/Toxic* pernicious anemia or folate deficiency, drugs (cancer chemotherapy, chloramphenicol), poisons (benzene); *Neoplastic* multiple myeloma, carcinomatous invasion, lymphoma, myelodysplasia, acute leukemia, myelofibrosis.

Increased Neutrophils: Leukocytosis, Neutrophilia. Leukocytosis usually represents a response to tissue injury or invasion by pathologic organisms. Always inspect the peripheral smear to detect band forms and toxic granulation. *CLINICAL OCCURRENCE: Endocrine* eclampsia; *Idiopathic* leukemoid reactions; *Infectious* acute pyogenic infections including pneumonia, meningitis, pyelonephritis, pelvic inflammatory disease, deep abscesses, endocarditis; *Inflammatory/Immune* acute necrotizing vasculitis; *Mechanical/Trauma* burns, acute hemolysis; *Metabolic/Toxic* exercise, uremia, diabetic acidosis, gout, drugs (granulocyte colony-stimulating factor, granulocyte-macrophage colony-stimulating factor, epinephrine, corticosteroids, lithium carbonate, parenteral foreign proteins, vaccines), poisons (venoms, mercury, black widow spider venom); *Neoplastic* myeloproliferative diseases (polycythemia vera, CML, myelofibrosis, idiopathic thrombocythemia); *Neurologic* seizures *Vascular* tissue necrosis, myocardial infarction, acute hemorrhage.

Decreased Neutrophils: Leukopenia or Neutropenia. *CLINICAL OCCURRENCE: Congenital* Gaucher disease; *Idiopathic* bone marrow failure (aplastic anemia), cyclic neutropenia; *Infectious* viral (infectious mononucleosis, hepatitis, HIV, influenza, rubeola, psittacosis), bacterial (streptococcal, staphylococcal diseases, sepsis, tularemia, brucellosis, tuberculosis), rickettsial disease (scrub typhus, sandfly fever); protozoa (malaria, kala-azar); *Inflammatory/Immune* hypersplenism, Felty syndrome, autoimmune neutropenia, SLE; *Mechanical/Trauma* portal hypertension; *Metabolic/Toxic* uremia, pernicious anemia/B_{12} deficiency, folate deficiency, cirrhosis, cachexia, drugs and therapy (cancer chemotherapy, sulfonamides, antibiotics, analgesics, antidepressants, arsenicals, antithyroid drugs, X-radiation), poisons (benzene); *Neoplastic* aleukemic leukemia, acute myeloblastic leukemia.

EOSINOPHIL COUNT Eosinophils are important in the defense against multicellular parasite infections.

Normal Eosinophil Count: 0% to 7% of WBCs.

Increased Eosinophils: Eosinophilia. *CLINICAL OCCURRENCE: Endocrine* adrenal insufficiency (Addison disease); *Idiopathic* Loeffler endocarditis, hypereosinophilic syndrome; Infectious scarlet fever, parasitic infestations (e.g., trichinosis, echinococcosis); *Inflammatory/Immune* asthma, hay fever, urticaria, drug reactions, erythema multiforme, pemphigus, dermatitis herpetiformis, eosinophilic gastroenteritis, ulcerative colitis, regional enteritis, polyarteritis nodosa, Churg-Strauss sarcoidosis pernicious anemia, eosinophilic fasciitis; *Mechanical/Trauma* postsplenectomy, black widow spider bite; *Metabolic/Toxic* poisons (phosphorus); *Neoplastic* metastatic carcinoma to bone, chronic myelocytic leukemia, polycythemia vera, Hodgkin disease; *Vascular* vasculitis (polyarteritis nodosa, Churg-Strauss).

Decreased Eosinophils: Eosinopenia. Bone marrow failure, corticosteroid treatment.

BASOPHIL COUNT The function of basophils is uncertain. They are similar to tissue mast cells.

Normal Basophil Count: 0% to 2.0% of WBCs.

Increased Basophils: Basophilia. *CLINICAL OCCURRENCE:* *Endocrine* hypothyroidism (myxedema); *Infectious* varicella, variola; *Inflammatory/ Immune* chronic hemolytic anemias; *Mechanical/Trauma* postsplenectomy; *Metabolic/Toxic* nephrotic syndrome; *Neoplastic* chronic myelocytic leukemia, polycythemia vera, myeloid metaplasia, Hodgkin disease.

Decreased Basophils. *CLINICAL OCCURRENCE:* *Endocrine* hyperthyroidism, pregnancy; *Idiopathic* bone marrow failure, aplastic anemia; *Metabolic/Toxic* drugs (chemotherapy, glucocorticoids).

LYMPHOCYTE COUNT   Most circulating lymphocytes are T cells, which traffic continuously between the blood, the tissues, and the lymph nodes until they become activated by exposure to specific antigen on antigen-presenting cells.

Normal Lymphocyte Count: 16% to 45% of WBCs.

Increased Lymphocytes: Lymphocytosis. *CLINICAL OCCURRENCE:* *Infectious* infectious mononucleosis, tuberculosis, viral pneumonia, infectious hepatitis, cholera, rubella, brucellosis, syphilis, toxoplasmosis, pertussis; *Neoplastic* lymphocytic leukemia, malignant lymphoma.

Decreased Lymphocytes: Lymphopenia. *CLINICAL OCCURRENCE:* *Idiopathic* idiopathic lymphopenia; *Infectious* acute infections (viral, HIV), chronic HIV; *Metabolic/Toxic* drugs (corticosteroids, irradiation therapy, cancer chemotherapy); *Neoplastic* carcinoma, lymphoma.

MONOCYTE COUNT   Monocytes circulate in the blood and then enter the tissue and terminally differentiate into tissue macrophages which are important antigen-presenting cells.

Normal Monocyte Count: 4% to 10% of WBCs.

Increased Monocytes: Monocytosis. *CLINICAL OCCURRENCE:* *Congenital* Gaucher disease; *Infectious* protozoal (malaria, kala-azar, trypanosomiasis), rickettsial (Rocky Mountain spotted fever, typhus), bacterial (subacute bacterial endocarditis, tuberculosis, brucellosis, syphilis); *Inflammatory/Immune* ulcerative colitis, regional enteritis, SLE, sarcoidosis; myeloproliferative diseases (polycythemia vera, essential thrombocythemia, CML, myeloid metaplasia), monocytic leukemia, recovery from agranulocytosis.

PLATELET COUNT (THROMBOCYTES)   Platelets are primarily responsible for initial hemostasis by adhesion and aggregation at the sites of endothelial damage. The platelet plug is then stabilized by fibrin deposition from activated coagulation.

Normal Platelet Count: 130 000 to 400 000/mm^3.

Increased Platelet Count: Thrombocytosis or Thrombocythemia. Platelets respond like an acute-phase reactant to tissue injury and many acute infections. *CLINICAL OCCURRENCE:* *Infectious* acute infections; *Inflammatory/Immune* RA; *Mechanical/Trauma* burns, postsplenectomy; *Metabolic/Toxic* exercise, cirrhosis, iron deficiency; *Neoplastic* myeloproliferative diseases (polycythemia vera, essential thrombocythemia, CML, myeloid metaplasia); *Vascular* hemorrhage.

Decreased Platelet Count: Thrombocytopenia. Think of the etiology in terms of decreased production, increased consumption or sequestration in the spleen.

CLINICAL OCCURRENCE: ***Congenital*** May-Hegglin anomaly, Gaucher disease, Kasabach-Merritt syndrome; ***Idiopathic*** aplastic anemia, marrow failure; ***Infectious*** subacute bacterial endocarditis, sepsis, AIDS, typhus; ***Inflammatory/Immune*** autoimmune thrombocytopenic purpura), hemolytic uremic syndrome, acquired hemolytic anemia, thrombotic thrombocytopenic purpura, DIC; ***Mechanical/Trauma*** hypersplenism (congestive splenomegaly, sarcoidosis, splenomegaly, Felty syndrome), massive blood transfusions, irradiation, heat stroke; ***Metabolic/Toxic*** uremia, pernicious anemia, folate deficiency, drugs (cancer chemotherapy, chloramphenicol, heparin induced thrombocytopenia, tranquilizers, antipyretics, heavy metals), poisons (benzol, snake bite, insect bites); ***Neoplastic*** polycythemia vera, myelocytic leukemia.

Coagulation

NORMAL COAGULATION Coagulation is a complex process involving many different blood proteins, platelets, calcium, and tissue factors. There is a constant balance between initiation of coagulation and coagulation inhibitors designed to protect against inappropriate coagulation while directing clot formation to the sites of vessel injury. Two major tests of the coagulation pathways are commonly used.

Prothrombin Time (PT). The PT is standardized by the International Normalized Ratio (INR), which adjusts the raw clotting time for the International Sensitivity Index of the particular thromboplastin used. It tests factors VII, V, X, thrombin (II), and fibrinogen (I) involved in the extrinsic coagulation pathway. The PT/INR is particularly sensitive to decreases in the vitamin K-dependent coagulation factors (II, VII, IX and X).

   Normal PT: 11 to 15 seconds (this is highly dependent upon the thromboplastin used).

   Normal INR: 1.0 to 1.2.

   Prolonged PT/INR: Deficiencies in factors I, II, V, VII, or X, liver disease, DIC, vitamin K deficiency, steatorrhea, idiopathic, hemodilution, warfarin administration, greatly decreased or abnormal fibrinogen. ***Technical Error*** incomplete filling of the Vacutainer tube during the blood draw.

Activated Partial Thromboplastin Time (aPTT). The aPTT assesses the intrinsic pathway of coagulation which uses factors XII, XI, IX, VIII, V, X, II and I.

   Normal aPTT: 22 to 39 seconds.

   Prolonged aPTT. Deficiency of any of the clotting factors—I, II, V, VIII, IX, X, XI, or XII; DIC, heparin, SLE (lupus anticoagulant), antiphospholipid syndrome, and antibody-mediated inhibitors of clotting factor activity.

Fibrinogen. The conversion of fibrinogen to fibrin by thrombin is the final pathway in clot formation. Abnormal fibrinogen levels indicate decreased synthesis or, more commonly, increased consumption because of diffuse activation of clotting.

   Normal Fibrinogen: 200 to 400 mg/dL.

   Increased Fibrinogen. Fibrinogen is an acute-phase reactant that increases during menstruation and pregnancy, infections, inflammation and hyperthyroidism.

Decreased Fibrinogen. Congenital afibrinogenemia, DIC, hemodilution, fibrinolysis.

Urinalysis

Considerable information can be rapidly obtained from examination of the urine. Optimally, urine is collected as a midstream specimen from the first morning voiding and is examined within 30 minutes. This tests renal-concentrating ability and permits identification of casts before they disintegrate. As with the peripheral smear, experience is required for interpretation. The clinician should establish the habit of examining the urine personally, especially in challenging cases.

COLOR Either clear or cloudy (from precipitated normally excreted urates, phosphates, or sulfates), the urine is usually yellow to amber. Other colors provide clues to the presence of abnormal substances for which chemical tests should be performed.

Abnormal-Colored Urine. Dark yellow to green (bilirubin); red to black (erythrocytes, hemoglobin, myoglobin); purple to brown on standing in the sunlight from porphyrins.

ACIDITY Normally the urine is acid, and the urine pH can reach 5.0 with an acid load. High urine pH suggests either an alkali load or inability to fully acidify the urine by distal tubular H^+ excretion. Interpretation of the urine pH requires an assessment of the serum or plasma acid-base status. Monitoring of urinary pH helps physicians attempting to alkalinize or acidify the urine to enhance the solubility and excretion of certain substances and drugs.

Normal Range of pH: 4.6–6.0.

Increased Urine pH. Infection with urea-splitting organisms (e.g., Proteus), systemic alkalosis, renal tubular acidosis, carbonic anhydrase inhibitors.

SPECIFIC GRAVITY An index of weight per unit volume, the specific gravity measures the kidney's ability to concentrate urine in response to the secretion of antidiuretic hormone, and to dilute the urine after a water load. Fasting during 8 hours of sleep should produce a first morning specimen with a specific gravity exceeding 1.018.

Normal Urine Specific Gravity Range: 1.003 to 1.030, achieved with forced water-drinking and fasting, respectively.

Increased Urine Specific Gravity. Fasting and dehydration, glycosuria, proteinuria, radiographic contrast media.

Decreased Urine Specific Gravity. Compulsive water drinking, diabetes insipidus.

Fixed Specific Gravity: Isosthenuria (1.010). This suggests inability to concentrate or dilute the urine, indicating damage to the renal medulla. *CLINICAL OCCURRENCE:* Severe renal parenchymal damage from many causes, for example, gout, prolonged potassium deficiency, hypercalcemia, myeloma kidney, sickle cell disease.

PROTEIN Normally, only the smallest protein molecules can pass the filtration barrier of the glomerulus, and most of these are reabsorbed by the tubules. Glomerular disease produces measurable proteinuria by allowing filtration of more and larger molecules than normal. Because of its low molecular weight, increased urinary albumin excretion is an early sign of glomerular injury. Tubular injury limits reabsorption of filtered proteins.

Normal Urine Protein: 5 to 15 mg/dL; males: 0 to 60 mg/d; females: 0 to 90 mg/d.

Elevated Urine Protein: Proteinuria. *CLINICAL OCCURRENCE:* *Mild Elevations* Pyelonephritis, fever, benign orthostatic proteinuria, idiopathic focal glomerulonephritis. *Severe Proteinuria* Nephrotic syndrome is defined as >3.5 g/d of proteinuria. Glomerulonephritis, diabetes mellitus, SLE, renal vein thrombosis, amyloidosis, and other causes of nephrotic syndrome.

GLUCOSE Glucose is normally filtered in the glomerulus and completely reabsorbed, mostly in the proximal tubule. Glucose in randomly collected fresh urine specimens is normally undetectable. When the serum glucose rises above 200 mg/dL, the filtered load will exceed the capacity for tubular reabsorption and glucose will appear in the urine. Dipsticks, impregnated with glucose oxidase and an indicator color, provide a convenient, rapid and semiquantitative estimate for the patient and physician.

Normal Glucose Excretion: 3 to 25 mg/dL; 50 to 300 mg/d.

Increased Urine Glucose: Glucosuria. *CLINICAL OCCURRENCE:* Hyperglycemia in diabetes mellitus; infrequently with renal abnormalities, including acute tubular damage, hereditary renal glycosuria, and proximal tubular dysfunction as in the Fanconi syndrome.

KETONES Ketones are the products of fatty acid metabolism. Increased ketones in the urine indicate that cellular metabolism is dependent upon fatty acids rather than glucose for energy. Progressively diminished glucose utilization in uncontrolled diabetes mellitus leads to lipolysis with increasing plasma and urinary concentrations of acetoacetic acid, β-hydroxybutyric acid, and ketones.

Increased Urinary Ketones: Ketonuria. *CLINICAL OCCURRENCE:* Diabetic acidosis, fasting, starvation, alcoholic ketoacidosis, isopropyl alcohol intoxication (the clue is an obtunded patient with normal glucose and acid-base status, urine tests positive for ketones and an osmolar gap).

URINARY SEDIMENT Normally, erythrocytes, leukocytes, hyaline casts, and crystals (urate, phosphate, oxalate) are found in the sediment of a fresh specimen collected after a night's fast.

Procedure For Examining the Urinary Sediment. Centrifuge, 10 mL of urine in a conical tube for 5 minutes, decant the supernatant, flick the tube to disperse formed elements in the remaining drop, and place it on a slide under a cover slip to be examined with the high-power field (hpf) objective of a microscope. Abnormal numbers of cells and casts or any bacteria reveal the presence of disease.

Erythrocytes: Hematuria. *Normal: 0 to 5 RBCs/hpf.* *CLINICAL OCCURRENCE:* Microscopic hematuria may occur with fever and exercise and many lesions of the urinary tract from the glomerulus to the urethral meatus [Cohen RA, Brown RS. Microscopic Hematuria. *NEJM.* 2003;348:2330–2338]. Causes of gross hematuria include coagulation defects, renal papillary necrosis, renal infarction, sickle cell disease, glomerulonephritis, Goodpasture syndrome, stone or carcinoma of the kidney, hemorrhagic cystitis, stone or carcinoma of the bladder, and prostatitis.

Leukocytes: Pyuria. *Normal: 0 to 10 WBCs/hpf. CLINICAL OCCURRENCE:* In addition to neutrophils excreted into the urine from the same anatomic sites as erythrocytes, leukocytes from vaginal exudates frequently contaminate routine specimens collected from women. When pyuria exceeding 10 WBCs/hpf is present in an uncontaminated specimen, a site of infection or inflammation in the urinary tract or kidney should be sought.

Casts. Occasional *hyalin casts,* arising from the normal renal tubular secretion of mucoproteins, are seen in fresh concentrated specimens. Finding many broad, fine, or coarse *granular casts* (composed of serum proteins like albumin, IgG, transferrin, haptoglobin) in urine containing excessive protein indicates renal parenchymal disease. *Red cell casts* generally indicate glomerular disease with RBCs passing the damaged glomeruli in large quantities. The urine of patients with the nephrotic syndrome, who exhibit glomerular proteinuria and hyperlipoproteinuria, contains *fatty casts,* casts with *doubly refractile fat bodies,* and *Maltese crosses* when examined in polarized light. *Red cell casts,* containing 10 to 50 distinct erythrocytes and doubly refractile fat bodies, indicate glomerular disease (glomerulonephritis). *White cell and/or renal tubular epithelial cell casts* are found in the urinary sediment of patients with pyelonephritis, polyarteritis, exudative glomerulonephritis, and renal infarction. *Bacteria* accompanying white cell casts indicate urinary tract infection. Broad orange or brown *hematin* casts occur in acute tubular injury and chronic renal failure.

Cerebrospinal Fluid

The brain and spinal cord are surrounded by, and suspended in, a clear, colorless fluid. Patients with acute CNS symptoms often require testing of the fluid. Below are the most commonly ordered tests, their reference ranges, and the more frequent causes of abnormality.

PROTEIN Normal CSF Protein: 20 to 50 mg/dL (SI Units: 0.5–2.0 g/L).

Increased CSF Protein. Traumatic tap, infection, hemorrhage, metabolic and demyelinating disorders.

Decreased CSF Protein. Young children, CSF leakage, water intoxication, CSF removal, hyperthyroidism.

GLUCOSE Normal CSF Glucose: 40 to 70 mg/dL (SI Units: 2.2–3/9 mmol/L).

Elevated CSF Glucose. Hyperglycemia.

Decreased CSF Glucose. Hypoglycemia, infection (especially bacterial or mycobacterial), meningeal malignancy.

CELL COUNT AND DIFFERENTIAL   Normal CSF Cell Count: Adult, 0 to 5 mononuclear cells per microliter; neonates, 0 to 30 mononuclear cells per microliter.

Increased CSF Leukocytes. *Mononuclear cells* increase in CNS infection (viral and early bacterial meningitis, meningoencephalitis, or abscess), neurologic disorders, and hematologic malignancies. *Neutrophils* increase in bacterial infection, hemorrhage, and meningeal malignancy. *Eosinophils* increase in shunt, parasitic infection, and allergic reactions.

Serous Body Fluids

Normally, a very small amount of fluid resides in the pleural, pericardial and peritoneal spaces. Any clinically detectable accumulation of fluid (effusion or ascites) in the cavity is caused by a pathologic condition. Effusions should be examined microscopically to determine the distribution of cells (differential count) and to detect malignant cells (cytology). Cell counts are useful in peritoneal fluid, but are less helpful in pleural fluid. Increased inflammatory cells have indications similar to those in other locations: *Neutrophils* (infection, neoplasm, leukemia); *lymphocytes* (infection, infarction, lymphoma, leukemia, neoplasm, rheumatologic serositis); *eosinophils* (air in cavity, infection, infarction, neoplasm, rheumatologic disease, CHF). Microbiologic examination, stains, and culture are indicated in exudates; cytologic examination will identify abnormal/malignant cells. Effusions are generally classified as *transudate* (low protein) or *exudate* (high protein).

Transudates. Transudates, commonly bilateral in the pleural cavities, are secondary to heart failure or medical conditions that cause a low serum albumin, for example, cirrhosis or nephrotic syndrome. Clear and pale, straw-colored fluids are usually transudates, and additional information is rarely provided by testing beyond that required to confirm that the fluid is a transudate. The few cells found in transudates are mesothelial cells and mononuclear cells (lymphocytes and monocytes) with very few neutrophils.

Exudates. Exudates are more frequently unilateral in the pleural cavities and secondary to localized disorders such as infection or neoplasm. Exudates can be cloudy from increased cellularity (leukocytes), red or pink from hemorrhage or trauma, green white from purulence, or milky from increased lipid.

PLEURAL EFFUSION   See page 352. Tests frequently useful in pleural effusions include gross appearance, fluid/serum protein ratios (<0.5 = transudate; >0.5 = exudate), fluid/serum LDH ratios (<0.6 = transudate; >0.6 = exudate), fluid/serum cholesterol ratio (<0.3 = transudate; >0.3 = exudate), morphologic exam (hematology and cytology), and pH (<7.20 with WBC count $>1000/mm^3$ and low glucose suggests empyema). Note: If the protein and LDH ratios are equivocal, the cholesterol ratios may help identify transudate/exudate. Transudates rarely benefit from further testing. Cell counts are rarely useful.

PERITONEAL EFFUSION: ASCITES   See page 473. Tests frequently useful in peritoneal effusion include gross appearance, serum/ascites albumin concentration gradient, cell count and differential, cytology and cultures for bacteria and mycobacteria.

Serum/Ascites Albumin Gradient. Subtracting peritoneal albumin from simultaneously determined serum albumin determines the *serum/ascites albumin gradient.* Values <1.1 indicate an exudate (bacterial peritonitis, neoplasm, nephrotic syndrome, pancreatitis, vasculitis); values >1.1 indicate a transudate (portal hypertension caused by cirrhosis, hepatic vein thrombosis, portal vein thrombosis, CHF). *Note: Protein and LDH ratios described above for pleural fluid are not reliable in peritoneal fluid to separate transudates from exudates.*

WBC Counts. Detection of spontaneous bacterial peritonitis in patients with transudative ascites is important. Neutrophil counts of >250/mm^3 indicate infection and the need for treatment and long-term prophylaxis. High leukocyte counts (>500/mm^3), mostly mononuclear cells, are also seen in malignancy.

ADDITIONAL READING

1. Fletcher RH, Fletcher SW, Wagner EH. *Clinical Epidemiology.* 3rd ed. Baltimore, MD: Williams & Wilkins; 1996.

2. Young DS, Huth EJ. *SI Units for Clinical Measurement.* Philadelphia, PA: American College of Physicians; 1998.

3. Black ER, Bordley DR, Tape TG, Panzer RJ, eds. *Diagnostic Strategies for Common Medical Problems.* 2nd ed. Philadelphia, PA: American College of Physicians; 1999.

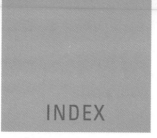

INDEX

Note: Page numbers followed by f indicate figures; those followed by t indicate tables.

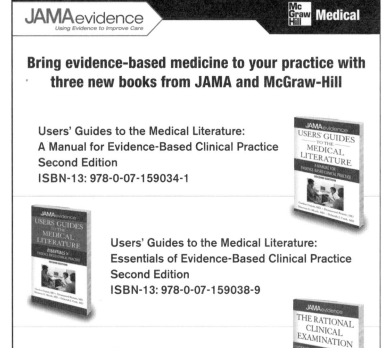

are present, they are swollen and stippled with prominent follicles. Tender, swollen cervical lymph nodes are common. This picture may be caused by *Staphylococcus*, but Group A *Streptococcus* is much more common. *Scarlet fever* presents as an extremely painful throat with few follicles but brilliant red mucosa in the oropharynx, which extends forward to end abruptly near the back of the soft palate and fauces as if red paint had been applied. This is streptococcal until proved otherwise [Ebell MH, Simth MA, Barry HC, et al. The rational clinical examination. Does this patient have strep throat? *JAMA*. 2000;284:2912–2918]. **DDX:** Hoarseness and cough are decidedly uncommon with bacterial pharyngitis; either argues strongly against empiric antibiotic therapy.

➤**Acute Epiglottitis.** Bacterial infection of the epiglottis produces severe edema which can compromise the airway leading to asphyxiation. The condition is both more common and more dangerous in children. Patients present with sore throat and painful swallowing, decreased voice and signs of pharyngitis. Stridor and the need to sit erect to breathe indicate impending airway compromise [Frantz TD, Rasgon BM, Quesenberry CP Jr. Acute epiglottitis in adults: Analysis of 129 cases. *JAMA*. 1994;272:1358–1360].

➤**Pharyngeal Diphtheria.** The fauces first become dull red and a patch of white membrane appears on the tonsil or oropharyngeal mucosa which is reddened, swollen, and edematous. The membrane becomes thick, gray or yellow and tenaciously adheres to the mucosa; when removed the mucosa bleeds. The membrane spreads rapidly to other structures including the larynx. The cervical lymph nodes are enlarged and tender, and the patient appears quite ill, with severe constitutional symptoms. A membrane in the pharynx requires culturing on media appropriate for the diphtheria bacillus. **DDX:** The throat is not nearly as sore as in streptococcal pharyngitis. A membrane limited to a tonsil must be distinguished from *Vincent angina* (acute necrotizing ulcerative stomatitis). In the latter, the membrane is limited to the tonsil and not tenacious; it is not accompanied by severe constitutional symptoms.

Oropharyngeal Candidiasis (Thrush). Shiny, raised white patches, surrounded by an erythematous rim, appear on the posterior pharynx, buccal mucosa, and tongue. They may be painful. An atrophic erythematous mucosal lesion without white exudate may occur also. Ask, if there is pain on swallowing, because *Candida* esophagitis may accompany pharyngitis, especially in the immunosuppressed or diabetic patient.

Infectious Mononucleosis. An acute acquired infection of lymphocytes with Epstein-Barr virus (EBV) leads to lymphadenopathy and atypical circulating lymphocytes. An identical clinical picture can be caused by acute HIV, CMV, and toxoplasma infections. Sore throat is the most common symptom, accompanied by slight fever, malaise, cough, and headache. The pharynx is red and edematous, often with enlarged tonsils coated with exudate, making distinction from streptococcal infection difficult. The tonsils may reach the midline and impair speech and, rarely, respirations. There may be petechiae on the palate and uvula. The cervical lymph nodes are usually enlarged and tender. Disproportionate cervical lymph node enlargement suggests a generalized disease, so the physician should search for axillary and inguinal lymphadenopathy and splenomegaly. A morbilliform rash, conjunctivitis, splenomegaly and occasionally jaundice with a tender, enlarged liver may be seen.

Larynx Syndromes

➤ **KEY SYNDROME** Acute Laryngeal Obstruction—Aphonia, Choking ("The Cafe Coronary")

This diagnosis calls for instant treatment. Even physicians may fail to recognize and treat laryngeal obstruction in time to save life. Usually during a meal, the victim rises suddenly with a look of panic or anguish, often with hand to throat, unable to speak or breathe. Ask the patient if he can speak. He may rush from the room, with face rapidly changing from pale to blue. This behavior is presumptive evidence of choking (in contrast, myocardial infarction permits speech and breathing), and there are fewer than 5 minutes in which to intervene before death.

The Heimlich Maneuver: With the Victim Standing (Fig. 7–69): Stand behind the victim wrapping your arms around their waist. Grasp your fist with the other hand, placing the thumb side of the fist against the victim's abdomen between the navel and the xiphoid. With a quick upward thrust press your fist deep into the abdomen; repeat several times, if necessary. Heimlich calculated that his maneuver could forcefully expel approximately 940 mL of residual and tidal air at an average pressure of 31 mm Hg, enough to force the bolus out.

KEY SYNDROME Acute Laryngitis

The most common cause of hoarseness, acute viral laryngitis, is often accompanied by an unproductive cough, producing pain or a burning dryness in the throat. Through the mirror, the true cords are reddened, their edges rounded by swelling. Erythema of the other laryngeal membranes is present; edema of the larynx is common.

Croup. An acute narrowing of the upper airway occurs with infection, allergy, foreign body, or neoplasm and is accompanied by a hoarse, brassy cough and dyspnea. Children are usually affected. Parainfluenza virus infection causing acute laryngotracheobronchitis is the most frequent cause in children. *Inflammatory croup* is actually acute laryngitis. The cords may appear normal and edema may be greatest in the sub-epiglottic region. An attack produces a danger of asphyxia. In *spasmodic croup*, the child is awakened with a barking cough, dyspnea, and stridor. Cyanosis from air hunger is frequent. Recovery is sudden and complete. Viewed in the mirror, the larynx looks normal. The cause of the condition is unknown.

KEY SYNDROME Chronic Laryngitis

Hoarseness and unproductive cough are usually present. Pain is negligible. The true cords may appear dull and thickened or edematous and polypoid. Frequently, the false cords are similarly affected. *CLINICAL OCCURRENCE:* Chronic overuse of the cords; tobacco smoking; syphilis; tuberculosis of the cords complicating cavitary pulmonary tuberculosis.

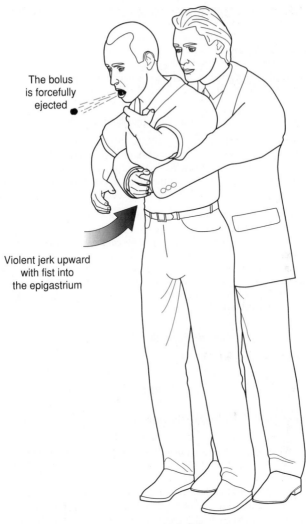

The bolus
is forcefully
ejected

Violent jerk upward
with fist into
the epigastrium

Heimlich maneuver

Fig. 7–69 *Heimlich Maneuver*. *This is used to dislodge foreign bodies from the larynx. Standing at the subject's back, encircle the subject's waist with your arms. Grasp your fist with the other hand and give it a sudden forceful jerk that thrusts the fist upward into the subject's epigastrium. Repeat until the obstructing bolus is forcefully expelled from the throat.*

Hysterical Aphonia: The organic causes of aphonia are readily diagnosed by inspection of the larynx. Even before laryngeal examination, hysterical aphonia may be distinguished by demonstrating that the patient can make a sharp normal cough. When viewed through the mirror, the cords are morphologically normal.

> ### KEY SYNDROME   Laryngeal Dyspnea

Shortness of breath has many causes (Chapter 8, page 335). In laryngeal disease, the occurrence of dyspnea is a mark of an advanced degree of obstruction, lesser degrees having been heralded by hoarseness and stridor. In laryngeal dyspnea, the harder the attempt to inhale, the greater the obstruction becomes. Exhalation is unopposed, so quiet breathing is more efficient.

> ### KEY SYNDROME   Paradoxical Vocal Cord Motion

During attempted inspiration the vocal cords paradoxically close narrowing the airway to produce wheezing. Patients often present with episodic wheezing and shortness of breath unresponsive to treatment appropriate for asthma. On auscultation, the wheeze is loudest over the larynx, not the lungs. Diagnosis requires direct visualization of the cords during an episode.

Dysphonia plicae ventricularis.   Intermittent or chronic hoarseness occurs when the false vocal cords close over the true cords instead of remaining passive during phonation. A single examination of the cords may disclose no abnormality; with repeated examinations, one eventually coincides with an the false cords closing partially or completely over the true cords. When this occurs, the voice breaks, as in a boy whose "voice is changing." The false cords may also be active when the true cords are separated by tumor, cricoarytenoid arthritis, voice abuse, or emotional instability.

> ### KEY SIGN   Disorders of Speech

See Chapter 14, page 760.

Salivary Gland Syndromes

> ### KEY SIGN   Dry Mouth—Xerostomia

Generalized abnormalities of salivary gland function result in inadequate wetting of the mucosa. The patient complains of a dry mouth and difficulty swallowing dry foods such as crackers. The patient often consumes large amounts of liquid in an attempt to keep the mouth wet. In addition to the dry mucosa, extensive caries are frequently seen, often leading to loss of all the teeth. The common causes are anticholinergic drugs, head and neck irradiation, and immune destruction of the salivary glands in Sjögren syndrome (page 282). Ask about dry eyes, xerophthalmia, which accompanies the latter.

> ### KEY SIGN   Parotid Tumors

Parotid neoplasia may be either benign or malignant.   *Pleomorphic Adenoma (Mixed Parotid Tumor*   presents as a firm, painless, nontender nodule, slightly above and in front of the mandibular angle. Less commonly, the site is just anterior to the tragus. It may remain benign for years, growing very slowly. Rarely, it suddenly becomes malignant, with rapid growth and metastases. The second most common benign neoplasm is the   *Warthin Tumor (Papillary Cystadenoma Lymphomatosum),*   which most commonly occurs in the tail of the parotid in older men and is bilateral more often than any other salivary gland tumor. Malignancy is suggested by pain and tenderness, rapid tumor growth, paralysis of a branch of the facial nerve, and fixation to the skin or underlying tissues. Biopsy is necessary because the biological behavior of the several tumor types requires different techniques for management.

KEY SYNDROME   Salivary Calculus—Sialolithiasis

Calcium phosphate stones frequently form in the salivary ducts. The cause is unknown. The stone is in the submandibular gland or duct in approximately 85% of patients with salivary calculi. The symptoms are pathognomonic: submandibular swelling, with or without pain, occurs suddenly while the patient is eating and subsides within 2 hours. The sequence may be invariable for several years. Occasionally, the gland becomes infected or the duct obstructed. In parotid duct stone, glandular swelling may persist for several days after onset. In all three glands, calculi are commonly identified by palpation. Approximately 80% of the calculi are calcified, so they can be seen by radiography without contrast. Intraoral dental radiographs are excellent for demonstrating the calculi because they can minimize the density of the mandible by positioning the film properly. A noncalcified impalpable stone must be detected by sialography.

Diseases of the Submaxillary and Sublingual Glands: These glands are subject to the same diseases as the parotid, with slight variations. Rarely, mumps involves the submandibular gland and not the parotid; it is more common to have the both involved. Ranula involving the sublingual or submaxillary gland is described on page 269.

Thyroid Goiters and Nodules

KEY SIGN   Hypothyroidism

See Chapter 5, page 109.

KEY SIGN   Hyperthyroidism

See Chapter 5, page 110.

KEY SYNDROME   Goiter

Enlargement of the thyroid gland is caused by hyperplasia of thyroid tissue, infiltration with foreign substances (e.g., amyloid), infection, or neoplastic growth (primary thyroid cancers, lymphoma, or metastatic disease). The patient may complain of fullness or a mass in the neck, but they are often unaware of the problem. The goiter may be evident as a bilobed fullness in the neck above the suprasternal notch that moves superiorly with swallowing; tangential light helps bring it out. Determine the size of each lobe and isthmus, its extent within the neck or retrosternal space, consistency (smooth, a single nodule, multinodular), fixation to surrounding structures, tenderness, and the presence or absence of regional lymph node enlargement, including Delphian nodes. Also assess the state of thyroid function: hypothyroid, euthyroid, or hyperthyroid (see page 110). Clinical classification of goiters is based upon whether the goiter is diffuse or nodular and the thyroid function: is it focal or diffuse, nodular or nonnodular, toxic (hyperthyroid) or nontoxic (euthyroid or hypothyroid) [Siminoski K. The rational clinical examination. Does this patient have a goiter? *JAMA.* 1995;273:813–817].

Diffuse Nontoxic Goiter. TSH stimulation of thyroid tissue leads to diffuse hyperplasia, while defects in thyroid hormone synthesis limit effective hormone production. All parts of the gland are smooth, enlarged, and firm. The surface may be slightly irregular (*bosselated*); but circumscribed nodules are absent. This is frequently termed *colloid goiter*, or *endemic goiter*, although the terms are not always applicable, because sporadic cases occur in nongoitrous regions. The gland is often more than twice normal size. This size goiter may result from any cause of smaller diffuse glands, except that physiologic hyperplasia rarely becomes so large. **CLINICAL OCCURRENCE:** **Physiologic Euthyroid Hyperplasia** before menstrual periods, females from puberty to 20 years of age, pregnancy; **Hypothyroid** iodine deficiency, antithyroid drugs, thiocyanates, paraaminosalicylic acid, phenylbutazone, lithium, amiodarone; rarely, iodides; inherited defects of thyroid enzymes; chronic thyroiditis.

Nontoxic Multinodular Goiter. The nodules are polyclonal proliferations, with less-efficient production of thyroid hormone than normal thyroid tissue. This is usually found in persons older than 30 years of age, most often women. The gland may be small or large. The significant feature is the presence of two or more distinct nodules in the parenchyma. The nodules may vary in consistency in the same goiter. Thyroid hormone secretion may be low or normal.

Diffuse Toxic Goiter—Graves' Disease. See page 110. The thyroid is smooth, diffusely enlarged and a bruit may be heard. The ophthalmopathy may occur independently of a goiter or any abnormality of thyroid function.

Toxic Multinodular Goiter. Autonomous function of one or more nodules produces elevated hormone levels. This often arises from a long-standing nontoxic multinodular gland. The onset is usually gradual with signs of hyperthyroidism (e.g., atrial fibrillation, weight loss, diarrhea) bringing the patient to the physician. The gland is bilaterally enlarged with multiple nodules apparent by palpation or ultrasound.

Retrosternal Goiter. When the lower border of a goiter cannot be palpated in the neck, consider the possibility of retrosternal extension, especially when the neck is short. Rarely, the goiter may be entirely retrosternal and rise only with increased intrathoracic pressure, as with Valsalva; this is called a *plunging goiter*. An increase in retromanubrial dullness seldom occurs. Compression of the trachea may be inferred from the history of dyspnea, or from the Kocher sign, in which pressure on the lateral lobe produces stridor. The trachea may be displaced laterally (Fig. 7–65, page 279).

A goiter in the superior thoracic aperture may compress other structures, causing (1) cough (2) dilated veins over the upper thorax from pressure on the internal jugular vein (Fig. 7–70) and, rarely, edema of the face; (2) dyspnea from a airway compression during sleep; (4) dyspnea when the head is tilted to the side or the arms are held up beside the head; and (5) hoarseness, from pressure on the recurrent laryngeal nerve. **Pemberton Sign.** Have the patient sit holding her arms up beside her head, for a few minutes. Facial venous suffusion and cyanosis with dyspnea imply an obstructed thoracic inlet [Wallace C, Siminoski K. The Pemberton sign. *Ann Intern Med.* 1996;125:568–569; Auwaerter PG. The Pemberton and Maroni signs. *Ann Intern Med.* 1997;126:916]. **DDX:** The internal jugular vein is rarely impaired,

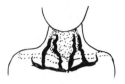

Venous engorgement
by retrosternal goiter

Fig. 7–70 *Venous Engorgement:* *compression of the external jugular vein by a retrosternal goiter produces engorgement of the superficial branches in the skin of the neck and clavicular regions.*

so the cyanosis of the face and edema of the neck associated with superior vena caval obstruction are not present. For unknown reasons, retrosternal goiter is associated with a high incidence of hyperthyroidism.

KEY SYNDROME   Solitary Thyroid Nodule

A solitary nodule may be a benign or malignant neoplasm, a cyst, or a dominant nodule in a multinodular gland. Many nodules thought to be solitary by palpation are found to be part of a multinodular process by ultrasound. Fine-needle aspiration of solitary nodules is the diagnostic procedure of choice. Irradiation of the thyroid in childhood increases the risk for carcinoma. Finding an isolated nodule in an atrophic thyroid gland suggests a Plummer nodule or toxic adenoma [Singer PA, Cooper DS, Daniels GH, et al. Treatment guidelines for patients with thyroid nodules and well-differentiated tyroid cancer. American Thyroid Association. *Arch Intern Med.* 1996;156:2165–2172; Mazzaferri EL. Management of a solitary thyroid nodule. *N Engl J Med.* 1993;328:553–559].

Toxic Adenoma. This benign tumor results when thyroid-stimulating hormone receptors are constitutively activated, with the resultant overproduction of thyroid hormone. The patient has symptoms and signs of hyperthyroidism, and examination shows a single nodule in an otherwise atrophic gland.

KEY DISEASE   Epithelial Carcinoma

Malignant thyroid cancers are classified as papillary, follicular, and anaplastic. Thyroid cancer is more common in women and in those exposed to radiation. It presents as a painless nodule in most cases. Anaplastic cancer spreads widely and rapidly, whereas papillary and follicular cancers spread regionally before widely metastasizing.

KEY DISEASE   Medullary Carcinoma

Neoplasia of the thyroid C cells, which produce calcitonin, is either sporadic or inherited alone or with multiple endocrine neoplasia syndromes (MEN) 2A or 2B. This should be sought in all patients with a family history of MEN-2A or MEN-2B or those with a family history of medullary carcinoma.

> **KEY SYNDROME** Thyroiditis

Inflammation, usually autoimmune, is common in the thyroid gland, especially in women after beginning childbearing. The inflammatory response may be antibody or cell mediated and damage to the thyroid may be by antibody- or cellular-cytotoxicity or via induction of apoptosis. Disrupted follicles release preformed thyroid hormones directly into the circulation resulting in clinical hyperthyroidism with suppression of TSH and iodine uptake. Several distinct syndromes are identified by their clinical pictures. Graves' disease, though not usually thought of as thyroiditis, is an immune mediated disease often leading to thyroid failure. In addition to autoimmunity, viral and bacterial infections may occur. **DDX:** The elevated T4 and T3, low TSH and low iodine uptake distinguish thyroiditis from Graves' disease, toxic adenomas and toxic multinodular goiter. Ingestion of exogenous thyroid hormone is distinguished by history and the finding of a diffuse, smooth goiter [Pearce EN, Farwell AP, Braverman LE. Thyroiditis. *N Engl J Med.* 2003;348:2646–2655].

Subacute Thyroiditis—De Quervain Thyroiditis, Viral Thyroiditis: Acute painful inflammation of the thyroid is caused by viral infection or postinfectious inflammation. Anterior neck pain is the presenting symptom, often aggravated by swallowing. The pain is frequently referred to the ear, so the physician may be consulted for earache. The gland is unusually firm and rather small (20–30 g), but it frequently contains one or more, often tender, nodules. The patient may be euthyroid or hyperthyroid in the acute phase.

Hashimoto Thyroiditis: Chronic lymphocytic infiltration of the gland leads to loss of functioning tissue and fibrosis. This is the most common cause of acquired hypothyroidism. It is more common in women and the prevalence increases with age. The gland may be diffusely enlarged, but is often normal in size or small. It is uniformly firm and nontender. The symptoms are related to hypothyroidism; neck symptoms are rare. Rarely encephalitis occurs in association, Hashimoto's encephalitis, which is not related to the state of thyroid function and responds to corticosteroids. Most patients become hypothyroid with time. **DDX:** Other autoimmune diseases are more common in patients with Hashimoto thyroiditis including type-1 diabetes, Addison disease, vitiligo, rheumatoid arthritis and systemic lupus.

Postpartum Thyroiditis: Inflammation of the thyroid in association with antibodies to thyroperoxidase occurs following delivery. Symptoms begin 2 to 6 months after delivery; hyperthyroidism is most common, often followed by a period of hypothyroidism. The condition is more common in patients with some thyroid autoimmunity before pregnancy. It is self limited, only requiring symptomatic therapy; it frequently recurs with subsequent pregnancies. **DDX:** Although a goiter may be present, the thyroid is nontender and may not appear a likely source of the problems. Mild symptoms of both hyper- and hypothyroidism are often misattributed to postpartum psychosocial stresses including inadequate sleep, mood changes and family stress.

Reidel Thyroiditis. The thyroid gland is densely fibrotic with fibrosis extending into the surrounding tissues; the cause is unknown. Patients may present with compressive symptoms of the esophagus, trachea, neck veins, or recurrent laryngeal nerves. Women in midlife are most often affected; thyroid function is usually preserved. The gland is hard and fixed.

Acute Suppurative Thyroiditis: Infection of the thyroid gland by bacteria or fungi often extends from branchial cleft remnants. There is acute pain and fever. The gland is slightly enlarged, asymmetric, and fluctuance may be noted.

ADDITIONAL READING

Jonathan D. Trobe. *The Physician's Guide to Eye Care.* 3rd Edition. San Francisco, CA: The American Academy of Ophthalmology; 2006.

The Chest: Chest Wall, Pulmonary, and Cardiovascular Systems; The Breasts

SECTION 1

CHEST WALL, PULMONARY, AND CARDIOVASCULAR SYSTEMS

Major Systems and Physiology

The Thoracic Wall

The skeletal and muscular shell of the thorax encloses the thoracic visceral organs, powers breathing and is the mechanical platform for arm and neck motion. It is bounded anteriorly by the sternum and ribs, laterally and posteriorly by the ribs, and supported posteriorly by the spine. The inferior boundary is the diaphragm and rib margins. Superiorly, it is bounded by the clavicles and soft tissues of the neck. The thoracic wall includes the bodies of the 12 thoracic vertebrae, the 12 pairs of ribs, and the sternum.

Bones of the Thorax

The thorax resembles a truncated cone, each pair of ribs having a greater diameter than that above, so the sternovertebral dimension is much smaller at the top than at the base. The ribs are separated by intercostal spaces, each space taking its numbers from the rib above. The first rib slopes slightly downward from vertebra to sternum; each succeeding rib has a greater slope increasing the width of the intercostal spaces progressively from top to bottom.

The **sternum** (Fig. 8–1) consists of the *manubrium*, the *gladiolus*, and the *xiphoid cartilage*. There is a fibrocartilage (rarely synovial) joint between the manubrium and gladiolus; mobility is slight. The xiphoid cartilage is either lance-shaped or bifid and may be mistaken for an abdominal mass when angulated forward; it usually calcifies in later life.

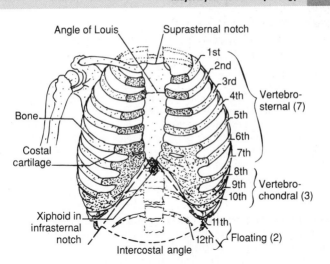

Fig. 8–1 *The Bony Thorax.* The left clavicle is removed exposing the underlying first rib. The cartilages of the xiphoid and ribs are stippled. Note the surface landmarks: the suprasternal notch, the angle of Louis, and the infrasternal notch. The two lower rib margins form the intercostal angle.

Each **rib** is a flattened arch. Each *typical rib* has two connections with the vertebral column: the head is bound to two adjacent vertebrae and their intervertebral disk at a gliding synovial joint; a second synovial joint on the articular tubercle of the rib's neck articulates with the transverse process of the upper vertebra. The sternal rib ends continue as costal cartilages. The first to seventh ribs are *true ribs* since their costal cartilages join the sternum. The costal cartilage of the first rib connects to the manubrium at a fibrous joint. The other six true ribs attach to the sternum by synovial joints. The second rib attaches to both the manubrium and gladiolus at their fibrocartilage with two synovial joints. The first, tenth, eleventh, and twelfth ribs are *atypical*, each articulating with a single vertebra. The eighth to twelfth ribs are *false ribs*. The eight, ninth, and tenth ribs are *vertebrochondral*, each costal cartilage usually joining the cartilage of the rib above; many variations are found. The eleventh and twelfth ribs are vertebral or floating ribs.

Muscles of the Thoracic Wall

The intercostal spaces contain the *intercostales externi and interni*. Each is a muscle sheet between adjacent edges of two ribs that draws the bones together. When the first rib is fixed by contraction of the scaleni, the externi and interni pull the ribs upward aided by the levatores costarum and the serratus posterior superior. When the last rib is fixed by contraction of the quadratus lumborum, the subcostales and the transversus thoracis draw the ribs downward.

The Respiratory System

The thoracic respiratory system is composed of the trachea entering superiorly, the lungs with their branching airways, arterial, venous and lymphatic vascular channels, and the *pleura*, which lines both the lung (*visceral pleura*) and the chest wall and mediastinum (*parietal pleura*).

Respiratory Excursions of the Thorax

At end expiration thoracic volume is at its normal minimum; inspiration increases the thoracic dimensions anteroposteriorly, transversely, and vertically, expanding lung volume. It is important to remember that volume varies as the third power of changes in linear dimension. Therefore, relatively small changes in the height, width, and depth of the thoracic cavity lead to large changes in its volume. Expiration is largely passive relying on the elastic recoil of the lung and chest wall; forced expiration by contraction of abdominal and chest wall muscles greatly accelerates airflow.

Increasing the anterior-posterior diameter of the thorax. The chest is like a cylindrical pail with its wire handle bowed in a semicircle of slightly greater diameter than the cylinder (Figure 8–2A). When the handle hangs obliquely, the distance from its center to the cylindric axis is the radius of the pail. Raising the handle toward the horizontal moves it away from the side of the pail. In the model in Figure 8–2B, a straight piece of wood represents the thoracic spine, a vertical stick is the sternum in the position of expiration (*dotted*) and the dotted hoop is a pair of ribs. When the sternum and first rib are pulled upward, the costal ring rotates pushing the sternum forward and upward. This is what occurs when the sternum and first rib are fixed by the scaleni while contraction of the external and internal intercostal muscles narrows the interspaces. The ribs are pulled upward and the sternum moves forward, increasing the anteroposterior dimension of the thoracic cavity.

Increasing the transverse diameter of the thorax. In a similar model (Figure 8–2C) the sternum and the first rib are fixed. Each rib of a pair is a separate semicircle rotating on an anteroposterior axis. During expiration, the planes of the hoops slant downward on either side of the axis. When the hoops are pulled upward toward the horizontal, each hoop acts as a pail handle by moving further from the center, increasing the transverse dimension. Anatomically, the narrowing of the interspaces by the intercostal muscles causes elevation of the rib curves increasing the transverse diameter of the thorax.

Thus, fixation of the first rib and manubrium and narrowing the interspaces causes rotation of each rib, except the first, on both an anteroposterior and a transverse axis, expanding the corresponding dimensions of the thoracic cavity. Because the lower ribs are longer and more oblique, and the interspaces wider, movement is greater in the lower thorax.

Increasing the vertical dimension of the thorax. The diaphragm is an elliptic muscular sheet with a fibrous aponeurosis at its center. Its edges are fixed to the lower ribs while the center domes into the thorax. At end expiration, the dome is high and the thoracic walls are closest together (Fig. 8–2D). During inspiration, the walls diverge and the muscular diaphragm contracts, both actions lowering the diaphragmatic dome and elongating the vertical dimension of the thoracic cavity and increasing its volume.

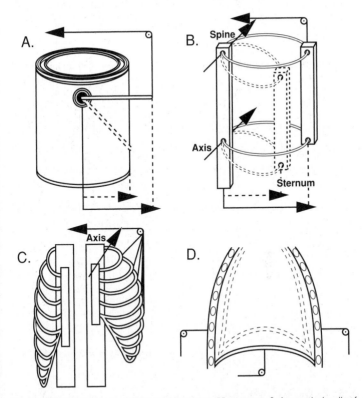

Fig. 8–2 *Models Illustrating Thoracic Respiratory Movements. **A***. At rest, the handle of a cylindric paint can hangs obliquely, so its center and the side of the pail are equidistant from the central axis of the cylinder. When the handle is raised to the horizontal, the center of the handle diverges from the side increasing the distance from the central axis. ***B***. In this model, two parallel rigid hoops pierce two vertical sticks. Elevation of the front stick (representing the sternum) will increase the distance between it and the other stick (representing the spine). The differences in the points of the arrows show this change in the anteroposterior diameter. ***C***. The semicircular ribs hang from the sternum and the spine, like the hoops in B and the bucket handle in A. The ribs move in such a way that elevation of the sternum and the lateral bows of the ribs during inspiration increases both the transverse (as in A) and the anteroposterior (as in B) diameters of the thorax. ***D***. Inspiratory volume further augmented by depression of the diaphragm.

The Lungs and Pleura

The airways include the nasal passages and nasopharynx, the mouth and oropharynx, the larynx, the trachea, and the branches of the bronchial tree supplying the pulmonary alveoli. The larynx is a frequent site of obstruction, either from intrinsic swelling or by paralysis of its vocal cords.

The Bronchial Tree

The trachea bifurcates asymmetrically into the *right and left mainstem bronchus* at the carina. The left bronchus diverges at a greater angle from the trachea than the right bronchus, explaining why foreign bodies are more likely to lodge in the right main stem bronchus. The right bronchus sends a *lobar bronchus* to each of three *pulmonary lobes*; the left bronchus forms two lobar bronchi. Each first branch of a lobar bronchus supplies a *bronchopulmonary lung segment*. The heart lies in front of the tracheal bifurcation and the aorta arches over the left bronchus from front to back. Interposed between the aorta and bronchus is the *left recurrent laryngeal nerve*, which descends in front of the aortic arch, loops under it, and ascends beside the trachea to the neck. The dilated aorta may produce a tracheal tug by pulsating against the left bronchus, or it may compress the left recurrent laryngeal nerve against the left bronchus, with resulting paralysis of the left vocal cord.

The Lungs

The lungs may be regarded as clusters of pulmonary alveoli around the subdivisions of the bronchial tree. The right lung has three lobes: the upper, middle, and lower lobes. The left lung has an upper and lower lobe. The lobes are separated by an infolding of visceral pleura; the *lobar fissures*. The shape of the lungs is molded by the rib cage; the medial edge of the left lung has an inferior-anterior indentation, the *cardiac notch*. Each lobe is divided into bronchopulmonary segments consisting of the cluster of alveoli supplied by a single first branch of the lobar bronchus (Figs. 8–3 and 8–4). Segments are not demarcated by fissures. However, if present, extra fissures do follow these boundaries. The lingula of the left upper lobe is homologous with the right middle lobe.

The Pleura

The relation of each lung to its pleura can be visualized by imagining a sphere of thin plastic material from which the air is being evacuated (Fig. 8–5). As the sphere collapses, one part invaginates to form a hollow hemisphere with convex and concave layers in apposition. The convex layer, representing the *parietal pleura*, is cemented to the inside of the thoracic cavity. The lung fills the

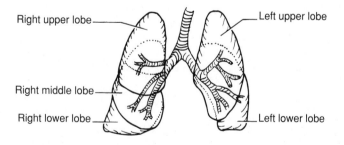

Fig. 8–3 *The Lobes of the Lungs.* The transparent diagram shows the anterior aspects of the pulmonary lobes and their main bronchi. Note the three divisions of the right main bronchus and the more direct line with the trachea on the right side. The dotted line shows the posterior extent of the lower lobes.

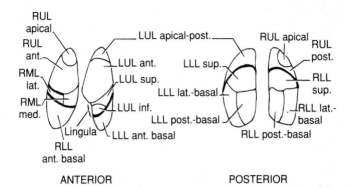

ANTERIOR   POSTERIOR

Fig. 8–4 Lung Segments. Each lobe is divided into segments. The thick lines are the anatomical fissures, readily identified on inspection of the lung and often in radiographs. The thinner lines are established only by careful dissections of injected preparations. In the abbreviations the first capital letter designates right or left; the second, upper, middle, or lower the third L is for lobe. Note that the lingula, composed of the superior and inferior segments of the left upper lobe, is near the heart and corresponds in many respects to the right middle lobe.

concavity, which represents the *visceral pleura*. The parietal pleura is adherent to the thoracic wall; the visceral pleura is fixed to the lung surface and also lines the interlobar fissures. The two apposing layers form the *pleural cavity*, devoid of air and containing only enough fluid for lubrication. The parietal pleura have the greater area, extending inferiorly on the ribs and diaphragm some distance below the lower tip of the lung to form the costophrenic sinus. This permits the lungs to move within the thoracic cavity, each descending part way into this sinus during deep inspiration. Between the two layers of pleura is a potential space, normally with a negative pressure relative to the atmospheric. This negative

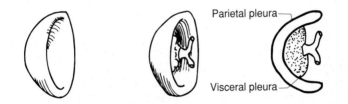

Fig. 8–5 Modelling the Relationship of the Pleura and Lung. Deflate a rubber or plastic sphere so that it assumes a hemisphere with a concave and convex surface. Place a model lung in the concavity and cement the lung surface to the inner surface of the hemisphere. On the right, in cross section, the parietal pleura is represented by the convex surface of the hemisphere; the cemented layers represent the visceral pleura. To complete the model, exhaust the hemisphere of air, replacing it with a little fluid to lubricate the inner surface. This geometry should be visualized in the examination of the chest and when looking at X-ray films, remembering that the pleural surfaces are anterior, lateral, medial, and inferior.

pressure maintains lung distention and transfers the inspiratory forces of diaphragm flattening and chest expansion to the lung. Introduction of air into this space (pneumothorax) destroys mechanical coupling of chest motion to lung expansion. The parietal pleura contains sensory nerve endings, but the visceral pleura is anesthetic. This is significant in performing thoracentesis.

Mechanics of the Lung and Pleura

When a normal lung is removed from the thoracic cavity, it partially collapses from the elastic recoil of its tissue. The volume of the collapsed lung is much smaller than its hemithorax. In the closed thorax, lung volume is much greater because it is held against the thoracic wall by the apposition of the parietal and visceral pleurae. Atmospheric pressure resists any force tending to separate the pleural layers. During expiration, about negative 25 cm of water intrapleural pressure is generated by the elastic recoil of the lung and thorax. During inspiration, the negative pressure increases to approximately 215 cm of water because additional elastic recoil is produced by stretching the lung as the thorax expands.

The Cardiovascular System
The Circulation

The circulatory system includes the heart, the blood and its conducting vessels, the lymph and its ducts, and the vessel walls. Since the heart and much of the aorta are intrathoracic, consideration of the circulatory system starts in the chest. Blood returning from the extremities enters the chest from the abdomen and lower extremities via the *inferior vena cava (IVC)*, and from the arms and head via the axillary and jugular veins, which merge into the *brachiocephalic veins* and *superior vena cava (SVC)* in the mediastinum. The heart is suspended from the great vessels (aorta, pulmonary artery, pulmonary veins, IVC, and SVC) within the pericardium, which allows free motion of the heart during ventricular contraction.

The Cardiac Conduction System

The normal pacemaker of the heart is the *sinoatrial (SA)* node located in the right atrial wall near the entrance of the SVC (Fig. 4–1, page 61). It originates rhythmic waves of excitation that spread quickly through both atria until they reach the *atrioventricular (AV) node* near the posterior margin of the interatrial septum. The AV node delays conduction during atrial systole. The impulse then passes down the *bundle of His*, which divides into *right and left bundle branches* to the muscle of the right and left ventricles via the *Purkinje network*. Conduction is normally very rapid, arriving nearly simultaneously in both atria, and, after AV delay, in both ventricles. Deviations in the timing or pathways taken by these electrical waves cause changes in rate, rhythm and electrical pattern of the P, QRS, and T waves that can be analyzed with considerable accuracy by the electrocardiogram (ECG). Normal cardiac function results when these electrical signals trigger mechanical muscular contraction via the cellular process of *electrical-mechanical coupling.*

Heart Movement and Function

The myocardial muscle fibers form a complete spiral, so contraction produces a decrease in all diameters during systole. The apex rotates forward and to the right, approaching the chest wall and frequently causing a visible and palpable thrust, the *apical impulse*. Occurring early in systole, this thrust is a marker for the onset of cardiac contraction.

The heart has extremely high oxygen and energy requirements and the highest oxygen extraction of any organ in the body. As a result, it is particularly sensitive to decreases in blood supply. Blood flow within the heart and lungs is dependent upon complete functional separation of the cardiac chambers by intact interatrial and interventricular septa and functional valves. Valve closure, turbulent blood flow, and the mechanical contraction of the heart can be felt and auscultated through the chest wall.

Peripheral Arteries

Blood is distributed to the body through the major branches of the aorta, which are easily examined where they leave the chest (carotid and axillary arteries) or abdomen (femoral arteries). Measurement of blood pressure and estimates of the blood flow within the arterial tree are easily performed on physical examination.

Leg Veins

Knowledge of the normal functional anatomy of the leg veins is essential: the *great saphenous vein* begins at the mediodorsal side of the foot continuing upward along the medial edge of the tibia, passing the knee behind the medial femoral condyle. In the thigh, it runs subcutaneously to the femoral canal, emptying into the *femoral vein*. The *small saphenous vein* begins at the lateral side of the foot, curving under and behind the lateral malleolus, continuing upward in the posterior midline and finally diving into the *popliteal vein*. Valved *communicating veins* connect the saphenous veins to the deep calf veins and the great saphenous to the femoral vein. Normal flow is from superficial to deep veins and thence proximally driven by the contraction of skeletal muscle resulting in compression of the veins within the muscle compartments (*the muscle pump*). Antegrade flow is assured by competant venous valves.

Superficial Thoracic Anatomy

The Chest Wall

The subcutaneous anterior surface of the sternum presents landmarks for inspection and palpation. The heads of the clavicles form the sides of the *suprasternal notch*; its base is the superior edge of the manubrium (Figs. 8–1, page 303 and 8–6). The junction of the manubrium and gladiolus, where the second rib articulates, forms the *angle of Louis* (sternal angle), a useful landmark for identifying ribs and interspaces. At the inferior end of the gladiolus a slight depression, the infrasternal notch, is formed by the junction of the 7th rib costal cartilages. The xiphoid cartilage may be felt below this notch.

The bony thorax is a truncated cone narrowing superiorly. This narrowing is partially obscured by the overlying clavicles, the shoulders, and muscles of the upper chest and arms, which give the body its broad shouldered, squared-off contour. The clavicles, sternum, and lower ribs are palpable throughout their extent; portions of most other ribs can be seen or palpated. The first rib is effectually overlaid by the clavicle. The pectoralis major and the female breasts obscure

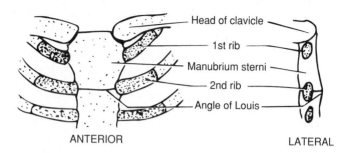

ANTERIOR   LATERAL

Fig. 8–6 *The Angle of Louis. The adjacent edges of the manubrium and gladiolus form the angle of Louis. This is a landmark for counting ribs anteriorly because the second rib abuts the junction that forms the angle. The costicartilage of the second rib articulates with the fibrocartilage between the manubrium and the gladiolus and with the edges of both bones.*

palpation of parts of the ribs anteriorly; the latissimus dorsi covers some ribs in the axillary line. Posteriorly, the scapulae overly the posterior chest wall lateral to the spine covering parts of the second thru seventh ribs. With the arms at the sides, the inferior border of the scapula is usually at the seventh or eighth intercostal space, serving as the usual landmark for counting ribs in the back (Fig. 8–7). The inferior margins of the seventh, eighth, and ninth costicartilages on the two sides meet in the midline to form the *infrasternal angle* (intercostal angle); the angle may be considerably more or less than 90 degrees. An oblique line drawn from the head of the clavicle to the anterior axillary line on the ninth rib approximately locates the *costochondral junctions* of the second to tenth ribs. The lower ribs with large radii, superficial location, and extensive anterior cartilage are vulnerable to injury; the upper ribs are much less susceptible to mechanical injury because of their smaller radius of curvature and overlying muscles.

The *scapula* is overlaid with skeletal muscle and glides on the chest wall. Its medial border, inferior angle, lateral border, *spine, acromion* and *coracoid process* are easily palpable. The lungs extend to the thoracic apex and may extend superiorly into the base of the neck where they are vulnerable to penetrating injury. The pleural spaces coapt in the anterior superior mediastinum, but are separated

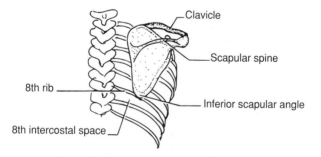

Fig. 8–7 *Surface Landmarks of the Posterior Thorax. Note the relation of the scapulae to the ribs. The inferior angle of the scapula is usually at the eighth interspace; this allows one to identify the eighth rib posteriorly to count ribs in the back.*

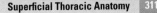

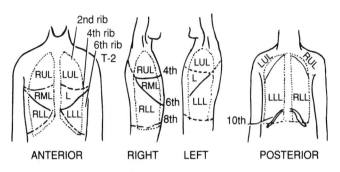

Fig. 8–8 *Topography of the Five Lobes of the Lungs.* The solid lines are the pulmonary fissures; the broken lines are projections. The boundary of the lingula (L) is hypothetical.

posteriorly by the spine and mediastinum and anteriorly and inferiorly by the pericardial sack and heart. The heart lays retrosternally and to the left with the right ventricle in the retrosternal position and the left ventricle left lateral and posterior. The liver and spleen are positioned inferior to the diaphragm deep to the inferior ribs. Deep inspiration with flattening of the diaphragm pushes them toward the costal margins where the normal liver and enlarged spleen can be palpated. The axillary folds are formed by the pectoralis major anteriorly and the subscapularis and latissimus dorsi posteriorly.

The Lungs and Pleura

The topography of the five lung lobes has some clinical applications. In Fig. 8–8, note that the anterior aspect of the right lung is formed almost entirely of the right upper and middle lobes; the posterior aspect contains only the upper and lower lobes. In the left lung, the upper and lower lobes present both back and front.

The Heart and Precordium

The anterior surface of the chest closest to the heart and aorta is termed the *precordium*. Normally, this area extends vertically from the second to the fifth intercostal space, transversely from the right border of the sternum to the left midclavicular line in the fifth and sixth interspaces. The upper epigastrium is occasionally included. When the heart is enlarged or displaced, the boundaries of the precordium shift accordingly. In *dextrocardia*, all signs described herein are located in the opposite hemithorax.

The projections of the normal heart upon the precordium are depicted in Fig. 8–9 and their projections on a chest radiograph are depicted in Fig. 8–10. Behind the manubrium sterni are the arch of the aorta and other mediastinal structures. The right border of the heart corresponds roughly to the right edge of the sternum from the third to fifth interspaces. The right atrium forms the right border with the right ventricle anterior under the sternum and left lower ribs. The left ventricle forms the cardiac apex and a slender area of the left border, and sits posteriorly to the right ventricle. Thus, the right ventricle forms most of the anterior surface of the heart even although it forms neither lateral border.

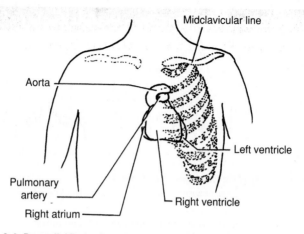

Fig. 8–9 *Precordial Projections of the Anterior Surface of the Heart.* *The entire central area of the precordium is a projection of the right ventricle. The left border and apex are formed by the left ventricle; the right atrium is the right border.*

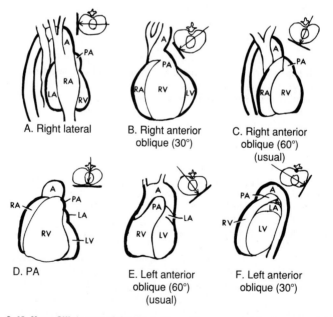

Fig. 8–10 *X-ray Silhouettes of the Heart.* *The positions are named for the aspect of the patient's thorax that faces the cassette (except for the PA view). Angles are measured between the direction of the X-ray beam and the plane of the patient's back. The heavy lines on the silhouettes indicate distinctive segments used in diagnosis.*

Physical Examination of the Chest and Major Vessels

Examination of the Rib Cage and Thoracic Musculature

Inspection

Thoracic wall. Inspect for structural deformities of the thorax and skin lesions that might restrict respiratory excursion. Observe several respiratory cycles noting the respiratory rate, amplitude, rhythm, and movements of the chest. Look for labored inspiration, intercostal retraction, and forced expiration, while noting cough or noisy breathing. Palpate with the palms of the hands to confirm areas of dyskinetic chest wall motion. Inspect the chest wall of the supine patient from the foot of the bed.

Thoracic spine. Have the patient stand or sit; inspect the profile of the spine from the side for kyphosis, lordosis, and gibbus. From the back, look for lateral deviation of the spinous processes indicating scoliosis. To detect scoliosis when the patient is obese, palpate and mark each spinous process. Observe of exaggerated thoracic kyphosis or kyphoscoliosis. The complete spinal examination is described in Chapter 13 on page 599.

Palpation

Trachea. Check the position of the trachea. Place your forefinger in the suprasternal notch and feel the space between the heads of the clavicles and the lateral border of the trachea. Alternatively, direct the finger posteriorly through the middle of the suprasternal notch until the fingertip touches the tracheal rings. If the apex of the rings touches the finger on the center of its tip, the trachea is in the midline.

Thoracic wall. Palpation is indicated if there is chest pain, a mass seen on inspection, breast masses or draining sinuses. Examine the soft tissues including the large muscles of the thorax to elicit tenderness; if tender, try to determine the movements that elicit pain. Feel for soft-tissue crepitus. Palpate the intercostal spaces for tenderness and masses. Examine the costal cartilages and palpate the costochondral junctions. Palpate the ribs for point tenderness, swelling, bone crepitus, and remote pain on compression. Palpate the xiphisternal joint for tenderness.

Testing excursion of the upper thorax. Place a hand on each side of the patient's neck with palms against the upper anterior thoracic wall. Curl the fingers firmly over the superior edges of the trapezii. Move the palms downward against the skin, to provide slack, until the palms lie in the infraclavicular fossae. Then extend your thumbs so their tips meet in the midline (Fig. 8–11A). Have the patient inspire deeply, which permits your palms to move freely with the chest while your fingers are anchored firmly on the trapezii. The upper four ribs move forward with inspiration, so your thumbs diverge from the midline. Normally, the thumbs move laterally for equal distances. Asymmetric excursions suggest a lesion on the lagging side in the chest wall, the pleura, or the upper lobe of the lung.

Testing excursion of the anterior middle thorax. With your fingers high in each axilla and your thumbs abducted, place the palms on the anterior chest. Move the hands medially, dragging skin to provide slack, until the thumb tips meet in the midline at the level of the sixth ribs (Fig. 8–11B). Have the patient inspire deeply

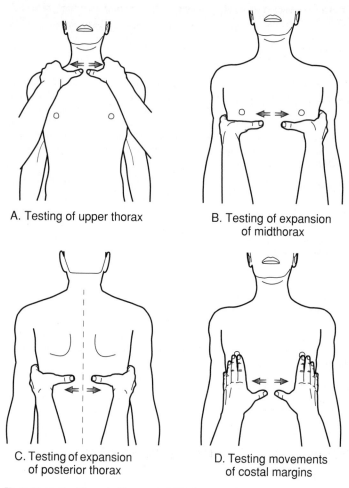

A. Testing of upper thorax

B. Testing of expansion of midthorax

C. Testing of expansion of posterior thorax

D. Testing movements of costal margins

Fig. 8–11 *Testing Thoracic Movement. A. The Upper Anterior Thorax. B. Expansion of the Anterior Mid-Thorax. C. Expansion of the Posterior Thorax. D. Movement of Costal Margins.*

letting your hands follow the chest movements. The thumbs should move apart. A unilateral lag indicates a nearby lesion in the wall, pleura, middle lobe of the right lung, or lingula of the left lung.

Testing excursion of the posterior lower chest. Have the patient sit or stand with his back toward you. Place your fingers in each axilla, with the palms applied firmly to the patient's chest, so your forefingers are one or two ribs below the inferior angles of the scapulae. To provide slack, press the soft tissues and pull your hands medially until your thumbs meet over the vertebral spines (Fig. 8–11C). Have the patient inspire deeply, following the lateral movements of the chest with your hands; your thumbs should move apart. A unilateral lag indicates a lesion in the nearby wall, pleura, or lower lobes of the lung.

Testing excursion of the costal margins. With the patient supine, place your hands so the extended thumbs lie along the inferior edges of the costal margins, with their tips nearly touching (Fig. 8–11D). Have the patient inspire deeply, letting your thumbs follow the costal margins. Normally, the thumbs diverge. Diminished divergence indicates depression of the dome of the diaphragm; convergence results when the dome is considerably flattened.

Examination of the Lungs and Pleura

Some argue that physical examination of the lungs and pleura is no longer necessary, because X-ray examination is readily available and discloses many lesions without physical signs. While the usefulness of X-ray examination is acknowledged, it does not replace the physical examination of the lungs. Physical examination is rapid, can be performed in all clinical situations, and does not require additional equipment or remove caregivers from the patient. In addition, some clinical conditions are diagnosed only by physical examination, or may be apparent on examination before radiographic signs appear: for example, early pneumonia can be diagnosed by the clinician before X-ray signs appear; a fractured rib may be obvious to palpation weeks before callus is evident in the X-ray film; the radiologist cannot diagnose asthma; the friction rub of pleurisy can appear and subside without X-ray signs; and pulmonary emphysema may be evident clinically before the radiologist can recognize it.

The physical examination of the pleura seeks to detect evidence of pleural inflammation, pleural adhesions, increases in pleural thickness, and the presence of air or excessive fluid in the pleural cavity. The lungs are examined to judge their volume, distensibility, density, changes in airway caliber, and abnormal secretions in the airways. Inspection and tactile palpation give some information. Vibratory qualities of the thorax and its contents yield significant information. Some vibrations are palpated; others are heard by the unaided ear, as in sonorous and definitive percussion, or through the stethoscope in auscultation. Vibrations are produced by the patient's spoken voice and by the examiner tapping the patient's chest. The caliber of the airways and their contained secretions modify the breath sounds or produce extraneous noises heard through the stethoscope.

Examination of the Lungs and Pleura by Palpation

Vibratory palpation of the lungs and pleura. *Vibratory palpation* uses the examiner's vibratory sense, which is most acute over the joints. To test this, apply the handle of a vibrating tuning fork first to the fingertip and then to volar surface of the metacarpophalangeal joint; this demonstrates the superior sensitivity of the basal part of the finger to vibrations (Fig. 8–12).

Speech produces vibrations in the bronchial air column that are conducted to the chest wall through the lung septa where they are felt by vibratory palpation as ***vocal fremitus***. Diminished vocal fremitus can be caused by airway obstruction, by sound screens of fluid or air in the pleural cavity, or by pleural fibrosis. Increased vocal fremitus occurs with lung consolidation; the density of the tissues is determined by percussion (see pages 38ff.). To compare vocal fremitus in different regions of the chest, each test word must be spoken with equal pitch and loudness. Vocal fremitus is normally more intense in the parasternal region in the right second interspace where it is closest to the bronchial bifurcation. The interscapular region is also near the bronchi and registers increased fremitus. Use the same technique to feel for pleural friction rubs (***friction fremitus***).

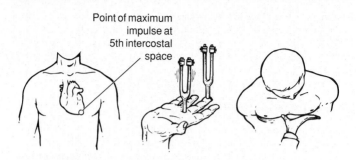

Fig. 8–12 *Vibratory Acuity in Various Parts of the Hand.* *Place the handle of a vibrating tuning fork sequentially on the fingertip and the palmar aspect of the metacarpophalangeal joint: the palmar base is more sensitive. This part of the hand should be applied to the precordium to detect thrills.*

Procedure for vibratory palpation. If able, have the patient sit or stand. Place the palmar bases of the fingers on to the interspaces (Fig. 8–13). Alternatively, the ulnar side of the hand and fifth finger may be used. Ask the patient to repeat the test words "ninety-nine" or "one-two-three," using the same pitch and intensity of voice each time. If vibrations are not felt, have the patient lower the pitch of their voice. Compare symmetrical parts of the chest sequentially with the same hand. It is better to compare two sensations sequentially with the same hand than to compare simultaneous sensations from two hands. When the lower thorax is reached, ascertain the point at which fremitus is lost. In the absence of a pleural lesion, this indicates the lung bases. Compare this with the position obtained by percussion and auscultation.

Percussion of the Lungs and Pleura

Thoracic percussion. See Chapter 3, page 38ff for a discussion of percussion techniques. For best results, press the pleximeter finger into the intercostal spaces between and parallel to the ribs, then strike a series of blows with the plexor. Percuss the back with the patient sitting and the anterior chest with the patient sitting and supine. The borders of the heart are outlined, and both sonorous and

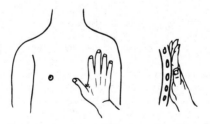

Fig. 8–13 *Detection of Vocal Fremitus by Vibratory Palpation.* *Symmetrical points on the chest are palpated sequentially with the same hand and the strength of vocal fremitus is compared in different regions. The palpating hand is applied firmly to the chest wall with palm in contact with the wall, and vibrations are sensed with the bases of the fingers.*

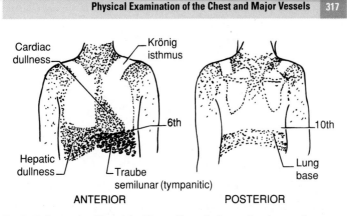

Fig. 8–14 *Percussion Map of the Thorax.* *The entire lung surface is normally resonant. At the apices, a band of resonance, known as the Krönig isthmus, runs over the shoulders like shoulder straps. Hepatic dullness ranges downward from the right sixth rib to merge into hepatic flatness. The Traube semilunar space of tympany extends downward from the left sixth rib; it is variable in extent, depending upon the amount of gas in the stomach. Posteriorly, the dullness below the lung bases begins at about the tenth rib.*

definitive percussion are applied to the back (Fig. 8–14). When the patient is ill in bed and unable to sit, he must be examined in the right and left lateral decubitus position which introduces problems in the interpretation of percussion sounds (see page 347 and Fig. 8–31).

Definitive chest percussion.   Definitive thoracic percussion is used to outline the borders between lung resonance and dullness of the heart, the spleen, the upper border of the liver, and the lumbar muscles below the lung bases. The boundary between resonant lung and tympanitic gastric bubble outlines the *Traube semilunar space*. The *Krönig isthmus* over the lung apices is defined by percussing the area of resonance in the supraclavicular fossae.

Cardiac dullness.   See page 320.

Anterior lungs.   Use sonorous percussion with heavy indirect bimanual percussion. Starting under the clavicles, compare the percussion sound from each interspace sequentially with that from the contralateral region. Work downward to the region of hepatic dullness on the right and the Traube semilunar space on the left (Fig. 8–14). Also, percuss the lateral thorax. Except for the area of cardiac dullness, the entire anterior region should be resonant.

Hepatic dullness.   The domed superior aspect of the liver normally produces a transverse zone of dullness from the fourth to the sixth interspaces in the right midclavicular line. Because a wedge of lung, edge downward, intervenes between the upper border of the liver and the chest wall, the transition from lung resonance to hepatic dullness is subtle and gradual. The dull zone merges into hepatic flatness as percussion is carried below the lung base.

Gastric tympany.   The stomach usually contains an air bubble that produces tympany in the Traube semilunar space. Because the left diaphragm is lower,

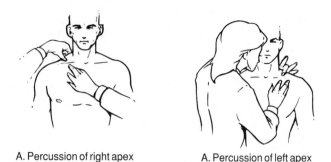

A. Percussion of right apex   A. Percussion of left apex

Fig. 8–15 *Percussion of the Lung Apices. Bimanual indirect percussion is applied in the usual fashion, except for the use of the pleximeter. See the text for descriptions.*

the upper tympanitic border is somewhat lower than the upper border of liver flatness on the opposite side.

Splenic dullness. The spleen produces an oval of dullness between the ninth and eleventh ribs in the left midaxillary line. Gastric or colonic tympany often obscures it completely. Dullness in this region may be enlarged by fluid or solids in the stomach or colon or by pleural effusion. An enlarged spleen is seldom obscured by gas; an increased area of splenic dullness or dullness in Traube's space should prompt careful palpation for the spleen.

Lung apices. The lung apices normally extend slightly above the clavicles, producing a band of resonance over each shoulder, widening at its scapular and clavicular ends. The narrowest part, the *Krönig isthmus*, lies atop the shoulder. Reproducibility of this finding is low. With the patient sitting or standing, sound each supraclavicular fossa. On the right place the examiner's left thumb in the right supraclavicular fossa (Fig. 8–15A) where it is struck by the plexor finger of the right hand. For the pleximeter in the left fossa, the examiner's left arm is put around the patient's back, and the left long finger is curled anteriorly over the trapezius muscle into the fossa (Fig. 8–15B). Fibrosis or infiltration of the lung narrows or obliterates the resonance.

Posterior lung. Use sonorous percussion with the patient sitting or standing. The patient's arms are folded in front with the shoulders forward ("hump the shoulders"), and the spine slightly flexed. Percussion is begun at the top, working downward comparing symmetrical regions sequentially. The scapular muscles and bones impair resonance in proportion to their mass, so interpretation of percussion notes is difficult, but symmetry should be preserved. Resonance ends inferiorly at about the ninth rib, the left lower than the right (see Fig. 8–14).

Diaphragm excursion. During quiet respiration, the inferior lung edges are relatively high in the costophrenic sulci, usually at about the ninth rib on the left and the eighth interspace on the right. The transition between lung resonance and muscle dullness (or flatness) is gradual. Light percussion is required. Mark the lung bases, during quiet respiration, then have the patient inspire deeply and hold the breath while you percuss the full inspiratory level. The bases should move downward 5 or 6 cm reflecting flattening of the diaphragm.

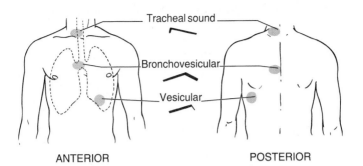

Fig. 8–16 *Breath Sounds Map in the Normal Chest.* The areas of the lungs that are unlabeled have normal vesicular breathing.

Auscultation of the Lungs and Pleura

Movements of the tracheobronchial air column produces vibrations that are perceived as sounds. Sounds from the lungs and heart have a frequency range between 60 and 3000 cycles per second. Vibrations may occur from air eddies in quiet breathing through normal airways, from air moving in dilated or constricted tubes, from the behavior of fluid moved by the air, or from the vocal cords. The absence of the sounds normally produced by the tracheobronchial air column indicates blockage in the airways or an abnormal screening of sound in the pleural cavity.

Auscultation of the lungs.   If possible, have the patient sit. When recumbent, the back should be examined by turning the patient from side to side. Demonstrate breathing through the mouth, deeper and slightly more forcefully than usual. Start by listening with the stethoscope diaphragm anteriorly at the apices and working downward, comparing symmetrical points sequentially. Next, listen to the back, starting at the apices and working downward. Note where breath sounds disappear inferiorly, compared with those determined by vocal fremitus and percussion.

Identify the breath sounds at each point as *vesicular, bronchovesicular, bronchial, asthmatic, cavernous,* or *absent* and their quality and pitch; note also the duration of inspiration and expiration (Fig. 8–16). If *crackles* are heard, note whether they persist or disappear after a few deep breaths. If crackles are not heard, test for *posttussive crackles* by listening to inspiration after the patient coughs at the end of expiration. If any abnormality is noted, go over the front and back again while the patient whispers test words, such as "one-two-three" or "ninety-nine," to determine the absence or the presence of **whispered pectoriloquy** (page 350). Test similarly with the spoken voice for **bronchophony** (page 350). Be alert for friction rubs, bone crepitus, and other unusual sounds.

Bedside Inspection of the Sputum

Inspection of the sputum discloses many valuable diagnostic clues to pulmonary disease. Have a clear plastic sputum cup on the bedside stand. Estimate the daily volume. Note the color, turbidity, and viscosity. Ascertain if it is bloody, frothy, or odoriferous. Look for caseous masses, mucous plugs, Curschmann spirals, bronchial casts, and concretions.

Examination of the Cardiovascular System

The examination of the cardiovascular system is presented here in a convenient sequence. The heart and blood vessels are examined sequentially with special emphasis on the precordium and careful examination of the neck and extremities for signs of cardiovascular dysfunction. A complete cardiovascular examination includes history taking, physical examination and, if indicated, supplementary procedures such as electrocardiography, echocardiography, CT and cine-CT, MRI, scintigraphy and cardiac catheterization to measure hemodynamics, perform angiography or perform electrophysiologic studies and interventions.

Physical Examination of the Heart and Precordium

Despite the vast improvements in diagnostic technology, the physical examination of the cardiovascular system remains an essential skill for the expert physician. It seems that practice under the mentorship of an expert is still critical to learn heart examination, although technologic advances are facilitating training [Issenberg SB, McGaghie WC, Hart IR, et al. Simulation technology for health care professional skills, training, and assessment. *JAMA.* 1999;282:861–866]. The physical examination is both sensitive and relatively specific for the diagnosis of valvular heart disease [Roldan CA, Shively BK, Crawford MH. Value of the cardiovascular physical examination for detecting valvular heart disease in asymptomatic subjects. *Am J Cardiol.* 1996;77:1327–1331].

Precordial inspection. The examiner should stand or sit at the patient's right side. Illuminate the precordium from a single source, shining transversely toward the examiner across the anterior chest surface. Alternatively, have the single light source shining from the head or foot. When possible, the patient should be examined both supine and erect. First, look for an *apical impulse*, it is visible in 20% of normal people; then shift your head so your line of sight is across the sternum to detect heaving of the precordium. Finally, inspect the manubrial area.

Precordial palpation. Pulsations, lifts, heaves and thrills can be felt in the precordium. Palpate the precordium with the palm of the hand, first examining areas of visible pulsations. If not visible, try to identify the *apical impulse* by palpation in the left fifth interspace 7 to 9 cm from the midsternal line (MSL), or approximately 1 to 2 cm medial from the midclavicular line. The impulse is synchronous with early ventricular systole; it should be no larger than 2 cm in diameter. The strength of the normal impulse must be learned by examining many hearts. Next, feel each part of the precordium. Determine the presence and strength of right and left ventricular (LV) thrusts. Pulsations at the base of the heart should be carefully felt. Thrills should be identified and timed by their relation to the apical impulse as systolic or diastolic. Recognize and time pleural and pericardial friction rubs.

Precordial percussion. The precordium is percussed to define the cardiac borders (*definitive percussion*). This is helpful in the absence of a palpable apical impulse. The left arm of the supine patient is abducted; the erect patient is asked to put her left hand on the hip. The sitting woman is requested to hold her left breast up with the left hand. Locate the *left border of cardiac dullness* (*LBCD*) by

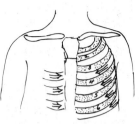

Fig. 8–17 *Pattern of Precordial Percussion.* The fifth, fourth, and third intercostal spaces on the left are percussed sequentially, as indicated by the arrows, starting near the axilla and moving medially until cardiac dullness is encountered.

percussing in the fifth, fourth, and third left interspaces sequentially, starting over resonant lung near the axilla and moving medially until cardiac dullness is encountered (Fig. 8–17). Measure the distance from the mid-sternum to the LBCD in the fifth interspace along a line perpendicular to the sternum; this measurement can be directly compared with posteroanterior (PA) film of the chest.

Percuss the *right border of cardiac dullness* (*RBCD*) the change from resonant lung to cardiac dullness is normally not apparent as the RBCD is behind the sternum. The examiner cannot be certain of its position; it may even be displaced leftward. When the right border is displaced rightward, the change in percussion note in the right hemithorax is definite. No conclusion about the size of the heart should be made by percussing only the left border. In the presence of hydrothorax or thickened pleura, percussion of the heart border may be impossible. Measure the width of the *retromanubrial dullness*; in the adult a width exceeding 6 cm suggests an anterior mediastinal mass.

Precordial auscultation.   The stethoscope and its proper use are described in Chapter 3 on pages 40ff. The same principles apply to auscultation of the heart as to lung auscultation. Listen in each of the primary valve areas (Fig. 8–18). Timing of cardiac sounds is especially important; use the apical impulse, or, if absent, the

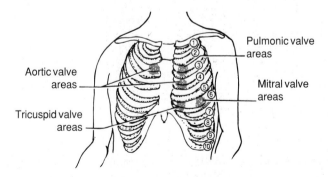

Aortic valve areas

Tricuspid valve areas

Pulmonic valve areas

Mitral valve areas

Fig. 8–18 *Cardiac Valve Areas for Precordial Auscultation.* These are the areas where the sounds originating from each valve is best heard; the areas are not necessarily closest to the anatomic location of the valves.

carotid upstroke to mark the onset of ventricular systole. Map the strength and radiation of abnormal sounds across the precordium.

Auscultation for cardiac rate and rhythm.   Guessing at the heart rate is fraught with error. Auscultate the precordium to determine the apical ventricular rate. It should be compared to the arterial pulse rate counted by palpating a peripheral artery. If the rate is regular and not very slow, counting for 15 seconds and multiplying by 4 is sufficiently accurate. If there is a difference between the auscultated apical and palpated arterial rates, it is termed a *pulse deficit*. Pulse deficit occurs whenever ventricular systole generates a stroke volume insufficient to produce a pulse wave in the arteries; it is frequent with premature beats, bigeminal rhythm and atrial fibrillation. **The ECG is the gold standard for heart rate, as not all electrical events produce an audible mechanical event, especially at high heart rates.**

After counting the heart rate, listen carefully for an *irregularity of rhythm*. Dysrhythmias are harder to detect when the diastolic intervals are either very long or very short, that is, with particularly slow or fast heart rates, respectively. Therefore, one should listen more intently under these conditions for irregularities of rhythm. If there is irregularity, determine if there is a relation to respiratory movements or if there are repeating patterns of beats.

Auscultation of the heart sounds S1 and S2.   Precordial auscultation reveals paired sounds, each usually distinct in intensity and pitch. The pair correlates with a single cardiac cycle (see Fig. 8–19). Definite identification of the first heart sound (S1) and second heart sound (S2) sounds is essential because they are audible markers for the beginning and end of ventricular systole. When an apical impulse is visible or palpable, the sound synchronous with it is S1. In the absence of an apical impulse, palpate the carotid pulse wave, allowing for a slight interval between the onset of cardiac systole and the arrival of the resulting wave in the neck. Never use the radial pulse for timing; it is too far from the heart to reliably distinguish the heart sounds. If the ventricular rate is less than 100 bpm, diastole is longer than systole, so the first sound can be accepted as the first of the pair. When identification of the heart sounds or timing of murmurs is difficult because the tones are muffled or the rate is fast, slow the heart for a few beats by having the patient perform a Valsalva maneuver or by gently massaging either carotid sinus. The initial sound after a long pause must be the first sound. Finally, at the base of the heart the second sound is almost invariably louder than the first.

After identifying S1 and S2 at the apex, move the stethoscope short distances along the left sternal border and toward the base (*inching*) tracing each sound across the precordium. Use separate passes concentrating sequentially on the intensity (accentuated or diminished), the quality, the duration and the presence of splitting of the sounds. Prolonged sounds can be differentiated from murmurs by their abrupt beginning and ending, whereas murmurs have gradual onset and end. A sound that begins abruptly but ends gradually is probably a heart sound followed by a murmur. It takes considerable experience listening to many normal and abnormal hearts to master cardiac auscultation, to learn to recognize ranges of normal and be able to identify the presence or absence of abnormal sounds.

Auscultation of cardiac murmurs.   Listen for cardiac murmurs only after S1 and S2 have been positively identified. Decide whether a sound of abnormal length is a split heart sound or a heart sound *and* murmur. Now turn your attention to the systolic interval between S1 and S2. Decide if there is any audible sound in this interval, by assuming that a heart sound is the shortest perceptible sound

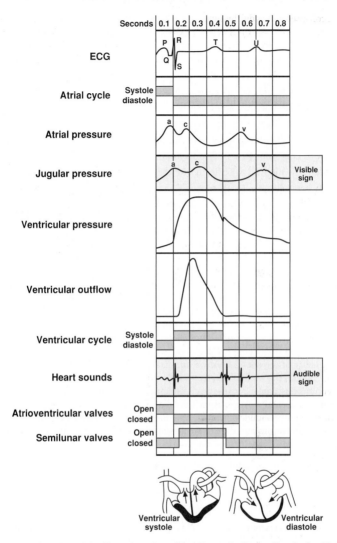

Fig. 8–19 *Relation of the Heart Sounds to Other Events in the Cardiac Cycle.* *Of all these phenomena, only one visible and one audible sign are produced.*

and that anything appreciably longer may be heart sound and murmur. In such a combination, remember that a heart sound begins and ends abruptly. A prolonged sound starting abruptly and dwindling is probably a heart sound followed by murmur; one developing gradually and ending abruptly is likely murmur and heart sound. Carefully examine each valve area with bell and diaphragm of the stethoscope. Cover the intervening spaces only moving the stethoscope short distances each time, "inching." Once the presence of a murmur is established, ascertain the following characteristics: *Timing:* Determine in what part of the cardiac cycle the murmur occurs, and whether it is early, middle, or late in the interval, by reference to the first and second heart sounds. *Location:* Ascertain where on the precordium the murmur exhibits maximum intensity. *Intensity:* Grade intensity by the following scale:

Grade I: Barely audible with greatest difficulty

Grade II: Faint but heard immediately upon listening

Grades III, IV, V and VI: Progressively louder

Grade IV: Characterized by the presence of a thrill

Grade V: Loud enough to be heard with the stethoscope placed on its edge

Grade VI: So loud; it can be heard with the stethoscope off the chest

The recording of grade III, for example, should be grade III/VI to show that the scale of VI is being used. *Pattern or Configuration:* Decide if the murmur is uniform in intensity throughout or whether the loudness increases (*crescendo*), or diminishes (*decrescendo*), or both (*crescendo-decrescendo*). The term *diamond-shaped murmur* is taken from the graphic representation on the screen of the phonocardiograph; the maximum intensity is midsystolic, with a crescendo preceding and decrescendo following the peak. *Pitch:* Determine whether the murmur is high or low pitched. To the inexperienced and nonmusical examiner, the simplest method is to determine whether the murmur is better heard with the bell (low pitched) or the diaphragm (high pitched). Remember, the bell should be applied lightly and the diaphragm should be pressed firmly against the skin. Determine whether the pitch is more like a murmur or a friction rub. The latter, being rare, is frequently misdiagnosed as a murmur; the only distinction is by the quality of the sound. *Posture and Exercise:* When possible, auscultate the heart in both the supine and erect positions. In addition, employ the left lateral decubitus position, especially when listening at the cardiac apex to demonstrate the murmur of mitral stenosis and the gallop rhythms. Exercise sometimes brings out otherwise inaudible murmurs. After the systolic interval has been thoroughly explored, turn your attention to the diastolic interval carrying out the same procedures while asking the same questions.

Listening for extra systolic sounds. After identifying systole and diastole by using S1 and S2 as markers and noting any murmurs, the examiner listens for extra sounds in the systolic interval. Any abnormal sound must be either a murmur or a systolic click (Fig. 8–20).

Listening for diastolic sounds. After the systolic interval has been examined, examine the diastolic interval between S2 and S1. Sounds in diastole can be murmurs, opening snaps, third heart sounds (S3), fourth heart sounds (S4), or pericardial knocks (Fig. 8–20).

Physical Examination of the Blood Vessels

Clinicians must have precise knowledge of the location of the accessible arteries and veins, their relations to other parts of the vascular system, and their responses to cardiac contraction. The following arteries are usually palpable: temporal, common and external carotid, axillary, brachial, radial, ulnar, common iliac, femoral, popliteal, dorsalis pedis, and posterior tibial (see Fig. 4–2). The abdominal aorta is palpable in slender individuals. The veins that are frequently visible are the

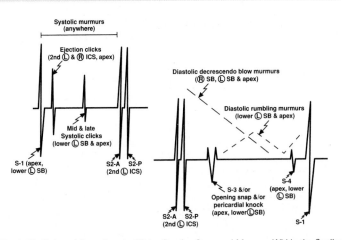

Fig. 8–20 *Timing of Heart Sounds, Clicks, Opening Snap, and Murmurs Within the Cardiac Cycle. ICS, intercostal space; SB, sternal border; S2-A, S2-in aortic area; S2-P, S2 in pulmonic area.*

external jugular, cephalic, basilic, median basilic, great saphenous, and the veins on the dorsa of the hands and feet.

Measurement of arterial blood pressure.   See Chapter 4, page 72ff.

Venous pressure.   *Central venous pressure (CVP)* is measured at the level of the right atrium. In the erect position, the level of the right atrium is at the fourth intercostal space. Vertically from this point, a direct venous channel extends through the SVC, the two subclavian veins, and then to the two *external jugular veins* that emerge from the thorax at the superior borders of the clavicles to become subcutaneous and visible in the neck. With normal venous pressure in the erect position, a column of blood distends the SVC to a height of approximately 10 cm above the right atrium (Fig. 8–21A). Any peripheral veins anatomically below this level are normally filled with blood; those above are collapsed. In most adults, the upper border of the clavicles is from 13 to 18 cm above the right atrium, so the visible segment of the external jugular veins in the neck is collapsed when the patient is erect (Fig. 8–21C). The visible veins in the dependent arms and forearms are distended with blood up to the same level as in the vena cava. When the thorax reclines at 45 degrees the column of blood rises higher in the neck veins, so the head of the column may be visible in the jugulars (Fig. 8–21B). In the horizontal position, all peripheral veins are filled (Fig. 8–21A). If the arm is raised slowly, the distal portions of the veins collapse as they attain the height of 10 cm above the level of the right atrium.

Estimating CVP.   Because the superior border of the clavicle in the adult is usually from 13 to 18 cm above the right atrium, distention of the external jugular vein in the neck when the body is vertical is valid evidence of increased CVP, provided that there is no compression of the venous channel proximal to the atrium. Factors that increase intrathoracic pressure must be excluded, for example, coughing, laughing, crying, and movements involving a Valsalva maneuver. A large cervical

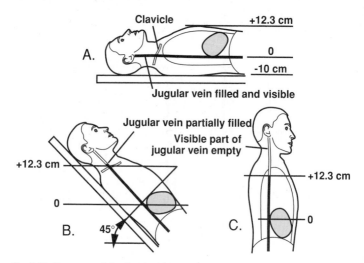

Fig. 8–21 *Response of the Jugular Blood Column to Changes in Posture.* *The antero-posterior diameter of the thorax at the fourth interspace is 20 cm; from this point, the vertical distance to the superior border of the clavicle is 15 cm in the erect position. The right atrium is located at the midpoint of an anteroposterior line from the fourth interspace to the back. In any posture, a horizontal plane through this point is the ÒphlebostaticÓ or Òzero level.Ó In this figure, a slightly elevated venous pressure of 12.3 cm is assumed. **A.** With the patient supine, the horizontal plane 12.3 cm above the zero level is above the neck; at normal venous pressure the jugular vein is filled. **B.** With the thorax at 45 degrees, the blood column extends midway up the jugular, so the head of the column is visible. **C.** In the erect position, the head of the column is concealed within the thorax, 2.7 cm below the upper border of the clavicle.*

or retrosternal goiter may cause venous obstruction. The presence of venous waves in the jugular veins excludes obstruction centrally; however, tense distention of the jugulars may prevent visualization of the venous waves. Venous pulsations transmitted from the *internal jugular veins* are easily visible in the base of the neck; the height of this pulsation may be used to estimate CVP.

Indirect measurement of CVP. The vertical distance in centimeters from the head of the jugular blood column to the right atrium is an approximate measure of CVP. When identifiable, the internal jugular vein provides a more accurate estimation of this pressure than the external jugular veins, and the veins on the right side of the neck are more reliable than those on the left. If the jugular veins are collapsed in the vertical position, slowly lower the thorax until the head of the blood column appears. The right atrial position is estimated by running an imaginary anteroposterior line from the anterior fourth interspace halfway to the back; a horizontal plane through this point is the zero level for measurement of venous pressure (Fig. 8–21B). The vertical distance in centimeters from this plane to the head of the blood column gives an approximation of the venous pressure. Another standard reference point in estimating the height of the jugular venous column is the angle of Louis (sternal angle); this is assumed to be approximately 6 cm above the atrium in most positions, although this is not always the case

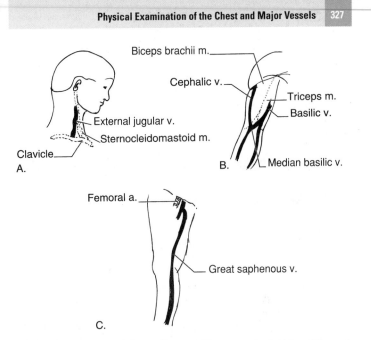

Fig. 8–22 *Visible Veins and Venous Pressure Measurements. A. Veins of the neck. B. Veins of the arm. C. Veins of the thigh and leg.*

[Seth R, Magner P, Matzinger F, van Walraven C. How far is the sternal angle from the mid-right atrium? *J Gen Intern Med*. 2002;17:852–856]. Jugular venous pulsations >3 cm vertically above this landmark indicate elevated venous pressure [McGee SR. Physical examination of venous pressure: A critical review. *Am Heart J*. 1998;136:10–18].

Alternate indirect measurement of CVP. Place the patient supine with the arm hanging down over the bedside. Raise the patient's arm slowly until a position is found where the distended veins in the arm or hand collapse. The vertical distance from the zero level to the point of collapse should give the venous pressure. Unfortunately, there is great individual variation in the caliber and superficiality of the veins of the arms. For observation, veins should be selected as close to the heart as possible so as to exclude blockage by valves; this is less likely in the cephalic, basilic, or median basilic veins (Fig. 8–22).

Venous pulsations. Under ideal conditions, one can see three upward components of the wave (Fig. 8–23) and two prominent descents. The rise of *the "a" wave* results from right atrial systole; the *"c" wave* is caused principally, if not entirely, by expansion of the underlying carotid artery and is usually not visible. The peak of the "a" wave is followed by an *"x" descent* initially related to atrial relaxation and later to downward movement of the tricuspid valve with right ventricular systole. The rising *"v" wave* is produced by filling of the right atrium from the systemic veins while the tricuspid valve is closed. The peak of the "v" wave is followed by the *y descent* associated with opening of the tricuspid valve with onset of right ventricular diastole. Proper identification of the waves and descents requires careful correlation with the cardiac cycle. The rapid descents

Jugular pulse (sphygmogram)

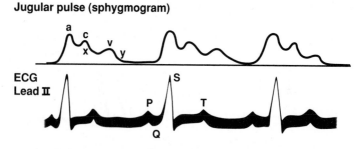

Fig. 8–23 *Jugular Veinous Pulse Waves. Heart action is reflected in the jugular vein. The waves should be timed with the apical impulse or heart sounds, remembering that a perceptible time elapses between cardiac events and their signs in the neck. The "a" wave is the rebound from atrial systole. The bulging of the tricuspid valve cusps early in ventricular systole produces the c deflection. The "v" wave results from atrial filling while the valve is closed, together with an upward movement of the AV valve ring at the end of ventricular systole. The x descent comes with atrial relaxation and the y descent with opening of the tricuspid valve.*

are usually better appreciated than the slowly rising waves. The *"x" descent* is normally the most readily observed portion of the jugular pulse, and its nadir is approximated by S2. The peak of "a" wave is normally the most prominent wave and should occur at about S1.

The venous pulse wave is a normal phenomenon that can be demonstrated in the external jugular veins. Venous pulsations can also be seen by the expansion of the neck, which occurs with filling and collapse of the internal jugular veins and their tributaries. This is best seen from the foot of the bed. In a few persons, pulsations occur in the superficial veins of the arms, forearms, and hands. Venous pulsation is readily distinguished from an arterial pulse by being impalpable. Venous pulses are best seen at the head of a blood column, but visibility depends on the amount of overlying tissue. Occasionally, a disproportion in the number of "a" waves and ventricular systoles gives direct indication of a dysrhythmia; but the waves are difficult to see consistently. When the geometry of posture has been so arranged as to expect a normal pulse wave, the absence of venous pulse is a sign of obstruction of the channel to the right atrium.

Capillary pulsation.   This has been widely advertised as a sign of aortic regurgitation, despite the repeated demonstrations of Thomas Lewis and others that it is a normal phenomenon, seen in most normal persons. To elicit it, press down on the tip of the fingernail until the distal third of the pink nail bed has paled: with each heartbeat, the border of pink extends and recedes. When seen in aortic regurgitation, it is known as *Quincke pulse*.

Physical Examination of Arterial Circulation in the Extremities

We consider large arteries as those with anatomic names and normally visible or palpable pulses whose occlusion can be recognized by the region of ischemia produced. Because smaller arteries and the arterioles are observable only in the superficial layers of the skin or in the retina, methods for their examination are quite different. In the routine physical examination, most physicians assess the circulation by (1) palpation of the pulse volume in the pairs of brachial, radial, femoral, dorsalis pedis, and posterior tibial arteries; (2) palpation for temperature changes; (3) inspection for varicose veins, edema, pallor, cyanosis, and ulceration of the arms and legs; and (4) inspection of the retinal vessels. Complaints of pain, coolness, or numbness in an extremity or signs of enlarged veins, masses, swellings, localized pallor, redness, or cyanosis lead to special examinations of the peripheral circulation. The cause of a circulatory deficit is frequently revealed by the history, the distribution of the deficit, and the state of the vessel wall.

When the affected part is below heart level, pooled venous blood obscures evidence of arterial flow. Normally, venous pressure rarely exceeds 30 cm above that of the right atrium, whereas the systolic arterial pressure produces a pressure more than 150 cm above the same reference point. Thus, when the hand or foot is lifted above the right atrium to a height exceeding the venous pressure, the masking venous blood pool is drained, permitting evaluation of the tissue color produced by the arterial blood. The most reliable sign of regional perfusion abnormality is a temperature or perfusion discrepancy between symmetrical parts at the same external temperature. If the pair is affected equally, the change in color is judged from experience with other patients.

Skin Color is imparted by the blood in the venules of the subpapillary layer and the melanin content of the skin. Examination for circulatory changes in dark-skinned individuals is difficult; focus attention on the mucous membranes, nail beds, and the palms of the hands. When the arterial flow is nil and the veins empty, the skin is chalky white. Partial but inadequate arterial supply may produce red or cyanotic skin, depending on the effect of external temperature and amount of pooled blood in the venules.

Skin Temperature is a reliable indicator of dermal perfusion. Normally, flow is governed principally by the constriction or dilatation of the arterioles. The internal body temperature is maintained within narrow limits, partly by the regulated dissipation of heat from the dermal vessels. In clothed persons, the skin of the head, neck, and trunk is warmer than that of the extremities and the digits are colder than their respective hands and feet. Peculiarly, the normal digits adjust their temperature to only one of two levels. The fingers are somewhat cooler ($32°C$ [$90°F$]) than blood temperature ($37°C$ [$98°F$]) when the air temperature exceeds $20°C$ ($68°F$). If the room temperature is below $16°C$ ($60°F$), the fingers adjust to a level of approximately $22°C$ ($72°F$); there are no intermediate levels of adjustment.

Dermal examination for arterial deficit. In a draft-less room at approximately $22°C$ ($72°F$) place the patient on an examining table or bed and expose the extremities for 10 minutes. If the room temperature much exceeds $26°C$ ($78°F$), coldness in the skin should not be demonstrable. Have the patient sit, hanging the legs from the table or bed; compare the skin color of both feet looking for pallor, deep redness, pale blueness, deep blueness, or a violaceous color (see Fig. 6–14, page 145 and Fig. 8–24A). With the back of your hand or fingers, feel the *skin temperature* from the feet up the legs. Compare similar sites on each leg in sequence; in moving proximally, note whether the increase in temperature is gradual or sharply demarcated. Have the patient lie supine. Grasp both of the patient's ankles and elevate the feet more than 30 cm (12 in) above the right atrium. Note any change in the color of the feet (Fig. 8–24C). If the color does not change, have the patient dorsiflex the feet five or six times, wait several minutes, then observe the feet for latent color changes induced by exercise. Allow the feet

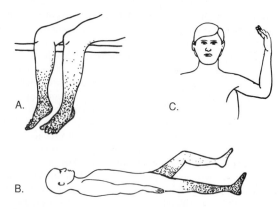

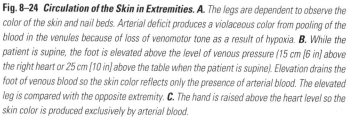

Fig. 8–24 *Circulation of the Skin in Extremities. **A.** The legs are dependent to observe the color of the skin and nail beds. Arterial deficit produces a violaceous color from pooling of the blood in the venules because of loss of venomotor tone as a result of hypoxia. **B.** While the patient is supine, the foot is elevated above the level of venous pressure (15 cm [6 in] above the right heart or 25 cm [10 in] above the table when the patient is supine). Elevation drains the foot of venous blood so the skin color reflects only the presence of arterial blood. The elevated leg is compared with the opposite extremity. **C.** The hand is raised above the heart level so the skin color is produced exclusively by arterial blood.*

to hang down again and note the time for the return of color to the skin. Note rapidity of return of color to an area blanched by finger pressure. Inspect the feet carefully for ***evidence of malnutrition***, for example, atrophy of the skin, loss of lanugo hair on the dorsa of the toes, thickening or transverse ridging of the nails, ulceration or patches of gangrene. Apply the same methods in examining the upper extremities. Expose the hands for 10 minutes and then observe the color in dependency and when elevated well above heart level (Fig. 8–24B). Have the hands opened and closed to disclose latent color changes. Note the time of return of color in dependency. Seek evidence of dermal malnutrition.

Examination of large arm and leg arteries. Palpate the walls of accessible arteries for increased thickness, tortuosity, and beading. A spastic artery feels like a small cord. Systematically compare the pulse volumes at symmetric levels of the arteries.

Upper extremities. Listen for a bruit over the *subclavian artery* in the supraclavicular fossa. The arteries of the arm and forearm are palpable only in a segment of the brachial artery in the upper arm and segments of the radial and ulnar arteries in the wrist. With the forearm in about 90 degrees of flexion, palpate the *brachial artery* on the medial aspect of the arm, in the groove between the biceps and triceps muscles (Fig. 8–25A). Feel the *radial artery* on the flexor surface of the wrist just medial to the distal end of the radius. Palpate the *ulnar artery* on the flexor surface of the wrist just lateral to the lower end of the ulna; it lies deeper than the radial artery and frequently it is impalpable in the normal subject. Examine the patency of the radial and ulnar arteries with the ***Allen test*** (Fig. 8–25B): Have the patient sit with her hands supinated on her knees; stand at the patient's side with your fingers around each of her wrists and your thumbs on the flexor

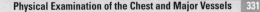

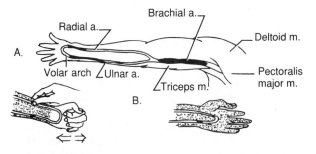

Fig. 8–25 *Testing Patency Arm Arteries. A. Palpable segments of the arm arteries* *(segments in solid black). Frequently the ulnar pulse is not palpable in normal persons.* **B.** **Allen test.** *See the text for details.*

surfaces of her wrists. Have the patient make a tight fist, and then compress the tissue over both the radial and ulnar arteries with your thumbs. Have the patient open the hand; the skin should be pale and remain so if both arteries are compressed. Take your thumb off the radial artery; the palm and fingers should quickly turn pink as flow returns. Delayed flush or no flush indicates partial or complete obstruction of the radial artery. Repeat the process, this time removing pressure from the ulnar artery. Return of flow is normally somewhat slower from the ulnar artery, but absence of flush is pathologic. Repeat this sequence on the other hand.

Lower extremities. Palpate the *abdominal aorta* deeply between the xiphoid and the umbilicus, where the aorta bifurcates. Palpate the *common femoral arteries* just below the inguinal ligaments, equidistant between the anterior superior iliac spines and the pubic tubercles (Fig. 8–26). Feel for the pulse of the *popliteal arteries* with the patient supine and the legs extended. Place a hand on each side of the patient's knee with your thumbs anteriorly near the patella and the fingers curling around each side of the knee so the tips rest in the popliteal fossa. Firmly press the fingers of both hands forward to compress the tissues and the artery against the lower end of the femur or the upper part of the tibia; feel for pulsation of the artery. Frequently, the pulse of a normal popliteal artery is impalpable. For the pulse of the *posterior tibial artery*, feel in the groove between the medial malleolus and the Achilles tendon. It may be more accessible with passive dorsiflexion of the foot. Locate the *dorsalis pedis artery* on the dorsum of the foot, just lateral to and parallel with the tendon of the extensor hallucis longus. In apparently normal persons older than age 45 years, either the dorsalis pedis or the posterior tibial pulses frequently will be impalpable, but not both on the same foot. In feeling for the patient's pulse, carefully guard against mistaking the pulse in your own fingertips for that of the patient. Check the **ankle-brachial index (ABI)** by measuring the systolic blood pressure in the brachial artery and the posterior tibial and/or the dorsalis pedis artery. The ABI is the ratio of the ankle systolic pressure to the brachial systolic pressure. Normal is >0.9, 0.75 to 0.9 is mild, 0.6 to 0.75 is moderate, and <0.6 is severe ischemia. ABI <0.5 is limb threatening. Use of Doppler (see Doppler Ultrasound Examination below) may be necessary. With the dorsal aspects of your fingers, palpate the skin of the thighs and legs for abnormal distribution of *skin temperature*, comparing symmetric areas. If the feet are abnormally cold, look for a sharp line demarcating a proximal region of

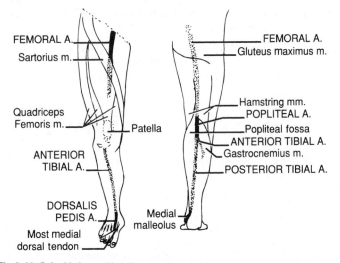

Fig. 8–26 Palpable Lower Limb Arteries. *The palpable segments of the arteries are in solid black. The femoral artery is palpable only a short distance below the inguinal ligament at the midpoint between the anterior superior iliac spine and the pubic tubercle. The popliteal artery lies vertically in the popliteal fossa; it can be felt only by compressing the contents of the fossa from behind against the bone. The posterior tibial artery can be felt as it curls forward and under the medial malleolus. The palpable segment of the dorsalis pedis artery lies just lateral to the most medial of the dorsal tendons of the foot (the flexor of the great toe) over the arch of the foot.*

normal temperature. Feel for a warm area over the knees or the anteromedial aspect of the thighs indicating collateral circulation via the *geniculate artery*.

Doppler ultrasound examination.   Small portable instruments for use at the bedside make it possible to evaluate the arterial circulation more precisely, especially when the pulses are not readily palpable.

Examination of the Large Limb Veins

Adequate drainage of blood from the extremities requires (1) patency of the venous lumina, (2) voluntary muscle contractions to furnish the pumping action by compressing the adjacent veins, and (3) competent valves in the perforating and deep veins so that venous compression moves the blood proximally. A defect in any of these may result in venous stasis with increased filtration pressure in the distal capillaries and post-capillary venules producing edema of the extremities, stasis pigmentation of the skin, and/or skin ulceration.

Examination of large arm and leg veins.   With the patient supine, look for signs of venous stasis. Have the patient stand, and look for dilated veins in the arms and legs. Demonstrate venous occlusion by elevating the extremity to determine whether the veins collapse promptly. If occlusion is present, palpate the venous walls for hard plugs of thrombus or hard cords of fibrosis. If patent varicose veins are present, use the special tests for incompetency of valves.

Laboratory examination of the large limb veins. Techniques such as ultrasonic Doppler, impedance plethysmography, venography, and MRI permit experienced laboratory personnel to determine the patency and competence of the large limb veins.

Chest, Cardiovascular and Respiratory Symptoms

General Symptoms

KEY SYMPTOM Pain in the Chest

Thoracic pain has many causes and, unless obviously the result of trauma, is likely to be accompanied by fear of heart disease. Chest pain often occurs without physical signs, so diagnostic accuracy requires careful attention to history, especially the attributes of pain (*PQRST: provocative-palliative factors, quality, region-referral, severity, and timing*). Always have the patient demonstrate the entire area where they perceive pain and the location of maximal intensity. The diagnostic approach is twofold: first to assess the risk for major vascular disease and acute coronary events, and second, to develop the differential diagnosis of noncardiovascular explanations [Lee TH, Goldman L. Evaluation of the patient with acute chest pain. *N Engl J Med.* 2000;342:1187–1195]. Acute coronary events may be missed in younger patients, women, and people with normal ECGs, so careful risk factor assessment and a high index of suspicion are necessary. Reassurance based upon the exclusion of cardiovascular disease is often the most effective therapy [Swap CJ, Nagurney JT. Value and limitations of chest pain history in the evaluation of patients with suspected acute coronary syndromes. *JAMA.* 2005;294:2623–2629]. See Six-Dermatome Pain Syndromes, page 400.

KEY SYMPTOM Deep Retrosternal or Precordial Pain and the Six-Dermatome Band

Dermatomes T1 to T6 cover the thoracic surface from the neck to beneath the xiphoid process and extend down the anteromedial aspects of the arms and forearms (Fig. 8–27). The upper four spinal segments are supplied by sensory afferent fibers from the dorsal roots of T1 to T4, and the lower cervical and upper thoracic sympathetic ganglia. In the ganglia and spinal cord, the fibers communicate with one another superiorly and inferiorly. The mediastinal, thoracic and abdominal organs are also supplied by sensory afferents and parasympathetic efferents via the vagus nerve (CNX). Practically, all the thoracic viscera are served by sensory fibers in these pathways: myocardium, pericardium, aorta, pulmonary artery, esophagus, and mediastinum. Lesions in any of these structures produce pain of the same quality: deep, visceral, and poorly localized. Spinal segments, T5 and T6 receive sensory fibers from the lower thoracic wall, the diaphragmatic muscles and their peritoneal surfaces, the gallbladder, the pancreas, the duodenum, and the stomach. Inflammation in these structures causes deep, visceral, poorly localized pain precisely similar in quality to that from the upper band. **Deep visceral pain behind the sternum, in the precordial region or epigastrium is typical for pain**

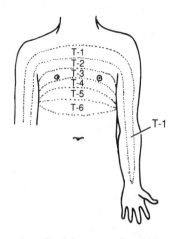

Fig. 8–27 *The Six-Dermatome Band.* *Dermatomes T1 to T6 form a band that covers most of the thorax and extends down the anteromedial aspect of the arms and forearms. Sensory pathways from the viscera of this entire region are so interconnected axially that stimulation of any part can produce the same patterns of chest pain.*

from the entire region supplied by spinal segments T1 to T6, including the sympathetics. It is *not* specific for heart disorders. The neuroanatomy of the region explains the structural basis for this clinical observation. Usually pain arising from T1 to T4 is maximal in the retrosternal region or the precordium; it often extends with lesser intensity upward into the neck and downward on the anteromedial aspects of one or both arms and forearms. Pain arising in T5 or T6 is maximally intense in the xiphoid region and in the back, inferior to the right scapula, but the pain may extend to the upper band of T1 to T4 through posterior connections in the sympathetics, so that the pattern may be indistinguishable from that arising above the diaphragm. **Accept the location of the pain as indicating only that the source is somewhere in the six-dermatome band (the myocardium, pericardium, aorta, pulmonary artery, mediastinum, esophagus, gallbladder, pancreas, duodenum, stomach, or subphrenic region).** Have the patient rate the pain intensity on a scale of 1 to 10. Shorten the list of possibilities by carefully searching for provocative-palliative factors and timing and do appropriate tests to distinguish between the disorders on the shortened list.

PRECORDIAL PAIN—CLINICAL OCCURRENCE: *Congenital* hypertrophic cardiomyopathy; *Endocrine* retrosternal thyroid; *Idiopathic* esophageal spasm, gastroesophageal reflux; *Inflammatory/Immune* esophagitis, pericarditis, pleuritis, myocarditis, postcardiotomy syndrome, pancreatitis, cholecystitis, gastritis; *Infectious* infectious pericarditis and pleuritis, myocarditis, subphrenic abscess; *Metabolic/Toxic* acid or alkali ingestion; *Mechanical/Trauma* pneumothorax, esophageal rupture, esophageal obstruction (extrinsic, foreign body, neoplasm, web, or ring), esophageal diverticulum, gastric perforation; *Neoplastic* carcinoma (primary or metastatic) of the esophagus, pericardium, lung, mediastinum, pleura; lymphoma; thymoma; teratoma; testicular cancer; *Neurologic* postherpetic neuralgia, diabetic radiculopathy, intercostal neuritis; *Psychosocial* somatization disorder, panic attack, hypochondriasis, malingering, Munchausen syndrome; *Vascular* myocardial ischemia (coronary atherosclerosis, spasm, embolism, thrombosis, vasculitis), pulmonary embolism and infarction, aortic dissection.

> **KEY SIGN** Shortness of Breath—Dyspnea

Dyspnea results from abnormalities of gas exchange (decreased oxygenation, hypoventilation, hyperventilation), and increased work of breathing because of changes in respiratory mechanics and/or anxiety. Dyspnea means difficult breathing; it is both a symptom and a sign. The patient's complaint is likely to be "shortness of breath," "quickly out of breath," "can't take a deep breath," "smothering," or "tightness in the chest." Dyspnea is often accompanied by tachypnea, increased respiratory excursions (hyperpnea), tensing of the scaleni and sternocleidomastoidei, flaring of the alae nasi, and facial expressions of distress. Sometimes, the patient seems unaware of being dyspneic although the examiner notes that the patient pauses for breath in the middle of a sentence. It is essential to identify the situational precipitants of dyspnea such as exertional dyspnea versus dyspnea at rest and dyspnea on standing or lying down. A diagnostic classification of the causes of dyspnea can be based on anatomic or physiologic criteria. Often more than one mechanism is involved, for example, pneumonia causes hypoxia and increases the work of breathing. Patients may complain of dyspnea disproportionate to any identifiable physiologic or anatomic abnormality: anxiety with hyperventilation or unsuspected decreases in respiratory compliance should be suspected.

✔ *DYSPNEA—CLINICAL OCCURRENCE:* **Decreased Fraction of Inspired Oxygen** high altitudes; **Airway Obstruction** *Larynx and Trachea* infections (laryngeal diphtheria, acute laryngitis, epiglottitis, Ludwig angina), angioedema, trauma (hematoma or laryngeal edema), neuropathic (abductor paralysis of vocal cords), foreign body, tumors of the neck (goiter, carcinoma, lymphoma, aortic aneurysm), ankylosis of the cricoarytenoid joints; *Bronchi and Bronchioles* acute and chronic bronchitis, asthma, retrosternal goiter, aspirated foreign bodies, extensive bronchiectasis, bronchial stenosis. **Abnormal Alveoli** *Alveolar Filling* pulmonary edema, pulmonary infiltration (infectious and aspiration pneumonia, carcinoma, sarcoidosis, pneumoconioses), pulmonary hemorrhage, pulmonary alveolar proteinosis; *Alveolar Destruction* pulmonary emphysema, pulmonary fibrosis, cystic disease of the lungs; *Compression of the Alveoli* atelectasis, pneumothorax, hydrothorax, abdominal distention; **Restrictive Chest and Lung Disease** paralysis of the respiratory muscles (especially the intercostals and the diaphragm), myasthenia gravis thoracic deformities (kyphoscoliosis, thoracoplasty), scleroderma or burns of the thoracic wall, pulmonary fibrosis; **Abnormal Pulmonary Circulation** pericardial tamponade, pulmonary artery stenosis, arteriovenous shunts in heart and lungs, pulmonary thromboembolism and infarction, other emboli (fat, air, amniotic fluid), arteriolar stenosis (primary pulmonary hypertension, irradiation); **Oxyhemoglobin Deficiency** anemia, carbon monoxide poisoning (carboxyhemoglobinemia), methemoglobinemia and sulfhemoglobinemia, cyanide and cobalt poisoning; **Abnormal Respiratory Stimuli pain** from respiratory movements, exaggerated consciousness of respiration (effort syndrome), hyperventilation syndrome, secondary respiratory alkalosis (increased intracranial pressure, metabolic acidosis).

> **KEY SYMPTOM   Paroxysmal Dyspnea**

There is a transient increase in pulmonary capillary pressure associated with re-distribution of fluid from edematous extremities to the lungs with recumbency, or ischemia-induced transient decreases in LV performance. This is characterized by sudden paroxysms of breathlessness. When sleep is interrupted, it is termed *parox-ysmal nocturnal dyspnea*. These attacks are attended by orthopnea and coughing. The patient often finds that sitting or walking a few minutes relieves the dyspnea, permitting the patient to resume sleep.

> **KEY SYMPTOM   Shortness of Breath When Lying Down—Orthopnea**

Redistribution of extracellular fluid from the periphery to the lungs, elevation of the diaphragm from obesity or ascites, and muscular weakness all contribute to dyspnea when lying flat. The patient assumes a resting position with the head and chest elevated; the severity is estimated by the number of pillows required to achieve a comfortable position for sleep. Many patients awaken from sleep in the supine position severely short of breath (*paroxysmal nocturnal dyspnea*). Orthopnea is easily overlooked, if the physician does not specifically ask about it or observe the patient supine.

> **KEY SYMPTOM   Shortness of Breath When Standing Up—Platypnea**

Enlargement of arteriovenous shunts within the pulmonary circulation leads to increased right to left shunts with standing. The results are decreased oxygen saturation on standing (*orthodeoxia*) and shortness of breath. This is part of the *hepatopulmonary syndrome* (see page 396) seen in patients with advanced liver disease. Patients complain of shortness of breath and weakness on standing, relieved by sitting, or lying they have stigmata of advanced liver disease including cutaneous spiders and ascites due to portal hypertension.

Chest Wall Symptoms

> **KEY SYMPTOM   Chest Pain with Tenderness**

See Chest Wall Signs, pages 340.

Lung and Pleural Symptoms

> **KEY SYMPTOM   Shortness of Breath—Dyspnea**

See page 335.

> **KEY SYMPTOM   Respiratory Pain—Intercostal Neuralgia**

Irritation of an intercostal nerve produces sharp, lancinating, stabbing pain along the nerve's course. The pain is frequently intensified by respiratory motion, trunk movements or exposure to cold. Tenderness along the nerve is diagnostic. Usually the tenderness is maximal near the vertebral foramen, in the axilla, or at the parasternal line; these points correspond to the major cutaneous branches of the nerve. *CLINICAL OCCURRENCE:* Herpes zoster, diabetes mellitus, tabes dorsalis, mediastinal neoplasm, neurofibroma (an intercostal mass may be felt), vertebral tuberculosis or obesity with nerve stretching.

> **KEY SYMPTOM** Herpes Zoster (Shingles)

See Chapter 6, page 165. Zoster produces a specific type of intercostal neuralgia. There is sudden onset of the neuralgic pain followed by the appearance of vesicular skin lesions on an erythematous base.

> **KEY SYMPTOM** Cough

A cough is a sudden, forceful, noisy expulsion of air from the lungs. The three stages of coughing are preliminary inspiration, glottal closure and contraction of respiratory muscles, followed by sudden glottal opening to produce the outward blast of air. The sensory nerve endings for the cough reflex are branches of the vagus (CNX) in the larynx, trachea, and bronchi; but cough may also be induced by stimulation in the external acoustic meatus that is supplied by the auricular nerve (Arnold nerve), a branch of the vagus, or by esophageal stimulation by acid reflux. Stimuli for coughing include exudates in the pharynx or bronchial tree, irritation of foreign bodies, and inflammation. Coughing may be voluntary or involuntary, single or paroxysmal. A *productive cough* raises sputum. Chronic unexplained coughs are most commonly related to one or a combination of chronic post-nasal drip, gastroesophageal reflux or cough-variant asthma [Irwin RS, Madison JM. The diagnosis and treatment of cough. *N Engl J Med.* 2000;343:1715–1721]. **DDX:** A *brassy cough* is nonproductive with a strident quality; it occurs with narrowing of the trachea or glottal space, most commonly laryngitis or epiglottitis, but also laryngeal paralysis, neoplasm of the vocal cord, or aortic aneurysm. In pertussis, the cough is characterized by a long strident inspiratory noise, a *whoop*, preceding the cough.

✔ **COUGH—CLINICAL OCCURRENCE:** *Congenital* tracheoesophageal fistula, mediastinal teratoma; *Endocrine* substernal thyroid; *Idiopathic* emphysema; *Inflammatory/Immune* inhaled allergens, asthma, chronic bronchitis, vasculitis, Goodpasture syndrome, relapsing polychondritis, endobronchial amyloidoma; *Infectious* sinusitis, pharyngitis, laryngitis, epiglottitis, tracheobronchitis, pneumonia, bronchiectasis, lung abscess, subphrenic abscess, typhoid; *Metabolic/Toxic* tobacco smoking, inhaled irritants, angiotensin-converting enzyme inhibitors; *Mechanical/Trauma* cervical osteophytes, inhaled foreign bodies, acute and chronic aspiration, mediastinal mass and lymphadenopathy; *Neoplastic* cancer of the larynx and lung, endobronchial adenoma, thymoma, mediastinal lymphoma, metastases to the lung; *Neurologic* gastroesophageal reflux, tympanic membrane irritation; *Psychosocial* cough tics and habits; *Vascular* congestive heart failure (CHF), vasculitis (Wegener, Churg-Strauss), aortic aneurysm, pulmonary embolism and infarction, pulmonary hemorrhage.

> **KEY SYMPTOM** Chest Pain Intensified by Respiratory Motion

See Chest Syndromes, page 388.

Cardiovascular Symptoms

KEY SYMPTOM **Chest Pain**

See pages 333 and 400.

KEY SYMPTOM **Palpitation**

When the patient is conscious of heart action, whether fast or slow, regular or irregular, the term palpitation is applied. The sensation is usually described as "pounding," "fluttering," "flip-flopping," "skipping a beat," "missing a beat," "stopping," "jumping," or "turning over." The frequency, regularity, rate, and intensity depend on the underlying cause. The evaluation of palpitations begins with a detailed history. Have the patient indicate whether the sensation is a single "extra beat or pause" or a series of beats. If the latter, ask them to describe whether it starts and ends abruptly or gradually, whether it is fast or slow, and whether it is regular or irregular. Ask them to tap out the rhythm with their finger. Determine the circumstances when the palpitations occur and any associated symptoms that precede, accompany or follow the palpitations. Next, perform a physical examination and obtain an ECG. If you find no evidence of heart disease and the palpitations are well tolerated and not sustained, reassure your patient. Ambulatory monitoring is recommended in patients who tolerate the palpitations poorly, have heart disease or sustained palpitations. Although often caused by trivial disorders, palpitations often frighten the patient. Identification of the cause and careful explanation are often the only treatment necessary.

KEY SYMPTOM **Exertional Limb Pain—Claudication**

Exercising muscle has high oxygen and energy requirements; energy is stored, but oxygen must be continuously delivered to meet the increased demand. Inability to increase blood flow during exertion produces ischemic muscle pain relieved by rest. Anemia increases symptoms by loss of oxygen-carrying capacity, while polycythemia increases blood viscosity slowing capillary flow. The patient usually complains of calf pain at a fixed distance of walking that requires him to stop or sit for relief. It is consistently reproducible. Claudication can occur in any exercising muscle; be alert for reproducible exertional extremity or gluteal pain. Pulses are usually diminished or absent in the popliteal, dorsalis pedis, and/or posterior tibial arteries of the affected leg. **CLINICAL OCCURRENCE:** Atherosclerotic, thrombotic or embolic obstruction of major arteries to the lower extremity is most common. Exertional pain in the buttocks and/or thighs may represent true claudication or pseudoclaudication because of spinal stenosis. Predisposing factors are tobacco use and diabetes.

Unilateral Claudication in the Young—Popliteal Artery Entrapment Syndrome: Entrapment of the popliteal artery by the medial head of the gastrocnemius muscle is a congenital anomaly. A young person develops unilateral claudication, with absence of or diminished pulses in the ipsilateral popliteal and dorsalis pedis arteries.

Cold hands and/or feet. This common problem is probably caused by regional vasoconstriction to conserve heat. Examine carefully, for any diminution in the peripheral pulses or skin changes suggesting decreased nutrition. Absent of these findings, the patient can be reassured. The head is the greatest site of heat loss; have the patient wear a warm hat.

Chest, Cardiovascular and Respiratory Signs

Chest Wall Signs

> **KEY SIGN** **Abnormalities of the Thoracic Spine**

See Musculoskeletal Signs, Chapter 13, page 623, for a complete discussion. It is important to remember that deformities of the thoracic spine and chest wall may decrease chest compliance, severely limit respiratory excursions, and increase the work of breathing. In either *curved or angular kyphosis* (Fig. 8–28A), the spinal flexion may force the thorax to assume permanently the inspiratory position, with increased anteroposterior diameter and horizontal ribs. Although the thoracic distortion is identical to the barrel chest of pulmonary emphysema, the auscultatory signs of emphysema are absent. Conversely, accentuation of the lumbar curve throws the thoracic spine backward and the thoracic cage becomes flattened from the pull of the abdomen, causing an expiratory position to be assumed (Fig. 8–28B). Lateral curvature of the thoracic spine is usually accompanied by some rotation of the vertebral bodies, but only the lateral deviations of the spinous processes are visible (Fig. 8–28C). Minor functional scoliosis forms a single lateral curve, usually with convexity to the right. With

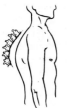
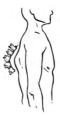
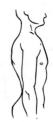

Curved Angular

A. Kyphosis

B. Lordosis

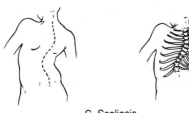

C. Scoliosis

Fig. 8–28 *Curvatures of the Spine Affecting the Thorax. A. Kyphotic thorax. B. Lordotic thorax. C. Scoliotic thorax.* Note the narrowing of the rib interspaces on the right and the accentuation of the interspaces, posterior humping of the chest, and elevation of the shoulder on the left.

structural changes, the lateral curve in the thorax produces an opposite compensatory curve inferiorly, so the line of spinous processes forms an S-shaped curve. The spinous processes always rotate toward the concave side. On the convex side, rotation of the vertebral bodies causes flattening of the ribs anteriorly and bulging of the chest posteriorly, lifting the shoulder and lowering the hip. Viewed from the patient's back, the posterior bulge is augmented with anteflexion of the spine.

> **KEY SIGN**   **Chest and Respiratory Pain with Tenderness**

The distinction between respiratory pain with tenderness and chest pain with tenderness is artificial; many conditions present in either manner, or with both pain at rest and with respirations. The patient may recognize the pain as superficial, sharp, and well localized. Almost always, this type of pain is accompanied by localized tenderness. The structures involved are the skin and subcutaneous tissues, the fat, skeleton, or the breasts. Careful examination of the chest discloses tenderness of specific structures.

Skin and Subcutaneous Structures: Inflammation, trauma, and neoplasm in these tissues offer no special diagnostic problems, provided that they are considered and searched for. The presence of bruises, lacerations, ulcers, hematomas, masses, trigger points or tenderness is usually diagnostic.

Chest wall pain.   Ask your patient to point to the region of pain. Next, perform four maneuvers: (1) Palpate the chest wall for tenderness by applying firm, steady pressure to the sternum, the costosternal junctions, the intercostal spaces, the ribs, and the pectoralis major muscles and their insertions; (2) adduct the arms horizontally by lifting one arm after the other by the elbow and pulling it across the chest toward the contralateral side, with the head rotated toward the ipsilateral side; (3) extend the neck by having the patient look toward the ceiling as the arms are pulled backward and slightly upward; and (4) exert vertical pressure on the head. If any of these tests reproduces the patient's pain, the problem is in the chest wall.

Costochondritis and Tietze Syndrome: This is a common cause of chest pain. The onset may be sudden or gradual. The pain is usually dull and may be intensified by respiratory motion and shoulder movements. The sole physical sign is tenderness at the costochondral junction. There is no swelling and there are no X-ray findings. In **Tietze syndrome**, the pain is accompanied by tender, fusiform swelling of one or more costicartilages, often that attached to the second rib. The overlying skin is reddened. Pain may radiate to the shoulder, neck, or arm. There is no lymphadenopathy. The pain may subside in a few weeks or persist for months while the swelling may persist after the pain and tenderness subside. The cause is unknown and the condition must be distinguished from osteitis, periostitis, rheumatic chondritis, and neoplasm of the ribs.

Rib Fracture: The diagnosis is readily made when the patient gives a history of trauma to the thorax, otherwise, the history may suggest pleurisy; ask about recent severe coughing. The patient complains of chest pain with breathing. Movement of rib fragments causes well-localized, sharp, lancinating pain. Inspiration is limited and palpation discloses point tenderness on a rib.

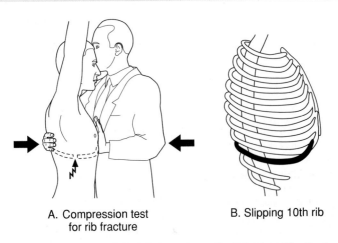

A. Compression test   B. Slipping 10th rib
for rib fracture

Fig. 8–29 *Examining for Rib Pain. A. Compression test for rib fracture. When the site of suspected rib fracture is located by point tenderness, the sternum is pushed toward the spine with one hand while the other hand supports the patient's back. The maneuver will elicit pain at the untouched fracture site. B. Slipping tenth rib. When the tenth rib lacks an anterior attachment, it can slip forward upon the ninth rib during respiratory movements and cause pain.*

The edges of the fracture may be felt, but bone crepitus is absent when the fragments are well opposed. With one hand supporting the back, compression of the sternum with the other elicits pain at the untouched fracture site (Fig. 8–29A).

Cough Fracture: Any rib from the second to the eleventh, most commonly the sixth, may break. The fracture is usually caused by a shearing force on the rib anterior to the serratus anterior attachment that pulls the rib upward, and posterior to the abdominal external oblique attachment that pulls the rib downward. Fracture results from structural fatigue (stress fracture) from repeated coughing. A patient who has been coughing for some time begins to experience pain with respiratory movements and coughing. The typical signs of fracture of a rib are present. If rib palpation is not performed, the condition may be misdiagnosed as pleurisy [Hanak V, Hartman TE, Ryu JH. Cough-induced rib fractures. *Mayo Clin Proc.* 2005;80:879–882].

Thrombophlebitis of the Thoracoepigastric Vein (Mondor Disease): The pain is felt along the anterolateral chest wall with radiation to the axilla or inguinal region. A tender cord, 3 to 4 mm in diameter, is usually palpable and often visible when the skin is stretched. The condition is self-limited and lasts 2 to 4 weeks.

Tender Muscle in the Thorax: Frequently, a tender muscle is mistaken by the patient and the physician for intrathoracic disease.

Adiposis Dolorosa (Dercum Disease) and Panniculitis: See Chapter 6, page 170.

Xiphisternal Arthritis: The pain may be ascribed to myocardial ischemia unless the xiphoid cartilage is palpated and the pain reproduced.

Periosteal Hematoma of Rib: There is well-localized severe pain and tenderness following direct trauma; fracture is expected, but not found on X-ray.

Periostitis of Ribs: Inflammation of the periosteum is extremely painful. Trauma or acute osteomyelitis produces periostitis with exquisite tenderness and severe sharp pain, often affected by motion and worse at night.

Slipping Cartilage: The interchondral ligament, most commonly between the ninth and tenth costicartilages, becomes weakened and elongated, or has been fractured, permitting the tenth rib to override the nineth with respiratory motion or movement. The slipping may be accompanied by an audible or palpable click (Fig. 8–29B). The slipping rib may cause pain, falsely attributed to intraabdominal disease.

Stitch Of The Intercostal Muscles: A sharp pain in the chest wall following severe exercise may be relieved by rest. The mechanism is unknown; it has been attributed to spasm of the diaphragm.

Intercostal Myositis: Severe aching pain, intensified by thoracic motion, results from inflammation of the intercostal muscles. The muscles are tender; induration and palpable nodules may ultimately appear.

Strain of the Pectoralis Minor: Irritation of this muscle from overuse, such as elevation of the arm, carrying a backpack, or lifting a baby, causes pain in the upper anterior lateral chest. The muscle is tender.

Shoulder Girdle Disorders: Shoulder disease may cause pain in the upper chest, augmented by arm and chest motion.

> **KEY SIGN** **Chest Pain with Dysesthesia—Herpes Zoster (Shingles)**

See page 165. The pain of zoster always precedes the rash by 2 to 3 days. Other causes of intercostal neuritis need to be considered until the diagnostic rash appears.

> **KEY SIGN** **Palpable Pleural Friction Rub**

The inflamed pleural surfaces lose their lubricating fluid ("dry pleurisy") and rub together during movements of the lungs. Sometimes the vibrations from the two rubbing surfaces can be felt, similar to that of two pieces of dry leather rubbing together. The rub is also heard with the stethoscope or the unaided ear as a creaking sound.

Rachitic rosary. The sternal ends of rachitic ribs bulge at their costochondral junctions. In severe cases of rickets, the outward bulging produces knobs at the costochondral junctions (Fig. 8–30A). The condition resolves completely with treatment.

Pigeon breast (pectus carinatum). During active rickets, the softened upper ribs bend inward, forcing the sternum forward increasing the anteroposterior dimension at the expense of the width. The sternum protrudes from the narrowed thorax like the keel of a ship (Fig. 8–30B). Vertical grooves are formed in the line of the costochondral junctions. This deformity persists after healing of the rickets. Pigeon breast also occurs in Marfan syndrome. Similar distortion occurs in severe primary kyphoscoliosis, but the sides of the thorax are not symmetric. Fusion

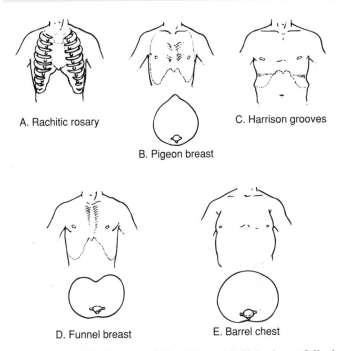

A. Rachitic rosary

B. Pigeon breast

C. Harrison grooves

D. Funnel breast

E. Barrel chest

Fig. 8–30 *Deformities of the Thorax. A. Rachitic rosary. B. Pigeon breast. C. Harrison grooves. D. Funnel breast. E. Barrel chest.*

abnormalities in the midline resembling pectus carinatum also occur in some forms of congenital heart disease.

Harrison Groove (Harrison Sulcus): During active rickets, the protuberant rachitic abdomen pushes the plastic lower ribs outward on a fulcrum formed by the costal attachments of the diaphragm. The line of bending forms a groove or sulcus in the rib cage, extending laterally from the xiphoid process, with flaring of the cage below the groove (Fig. 8–30C). The deformity remains when the rickets heals.

Funnel breast (pectus excavatum). The reverse of the pigeon breast, the lower costal cartilages, inferior sternum and xiphoid process are retracted toward the spine. In its rudimentary form, an oval pit occurs near the infrasternal notch. A more extensive distortion (Fig. 8–30D) is formed when the entire lower sternum sinks, significantly diminishing the anteroposterior dimension of the thoracic cavity. Rickets and Marfan syndrome are known causes, but many cases are unexplained.

Barrel chest. Both the anteroposterior and transverse dimensions of the thorax are enlarged, so the ribs become nearly perfect circles (Fig. 8–30E). Emphysema causes increased residual volume evident by increased anteroposterior diameter of the chest, horizontal ribs, depressed diaphragm, prolonged expiration, and decreased breath sounds. Kyphosis of the thoracic spine produces a similar position of the ribs, but lacks the lung signs of emphysema.

KEY SIGN Inspiratory Retraction of Interspaces

Airway obstruction or decreased lung compliance leads to inspiratory collapse of the intercostal spaces because of the excessively negative inspiratory intrapleural pressure. The inward intercostal movement is usually more evident in the lower thorax. Sudden, violent retractions occur in tracheal obstruction and severe paroxysms of asthma.

KEY SIGN Diminished Local Excursion of the Thorax

This points to a lesion in the underlying chest wall, pleura, or lung; causes include pain, fibrosis, or consolidation. The restricted movement may be best observed from the foot of the bed.

Diminished Local Excursion of the Thorax—Tension Pneumothorax: See page 390.

KEY SIGN Localized Bulging of the Thorax During Expiration—Flail Chest

Fracture of several contiguous ribs or the separation of several contiguous costal cartilages results in loss of chest wall integrity. The negative intrathoracic pressure during inspiration pulls the injured segment inward while the rise in intrathoracic pressure during expiration causes it to bulge outwards. The paradoxical chest movements decrease minute ventilation, and if extensive produces respiratory failure.

KEY SIGN Inspiratory Convergence of Costal Margins

When the dome of the diaphragm is flattened, the direction of its pull on the costal margins is changed from upward to inward. The degree of outward flare of the margins is lessened or, in extreme cases, the margins are pulled inward. Lowering of the diaphragm may be caused by pulmonary emphysema or by accumulations of fluid or air in the pleural space.

Exaggerated Costal Margin Flare During Inspiration: Elevation of the dome of the diaphragm increases the upward pull of the diaphragm during inspiration. The most common causes are hepatomegaly and subphrenic abscess.

KEY SIGN Lateral Deviations of the Trachea

Lateral tracheal deviation at the level of the suprasternal notch can be caused by a mass higher in the neck, such as cervical goiter or enlarged lymph nodes (see Fig. 7–64, page 279), or by mediastinal shifts within the chest. Below the suprasternal notch, a retrosternal goiter, eccentrically located, may push the trachea to one side. The trachea and mediastinum deviate to the opposite side with pleural effusion and tension pneumothorax. Displacement of the trachea to the ipsilateral side occurs in pulmonary atelectasis or fibrosis of the lung or pleura reducing lung volume.

KEY SIGN Fixation of the Trachea

While the patient's head is held in the customary position, the examiner palpates the cricoid cartilage or tracheal rings with the thumb and index finger and asks the patient to swallow. Normally, this lifts the larynx and trachea cephalad and there is considerable axial mobility. Grasp the trachea gently and move it side to side;

usually, it is easily mobile. Fixation of the trachea occurs normally when the neck is dorsiflexed, and abnormally in pulmonary emphysema, adhesive mediastinitis, aortic aneurysm, and mediastinal neoplasm.

➤ **KEY SIGN** **Subcutaneous and Mediastinal Emphysema**

Chest trauma may produce subcutaneous emphysema of the thoracic wall. Air may invade the chest wall from the neck or directly from the lung. Rupture of alveoli permits air to travel beneath the visceral pleura to the hilum of the lung, then along the trachea to the neck. The thoracic wall is involved secondarily by migration from the neck. When a fractured rib or penetrating foreign body punctures the pleura, air travels across the pleura to the thoracic wall causing emphysema in the deep muscle layers and later the subcutaneous tissues. Soft-tissue crepitus may be the first clue to rupture of the alveoli, pleura or esophagus. Crepitus is a sensation imparted to the pressing finger by small globules of air moving in the tissues. The air may invade the mediastinum, where it produces a distinctive systolic crunching in the precordium known as *Hamman sign*. Vomiting with esophageal rupture produces this sign. Compression of the soft tissues of the neck can occur, producing massive swelling of the neck and face accompanied by cyanosis.

Fluctuant intercostal masses.   These are usually abscesses. A cold abscess, so named because it lacks surrounding inflammation, is usually tuberculosis arising from a nearby rib. Actinomycosis frequently produces abscesses in the lung that burrow through the chest wall. An abscess may result when an untreated pleural empyema points through the interspaces, termed empyema necessitatis.

Rib mass.   Some causes of masses on ribs are callus around an old fracture or fibrous dysplasia, neoplasm of ribs (e.g., chondrosarcoma), myeloma, desmoid tumor, metastasis of carcinoma, angioma, eosinophilic granuloma, and bone cysts, including osteitis fibrosa cystica. A neurofibroma arising from an intercostal nerve causes a swelling near the neck of the rib. Imaging usually distinguishes the various lesions.

Thoracic wall sinuses.   Chronic sinuses discharging through the intercostal spaces may result from a variety of conditions, including empyema, tuberculosis, actinomycosis, and rib necrosis. Actinomycosis produces a sinus with a peculiar dusky color around its mouth.

Pulsating sternoclavicular joint.   This sign denotes an enlarged major vascular structure impinging on the manubrium posteriorly. It is seen with dissection of the aortic arch, ruptured saccular aortic aneurysm, persistent right aortic arch or fusiform aneurysms of the innominate, carotid, or subclavian artery.

Lung, Pleura, and Respiratory Signs
Inspection

KEY SIGN **Shortness of Breath—Dyspnea**

See page 335.

KEY SIGN **Hiccup**

Hiccup is a sudden, involuntary diaphragmatic contraction producing an inspiration interrupted by glottal closure causing a characteristic sharp sound. It is thought to be mediated centrally through the phrenic nerve, by direct stimulation of the phrenic nerve, or by direct irritation of the diaphragm. The contractions occur two or three times each minute. A variety of clinical conditions are associated with hiccup prompting the inference that it may be initiated centrally or peripherally.

✔ *HICCOUGH—CLINICAL OCCURRENCE:*   *Hiccough Without Organic Disease*   excessive laughter, tickling, aerophagia, tobacco smoking, intake of alcohol, hysteria (persisting for weeks, but ceasing during sleep); *Diseases of the Central Nervous System*   encephalitis, meningitis, vertebrobasilar ischemia, intracranial hemorrhage, intracranial tumor, uremia, degenerative changes in brain and medulla, tabes dorsalis; *Mediastinal Disorders*   trauma to phrenic nerve, enlargement of mediastinal lymph nodes (tuberculosis, malignant neoplasm, fibrosis), bronchial obstruction, adherent pericardium, cardiac enlargement, myocardial infarction, esophageal obstruction; *Pleural Irritation*   pneumonia with pleurisy; *Diaphragmatic and Abdominal Disorders*   diaphragmatic hernia of stomach, subphrenic abscess, subphrenic peritonitis, hepatic neoplasm, gumma or abscess, carcinoma of stomach, splenic infarction, acute intestinal obstruction, acute hemorrhagic pancreatitis, after operations in the upper abdomen, diaphragmatic stimulation by an implanted cardiac pacemaker.

KEY SIGN   Hemoptysis

Spitting or coughing of blood is hemoptysis. The bleeding lesion may be anywhere from the nose to the alveoli. Expectorated blood usually comes from the upper respiratory tract while blood in the bronchial tree induces coughing. However, the patient may not be able to distinguish which of the two is occurring, so both upper and lower respiratory tract disorders must be considered.

✔ *HEMOPTYSIS—CLINICAL OCCURRENCE:*   *Upper Respiratory Tract*   epistaxis, bleeding from the oropharynx, gum bleeding, laryngitis, laryngeal carcinoma, hereditary hemorrhagic telangiectasia; *Bronchial Tree*   acute and chronic bronchitis, trauma from coughing, bronchiectasis, bronchial carcinoma, broncholiths, foreign body aspiration, erosion by aortic aneurysms; *Lungs*   infections (pneumonia, especially caused by *Klebsiella*, lung abscess, tuberculosis, fungal infections, amebiasis, hydatid cyst), pulmonary embolism with infarction, trauma, pulmonary hemorrhage (vasculitis especially Wegener, Goodpasture syndrome), idiopathic pulmonary hemosiderosis, lipoid pneumonia; *Cardiovascular*   mitral stenosis, CHF, arteriovenous fistula, anomalous pulmonary artery, hypertension; *Hematologic*   thrombocytopenia, leukemia, hemophilia.

KEY SIGN   Snoring

Snoring is the common and harmless noise produced by vibrations of the lax soft palate during sleep. It also occurs in association with obstructive sleep apnea (see Chapter 5, page 72). A similar sound results from vibrations of secretions in the upper respiratory tract. When this occurs during severe illness, it is frequently a grave prognostic sign, the "death rattle."

➤ KEY SIGN   Stridor

A high-pitched whistling or crowing sound is caused by passage of air through the partly closed glottis. It occurs in edema of the vocal cords, neoplasm, diphtheritic membrane, abscess of the pharynx, and foreign body in the larynx or trachea. It may signal impending airway closure and asphyxiation.

Vibratory Palpation

> **KEY SIGN** **Diminished or Absent Vocal Fremitus**

Damped transmission of vibrations occurs when lung tissue is destroyed, the pleura is thickened or the pleural surfaces are separated by air or fluid. Blockage of the airways results in absent vocal fremitus. The interposition of filters of variable quality such as thickened pleura, pleural effusion, pneumothorax or loss of lung parenchyma (e.g., emphysema) obstructs transmission of vibration through the chest wall, with diminished or absent vocal fremitus.

> **KEY SIGN** **Increased Vocal Fremitus**

Increased tension in the lung septa increases transmission of vibrations. Consolidated tissue in pneumonia or inflammation around a lung abscess, when in contact with a bronchus or cavity in the lung, transmits bronchotracheal air vibrations with greater efficiency than do the air-filled pulmonary alveoli; hence, vocal fremitus is increased.

Sonorous Percussion

> **KEY SIGN** **Normal Dullness in the Lateral Decubitus Position**

When the patient cannot sit, percuss the back with the patient on one side then the other. The position is not optimal because it is difficult to interpret the percussion sounds. The damping effect of the mattress causes a band of dullness in the part of the thorax nearest the bed (Fig. 8–31). Directly above this band is an irregular area of dullness caused by compression of the downward lung by the body weight. If there is a lengthwise sag of the mattress from the body weight, it flexes the spine laterally compressing the thoracic wall and lung in the upward hemithorax, producing another area of dullness.

> **KEY SIGN** **Abnormal Sonorous Percussion**

An abnormal distribution of sounds of normal quality can be pathologic. The lung is normally resonant. As consolidation occurs its density increases to yield,

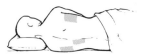

Fig. 8–31 *Areas of Percussion Dullness Created by the Lateral Decubitus Position.* *The lowest blue-shaded area is dull from compression of the thorax against the mattress. Immediately above, dullness is produced by compression of the lung from the body weight. In the opposite lung, dullness results by lateral deviation of the spine as it follows the sag in the mattress and compresses the lung.*

successively, impaired resonance, dullness, and flatness. The normal pleura contributes little to the percussion note, but a thickened pleura produces dullness. Fluid in the pleural cavity gives dullness to flatness in a dependent distribution.

Dullness Replacing Resonance in the Upper Lung: This finding suggests neoplasm, atelectasis or consolidation.

Dullness Replacing Resonance in the Lower Lung: Pleural effusion, pleural thickening, and elevation of the diaphragm are specific to this area; neoplasm, atelectasis and consolidation are other causes.

Flatness Replacing Resonance or Dullness: Almost invariably, flatness in the thorax results from massive pleural effusion.

Hyperresonance Replacing Resonance or Dullness: When hyperresonance replaces resonance or the area of hepatic and cardiac dullness is resonant or hyperresonant, emphysema, pneumothorax or the interposition of gas filled gut are suggested.

Tympany Replacing Resonance: This occurs almost exclusively with a large pneumothorax.

Auscultation of Breath Sounds

Several types of breath sounds with distinctive qualities are recognized. All are characterized by rising pitch during inspiration and falling pitch during expiration (Doppler effect). The duration and force of inspiration and expiration affect the breath sounds.

> **KEY SIGN** **Normal Breath Sounds—Vesicular Breathing**

Tidal breathing during quiet respirations produces vesicular breath sounds characterized by a longer inspiratory than expiratory phase (Fig. 8–32). They are heard normally over the entire lung surface, except beneath the manubrium and in the upper interscapular region, where we hear bronchovesicular sounds. The breath sounds are faintest over the thinner portions of the lungs.

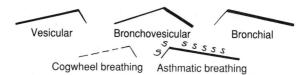

Fig. 8–32 _Distinguishing Features of Breath Sounds._ _In the diagrams, the vertical component indicates rising and falling pitch, the thickness of the lines indicates loudness, and the horizontal distance represents duration. Inspiration is longer in vesicular breathing, expiration in bronchial breathing. Bronchovesicular breathing is a mixture of the two. Normally vesicular breathing is heard over most of the lungs, except that bronchovesicular breathing occurs over the thoracic portion of the trachea, anteriorly and posteriorly. Bronchial breathing does not occur in the normal lung. In cogwheel breathing, the inspiratory sound is interrupted with multiple breaks. Asthmatic breathing is characterized by a much prolonged and higher-pitched expiratory sound than is found in bronchial breathing. Asthmatic breathing is usually, but not always, accompanied by wheezes._

Cogwheel Breathing: This is identical with vesicular breathing except that the inspiratory phase is broken by short pauses, giving the impression of jerkiness (Fig. 8–32). The pauses are attributed to irregular inflation of the alveoli; it has no pathologic significance.

KEY SIGN   Bronchovesicular Breathing

Bronchovesicular breathing is pathologic and indicates a small degree of pulmonary consolidation or compression that transmits sounds from the bronchial tree with increased facility. As the name indicates, this is intermediate between vesicular and bronchial breathing. The two respiratory phases are about equal in duration (Fig. 8–32), although expiration is frequently a bit longer. Normally, it is heard at the manubrium and in the upper interscapular region. As the degree of compression or consolidation increases, bronchovesicular breathing becomes bronchial.

KEY SIGN   Bronchial Breathing (Tubular Breathing)

This results from consolidation or compression of lung facilitating sound transmission from the bronchi. In contrast to vesicular breathing, bronchial breath sounds have a shorter inspiratory than expiratory phase (Fig. 8–32). They are usually louder, but this is not diagnostic. Bronchial breathing does not occur in the normal lung. The closest normal counterpart is tracheal breathing, heard in the suprasternal notch and over the sixth and seventh cervical spines; it is harsher and hollower than true bronchial breathing.

KEY SIGN   Wheezes

Wheezes arise from turbulent airflow and the vibration of small airways in which there is partial obstruction to airflow. Wheezes are heard predominantly during expiration. They occur when airways are narrowed by bronchospasm, edema, collapse, or by intraluminal secretions, neoplasm, or foreign body. They are diffuse in asthma and bronchitis, usually accompanying a prolonged expiratory phase of respiration. An isolated wheeze heard in just one area may signal bronchial obstruction by a tumor or foreign body. Wheezing is neither sensitive nor specific for detecting airflow obstruction.

Asthmatic or Obstructive Breathing: Like bronchial breathing, inspiration is short and expiration prolonged, but there is no confusing the two (Fig. 8–33). In asthma, the expiratory phase is several times longer than in bronchial breathing, and the pitch is much higher. The listener is aware that expiration is active, not passive, and may require significant effort. Frequently, but not always, asthmatic breathing is accompanied by wheezes audible without the stethoscope. Emphysema produces a similar pattern of breath sounds, but wheezing is absent and the sound intensity is diminished.

KEY SIGN   Crackles (Rales)

Crackles result from the opening and closing of alveoli and small airways during respiration. In pulmonary edema, fine crackles may be produced by air bubbling through fluid in the distal small airways. Inspiratory crackles resemble the sound of several hairs being rubbed together between thumb and forefinger. They are heard in the bases of patients with interstitial lung disease, fibrosing alveolitis, atelectasis, pneumonia, bronchiectasis, and pulmonary edema, and in the apices with tuberculosis.

KEY SIGN   Rhonchus

Rhonchi occur as low-pitched gurgling sounds when there is liquid within the larger airways from inflammatory secretions or drowning and in agonal states (death rattle). They clear or change significantly after an effective cough.

Metamorphosing Breathing: The breath sounds suddenly change in intensity during different parts of the respiratory cycle. This is usually caused by movement of a loose bronchial plug.

KEY SIGN   Amphoric Breathing

This sound is produced by a large empty superficial cavity communicating with a bronchus or an open pneumothorax. Amphoric breath sounds sound like blowing air over the mouth of a large bottle. When the pitch is relatively low and the sound hollow, it is called cavernous breathing.

Auscultation of Voice Sounds

KEY SIGN   Voice Sounds

In the normal lungs whispered words are faint and their syllables indistinct, except over the main bronchi. Increasing loudness and distinctness indicate consolidation, atelectasis, or fibrosis, all of which improve sound transmission. Because of their pitch and loudness, whispered and spoken voice sounds are more useful than breath sounds in detecting pulmonary consolidation, infarction, and atelectasis. Spoken voice sounds are not as useful as whispered sounds since they are too loud for careful discrimination.

Whispered Pectoriloquy: Consolidated lung transmits whispered syllables distinctly, even when the pathologic process is too small to produce bronchial breathing. This sign is particularly valuable in detecting early pneumonia, infarction, and pulmonary atelectasis.

Bronchophony: Spoken syllables are normally heard indistinctly. With lung consolidation syllables are distinct and sound close to the ear.

Egophony: This is a form of bronchophony in which the spoken "Eee" is changed to "Ay," with a peculiar nasal or bleating quality. This arises from compressed lung below a pleural effusion, and occasionally with lung consolidation.

Auscultation of Abnormal Sounds

Abnormal sounds, including crackles (rales), wheezes, rhonchi, rubs, and bruits, are heard in the lungs of patients with various illnesses. In patients with pulmonary complaints, they should be actively searched for with normal and deep breathing, both before and after coughing, and with forced expiration.

> **KEY SIGN** Rubs (Pleural Friction Rub)

Pleural friction rubs occur when inflamed, surfaces of pleurae rub together during respiration. They are characterized as the "creaking of new leather." Listen at the spot where the patient feels pleuritic pain. Rubs may be ephemeral and disappear after several respiratory cycles.

> **KEY SIGN** Continuous Murmur

The continuous murmur of a pulmonary arteriovenous fistula increases in intensity with inspiration. In patients with coarctation of the aorta, continuous murmurs may be heard below the left scapula and over the intercostal and internal mammary arteries from the collateral circulation. These are rare findings.

Bone crepitus. The movements of fractured ends of a rib may produce a grating sound, leading to a correct diagnosis.

Systolic Popping, Clicking, or Crunching Sounds: Hamman Sign; see page 406.

Interpretation of Pulmonary and Pleural Signs

The findings of thoracic inspection, palpation, percussion, and auscultation must be synthesized to suggest a pathophysiologic process or diagnosis. The signs of altered lung density serve as a starting point for the differential diagnosis. It is especially useful to draw a chest diagram like those in Figures 8–33 and 8–34 to help synthesize your findings and hypotheses.

> **KEY SIGN** Dullness and Diminished Vibrations—Pleural Effusion or Pleural Thickening

Unless the fluid is loculated, dullness always occurs in the lowermost part of the thorax (Fig. 8–33, left). Because the costophrenic sulcus is higher in front, the dull region is a transverse band broadest posteriorly and laterally. The superior border of the dullness may be difficult to percuss accurately because the fluid

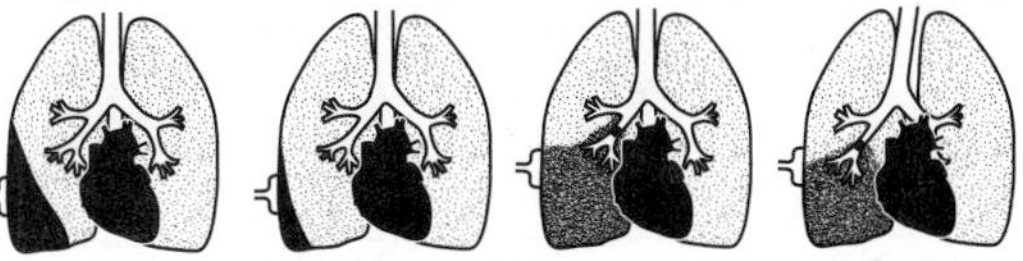

	Small pleural effusion	Pleural thickening	Consolidation and bronchial plug	Atelectasis and bronchial plug
Tracheal deviation	O	O or ←	O	←
Fremitus	V or O	V	O	O
Percussion	Dull	Dull	Dull	Dull
Breath sounds	V	V	V or O	O
Whisper sounds	V	V	V or O	O
Voice sounds	V	V	V or O	O
Rales	O	O	O	O

Fig. 8–33 *Thoracic Disorders with Dullness and Diminished Vibration.* ◯, absent; ∨, diminished; ∧, increased; ←, direction of deviation.

layer is an upward-pointing wedge. Shifting dullness is not usually demonstrable. Since air is absent, there is no succession splash. With a small amount of fluid, thoracic respiratory excursions are normal. In pleurisy, an antecedent friction rub disappears when fluid forms. Pleural fluid baffles vibrations from the bronchotracheal air column, so vocal fremitus, breath sounds, whispered and spoken voice are transmitted poorly to the stethoscope. The mediastinum is not shifted with small pleural effusions. Unless the fluid has recently appeared, the signs cannot be distinguished from thickened pleura. Because pleural fibrosis results from the organization of pleural effusion, the distribution of dullness is the same. The pleura may attain a thickness of 5 or 6 cm. The thicker it is, the more it obstructs sound transmission and the more the percussion note indicates denseness. Extensive fibrosis may pull the trachea to the affected side. Ultrasound and decubitus radiography distinguish the two. Any longstanding pleural effusion may organize. Neoplastic involvement may simulate thickening. Asbestosis and/or mesothelioma may cause thickening.

KEY SIGN   Dullness and Diminished Vibrations—Pleural Fluid

Fluid accumulates in the pleural space due to transudation of fluid from the pleural and pulmonary vessels (increased venous hydrostatic pressure, decreased oncotic pressure, capillary leak), increased production of pleural fluid (inflamed pleura or pleural neoplasm), decreased pleural absorption of fluid (lymphatic obstruction, systemic venous hypertension), or by bleeding into the pleural space. The pleural fluid produces a dull or flat note to percussion. The lung immediately over the fluid may be hyperresonant (*skodaic resonance*) from distention of the alveoli above a compressed region. The distribution of dullness is dependent. With large amounts of fluid, the trachea may be pushed to the unaffected side (Fig. 8–34). Vocal fremitus is absent. Occasionally, loud bronchial breathing is heard through the fluid from the compressed lung; the unwary mistake it for consolidation. Fluid is distinguished from consolidation by noting diminished breath sounds and absence of fremitus with fluid, and bronchial breath sounds

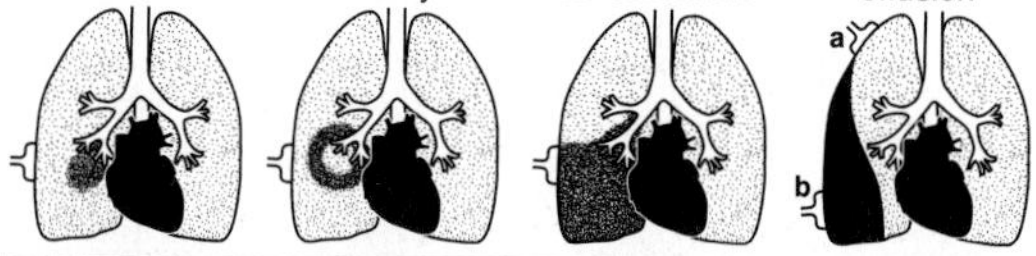

	Small consolidation	Thick-walled cavity	Massive consolidation	Large pleural effusion
Tracheal deviation	O	O	O	→
Fremitus	N or ∧	N or ∧	∧	O
Percussion	Slight dullness	Slight dullness	Dull or flat	(a) Hyperresonant (b) Flat
Breath sounds	Bronchovescular or bronchial	Bronchovescular or amorphic	Bronchial	O or loud bronchial
Whisper sounds	N, O, or ∧	Pectoriloquy	∧	O or ∧
Voice sounds	N, O, or ∧	∧	∧	O or ∧
Rales	+ or O	+	+	O

Fig. 8–34 *Thoracic Disorders with Dullness and Accentuated Vibration.* *O, absent; N, normal; +, present; , increased; →, direction of deviation.*

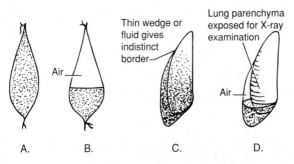

Fig. 8–35 *Models Illustrating Pleural Effusion and Pneumothorax. **A.** Suspend a plastic bag filled with water, noting its contour. **B.** When air is introduced, a fluid level forms, the contour changes, and a succussion splash occurs with shaking. **C.** An Uncomplicated Pleural Effusion: Note the tapering upper wedge, or meniscus, of fluid. **D.** Hydropneumothorax: When air is introduced, a fluid level forms and the meniscus largely disappears.*

with "E" to "A" changes in consolidation. Massive pleural effusion obscures the lung fields on radiographs, so that no appraisal of the parenchyma is possible. With a hydropneumothorax, when the patient stands, the fluid level falls below much of the lung, permitting visualization of the lung (Fig. 8–35) [Case with differential diagnosis: Case records of the Massachusetts General Hospital. Case 8-2002. *N Engl J Med.* 2002;346:843–850]. ***CLINICAL OCCURRENCE:*** *Increased Transudation* CHF, hypoalbuminemia (cirrhosis, nephrotic syndrome), pulmonary embolism, SVC syndrome; *Increased Production* mesothelioma, metastatic cancer, infections (bacteria, mycobacteria, viral, parasites, fungi), pulmonary infarction, pancreatitis, mediastinitis, collagen-vascular diseases (e.g., RA, systemic lupus erythematosus [SLE], drug-induced lupus, vasculitis), after heart or lung surgery, uremia, Meigs syndrome, pleuropericarditis peritoneal dialysis; *Decreased Absorption* lymphatic obstruction (lymphoma, lymphatic carcinomatosis, irradiation, surgical injury), CHF, SVC syndrome; *Bleeding* ruptured aortic aneurysm or dissection, trauma, postoperative.

KEY SIGN **Dullness and Diminished Vibration—Pulmonary Consolidation with Bronchial Plugging**

The consolidated lung produces dullness. Bronchial plugging blocks vibrations from the air column, so there is absence of vocal fremitus, breath sounds, whispered and spoken voice (Fig. 8–33, middle right). The trachea is not displaced. Plugging of a bronchus is usually a transitory occurrence in lobar pneumonia, so it is recognized by the sudden loss of air transmission. Imaging can distinguish between pleural effusion and pulmonary consolidation. If the dullness is in the upper lobe, effusion is excluded on physical examination.

KEY SIGN **Dullness with Diminished Vibration—Atelectasis with Bronchial Plug**

The volume of the atelectatic lung is diminished; with considerable lung involvement, the dense mass is pulled toward the chest wall by the negative intrapleural pressure shifting the trachea to the affected side. The collapsed lung is dull because its density is increased. The bronchial plug prevents transmission of air vibration, so vocal fremitus and breath and voice sounds are absent (Fig. 8–33, right). The tracheal deviation distinguishes atelectasis from consolidation with bronchial plug and from pleural effusion. Often, atelectasis is accompanied by fever that distinguishes it from thickened pleura with fibrotic traction on the mediastinum. Similar findings of dullness and decreased breath sounds at the tip of the left scapula can be caused by a large pericardial effusion compressing the LLL (*Ewart's sign*).

> **KEY SIGN**   **Dullness with Accentuated Vibration—Pneumonia with Small Consolidation**

A small, deeply placed region of consolidation may produce impaired resonance or dullness, depending on its size and depth from the chest wall. The dense lung transmits the air column with increased facility, so vocal fremitus is increased and bronchovesicular or bronchial breathing and crackles may be heard (Fig. 8–34, left). Symptoms of fever, chills, and productive cough are accompanied by tachypnea and tachycardia. Whispered pectoriloquy and bronchophony are produced by the consolidation. Small regions of consolidation must be distinguished from a small cavity lying near a bronchus. Imaging is required for definitive diagnosis. Pneumonia, granulomatous infiltrates of the lung, neoplasm about a bronchus, rheumatoid arthritis (RA), and sarcoidosis may all produce these findings.

> **KEY SIGN**   **Dullness with Accentuated Vibration—Pneumonia with Lobar Consolidation**

The dense lung yields dullness or flatness on percussion. The consolidated lung in contact with a bronchus transmits vibrations with increased facility, so vocal fremitus is pronounced, there is bronchial breathing, and whispered and spoken voice produce pectoriloquy and bronchophony (Fig. 8–34, middle right). Crackles (rales) are frequently present. The lung volume is unchanged, so the trachea remains in the midline. Occasionally consolidation may be confused with a thick-walled cavity, and the distinction must be made by imaging. These finding are seen classically in lobar pneumonia but occasionally in neoplasms of the lung and pulmonary infarction. Massive pleural effusion gives dullness and may transmit loud bronchial breath sounds above the effusion, but the trachea is usually displaced to the unaffected side.

> **KEY SIGN**   **Dullness with Accentuated Vibration—Thick-walled Cavity**

The signs of pulmonary consolidation are present: dullness, increased vocal fremitus, bronchovesicular breathing, and pectoriloquy (Fig. 8–34, middle left). Usually distinctive, but most infrequent, is amphoric breathing or cracked-pot resonance. Even these signs may be present in consolidation without cavity.

> **KEY SIGN**   **Resonance and Hyperresonance—Pulmonary Emphysema**

Loss of interstitial elasticity and interalveolar septa leads to air trapping, so the volume of the lungs is increased. The air trapping holds the chest in the inspiratory position, producing a barrel chest. The diaphragm is flattened, so the costal margins move out sluggishly or actually converge during inspiration (Fig. 8–36, left). The lungs are hyperresonant throughout because of their low density. Air pockets are poor transmitters of vibrations; thus vocal fremitus, breath sounds, heart sounds, and whispered and spoken voice are impaired or absent. When the breath sounds are audible, they are faint and harsh, distinctively lacking the rustling quality of vesicular breathing; this may antedate recognizable X-ray evidence of emphysema. The expiratory phase of respiration usually exceeds the inspiratory phase. Rales are not necessarily present and wheezes are not heard. The elevated clavicles and flattened diaphragm grue rise to two signs: the thyroid cartilege appears to be low in a shortened neck and it descends less than 4 cm toward the suprasternal notch with full inspiration. Also the thyroid is often in a retrosternal position and not palpable.

KEY SIGN   Resonance or Hyperresonance—Closed Pneumothorax

When the air leak between lung and pleura becomes sealed a closed pneumothorax is formed. If the volume of enclosed air is small, the lung remains partially inflated and the mediastinum is not displaced (Fig. 8–36, middle left). In an open pneumothorax, a similar situation may be created by pleural adhesions, which prevent collapse of the lung and displacement of the trachea. Vocal fremitus, breath sounds, and whispered and spoken voice are usually inaudible or impaired. The chest wall is resonant or hyperresonant. Frequently, pneumothorax cannot be distinguished from a normal or emphysematous chest by percussion. A disparity between the breath sounds on the two sides suggests pneumothorax on the quieter side. There may be a pendular deviation of the trachea toward the affected side during inspiration. The tear in the pleura may be spontaneous or the

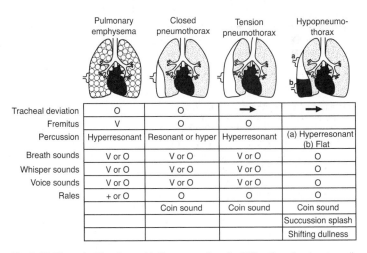

	Pulmonary emphysema	Closed pneumothorax	Tension pneumothorax	Hypopneumothorax
Tracheal deviation	O	O	→	→
Fremitus	V	O	O	
Percussion	Hyperresonant	Resonant or hyper	Hyperresonant	(a) Hyperresonant (b) Flat
Breath sounds	V or O	V or O	V or O	O
Whisper sounds	V or O	V or O	V or O	O
Voice sounds	V or O	V or O	V or O	O
Rales	+ or O	O	O	O
		Coin sound	Coin sound	Coin sound
				Succussion splash
				Shifting dullness

Fig. 8–36 *Thoracic Disorders with Resonance Impaired Vibration.* ◯, *absent;* ∨, *diminished;* +, *present;* →, *direction of deviation.*

result of trauma to the thorax [Sahn SA, Heffner JE. Spontaneous pneumothorax. *N Engl J Med*. 2000;342:868–874].

➤   **KEY SIGN**   **Resonance or Hyperresonance—Open Pneumothorax**

With continual communication between lung and pleural cavity, the air in the open pneumothorax is under atmospheric pressure. The collapse of the affected lung is complete, and the mediastinum may be drawn toward the unaffected side by the contraction of the normal lung. Overlying the pneumothorax, the chest wall is hyperresonant or tympanitic. Fremitus and breath and voice sounds are absent. Usually, the patient is severely dyspneic and may be cyanotic.

➤   **KEY SIGN**   **Resonance or Hyperresonance—Tension Pneumothorax**

A one-way tissue valve permits air to be forced into the pleural space during inspiration and prevents its expulsion during expiration. Thus, the pressure in the cavity builds up in excess of the atmosphere. The affected lung is collapsed and the increasing intrapleural pressure causes extreme tracheal deviation, compression of the unaffected lung, and decreased venous return to the heart (Fig. 8–36, middle left). The signs of decreased respiratory excursion of a distended tympanitic hemithorax combined with tracheal deviation away from the immobile side are diagnostic of pneumothorax with tension. This situation is accompanied by deep cyanosis, severe dyspnea, and shock that demands aspiration of air from the cavity as a lifesaving measure.

KEY SIGN   **Resonance and Hyperresonance—Hydropneumothorax**

Hyperresonance or tympany in the upper part of the thorax, with dullness inferiorly, suggests either hydropneumothorax or a massive pleural effusion (Fig. 8–36, right). In either case, the trachea may be displaced to the unaffected side. In hydropneumothorax, the hyperresonant region does not transmit fremitus, breath sounds, or voice sounds, whereas the lung over a simple hydrothorax transmits well. When hydropneumothorax is present, the fluid level can be sharply demarcated by percussion; the level is vague in simple effusion. Shifting dullness is readily demonstrated by percussion in the presence of hydropneumothorax; this is not the case in hydrothorax. The air-filled cavity carries bell tympany, and a succession splash may be demonstrated.

Special Sounds in Hydropneumothorax: Fluid movement is silent in a cavity devoid of air. When the cavity contains both air and fluid, body movements cause a succussion splash, audible to the patient and the examiner. Grasp the patient's shoulders shaking the thorax while listening with and without a stethoscope. An abdominal *succussion splash* is present in the normal and dilated stomach. A thoracic succussion splash suggests a hydropneumothorax, but a fluid-filled stomach herniating into the thorax through a diaphragmatic hernia may also produce the splash. Occasionally, one hears a *falling-drop sound,* resembling a drop of water hitting the surface of fluid; it is occasionally encountered in the collapsed lung. A metallic tinkle may be heard when air bubbles emerge through a small bronchopleural fistula below the fluid level; when the fistula is larger, the air may gurgle, a *lung-fistula sound.*

Sputum Signs

KEY SIGN   Bloody Sputum: Hemoptysis

Blood in the sputum usually impresses patients enough to bring them to the physician. First identify the anatomic site of hemorrhage.   *Blood-Streaked Sputum* is usually caused by inflammation in the nose, nasopharynx, gums, larynx, or bronchi. Sometimes it occurs only after severe paroxysms of coughing and is attributed airway trauma. Pink Sputum results from blood mixing with secretions in the alveoli or smaller bronchioles; it is most characteristic of pneumonia and pulmonary edema.   *Massive Bleeding*   occurs with erosion of a bronchial artery by cavitary tuberculosis, aspergilloma, lung abscess, bronchiectasis, embolism with infarction, bronchogenic carcinoma or a broncholith.   *Alveolar Hemorrhage* does not produce bloody sputum in all cases; it results from pulmonary vasculitis of any cause and blunt chest trauma.

Bloody Gelatinous (Currant-Jelly) Sputum: Copious quantities of tenacious, bloody sputum are almost pathognomonic for pneumonia caused by *Klebsiella pneumoniae* or *Streptococcus pneumoniae*.

Rusty Sputum: Purulent sputum containing degraded blood pigment is typical of pneumococcal pneumonia but it is frequently preceded by small amounts of frank blood.

KEY SIGN   Frothy Sputum—Pulmonary Edema

Fluid from the pulmonary capillaries enters the alveoli and is expectorated. A thin secretion containing air bubbles, frequently colored with hemoglobin, is typical of pulmonary edema. Both acute lung injury and LV failure produce this sign.

KEY SIGN   Purulent Sputum

Inflammatory cells, predominately polymorphonuclear leukocytes, enter the airways and alveoli in response to lower airway infection. The exudate may be yellow, green, or dirty gray. Small amounts are typical of acute bronchitis, pneumonia during resolution, small tuberculous cavities or lung abscess. Copious purulent sputum occurs with lung abscess, bronchiectasis, or bronchopleural fistula communicating with an empyema. Fetid sputum is characteristic of anaerobic infection and/or lung abscess. Many lung abscesses do not yield much sputum because their bronchial communications are inadequate for complete drainage. In bronchiectasis, the daily volume is often from 200 to 500 mL. On standing, bronchiectatic sputum typically separates into three layers, with mucus on top separated by clear fluid from pus on the bottom. Copious sputum from a patient with signs of pleural effusion suggests a bronchopleural fistula.

Stringy mucoid sputum.   Increased mucous production and formation of mucous plugs occur in asthma; during resolution of an acute attack, retained mucous and mucous plugs are mobilized.

Broncholiths.   Calcified particles found in the sputum are usually broncholiths. They are derived from calcified lymph nodes eroding the bronchi or from calcareous granulomas in silicosis, tuberculosis, or histoplasmosis. They may explain the source of pulmonary hemorrhage [Harris NL, McNeely WF, et al.

Case 14-2002. Case Records of the Massachusetts General Hospital. *N Engl J Med.* 2002;346:1475–1482].

Cardiovascular Signs

The physical signs from inspection, palpation, and percussion of the precordium depend for their interpretation on relatively normal anatomic relations between the heart and the chest wall. In gross distortions of the thoracic cage, such as kyphoscoliosis, funnel breast, or thoracoplasty, conclusions must be formed cautiously.

Inspection

> **KEY SIGN** **Dyspnea (Shortness of Breath)**

See page 355.

> **KEY SIGN** **Pallor**

See Chapter 6, page 144.

> **KEY SIGN** **Cyanosis**

See Chapter 6, page 144.

Palpation

> **KEY SIGN** **Edema**

Extracellular fluid (saline) is partitioned between blood and interstitial tissues by a net equilibrium between hydrostatic and oncotic pressures. Normally, fluid flows into the extravascular interstitial space in response to hydrostatic pressure in the precapillary arterioles and capillaries (intravascular > interstitial), which is only partially offset by the opposing oncotic pressure (intravascular > interstitial). In the postcapillary venules, the lowered intravascular hydrostatic pressure is more than compensated by the intravascular oncotic pressure, resulting in return of interstitial saline to the intravascular space. Interstitial fluid, proteins, and cells are also removed from the interstitial space and, ultimately, returned to the blood through the lymphatics. Alteration of any of these forces upsets the equilibrium. An increase in the systemic venous pressure in CHF produces dependent edema; occlusion of a vein may result in localized edema. Obstruction of lymphatic channels produces lymphedema. Reduction in the plasma albumin (the plasma protein with the highest contribution to oncotic pressure) results in lowering the oncotic pressure of the plasma, permitting edema to form; this type of edema may first appear in areas of decreased tissue pressure such as the periorbital tissues. Increased capillary permeability may cause edema that is not dependent. Tissue inflammation by bacterial, chemical, thermal, or mechanical means increases capillary permeability to make localized edema. Excessive accumulation of interstitial fluid, either localized or generalized, is termed *edema.* When the amount of generalized edema is great, the condition is termed *anasarca* or dropsy. In the adult, approximately 4.5 kg (10 lb) of fluid accumulates before it is detectable as pitting edema. To demonstrate the presence of edema, gently press your thumb into the skin against a bony surface, such as the anterior tibia, fibula, dorsum of the foot, or sacrum. When the thumb is withdrawn, an indentation persists.

The *distribution of edema* should be noted; the amount of fluid is roughly proportional to its extent and thickness. Because dependent edema responds to gravity, it first appears in the feet and ankles of the ambulatory patient or over the posterior calves or sacrum of the supine patient. As the amount of dependent fluid increases, a fluid level may be detected; seldom does dependent edema rise higher than the heart. Anasarca can be recognized at a glance by the obliteration of subcutaneous superficial landmarks. Chronic edema leads to fibrosis of the subcutaneous tissues and skin, so they no longer pit on pressure; this is sometimes called *brawny edema*. Symmetric edema affecting both legs suggests that the problem is in the pelvis or more proximally, while edema, limited to the arms and head suggests SVC obstruction. Edema limited to one extremity suggests a local problem with vascular channels or local inflammation.

The processes involved in edema formation are the same whether the edema is generalized or local. To evaluate local edema, the examiner must consider the local anatomy of the arteries, veins, lymphatics and soft tissues, the presence of any local inflammatory or structural disease and then form hypotheses as to the likely mechanism and anatomic site of the problem.

Exclusive dependence upon clinical information may miss cardiovascular causes of bilateral leg edema, so consider measurement of B-type natruretic peptide and/or echocardiographic evaluation with estimation of pulmonary artery and right atrial pressure, right and LV size and function and tricuspid valve function [Blankfield RP, Finkelhor RS, Alexander JJ, et al. Etiology and diagnosis of bilateral leg edema in primary care. *Am J Med*. 1998;105:192–197]. The following approach, based upon the anatomic distribution of edema, is diagnostically useful.

✔ *EDEMA—CLINICAL OCCURRENCE: Localized Edema* **Inflammation** infection, angioedema, contact allergy; *Metabolic Causes* gout; *Insufficiency of the Venous Valves* (with or without varicosities); *Venous Thrombosis* postoperative, prolonged air or automobile travel; *Venous or Lymphatic Compression* malignancies, constricting garments; *Chemical or Physical Injuries* burns, irritants and corrosives, frostbite, chilblain, envenomation (insects, snakes, spiders); *Congenital* amniotic bands, arteriovenous fistulas, Milroy disease; *Bilateral Edema Above the Diaphragm* SVC obstruction; *Bilateral Edema Below the Diaphragm* *Congestive Cardiac Failure* with elevated jugular venous pressure including elevated pulmonary artery pressures caused by left heart abnormalities, intrinsic pulmonary disorders, right heart abnormalities, and constrictive pericarditis; *Portal Vein Hypertension or Obstruction* cirrhosis, portal vein thrombosis, schistosomiasis; *IVC Obstruction* thrombosis, extrinsic compression, pregnancy; *Loss of Venous Tone* drugs (calcium channel blockers, angiotensin-converting enzyme inhibitors, other vasodilators), convalescence, lack of exercise; *Generalized Edema* *Hypoalbuminemia* nephrotic syndrome, cirrhosis, chronic liver disease, protein losing conditions (e.g., enteropathy, burns, fistulas); *Renal Retention of Salt and Water* corticosteroids, nonsteroidal anti-inflammatory drugs; *Increased Capillary Permeability* sepsis, systemic inflammatory response syndrome, interleukin-2, idiopathic capillary leak syndrome.

Idiopathic Edema: Recurrent and chronic edema may be observed in women in the third to fifth decades in the absence of cardiac, hepatic, or renal abnormalities or of venous or lymphatic obstruction. Affective disorders and obesity may coexist. Possible mechanisms include mild persistent precapillary arteriolor dilatation, exaggerated capillary leakage on assuming the upright posture and inappropriate chronic diuretic administration started initially for minor degrees of peripheral edema (*diuretic-induced edema*). Each mechanism probably lead to inappropriate activation of renin-aldosterone leading to salt and water retention.

Heat Related Edema: Pitting edema of the ankles often occurs abruptly in normal adults within 48 h after they have traveled from a temperate climate to the heat of the tropics or in temperate zones when weather changes from cool and dry to warm and humid. It spontaneously resolves in a few days of acclimatization.

Angioedema: Painless subcutaneous soft-tissue edema begins abruptly and spreads to involve several centimeters of tissue with diffuse borders. Erythema is not prominent. Angioedema often involves the face, lips, or tongue, and is life-threatening when the larynx is involved. Causes include hereditary absence of C1 esterase, exposure to allergen, and angiotensin-converting enzyme inhibitors.

KEY SIGN   Apical Impulse

Careful examination of the apical impulse yields useful information about the heart size, the force of LV contraction, the presence of obstruction to LV ejection, and the stroke volume.

Increased Amplitude: Increased force of LV contraction increases the apical impulse amplitude. This may be caused by LV hypertrophy (arterial hypertension, aortic stenosis, aortic regurgitation, mitral regurgitation). An increased impulse is also associated with heightened myocardial contractility (exertion, emotion, hyperthyroidism).

Enlarged, Sustained Apical Impulse: A left ventricle ejecting against increased afterload ejects more slowly than normal. Aortic valvular stenosis and arterial hypertension produces an enlarged sustained impulse rather than the normal brief tapping impulse.

Displaced to the Left: Volume overload of the left ventricle leads to LV dilation, but does not interfere with ejection. Volume overload from aortic or mitral regurgitation or from cardiac shunts produces ventricular impulses that are enlarged, brisk, and displaced laterally but are not sustained. A weak myocardium produces an apical impulse of lesser intensity, although dilatation of the heart may cause it to be perceived over a wider area than normal. Other causes of leftward displacement are right pneumothorax, left pleural adhesions, or volume loss in the left lung.

Displaced to the Right: This occurs with left pneumothorax, right pleural adhesions, volume loss of the right lung, and dextrocardia.

Shifted to Downward: Severe pulmonary emphysema flattens the diaphragm drawing the heart and mediastinum downward. The impulse may be felt in the epigastrium just inferior to the xiphoid.

KEY SIGN   Right Ventricular Impulse

Contraction of the normal right ventricle does not produce a palpable impulse; a dilated, hypertrophied or forward displaced right ventricle may produce a palpable impulse. Any palpable impulse in the precordium medial to the apex impulse and near the left edge of the sternum in the third, fourth or fifth interspace almost always originates in a pressure or volume overloaded right ventricle. It is nearly always abnormal. An exception is seen with severe mitral insufficiency where the expanding the left atrium forces the right ventricle forward producing a sternal or parasternal impulse. The latter impulse peaks with S2 whereas true right ventricular impulses peak during systole. Slight impulses only move the interspaces; with more advanced disease the lower sternum lifts with each beat. *CLINICAL OCCURRENCE:*   *Right Ventricular Hypertrophy (Pressure Overload)* pulmonic stenosis, pulmonary hypertension, mitral stenosis;   *Right Ventricular Dilation (Volume Overload)*   tricuspid or pulmonary valve insufficiency, left-to-right intracardiac shunts;   *Forward Displacement of the Heart*   tumors behind the heart, enlarged left atrium;   *Protuberance of the Right Ventricle*   aneurysm of the right ventricular wall;   *Hyperdynamic Circulation*   exertion, emotion, hyperthyroidism.

Precordial Bulge: In both children and adults, a protrusion of the bony thorax over the right ventricle may result from marked cardiac enlargement in some forms of congenital heart disease. In the adult, a bulge near the upper sternum may be produced by erosion from a syphilitic aortic aneurysm.

Retraction of the Fifth Interspace: In some normal persons, a systolic retraction of the fifth interspace near the apex can be noted. This is not a reliable sign of disease. It is often present with considerable right ventricular hypertrophy.

Epigastric Pulsation: This occurs in many normal persons, especially after exertion. Occasionally, displacement of the heart in pulmonary emphysema causes it. Most frequently, it is produced by pulsation of a normal abdominal aorta; aneurysmal dilation should be excluded.

Pulsations at the Base: In pulmonary hypertension and/or with increased pulmonary blood flow as might occur with a large left to right shunt an impulse may be felt over the pulmonary conus in the second or third interspace just to the left of the sternum. Pulsations in the right second interspace may occur from an aneurysm at the base of the aorta.

KEY SIGN   Thrills

Turbulent blood flow produces vibrations that are audible as murmurs and palpable as thrills when transmitted to peripheral structures. The vibrations feel similar to the sensation of holding a purring cat. The closest normal analogue is the tactile chest fremitus produced when a person is speaking. Since the ear is more sensitive to vibrations than the hand, thrills are associated with murmurs and indicate greater intensity (grade IV/VI). Thrills must be accurately localized and timed to the cardiac cycle. **DDX:** In mitral stenosis, diastolic and presystolic thrills may be felt at the apex. Severe aortic stenosis causes a systolic thrill in the second right interspace and in the carotid arteries. Thrills may accompany other organic murmurs, such as a ventricular septal defect (VSD) felt at the fourth and fifth interspaces near the left edge of the sternum. Thrills may be produced by a ruptured chorda tendinea or valve leaflet.

Palpable Friction Rubs (Friction Fremitus): Although auscultation is more sensitive, a friction rub occasionally will be felt. The tactile sensation is like two pieces of leather being rubbed together. See Pleural Rub (page 351) and Pericardial Rub (page 368).

Percussion

> **KEY SIGN** Shifted Borders of Cardiac Dullness

Although precordial percussion can estimate the distance of the cardiac apex from the midsternal line (MSL) in the fifth interspace with fair accuracy, only gross changes in cardiac size can be detected.

Left Border Shifted to Left: The LBCD is normally 7 to 9 cm to the left of the MSL. DDX: Causes of a leftward shift include dilatation of the left ventricle (RBCD normally placed or shifted to right), pericardial effusion (RBCD shifted to right, muffled heart sounds, paradoxical pulse), and displacement of a normal-sized heart to left by right pneumothorax, right hydrothorax, left pleural adhesions, or atelectasis of left lung with mediastinal shift to left.

Left Border Shifted to Right: Consider pulmonary emphysema with a normal heart in the midline, a prominent lingula anterior to the heart preventing accurate percussion of LBCD, and displacement rightward from right lung fibrosis or atelectasis, left pneumothorax, or left hydrothorax.

Right Border Shifted to Right: Causes include cardiac dilatation, pericardial effusion, left pneumothorax, left hydrothorax, right lung atelectasis, right pleural adhesions, and dextrocardia.

Right Border Shifted to Left: Causes include left lung atelectasis, left pleural adhesions, right pneumothorax, and right hydrothorax.

> **KEY SIGN** Enlarged Area of Cardiac Dullness

The area of cardiac dullness is judged to be expanded when you find (1) lateral displacement of the right or left border with the opposite border normally situated or (2) lateral displacement of both borders in opposite directions. An enlarged area of cardiac dullness is caused by either cardiac dilatation or pericardial effusion. Indirect definitive percussion is accurate when compared to CT [Heckerling PS, Weiner SL, Wolfkiel CJ, et al. Accuracy and reproducibility of precordial percussion and palpation for detecting increased left ventricular end-diastolic volume and mass. *JAMA*. 1993;270:1943–1948].

Widened Retromanubrial Dullness: Width in excess of 6 cm suggests aortic aneurysm, retrosternal goiter, thymic tumor, lymphoma, or metastatic carcinoma.

Auscultation of Heart Sounds

In writing this section, the authors have depended heavily on several publications to which you are referred for more details [Shaver JL, Leonard JJ, Leon DF. Examination of the Heart, Part IV: Auscultation of the Heart. Dallas, TX, American

Heart Association, 1990; Perloff JK. The physiologic mechanisms of cardiac and vascular physical signs. *J Am Coll Cardiol.* 1983;1:184–198].

KEY SIGN   First and Second Heart Sounds

At the onset of ventricular systole, ventricular contraction rapidly increases intraventricular pressure, closing the AV valves (mitral and tricuspid) and, shortly thereafter, opening the aortic and pulmonic valves (Fig. 8–19). Tensing of the AV valves is associated with the S1; tensing of the aortic and pulmonic valves is associated with the S2. *The normal heart sounds are NOT caused by slapping together of the leaflets.* Rather, the high-frequency components of these sounds are probably caused by tensing of the closed valves producing abrupt deceleration of blood with vibrations of the heart, vessels and blood column. Ventricular contraction forces blood silently into the aorta and pulmonary artery until the ventricles relax and the intraventricular pressure falls. Initial apposition of the aortic and pulmonic valve leaflets occurs prior to the high-frequency components of the second heart sound. The gradient of pressure between the artery and the more rapidly declining intraventricular pressures leads to an abrupt stretching of the elastic leaflet tissue producing the second heart sound. The sound occurs when flow in the artery has fallen to near zero but just before brief retrograde flow occurs [Sabbah HN, Stein PD. Investigation of the theory and mechanism of the origin of the second heart sound. *Circ Res.* 1976;39:874–882]. The heart sounds are usually loudest in the precordium nearest their point of origin: the first sound from the AV valves at the apex and lower left sternal border; the second sound from the semilunar valves at the base. Invariably, the second sound is louder than the first at the base. Occasionally, S2 at the apex may be as loud as or louder than S1. The intensity of the heart sounds changes when more or less stress is put on the valve leaflets.

Prosthetic Heart Valves: Prosthetic heart valves are very common. It is advisable for the clinician to be familiar with the various types of valves and their auscultatory features [Vongpatanasin W, Hillis LD, Lange RA. Prosthetic heart valves. *N Engl J Med.* 1996;335:407–416].

KEY SIGN   First Heart Sound—Onset of Ventricular Systole

Normally heard over the entire precordium, S1 is usually louder than S2 at the cardiac apex (left fifth interspace near the midclavicular line). At the base, it is fainter than S2. S1 marks the beginning of ventricular systole and is approximately synchronous with the visible apical impulse and the palpable precordial thrust.

Splitting of the S1: S1 splits when tensing of the tricuspid and mitral valves are asynchronous. Slight splitting of S1 is a common normal finding. Wide splitting classically occurs with right bundle-branch block, which delays onset of right ventricular contraction.

Accentuated S1: Thickening with preserved mobility of the bellies of the mitral valve leaflets or increased force of LV contraction accentuate S1. This occurs in mitral stenosis, tachycardia from fever, hyperthyroidism, exercise, emotion, and hypertension.

Diminished S1: When the mitral and tricuspid valves are more closely approximated at the onset of systole, their tensing is less forceful. Attenuation of heart sounds by chest wall soft tissues also diminishes the sound. This occurs with the thick chest wall of an obese person, pulmonary emphysema, pericardial effusion and pleural effusion. Other causes include weak ventricular contraction, aortic insufficiency, prolonged PR intervals, and heavily calcified mitral valve leaflets.

Variable and intermittently very loud S1 (Bruit de Canon). Variable ventricular diastolic filling and asynchrony of atrial and ventricular contraction change the intensity of valve tensing from beat to beat. Atrial fibrillation, atrial flutter with varying degrees of block, complete AV block, frequent premature beats, and ventricular tachycardia can each be a cause.

> **KEY SIGN** **Second Heart Sound—Onset of Ventricular Diastole**

Tensing of the closed semilunar aortic (A2) and pulmonic (P2) valves produces the second heart sound; normally, A2 slightly precedes P2. The relatively increased compliance of the pulmonary artery compared to the aorta and the effect of respiration on right heart filling and pulmonary artery compliance accounts for the fact that A2 precedes P2 and that normally the interval between the two (splitting) widens during inspiration. The more compliant or distensible an artery is, the less faithfully the pressure in the artery will follow temporally the rise and fall of the pressure in the ventricle ejecting into that artery, a phenomenon known as *hangout* [Curtiss EI, Matthews RF, Shaver JA. Mechanism of normal splitting of the second heart sound. *Circulation*. 1975;51:157–164]. Thus, the lesser compliance of the aorta as compared with the usually greater compliance of the pulmonary artery causes the interval between the completion of LV systole and A2 to be much shorter than that between the completion of right ventricular systole and P2; therefore, A2 precedes P2 (Fig. 8–37). The intensity of A2 normally

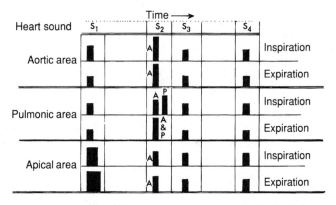

Fig. 8–37 ***Normal Physiologic Variations in the Heart Sounds.*** *Duration is represented on the horizontal axis, and intensity of the heart sounds on the vertical axis. The S1 is prolonged during inspiration. The aortic component of the second sound (A2) is audible over the entire precordium, but (P2) the weaker pulmonic component is heard only in the left second intercostal space. During expiration, the aortic and pulmonic components of are fused. With inspiration the splitting of S2 widens. Splitting of S2 is normal only in this pulmonic area; it is pathologic elsewhere.*

should be greater than that of P2. This follows logically from the normally much higher pressures in the aorta distending the aortic leaflets compared with the pressure in the pulmonary artery. The only truly reliable way to judge the relative intensities is by comparing the relative intensities of the two components when heard in the second left intercostal space. In adults, only A2 is present at the cardiac apex; if both components are heard at the apex, this should suggest that P2 is abnormally loud. *Respiratory Effect* The pulmonary valve closes later during inspiration than during expiration because of the increased venous return to the right heart and change in pulmonary compliance created by the negative intrathoracic pressure. This produces inspiratory splitting of S2. In children and adolescents, the normal respiratory splitting of S2 is wider than that in older adults, probably as a result of reduced aortic compliance as we age. In recumbent young persons, the split S2 may not fuse into a single sound with expiration. In the sitting position, fusion should occur during expiration; failure to fuse suggests that the splitting is unusually wide. With advancing age, the splitting of S2 with inspiration may not be detectable even in recumbency due to the narrowness of the normal split.

Accentuated A2: Increased pressure against the closed aortic valve increases A2. Arterial hypertension is most common, but aneurysm of the ascending aorta can be associated.

Diminished A2: A2 is decreased when the valve is rigid and immobile or decreased forces are applied to the valve and aortic root at end systole. Heavily calcified aortic valves as occur in aortic stenosis diminish A2. It is also diminished with systemic arterial hypotension.

Accentuated P2: An accentuated P2 is seen in primary or secondary pulmonary hypertension, atrial septal defect (ASD), truncus arteriosus and in adolescence (Fig. 8–21A).

Diminished P2: Diminished pulmonary artery pressure reduces tension on the pulmonic valve. Pulmonic stenosis is the most common cause (Fig. 8–38).

Widened inspiratory splitting of S2: This means either delayed tensing of the pulmonic valve or early aortic valve tensing. P2 delay occurs with right bundle-branch block, ASD and pulmonic stenosis. Early closure of the aortic valve occurs with severe mitral regurgitation (Fig. 8–38).

Reversed or Paradoxic Splitting of S2: A delay of LV ejection causes A2 to coincide with or occur after P2. There is a single sound, or more closely approximated sounds, during inspiration; expiration is associated with increased splitting of the second heart sound. It is seen in hypertrophic cardiomyopathy with LV outflow obstruction (idiopathic hypertrophic subaortic stenosis [IHSS]), valvular aortic stenosis or left bundle-branch block (Fig. 8–38).

> **KEY SIGN** **Triple Rhythms and Gallops**

These low-pitched sounds are easily missed unless specifically listened for in a quiet room. Listen for triple heart sounds: couplets alternating with single sounds resembling a horse's gallop. The couplet may be either a normal S2 followed closely by an audible S3 or an audible S4 preceding a normal S1. Differentiating S3 from S4 requires accurate identification of S1 and S2. The gallop rhythm will become most evident at rates > 100 bpm and some would reserve the term "gallop" for the presence of an S3 and/or S4 *and* a rate >100 bpm. At very fast rates, S3 and S4 fuse creating a *summation gallop* in the middle of diastole.

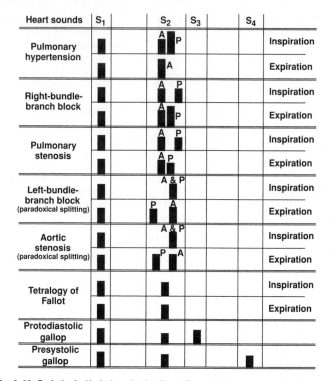

Heart sounds	S_1		S_2	S_3		S_4	
Pulmonary hypertension			A P				Inspiration
			A				Expiration
Right-bundle-branch block			A P				Inspiration
			A P				Expiration
Pulmonary stenosis			A P				Inspiration
			A P				Expiration
Left-bundle-branch block (paradoxical splitting)			A & P				Inspiration
			P A				Expiration
Aortic stenosis (paradoxical splitting)			A & P				Inspiration
			P A				Expiration
Tetralogy of Fallot							Inspiration
							Expiration
Protodiastolic gallop							
Presystolic gallop							

Fig. 8–38 *Pathologic Variations in the Heart Sounds.* *Pulmonary hypertension causes an increased P2. Right bundle-branch block delays right ventricular emptying, increasing the normal split and accentuating P2. Pulmonic stenosis also delays P2, but decreases its intensity. In left bundle-branch block and aortic stenosis, LV ejection is delayed so A2 coincides with P2 and the normal expiratory movement of P2 causes paradoxic splitting during expiration.*

S3, Ventricular or Protodiastolic Gallop: S3 occurs at the transition from the rapid phase of ventricular filling to the slow-filling phase, as the walls reach the limits of early diastolic excursion. The resulting reverberations of ventricular muscle and blood mass cause the sound (Fig. 8–20, page 325 and 8–38). An audible S3 closely follows S2 in early diastole. It has the cadence of Kentucky: ken....TUCK..eh. By whispering "ken....TUCK..eh" to yourself as you listen, timing "ken" to S1 and "TUCK" to S2 you can train your ear to listen for the low pitched S3 coincident with "eh." If the S3 is from the left ventricle, it is best heard at the apex with the patient lying 45 degrees to the left side; if from the right ventricle it is best heart near the lower left sternal border. S3 are best heard in expiration and are accentuated by exercise, abdominal pressure, or flexing the knees on the abdomen, all of which increase venous return. An S3 is normal in children, young adults and with pregnancy. After the third decade, it may indicate myocardial systolic dysfunction, with increased LV end-diastolic pressure and elevated left atrial pressure. It is also seen, although of less concern, when caused by a hyperkinetic circulatory state as with fever, anemia, hyperthyroidism, or by excessively rapid ventricular filling from mitral regurgitation or a large left to right shunt due to a VSD.

S4, Presystolic or Atrial Gallop: S4 is caused by vibrations of the LV muscle, the mitral valve apparatus, and the LV outflow tract as a result of atrial contraction (Fig. 8–20, page 325 and 8–38). S4 occur after atrial contraction but before S1. They have the cadence of Tennessee: "te..NUH . . . . .see." These are the most difficult to hear of all heart sounds; listening at apex with patient in left lateral decubitus position is mandatory. As you listen, whisper to yourself "te..NUH . . . .see," timing "NUH" to S1 and "see" to S2; train your ear for the S4 coincident with "te." S4 is low-pitched, essentially identical to S3. The S4 always indicates a high pressure, powerful atrial contraction, most often associated with a decrease in ventricular compliance. S4 is heard with a thickened, noncompliant left ventricle, as occurs with aortic stenosis, subaortic stenosis, hypertension, and acute ischemia or infarction from coronary artery disease (CAD).

Diastolic Sound—Summation Gallop, Mesodiastolic Gallop: The sounds of S3 and S4 are so close together that they give the impression of a single sound or a rumbling murmur. Vagus stimulation by carotid pressure may slow the rate enough to distinguish four sounds per cycle.

Auscultation of Extracardiac Sounds

Because they are relatively uncommon and are heard in the precordial region, the extracardiac sounds are very often mistaken for murmurs. Once their possibility is considered, the discrimination can usually be made. The decisive difference is that extracardiac sounds may move about within a specific part of the cardiac cycle.

Early Systolic Ejection Sound (formerly called Ejection Click)—Aortic Ejection Sound: This is attributed to sudden tensing of the root of the aorta at the onset of ejection. In other cases, sudden doming of a stenotic yet flexible aortic valve may be the cause (Fig. 8–20, page 325). A click is heard in early systole, at the onset of LV ejection. It is heard at the base and apex, although usually louder at the base, and is unaffected by respirations. Ejection clicks occur with dilation of the aortic root due to aneurysm of the ascending aorta, coarctation of the aorta, hypertension, valvular aortic stenosis (with flexible, noncalcified leaflets), a bicuspid aortic valve or aortic regurgitation.

Early Systolic Ejection Sound (formerly called Ejection Click)—Pulmonic Ejection Sound: See Aortic Ejection Sound above and Fig. 8–20, page 325. This is a click at the onset of right ventricular ejection, occurring when there is pulmonary valve stenosis or when the pulmonary artery is dilated. It is best heard early in systole in the left second interspace. In some cases, a loud click is fused with S1 and S1 is interpreted as loud. The closer the sound to S1, the more severe is the stenosis. Pulmonic clicks may decrease or disappear with inspiration.

> **KEY SIGN** **Mid or Late Systolic Click—Mitral Valve Prolapse**

This click is heard at the apex in mid or late systole; it may be intermittent (Fig. 8–20, page 325). It is unchanged by respiration, but can be delayed or abolished with increased LV cavity dimension following a squat from standing or raising the legs of a supine patient. The click may first become apparent or, if already audible, will move toward the S1 as the LV cavity dimension decreases with standing or a Valsalva. It is sometimes associated with a late systolic murmur of mitral insufficiency. Most individuals are otherwise normal, although mitral prolapse occurs with increased frequency in Marfan syndrome and myxomatous mitral valve changes (see also page 380).

KEY SIGN   Diastolic Snap—Mitral Opening Snap

When stenotic mitral valve leaflets are tethered at their commissures but still flexible (noncalcified), they buckle or bow outward into the left ventricle when ventricular pressure drops below left atrial pressure, producing a snap. The diastolic rumble begins a few hundredths of a second later (Fig. 8–20, page 325). The snap is best heard at the apex, but may radiate to base and left sternal border, where it may simulate a widely split S2. This sign is characteristic of rheumatic mitral stenosis.

Diastolic Snap—Tricuspid Opening Snap: See Mitral Opening Snap above. Because it is associated with other rheumatic valvular abnormalities, this snap is usually difficult to identify.

KEY SIGN   Diastolic Sound—Pericardial Knock

With constrictive pericarditis, abrupt termination of ventricular filling occurs early in diastole, producing the vibrations known as a pericardial knock. Knocks are heard widely over the precordium and are more high-pitched than the S3, similar in pitch to an opening snap. They may occur slightly earlier in diastole than an S3 and may increase with inspiration (Fig. 8–20, page 329).

KEY SIGN   Pericardial Friction Rub

The sound arises from two inflamed pericardial surfaces rubbing together. Rubs may occur with a pericardial effusion since effusions often do not cover the entire pericardium. Listen to the precordium during deep expiration with the patient prone or sitting and leaning forward. Rubs are scratchy, grating, rasping, or squeaky. In approximately half the cases, the sound is triphasic, heard in systole and early and late diastole. In approximately one-third of patients it is systolic and late diastolic. In the remainder, it is heard only in systole; often it is intermittent. Rubs seem closer to the ear than murmurs. Causes are infectious pericarditis, myocardial infarction or cardiac surgery, uremia, carcinoma metastatic to pericardium, and, rarely, pulmonary infarction.

KEY SIGN   Mediastinal Crunch (Hamman Sign)

See page 406.

KEY SIGN   Venous Hum

High-velocity flow in the internal jugular veins, especially the right, produces a humming sound. Hums are usually heard in both supraclavicular fossae and often in the second and third interspaces near the sternum. They are low pitched, persist throughout the cardiac cycle, and frequently increase during diastole. Hums are intensified by having the patient sit or stand; they do not vary with respirations. The hum is readily abolished by light pressure on the jugular veins beside the trachea. The hum is frequently mistaken for an intracardiac murmur. Venous hums occur in some normal children and adults. They are more common with hyperthyroidism and anemia. The combination of a venous hum and an intracranial bruit suggests the presence of intracranial arteriovenous malformation.

Auscultation of Heart Murmurs

> **KEY SIGN** **Heart Murmurs**

In normal vessels and heart chambers, blood flow at rest is laminar and silent. Murmurs result from vibrations due to turbulence (vortices) developing near the vessel wall-bloodstream interface as the blood passes an obstruction or dilatation (vortex-shedding theory). For a model, attach 60 cm (24 in) of pliable rubber tubing to a laboratory water faucet. Palpate the tubing with the thumb and finger of one hand and turn on the water with the other. A velocity can be attained that will not vibrate the walls of the tubing, because the flow is laminar and smooth. At this velocity, constricting the tubing slightly with the fingers will cause vibrations distally. Also, with no constriction, increasing the velocity of flow will induce turbulence. One can also demonstrate that a less-viscous fluid will set up vibrations at less velocity than water. In a normal heart, murmurs may be induced when the velocity of normal blood is increased by high output states such as exercise, anemia, pregnancy or hyperthyroidism, that is, a flow murmur. Normal blood flowing over obstructions or through unusual openings in the circulation sets up turbulence and collision currents that result in murmurs. Careful observation of murmurs for their location, pitch, and relations to the cardiac cycle can lead to remarkably accurate diagnoses of the anatomic derangements within the heart and vessels. The quality of murmurs is of some diagnostic value. Ventricular filling murmurs (for instance those involving diastolic flow across the AV valves) are relatively low pitched because they are produced by blood flowing under relatively low pressure gradients; blood flowing through narrow orifices under higher pressure gradients cause high-pitched murmurs.

Study Figures 8–39, 8–40 and 8–41 to familiarize yourself with anatomic correlates and pattern of the murmurs for each of the major conditions.

Systolic Murmurs

Systolic murmurs are described according to the part of the systolic interval in which they occur: early, mid, and late systolic. When the murmur is heard throughout systole, it is termed *pansystolic* or *holosystolic.* Blood moving across a rising then falling pressure gradient produces a *crescendo-decrescendo* "ejection murmur," as the flow initially accelerates then slows. An example is aortic stenosis, where the murmur starts soon after S1, intensifies to a maximum at mid-systole, and tapers off to disappear before S2 when the intraventricular pressure equals that in the aorta. In contrast, regurgitant murmurs occur when blood flows continuously from a high-pressure region to one of low pressure producing a pansystolic murmur of almost uniform intensity. This is typical of mitral regurgitation. Using these criteria, it is usually possible to distinguish the systolic murmurs of organic disease from those occurring only in early systole or

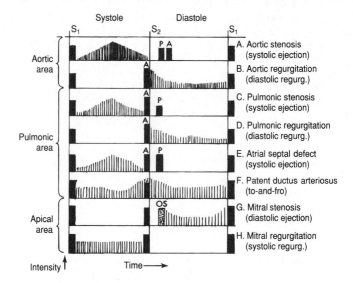

Fig. 8–39 *Common Pathologic Heart Murmurs.* *The diagrams are drawn to represent intensity of the heart sounds and murmurs on the vertical axis and duration on the horizontal axis. Pitch is depicted by the spacing of the shading: wider spacing lower pitch. ÒAÓ and ÒPÓ refer to the aortic and pulmonic components of the S2. ÒOSÓ indicates the opening snap of the mitral valve in mitral stenosis. Note that the systolic ejection murmurs are inaudible at either end of systole and attain maximum intensity at mid-systole (in this diagram they form the upper halves of Òdiamond-shapedÓ figures of the phonocardiogram). Systolic regurgitant murmurs are pansystolic. The configuration of the diastolic ejection murmur of mitral stenosis terminates in a crescendo caused by superimposition of atrial contraction. Although the diastolic regurgitant murmurs are pandiastolic, in aortic and pulmonic regurgitation, the late diastolic part is seldom heard.*

mid-systole that are of little significance [Etchells E, Bell C, Robb K. The rational clinical examination. Does this patient have an abnormal systolic murmur? *JAMA.* 1997;277:564–571]. Echocardiography is an important adjunct to the evaluation of patients with organic systolic murmurs as some important lesions can be missed even by experienced observers. Common errors are underestimating the severity of aortic stenosis due to decreased LV function, failing to identify combined mitral and aortic murmurs and missing aortic insufficiency in association with aortic systolic murmurs [Jost CHA, Turina J, et al. Echocardiography in the evaluation of systolic murmurs of unknown cause. *Am J Med.* 2000;108:614–620].

KEY SIGN **Basal Systolic Murmurs—Benign Murmurs (Innocent, Physiologic, Functional, Nonpathologic)**

Some authors believe that most of these murmurs are produced by increases in velocity or decreases in viscosity of the blood. Most common in the second left interspace, they are characterized as medium-pitched and generally grade I or II, although occasionally louder. When maximum in the second interspace, they are

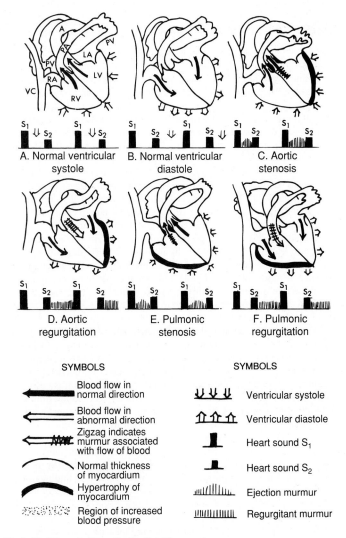

Fig. 8–40 *Anatomic Bases for Cardiac Murmurs I.*

infrequently transmitted to the neck. They are best heard in the supine position and tend to disappear with sitting or standing. Have the patient sit upright with the shoulders back. The murmur may persist if the patient sits in a slouched position. Functional murmurs occur in normal adults with anemia, fever, anxiety, exercise, hyperthyroidism, or pregnancy. Approximately 50% of normal children have functional systolic murmurs. **DDX:** Usually they are short, occurring early in systole. Their short duration without accompanying abnormalities of history and cardiovascular examination assists to distinguish them from murmurs of organic disease.

Progressive commissural fusion and leaflet fibrosis results in narrowing of the valve orifice and impedance to LV ejection (Fig. 8–40C). *The Murmur* Classically the murmur is heard in the second right interspace, but almost as often it is audible along the left sternal border in the third and fourth interspaces and at the apex. In approximately 15% of cases, it is loudest at the apex. Regardless of the area of maximal intensity, it is transmitted to the carotid arteries. Loud murmurs are often accompanied by systolic thrills over the base and in the carotids. It is a typical ejection murmur with onset a very short interval after S1, when intraventricular pressure first exceeds aortic pressure; it ceases before the second sound, when the intraventricular pressure falls below aortic pressure. Its configuration is diamond-shaped, initially rising (crescendo) then falling (decrescendo) in intensity (Fig. 8–39). The murmur is usually medium-pitched, so it is audible with either the bell or the diaphragm. Although usually harsh, occasionally it has a peculiar quality that prompts the term seagull murmur, like the call of a gull or the cooing of a dove. With a decrease in LV contractility, the murmur may decrease in intensity. *Heart Sounds* In moderate or severe stenosis accompanied by significant valvular calcification, A2 is diminished or absent. This is best appreciated by noting the second heart sounds at the apex to be faint or absent. If the valve is stenotic but not calcified (as in congenital aortic stenosis), S2 may be split during expiration (paradoxically) from delayed closure of the aortic valve (Fig. 8–38). Normal inspiratory splitting of S2 suggests that the stenosis is not severe. When the valve remains flexible although stenotic, the murmur is preceded by an ejection or early systolic sound caused by doming of the valve in early systole; this disappears when the valve becomes calcified. An S4 is frequently audible at the apex. *Precordial Thrust* Hypertrophy of the left ventricle produces an accentuated precordial apical thrust. In the left lateral decubitus position, a double (bifid) apical thrust is sometimes felt; the first impact comes from atrial contraction, the second from LV systole. *Arterial Pulse* Severe aortic stenosis produces a slowly rising carotid pulse contour (tardus or anacrotic pulse, Fig. 8–42D, page 383) and diminished pulse pressure. A decrease in the rate of rise is appreciated as a "sustained caress" to the finger rather than the normal brief "tap." A decrease in amplitude is often perceptible but is best judged by the pulse pressure noted when taking the arterial blood pressure. Physical findings do not always allow precise estimation of the severity of aortic stenosis [Munt B, O'Legget ME, Draft CD, et al. Physical examination in valvular aortic stenosis: Correlation with stenosis severity and prediction of outcome. *Am Heart J.* 1999;137:298–306]. *Symptoms* Aortic stenosis may be asymptomatic until constriction of the orifice is severe, when exercise induces dyspnea, angina, or syncope. The most common etiologies for aortic stenosis are rheumatic valvulitis, calcific disease of the aortic valve, and congenital bicuspid valve. *X-Ray Findings* Calcification of the aortic valve may be seen on the films. DDX: The systolic murmur of aortic sclerosis (atherosclerosis of the aortic valve) is accompanied by normal heart sounds at the base and is briefer. The apical systolic murmur of mitral regurgitation is of a "blowing" quality and is often pansystolic or holosystolic. A systolic diamond-shaped murmur may occur in valvular aortic stenosis or hypertrophic subaortic stenosis [Carabello BA. Aortic stenosis. *N Engl J Med.* 2002;346:677–682].

> **KEY SIGN   Hypertrophic Obstructive Cardiomyopathy (IHSS)**

This results from asymmetric hypertrophy of the left ventricle with prominent hypertrophy of the basal interventricular septum. Dynamic obstruction occurs shortly after the onset of systole from apposition of the anterior leaflet of the mitral valve to the hypertrophied septum, which may cause mitral insufficiency. A family history with autosomal dominant inheritance is often present; unexplained sudden deaths in the family should suggest the diagnosis of hypertrophic cardiomyopathy, with or without obstruction. The condition should be suspected when the signs of aortic stenosis are atypical. The apical impulse is often double. *The Murmur*   A systolic ejection murmur begins well after S1 and is best heard along the left sternal border and at the apex. It is less intense in the right second interspace and usually does not radiate to the carotids. At the apex, the murmur may have the blowing holosystolic quality of mitral regurgitation. The murmur varies with changes in ventricular volume, peripheral resistance and contractility. The dynamic outflow obstruction and murmur are intensified by maneuvers which reduce LV filling (standing and/or the Valsalva maneuver), whereas the murmur of valvular aortic stenosis diminishes under such circumstances. Handgrip, by raising diastolic blood pressure reduces the dynamic obstruction and murmur. Squatting or lifting the legs increases venous return and LV end-diastolic volume, reducing the obstruction and murmur.   *Arterial Pulse*   In contrast to the pulse of valvular stenosis with its diminished amplitude and delayed upstroke, the arterial pulse wave has a sharp upstroke. Bisferiens pulse may be present (Fig. 8–42B, page 383).   *Heart Sounds*   As in valvular stenosis, an S4 is frequent. Absence of a systolic ejection click is distinctive of subaortic stenosis.   *Symptoms*   The symptoms are identical to those of severe aortic valvular stenosis. The diagnosis is confirmed by echocardiography.

Supravalvular Aortic Stenosis: A rare congenital anomaly, this is the result of narrowing of the ascending aorta, or a small-holed diaphragm distal to the valve. It produces most of the signs of valvular stenosis, but A2 is accentuated and the carotid murmurs are unusually loud. The finding of a systolic blood pressure that is more than 10 mm Hg greater in the right arm than the left is typical of supravalvular aortic stenosis. The diagnosis is confirmed by cardiac catheterization.

> **KEY SIGN   Aortic Valve Sclerosis**

Aortic sclerosis is caused by the thickening of the aortic leaflet (sclerosis) without significant obstruction (stenosis). A murmur of medium pitch and moderate intensity is frequently heard in the aortic region of persons with hypertension or arteriosclerosis. It may be transmitted to the apex. It is usually softer than murmurs of aortic stenosis. It is often brief and confined to early systole. The murmur may be faintly heard in the carotids. A2 is usually present at the apex. DDX: Aortic stenosis is easily excluded, because the murmur is seldom loud or long, or accompanied by abnormality of the carotid pulse. Preservation of A2 at the apex speaks against severe calcific aortic valvular stenosis.

> **KEY SIGN   Valvular Pulmonic Stenosis**

The Murmur   This is a systolic ejection murmur, with diamond-shaped contour, maximal in the second left interspace (Figs. 8–40E and 8–39C, page 371). It is otherwise similar to an aortic stenosis murmur in intensity, configuration, and pitch. Carotid transmission may occur (left > right). *Heart Sounds* Slowed ejection through the pulmonic orifice delays P2 and the decreased pulmonary arterial pressure decreases its intensity; the S2 is widely split, but the pulmonic component is difficult to hear (Figs. 8–20 and 8–39C, page 374). There is often an early ejection sound, marking the lesion as valvular rather than infundibular pulmonic stenosis. *Palpation* Right ventricular hypertrophy may be detectable as an accentuated precordial thrust or sternal lift. DDX: The murmur is similar to the pulmonary flow murmur with ASD. In ASD, the wide splitting of S2 is fixed and P2 is not diminished in intensity. Pulmonary stenosis is usually congenital, either alone or in the tetralogy of Fallot. It can be acquired with carcinoid tumors.

Infundibular Pulmonic Stenosis: The infundibulum is the funnel-shaped portion of the right ventricular chamber leading to the pulmonary artery. Congenital narrowing produces a form of pulmonic stenosis. *The Murmur* In contrast to valvular stenosis, the ejection murmur and the systolic thrill are usually in the third left interspace and there is no ejection click. Although this lesion may be isolated, it is usually accompanied by a VSD, as in the tetralogy of Fallot.

Ostium Secundum ASD: The systolic murmur is produced by the high-volume, high-velocity flow across the pulmonic valve due to right ventricle overfilling from the congenital left-to-right interatrial shunt (Fig. 8–41A). *The Murmur* A medium-pitched murmur is nearly always heard in the second or third left interspace. The configuration frequently resembles that of pulmonic stenosis, with maximum intensity a little before mid-systole (Fig. 8–39E, page 370). The pulmonary outflow tract murmur is sometimes accompanied by a low-pitched diastolic flow murmur heard along the lower left sternal border, resulting from increased flow through the tricuspid valve. *Heart Sounds* S2 is widely split and fixed. P2 is not diminished. DDX: Sometimes the murmur is indistinguishable from pulmonic stenosis, though it usually is lower-pitched and peaks earlier in systole, leaving a longer pause before the second sound. The murmur rarely becomes very loud, in contrast to that of pulmonic stenosis. The wide splitting of S2 is the same during inspiration and expiration (the split is fixed) with a normal or accentuated intensity of the pulmonic component of S2.

Ostium Primum ASD: A congenital opening in septum near AV valves is often associated with a cleft mitral valve leaflet. *The Murmur* There is a harsh systolic murmur at left sternal border and an apical systolic murmur transmitted to axilla if mitral regurgitation is present. Sometimes a mid-diastolic murmur is heard at the lower left sternal border. *Heart Sounds* S2 is accentuated with fixed splitting during inspiration and expiration. The chest may be rounded, rarely with a precordial bulge. The sternal-parasternal right ventriclar impulse is prominent; the LV apical impulse may be accentuated and laterally displaced due to mitral regurgitation.

> **KEY SIGN** **Coarctation of the Aorta**

See also page 421. The site of constriction is remote from the precordium, so the murmur is faintly heard, if at all, on the anterior chest. The murmur of the

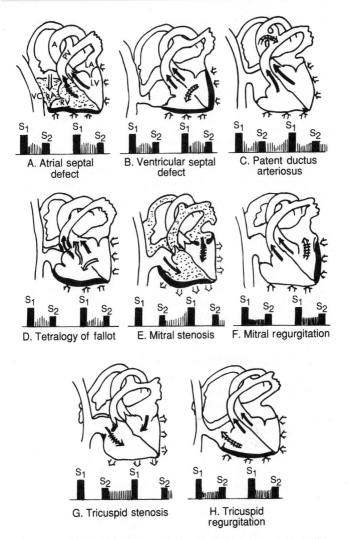

Fig. 8–41 *Anatomic Basis for Cardiac Murmurs II.* *(Same symbols as in Fig. 8–40.)*

coarctation is heard best in the interscapular area posteriorly. A continuous bruit can sometimes be heard over the sternum from the dilated internal mammary arteries.

Benign Thoracic Outlet Bruit: Most common in well-developed, muscular young men, this systolic bruit is maximal in the supraclavicular fossa. It is usually heard in the first right intercostal space as well, but attenuates as the aortic area is approached. It may also radiate to the right carotid. Having the patient sit with elbows placed to the scapular tips usually decreases the bruit. It has no clinical significance, but has been confused with aortic stenosis.

Mid-Precordial Systolic Murmurs

> **KEY SIGN** **Ventricular Septal Defect**

Blood flows from the left ventricle into the much lower pressure right ventricle through an opening in the interventricular septum (Fig. 8–41B). VSD is more common in the membranous than muscular septum. ***The Murmur*** Typically, the high-pitched murmur is pansystolic with peak intensity in the fourth and fifth left interspace. The murmur may be transmitted over the entire precordium and to the interscapular region. With muscular septal defects, the murmur may not persist throughout systole. ***Palpation*** Loud murmurs may be accompanied by a thrill. With the development of pulmonary hypertension, intensity and harshness diminish and the midsystolic accentuation is lost. ***Heart Sounds When*** the defect is large, S2 may be accentuated. **DDX:** With pulmonary hypertension, imaging may be needed to distinguish VSD from patent ductus arteriosus. Faint murmurs must be distinguished from benign systolic murmurs [Ammash NM, Warnes CA. Ventricular septal defects in adults. *Ann Intern Med.* 2001;135:812–824]. **CLINICAL OCCURRENCE:** Congenital septal defects occur alone and in the syndromes of Eisenmenger and Fallot. VSD may complicate myocardial infarction, typically at the cardiac apex; large acquired defects are rapidly fatal.

> **KEY SIGN** **Tricuspid Regurgitation (TR)**

Right ventricular contraction produces backflow of blood into the right atrium and major veins, with a pulsatile increase in CVP (Fig. 8–41H). ***The Murmur*** Faint murmurs are early systolic, loud murmurs are heard throughout systole; both are augmented during inspiration. They are high pitched and blowing, best heard with the diaphragm. The point of maximum intensity is nearly always along the lower left sternal border. It may be sharply localized or transmitted to the apex. ***Palpation*** Right ventricular hypertrophy may be present with a palpable right ventricular precordial thrust. When severe, tricuspid insufficiency produces prominent jugular "v" waves, neck vein engorgement and hepatic pulsations. ***Heart Sounds*** There are no characteristic changes in the heart sounds. **DDX:** The location of maximum intensity, large "v" waves and the effect of inspiration are diagnostic. **CLINICAL OCCURRENCE:** Congenital TR occurs with Ebstein anomaly. It is acquired in rheumatic heart disease, right ventricular failure from any cause, endocarditis, carcinoid tumor, and pulmonary embolism.

Apical Systolic Murmurs

> **KEY SIGN** **Mitral Regurgitation (MR)**

Blood is forced backward through the mitral orifice with almost constant velocity during the entire systolic interval (Fig. 8–41F). With severe MR, the left ventricle empties prematurely, so A2 is early, causing wide splitting of S2. ***The Murmur*** This is the prototypic systolic regurgitant murmur: loud, high-pitched, pansystolic with maximum intensity at the apex, beginning with S1 and continuing throughout systole to end at or near S2 (Fig. 8–39H, page 370). Many variations exist: The murmur may mask S1, begin with S1 and decrescendo to end in early to mid-systole or begin in mid-to-late systole and crescendo to end with, or even after, S2. Faint murmurs are well localized; loud murmurs are transmitted to the axilla. Murmurs from eccentric jets may produce unusual radiation to the base and carotids or to the lung bases and spine. There is little variation with phases of respiration or rhythm irregularities. An early diastolic murmur may be heard from the increased flow volume across the mitral valve. **Heart Sounds** S1 is often diminished; there may be wide splitting of S2 with severe regurgitation. An S3 is sometimes heard with moderate or severe MR. **Palpation** Accentuation and lateral displacement of the apical thrust suggest LV hypertrophy and dilatation, respectively. An increased left parasternal thrust or lift may indicate systolic expansion of the left atrium rather than right ventricular disease. **DDX:** The murmur must be distinguished from aortic stenosis, which is often loud at the apex, as well as at the base. The duration and quality and comparison at the apex and base make differentiation possible. Benign murmurs at the apex are usually short, medium-pitched and limited to only a part of systole [Otto CM. Evaluation and management of chronic mitral regurgitation. *N Engl J Med.* 2001;345:740–746]. **CLINICAL OCCURRENCE:** MR results from myxomatous change in the valve, endocarditis, rheumatic valvulitis, ruptured chordae, papillary muscles ischemia or rupture, myocardial infarction, and dilatation of the mitral valve ring by any condition producing LV dilatation.

KEY SIGN   **Mitral Valve Prolapse—Midsystolic Click and Apical Late Systolic Murmur**

The valve undergoes myxomatous degeneration, producing redundant valve tissue (especially the posterior leaflet), enlargement of the valve annulus and elongation of the chordae tendineae. During systole, as the ventricular volume is reduced, one or more scallops of the valve leaflets billows and prolapses backward into the atrium, losing coaptation and producing mitral regurgitation. This is a very common condition (perhaps 2%-5% of the population) and more frequent in women. It can be inherited, probably as an autosomal dominant with reduced male expressivity. **The Murmur** The systolic crescendo murmur classically occurs late in systole, heard best at the apex. It is usually short, relatively high-pitched and blowing, persisting into S2. It may be transmitted to the back, left of the spine. In unusual cases, it is described as cooing, honking, or whooping. It may be inaudible or so loud as to be heard without a stethoscope. It typically moves closer to S1 with standing (decreased venous return, smaller LV volume), and becomes shorter and later in systole with the patient squatting or recumbent (increased venous return, larger LV volume). Auscultation in the erect position during a Valsalva maneuver may elicit a murmur that could not be heard at rest with the patient supine. **Heart Sounds** A clicking sound is sometimes heard during mid-systole, coincident with the onset of the murmur; the click may occur without a murmur. **Associated Dysrhythmias** Ventricular premature beats, paroxysmal atrial tachycardia, atrial fibrillation, sinus bradycardia, periods of sinus arrest and positional atrial flutter can all occur in association. **Noncardiac Signs** Most patients are otherwise normal; there is an increase incidence of chest wall abnormalities, particularly pectus excavatum. Mitral valve prolapse is common in Marfan syndrome with arachnodactyly, hyperextensible joints, and ectomorph build. *Symptoms* Most persons are without symptoms. The minority develops easy fatigue, shortness of breath, nonanginal chest pain, palpitation, or syncope. There is an increased relative risk for cerebral transient ischemic attacks, rupture of chordae tendineae, congestive cardiac failure, endocarditis, and sudden death, but these are still quite rare.

➤　　KEY SIGN　**Sudden Onset of Loud Systolic Murmurs—Rupture of Interventricular Septum, Papillary Muscle or Chordae Tendineae**

Sudden appearance of a loud pansystolic murmur suggests rupture of the interventricular septum, a chordae, or papillary muscle, or severe papillary muscle dysfunction. There may be a precordial thrill; severe pulmonary edema occurs with chordae or papillary muscle injury. The murmur is usually grade II-IV/VI; however, severe mitral insufficiency may be associated with a surprisingly soft murmur. With a ruptured septum, there are signs of right-sided failure, low cardiac output and poor peripheral perfusion. Prompt recognition and treatment may be life saving.

Diastolic Murmurs

Diastolic murmurs are practically always pathologic. They are classified as early, mid, and late diastolic. Diastolic regurgitant murmurs due to flow from the aorta or pulmonary arteries back into a ventricle begin with the second heart sound and many are prolonged since the pressure in the great vessels exceeds that in the ventricles throughout diastole. The diastolic murmur of mitral stenosis does not start with the second heart sound because pressure in the ventricle must continue to fall before becoming less than atrial pressure (the period of isovolumic relaxation).

Basal Diastolic Murmurs

KEY SIGN　**Aortic Insufficiency (AI, Aortic Regurgitation)**

The decrescendo murmur contour is the result of a decreasing transvalvular pressure gradient as aortic diastolic pressure falls from beginning to end diastole. The high pitch is caused by blood being forced through a relatively small orifice at high pressure (Fig. 8–40D). *The Murmur* The murmur is best heard with the diaphragm held firmly against the chest while the patient is leaning forward in full expiration. The point of maximum intensity is in either the right second or left third interspace. The high-pitched blowing murmur immediately follows S2 and exhibits a rapid decrescendo; it may not last throughout diastole (Fig. 8–39B, page 370). There is often an accompanying aortic systolic murmur. Transmission down the right rather than the left sternal border should suggest aneurysmal dilatation of the aortic root. *Heart Sounds* The S1 is usually normal; A2 may be accentuated. *Palpation* Accentuation and lateral displacement of the apical thrust suggest LV hypertrophy and dilatation. *Arterial Pulses* The pulse has a collapsing quality. Vasodilatation, high pulse pressure, and pistol-shot sounds may be found; nailbed pulsation is easily seen. DDX: The quality and location of the murmur do not distinguish AI from pulmonic regurgitation, but maximal intensity in the aortic area, an accentuated and displaced apical thrust, increased pulse pressure, brisk carotid upstrokes, pulsus bisferiens, and Duroziez sign all favor AI [Choudhry NK, Etchells EE. The rational clinical examination. Does this patient have aortic regurgitation? *JAMA*. 1999;281:2231–2238]. *CLINICAL OCCURRENCE:* Common causes are rheumatic valvulitis, congenitally bicuspid aortic valve, and endocarditis. Marfan syndrome, aortic dissection, aneurysm of the sinus of Valsalva, and annular ectasia of the aorta are less common. Syphilitic aortitis is increasingly uncommon.

KEY SIGN   Pulmonic Regurgitation

This most commonly results from dilation of the pulmonic valve ring in pulmonary hypertension leading to backflow of blood from the pulmonary artery into the right ventricle resulting in RV volume overload as well as pressure overload (Fig. 8–40F). *The Murmur* This is frequently termed the Graham Steell murmur. It is indistinguishable in quality and timing from the high-pitched murmur of aortic regurgitation (Fig. 8–39D, page 370). It is usually less loud and transmitted less widely than the AI murmur. The point of maximum intensity is usually in the second or third left interspace. In the absence of pulmonary hypertension, as occurs after pulmonary valvotomy for congenital pulmonic stenosis, the murmur of pulmonary regurgitation is medium- to low-pitched. *Heart Sounds* P2 may be accentuated. *Palpation* A precordial thrust of the right ventricle may be palpated. **DDX:** Usually the diagnosis is made by the signs of right ventricular hypertrophy and the absence of peripheral signs of aortic regurgitation. *CLINICAL OCCURRENCE:* This occurs with pulmonary hypertension from any cause (mitral stenosis, left-sided heart failure, pulmonary emphysema, idiopathic pulmonary hypertension, congenital heart lesions, obstructive sleep apnea, chronic pulmonary emboli) or after pulmonary valvotomy.

Mid-Precordial Diastolic Murmur

KEY SIGN   Tricuspid Stenosis

Right atrial contraction against the stenotic valve orifice causes presystolic accentuation of the murmur and giant "a" waves. Impedance to right ventricular filling leads to elevated CVP. (Fig. 8–41G). *The Murmur* The diastolic murmur is low-pitched and rumbling with a presystolic crescendo when atrial fibrillation is absent. It is best heard with the bell lightly placed. When mild, the murmur is late diastolic; with increasing severity, it occupies mid and even early diastole. The murmur becomes louder during inspiration due to increased venous return. *Venous Pulse* Giant "a" waves are present; the CVP will progressively elevate as stenosis worsens. *Heart Sounds* S1 is accentuated. Sometimes an opening snap of the tricuspid valve can be identified. *Palpation* The point of maximum intensity is quite sharply localized at the lower-left sternal border in the fourth or fifth interspace. In severe stenosis, signs of central venous congestion (elevated CVP, hepatomegaly, ascites, edema) are found, mimicking right ventricular failure. **DDX:** The murmur can usually be distinguished from that of mitral stenosis by its location and accentuation during inspiration. A murmur identical to the mid-diastolic rumble of tricuspid stenosis is the diastolic flow rumble that accompanies severe TR or a large ASD. *CLINICAL OCCURRENCE:* Rheumatic valvulitis, congenital heart disease, and carcinoid tumor produce this lesion.

Apical Diastolic Murmurs

> **KEY SIGN** **Mitral Stenosis**

In mild mitral stenosis, ventricular filling is only slightly delayed and the period of rapid filling is shortened, so a mid-diastolic murmur is produced; with moderate or severe stenosis, ventricular filling is prolonged, so atrial systole increases the pressure gradient across the valve, producing a presystolic crescendo murmur. This presystolic accentuation is absent in atrial fibrillation. The accentuated S1 is caused by the prolonged filling time, which places the valves low in the ventricle at the onset of systole. Pulmonary hypertension produces the accentuated P2. The opening snap is attributed to the thickened but flexible leaflets, tethered at their commissures, bulging forward into the left ventricle when the elevated atrial pressure exceeds LV pressure; the snap is absent with immobile leaflets (Fig. 8–41E).   *The Murmur*   This murmur is heard best in the left lateral position near the apex. It is usually sharply localized, so the bell must be placed directly on the apex. Sometimes, only by carefully inching the bell over the entire apex will a loud murmur be discovered. The murmur is low-pitched and rumbling, sometimes only heard with the bell held lightly. The sound may resemble the roll of a drum. In mild stenosis, the murmur occurs in mid-diastole. As the orifice narrows, the murmur starts earlier and ends later, until it almost covers the diastolic interval. There is always a pause after S2 before the murmur begins. A long murmur often has a presystolic crescendo (Fig. 8–39G, page 370).   *Heart Sounds*   S1 at the apex is accentuated so long as the leaflets are mobile. If there is pulmonary hypertension, P2 is accentuated and occurs early but is normally delayed by inspiration. When the murmur is loud, there is usually a mitral opening snap shortly after A2, heard best at the left sternal border between the second and fourth interspaces. This is commonly mistaken for a split second sound. The opening snap disappears when the mitral cusps become rigid due to calcification.   *Palpation* The murmur is often accompanied by a thrill at the apex when the patient is in the left decubitus position. Often there is a palpable right ventricular thrust indicating right ventricular hypertrophy. **DDX:** Tricuspid stenosis produces a similar murmur, but it is localized nearer the sternum. A similar diastolic apical rumble may be heard with increased mitral diastolic flow due to severe mitral regurgitation. The murmurs of aortic and pulmonic regurgitation also occur at the apex [Thibault GE. Studying the classics. *N Engl J Med.* 1995;333:648–653]. *CLINICAL OCCURRENCE:*   This nearly always results from rheumatic heart disease, but is rarely congenital.

> **KEY SIGN** **Austin Flint Murmur**

Aortic insufficiency is often associated with fluttering of the anterior mitral valve leaflet. However, neither this phenomenon nor others accompanying chronic aortic regurgitation seem consistently to correlate with the murmur. The examiner confronted with a combination of aortic and mitral murmurs must decide if the mitral valve is normal. Authors vary on the criteria for diagnosis; the methods of Levine and Harvey are cited here.   *The Murmur*   Some patients with severe AI and normal mitral valves have murmurs at the cardiac apex similar in pitch and timing to that produced by mitral stenosis. When the aortic lesion is undoubtedly syphilitic, the murmur is the Flint type. The presence of atrial fibrillation favors an organic lesion of the mitral valve, as the dysrhythmia is rarely associated with an aortic lesion. *Heart Sounds* S1 is not accentuated with the Flint murmur. Accentuation of S1 or P2 favors organic mitral stenosis. The opening snap of the mitral valve is absent in the Flint murmur. *ECG* Notching of the P waves in the ECG favors an organic lesion of the mitral valve. *Amyl Nitrite Test* When tachycardia and diminished systolic blood pressure have been produced by the inhalation of amyl nitrite, the apical diastolic rumbling of the Flint murmur becomes fainter, but the murmur of organic mitral stenosis becomes louder. *CLINICAL OCCURRENCE:* Aortic regurgitation from rheumatic valvulitis, syphilis, or acute endocarditis.

Continuous Murmurs

Murmurs heard throughout the cardiac cycle indicate that turbulent flow is occurring without interruption. Therefore, the flow must be from a continuous high-pressure source to a low-pressure sump, that is, from the aorta to the pulmonary artery or a vein, or across a fixed obstruction in the aorta.

KEY SIGN Patent Ductus Arteriosus

A patent ductus is an arteriovenous fistula between an arterial circuit of high pressure (aorta) and an arterial system of lesser pressure (pulmonary artery) (Fig. 8–41C). The continuous murmur results from blood flowing continuously into the pulmonary artery during the entire heart cycle. The higher pressure during ventricular systole increases murmur's pitch. Uncorrected, the increased PA pressure leads to RVH and eventually right-to-left shunting with peripheral cyanosis confined to the lower extremities (*Eisenmenger physiology*). *The Murmur* A murmur heard in the first and second left interspace continuously through systole and diastole is usually caused by a patent ductus. The murmur is medium-pitched and rough, heard with either bell or diaphragm. Louder murmurs are harsh. There is typically a crescendo late in systole and a decrescendo after S2, producing a machinery murmur (Fig. 8–39F, page 370). Most frequently, transmission is to the interscapular region; occasionally it is transmitted down the left sternal border, sometimes to the apex. As pulmonary artery pressures approach aortic pressure, the diastolic portion of the murmur may disappear. TR may develop from the pulmonary hypertension. Increased flow through the mitral orifice may produce a diastolic rumble simulating mitral stenosis. *Heart Sounds* S2 may be buried in the crescendo portion of the murmur. Frequently there is a short pause between S1 and the murmur. *Palpation* The precordial thrust of both ventricles may be accentuated. *Arterial Pulses* With large shunts the peripheral pulse may have a collapsing quality, similar to AI. DDX: Clubbing may be present in the toes but spare the fingers when persistent right to left shunt occurs late. The continuous murmur must be distinguished from a venous hum.

KEY SIGN Coarctation of Aorta

See pages 374 and 421.

Mid-precordial continuous murmur—coronary arteriovenous fistula or ruptured sinus of valsalva aneurysm. Similar physical signs in these two conditions require diagnostic imaging for differentiation. *The Murmur* A continuous murmur with late systolic accentuation (machinery or to-and-fro) is audible at the lower portion of the sternum, on either or both sides. It is often accompanied by a systolic or continuous thrill. DDX: Although the to-and-fro murmur has the same quality as that in ductus arteriosus, the location is sufficiently different to be distinctive. A mid-precordial to-and-fro murmur can occur with the combination of interventricular septal defect and aortic regurgitation, but this murmur lacks the late systolic accentuation. Although a venous hum may be audible behind the upper sternum, its accentuation is diastolic and it is abolished by pressure on the internal jugular vein.

Vascular Signs of Cardiac Activity

LV contraction maintains arterial blood pressure and produces pulsations in all accessible arteries. Right atrial and ventricular contractions generate venous pulsations in the upper body. Because arterial pressure is normally approximately 16 times higher than CVP, arterial pulsations are palpable whereas venous pulsations are not. This is useful in determining the origin of visible pulsations.

Arterial signs of cardiac action. The contour of the arterial pulse wave is affected by the contractility of the left ventricle, the distensibility of the aorta, the size of the aortic valve orifice and the LV outflow tract. The carotid pulse most accurately reflects the contour of the aortic pulse wave. Alterations of the normal pulse contour and volume are diagnostically significant.

Pulse Contour

> **KEY SIGN** **Normal Arterial Pulse**

The palpable primary wave starts with a swift upstroke to the peak systolic pressure, followed by a more gradual decline. A second, and normally smaller, upstroke, *the dicrotic wave*, occurs at approximately the end of ventricular systole, but is not usually palpable. It is caused by the blood column; rebounding off the closed aortic valve (Fig. 8–42A).

> **KEY SIGN** **Twice Peaking (Dicrotic) Pulses**

There are two types of twice peaking arterial pulses (Fig. 8–42B). Most common is pulsus bisferiens with two palpable waves during systole. Less common is the dicrotic pulse, which has one wave palpable in systole and a second in diastole. *CLINICAL OCCURRENCE:* *Pulsus Bisferiens* severe aortic regurgitation especially when associated with moderate aortic stenosis, hypertrophic subaortic stenosis, and hyperkinetic circulatory states such as hyperthyroidism; *Dicrotic Pulse* very low cardiac output as with dilated cardiomyopathy or cardiac tamponade, especially in patients with normal aortic compliance.

> **KEY SIGN** **Bounding or Collapsing Pulse (Corrigan Pulse, Water-Hammer Pulse)**

A large stroke volume and/or vigorous LV contraction generates a rapid upstroke of the pulse wave followed by a rapid runoff of blood from the aorta. With high pulse pressure, the upstroke may be very sharp, while the downward slope is precipitous (Fig. 8–42C). It may be accompanied by the pistol-shot sound.

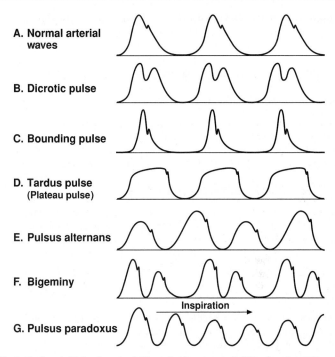

A. Normal arterial
   waves

B. Dicrotic pulse

C. Bounding pulse

D. Tardus pulse
   (Plateau pulse)

E. Pulsus alternans

F. Bigeminy

Inspiration

G. Pulsus paradoxus

Fig. 8–42 *Arterial Pulse Contour. A. Normal pulse contour. B. Dicrotic pulse. C. Bounding or collapsing pulse. D. Plateau pulse. E. Pulsus alternans. F. Pulsus bigeminus. G. Pulsus paradoxus.*

CLINICAL OCCURRENCE: This is encountered in hyperthyroidism, anxiety, aortic regurgitation, patent ductus arteriosus, and arteriovenous fistula.

> **KEY SIGN Plateau Pulse (Pulsus Tardus)**

The upstroke is gradual and the peak delayed toward late systole (Fig. 8–42D). Carotid palpation reveals a gentle, sustained caress, lifting the palpating finger, in contrast to the normal brief pulsatile tap. This occurs in severe aortic stenosis.

Pulse Volume

> **KEY SIGN Absent Pulses, Pulseless Disease**

See Takayasu Aortitis, page 414.

> **KEY SIGN Pulsus Alternans**

The pulse waves alternate between greater and lesser volume, despite a normal rhythm and a constant rate (Fig. 8–42E). The differences may not be palpable but are readily detected while measuring the blood pressure by auscultation: as the cuff is slowly deflated, the sounds from every other beat are audible first, then, with further deflation, the beats double. This is a sign of LV dysfunction. DDX: This must be distinguished from bigeminal rhythm, in which a normal beat is followed by a premature beat.

KEY SIGN   Bigeminy (Coupled Rhythm)

If the second or premature beat occurs before ventricular filling is complete, it has a smaller stroke volume than the preceding normal beat. A normal beat is followed by a premature beat and a pause (Fig. 8–42F). If the premature beats occur with a very short coupling interval they do not produce a palpable arterial pulsation and the radial pulse rate is half the ventricular rate. Diagnostic errors can be avoided by assessing the rhythm over the precordium by auscultation.

KEY SIGN   Pulsus Paradoxus

Inspiration decreases intrathoracic pressure, normally increasing blood flow into the chest and right ventricle. Despite the increased right ventricular stroke volume, inspiratory dilation of the pulmonary vasculature decreases LV filling resulting in decreased LV stroke volume and systolic blood pressure. In pericardial tamponade total heart volume is limited, and further reduced during inspiration, so that LV filling, LV stroke volume and systolic blood pressure all fall dramatically with inspiration. Labored breathing associated with exacerbations of obstructive airway disease also produce a paradoxical pulse. Under normal resting conditions, there is an inspiratory fall of less than 10 mm Hg in the arterial systolic pressure and an accompanying inspiratory fall in venous pressure. A paradoxical pulse exists when inspiration creates more than a 10 mm Hg drop in systolic arterial pressure. The exaggerated waxing and waning in the pulse volume may be detected by palpation (Fig. 8–42G); more often, it can only be detected by use of the sphygmomanometer. DDX: Similar findings can be seen with an irregular rhythm or AV asynchrony. *CLINICAL OCCURRENCE:*   Pericardial tamponade, pulmonary emphysema, severe asthma.

KEY SIGN   Inequality of Pulses

Disparity between the right and left arterial pulse volumes are detected by simultaneous palpation. If possible, confirm the finding by taking the blood pressure at both sites. Arterial pressure differences between the two arms must be considered with circumspection: pressures not measured precisely simultaneously are >10 mm Hg different in up to 20% of normal individuals, whereas, when measured simultaneously by cuff, 5% or less show the same difference. Nonsimultaneously measured systolic pressure differences of >10 mm Hg occur in almost 30% of hypertensive patients [Harrison EG Jr, Roth GM, Hines EA. Bilateral indirect and direct arterial pressures. *Circulaton.* 1960;22:419–436]. Asymmetry suggests atherosclerosis, dissecting aneurysm or another arterial disease.

Dysrhythmias. See Chapter 4, page 64ff. Many dysrhythmias produce arterial beats of greater or lesser volume and disordered timing. It is preferable to evaluate the disturbance from the precordial findings rather than attempting a judgment from the peripheral pulse alone. You should realize that any ventricular contraction occurring before the ventricle has had time to fill will produce a peripheral pulse wave of diminished volume, or none at all. The ECG, not palpation or auscultation, is the only way to accurately diagnose rhythm disturbances.

Arterial Sounds

Arteries are normally silent when auscultated. Turbulence is heard as a murmur and palpated as a thrill. Although murmur and bruit are literally synonymous, there is a tendency among Americans to reserve bruit for arterial sounds. The presence of a bruit does not necessarily indicate limitation of flow.   *CLINICAL OCCURRENCE:*   Arteries become tortuous from arteriosclerosis or other circumstances or dilate with aneurysm. They may be constricted congenitally, by intimal proliferation, or by an atherosclerotic plaque. Dilatation of the thyroid arteries with increased blood flow occurs in Graves' disease (here, the word bruit is often used). Blood flow through an arteriovenous fistula or large arterial collaterals, as in aortic coarctation, is often accompanied by bruits. A continuous murmur is produced by an arteriovenous fistula or a partially obstructed artery when the collateral circulation is poor and the diastolic pressure is quite low distal to the obstruction.

Carotid Bruit: Most of the blood flow to the brain, and virtually all to the cerebral cortex comes via the internal carotid arteries. Despite collateral flow through the circle of Willis from the contralateral carotid and vertebrobasilar system, high grade obstruction of one common and/or internal carotid artery is associated with a high risk for disabling stroke. The neck should always be auscultated for bruits, and any bruit should be evaluated by imaging. The degree of stenosis cannot be estimated by physical examination findings. The presence of cerebral symptoms in the distribution of the affected artery significantly increases the risk for stroke within hours to days.

Arterial Sound—Pistol-Shot Sound: This is produced by the wave front of an arterial pulse wave of higher than normal pulse pressure striking the arterial wall in the region of auscultation. When the stethoscope bell is placed lightly over an artery, particularly the femoral, a sharp sound like a gunshot may be heard.   *CLINICAL OCCURRENCE:*   Although commonly associated with aortic regurgitation, it also occurs in other conditions with high pulse pressure, such as hyperthyroidism, and anemia.

Duroziez Sign: Formerly attributed to retrograde flow of blood in the vessel, the second murmur only occurs when the second or diastolic murmur is associated with an exaggerated onward acceleration of blood flow. Compressing the femoral artery with the stethoscope bell produces eddies and a systolic bruit. If this compression produces a second murmur closely following the first but in diastole, giving the impression of a to-and-fro murmur, it is Duroziez sign. Listen while pressure on the bell is gradually increased. First, the normal systolic murmur appears; with further pressure, a critical point is reached when the second murmur becomes audible. Most commonly encountered in severe aortic regurgitation, it occurs in other conditions with a high pulse pressure (see Chapter 4, page 78).

Venous Signs of Cardiac Action

Cardiac action produces physical signs in the venous system by: (1) alteration of the venous pressure in the periphery, (2) production of venous congestion in the viscera, or (3) alteration of the venous pulse waves.

> ### KEY SIGN Elevated Central Venous Pressure (CVP)

Elevated CVP indicates overfilling of the intravascular space, exceeding venous capacitance, and/or impedance to filling of the right atrium or right ventricle. Impedance to right ventricular filling often occurs as a result of impaired outflow from the right ventricle causing elevated right ventricular end-diastolic pressure. When the venous pressure exceeds 10 or 12 cm of water under resting conditions, it should be considered elevated. **DDX:** A generalized increase in venous pressure must be distinguished from superior and/or IVC obstruction. Always assess whether the venous pressure appears uniformly elevated above and below the diaphragm; it must be if the *CVP* is elevated. Absence of signs below the diaphragm suggests SVC obstruction [Cook DJ, Simel DL. The rational clinical examination. Does this patient have abnormal central venous pressure? *JAMA.* 1996;275:630–634; Vinayak AG, Levitt J, Gehlbach B, et al. Usefulness of the external jugular vein examination in detecting abnormal central venous pressure in critically ill patients. *Arch Intern Med.* 2006;166:2132–2137]. *CLINICAL OC-CURRENCE: Overfilling of the Vascular Space* kidney failure, rapid infusion of fluids and blood products, chronic CHF with edema; *Impedance to Right Heart Filling* tricuspid stenosis, TR, pericardial tamponade, constrictive pericarditis; *Impaired Outflow from the Right Ventricle* pulmonary hypertension, pulmonary embolus, pulmonic stenosis, right ventricular infarction.

> ### KEY SIGN Diminished Venous Pressure

This occurs in peripheral circulatory failure that is part of the shock syndrome, usually associated with intravascular hypovolemia, diminished venous tone and/or peripheral pooling. The peripheral veins are collapsed when the patient is supine. See the discussion of Hypotension, Chapter 4, page 76.

> ### KEY SIGN Giant "a" Waves—Tricuspid Stenosis

See page 379.

> ### KEY SIGN Cannon "a" Waves—AV Asynchrony

As in tricuspid stenosis, atrial contraction against a closed tricuspid valve produces retrograde ejection of atrial blood into the central venous channels. Intermittent prominent venous pulsations are visible in the neck veins, *cannon "a" waves*. They are identified as "a" waves, since they are asynchronous with the apical impulse and carotid upstroke. They are easily obliterated by gentle pressure at the base of the neck insufficient to diminish the carotid pulse. **DDX:** Irregular cannon "a" waves suggest that at least some atrial contractions are occurring simultaneously with ventricular contraction. A regular pattern of cannon "a" waves suggests a fixed pattern of AV block, for example, atrial flutter with 2:1 block. An irregular pattern with variable "a" waves volume suggests AV dissociation, for example, complete heart block. *An ECG is required to diagnose the rhythm*. Regular giant "a" waves occurring consistently in synchrony with the heart sounds and arterial pulse suggests impedance to right atrial outflow, for example, a noncompliant right ventricle or tricuspid stenosis.

> **KEY SIGN** Large "v" Waves in the Venous Pulse—TR

Tricuspid insufficiency allows the right ventricle to eject blood retrograde into the central venous channels. Large "v" waves are visible in the jugular veins and there may be palpable pulsation of the liver. The waves are identified as "v" waves since they are synchronous with the apical impulse and carotid upstroke. There may be a right ventricular thrust reflecting the pressure overload on the right ventricle.

> **KEY SIGN** Hepatojugular Reflux and Kussmaul Sign

These phenomena are caused by inability of the right heart to accommodate increased venous return. Position the patient so the blood column is just visible in the jugular veins above the clavicle. With the patient breathing normally, place the right hand on the right upper abdominal quadrant and press firmly upward under the costal margin for at least 10 to 15 seconds. The *hepatojugular reflux* sign is present if the top of the jugular venous column in the neck rises and persists as long as the abdominal pressure is continued. *Kussmaul sign* is present when the jugular venous column fails to collapse during inspiration due to increased intraabdominal pressure created by the diaphragm during inspiration. **CLINICAL OCCURRENCE:** The hepatojugular reflux sign is most commonly seen with early right heart failure. Both signs may be seen with severe right heart failure, constrictive pericarditis, and right ventricular infarction [Bilchick KD, Wise RA. Paradoxical physical findings described by Kussmaul: Pulsus paradoxus and Kussmaul's sign. *Lancet.* 2002;359:1940–1942; Wiese J. The abdominojugular reflux sign. *Am J Med.* 2000;109:59–61].

Arterial Circulation Signs

The tissue effects of arterial blood flow must be distinguished from those of venous drainage. Arterial deficits cause dermal pallor, coldness, and tissue atrophy. Small-vessel disturbances are recognizable as patterns in the skin and are detected by the methods of dermatologic description. Diseases of the larger vessels cause regional hypoperfusion syndromes; diseases, such as the vasculitides, which affect smaller vessels, tend to be more diffuse. For signs in the skin see also Chapter 6, pages 144 and 174.

Warm Skin: Normal skin temperature indicates adequate arterial flow. The normal color of the nail beds is red or pink. If warm feet have blue nail beds, the warmth has been externally applied to feet with inadequate arterial flow.

> **KEY SIGN** Atheroembolic Disease

See Chapter 6, page. Embolization of cholesterol-rich atheroma to the small arteries produces hemorrhagic cutaneous infarcts and livedo.

> **KEY SIGN** Palpable Purpura—Vasculitis

See page 415ff and Chapter 6, page 149.

KEY SIGN   Skin Pallor and Coldness—Chronic Arterial Obstruction

Chronic progressive arterial obstruction allows development of collateral circulation and tissue accommodation to ischemia. Pallid cool skin strongly suggests regional hypoperfusion. It is normal in a cold environment, but should rapidly resolve on exposure to warm air or water. Failure to do so suggests that the problem is not limited to the skin vessels but involves a major trunk artery. Pain may be present with exertion (*claudication*). The distribution of the arterial deficit will depend upon the site of the obstruction and the presence and extent of collateral circulation. Other useful signs are prolonged venous filling time; abnormal pedal pulses and a femoral bruit [McGee SR, Boyko EJ. Physical examination and chronic lower-extremity ischemia: A critical review. *Arch Intern Med.* 1998;158:1357–1364].   *CLINICAL OCCURRENCE:* Atherosclerosis is most common; less common causes are large vessel vasculitis (Takayasu aortitis, giant cell arteritis), Buerger disease, vasospastic disorders, and ergotism.

KEY SIGN   Dependent Rubor and Coldness—Chronic Arterial Obstruction

See Chapter 6, page 145 and page 427.

► KEY SIGN   Acute Pain with Skin Pallor and Coolness—Arterial Embolus or Thrombosis

Acute occlusion of a major peripheral artery causes cutaneous and muscular ischemia producing skin and nail bed pallor, decreased temperature, and ischemic pain. The pain is severe and unremitting with changes in position. Embolic arterial occlusion is most common in native vessels, whereas thrombus is more common in prosthetic vascular channels. Urgent relief of the obstruction is necessary to preserve the part. See page 427.   *CLINICAL OCCURRENCE:*   The heart is the most common source for emboli (endocarditis, prosthetic valve, atrial fibrillation); less commonly, it may arise from thrombus within an aortic aneurysm or paradoxical embolism via a patent foramen ovale.

KEY SIGN   Nodular Vessels—Polyarteritis Nodosa

See page 414.

Chest, Cardiovascular and Respiratory Syndromes

Chest Wall Syndromes
Chest Pain Intensified by Respiratory Motion

Pain accentuated by breathing, coughing, laughing, or sneezing usually indicates inflammation or injury to the ribs, cartilages, muscles, nerves, and pleurae of the chest wall. The causes of pain in each of these tissues should be considered in the examination. The specific area may also be tender, so see Chest Wall Pain with Tenderness, page 340, as there is significant overlap between these categories.

KEY SYNDROME   Pleuritis and Pleurisy

The parietal pleura has sensory fibers from the intercostal nerves that also give off twigs to the skin. The visceral pleura is anesthetic. Pleural pain is caused either by stretching of the inflamed parietal pleura or by separation of fibrous adhesions between two pleural surfaces. It is difficult to accept that pain is produced by rubbing the two pleural surfaces together: pain often occurs without a friction rub, and a rub is often present without pain. Pleural inflammation (*pleuritis*) produces knife-like shooting pains in the thoracic wall, intensified by breathing, coughing, and laughing. Feel and listen for a friction rub; rubs are not constantly present, so repeat your examination. Pleural effusion may develop. The diagnosis of *pleurisy* is made from the typical pain history or the presence of a friction rub after excluding other causes of pleuritis, rib fractures, myositis, and neuritis. Pleurisy and a rub may precede radiographic evidence of pneumonia.   *CLINICAL OCCURRENCE:* Bacterial and viral pneumonia, tuberculosis, empyema, viral pleuritis, pulmonary infarction from embolus, mesothelioma, primary and metastatic lung neoplasm, and connective-tissue diseases.

Diaphragmatic Pleuritis and Pleurisy: The periphery of the diaphragmatic pleura is supplied by the fifth and sixth intercostal nerves, which give pain near the costal margins. The central diaphragm (thoracic and peritoneal) is innervated by the phrenic nerve (C3–4), which also innervates the neck and supraclavicular fossae. Thus, pain in the neck may result from irritation of the diaphragmatic pleura (Fig. 8–43). There is sharp shooting pain intensified by deep breathing, coughing, or laughing. Pain may be localized along the costal margins, epigastrium, lumbar region, or neck at the superior border of the trapezius or the supraclavicular fossa, always on the same side. A pleural or pericardial friction rub may be present. **DDX:** The diagnosis of pleurisy is suggested when pain is accompanied by fever and a friction rub; later, pleural effusion may appear. A history of dysphagia or intraabdominal disease should suggest disorders of the esophagus, subphrenic abscess, peptic ulcer, splenic infarction, splenic rupture or pancreatitis. Hiatal hernia may produce similar pain. Pericarditis with pleuritic pain (*pleuropericarditis*) should be considered.

Epidemic Pleurodynia (Bornholm Disease, Devil's Grip): Infection with group B coxsackievirus is the common cause. After a nondescript prodrome, the patient is suddenly seized with sharp, knife-like thoracic or abdominal pains intensified by breathing and other bodily motions and accompanied by fever;

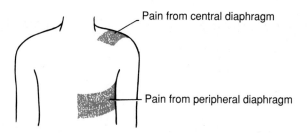

Pain from central diaphragm

Pain from peripheral diaphragm

Fig. 8–43 *Referral of Left Diaphragmatic Pain.*

the thorax may be splinted and the thighs flexed on the belly. Paroxysms of intense pain are separated by intervals of complete comfort. Cases may be sporadic or epidemic. Mild pharyngitis and myalgias with tenderness of the neck, trunk, and limbs may be noted. A friction rub is detected in 25% of cases. The sudden retrosternal pain suggests myocardial infarction or dissecting aneurysm. A period of several days of worried observation, until symptoms subside, is the usual method of diagnosis.

Chest Wall Twinge Syndrome (Precordial Catch): The patient experiences brief episodes of nonexertional sharp pain or "catches" in the anterior chest, usually on the left side. Some patients report onset while bending over. The pains last from seconds to minutes and are aggravated by deep breathing and relieved by shallow respirations. The cause is unknown. The condition is common and harmless.

Rib Fracture, Periosteal Hematoma, Periostitis, Intercostal Myositis. See page 340.

Respiratory Syndromes

> **KEY SYNDROME** Pneumothorax

Rupture of a subpleural bleb or penetrating chest trauma allows air to enter the pleural space separating the lung from the chest wall leading to failure of respiratory mechanics and lung collapse. *Symptoms* There is usually sudden severe chest pain, often unilateral, rarely localized, followed immediately by increasing dyspnea. *Signs* See page 355. With a large pneumothorax, the physical signs are distinctive: hyperresonant percussion, decreased fremitus, voice transmission and breath sounds on the affected side, and tracheal deviation away from the affected side. Respiratory movements of the ribs are decreased with persistent expiratory distention of the hemithorax. When tension pneumothorax develops, urgent diagnosis and treatment are necessary to prevent suffocation. With a small pneumothorax, the only sign may be decreased breath sounds. *Chest X-Ray* Lung markings are absent and often, the line of the visceral pleura can be identified. *CLINICAL OCCURRENCE:* Pneumothorax results from rupture of a pleural bleb in pulmonary emphysema, and, occasionally, from nonsuppurative lung disease, such as sarcoidosis, fibrosis, or silicosis. Puncture of the lung by a fractured rib is the most common traumatic cause. It is not rare in slender, healthy young persons with no discernible pulmonary lesion. The sudden pain must be distinguished from pulmonary embolism, myocardial infarction, and acute pericarditis.

> **KEY SYNDROME** Acute Bronchitis

Acute infection is usually viral; less commonly, it is an atypical organism. Airway inflammation produces persistent cough and often retrosternal burning pain. Fever is absent. Secretions in the bronchi and trachea produce rhonchi and, occasionally, wheezing. Secretions high in the trachea produce rhonchi that are heard throughout the thorax. The cough may be unproductive or tenacious, mucoid sputum may be raised. Usually, there is no impairment of the airways, so breath sounds are normal. **DDX:** In epidemics, influenza and respiratory syncytial virus should be considered. Chest X-rays are normal.

KEY SYNDROME   Pneumonia

Infection or inflammation of the lung is called pneumonitis or pneumonia. The process may be limited to the airways and alveolar airspaces, or involve the pulmonary interstitium and vascular channels. The diagnostic challenges are to separate infectious from noninfectious forms of pneumonia, and then to identify the specific etiology. Onset may be sudden or gradual, depending upon the etiology. Patients present with cough, dyspnea, fatigue, and, especially with infection, high fever, often with rigors. Physical findings range from minimal signs of airspace disease (bronchophony, whispered pectoriloquy) to respiratory failure with multilobar consolidation. Infectious pneumonia is separated into community-acquired or hospital-healthcare-associated categories. An approach to the diagnosis of specific etiologies of pneumonia is beyond the scope of this text [Metlay JP, Kapoor WN, Fine MJ. The rational clinical examination. Does this patient have community-acquired pneumonia? Diagnosing pneumonia by history and physical examination. *JAMA*. 1997;278:1440–1445; File TM. Community-acquired pneumonia. *Lancet*. 2003;362:1991–2001].

✔ *PNEUMONIA—CLINICAL OCCURRENCE:* **Congenital** pulmonary sequestration (may be confused with pneumonia on chest X-ray); **Idiopathic** idiopathic interstitial pneumonia, eosinophilic pneumonia (acute and chronic primary alveolar proteinosis); **Inflammatory/Immune** hypersensitivity pneumonitis, vasculitis, lymphomatoid granulomatosis, Goodpasture syndrome, lipoid pneumonia, collagen vascular diseases; **Infectious** bacterial, viral, tuberculosis, nontuberculous mycobacteria, rickettsia, fungi, Nocardia, pneumocystis, parasites, **Metabolic/Toxic** inhalational injury, drug reactions, pneumoconioses; **Mechanical/Trauma** aspiration; **Neoplastic** endobronchial neoplasm with post obstructive infection, bronchioloalveolar cell carcinoma; **Vascular** vasculitis (Churg-Strauss, Wegener).

KEY SYNDROME   Severe Acute Respiratory Syndrome (SARS)

Infection with a novel coronavirus causes severe lung inflammation leading to hypoxia and respiratory failure. First recognized in early 2003, this virus appears to have originated in China and spread rapidly to other countries. The initial symptoms are those of a flu-like illness, followed by rapidly progressive pneumonia. The case fatality rate is approximately 15%, higher in patients over age 50. Spread is by droplets and contact with infected persons and contaminated surfaces. To make the diagnosis, a high index of suspicion is necessary with careful questioning about contact with infected or potentially infected people and travel to known areas of ongoing transmission. Current information is available at the Centers for Disease Control web site, www.cdc.gov.

KEY SYNDROME   Aspiration Pneumonia

Aspiration of oral secretions, food, or regurgitated stomach contents causes mechanical obstruction of the airways with secondary inflammation (especially with gastric contents at low pH) and secondary infection often with anaerobic flora from the oral cavity. The right middle and apical segment of the right lower lobe are commonly affected. Aspiration is common in association with reduced consciousness of any cause and with impaired oropharyngeal function. Coughing in association with meals and nocturnal regurgitation with cough and dyspnea are suggestive of chronic aspiration. Necrotizing anaerobic infections may lead to lung abscess with fetid sputum. Aspiration should be suspected in any patient with a history of impaired consciousness or oropharyngeal neurologic dysfunction who presents with pneumonia [Marik PE. Aspiration pneumonitis and aspiration pneumonia. *N Engl J Med*. 2001;344:665–671].

KEY SYNDROME   Lung Abscess

Infection with necrotizing organisms destroys lung tissue creating cavities with low oxygen tension, ideal for growth of microaerophilic or anaerobic organisms. A history compatible with aspiration is often present. The sputum is scant to intermittently copious, purulent, and foul smelling. Signs of consolidation may be present; amphoric breath sounds may be heard if the cavity communicates with a bronchus and is only partially filled (see page 354). Old abscess cavities may become colonized with *Aspergillus* producing a fungus ball.

Bronchopleural Fistula: A communication between a bronchus and the pleural cavity is usually caused by an empyema draining through a bronchus or a lung abscess invading the pleural cavity. Patients present with chronic cough producing a large volume of purulent sputum. The sudden drainage of pus into the pleural cavity produces severe prostration, chills, fever, or shock. Dullness and absent breath sounds in lower hemithorax, with a resonant region above—the whole devoid of breath sounds—suggest the diagnosis. A succussion splash may be heard.

KEY SYNDROME   Pulmonary Embolism

Thrombus dislodged from a site of deep venous thrombosis occludes the main pulmonary artery bifurcation or one of its branches. Deep venous thrombosis develops after surgery (particularly total hip and knee replacement), prolonged bed rest and air travel, immobilization by a cast, and venous stasis from venous insufficiency or CHF. Thrombophilia (factor V Leiden, prothrombin gene mutations, antiphospholipid syndrome, protein C or S deficiency, mucinous adenocarcinomas, estrogens, pregnancy, etc.) increases the risks of deep venous thrombosis. Large emboli obstruct the pulmonary circulation producing acute pulmonary hypertension, right ventricular pressure overload and failure with circulatory collapse. Infarction of lung tissue results in local inflammation. Hypoxia occurs from ventilation-perfusion mismatching and intrapulmonary shunts. Less-commonly embolized material are fat (from the marrow of fractured bones), air, amniotic fluid (when the fluid contains meconium, it is especially dangerous), and tumor tissue. Patients may be minimally symptomatic or present with sudden dyspnea, chest pain and circulatory failure. *Symptoms* Sudden dyspnea, with or without pain or tachypnea, is the key symptom. The pain is either pleuritic or a deep, crushing sensation in the six-dermatome band. Sometimes painless dyspnea resembles asthma due to the release of serotonin from platelets in the blood clot. Massive pulmonary embolus may present with syncope and no other symptoms [Goldhaber SZ, Nadel ES, King ME, et al. *NEJM*. 2004;350:2281–2290, Case 17-2004]. *Signs* Systemic effects may predominate, with weakness, prostration, sweating, nausea, and vomiting. Tachycardia is constant and fever occurs with infarction. Dyspnea, tachypnea, and cyanosis may be extreme. When present, hemoptysis, a pleural friction rub, and bloody pleural effusion strongly support the diagnosis. Massive